Pathogenesis and Management of Atopic Dermatitis

Current Problems in Dermatology

Vol. 41

Pathogenesis and Management of Atopic Dermatitis

Volume Editor

Tetsuo Shiohara Tokyo

26 figures, 20 in color, and 9 tables, 2011

KARGER

Basel · Freiburg · Paris · London · New York · New Delhi · Bangkok · Beijing · Tokyo · Kuala Lumpur · Singapore · Sydney

Current Problems in Dermatology

Tetsuo Shiohara
Department of Dermatology
Kyorin University School of Medicine
6-20-2 Shinkawa, Mitaka
Tokyo 181-8611
Japan

Library of Congress Cataloging-in-Publication Data

Pathogenesis and management of atopic dermatitis / volume editor, Tetsuo Shiohara.
p. ; cm. -- (Current problems in dermatology, ISSN 1421-5721; vol. 41)
Includes bibliographical references and indexes.
ISBN 978-3-8055-9686-2 (hard cover : alk. paper) -- ISBN 978-3-8055-9687-9 (electronic)
1. Atopic dermatitis. I. Shiohara, Tetsuo. II. Series: Current problems in dermatology ; v. 41.
[DNLM: 1. Dermatitis, Atopic. W1 CU804L v.41 2011 / WR 160]
RL243.P38 2011
616.5'1--dc22
2011003457

Bibliographic Indices. This publication is listed in bibliographic services, including MEDLINE/Pubmed.

Drug Dosage. The authors and the publisher have exerted every effort to ensure that drug selection and dosage set forth in this text are in accord with current recommendations and practice at the time of publication. However, in view of ongoing research, changes in government regulations, and the constant flow of information relating to drug therapy and drug reactions, the reader is urged to check the package insert for each drug for any change in indications and dosage and for added warnings and precautions. This is particularly important when the recommended agent is a new and/or infrequently employed drug.

www.karger.com
Printed in Switzerland on acid-free and non-aging paper (ISO 9706) by Reinhardt Druck, Basel
ISSN 1421–5721
ISBN 978–3–8055–9686–2
e-ISBN 978–3–8055–9687–9

Contents

Preface

Atopic dermatitis (AD) is indeed a multifactorial genetic disease arising as a result of the complicated interaction of many genes with environmental factors. It has long been thought that a genetic predisposition to a defective skin barrier represents a primary event that can favor the increased penetration of allergens, thereby facilitating the occurrence of allergic inflammatory responses. A recent breakthrough in the understanding of AD pathogenesis has been made with the studies successfully linking loss-of-function mutations in the genes encoding the epidermal structure protein filaggrin with the subsequent risk of developing AD. Another area of AD research apparently points us to the importance of the increase in exposure to various environmental agents, particularly deprived of microbial stimuli, which is known as the 'hygiene hypothesis'. Recent studies also suggest specific mechanisms whereby innate immune responses are functionally defective in AD. After a long period of neglect, sweating disturbance in AD has recently received increasing attention, because sweat is now recognized as the first element of the innate immune system. Nevertheless, the most common emergent theme has been the role of adaptive immunity in providing cytokines and chemokines that sustain the recruitment, retention and activation of allergen-specific T cells, dendritic cells, eosinophils, basophils and mast cells in the involved tissues.

However, no single text concerning the entire spectrum has been available. The key message of this book is to address the questions raised by dermatologists, pediatricians, practicing physicians, basic immunologists, biologists, pharmacologists and students studying medicine on the pathogenesis, management and therapies of AD. To this end, virtually all chapters have been authored by original investigators who have contributed significantly to the establishment of current concepts. I would like to thank the distinguished authors who made tremendous efforts to make this book very useful, and I am also very thankful to the staff of Karger AG, in particular Ms. Tanja Sebuk.

Tetsuo Shiohara, Tokyo

Shiohara T (ed): Pathogenesis and Management of Atopic Dermatitis.
Curr Probl Dermatol. Basel, Karger, 2011, vol 41, pp 1–34

Atopic Dermatitis and the Hygiene Hypothesis Revisited

Carsten Flohr · Lindsey Yeo

Department of Paediatric Dermatology, St. John's Institute of Dermatology, Guy's and St. Thomas' Hospital NHS Foundation Trust and King's College London, London, UK

Abstract

Background: We published a systematic review on atopic dermatitis (AD) and the hygiene hypothesis in 2005. Since then, the body of literature has grown significantly. **Objectives:** We therefore repeated our systematic review to examine the evidence from population-based studies for an association between AD risk and specific infections, childhood immunizations, the use of antibiotics and environmental exposures that lead to a change in microbial burden. **Methods:** Medline was searched from 1966 until June 2010 to identify relevant studies. **Results:** We found an additional 49 papers suitable for inclusion. There is evidence to support an inverse relationship between AD and endotoxin, early day care, farm animal and dog exposure in early life. Cat exposure in the presence of skin barrier impairment is positively associated with AD. Helminth infection at least partially protects against AD. This is not the case for viral and bacterial infections, but consumption of unpasteurized farm milk seems protective. Routine childhood vaccinations have no effect on AD risk. The positive association between viral infections and AD found in some studies appears confounded by antibiotic prescription, which has been consistently associated with an increase in AD risk. **Conclusions:** There is convincing evidence for an inverse relationship between helminth infections and AD but no other pathogens. The protective effect seen with early day care, endotoxin, unpasteurized farm milk and animal exposure is likely to be due to a general increase in exposure to non-pathogenic microbes. This would also explain the risk increase associated with the use of broad-spectrum antibiotics. Future studies should assess skin barrier gene mutation carriage and phenotypic skin barrier impairment, as gene-environment interactions are likely to impact on AD risk.

There has been a dramatic increase in the prevalence of atopic dermatitis (AD) over past decades, currently affecting around 20% of children in developed countries [1]. Although family history plays an important role in AD susceptibility, probably at least partly explained by skin barrier gene mutation carriage, genetics alone cannot explain the increase in AD prevalence [2, 3]. Epidemiological research has therefore focused on identifying possible environmental and lifestyle-related factors that are associated with an increased AD risk. For instance, AD is more common in urban than in rural communities [4]. In addition, migrant studies have demonstrated that immigrants take on the risk of the community to which they move, with AD being more prevalent in western industrialized countries than developing nations [5, 6]. The risk of developing AD is also higher in children growing up in smaller families and families of higher socio-economic status [7–9]. All this strongly suggests an environmental aetiology.

The so-called 'hygiene hypothesis' was formulated in the late 1980s, based on the observation that AD and hay fever were noted to be less common among UK children growing up with larger numbers of older siblings [10]. At the time, this was thought to be due to a higher exposure to certain viral and bacterial pathogens in larger families. The hygiene hypothesis has stimulated a large body of both epidemiological and immunological research. For instance, there is evidence from animal models that allergic disease occurs when the developing immune system is deprived of the obligatory stimulation through certain microbial antigens, especially when this happens directly postnatally or even already in utero [11]. Immunologically, this seems partly due to an imbalance between type 1 and type 2 T helper cells and their cytokines. However, the immunological processes ultimately leading to allergic disease are more complex than this. The current hypothesis is that regulatory T cells and anti-inflammatory cytokines such as interleukin 10 and transforming growth factor β play an important role in the protection against clinical allergy, possibly induced by microbial stimulation of dendritic cells via Toll-like receptors at the level of the gastrointestinal mucosa or other lymphoid tissues (fig. 1a, b) [12–15].

Since our original systematic review on AD and the hygiene hypothesis in 2005, the body of literature has grown significantly, and we therefore decided to revisit this fascinating topic for a second time [16]. We performed a systematic Medline search from inception until June 2010 to address the following questions at the population level: (1) Is there any evidence that the risk of AD is related to environmental exposures that alter microbial burden? (2) Which specific infections have been associated with a reduced AD risk? (3) Is there a link between immunizations, use of antibiotics and AD risk? The online search strategy is available on request from the corresponding author and was supplemented by an extensive hand search of the literature through references identified from retrieved articles. Overall, we identified 49 new studies suitable for inclusion. All studies were analysed qualitatively, and results are presented in summary tables. Where appropriate, we also conducted meta-analyses, namely for pet and antibiotic exposure.

The Link between AD and Environmental Exposures That Can Alter Microbial Burden

Basic hygiene, day care attendance, anthroposophic lifestyle, living on a farm and pets have all been examined as potential risk factors for allergic disease, including AD, since they at least theoretically increase exposure to microbes.

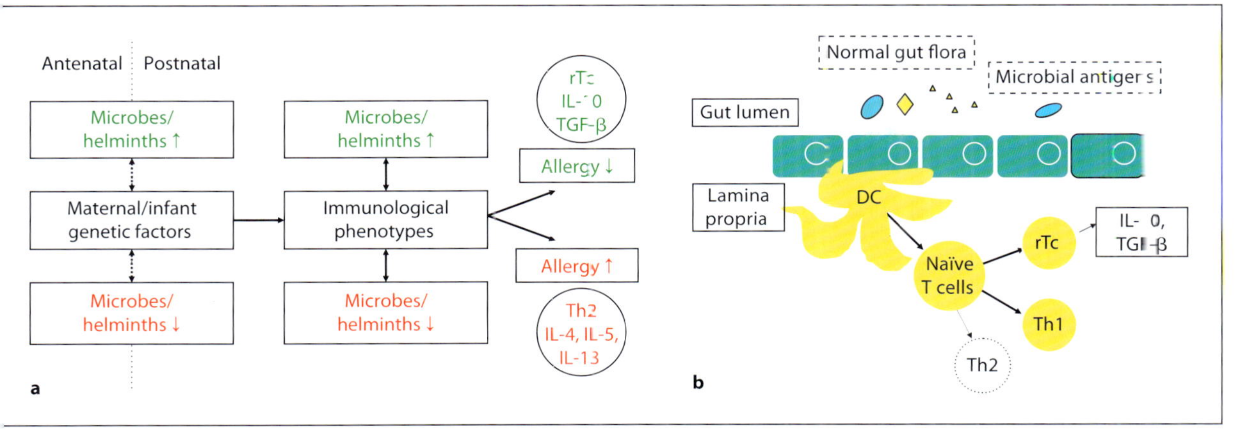

Fig. 1. a Microbial and helminth exposure in utero and postnatally is likely to play an important role in the development of AD. In this model, high exposure burden, probably in interaction with maternal and infant genetic factors, reduces AD risk, whereas AD risk increases if the fetal and/or infantile immune system is deprived of microbial stimulation. The gut mucosa is likely to be a key site for the priming of the immune system (see **b**). rTc = Regulatory T cells; Th2 = type 2 T helper cells; IL = interleukin; TGF-β = transforming growth factor β. **b** The postulated link between allergic disease and the gut microflora. Chronic stimulation of gut-associated lymphoid tissue through normal gut flora and other non-/pathogenic microbial antigens might ensure the development of a Th1/regulatory T cell-dominated cytokine milieu and therefore prevent clinical expression of allergic disease. Regulatory T cells may have a role in this by the production of anti-inflammatory cytokines, such as IL-10 and TGF-β. DC = Dendritic cell; Th = T helper cell; rTc = regulatory T cell.

Basic Hygiene

Only one large birth cohort study, the Avon Longitudinal Study of Parents and Children, has so far addressed the question whether cleanliness in terms of general hygiene measures, such as frequency of washing, is associated with an increase in AD risk. Children were seen at 6 and 30–42 months of age, and a moderate increase in AD risk was found with higher levels of personal hygiene, measured as an empirical hygiene score from 1 to 14 (baseline adjusted odds ratio, adj. OR = 1.04, 95% confidence interval, CI = 1.01–1.07; table 1) [17].

Day Care

Three birth cohort studies, one from the USA, one from Denmark and one from Germany, found an inverse relationship between day care attendance and AD, with risk reductions up to 88% (German study adj. OR = 0.12, 95% CI = 0.04–0.31) [18–20]. One substantial questionnaire-based cross-sectional study from Sweden

Table 1. Environmental exposures that may alter microbial burden and their association with AD risk

Study	Study type and country	Number of participants	Age	Diagnostic criteria (D) and exposure measures (E)	Outcome measure(s) and comments
Basic hygiene					
Sherriff and Golding [17], 2002	Birth cohort UK	14,541	30–42 months	Questionnaire (D) Hygiene score 1–14 (E)	Baseline adj. OR = 1.04 (1.01–1.07), i.e. someone with a hygiene score of 14 will have a 14 times higher OR compared with baseline (OR = 1.56)
Day care					
Celedón et al. [18], 2003	Birth cohort USA	453	6 years	Questionnaire (D) Questionnaire (E)	adj. OR = 0.30 (0.10–0.80)
Benn et al. [19], 2004	Birth cohort Denmark	13,070	0–18 months	Questionnaire and subgroup physical examination (D) Questionnaire (E)	Day care before the age of 6 months adj. IRR = 0.82 (0.70–0.96)
Hagerhed-Engman et al. [21], 2006	Cross-sectional Sweden	10,851	1–6 years	Questionnaire (D) Questionnaire (E)	Age 1–4 years adj. OR = 1.44 (1.17–1.78) Age 4–6 years adj. OR = 1.32 (0.92–1.89)
Dunder et al. [22], 2007	RCT Finland	928	12 years	Hygiene intervention Physician (D)	OR = 1.1 (0.9–1.4)
Dom et al. [20], 2010	Birth cohort Germany	773	0–4 years	Questionnaire (D) Questionnaire (E)	adj. OR = 0.12 (0.04–0.31)
Anthroposophic lifestyle					
Alm et al. [23], 1999	Case-control Sweden	295 anthroposophic school 380 control school	5–13 years	Physician (D) Questionnaire (E)	OR = 0.28 (0.13–0.61)
Floistrup et al. [26], 2006	Cross-sectional Germany, Switzerland, Sweden, the Netherlands and Austria	4,606 Steiner schools, 2,024 control schools	5–13 years	Questionnaire (D) Questionnaire (E)	Current eczema symptoms adj. OR = 0.70 (0.58–0.83) Doctor's diagnosis adj. OR = 0.90 (0.75–1.08)

Table 1. Continued

Study	Study type and country	Number of participants	Age	Diagnostic criteria (D) and exposure measures (E)	Outcome measure(s) and comments
Farming					
Braun-Fahrländer et al. [27], 1999	Case-control Switzerland	1,619	6–7, 9–11, 13–15 years	Questionnaire (D) Questionnaire (E)	adj. OR = 0.86 (0.49–1.50)
Von Ehrenstein et al. [28], 2000	Cross-sectional Germany	10,163	5–7 years	Questionnaire (D) Questionnaire (E)	adj. OR = 0.87 (0.73–1.04)
Riedler et al. [29], 2000	Cross-sectional Austria	2,283	8–10 years	Questionnaire (D) Questionnaire (E)	adj. OR = 0.81 (0.52–1.26)
Kilpeläinen et al. [30], 2000	Cross-sectional Finland	10,667	18–24 years	Questionnaire (D) Questionnaire (E)	adj. OR = 0.93 (0.75–1.17)
Wickens et al. [31], 2002	Cross-sectional New Zealand	293	7–10 years	Questionnaire (D) Questionnaire (E)	*Eczema ever* and farm exposure First year of life adj. OR = 0.7 (0.3–1.8) Current exposure adj. OR = 1.7 (0.7–4.1) Unpasteurized farm milk <2 years adj. OR = 0.2 (0.1–0.8)
Bråbäck et al. [32], 2004	Cohort of conscripts Sweden	1,309,652	17–20 years	Physician (D) Population register (E)	adj. RR = 0.93 (0.89–0.98) for 1972–1981 cohort only
Benn et al. [19], 2004	Birth cohort Denmark	13,070	0–18 months	Questionnaire and subgroup physical examination (D) Questionnaire (E)	adj. IRR = 0.90 (0.74–1.10)
Perkin and Strachan [33], 2006	Cross-sectional UK	4,647	5–10 years	Questionnaire (D) Questionnaire (E)	adj. OR = 0.91 (0.68–1.21) Current eczema symptoms and current unpasteurized milk consumption adj. OR = 0.59 (0.40–0.87)

Table 1. Continued

Study	Study type and country	Number of participants	Age	Diagnostic criteria (D) and exposure measures (E)	Outcome measure(s) and comments
Douwes et al. [34], 2007	Case-control New Zealand	2,509 farming and 1,001 non-farming families	Children and adults for cases (but age not specified); 25–49 years for controls	Questionnaire (D) Questionnaire (E)	Current eczema symptoms adj. OR = 0.73 (0.64–0.85), disregard of whether exposure was only during childhood or current or both
Karadag et al. [35], 2007	Cross-sectional Austria, Germany, the Netherlands, Sweden, Switzerland	14,893	5–13 years	Questionnaire (D) Questionnaire (E) Endotoxin and allergens in house dust (E)	No overall association Helping with haying and current eczema symptoms adj. OR = 0.65 (0.46–0.93) or doctor's diagnosis adj. OR = 0.73 (0.51–1.05) *only* in the presence of asthma phenotype
Douwes et al. [36], 2008	Cross-sectional New Zealand	3,510 (1,333 farmer's children, 566 reference children)	5–17 years	Questionnaire (D) Questionnaire (E)	No significant association for current/lifetime exposure to farm or unpasteurized farm milk Daily farm exposure of mother during pregnancy protective for eczema ever adj. OR = 0.58 (0.40–0.84) Combined prenatal and current exposure adj. OR = 0.46 (0.30–0.70)
Pets					
Hesselmar et al. [37], 1999	Cross-sectional Sweden	2,481	7–8 years	Questionnaire (D) Questionnaire (E)	NS, OR could not be calculated from the data presented
Bråbäck et al. [38], 2001	Cross-sectional Sweden	2,505	10–11 years	Questionnaire (D) Questionnaire (E)	NS, OR could not be calculated from the data presented
Nafstad et al. [39], 2001	Birth cohort Norway	2,531	0–6 months	Questionnaire (D) Questionnaire and collection of dust samples for allergen exposure (E)	Dog at birth adj. OR = 0.70 (0.40–1.00) Cat at birth adj. OR = 0.50 (0.30–0.90)

Table 1. Continued

Study	Study type and country	Number of participants	Age	Diagnostic criteria (D) and exposure measures (E)	Outcome measure(s) and comments
Zirngibl et al. [40], 2002	Birth cohort Germany	4,578	0–2 years	Questionnaire (D) Questionnaire (E)	Any pet first year adj. OR = 0.71 (0.55–0.92) Dog first year adj. OR = 0.62 (0.39–0.98)
Kerkhof et al. [41], 2003	Birth cohort Netherlands	708	0–12 months	Questionnaire (D) Questionnaire (E)	Dog at birth adj. OR = 1.1 (0.4–3.1) Cat at birth adj. OR = 0.5 (0.2–1.1)
Phipatanakul et al. [42], 2004	Birth cohort USA	498	0–12 months	Questionnaire (D) Questionnaire (E)	Dog at 2–3 months OR = 0.60 (0.34–1.09) Cat at 2–3 months OR = 1.05 (0.65–1.69)
Illi et al. [43], 2004	Birth cohort Germany	858	0–7 years	Questionnaire (D) Questionnaire (E)	Cat in early life adj. OR = 2.33 (0.85–6.33)
Benn et al. [19], 2004	Birth cohort Denmark	13,070	0–18 months	Questionnaire and subgroup physical examination (D) Questionnaire (E)	Any pet adj. IRR = 0.87 (0.79–0.95)
Gern et al. [44], 2004	Birth cohort USA	285	0, 2, 4, 6, 9, 12 months	Questionnaire (D) Questionnaire at birth and at 2 years (E)	Dog at birth and current adj. OR = 0.40 (0.24–0.67)
Yemaneberhan et al. [45], 2004	Cross-sectional Ethiopia	12,876	1–65 years and above	Questionnaire (D) Questionnaire (E)	Any animal inside the house adj. OR = 1.35 (0.97–1.88)
Purvis et al. [47], 2005	Case-control New Zealand	550	3.5 years	Questionnaire (D) Questionnaire (E)	Current cat exposure adj. OR = 0.45 (0.21–0.97) Current dog exposure adj. OR = 1.25 (0.63–2.46)
Hagendorens et al. [48], 2005	Birth cohort Germany	1,084	0–1 year	Questionnaire (D) Questionnaire (E)	Cat first year adj. OR = 0.68 (0.47–0.97)
Kurosaka et al. [46], 2006	Cross-sectional Japan	35,552	6 years	Questionnaire (D) Questionnaire (E)	Current cat exposure adj. OR = 0.79 (0.67–0.93)

Table 1. Continued

Study	Study type and country	Number of participants	Age	Diagnostic criteria (D) and exposure measures (E)	Outcome measure(s) and comments
Pohlabeln et al. [49], 2007	Birth cohort Germany	1,881	0–2 years	Questionnaire (D) Questionnaire (E)	Dog at birth without family history of atopic disease adj. OR = 0.52 (0.33–0.83) Dog at birth with family history of atopic disease adj. OR = 1.43 (0.95–2.15) Cat at birth adj. OR = 1.17 (0.82–1.68)
Bufford et al. [50], 2008	Birth cohort USA	275	0–3 years	Questionnaire (D) Questionnaire (E)	*Eczema ever* Dog at birth adj. OR = 0.24 (0.11–0.53) Dog at the age of 3 adj. OR = 0.42 (0.20–0.88)
Bisgaard et al. [51], 2008	Birth cohort UK and Denmark	503 (UK) 379 (Denmark)	0–12 months	UK cohort: Questionnaire (D) Questionnaire (E) Danish cohort: Skin examination (D) Questionnaire (E) FLG genotyping	*FLG mutation and cat at birt* Denmark HR = 11.11 (3.79–32.60) UK HR = 3.82 (1.35–10.81) *Dog at birth* Denmark HR = 0.49 (0.24–1.01) UK HR = 0.59 (0.16–2.20) no association with FLG status
Schuttelaar et al. [52], 2009	Birth cohort Netherlands	934	0–8 years	Questionnaire (D) Questionnaire (E) FLG genotyping	FLG mutation and cat first year adj. OR = 6.0 (3.2–11.3)
Schäfer et al. [53], 2009	Birth cohort Germany	606	5–6 years	Questionnaire and physical examination (D) Questionnaire (E)	Current cat exposure adj. OR = 3.8 (1.4–10.8)
Dom et al. [20], 2010	Birth cohort Germany	773	0–4 years	Questionnaire (D) Questionnaire (E)	Postnatal exposure to cat o dog adj. OR = 0.42 (0.25–0.69)
Endotoxin					
Gehring et al. [54], 2001	Birth cohort Germany	1,884	6 and 12 months	Questionnaire (D) Endotoxin and allergens in house dust (E)	Only very high exposure protective at 6 months adj. OR = 0.50 (0.28–0.88)

Table 1. Continued

Study	Study type and country	Number of participants	Age	Diagnostic criteria (D) and exposure measures (E)	Outcome measure(s and comments
Bolte et al. [55], 2003	Birth cohort Germany	1,942	2 years	Questionnaire (D) Endotoxin and allergens in house dust (E)	First to fourth quartiles of endotoxin exposure not associated with AD OR fourth quartile = 1.04 (0.73–1.47)
Phipatanakul et al. [42], 2004	Birth cohort USA	498	2, 4, 6, 8, 10, 12 months	Questionnaire (D) Endotoxin and allergens in house dust (E)	Third and fourth quartiles of endotoxin exposure associated with AD adj. OR = 0.76 (0.61–0.96)
Perzanowski et al. [56], 2006	Birth cohort USA	301	12–36 months	Questionnaire (D) Endotoxin and allergens in house dust (E)	*Doctor-diagnosed eczema* and current endotoxin exposure 1 year adj. OR = 0.70 (0.53–0.93) 2 years adj. OR = 0.86 (0.64–1.20) 3 years adj. OR = 0.74 (0.52–1.05)
Simpson et al. [57], 2006	Birth cohort UK	442	0–5 years	Skin examination (D) Endotoxin and allergens in house dust (E) CD14 genotyping	Current eczema (CD14 CC) adj. OR = 0.73 (0.56–0.95) No association with other genotypes
Karadag et al. [35], 2007	Cross-sectional Austria, Germany, the Netherlands, Sweden and Switzerland	14,893	5–13 years	Questionnaire (D) Endotoxin and allergens in house dust (E)	adj. OR = 0.72 (0.56–0.93)
Chen et al. [58], 2009	Birth cohort Germany	2,166	0–6 years	Questionnaire (D) Endotoxin and allergens in house dust (E)	Eczema symptoms adj. OR = 1.1 (0.5–2.3) Doctor-diagnosed eczema adj. OR = 1.1 (0.4–3.3)

Figures in parentheses indicate 95% CI. IRR = incidence rate ratio; RCT = randomized controlled trial; RR = relative risk; NS = not shown; FLG = filaggrin; HR = hazard ratio.

however suggested a slight risk increase associated with attendance of day care facilities compared to being at home during preschool years (AD age 4–6 years: adj. OR = 1.32, 95% CI = 0.92–1.89), but only 5% of children in this cohort were in day care before their first birthday [21]. This suggests that day care attendance may only be protective during infancy. Finally, a randomized, controlled hygiene intervention, involving more frequent hand washing and use of antiseptics among 928 Finnish day care children, did not result in an increase in clinical allergy among the intervention group children by the age of 12 years (OR = 1.1, 95% CI = 0.9–1.4), but episodes of infection were purely based on parental report, and the hygiene intervention did not reduce the frequency of infections to home care levels [22].

Anthroposophic Lifestyle

Current AD has been shown to be more than 70% less common among 5- to 15-year-old children growing up in anthroposophic communities[1] in comparison to schoolchildren from a non-anthroposophic background in a Swedish case-control study (OR = 0.28, 95% CI = 0.13–0.61; table 1) [23]. The authors speculated that the risk differences may be due to the restricted prescribing of antibiotics and vaccinations by anthroposophic doctors, potentially resulting in a higher exposure to microbes. In addition, dietary factors could play an important role in AD risk reduction, as anthroposophic families frequently consume fermented vegetables rich in lactobacilli, and dietary supplementation with *Lactobacillus* GG has previously been shown to change the gut microflora and to reduce AD risk [24, 25].

Floistrup et al. [26] consequently conducted an in-depth cross-sectional risk factor analysis among 4,606 Steiner school children and 2,024 controls from 5 European countries. Again, AD risk was reduced among those attending anthroposophic schools, but the protective effect was weaker and only significant for reported AD symptoms (adj. OR = 0.70, 95% CI = 0.58–0.83) and not for a physician diagnosis (adj. OR = 0.90, 95% CI = 0.75–1.08). The risk differences were partly explained by differences in the use of antibiotics and antipyretics in early life (antibiotics: current AD symptoms adj. OR = 1.61, 95% CI = 1.21–2.15, physician diagnosis adj. OR = 1.63, 95% CI = 1.22–2.17; antipyretics: current AD symptoms adj. OR = 1.59, 95% CI = 1.17–2.15, physician diagnosis adj. OR = 1.30, 95% CI = 0.96–1.76). Diet, past measles infection and measles-mumps-rubella (MMR) vaccination showed no significant associations.

[1] The anthroposophic movement ('anthroposophy', Greek for 'wisdom of man') was founded by Rudolf Steiner in the early twentieth century. Anthroposophical philosophy has been applied to many domains of life since then, including agriculture and medicine.

Farm Environment

As yet another extension of the hygiene hypothesis, it has been postulated that children growing up on farms are at a reduced risk of developing allergic disease, possibly due to consumption of unpasteurized farm milk rich in lactobacilli and frequent contact with farm animals. While no convincing protective effect of children's farm exposure per se has been found [19, 27–36], there is evidence from a cross-sectional study to suggest that daily farm exposure of the mother during pregnancy can reduce AD risk by 42% (adj. OR = 0.58, 95% CI = 0.40–0.84), and this protective effect was even stronger in those with both pre- and postnatal exposure (adj. OR = 0.46, 95% CI = 0.30–0.70; table 1) [36]. In addition, the same research group conducted an earlier survey that found an 80% risk reduction in AD if children had consumed unpasteurized farm milk during the first 2 years of life (adj. OR = 0.2, 95% CI = 0.1–0.8), and this has been confirmed in a similar cross-sectional survey among children in a rural area in the UK (adj. OR = 0.59, 95% CI = 0.40–0.87) [31, 33].

Pets

Like farm animals, pets have been implicated as potentially protective against AD. Overall, 5 cross-sectional and 13 birth cohort studies have looked at this question (table 1) [19, 20, 37–53]. A meta-analysis of studies reveals an almost uniform protective effect of dog exposure (pooled OR = 0.61, 95% CI = 0.50–0.74; fig. 2), especially where exposure occurs in early life. The picture is less clear for cats. Meta-analysis again showed a protective effect (pooled OR = 0.83, 95% CI = 0.74–0.95), but study heterogeneity was significant ($I^2 = 66\%$, $p = 0.003$; fig. 2). It is interesting to note that where filaggrin skin barrier mutation carriage was taken into the equation, there was a significantly higher risk of AD in those with filaggrin mutations compared to wild-type children, suggesting that cat sensitization is facilitated by an impaired skin barrier and can be a risk factor for AD [51, 52].

Endotoxin

Some have argued that the risk reduction seen with dog exposure and farm exposure during pregnancy is due to endotoxins, a group of lipopolysaccharides found on the cell surface of Gram-negative bacteria, not least because endotoxins are known to be inducers of interleukin 10 and γ-interferon [15]. Five out of 7 birth cohort studies have suggested an up to 50% reduction in AD risk associated with endotoxin exposure (table 1) [35, 42, 54–58]. However, this effect tended to be confined to high endotoxin exposure levels [42, 54] and/or the first year of life [55, 56]. One possible explanation for these partly conflicting results are differences in the lipopolysaccharide receptor complex encoded on chromosome 5q31.1 (CD14), as a UK birth cohort found that only the CD14 CC genotype was associated with a significant reduction in AD risk (OR = 0.73, 95% CI = 0.56–0.95) [57].

Specific Infections and Risk of Atopic Dermatitis

More direct evidence for and against the hygiene hypothesis in AD comes from studies that have examined the relationship between specific infections and AD.

Prenatal Infections

A large British historical cohort study, using a general practitioner research database, examined the effect of infections during pregnancy on AD in the offspring and found a small increase in AD risk associated with 2 or more antenatal infections (adj. hazard ratio, HR = 1.16, 95% CI = 1.07–1.26; table 2) [59]. However, a more recent analysis based on historical data on acute viral respiratory infection notifications in former Eastern Germany suggested the opposite: a reduction in AD risk associated with exposure to prenatal viral respiratory infections. This effect was particularly strong for exposures during the last trimester (adj. HR = 0.70, 95% CI = 0.52–0.95) and extended into the postnatal period up to 7 months of age [60].

Childhood Infections

More work has been done on common viral and bacterial childhood infections, such as chickenpox, mumps, whooping cough, measles, diarrhoeal disease and pneumonia. All studies except one that looked at past childhood infections as a surrogate marker found a positive association with AD, although results in some studies did not reach conventional statistical significance (table 2) [19, 61–71]. However, these studies tended to ignore concomitant antibiotic prescribing as a potential confounding factor. Schmitt et al. [72] examined the complex relationship between respiratory, gastrointestinal and ear infections, as well as antibiotic prescribing and AD risk, and found that it was the antibiotics that seemed causally linked to an increased risk in developing AD rather than the infections themselves (table 3).

As for individual infections, a case-control study among 778 US children found a 44% AD risk reduction associated with past chickenpox infection (adj. OR = 0.56, 95% CI = 0.35–0.90). The protective effect was seen with chickenpox exposure up to

Dog exposure and AD risk

Study or subgroup	log [OR]	SE	Weight	OR IV, fixed, 95% CI
Bisgaard et al. [51], 2008	−0.5276	0.6686	2.2%	0.59; 0.16–2.19
Bufford et al. [50], 2008	−0.8675	0.4011	6.2%	0.42; 0.19–0.92
Gern et al. [44], 2004	−0.9163	0.2619	14.5%	0.40; 0.24–0.67
Kerkhof et al. [41], 2003	0.0953	0.5223	3.6%	1.10; 0.40–3.06
Nafstad et al. [39], 2001	−0.3567	0.2338	18.2%	0.70; 0.44–1.11
Phipatanakul et al. [42], 2004	−0.5108	0.2972	11.2%	0.60; 0.34–1.07
Pohlabeln et al. [49], 2007	−0.6539	0.2353	17.9%	0.52; 0.33–0.82
Purvis et al. [47], 2005	0.2231	0.3475	8.2%	1.25; 0.63–2.47
Zirngibl et al. [40], 2002	−0.478	0.2351	18.0%	0.62; 0.39–0.98
Total			100.0%	0.61; 0.50–0.74

Heterogeneity: $\chi^2 = 9.81$, d.f. = 8 ($p = 0.28$); $I^2 = 18\%$
Test for overall effect: $Z = 5.03$ ($p < 0.00001$)

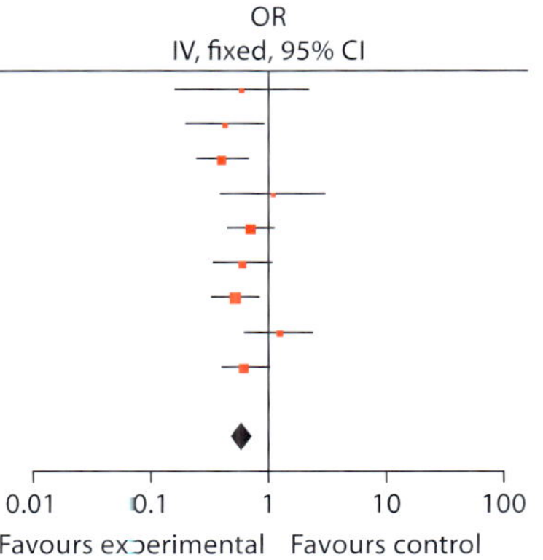

Cat exposure and AD risk

Study or subgroup	log [OR]	SE	Weight	OR IV, fixed, 95% CI
Hagendorens et al. [48], 2005	−0.3857	0.1848	12.0%	0.68; 0.47–0.98
Illi et al. [43], 2004	0.8459	0.5142	1.5%	2.33; 0.85–6.38
Kerkhof et al. [41], 2003	−0.6931	0.4348	2.2%	0.50; 0.21–1.17
Kurosaka et al. [46], 2005	−0.2357	0.0836	58.4%	0.79; 0.67–0.93
Nafstad et al. [39], 2001	−0.6931	0.2802	5.2%	0.50; 0.29–0.87
Phipatanakul et al. [42], 2004	0.0488	0.2438	6.9%	1.05; 0.65–1.69
Pohlabeln et al. [49], 2007	0.157	0.1829	12.2%	1.17; 0.82–1.67
Purvis et al. [47], 2005	−0.7985	1.5301	0.2%	0.45; 0.02–9.03
Schäfer et al. [53], 2009	1.335	0.5212	1.5%	3.80; 1.37–10.55
Total			100.0%	0.83; 0.74–0.95

Heterogeneity: $\chi^2 = 23.30$, d.f. = 8 ($p = 0.003$); $I^2 = 66\%$
Test for overall effect: $Z = 2.83$ ($p = 0.005$)

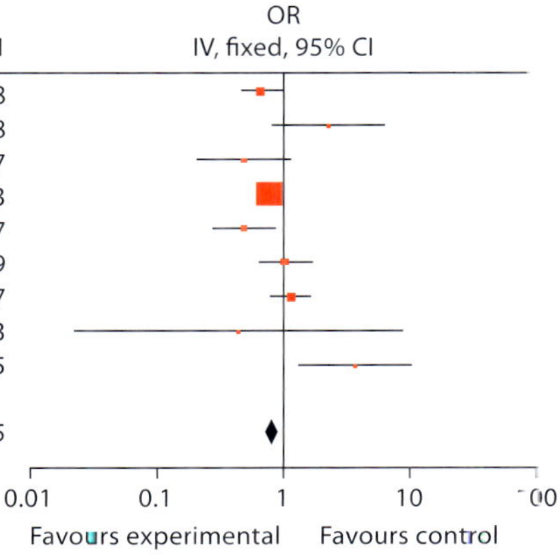

Fig. 2. The protective effect of dog exposure in early life; the effect is less clear for cats.

8 years of age and was strongest for moderate and severe AD (adj. OR = 0.08, 95% CI = 0.04–0.15, and adj. OR = 0.04, 95% CI = 0.01–0.13, respectively) [73]. However, in a similar study Farooqi and Hopkin [62] found a positive association between past chickenpox infection and AD risk among 1,934 UK children (OR = 1.40, 95% CI = 1.09–1.81). Indeed, all other individual viral childhood infections tended to yield ORs close to 1 with a trend towards an increase in risk (table 2). It may therefore not be a specific pathogen but non-pathogenic microbial burden per se that has an impact on AD development. There was also a significant sibling effect where examined, in that higher numbers of older siblings reduced AD risk, and this effect remained after adjustment for infections, suggesting that the sibling effect was early and independent of infections [19, 66].

Table 2. Infection and AD risk

Study	Study type and country	Number of participants	Age	Diagnostic criteria (D) and exposure measures (E)	Outcome measure(s) and comments
Perinatal infection					
McKeever et al. [59], 2002	Birth cohort UK	29,238	0–11 years	Physician (D) General practitioner research database (E)	≥2 antenatal infections adj. HR = 1.16 (1.07–1.26)
Zutavern et al. [60], 2006	Birth cohort Germany	4,672	5–14 years	Questionnaire (D) National database (E)	Exposure to acute respiratory infection during pregnancy and the first year of life showed reduced odds for AD up to the seventh month of life; the protective effect was lost afterwards Lifetime AD and ARI last trimester adj. HR = 0.70 (0.52–0.95) Lifetime AD and ARI 7 months adj. HR = 0.72 (0.52–0.98) Lifetime AD and ARI 1 year adj. HR = 1.24 (0.73–2.10)
Childhood infections					
Shirakawa et al. [61], 1997	Cross-sectional Japan	867	12–13 years	Questionnaire (D) Questionnaire (E)	Measles NS, data not presented
Farooqi and Hopkin [62], 1998	Cross-sectional UK	1,934	0–12 years	Physician (D) General practitioner database (E)	Mumps OR = 1.43 (1.07–1.91) Chickenpox OR = 1.40 (1.09–1.81) Croup OR = 1.75 (1.16–2.64) Measles OR = 1.12 (0.74–1.68) Whooping cough OR = 1.51 (0.94–2.44)

Table 2. Continued

Study	Study type and country	Number of participants	Age	Diagnostic criteria (D) and exposure measures (E)	Outcome measure(s) and comments
Bodner et al. [63], 1998	Cross-sectional UK	2,743	10–14 years	Questionnaire (D) Questionnaire (E)	Rubella, mumps and varicella adj. OR = 3.10 (1.40–6.70) Rubella ≤3 years adj. OR = 2.00 (1.00–4.00) Pertussis >3 years adj. OR = 2.00 (1.20–3.50)
Von Mutius et al. [64], 1999	Cross-sectional Germany	15,043	5–7 years 9–11 years	Questionnaire (D) Questionnaire (E)	≥5 fever episodes adj. OR = 1.49 (1.16–1.92)
Paunio et al. [65], 2000	Cross-sectional Finland	547,910	14 months to 19 years	Questionnaire (D) Questionnaire (E) at time of MMR vaccination	Measles adj. OR = 1.32 (1.27–1.36)
McKeever et al. [66], 2002	Birth cohort UK	29,238	0–11 years	Physician (D) General practitioner research database (E)	Bacterial infections (any) adj. HR = 1.33 (1.14–1.56) Viral infections (any) adj. HR = 0.98 (0.85–1.14) No significant association between infections in siblings and AD No significant association between number of infections, number of siblings and AD
Olesen et al. [67], 2003	Cross-sectional Denmark	9,744	3–15 years	Questionnaire (D) Questionnaire (E)	Measles adj. RR = 2.08 (0.98–4.42)
Gibbs et al. [68], 2004	Case-control UK	602	1–5 years	Physician (D) Questionnaire, general practitioner records and salivary IgG antibodies to EBV and VZV (E)	VZV antibodies adj. OR = 1.30 (0.90–1.39) EBV antibodies adj. OR = 0.71 (0.46–1.09) Also examined: coughs and colds, diarrhoea, ear infections, bronchiolitis, chickenpox, pneumonia; ORs either close to 1 or non-significant trend for exposure to increase AD risk

Table 2. Continued

Study	Study type and country	Number of participants	Age	Diagnostic criteria (D) and exposure measures (E)	Outcome measure(s) and comments
Benn et al. [19], 2004	Birth cohort Denmark	13,070	0–18 months	Questionnaire and subgroup physical examination (D) Questionnaire (E)	Total number of infections ≥3 adj. IRR = 1.33 (1.16–1.53) Also examined: colds, diarrhoea, otitis media, pneumonia, chickenpox, exanthema subitum; ORs either close to 1 or non-significant trend for exposure to increase AD risk No link between sibling effect and infections
Herbarth et al. [69], 2007	Cross-sectional Germany	2,487	mean age 6.3 years	Questionnaire (D) Questionnaire (E)	*Lifetime doctor-diagnosed AD* Bronchitis adj. OR = 1.99, $p < 0.001$ Frequent colds adj. OR = 1.09, $p < 0.493$
Reimerink et al. [70], 2009	Birth cohort The Netherlands	612	0–24 months	Questionnaire (D) Questionnaire (E)	AD first year of life and rotavirus adj. OR = 0.9 (0.5–1.7) Norovirus IgG (GGII.4) adj. OR = 1.1 (0.6–1.9) Norovirus IgG (GGI.1) adj. OR = 1.3 (0.7–2.5)
Rosenlund et al. [71], 2009	Cross-sectional Austria, Germany, the Netherlands, Sweden, Switzerland	9,136	5–13 years	Questionnaire (D) Questionnaire (E)	Measles adj. OR = 1.08 (0.85–1.36)
Silverberg et al. [73], 2010	Case-control USA	256 cases, 422 controls	1–18 years	General practitioner database (D + E)	Chickenpox adj. OR = 0.56 (0.35–0.90) *Chickenpox and AD severity* Moderate AD adj. OR = 0.08 (0.04–0.15) Severe AD adj. OR = 0.04 (0.01–0.13)

Table 2. Continued

Study	Study type and country	Number of participants	Age	Diagnostic criteria (D) and exposure measures (E)	Outcome measure(s) and comments
Hepatitis A, B, HSV and Helicobacter pylori					
Uter et al. [74], 2003	Cross-sectional Germany/Spain	1,368	First-year university students	Questionnaire (D) Anti-hepatitis-A, -B and Anti-HSV-1 IgG antibodies Anti-*Helicobacter* IgG and IgA antibodies (E)	Anti-HAV+ adj. OR = 0.61 (0.27–1.22) Anti-HBc+ adj. OR = 1.24 (0.58–2.13) Anti-HSV+ adj. OR = 1.02 (0.58–1.54) *H. pylori* adj. OR = 1.05 (0.63–1.70)
McCune et al. [75], 2003	Cross-sectional UK	3,244	20–59 years	Use of topical steroids (D) ^{13}C urea breath test (E)	adj. OR = 0.70 (0.54–0.91)
Herbarth et al. [69], 2007	Cross-sectional Germany	3,347	mean age 6.3 years	Questionnaire (D) ^{13}C urea breath test (E)	adj. OR = 0.31, p = 0.006
Endoparasites					
Huang et al. [78], 2002	Cross-sectional Taiwan	3,110	First to sixth grade	Questionnaire (D) Tape test parasite eggs (E)	*Enterobius vermicularis* NS, data does not allow calculation of OR
Cooper et al. [79], 2003	Cross-sectional Ecuador	4,433	5–18 years	Questionnaire (D) Parasite stool analysis (E)	Any geohelminth infection adj. OR = 0.85 (0.50–1.46)
Schäfer et al. [82], 2005	Cross-sectional Germany	4,169	mean age 9.2 years	Questionnaire (D) Questionnaire (E)	Worm infection prior to AD adj. OR = 0.45 (0.33–0.60)
Haileamlak et al. [80], 2005	Cross-sectional Ethiopia	732	1–5 years	Skin examination (D) Parasite stool analysis (E)	Any helminth infection adj. OR = 1.58 (1.16–2.15) *Trichuris* infection adj. OR = 1.61 (1.14–2.26) *Ascaris* and hookworm NS
Elliott et al. [81], 2005	Birth cohort Uganda	103	0–15 months	Skin examination (D) Parasite stool analysis (E)	Maternal helminth infection during last trimester and at delivery (predominantly hookworm) adj. RR = 0.26 (0.08–0.83)

Table 2. Continued

Study	Study type and country	Number of participants	Age	Diagnostic criteria (D) and exposure measures (E)	Outcome measure(s) and comments
Cooper et al. [84], 2006	Cluster randomized trial Antihelminthic treatment	2,373	mean age 9.4 years	Skin examination (D) Parasite stool analysis (E)	AD after 1 year of antihelminthic treatment with albendazole adj. OR = 0.86 (0.53–1.39)
Mpairwe et al. [83], 2009	RCT Antihelminthic treatment of the mother during the last trimester	2,507	1 year	Skin examination (D) Parasite stool analysis (E)	*AD in children at 1 year* Albendazole group (all) Cox HR = 1.82 (1.26–2.64) Praziquantel group (only if mother infected with schistosomiasis) Cox HR = 2.65 (1.16–6.08)
Flohr et al. [85], 2010	RCT Antihelminthic treatment	1,566	6–17 years	Skin examination (D) Parasite stool analysis (E)	AD after 1 year of antihelminthic treatment with albendazole adj. OR = 1.15 (0.39–3.45)
Tuberculosis					
Von Mutius et al. [64], 1999	Ecological ISAAC	235,477; 85 centres	13–14 years	Questionnaire (D) Annual tuberculosis notification rate per 100,000 per country from WHO data (E)	correlation r = 0.061, p = 0.278
Tuberculin skin response					
Shirakawa et al. [61], 1997	Cross-sectional Japan	867	12–13 years	Questionnaire (D) Tuberculin test (E)	adj. OR = 0.50 (0.33–0.91)
Yilmaz et al. [87], 2000	Case-control Turkey	538 cases, 198 controls	3–16 years	Physician (D) Tuberculin test (E)	NS, data does not allow calculation of OR
Grüber et al. [88], 2001	Birth cohort Germany	774	3, 6, 12, 18 months, 2, 3, 4, 5, 6 and 7 years	Questionnaire, physician (D) Tuberculin test (E)	NS, data does not allow calculation of OR
Wong et al. [89], 2001	Cross-sectional Hong Kong	3,110	10 years	Questionnaire (D) Tuberculin test (E)	adj. OR = 0.58 (0.30–1.15)
Miyake et al. [86], 2008	Cross-sectional Japan	5,717	8–11 years	Questionnaire (E) Immunization records (E)	adj. OR = 0.77 (0.62–0.95)
Eifan et al. [90], 2009	Birth cohort Turkey	399	0–5 years	Questionnaire (D) Tuberculin test (E)	No association between AD and tuberculin skin tes

Table 2. Continued

Study	Study type and country	Number of participants	Age	Diagnostic criteria (D) and exposure measures (E)	Outcome measure(s) and comments
BCG vaccination					
Alm et al. [91], 1997	Birth cohort Sweden	216 cases, 358 controls	2–7 years	Questionnaire (D) BCG scar (E)	OR = 0.86 (0.59–1.25)
Anderson et al. [92], 2001	Ecological ISAAC	235,477; 85 centres	13–14 years	Questionnaire (D) National immunization data from WHO (E)	Results were statistically not significant and not separately shown
Grüber et al. [93], 2002	Cross-sectional Germany	38,808	mean age 6 years	Questionnaire (D) Official vaccination documents (E)	adj. OR = 0.99 (0.87–1.13)
Yemaneberhan et al. [45], 2004	Cross-sectional Ethiopia	12,876	1–65 years and above	Questionnaire (D) Questionnaire (E)	adj. OR = 0.81 (0.51–1.28)
Garcia-Marcos et al. [94], 2005	Cross-sectional Spain	9,590	6–7 years	Questionnaire (D) Questionnaire (E)	adj. OR = 0.89 (0.76–1.05)
Steenhuis et al. [95], 2008	Prospective single-blind placebo-controlled BCG vaccination at 6 weeks of age	121	0–13 months	Skin examination(D) Questionnaire (E)	AD at 18 months RR = 0.77 (0.4–1.4) AD 'ever' by 18 months RR = 0.58 (0.3–1.0)
Möhrenschlager et al. [96], 2007	Cross-sectional Germany	1,673	5–7 years	Questionnaire and skin examination(D) Official vaccination documents (E)	AD preschool examination adj. OR = 1.67 (0.74–3.87) AD 'ever' (questionnaire) adj. OR = 0.76 (0.49–1.16)

ARI = Acute respiratory infection; EBV = Epstein-Barr virus; VZV = varizella-zoster virus; HSV = herpes simplex virus; HAV = hepatitis A virus; ISAAC = International Study of Asthma and Allergies in Childhood; BCG = bacille Calmette-Guérin. For additional explanations, see table 1.

Hepatitis, Herpes simplex virus and Helicobacter pylori

Although extremely common across the world, hepatitis, herpes virus and *Helicobacter pylori* infection have received little attention from the allergy community. A large cross-sectional questionnaire survey among first-year university students in Spain and Germany found no association with AD [74]. However, 2 cross-sectional surveys, one from the UK and the other from Germany, suggested an up to 70% reduction in AD risk in those with *H. pylori* infection (adj. OR = 0.70, 95% CI = 0.54–0.91, and adj. OR = 0.31, p = 0.006, respectively), and this area clearly warrants further research (table 2) [69, 75].

Helminth Infections

There is evidence from observational studies that eczema is common in populations with low parasite burden [12, 76, 77]. However, cross-sectional studies have not provided strong evidence for an effect of helminth infection on eczema, with both negative and positive associations reported (table 2) [78–81]. In 2005, Schäfer et al. [82] showed an independent inverse association between reported worm infection and AD in a population-based questionnaire study of 4,169 East German children (adj. OR = 0.45, 95% CI = 0.33–0.60). Further supporting evidence for an inverse relationship between AD and helminth infection comes from a small birth cohort study among 103 mother-infant pairs in Uganda, where the cumulative AD risk was decreased by 74% until the age of 15 months among children whose mothers were infected with helminths during the last trimester of pregnancy (adj. relative risk = 0.26, 95% CI = 0.08–0.83) [81]. Even stronger evidence comes from a double-blind randomized controlled trial conducted by the same group among 2,507 pregnant mothers in a helminth-endemic area (mainly hookworm and schistosomiasis). Albendazole and praziquantel were given in a 2 × 2 factorial design during the last trimester of pregnancy, and the risk of developing AD up to 1 year of age was significantly increased in the intervention groups (albendazole group, all children: Cox HR = 1.82, 95% CI = 1.26–2.64; praziquantel group, schistosomiasis-infected children only: Cox HR = 2.65, 95% CI = 1.16–6.08; table 2) [83]. This suggests that antenatal exposure to helminth parasites can protect against AD in the offspring. Interestingly, loss of helminth exposure does not appear to affect AD risk later on in life [84, 85], further supporting the notion that especially prenatal priming of the immune system exercises protection, with more host-invasive helminth species, such as hookworm and schistosomiasis, showing the strongest effects [77].

Tuberculosis, Tuberculin Responses and Bacille Calmette-Guérin Vaccination

The decline in tuberculosis infection in western industrialized countries a few decades ago preceded the recent epidemic of allergic disease and is therefore an important candidate for investigation. However, the only study to date, a worldwide ecological survey among 13- to 14-year-old schoolchildren, found no association between AD and tuberculosis [64].

Two Japanese cross-sectional surveys reported an up to 50% risk reduction in AD associated with positive tuberculin skin responses (>10 mm) in a setting where bacille Calmette-Guérin vaccination in infants is universal (table 2) [61, 86]. However, these findings could not be replicated elsewhere [87–90]. In addition, none out of 7 studies found a significant protective effect of bacille Calmette-Guérin vaccination on AD risk, although there was a trend towards protection (table 2) [45, 91–96].

Routine Childhood Vaccinations, Antibiotics and Atopic Dermatitis Risk

Two other factors that may profoundly affect the child's immune system in early life are childhood vaccination programmes and prescribing of antibiotics. Vaccinations expose infants and children to antigens of infectious agents that may lead to Th2-dominated immune responses, as has been shown in animal and clinical studies, and there is therefore concern that these might lead to an increase in allergic disease [97, 98]. Vaccines also contain adjuvants and stabilizers, which could conceivably enhance allergenicity [99]. Antibiotics may lead to a reduction in microbial burden, but are also known to alter the gut microflora and thus have an effect on the child's immune system at the level of the gut mucosa [100].

Routine Childhood Vaccinations

A cross-sectional study based on a UK general practice cohort indicated a slight increase in AD risk at 12 years of age in those who had received the combined diphtheria-pertussis-tetanus vaccine (OR = 1.37, 95% CI = 1.12–2.01) [62]. Only univariate analysis results were presented, however, and no significant associations with other vaccines were found. A Danish population-based cross-sectional study, assessing the risk of the MMR vaccine, demonstrated an almost twofold increase in AD risk in 3- to 15-year-old children (adj. OR = 1.86, 95% CI = 1.25–2.79) [67]. Significant positive associations between AD risk and the MMR as well as diphtheria-pertussis-polio-tetanus vaccines have also been found in a substantial UK general practice cohort of 29,238 children (adj. HR diphtheria-pertussis-polio-tetanus = 7.51, 95% CI = 5.27–10 70; adj. HR MMR = 3.50, 95% CI = 2.38–5.15; table 3) [101]. However, the latter study noted that the significant positive associations were confined to children in the lowest category of consultation frequency, suggesting that ascertainment bias rather than a true causal relationship was responsible. Six further studies have also not found any evidence for an increase in AD risk (1 ecological, 3 cross-sectional, 1 birth cohort and 1 randomized controlled trial [45, 71, 92, 96, 102, 103]). In addition, a cross-sectional study by Grüber et al. [104] among 2,184 children aged 1–2 years with established mild to severe AD suggested that a broad range of childhood vaccinations protects against severer disease (table 3).

Antibiotics

The vast majority of studies on the association between antibiotic use and AD risk have shown significant positive associations (pooled OR = 1.43, 95% CI = 1.36–1.49), especially if prescribed more frequently and during early life (fig. 3) [20, 59, 62, 64, 66, 72, 105–113]. Where examined, a dose-response relationship was seen (table 3) [72, 112]. Schmitt et al. [72] found among 487 German children that the risk was

Table 3. Exposure to vaccinations and antibiotics and AD risk

Study	Study type and country	Number of participants	Age	Diagnostic criteria (D) and exposure measures (E)	Outcome measure(s) and comments
Vaccinations					
Kemp et al. [102], 1997	Birth cohort New Zealand	1,265	5, 10 and 16 years	Questionnaire (D) Questionnaire (E)	*DPT vaccine at ages of 3 and 5 months and measles vaccine at 12–15 months* Age of 0–5 years OR = 1.30 (0.50–4.90) Age of 0–10 years OR = 1.20 (0.50–3.70) Age of 0–16 years OR = 1.30 (0.50–2.80)
Nilsson et al. [103], 1998	RCT Sweden	669	2 months to 2.5 years	Questionnaire (D) Several pertussis vaccines versus DT vaccine (E)	NS, data does not allow calculation of OR
Farooqi and Hopkin [62], 1998	Cross-sectional UK	1,934	0–12 years	Physician (D) General practitioner database (E)	Pertussis OR = 1.37 (1.12–2.01) Measles OR = 1.12 (0.74–1.68)
Anderson et al. [92], 2001	Ecological ISAAC	92 ISAAC centres	13–14 years	Questionnaire (D) National immunization data from WHO (E)	DPT r = –0.27 (–0.76 to 0.21) Measles r = –0.42 (–0.98 to 0.13), both adjusted for GNP
Olesen et al. [67], 2003	Cross-sectional Denmark	9,744	3–15 years	Questionnaire (D) Questionnaire (E)	MMR adj. OR = 1.86 (1.25–2.79)
Yemaneberhan et al. [45], 2004	Cross-sectional Ethiopia	12,876	1–65 years and above	Questionnaire (D) Questionnaire (E)	Measles adj. OR = 0.79 (0.49–1.28) Pertussis adj. OR = 0.60 (0.37–0.99) Diphtheria adj. OR = 0.72 (0.44–1.18) Tetanus adj. OR = 0.98 (0.65–1.47)

Table 3. Continued

Study	Study type and country	Number of participants	Age	Diagnostic criteria (D) and exposure measures (E)	Outcome measure(s) and comments
McKeever et al. [101], 2004	Birth cohort UK	29,238	0–11 years	General practitioner database (D + E)	Results only significant in group of children with lowest general practitioner consultation frequency, i.e. most likely due to bias rather than direct causality DPPT adj. HR = 7.51 (5.27–10.70) MMR adj. HR = 3.50 (2.38–5.15)
Möhrenschlager et al. [96], 2007	Cross-sectional Germany	1,673	5–7 years	Questionnaire (D) Questionnaire (E)	Physician-diagnosed AD Pertussis adj. OR = 1.22 (0.69–2.15)
Grüber et al. [104], 2008	Cross-sectional Australia, Austria, Belgium, Czech Republic, France, Germany, Italy, the Netherlands, Poland, South Africa, Spain and the UK	2,184	1–2 years, infants with active AD	Questionnaire (D) Questionnaire (E) Immunization cards	Mild versus moderate-severe AD Polio in first 6 months adj. OR = 0.66 (0.45–0.97) Pertussis in first year adj. OR = 0.30 (0.10–0.89) Varicella in first year adj. OR = 0.34 (0.12–0.93) Measles since birth adj. OR = 0.63 (0.49–0.80) Mumps since birth adj. OR = 0.68 (0.54–0.86) Rubella since birth adj. OR = 0.69 (0.55–0.87)
Rosenlund et al. [71], 2009	Cross-sectional Austria, Germany, the Netherlands, Sweden, Switzerland	14,893	5–13 years	Questionnaire (D) Questionnaire (E)	Physician-diagnosed AD Measles vaccination alone adj. OR = 0.94 (0.77–1.15) Measles vaccination – infection adj. OR = 0.88 (0.64–1.20)

Table 3. Continued

Study	Study type and country	Number of participants	Age	Diagnostic criteria (D) and exposure measures (E)	Outcome measure(s) and comments
Antibiotics					
Farooqi and Hopkin [62], 1998	Cross-sectional UK	1,934	1975–1984 birth cohort	Physician (D) General practitioner database (E)	OR = 2.04 (1.53–2.73)
Von Mutius et al. [64], 1999	Cross-sectional Germany	7,545 7,498	5–7 years 9–11 years	Questionnaire (D) Questionnaire (E)	1–2 courses adj. OR = 1.26 (1.05–1.52) 3–5 courses adj. OR = 1.50 (1.23–1.82) >5 courses adj. OR = 1.57 (1.23–1.99)
Wickens et al. [105] 1999	Cross-sectional New Zealand	456	5–10 years	Questionnaire (D) Questionnaire (E)	adj. OR = 1.23 (0.71–2.13)
Droste et al. [106], 2000	Cross-sectional Belgium	1,592	7–8 years	Questionnaire (D) Questionnaire (E)	adj. OR = 1.60 (1.00–2.60)
McKeever et al. [59], 2002	Birth cohort UK	29,238	0–11 years	Physician (D) General practitioner research database(E)	adj. HR = 1.48 (1.31–1.68)
McKeever et al. [66], 2002	Birth cohort UK	29,238	0–11 years	Physician (D) General practitioner research database(E)	Prenatal antibiotics adj. HR = 1.17 (1.06–1.29)
Celedón et al. [107], 2002	Birth cohort USA	498	0–5 years	Questionnaire (D) Questionnaire (E)	adj. OR = 1.10 (0.40–3.10)
Foliaki et al. [113], 2009	Ecological ISAAC	99 centres	13–14 years	Questionnaire (D) Data on national antibiotic sales obtained from the Institute for Medical Statistics (E)	r = –0.16, p = 0.44

Table 3. Continued

Study	Study type and country	Number of participants	Age	Diagnostic criteria (D) and exposure measures (E)	Outcome measure(s) and comments
Cohet et al. [108], 2004	Case-control New Zealand	1,584 cases, 2,539 controls	6–7 years	Questionnaire (D) Questionnaire (E)	adj. OR = 1.40 (1.21–1.62)
edrychowski et al. [109], 2006	Birth cohort Poland	102	1 year	Questionnaire (D) Questionnaire (E)	Prenatal antibiotics adj. OR = 2.30 (0.91–5.80)
ummeling et al. [110], 2007	Birth cohort The Netherlands	2,583	0–24 months	Questionnaire (D) Questionnaire (E)	Through breastmilk adj. OR = 1.07 (0.80–1.42) Through medication adj. OR = 0.94 (0.75–1.18)
Wickens et al. [111], 2008	Birth cohort New Zealand	967	0–4 years	Questionnaire (D) Questionnaire (E)	Eczema <15 months adj. OR = 1.71 (1.26–2.33) Eczema 3–4 years adj. OR = 1.14 (0.87–1.51)
usel et al. [112], 2008	Birth cohort Australia	198	0–5 years	Physical examination (D) Daily diary for 5 years (E)	First year of life adj. OR = 1.5 (0.7–3.3) No association with number of courses of antibiotics either
oliaki et al. [113], 2009	Cross-sectional ISAAC phase III	193,412	6–7 years	Questionnaire (D) Questionnaire (E)	adj. OR = 1.42 (1.33–1.51)
om et al. [20], 2010	Birth cohort Germany	773	0–4 years	Questionnaire (D) Questionnaire (E)	*Prenatal antibiotics* adj. OR = 1.82 (1.14–2.92) *Postnatal antibiotics* through breastmilk adj. OR = 1.14 (0.55–2.35) through medication exposed first year of life adj. OR = 0.61 (0.36–1.01) exposed after first year of life adj. OR = 0.11 (0.05–0.23)

Table 3. Continued

Study	Study type and country	Number of participants	Age	Diagnostic criteria (D) and exposure measures (E)	Outcome measure(s) and comments
Schmitt et al. [72], 2010	Birth cohort Germany	487	0–2 years	Health insurance database (D + E)	Antibiotic exposure 'yes/no' RR = 1.66 (0.95–2.90) ≥2 courses of antibiotics RR = 2.11 (1.05–4.22) *Respiratory tract infections* treated with penicillin RR = 1.15 (0.48–2.75) treated with macrolides RR = 2.15 (1.18–3.91) treated with cephalosporins RR = 1.93 (1.07–3.49)

DPT = Diphtheria-pertussis-tetanus; DT = diphtheria-tetanus; GNP = gross national product; DPPT = diphtheria-pertussi polio-tetanus. For additional explanations, see tables 1 and 2.

highest with macrolides and cephalosporins, whereas the less broad-spectrum penicillins showed no significant association. The effect of antibiotics seems to extend into the antenatal period [20, 66, 109]. A recent ecological study could not find an association between antibiotic sales and AD risk at the population level [114].

Most authors have speculated that it is an antibiotic-induced alteration of the gut microflora, which promotes the development of allergic disease. Indeed, the gut of children with AD is less often colonized with lactobacilli. Instead, more coliform microbes and *Staphylococcus aureus* are found, and these changes can precede the clinical manifestation of AD [115–117].

Conclusions

Main Findings

Although a consistent association between a decreased risk of AD and a higher number of older siblings initially led to the hypothesis that such an association might be due to an increased exposure to certain infections, we found no convincing evidence to support this hypothesis in industrialized countries. However, birth cohort and intervention studies in developing nations suggest that helminths, in particular

Study or subgroup	log [OR]	SE	Weight	OR IV, fixed, 95% CI
Celedon et al. [107], 2002	0.0953	0.5224	0.2%	1.10; 0.40–3.06
Cohet et al. [108], 2004	0.3365	0.0744	10.1%	1.40; 1.21–1.62
Dom et al. [20], 2010	–0.4943	0.2632	0.8%	0.61; 0.36–1.02
Droste et al. [106], 2000	0.47	0.0986	5.8%	1.60; 1.32–1.94
Farooqi and Hophin [62], 1998	0.7129	0.1486	2.5%	2.04; 1.52–2.73
Foliaki et al. [113], 2009	0.3507	0.0324	53.3%	1.42; 1.33–1.51
Kummeling et al. [110], 2007	–0.06	0.1156	4.2%	0.94; 0.75–1.18
Kusel et al. [112], 2008	0.4055	0.3956	0.4%	1.50; 0.69–3.26
McKeever et al. [59], 2002	0.392	0.0646	13.4%	1.48; 1.30–1.68
Schmitt et al. [72], 2010	0.7655	0.3056	0.5%	2.15; 1.18–3.91
Von Mutius et al. [64], 1999	0.4054	0.0986	5.3%	1.50; 1.24–1.82
Wickens et al. [105], 1999	0.207	0.2801	0.7%	1.23; 0.71–2.13
Wickens et al. [111], 2008	0.5365	0.1568	2.3%	1.71; 1.26–2.33
Total			100.0%	1.43; 1.36–1.49

Heterogeneity: $\chi^2 = 34.82$, d.f. = 12 ($p = 0.0005$); $I^2 = 66\%$
Test for overall effect: $Z = 15.02$ ($p < 0.00001$)

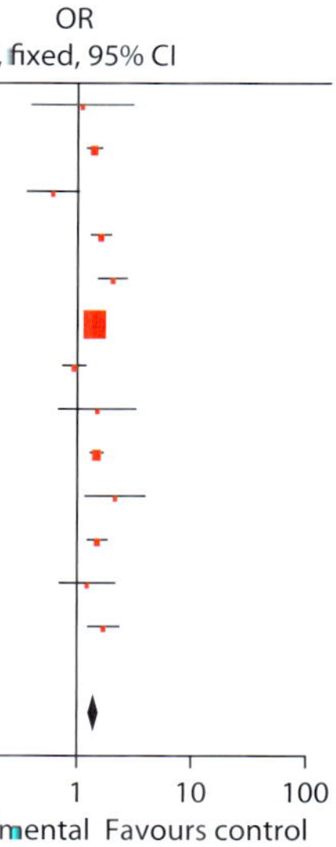

Fig. 3. Antibiotics and AD risk.

hookworm and schistosomiasis, can protect against the development of AD, especially if such exposures occur already during pregnancy. Broad-spectrum antibiotics used both during pregnancy and infancy significantly increase the risk of AD, possibly due to modification of the gut microflora, which would also explain why probiotics can have a preventative effect on AD development [118]. Likewise, the protective effect associated with unpasteurized farm milk consumption, endotoxin exposure, day care during infancy and being brought up with a dog during early life could all be mediated by non-pathological microbial stimulation of the immune system [119]. The timing as well as the degree of exposure is likely to be important, as has for instance been shown for endotoxins, where only high exposure levels in early life appear protective. One study has found that children in families who wash more frequently have a higher AD risk, but this could be due to irritation of the skin barrier by increased soap usage rather than a reduction in pathogens, in particular in those with a genetic predisposition to skin barrier impairment, but this was not assessed as part of the study.

Gene-Environment Interaction

So far, only very few population-based studies have determined skin barrier gene mutation status and how this interacts with environmental factors. In the context of the hygiene hypothesis, it was interesting to note that the number of older siblings interacted positively with filaggrin skin barrier gene mutation carriage on AD risk in 2 German cohort studies, but this needs replication and further investigation [120]. In addition, children with filaggrin mutations who were exposed to a cat during the first year of life had an up to 11 times higher risk of developing AD compared to wild-type children [51, 52]. Another example of gene-environment interaction is that endotoxin exposure only reduced AD risk in those carrying a specific genotype of the CD14 lipopolysaccharide receptor complex encoded on chromosome 5q31.1 in a UK cohort [57]. Overall, there certainly is a need for further prospective population-based studies that carefully disentangle how genetic and environmental factors linked to the hygiene hypothesis interact on the path to clinical AD (fig. 1a).

Implications for Clinical Practice

It is reassuring that childhood vaccinations do not increase the risk of AD, but caution should prevail in the frequent prescribing of broad-spectrum antibiotics early in life, especially in children with a family history of atopic disease. So far, attempts to treat established allergic disease by voluntary helminth infection in asthmatics and hay fever sufferers have been disappointing [77]. Although no such trials exist in AD patients yet, rather than infecting ourselves with potentially harmful pathogens, success is more likely if we can find creative ways of mimicking what occurs in developing country settings through the development of parasite-derived drugs [121]. An example of such a target molecule is ES-62, a glycoprotein secreted by filarial worms that is able to inhibit mast cell degranulation, but clinical studies are still awaited [122].

Once our immune systems have lost balance and are on a track towards allergic tissue inflammation, such interventions are likely to come too late. A recent meta-analysis of intervention studies suggested that probiotics, such as live *Lactobacillus rhamnosus*, given to both pregnant mothers and their infants postnatally can reduce AD risk by around 40% [123]. Interestingly, similar therapeutic interventions in established AD have been disappointing [118, 123], as has the attempt to treat AD with subcutaneous injections of non-pathogenic mycobacteria, further suggesting that early priming of the immune system via the gut mucosa is key [124–128]. We should therefore focus our research efforts on developing preventative methods for high-risk children. This would certainly be a significant therapeutic step forward, given that our current treatments for AD and other allergies only achieve symptom control rather than cure.

References

1 Williams HC: Epidemiology of atopic dermatitis. Clin Exp Dermatol 2000;25:522–529.
2 Schultz Larsen F: Atopic dermatitis: a genetic-epidemiologic study in a population-based twin sample. J Am Acad Dermatol 1993;28:719–723.
3 McGrath JA, Uitto J: The filaggrin story: novel insights into skin-barrier function and disease. Trends Mol Med 2008;14:20–27.
4 Schram ME, Tedja AM, Spijker R, Bos JD, Williams HC, Spuls PI: Is there a rural/urban gradient in the prevalence of eczema? A systematic review. Br J Dermatol 2010;162:964–973.
5 Hjern A, Haglund B, Hedlin G: Ethnicity, childhood environment and atopic disorder. Clin Exp Allergy 2000;30:521–528.
6 Odhiambo JA, Williams HC, Clayton TO, Robertson CF, Asher MI: Global variations in prevalence of eczema symptoms in children from ISAAC Phase Three. J Allergy Clin Immunol 2009;124: 1251–1258.
7 Williams HC, Strachan DP, Hay RJ: Childhood eczema: disease of the advantaged? BMJ 1994;308: 1132–1135.
8 McKeever TM, Lewis SA, Smith C, Collins J, Heatlie H, Frischer M, Hubbard R: Siblings, multiple births, and the incidence of allergic disease: a birth cohort study using the West Midlands general practice research database. Thorax 2001;56:758–762.
9 Karmaus W, Botezan C: Does a higher number of siblings protect against the development of allergy and asthma? J Epidemiol Community Health 2002; 56:209–217.
10 Strachan DP: Hay fever, hygiene, and household size. BMJ 1989;299:1259–1260.
11 Bach JF: The protective effect of infections on immune disorders. J Pediatr Gastroenterol Nutr 2005;40(suppl 1):S8.
12 Yazdanbakhsh M, Kremsner PG, van Ree R: Allergy, parasites, and the hygiene hypothesis. Science 2002; 296:490–494.
13 Yazdanbakhsh M, Rodrigues LC: Allergy and the hygiene hypothesis: the Th1/Th2 counterregulation cannot provide an explanation. Wien Klin Wochenschr 2001;113:899–902.
14 Holt PG, Sly PD, Bjorksten B: Atopic versus infectious diseases in childhood: a question of balance? Pediatr Allergy Immunol 1997;8:53–58.
15 Okada H, Kuhn C, Feillet H, Bach JF: The 'hygiene hypothesis' for autoimmune and allergic disease: an update. Clin Exp Immunol 2010;160:1–9.
16 Flohr C, Pascoe D, Williams HC: Atopic dermatitis and the 'hygiene hypothesis': too clean to be true? Br J Dermatol 2005;152:202–216.
17 Sherriff A, Golding J: Hygiene levels in a contemporary population cohort are associated with wheezing and atopic eczema in preschool infants. Arch Dis Child 2002;87:26–29.
18 Celedón JC, Wright RJ, Litonjua AA, Sredl D, Ryan L, Weiss ST, Gold DR: Day care attendance in early life, maternal history of asthma, and asthma at the age of 6 years. Am J Respir Crit Care Med 2003;167: 1239–1243.
19 Benn CS, Melbye M, Wohlfahrt J, Bjorksten B, Aaby P: Cohort study of sibling effect, infectious diseases, and risk of atopic dermatitis during first 18 months of life. BMJ 2004;328:1223.
20 Dom S, Droste JH, Sariachvili MA, Hagendorens MM, Oostveen E, Bridts CH, Stevens WJ, Wieringa MH, Weyler JJ: Pre- and post-natal exposure to antibiotics and the development of eczema, recurrent wheezing and atopic sensitization in children up to the age of 4 years Clin Exp Allergy 2010;40: 1378–1387.
21 Hagerhed-Engman L, Bornehag CG, Sundell J, Aberg N: Day-care attendance and increased risk for respiratory and allergic symptoms in preschool age. Allergy 2006;61:447–453.
22 Dunder T, Tapiainen T, Pokka T, Uhari M: Infections in child day care centers and later development of asthma, allergic rhinitis, and atopic dermatitis: prospective follow-up survey 12 years after controlled randomized hygiene intervention. Arch Pediatr Adolesc Med 2007;161:972–977.
23 Alm JS, Swartz J, Lilja G, Scheynius A, Pershagen G: Atopy in children of families with an anthroposophic lifestyle. Lancet 1999;353:1485–1488.
24 Kirjavainen PV, Arvola T, Salminen SJ, Isolauri E: Aberrant composition of gut microbiota of allergic infants: a target of bifidobacterial therapy at weaning? Gut 2002;51:51–55.
25 Vaarala O: Immunological effects of probiotics with special reference to lactobacilli. Clin Exp Allergy 2003;33:1634–1640.
26 Floistrup H, Swartz J, Bergstrom A, Alm JS, Scheynius A, van Hage M, Waser M, Braun-Fahrlander C, Schram-Bijkerk D, Huber M, Zutavern A, von Mutius E, Ublagger E, Riedler J, Michaels KB, Pershagen G: Allergic disease and sensitization in Steiner school children. J Allergy Clin Immunol 2006;117:59–66.

27 Braun-Fahrlander C, Gassner M, Grize L, Neu U, Sennhauser FH, Varonier HS, Vuille JC, Wuthrich B: Prevalence of hay fever and allergic sensitization in farmer's children and their peers living in the same rural community. SCARPOL team. Swiss Study on Childhood Allergy and Respiratory Symptoms with Respect to Air Pollution. Clin Exp Allergy 1999;29:28–34.

28 Von Ehrenstein OS, von Mutius E, Illi S, Baumann L, Bohm O, von Kries R: Reduced risk of hay fever and asthma among children of farmers. Clin Exp Allergy 2000;30:187–193.

29 Riedler J, Eder W, Oberfeld G, Schreuer M: Austrian children living on a farm have less hay fever, asthma and allergic sensitization. Clin Exp Allergy 2000;30: 194–200.

30 Kilpelainen M, Terho EO, Helenius H, Koskenvuo M: Farm environment in childhood prevents the development of allergies. Clin Exp Allergy 2000;30: 201–208.

31 Wickens K, Lane JM, Fitzharris P, Siebers R, Riley G, Douwes J, Smith T, Crane J: Farm residence and exposures and the risk of allergic diseases in New Zealand children. Allergy 2002;57:1171–1179.

32 Bråbäck L, Hjern A, Rasmussen F: Trends in asthma, allergic rhinitis and eczema among Swedish conscripts from farming and non-farming environments: a nationwide study over three decades. Clin Exp Allergy 2004;34:38–43.

33 Perkin MR, Strachan DP: Which aspects of the farming lifestyle explain the inverse association with childhood allergy? J Allergy Clin Immunol 2006; 117:1374–1381.

34 Douwes J, Travier N, Huang K, Cheng S, McKenzie J, Le Gros G, von Mutius E, Pearce N: Lifelong farm exposure may strongly reduce the risk of asthma in adults. Allergy 2007;62:1158–1165.

35 Karadag B, Ege MJ, Scheynius A, Waser M, Schram-Bijkerk D, van Hage M, Pershagen G, Brunekreef B, Riedler J, Braun-Fahrlander C, von Mutius E: Environmental determinants of atopic eczema phenotypes in relation to asthma and atopic sensitization. Allergy 2007;62:1387–1393.

36 Douwes J, Cheng S, Travier N, Cohet C, Niesink A, McKenzie J, Cunningham C, Le Gros G, von Mutius E, Pearce N: Farm exposure in utero may protect against asthma, hay fever and eczema. Eur Respir J 2008;32:603–611.

37 Hesselmar B, Aberg N, Aberg B, Eriksson B, Bjorksten B: Does early exposure to cat or dog protect against later allergy development? Clin Exp Allergy 1999;29:611–617.

38 Bråbäck L, Kjellman NI, Sandin A, Bjorksten B: Atopy among schoolchildren in northern and southern Sweden in relation to pet ownership and early life events. Pediatr Allergy Immunol 2001; 12:4–10.

39 Nafstad P, Magnus P, Gaarder PI, Jaakkola JJ: Exposure to pets and atopy-related diseases in the first 4 years of life. Allergy 2001;56:307–312.

40 Zirngibl A, Franke K, Gehring U, von Berg A, Berdel D, Bauer CP, Reinhardt D, Wichmann HE, Heinrich J: Exposure to pets and atopic dermatitis during the first two years of life: a cohort study. Pediatr Allergy Immunol 2002;13:394–401.

41 Kerkhof M, Koopman LP, van Strien RT, Wijga A, Smit HA, Aalberse RC, Neijens HJ, Brunekreef B, Postma DS, Gerritsen J: Risk factors for atopic dermatitis in infants at high risk of allergy: the PIAMA study. Clin Exp Allergy 2003;33: 1336–1341.

42 Phipatanakul W, Celedón JC, Raby BA, Litonjua AA, Milton DK, Sredl D, Weiss ST, Gold DR: Endotoxin exposure and eczema in the first year of life. Pediatrics 2004;114:13–18.

43 Illi S, von Mutius E, Lau S, Nickel R, Grüber C, Niggemann B, Wahn U: The natural course of atopic dermatitis from birth to age 7 years and the association with asthma. J Allergy Clin Immunol 2004;113: 925–931.

44 Gern JE, Reardon CL, Hoffjan S, Nicolae D, Li Z, Roberg KA, Neaville WA, Carlson-Dakes K, Adler K, Hamilton R, Anderson E, Gilbertson-White S, Tisler C, Dasilva D, Anklam K, Mikus LD, Rosenthal LA, Ober C, Gangnon R, Lemanske RF Jr: Effects of dog ownership and genotype on immune development and atopy in infancy. J Allergy Clin Immunol 2004;113:307–314.

45 Yemaneberhan H, Flohr C, Lewis SA, Bekele Z, Parry E, Williams HC, Britton J, Venn A: Prevalence and associated factors of atopic dermatitis symptoms in rural and urban Ethiopia. Clin Exp Allergy 2004;34:779–785.

46 Kurosaka F, Nakatani Y, Terada T, Tanaka A, Ikeuchi H, Hayakawa A, Konohana A, Oota K, Nishio H: Current cat ownership may be associated with the lower prevalence of atopic dermatitis, allergic rhinitis, and Japanese cedar pollinosis in schoolchildren in Himeji, Japan. Pediatr Allergy Immunol 2006;17: 22–28.

47 Purvis DJ, Thompson JM, Clark PM, Robinson E, Black PN, Wild CJ, Mitchell EA: Risk factors for atopic dermatitis in New Zealand children at 3.5 years of age. Br J Dermatol 2005;152:742–749.

48 Hagendorens MM, Bridts CH, Lauwers K, van Nuijs S, Ebo DG, Vellinga A, De Clerck LS, Van Bever HP, Weyler JJ, Stevens WJ: Perinatal risk factors for sensitization, atopic dermatitis and wheezing during the first year of life (PIPO study). Clin Exp Allergy 2005;35:733–740.

49 Pohlabeln H, Jacobs S, Böhmann J: Exposure to pets and the risk of allergic symptoms during the first 2 years of life. J Investig Allergol Clin Immunol 2007;17:302–308.

50 Bufford JD, Reardon CL, Li Z, Roberg KA, Da Silva D, Eggleston PA, Liu AH, Milton D, Alwis U, Gangnon R, Lemanske RF Jr, Gern JE: Effects of dog ownership in early childhood on immune development and atopic diseases. Clin Exp Allergy 2008;38:1635–1643.

51 Bisgaard H, Simpson A, Palmer CN, Bonnelykke K, McLean I, Mukhopadhyay S, Pipper CB, Halkjaer LB, Lipworth B, Hankinson J, Woodcock A, Custovic A: Gene-environment interaction in the onset of eczema in infancy: filaggrin loss-of-function mutations enhanced by neonatal cat exposure. PLoS Med 2008;5:e131.

52 Schuttelaar ML, Kerkhof M, Jonkman MF, Koppelman GH, Brunekreef B, de Jongste JC, Wijga A, McLean WH, Postma DS: Filaggrin mutations in the onset of eczema, sensitization, asthma, hay fever and the interaction with cat exposure. Allergy 2009;64:1758–1765.

53 Schäfer T, Stieger B, Polzius R, Krauspe A: Associations between cat keeping, allergen exposure, allergic sensitization and atopic diseases: results from the Children of Lubeck Allergy and Environment Study (KLAUS). Pediatr Allergy Immunol 2009;20:353–357.

54 Gehring U, Bolte G, Borte M, Bischof W, Fahlbusch B, Wichmann HE, Heinrich J: Exposure to endotoxin decreases the risk of atopic eczema in infancy: a cohort study. J Allergy Clin Immunol 2001;108:847–854.

55 Bolte G, Bischof W, Borte M, Lehmann I, Wichmann HE, Heinrich J: Early endotoxin exposure and atopy development in infants: results of a birth cohort study. Clin Exp Allergy 2003;33:770–776.

56 Perzanowski MS, Miller RL, Thorne PS, Barr RG, Divjan A, Sheares BJ, Garfinkel RS, Perera FP, Goldstein IF, Chew GL: Endotoxin in inner-city homes: associations with wheeze and eczema in early childhood. J Allergy Clin Immunol 2006;117:1082–1089.

57 Simpson A, John SL, Jury F, Niven R, Woodcock A, Ollier WE, Custovic A: Endotoxin exposure, CD14, and allergic disease: an interaction between genes and the environment. Am J Respir Crit Care Med 2006;174:386–392.

58 Chen CM, Sausenthaler S, Bischof W, Herbarth O, Borte M, Behrendt H Kramer U, Williams HC, Wichmann HE, Heinrich J: Perinatal exposure to endotoxin and the development of eczema during the first 6 years of life. Clin Exp Dermatol 2009;35:238–244.

59 McKeever TM, Lewis SA, Smith C, Hubbard R: The importance of prenatal exposures on the development of allergic disease: a birth cohort study using the West Midlands General Practice Database. Am J Respir Crit Care Med 2002;166:827–832.

60 Zutavern A, von Klot S, Gehring U, Krauss-Etschmann S, Heinrich J: Pre-natal and post-natal exposure to respiratory infection and atopic diseases development: a historical cohort study. Respir Res 2006;7:81.

61 Shirakawa T, Enomoto T, Shimazu S, Hopkin JM: The inverse association between tuberculin responses and atopic disorder. Science 1997;275:77–79.

62 Farooqi IS, Hopkin JM: Early childhood infection and atopic disorder. Thorax 1998;53:927–932.

63 Bodner C, Godden D, Seaton A: Family size, childhood infections and atopic diseases. The Aberdeen WHEASE Group. Thorax 1998;53:28–32.

64 Von Mutius E, Illi S, Hirsch T, Leupold W, Keil U, Weiland SK: Frequency of infections and risk of asthma, atopy and airway hyperresponsiveness in children. Eur Respir J 1999;14:4–11.

65 Paunio M, Heinonen OP, Virtanen M, Leinikki P, Patja A, Peltola H: Measles history and atopic diseases: a population-based cross-sectional study. JAMA 2000;283:343–346.

66 McKeever TM, Lewis SA, Smith C, Collins J, Heatlie H, Frischer M, Hubbard R: Early exposure to infections and antibiotics and the incidence of allergic disease: a birth cohort study with the West Midlands General Practice Research Database. J Allergy Clin Immunol 2002;109:43–50.

67 Olesen AB, Juul S, Thestrup-Pedersen K: Atopic dermatitis is increased following vaccination for measles, mumps and rubella or measles infection. Acta Derm Venereol 2003;83:445–450.

68 Gibbs S, Surridge H, Adamson R, Cohen B, Bentham G, Reading R: Atopic dermatitis and the hygiene hypothesis: a case-control study. Int J Epidemiol 2004;33:199–207.

69 Herbarth O, Bauer M, Fritz GJ, Herbarth P, Rolle-Kampczyk U, Krumbiegel P, Richter M, Richter T: *Helicobacter pylori* colonisation and eczema. J Epidemiol Community Health 2007;61:638–640.

70 Reimerink J, Stelma F, Rockx B, Brouwer D, Stobberingh E, van Ree R, Dompeling E, Mommers M, Thijs C, Koopmans M: Early-life rotavirus and norovirus infections in relation to development of atopic manifestation in infants. Clin Exp Allergy 2009;39:254–260.
71 Rosenlund H, Bergstrom A, Alm JS, Swartz J, Scheynius A, van Hage M, Johansen K, Brunekreef B, von Mutius E, Ege MJ, Riedler J, Braun-Fahrlander C, Waser M, Pershagen G: Allergic disease and atopic sensitization in children in relation to measles vaccination and measles infection. Pediatrics 2009;123:771–778.
72 Schmitt J, Schmitt NM, Kirch W, Meurer M: Early exposure to antibiotics and infections and the incidence of atopic eczema: a population-based cohort study. Pediatr Allergy Immunol 2010;21: 292–300.
73 Silverberg JI, Norowitz KB, Kleiman E, Silverberg NB, Durkin HG, Joks R, Smith-Norowitz TA: Association between varicella zoster virus infection and atopic dermatitis in early and late childhood: a case-control study. J Allergy Clin Immunol 2010; 126:300–305.
74 Uter W, Stock C, Pfahlberg A, Guillen-Grima F, Aguinaga-Ontoso I, Brun-Sandiumenge C, Kramer A: Association between infections and signs and symptoms of 'atopic' hypersensitivity – results of a cross-sectional survey among first-year university students in Germany and Spain. Allergy 2003;58: 580–584.
75 McCune A, Lane A, Murray L, Harvey I, Nair P, Donovan J, Harvey R: Reduced risk of atopic disorders in adults with *Helicobacter pylori* infection. Eur J Gastroenterol Hepatol 2003;15:637–640.
76 Flohr C: Dirt, worms and atopic dermatitis. Br J Dermatol 2003;148:871–877.
77 Flohr C, Quinnell RJ, Britton J: Do helminth parasites protect against atopy and allergic disease? Clin Exp Allergy 2009;39:20–32.
78 Huang SL, Tsai PF, Yeh YF: Negative association of *Enterobius* infestation with asthma and rhinitis in primary school children in Taipei. Clin Exp Allergy 2002;32:1029–1032.
79 Cooper PJ, Chico ME, Bland M, Griffin GE, Nutman TB: Allergic symptoms, atopy, and geohelminth infections in a rural area of Ecuador. Am J Respir Crit Care Med 2003;168:313–317.
80 Haileamlak A, Dagoye D, Williams H, Venn AJ, Hubbard R, Britton J, Lewis SA: Early life risk factors for atopic dermatitis in Ethiopian children. J Allergy Clin Immunol 2005;115:370–376.
81 Elliott AM, Mpairwe H, Quigley MA, Nampijja M, Muhangi L, Oweka-Onyee J, Muwanga M, Ndibazza J, Whitworth JA: Helminth infection during pregnancy and development of infantile eczema. JAMA 2005;294:2032–2034.
82 Schäfer T, Meyer T, Ring J, Wichmann HE, Heinrich J: Worm infestation and the negative association with eczema (atopic/nonatopic) and allergic sensitization. Allergy 2005;60:1014–1020.
83 Mpairwe H, Webb E, Muhangi L, Ndibazza J, Tumusiimo J, Rodrigues L, Elliott A: Effects of treatment of helminths with albendazole and praziquantel in pregnancy on the incidence of allergy in the first year of life: trial results. Allergy 2009;64:92.
84 Cooper PJ, Chico ME, Vaca MG, Moncayo AL, Bland JM, Mafla E, Sanchez F, Rodrigues LC, Strachan DP, Griffin GE: Effect of albendazole treatments on the prevalence of atopy in children living in communities endemic for geohelminth parasites: a cluster-randomised trial. Lancet 2006;367: 1598–1603.
85 Flohr C, Tuyen LN, Quinnell RJ, Lewis S, Minh TT, Campbell J, Simmons C, Telford G, Brown A, Hien TT, Farrar J, Williams H, Pritchard DI, Britton J: Reduced helminth burden increases allergen skin sensitization but not clinical allergy: a randomized, double-blind, placebo-controlled trial in Vietnam. Clin Exp Allergy 2010;40:131–142.
86 Miyake Y, Arakawa M, Tanaka K, Sasaki S, Ohya Y: Tuberculin reactivity and allergic disorders in schoolchildren, Okinawa, Japan. Clin Exp Allergy 2008;38:486–492.
87 Yilmaz M, Bingol G, Altintas D, Kendirli SG: Correlation between atopic diseases and tuberculin responses. Allergy 2000;55:664–667.
88 Grüber C, Kulig M, Bergmann R, Guggenmoos-Holzmann I, Wahn U: Delayed hypersensitivity to tuberculin, total immunoglobulin E, specific sensitization, and atopic manifestation in longitudinally followed early bacille Calmette-Guérin-vaccinated and nonvaccinated children. Pediatrics 2001;107: E36.
89 Wong GW, Hui DS, Tam CM, Chan HH, Fok TF, Chan-Yeung M, Lai CK: Asthma, atopy and tuberculin responses in Chinese schoolchildren in Hong Kong. Thorax 2001;56:770–773.
90 Eifan AO, Akkoc T, Ozdemir C, Bahceciler NN, Barlan IB: No association between tuberculin skin test and atopy in a bacillus Calmette-Guérin vaccinated birth cohort. Pediatr Allergy Immunol 2009; 20:545–550.
91 Alm JS, Lilja G, Pershagen G, Scheynius A: Early BCG vaccination and development of atopy. Lancet 1997;350:400–403.

92 Anderson HR, Poloniecki JD, Strachan DP, Beasley R, Bjorksten B, Asher MI: Immunization and symptoms of atopic disease in children: results from the International Study of Asthma and Allergies in Childhood. Am J Public Health 2001;91: 1126–1129.
93 Grüber C, Meinlschmidt G, Bergmann R, Wahn U, Stark K: Is early BCG vaccination associated with less atopic disease? An epidemiological study in German preschool children with different ethnic backgrounds. Pediatr Allergy Immunol 2002;13: 177–181.
94 Garcia-Marcos L, Suarez-Varela MM, Canflanca IM, Garrido JB, Quiros AB, Lopez-Silvarrey Varela A, Hernandez GG, Guillen-Grima F, Diaz CG, Gonzalez IH, Pena AA, Monge RB: BCG immunization at birth and atopic diseases in a homogeneous population of Spanish schoolchildren. Int Arch Allergy Immunol 2005;137:303–309.
95 Steenhuis TJ, van Aalderen WM, Bloksma N, Nijkamp FP, van der Laag J, van Loveren H, Rijkers GT, Kuis W Hoekstra MO: Bacille Calmette-Guérin vaccination and the development of allergic disease in children: a randomized, prospective, single-blind study. Clin Exp Allergy 2008;38:79–85.
96 Möhrenschlager M, Haberl VM, Kramer U, Behrendt H, Ring J: Early BCG and pertussis vaccination and atopic diseases in 5- to 7-year-old preschool children from Augsburg, Germany: results from the MIRIAM study. Pediatr Allergy Immunol 2007;18:5–9.
97 Lindsay DS, Parton R, Wardlaw AC: Adjuvant effect of pertussis toxin on the production of anti-ovalbumin IgE in mice and lack of direct correlation between PCA and ELISA. Int Arch Allergy Immunol 1994;105:281–288.
98 Pauwels R, van der Straeten M, Platteau B, Bazin H: The non-specific enhancement of allergy. I. In vivo effects of *Bordetella pertussis* vaccine on IgE synthesis. Allergy 1983;38:239–246.
99 Grüber C, Nilsson L, Bjorksten B: Do early childhood immunizations influence the development of atopy and do they cause allergic reactions? Pediatr Allergy Immunol 2001;12:296–311.
100 Guarner F, Malagelada JR: Gut flora in health and disease. Lancet 2003;361:512–519.
101 McKeever TM, Lewis SA, Smith C, Hubbard R: Vaccination and allergic disease: a birth cohort study. Am J Public Health 2004;94:985–989.
102 Kemp T, Pearce N, Fitzharris P, Crane J, Fergusson D, St George I, Wickens K, Beasley R: Is infant immunization a risk factor for childhood asthma or allergy? Epidemiology 1997;8:678–680.
103 Nilsson L, Kjellman NI, Bjorksten B: A randomized controlled trial of the effect of pertussis vaccines on atopic disease. Arch Pediatr Adolesc Med 1998;152: 734–738.
104 Grüber C, Warner J, Hill D, Bauchau V: Early atopic disease and early childhood immunization – is there a link? Allergy 2008;63 1464–1472.
105 Wickens K, Pearce N, Crane J, Beasley R: Antibiotic use in early childhood and the development of asthma. Clin Exp Allergy 1999;29:766–771.
106 Droste JH, Wieringa MH, Weyler JJ, Nelen VJ, Vermeire PA, van Bever HP: Does the use of antibiotics in early childhood increase the risk of asthma and allergic disease? Clin Exp Allergy 2000;30: 1547–1553.
107 Celedón JC, Litonjua AA, Ryan L, Weiss ST, Gold DR: Lack of association between antibiotic use in the first year of life and asthma, allergic rhinitis, or eczema at age 5 years. Am J Respir Crit Care Med 2002;166:72–75.
108 Cohet C, Cheng S, MacDonald C, Baker M, Foliaki S, Huntington N, Douwes J, Pearce N: Infections, medication use, and the prevalence of symptoms of asthma, rhinitis, and eczema in childhood. J Epidemiol Community Health 2004;58:852–857.
109 Jedrychowski W, Galas A, Whyatt R, Perera F: The prenatal use of antibiotics and the development of allergic disease in one year old infants: a preliminary study. Int J Occup Med Environ Health 2006; 19:70–76.
110 Kummeling I, Stelma FF, Dagnelie PC, Snijders BE, Penders J, Huber M, van Ree R, van den Brandt PA, Thijs C: Early life exposure to antibiotics and the subsequent development of eczema, wheeze, and allergic sensitization in the first 2 years of life: the KOALA Birth Cohort Study. Pediatrics 2007;119: e225–231.
111 Wickens K, Ingham T, Epton M, Pattemore P, Town I, Fishwick D, Crane J: The association of early life exposure to antibiotics and the development of asthma, eczema and atopy in a birth cohort: confounding or causality? Clin Exp Allergy 2008;38: 1318–1324.
112 Kusel MM, de Klerk N, Holt PG, Sly PD: Antibiotic use in the first year of life and risk of atopic disease in early childhood. Clin Exp Allergy 2008;38: 1921–1928.
113 Foliaki S, Pearce N, Bjorksten B, Mallol J, Montefort S, von Mutius E: Antibiotic use in infancy and symptoms of asthma, rhinoconjunctivitis, and eczema in children 6 and 7 years old: International Study of Asthma and Allergies in Childhood Phase III. J Allergy Clin Immunol 2009;124:982–989.

114 Foliaki S, Nielsen SK, Bjorksten B, von Mutius E, Cheng S, Pearce N: Antibiotic sales and the prevalence of symptoms of asthma, rhinitis, and eczema: the International Study of Asthma and Allergies in Childhood (ISAAC). Int J Epidemiol 2004;33:558–563.

115 Bjorksten B, Naaber P, Sepp E, Mikelsaar M: The intestinal microflora in allergic Estonian and Swedish 2-year-old children. Clin Exp Allergy 1999;29:342–346.

116 Bjorksten B, Sepp E, Julge K, Voor T, Mikelsaar M: Allergy development and the intestinal microflora during the first year of life. J Allergy Clin Immunol 2001;108:516–520.

117 Watanabe S, Narisawa Y, Arase S, Okamatsu H, Ikenaga T, Tajiri Y, Kumemura M: Differences in fecal microflora between patients with atopic dermatitis and healthy control subjects. J Allergy Clin Immunol 2003;111:587–591.

118 Boyle RJ, Leonardi-Bee J, Bath-Hextall FJ, Tang ML: Probiotics for the treatment or prevention of eczema. J Allergy Clin Immunol 2009;123:266–267, author reply 267.

119 Matricardi PM, Bonini S: High microbial turnover rate preventing atopy: a solution to inconsistencies impinging on the hygiene hypothesis? Clin Exp Allergy 2000;30:1506–1510.

120 Cramer C, Link E, Horster M, Koletzko S, Bauer CP, Berdel D, von Berg A, Lehmann I, Herbarth O, Borte M, Schaaf B, Behrendt H, Chen CM, Sausenthaler S, Illig T, Wichmann HE, Heinrich J, Kramer U: Elder siblings enhance the effect of filaggrin mutations on childhood eczema: results from the 2 birth cohort studies LISAplus and GINIplus. J Allergy Clin Immunol 2010;125:1254–1260.

121 Fallon PG, Mangan NE: Suppression of Th2-type allergic reactions by helminth infection. Nat Rev Immunol 2007;7:220–230.

122 Melendez AJ, Harnett MM, Pushparaj PN, Wong WS, Tay HK, McSharry CP, Harnett W: Inhibition of Fc epsilon RI-mediated mast cell responses by ES-62, a product of parasitic filarial nematodes. Nat Med 2007;13:1375–1381.

123 Lee J, Seto D, Bielory L: Meta-analysis of clinical trials of probiotics for prevention and treatment of pediatric atopic dermatitis. J Allergy Clin Immunol 2008;121:116–121.

124 Berth-Jones J, Arkwright PD, Marasovic D, Savani N, Aldridge CR, Leech SN, Morgan C, Clark SM, Ogilvie S, Chopra S, Harper JI, Smith CH, Rook GA, Friedmann PS: Killed *Mycobacterium vaccae* suspension in children with moderate-to-severe atopic dermatitis: a randomized, double-blind, placebo-controlled trial. Clin Exp Allergy 2006;36:1115–1121.

125 Arkwright PD, David TJ: Intradermal administration of a killed *Mycobacterium vaccae* suspension (SRL 172) is associated with improvement in atopic dermatitis in children with moderate-to-severe disease. J Allergy Clin Immunol 2001;107:531–534.

126 Arkwright PD, David TJ: Effect of *Mycobacterium vaccae* on atopic dermatitis in children of different ages. Br J Dermatol 2003;149:1029–1034.

127 Brothers S, Asher MI, Jaksic M, Stewart AW: Effect of a *Mycobacterium vaccae* derivative on paediatric atopic dermatitis: a randomized, controlled trial. Clin Exp Dermatol 2009;34:770–775.

128 Yu LC: The epithelial gatekeeper against food allergy. Pediatr Neonatol 2009;50:247–254.

Dr. Carsten Flohr
Department of Paediatric Dermatology
St. John's Institute of Dermatology, St. Thomas' Hospital
Lambeth Palace Road, London SE1 7EH (UK)
Tel. +44 20 7188 7188, ext. 51601, Fax +44 20 7188 9782, E-Mail carsten.flohr@kcl.ac.uk

Shiohara T (ed): Pathogenesis and Management of Atopic Dermatitis.
Curr Probl Dermatol. Basel, Karger, 2011, vol 41, pp 35–46

Loss-of-Function Mutations within the Filaggrin Gene and Atopic Dermatitis

Hiroshi Kawasaki[a] · Akiharu Kubo[a,b] · Takashi Sasaki[a,b] · Masayuki Amagai[a]

[a]Department of Dermatology and [b]Center for Integrated Medical Research, Keio University School of Medicine, Tokyo, Japan

Abstract

Atopic dermatitis (AD) is a chronic relapsing eczematous skin disorder that is frequently associated with elevated serum IgE levels and a personal or family history of AD, allergic rhinitis and/or asthma. Filaggrin is a major constituent of the stratum corneum (SC) and contributes to keratin filament aggregation. Its breakdown products form natural moisturizing factor, which plays a central role in hydration of the SC. Sequence analysis and epidemiological studies indicate that loss-of-function mutations in the filaggrin gene known to cause the autosomal dominant scaly skin disorder ichthyosis vulgaris are major genetic predisposing factors of AD. Mutations in filaggrin are also associated with atopic asthma. These findings established the 'filaggrin hypothesis,' which states that AD can be triggered by the chronic exposure of barrier-disrupted skin to percutaneous antigens due to abnormalities in filaggrin. In this chapter, we summarize the genome-wide screening of AD susceptibility loci, filaggrin biochemistry and recent epidemiological studies on filaggrin mutations and allergic diseases. We also summarize recent advances in the study of skin barrier mechanisms and filaggrin-associated skin barrier abnormalities in animal models. Taken together, these findings provide novel perspectives on the pathophysiology of AD and effective therapeutic methods for the treatment and/or prevention of AD through the modification of skin barrier dysfunction.

Atopic dermatitis (AD) is a chronic relapsing skin disorder that is frequently associated with elevated serum IgE levels and a personal or family history of AD, allergic rhinitis and/or asthma (fig. 1a). The clinical manifestations of AD, which vary with age, are divided into 3 stages: infancy, childhood and adulthood [1]. The disease usually presents during early infancy and childhood, but it can persist into or begin in adulthood [2]. AD is highly prevalent in industrialized countries, where it affects approximately 15–30% of children and 2–10% of adults [1]. The various observations

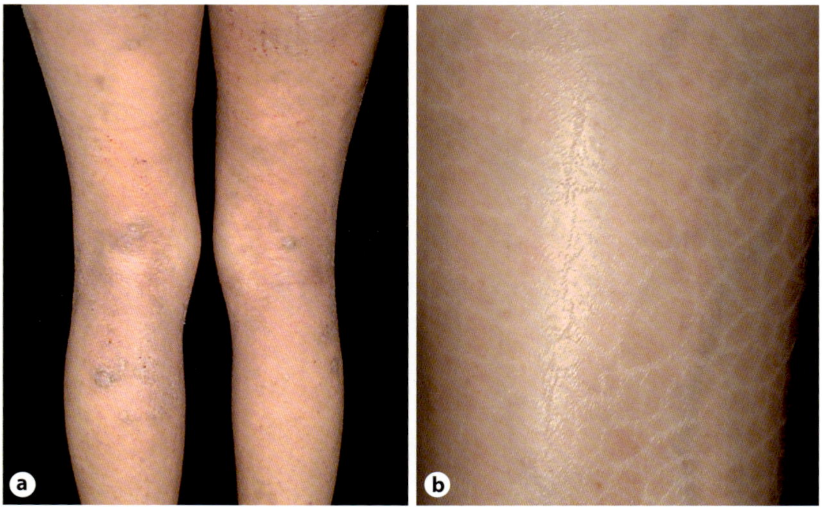

Fig. 1. Clinical features of AD and ichthyosis vulgaris. **a** Typical chronic, scaly, erythematous and lichenified flexural lesions in AD. **b** Ichthyosis vulgaris is characterized by dry, scaly skin on the extensor surfaces of the extremities; hyperlinearity is also involved.

of the disease indicate that AD has a complex etiology with genetic, immunological and environmental aspects.

Recent findings have revealed a major role for the epidermal protein filaggrin in the development of AD. Furthermore, a significant association has been demonstrated between filaggrin abnormalities and the combination of asthma and AD. Understanding the mutations involved may help explain the disease mechanism of AD and systemic allergic responses due to percutaneous antigen exposure, as well as lead to the development of an effective therapeutic strategy. In this chapter, we review the recent progress in filaggrin genetics and our understanding of the pathophysiology of filaggrin-associated AD.

Discovery of Susceptibility Loci for Atopic Dermatitis by Genome-Wide Linkage and Association Analyses

The genetic aspect of AD has long been recognized. Several studies have reported that a family history of AD is a strong risk factor [3], and twin studies of AD have shown higher concordant rates in monozygotic twins (57–86%) compared with dizygotic twins (21–23%) [4]. Current researches, mainly through genome-wide linkage studies, have identified major susceptibility loci for AD on chromosomes 3q21 (ATOD1), 1q21 (ATOD2), 20p (ATOD3), 17q25.3 (ATOD4), 13q12–q14 (ATOD5), 5q31–q33 (ATOD6), 11q13.5 (ATOD7), 4q22.1 (ATOD8) and 3p24 (ATOD9)

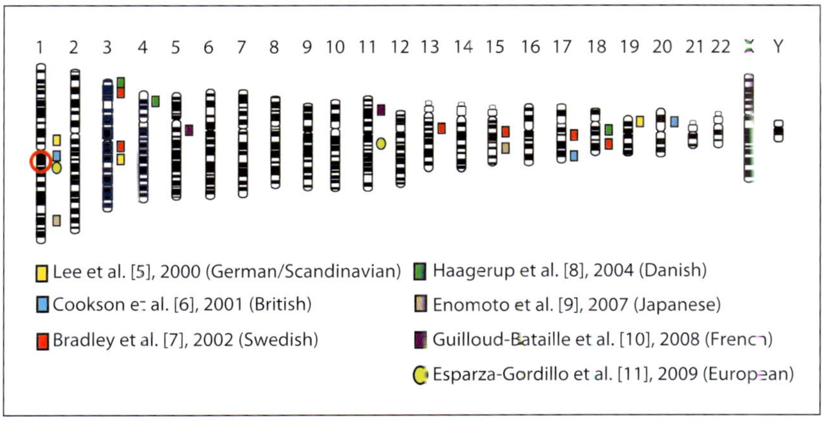

Fig. 2. Susceptibility loci identified by genome-wide linkage and association studies of AD. Representation of the 24 human chromosomes, highlighting those loci for which genome screens have identified linkage to AD. All loci are mapped to short or long chromosomal arms and color coded according to the studies listed in the legend. Chromosome 1q21 is shown as a red circle. Figure modified from Barnes [3].

(OMIM 603165) [3] (fig. 2). Furthermore, a recent genome-wide association study for *FLG* (gene symbol for filaggrin) revealed 2 single-nucleotide polymorphisms located on chromosomes 1q21 and 11q13 that are significantly associated with AD [11] (fig. 2).

The region of strong linkage was located on chromosome 1q21, which contains a very large and diverse family of genes associated with the epidermal differentiation complex [12], a group of epithelium-related genes. Among these epidermal differentiation complex genes, *FLG*, which encodes filaggrin, was reported to be an AD-associated gene in humans [13]. Therefore, *FLG* has been studied intensively as an AD-associated gene over the past decade.

Molecular Biological Studies of Filaggrin

Filaggrin is produced as the precursor profilaggrin (>400 kDa in humans), which is a major constituent of the keratohyalin granules in the granular layer of the epidermis [14]. Human profilaggrin is an insoluble, highly phosphorylated, histidine-rich protein comprised of 10–12 highly homologous tandem filaggrin monomer repeats, which are flanked on either side by 2 partial filaggrin repeats and N- and C-terminal domains [14]. During the later stages of epidermal terminal differentiation, profilaggrin is dephosphorylated and proteolyzed into filaggrin monomers (37 kDa in humans) at the border between the stratum granulosum and stratum corneum (SC)

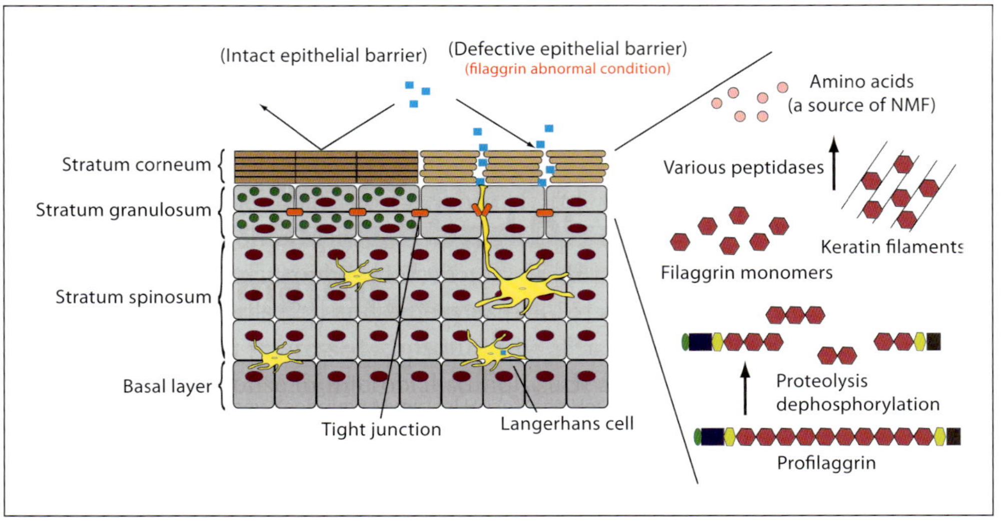

Fig. 3. Schematic representation of filaggrin expression and metabolism. The precursor protein profilaggrin is a major constituent of the keratohyalin granules in the stratum granulosum of the epidermis. During terminal differentiation of the epidermis, profilaggrin is dephosphorylated and proteolyzed into free filaggrin monomers, which associate specifically with intermediate filaments, particularly keratins, and contribute to aggregation of the keratin cytoskeleton. In the upper layers of the stratum corneum (SC), filaggrin monomers are further processed into hygroscopic amino acids and their derivatives by various proteases, including caspase 14. These are collectively referred to as natural moisturizing factor (NMF), which contributes to SC hydration. If there is a reduction in or absence of filaggrin, the SC barrier might be disorganized, resulting in the enhanced penetration of external antigens through the SC and increased antigen uptake by LCs outside the tight junction barrier. This potentially promotes Th2-polarized responses and the development of AD and secondary atopic disorders.

(fig. 3). These filaggrin monomers associate specifically with intermediate filaments, particularly keratins, but not with other filamentous cytoskeletal proteins such as actin and microtubules [15]. Filaggrin monomers have been shown to contribute to aggregation of the keratin cytoskeleton and to mediate cellular compaction into squames. In the upper layers of the SC, filaggrin monomers are processed further into hygroscopic amino acids and their derivatives by various proteases, including caspase 14 [16] (fig. 3). Together with certain ions, such as chloride, sodium, lactate and urate, these filaggrin breakdown products form natural moisturizing factor within the SC and play a central role in the hydration of the SC [17].

Although biochemical studies have improved our understanding of filaggrin biology and function, the molecular genetics of *FLG* have not been elucidated due to complicated genomic structures, including unusually large open reading frames, homology of the repeats and polymorphisms in the number of repeats. However, the use of advanced DNA sequencing techniques has enabled the comprehensive analysis of *FLG* [18, 19] and provided genetic evidence of the association between filaggrin abnormalities and inherited skin disease.

A Loss-of-Function Mutation in *FLG* Causes Ichthyosis Vulgaris

Ichthyosis vulgaris (IV) is a common autosomal dominant disorder of keratinization characterized by scaly skin, typically on the flexor limbs and with palmoplantar hyperlinearity [20] (fig. 1b). Early studies suggested that IV was associated with filaggrin abnormalities. Many reports have shown a histological reduction in or lack of keratohyalin granules in the epidermis as well as decreased filaggrin expression in IV patients [21]. Another study suggested that *FLG* is involved in the development of IV by mapping of the disorder to 1q21–q22 [22]. Smith et al. [23] finally demonstrated that loss-of-function mutations in *FLG* cause IV using improved sequencing techniques. Specifically, they surveyed 15 IV pedigrees and identified the homozygous and compound heterozygous mutations R501X and 2282del4 in *FLG* as the cause of moderate to severe IV. They also showed that these mutations have a semidominant inheritance pattern and that heterozygotes exhibited a mild phenotype with incomplete penetrance.

FLG Mutations Are Major Genetic Predisposing Factors of Atopic Dermatitis

The identification of *FLG* as the causative gene in IV has provided clues to the genetic defect in AD. Although the pathophysiological mechanism of IV and AD co-occurrence is unknown, the fact that AD often occurs in patients with IV is well established [24]. In addition, decreased filaggrin expression has been reported in the skin of patients with AD [21]. Furthermore, strong linkage with AD has been demonstrated for chromosome 1q21 [6, 11]. These observations indicate that *FLG* mutations in IV might be crucial for the development of AD. In fact, 2 common independent loss-of-function mutations (R510X and 2282del4) in *FLG*, which were initially identified in IV, are strongly associated with AD [13]. This association has been demonstrated in multiple populations worldwide. To date, more than 40 *FLG* mutations have been identified [24, 25] (fig. 4). Interestingly, these mutations may be ethnicity and region specific, since the mutations in European and non-European populations are distinct. Most *FLG* mutations in AD are heterozygous. A large, longitudinal population-based study showed the association of an AD-specific filaggrin abnormality with early onset of the disease and increased persistence into adulthood [14]. Although several clinical reports have revealed an association between transepidermal water loss and SC hydration as a parameter of skin barrier function in AD [26, 27], the influence of filaggrin abnormalities remains controversial [28–31]. Further evidence from human clinical findings and bench level studies is needed to elucidate the detailed mechanism of AD.

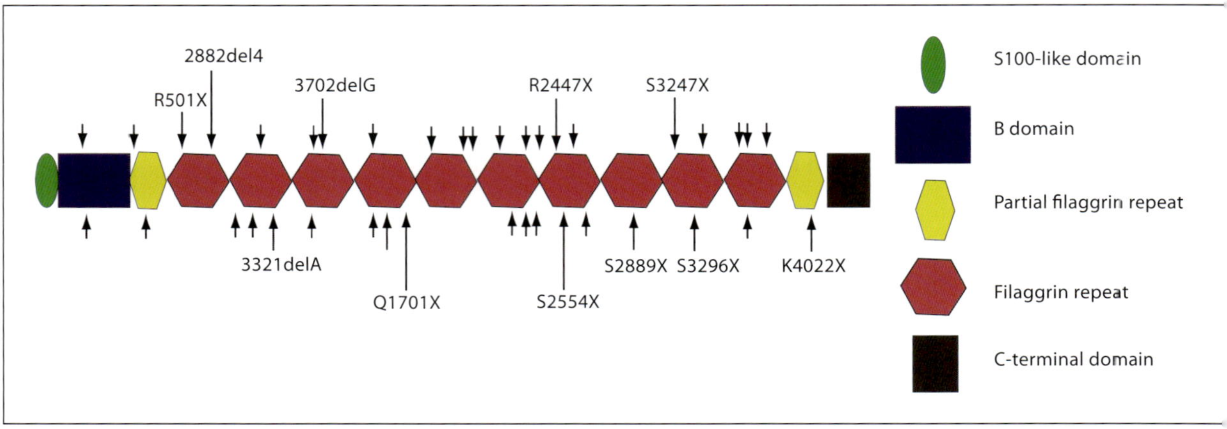

Fig. 4. Structure of profilaggrin and location of mutations. Profilaggrin is comprised of 10–12 highly homologous tandem filaggrin monomer repeats, which are flanked on either side by 2 partial filaggrin repeats and N- and C-terminal domains. The *FLG* mutations identified in European populations are shown above, while those in non-European populations are shown below. The prevalent *FLG* mutations are indicated above/below the arrow. Figure modified from O'Regan et al. [25].

FLG Mutations Are Associated with Atopic Disorders, such as Asthma and Allergic Rhinitis

AD is often associated with other atopic disorders, such as allergic rhinitis and asthma [1], which are characterized by elevated serum IgE levels and peripheral eosinophilia. A number of epidemiological studies showing *FLG* mutations in patients with AD also demonstrated a strong association with asthma. Importantly, this relationship has been reported with asthma in combination with AD (i.e. atopic asthma), but not with asthma alone [21]. Recent systemic reviews and meta-analyses strongly support this finding, adding to the evidence of a strong association with allergic rhinitis [32, 33]. These findings have also been confirmed in non-European populations [34]. Previous studies indicated that filaggrin deficiency in IV and AD might result in functional abnormalities in the epidermal barrier [35]. These results have provided us with an attractive hypothesis for the pathogenic mechanism of AD and secondary allergic conditions [21] (fig. 3). Because filaggrin might be crucial for the formation of a protective skin barrier against the external environment, its reduction or absence might lead to the increased entry of allergens and microbes, and make contact with antigen-presenting cells, e.g. Langerhans cells (LCs), present in the skin. As a consequence, chronic skin inflammation and systemic Th2-polarized responses might be initiated, followed by AD and secondary atopic disorders. This hypothesis is reasonable given that AD patients with a perturbed epidermal barrier are predisposed to asthma, even though the human mucosa lacks filaggrin [36]. Furthermore, these findings are supported by a mouse model of cutaneous sensitization showing that barrier-disrupted skin not only developed local inflammation, but also exhibited systemic allergic responses such as increased serum IgE levels and enhanced airway hypersensitivity [37].

Evaluation of Filaggrin Abnormalities in Other Skin Disorders

There have been several reports of an association between filaggrin abnormal conditions and other skin disorders. Psoriasis is a common chronic inflammatory skin disease involving abnormal keratinization. Psoriasis and AD share certain features, including chronic skin inflammation and disrupted skin barriers. In addition, a number of susceptibility loci for psoriasis, including chromosome 1q21, overlap with those for AD [12]. However, several current reports have shown no association between psoriasis and filaggrin null alleles (especially R501X and 2282del4) [21]. These results indicate that the genetic background involved in epidermal barrier abnormalities in AD differs from that in psoriasis. In contrast, contact dermatitis, hand eczema and alopecia areata are thought to be related to filaggrin abnormalities [38–42]. Additional studies are needed to reveal the association between filaggrin abnormalities and other diseases.

Analyses of Filaggrin-Deficient Conditions in a Mouse Model

Several recent studies have sought to explain the molecular mechanism of AD associated with filaggrin abnormalities using animal models. Flaky tail mice, which have 2 distinct mutations, *ft* and *ma*, and which develop spontaneous AD-like dermatitis in an autosomal recessive manner, were first described in 1958 [43] (fig. 5). These mice show large, disorganized scales and deep furrows (fig. 5). Biochemical and histological analyses have demonstrated that these mice possess mutant profilaggrin and significantly reduced profilaggrin/filaggrin expression, similar to human IV; thus, these mice are considered to be an IV model [44]. Fallon et al. [45] confirmed these findings at the molecular level by the detection of a 1-bp deletion (5303delA) in murine *Flg* gene in flaky tail mice. These investigators also showed that the topical application of an allergen to the mice resulted in enhanced percutaneous allergen priming with the development of allergen-specific antibody responses. The skin barrier phenotypes and cutaneous immune responses of these mice have been evaluated, and these mice have been concluded to be an attractive model for the development of AD [46–48]. Nevertheless, because flaky tail mice are spontaneously mutated animals, other unknown mutations may occur, including *ma*. Therefore, it could be advantageous to remove these alleles from flaky tail mice [45] or to generate pure filaggrin-deficient mice in order to evaluate the precise function of filaggrin itself.

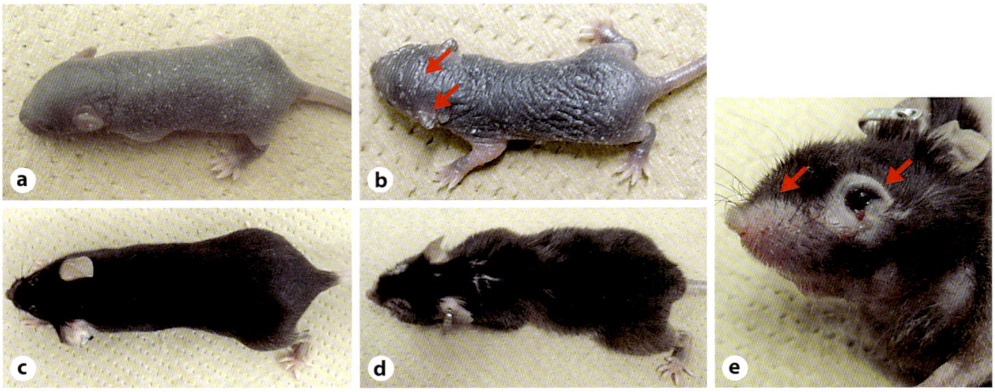

Fig. 5. Gross appearance of normal (**a**, **c**) and flaky tail (**b**, **d**, **e**) mice. Neonatal flaky tail mice exhibit large, disorganized scales (arrows) and deep furrows, which are seen in human IV patients (**a**, **b**). Adult flaky tail mice show matted hair and develop dermatitis (arrows) spontaneously under specific-pathogen-free conditions (**c**, **d**, **e**).

Analyses of (Pro)Filaggrin Degradation in a Mouse Model

Studies of caspase-14-deficient mice have indicated a role for caspase 14 in filaggrin monomer degradation [16]. Biochemical analyses have shown that an epidermal caspase 14 deficiency results in aberrant keratohyalin granules and profilaggrin storage, in addition to altered profilaggrin processing [16]. The same investigators also showed that recombinant caspase 14 could cleave profilaggrin directly in vitro and that caspase 14 has a role in the degradation of filaggrin monomers into free amino acids and their derivatives, although this may affect the degradation of other differentiation-associated proteins [16]. Caspase-14-deficient mice show shiny and lichenified phenotypes with reduced skin hydration levels and increased water loss; these same phenotypes are present in human IV [16]. Interestingly, these mice have not been reported as showing spontaneous dermatitis development.

Such animal models will produce useful data regarding the function of filaggrin and the pathogenic mechanism of AD induced by barrier-disrupted skin.

External Antigen Uptake by Langerhans Cells through Epidermal Tight Junction Barriers

The mammalian epidermis has another barrier system, tight junctions (TJs) [49], under the SC barrier; however, whether filaggrin deficiency affects epidermal TJs is unknown. How external antigens penetrate these 2 barriers and are captured by epidermal LCs or dermal dendritic cells also remains to be elucidated. Recently, we discovered that epidermal LCs gain access through epidermal TJs to external antigens that have violated the SC barrier [50]. We found that activated LCs, but not resting LCs, elongated their dendrites to dock with or penetrate TJs and survey the extra-TJ environment located outside the TJ barrier, just beneath the SC (fig. 3). TJ-penetrated dendrites take up external antigens from the tip and transport them to the cell body. During this phenomenon, the integrity of the epidermal TJ barrier is maintained by the dynamic rearrangement of claudin-based TJs between keratinocytes and LC dendrites. This discovery suggests that an impaired SC barrier due to filaggrin abnormalities results in the increased entry of external antigens through the SC and antigen uptake by LCs outside TJs, which would accelerate Th2-polarized responses and the development of AD [51]. Further investigation into the trans-TJ antigen uptake activity of LCs under filaggrin-deficient conditions will provide new insight into the pathogenic mechanism of AD, especially in percutaneous sensitization.

Future Clinical and Therapeutic Strategies Based on the Filaggrin Hypothesis

AD patients have a complex background with genetic, immunological and environmental aspects; thus, their phenotypes vary widely. An understanding of the factors that predispose to AD is crucial for the development of effective clinical and therapeutic strategies. *FLG* is not the only candidate gene in AD, but its abnormalities are clearly influenced by the pathogenesis of AD. Therefore, the identification of filaggrin mutations is important for developing preventive and therapeutic strategies for AD. It was recently suggested that natural moisturizing factor levels are associated with *FLG* mutations and can be used as a marker for the *FLG* genotype in patients with moderate to severe AD [31, 52]. Additional studies may produce more efficient methods for evaluating *FLG* genotypes.

In the near future, insight into AD associated with *FLG* abnormalities may lead to novel prevention strategies for restoring skin barrier function. Currently, moisturizers are widely used as a fundamental treatment for AD, and they have been shown to reduce topical steroid use [53]. In addition, specific lipid replacement therapy has been shown to promote normal epidermal function in both AD animal models and human patients [54]. However, once eczema has developed, it can be difficult to inhibit antigen penetration; this is followed by the development of cutaneous and systemic allergies (so-called atopic disease, which includes asthma). Therefore, in patients with a high risk of filaggrin abnormalities (e.g. family history), early intervention such as topical moisturizers or lipid replacement therapy may be effective in improving skin barrier function and decreasing antigen sensitization.

References

1 Bieber T: Atopic dermatitis. N Engl J Med 2008;358:1483–1494.

2 Leung DY, Boguniewicz M, Howell MD, Nomura I, Hamid QA: New insights into atopic dermatitis. J Clin Invest 2004;113:651–657.

3 Barnes KC: An update on the genetics of atopic dermatitis: scratching the surface in 2009. J Allergy Clin Immunol 2010;125:16–29.

4 Thomsen SF, Ulrik CS, Kyvik KO, Hjelmborg JB, Skadhauge LR, Steffensen I, Backer V: Importance of genetic factors in the etiology of atopic dermatitis: a twin study. Allergy Asthma Proc 2007;28:535–539.

5 Lee YA, Wahn U, Kehrt R, Tarani L, Businco L, Gustafsson D, Andersson F, Oranje AP, Wolkertstorfer A, v Berg A, Hoffmann U, Kuster W, Wienker T, Ruschendorf F, Reis A: A major susceptibility locus for atopic dermatitis maps to chromosome 3q21. Nat Genet 2000;26:470–473.

6 Cookson WO, Ubhi B, Lawrence R, Abecasis GR, Walley AJ, Cox HE, Coleman R, Leaves NI, Trembath RC, Moffatt MF, Harper JI: Genetic linkage of childhood atopic dermatitis to psoriasis susceptibility loci. Nat Genet 2001;27:372–373.

7 Bradley M, Soderhall C, Luthman H, Wahlgren CF, Kockum I, Nordenskjold M: Susceptibility loci for atopic dermatitis on chromosomes 3, 13, 15, 17 and 18 in a Swedish population. Hum Mol Genet 2002;11:1539–1548.

8 Haagerup A, Bjerke T, Schiotz PO, Dahl R, Binderup HG, Tan Q, Kruse TA: Atopic dermatitis – a total genome-scan for susceptibility genes. Acta Derm Venereol 2004;84:346–352.

9 Enomoto H, Noguchi E, Iijima S, Takahashi T, Hayakawa K, Ito M, Kano T, Aoki T, Suzuki Y, Koga M, Tamari M, Shiohara T, Otsuka F, Arinami T: Single nucleotide polymorphism-based genome-wide linkage analysis in Japanese atopic dermatitis families. BMC Dermatol 2007;7:5.

10 Guilloud-Bataille M, Bouzigon E, Annesi-Maesano I, Bousquet J, Charpin D, Gormand F, Hochez J, Just J, Lemainque A, Le Moual N, Matran R, Neukirch F, Oryszczyn MP, Paty E, Pin I, Vervloet D, Kauffmann F, Lathrop M, Demenais F, Dizier MH: Evidence for linkage of a new region (11p14) to eczema and allergic diseases. Hum Genet 2008;122:605–614.

11 Esparza-Gordillo J, Weidinger S, Folster-Holst R, Bauerfeind A, Ruschendorf F, Patone G, Rohde K, Marenholz I, Schulz F, Kerscher T, Hubner N, Wahn U, Schreiber S, Franke A, Vogler R, Heath S, Baurecht H, Novak N, Rodriguez E, Illig T, Lee-Kirsch MA, Ciechanowicz A, Kurek M, Piskackova T, Macek M, Lee YA, Ruether A: A common variant on chromosome 11q13 is associated with atopic dermatitis. Nat Genet 2009;41:596–601.

12 Cookson W: The immunogenetics of asthma and eczema: a new focus on the epithelium. Nat Rev Immunol 2004;4:978–988.

13 Palmer CN, Irvine AD, Terron-Kwiatkowski A, Zhao Y, Liao H, Lee SP, Goudie DR, Sandilands A, Campbell LE, Smith FJ, O'Regan GM, Watson RM, Cecil JE, Bale SJ, Compton JG, Di Giovanna JJ, Fleckman P, Lewis-Jones S, Arseculeratne G, Sergeant A, Munro CS, El Houate B, McElreavey K, Halkjaer LB, Bisgaard H, Mukhopadhyay S, McLean WH: Common loss-of-function variants of the epidermal barrier protein filaggrin are a major predisposing factor for atopic dermatitis. Nat Genet 2006;38:441–446.

14 Sandilands A, Sutherland C, Irvine AD, McLean WH: Filaggrin in the frontline: role in skin barrier function and disease. J Cell Sci 2009;122:1285–1294.

15 Steinert PM, Cantieri JS, Teller DC, Lonsdale-Eccles JD, Dale BA: Characterization of a class of cationic proteins that specifically interact with intermediate filaments. Proc Natl Acad Sci USA 1981;78:4097–4101.

16 Denecker G, Hoste E, Gilbert B, Hochepied T, Ovaere P, Lippens S, van den Broecke C, van Damme P, D'Herde K, Hachem JP, Borgonie G, Presland RB, Schoonjans L, Libert C, Vandekerckhove J, Gevaert K, Vandenabeele P, Declercq W: Caspase-14 protects against epidermal UVB photodamage and water loss. Nat Cell Biol 2007;9:666–674.

17 Rawlings AV, Harding CR: Moisturization and skin barrier function. Dermatol Ther 2004;17(suppl 1):43–48.

18 Sandilands A, Terron-Kwiatkowski A, Hull PR, O'Regan GM, Clayton TH, Watson RM, Carrick T, Evans AT, Liao H, Zhao Y, Campbell LE, Schmuth M, Gruber R, Janecke AR, Elias PM, van Steensel MA, Nagtzaam I, van Geel M, Steijlen PM, Munro CS, Bradley DG, Palmer CN, Smith FJ, McLean WH, Irvine AD: Comprehensive analysis of the gene encoding filaggrin uncovers prevalent and rare mutations in ichthyosis vulgaris and atopic eczema. Nat Genet 2007;39:650–654.

19 Sasaki T, Kudoh J, Ebihara T, Shiohama A, Asakawa S, Shimizu A, Takayanagi A, Dekio I, Sadahira C, Amagai M, Shimizu N: Sequence analysis of filaggrin gene by novel shotgun method in Japanese atopic dermatitis. J Dermatol Sci 2008;51:113–120.
20 Akiyama M, Shimizu H: An update on molecular aspects of the non-syndromic ichthyoses. Exp Dermatol 2008;17:373–382.
21 McGrath JA, Uitto J: The filaggrin story: novel insights into skin-barrier function and disease. Trends Mol Med 2008;14:20–27.
22 Zhong W, Cui B, Zhang Y, Jiang H, Wei S Bu L, Zhao G, Hu L, Kong X: Linkage analysis suggests a locus of ichthyosis vulgaris on 1q22. J Hum Genet 2003;48:390–392.
23 Smith FJ, Irvine AD, Terron-Kwiatkowski A, Sandilands A, Campbell LE, Zhao Y, Liao H, Evans AT, Goudie DR, Lewis-Jones S, Arseculeratne G, Munro CS, Sergeant A, O'Regan G, Bale SJ, Compton JG, Di Giovanna JJ, Presland RB, Fleckman P, McLean WH: Loss-of-function mutations in the gene encoding filaggrin cause ichthyosis vulgaris. Nat Genet 2006;38:337–342.
24 Akiyama M: *FLG* mutations in ichthyosis vulgaris and atopic eczema: spectrum of mutations and population genetics. Br J Dermatol 2010;162: 472–477.
25 O'Regan GM, Sandilands A, McLean WH, Irvine AD: Filaggrin in atopic dermatitis. J Allergy Clin Immunol 2008;122:689–693.
26 Holm EA, Wulf HC, Thomassen L, Jemec GB: Instrumental assessment of atopic eczema: validation of transepidermal water loss, stratum corneum hydration, erythema, scaling, and edema. J Am Acad Dermatol 2006;55:772–780.
27 Proksch E, Folster-Holst R, Jensen JM: Skin barrier function, epidermal proliferation and differentiation in eczema. J Dermatol Sci 2006;43:159–169.
28 Hubiche T, Ged C, Benard A, Leaute-Labreze C, McElreavey K, de Verneuil H, Taieb A, Boralevi F: Analysis of SPINK 5, KLK 7 and FLG genotypes in a French atopic dermatitis cohort. Acta Derm Venereol 2007;87:499–505.
29 Jungersted JM, Scheer H, Mempel M, Baurecht H, Cifuentes L, Hogh JK, Hellgren LI, Jemec GB, Agner T, Weidinger S: Stratum corneum lipids, skin barrier function and filaggrin mutations in patients with atopic eczema. Allergy 2010;65:911–918.
30 Nemoto-Hasebe I, Akiyama M, Nomura T, Sandilands A, McLean WH, Shimizu H: Clinical severity correlates with impaired barrier in filaggrin-related eczema. J Invest Dermatol 2009;129: 682–689.
31 O'Regan GM, Kemperman PM, Sandilands A, Chen H, Campbell LE, Kroboth K, Watson R, Rowland M, Puppels GJ, McLean WH, Caspers PJ, Irvine AD: Raman profiles of the stratum corneum define 3 filaggrin genotype-determined atopic dermatitis endophenotypes. J Allergy Clin Immunol 2010;126: 574–580.
32 Rodriguez E, Baurecht H, Herberich E, Wagenpfeil S, Brown SJ, Cordell HJ, Irvine AD, Weidinger S: Meta-analysis of filaggrin polymorphisms in eczema and asthma: robust risk factors in atopic disease. J Allergy Clin Immunol 2009;123:1361–1370, e1367.
33 Van den Oord RA, Sheikh A: Filaggrin gene defects and risk of developing allergic sensitisation and allergic disorders: systematic review and meta-analysis. BMJ 2009;339:b2433.
34 Osawa R, Konno S, Akiyama M, Nemoto-Hasebe I, Nomura T, Nomura Y, Abe R, Sandilands A, McLean WH, Hizawa N, Nishimura M, Shimizu H: Japanese-specific filaggrin gene mutations in Japanese patients suffering from atopic eczema and asthma. J Invest Dermatol 2010;130:2834–2836.
35 McLean WH, Hull PR: Breach delivery: increased solute uptake points to a defective skin barrier in atopic dermatitis. J Invest Dermatol 2007;127:8–10.
36 Ying S, Meng Q, Corrigan CJ, Lee TH: Lack of filaggrin expression in the human bronchial mucosa. J Allergy Clin Immunol 2006;118:1386–1388.
37 Spergel JM, Mizoguchi E, Brewer JP, Martin TR, Bhan AK, Geha RS: Epicutaneous sensitization with protein antigen induces localized allergic dermatitis and hyperresponsiveness to methacholine after single exposure to aerosolized antigen in mice. J Clin Invest 1998;101:1614–1622.
38 Betz RC, Pforr J, Flaquer A, Redler S, Hanneken S, Eigelshoven S, Kortum AK, Tuting T, Lambert J, De Weert J, Hillmer AM, Schmael C, Wienker TF, Kruse R, Lutz G, Blaumeiser B, Nothen MM: Loss-of-function mutations in the filaggrin gene and alopecia areata: strong risk factor for a severe course of disease in patients comorbid for atopic disease. J Invest Dermatol 2007;127:2539–2543.
39 Carlsen BC, Johansen JD, Menne T, Meldgaard M, Szecsi PB, Stender S, Thyssen JP: Filaggrin null mutations and association with contact allergy and allergic contact dermatitis: results from a tertiary dermatology clinic. Contact Dermatitis 2010;63: 89–95.
40 De Jongh CM, Khrenova L, Verberk MM, Calkoen F, van Dijk FJ, Voss H, John SM, Kezic S: Loss-of-function polymorphisms in the filaggrin gene are associated with an increased susceptibility to chronic irritant contact dermatitis: a case-control study. Br J Dermatol 2008;159:621–627.

41 Novak N, Baurecht H, Schafer T, Rodriguez E, Wagenpfeil S, Klopp N, Heinrich J, Behrendt H, Ring J, Wichmann E, Illig T, Weidinger S: Loss-of-function mutations in the filaggrin gene and allergic contact sensitization to nickel. J Invest Dermatol 2008;128:1430–1435.
42 Thyssen JP, Johansen JD, Linneberg A, Menne T, Nielsen NH, Meldgaard M, Szecsi PB, Stender S, Carlsen BC: The association between null mutations in the filaggrin gene and contact sensitization to nickel and other chemicals in the general population. Br J Dermatol 2010;162:1278–1285.
43 Lane PW: Two new mutations in linkage group XVI of the house mouse: flaky tail and varitint-waddler-J. J Hered 1972;63:135–140.
44 Presland RB, Boggess D, Lewis SP, Hull C, Fleckman P, Sundberg JP: Loss of normal profilaggrin and filaggrin in flaky tail (ft/ft) mice: an animal model for the filaggrin-deficient skin disease ichthyosis vulgaris. J Invest Dermatol 2000;115: 1072–1081.
45 Fallon PG, Sasaki T, Sandilands A, Campbell LE, Saunders SP, Mangan NE, Callanan JJ, Kawasaki H, Shiohama A, Kubo A, Sundberg JP, Presland RB, Fleckman P, Shimizu N, Kudoh J, Irvine AD, Amagai M, McLean WH: A homozygous frameshift mutation in the mouse Flg gene facilitates enhanced percutaneous allergen priming. Nat Genet 2009;41: 602–608.
46 Moniaga CS, Egawa G, Kawasaki H, Hara-Chikuma M, Honda T, Tanizaki H, Nakajima S, Otsuka A, Matsuoka H, Kubo A, Sakabe J, Tokura Y, Miyachi Y, Amagai M, Kabashima K: Flaky tail mouse denotes human atopic dermatitis in the steady state and by topical application with *Dermatophagoides pteronyssinus* extract. Am J Pathol 176:2385–2393.
47 Oyoshi MK, Murphy GF, Geha RS: Filaggrin-deficient mice exhibit TH17-dominated skin inflammation and permissiveness to epicutaneous sensitization with protein antigen. J Allergy Clin Immunol 2009;124:485–493.
48 Scharschmidt TC, Man MQ, Hatano Y, Crumrine D, Gunathilake R, Sundberg JP, Silva KA, Mauro TM, Hupe M, Cho S, Wu Y, Celli A, Schmuth M, Feingold KR, Elias PM: Filaggrin deficiency confers a paracellular barrier abnormality that reduces inflammatory thresholds to irritants and haptens. J Allergy Clin Immunol 2009;124:496–506.
49 Furuse M, Hata M, Furuse K, Yoshida Y, Haratake A, Sugitani Y, Noda T, Kubo A, Tsukita S: Claudin-based tight junctions are crucial for the mammalian epidermal barrier: a lesson from claudin-1-deficient mice. J Cell Biol 2002;156:1099–1111.
50 Kubo A, Nagao K, Yokouchi M, Sasaki H, Amagai M: External antigen uptake by Langerhans cells with reorganization of epidermal tight junction barriers. J Exp Med 2009;206:2937–2946.
51 Nagao K, Ginhoux F, Leitner WW, Motegi S, Bennett CL, Clausen BE, Merad M, Udey MC: Murine epidermal Langerhans cells and langerin-expressing dermal dendritic cells are unrelated and exhibit distinct functions. Proc Natl Acad Sci USA 2009;106: 3312–3317.
52 Kezic S, Kammeyer A, Calkoen F, Fluhr JW, Bos JD: Natural moisturizing factor components in the stratum corneum as biomarkers of filaggrin genotype: evaluation of minimally invasive methods. Br J Dermatol 2009;161:1098–1104.
53 Cork MJ, Britton J, Butler L, Young S, Murphy R, Keohane SG: Comparison of parent knowledge, therapy utilization and severity of atopic eczema before and after explanation and demonstration of topical therapies by a specialist dermatology nurse. Br J Dermatol 2003;149:582–589.
54 Elias PM: Therapeutic implications of a barrier-based pathogenesis of atopic dermatitis. Ann Dermatol 2010;22:245–254.

Prof. Masayuki Amagai, MD, PhD
Department of Dermatology
Keio University School of Medicine
35 Shinanomachi, Shinjuku-ku, Tokyo 160-8582 (Japan)
Tel. +81 3 3353 1211, Fax +81 3 3351 6880, E-Mail amagai@sc.itc.keio.ac.jp

Shiohara T (ed): Pathogenesis and Management of Atopic Dermatitis.
Curr Probl Dermatol. Basel, Karger, 2011, vol 41, pp 47–53

FcεRI-Toll-Like Receptor Interaction in Atopic Dermatitis

Natalija Novak · Thomas Bieber

Department of Dermatology and Allergy, University of Bonn, Bonn, Germany

Abstract

Exogenous factors such as allergens and microbial components play an important role as triggers of atopic dermatitis (AD). According to the current disease model, allergens as well as microbial antigens get into contact with surface receptors expressed by dendritic cells (DCs) in the skin of patients with AD. Allergen binding is most likely by the high-affinity receptor for IgE (FcεRI), which is highly expressed by epidermal DCs in AD. Beyond, pattern recognition receptors such as Toll-like receptors (TLRs) sense the environment for pathogen-associated molecular patterns. Combined stimulation of both receptor types by allergens and microbial antigens in the cellular micro-environment occurs frequently in AD. Modifications in the gene regions encoding those receptors as well as the pattern of DCs in the skin, the influence of the micro-environment together with the nature of incoming signals determine the type of immune response induced by FcεRI- and TLR-bearing DCs.

The high-affinity receptor for IgE (FcεRI) binds immunoglobulin E (IgE) and plays a major role in allergic diseases [1]. The extracellular part of the α-chain is responsible for IgE binding, while the covalently bound γ-chain dimers, which contain immunoreceptor tyrosine-based activation motifs, are essential for downstream signalling. The β-chain stabilizes the receptor complex on the cell surface and acts as an amplifier of FcεRI-mediated signalling [2]. The tetrameric FcεRI (αβ2γ)-chain complex is expressed by effector cells, while a trimeric (α2γ) variant, which lacks the β-chain, is expressed by monocytes, myeloid dendritic cells (DCs), plasmacytoid DCs (PDCs) and eosinophils [1]. FcεRI expression by DCs depends on the maturation stage and type of DCs, the type of tissue they are located in [3–5], total IgE serum levels as well as different cofactors in the cellular micromilieu, such as IgE, interleukin (IL) 4 and transforming growth factor β during in vitro culture of DCs [6–8]. Additionally, FcεRI surface expression is distinctly regulated in atopic and non-atopic donors and depends on the amount of the FcεRI γ-chain as well as the presence of a structurally modified, so-called mature variant of the FcεRI α-chain [8].

Moreover, genetic factors seem to play a role. In this regard, with the help of a genome-wide scan it was found that functional variants in the gene region on chromosome 1q23, which encodes the FcεRI α-chain, were significantly associated with elevated total serum IgE levels in atopic individuals [9, 10]. Furthermore, a polymorphism in the gene region of *FCER1A* (–344C→T) was shown to be associated with high IgE serum levels in another study [11]. Together, these data imply a genetically predetermined susceptibility for high serum IgE levels and allergic sensitizations, regulated by *FCER1A* gene modifications, which might also be of relevance for patients with atopic dermatitis (AD).

In the epidermal and dermal compartment of lesional and non-lesional AD skin, a high number of FcεRI-bearing DC subtypes is present. In terms of DCs of the myeloid type, CD207+/CD1a+, i.e. Langerhans cells (LCs) as well as CD207–/CD1a+/FcεRI+ DCs have been observed in the epidermis [12]. In contrast, only a few CD207+/FcεRI+/CD1a+ DCs populate the dermal compartment. The main DC subpopulation of the dermis is represented by CD1c+/FcεRI+ DCs [13].

IgE-receptor-bearing epidermal LCs, which are characterized by their Birbeck granules, are the major epidermal DC population in non-lesional AD, whereas a subtype of DCs without Birbeck granules, the so-called inflammatory dendritic epidermal cells (IDECs), migrates to the epidermal compartment of the skin in the acute phase of AD [14]. Analysis of DC subtypes in biopsies taken before and after atopy patch testing demonstrated an increase in chemotactic signals in the skin [15–18] and a concomitant increase in IDECs and other pro-inflammatory cell subtypes, which migrate to the epidermis 24–48 h after allergen application. In contrast, the number of IDECs in the epidermis decreases markedly after successful topical treatment of the skin lesions with the topical calcineurin inhibitor tacrolimus [19–21]. Despite differences in their phenotype and presence related to the disease state, LCs and IDECs seem to play different roles in AD [22]: LCs are in particular important in the initial phase, when they take up allergens, release chemotactic signals and migrate to the lymph nodes to prime first T cells of the Th2 type [23]. The number of IDECs in non-lesional AD skin is low; IDECs are recruited at the initiation of skin inflammation by chemotactic signals [13]. IDECs release pro-inflammatory cytokines and chemokines upon FcεRI cross-linking in vitro and might contribute to the switch of the initial Th2 immune response into an immune response of the Th1 type in vivo. Thereby, IDECs act as important amplifiers of the inflammatory reaction and target cells for therapeutic approaches in AD.

The Role of Toll-Like Receptors in Atopic Dermatitis

So far, 10 different TLRs were identified in humans [24]: TLR1, TLR2, TLR4, TLR6 and TLR10 detect extracellular pathogen-associated molecular patterns, while TLR3,

TLR7, TLR8 and TLR9 are expressed on endosomal membranes and recognize nucleosides, nucleotides and oligo- and polynucleotides derived from viral and bacterial pathogens in the intracellular space [25]. TLR activation and downstream signalling are achievable by several natural and synthetic TLR ligands [26].

TLRs contain an extracellular part, with leucin-rich repeats, which allow binding of pathogen-associated molecular patterns. Further on, TLRs consist of a transmembrane domain and an intracellular Toll/IL-1 receptor domain, which is responsible for cell signalling [27]. TLR2 builds a complex with TLR1 or TLR6 and recognizes bacterial lipopeptides, peptidoglycans and zymosan. TLR4 recognizes lipopolysaccharides and TLR5 bacterial flagellins. TLR3 detects double-stranded viral RNA, while single-stranded viral RNA is recognized by TLR7 and TLR8 and microbial DNA by TLR9 [26]. Intensive interaction and cross-talk among TLRs and other surface receptors is a characteristic feature of TLRs [28]. Several studies have investigated the association of polymorphisms in gene regions encoding different TLRs with AD.

An association of a single nucleotide polymorphism (SNP) in the *TLR2* gene with AD has been reported [29]. This SNP has been further linked to functional impairment including lower TLR2 protein expression by monocytes and macrophages in AD [29, 30]. Consequently, monocytes from patients with AD carrying the *TLR2* R753Q polymorphism produced significantly more IL-6 and IL-12 upon TLR2 stimulation than monocytes of patients with the wild-type TLR2 variant [31]. Lower release of IL-6, IL-8 and IL-1β by monocytes and macrophages of *TLR2* R753Q polymorph AD patients has been observed as well (fig. 1, mechanism A) [30]. Moreover, expression of CD36 was less downregulated in response to stimulation of monocytes of *TLR2* R753Q polymorph AD patients with peptidoglycan or lipoteichoic acid [32]. However, the association of TLR2/TLR4 SNPs with AD was not found in another study [33]. Furthermore, no association of SNPs in the *TLR3* gene with AD has been detected [34]. In contrast, the association of an SNP in the *TLR9* promoter region, which impacted on the promoter activity in functional assays, has been observed to be associated with pure AD [35]. Additionally, in vitro generated monocyte-derived DCs of patients with AD did not show any difference in their capacity to release pro-inflammatory cytokines upon stimulation with TLR ligands [34]. Furthermore, no evidence was detected for an association of SNPs in the IL-1-receptor-associated kinase M gene, which encodes an IL-2-receptor-associated kinase M negatively regulating TLR signalling with AD [36]. Additionally, a very weak association of an SNP was found in a gene region encoding the Toll-interacting protein, an inhibitory adaptor protein of the TLR pathway with AD [37]. Impaired TLR2-mediated production of pro-inflammatory cytokines by monocytes isolated from the peripheral blood of patients with AD went along with a higher expression of the high-affinity receptor for IgE (FcεRI) of these cells [38]. In contrast to TLR2, cytokine response after TLR4 ligation on monocytes of AD patients did not differ significantly from cytokine responses observed in healthy controls [38].

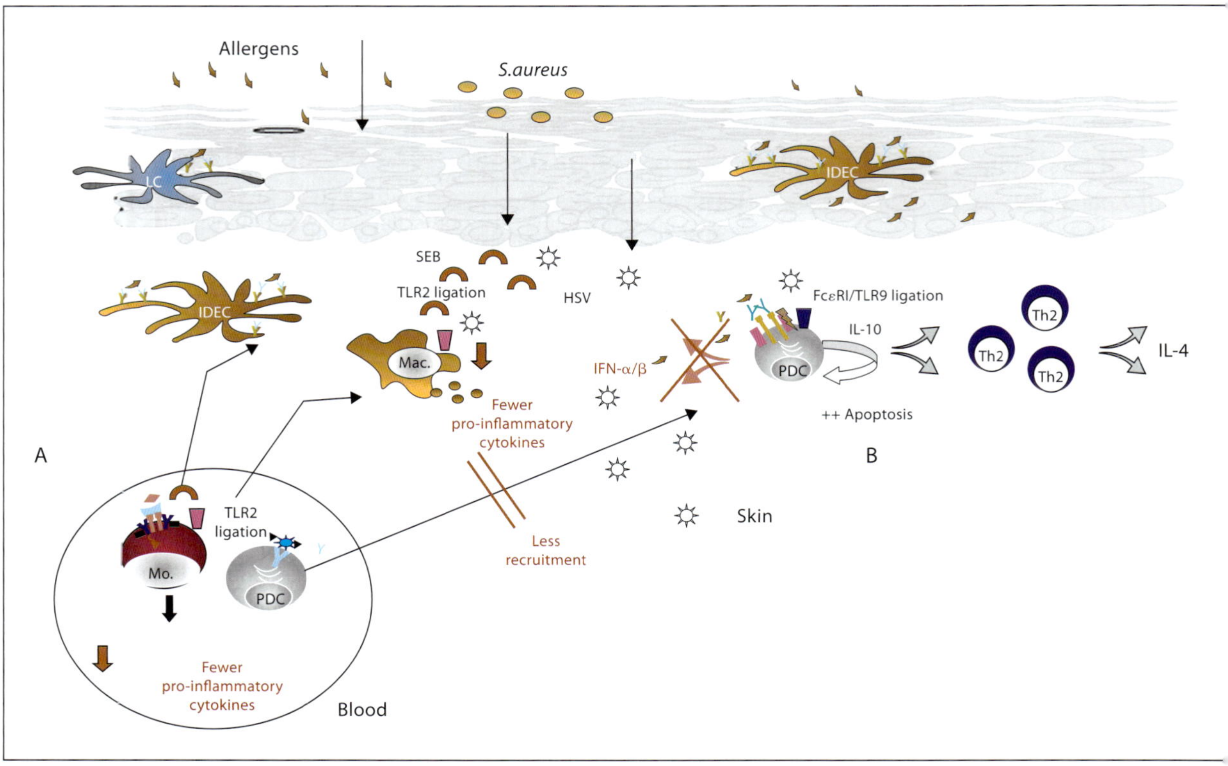

Fig. 1. Summary of the putative mechanisms of modified TLR/FcεRI signalling in AD. Mechanism A: monocytes and macrophages of genetically susceptible patients with AD show lower production of pro-inflammatory cytokines after TLR2 stimulation. Mechanism B: lower recruitment and viability of PDCs in epidermal skin of AD due to Th2 cytokines in the micromilieu as well as combined FcεRI/TLR9 stimulation might impair the capacity of PDCs to produce IFN-α/β in response to HSV in AD. Mo. = Monocyte; Mac. = macrophage; *S. aureus* = *Staphylococcus aureus;* SEB = *S. aureus* enterotoxin B; IFN = interferon; HSV = herpes simplex virus.

Interaction of FcεRI with Toll-Like Receptors on Dendritic Cells

Our insight into the putative interaction between both structures on DCs is still very limited and mostly confined to PDCs. Expression of FcεRI on the surface of PDCs, a subtype of DCs characterized by the expression of the blood-derived dendritic cell antigen 2/4, correlates positively with the IgE serum level [39]. PDCs are important interferon (IFN)-α/β-producing cells, link the innate and the adaptive immune system and play a major role in the defence of virus infections [40]. The function of FcεRI on PDCs has not been elucidated in detail yet, but a counterregulation between FcεRI and TLR9 has been described, which implies that allergen contact closely modifies the capability of PDCs to release IFN-α/β [41]. While PDCs are detectable in the dermis and in the epidermis of patients with chronic inflammatory skin diseases such as psoriasis or contact dermatitis, PDCs are nearly absent from the epidermis of lesional AD skin [42]. Aggregation of FcεRI on PDCs induces the release of IL-10 and increases in an endogenous loop IL-10-mediated apoptosis of PDCs in vitro. Further on, the pre-activation of PDCs via allergen challenge significantly reduces the capacity of PDCs to produce IFN-α and IFN-β in response to subsequent stimulation with viral DNA motifs in vitro (fig. 1, mechanism B) [39]. The reduced capacity of PDCs to produce type I IFN after allergen challenge together with a decreased number of PDCs in the epidermal skin, which is most likely caused by the Th2-dominated micromilieu, might be one of the reasons for the high susceptibility of AD patients to viral infections [43–45].

Conclusion

Stimulation of both FcεRI and TLRs on DCs by distinct ligands plays without any doubt an important role in AD. Thus, genetically predetermined modifications in gene regions encoding both FcεRI and TLRs, which have been shown to be associated with subtypes of AD or high serum IgE levels, cofactors of the cellular micromilieu and pattern of cells in the skin, as well as the strength and the mode of stimulation might direct the nature of the immune response primed by FcεRI/TLR-stimulated DCs.

References

1 Kraft S, Kinet JP: New developments in FcepsilonRI regulation, function and inhibition. Nat Rev Immunol 2007;7:365–378.
2 Lin S, Cicala C, Scharenberg AM, Kinet JP: The Fc(epsilon)RIbeta subunit functions as an amplifier of Fc(epsilon)RIgamma-mediated cell activation signals. Cell 1996;85:985–995.
3 Novak N, Allam JP, Betten H, Haberstok J, Bieber T: The role of antigen presenting cells at distinct anatomic sites: they accelerate and they slow down allergies. Allergy 2004;59:5–14.
4 Novak N, Bieber T: 2. Dendritic cells as regulators of immunity and tolerance. J Allergy Clin Immunol 2008;121(suppl):S370–S374.
5 Allam JP, Novak N, Fuchs C, Asen S, Berge S, Appel T, et al: Characterization of dendritic cells from human oral mucosa: a new Langerhans' cell type with high constitutive FcepsilonRI expression. J Allergy Clin Immunol 2003;112:141–148.
6 Allam JP, Klein E, Bieber T, Novak N: Transforming growth factor-beta1 regulates the expression of the high-affinity receptor for IgE on CD34 stem cell-derived CD1a dendritic cells in vitro. J Invest Dermatol 2004;123:676–682.
7 Geiger E, Magerstaedt R, Wessendorf JH, Kraft S, Hanau D, Bieber T: IL-4 induces the intracellular expression of the alpha chain of the high-affinity receptor for IgE in in vitro-generated dendritic cells. J Allergy Clin Immunol 2000;105:150–156.
8 Novak N, Tepel C, Koch S, Brix K, Bieber T, Kraft S: Evidence for a differential expression of the FcepsilonRIgamma chain in dendritic cells of atopic and nonatopic donors. J Clin Invest 2003;111:1047–1056.
9 Weidinger S, Gieger C, Rodriguez E, Baurecht H, Mempel M, Klopp N, et al: Genome-wide scan on total serum IgE levels identifies FCER1A as novel susceptibility locus. PLoS Genet 2008;4:e1000166.
10 Mahachie John JM, Baurecht H, Rodriguez E, Naumann A, Wagenpfeil S, Klopp N, et al: Analysis of the high affinity IgE receptor genes reveals epistatic effects of FCER1A variants on eczema risk. Allergy 2010;65:875–882.
11 Potaczek DP, Sanak M, Mastalerz L, Setkowicz M, Kaczor M, Nizankowska E, et al: The alpha-chain of high-affinity receptor for IgE (FcepsilonRIalpha) gene polymorphisms and serum IgE levels. Allergy 2006;61:1230–1233.

12 Wollenberg A, Kraft S, Hanau D, Bieber T: Immunomorphological and ultrastructural characterization of Langerhans cells and a novel, inflammatory dendritic epidermal cell (IDEC) population in lesional skin of atopic eczema. J Invest Dermatol 1996;106:446–453.

13 Stary G, Bangert C, Stingl G, Kopp T: Dendritic cells in atopic dermatitis: expression of FcepsilonRI on two distinct inflammation-associated subsets. Int Arch Allergy Immunol 2005;138:278–290.

14 Wollenberg A, Wen S, Bieber T: Langerhans cell phenotyping: a new tool for differential diagnosis of inflammatory skin diseases (letter). Lancet 1995;346:1626–1627.

15 Gombert M, Dieu-Nosjean MC, Winterberg F, Bunemann E, Kubitza RC, Da Cunha L, et al: CCL1-CCR8 interactions: an axis mediating the recruitment of T cells and Langerhans-type dendritic cells to sites of atopic skin inflammation. J Immunol 2005;174:5082–5091.

16 Gunther C, Bello-Fernandez C, Kopp T, Kund J, Carballido-Perrig N, Hinteregger S, et al: CCL18 is expressed in atopic dermatitis and mediates skin homing of human memory T cells. J Immunol 2005;174:1723–1728.

17 Pivarcsi A, Gombert M, DIeu-Nosjean MC, Lauerma A, Kubitza R, Meller S, et al: CC chemokine ligand 18, an atopic dermatitis-associated and dendritic cell-derived chemokine, is regulated by staphylococcal products and allergen exposure. J Immunol 2004;173:5810–5817.

18 Gros E, Bussmann C, Bieber T, Forster I, Novak N: Expression of chemokines and chemokine receptors in lesional and nonlesional upper skin of patients with atopic dermatitis. J Allergy Clin Immunol 2009;124:753–760.

19 Schuller E, Oppel T, Bornhovd E, Wetzel S, Wollenberg A: Tacrolimus ointment causes inflammatory dendritic epidermal cell depletion but no Langerhans cell apoptosis in patients with atopic dermatitis. J Allergy Clin Immunol 2004;114:137–143.

20 Simon D, Vassina E, Yousefi S, Kozlowski E, Braathen LR, Simon HU: Reduced dermal infiltration of cytokine-expressing inflammatory cells in atopic dermatitis after short-term topical tacrolimus treatment. J Allergy Clin Immunol 2004;114:887–895.

21 Kwiek B, Peng WM, Allam JP, Langner A, Bieber T, Novak N: Tacrolimus and TGF-beta act synergistically on the generation of Langerhans cells. J Allergy Clin Immunol 2008;122:126–132.

22 Novak N, Bieber T: The role of dendritic cell subtypes in the pathophysiology of atopic dermatitis. J Am Acad Dermatol 2005;53(suppl 2):S171–S176.

23 Novak N, Valenta R, Bohle B, Laffer S, Haberstok J, Kraft S, et al: FcepsilonRI engagement of Langerhans cell-like dendritic cells and inflammatory dendritic epidermal cell-like dendritic cells induces chemotactic signals and different T-cell phenotypes in vitro. J Allergy Clin Immunol 2004;113:949–957.

24 Iwasaki A, Medzhitov R: Toll-like receptor control of the adaptive immune responses. Nat Immunol 2004;5:987–995.

25 Agrawal S, Kandimalla ER: Synthetic agonists of Toll-like receptors 7, 8 and 9. Biochem Soc Trans 2007;35:1461–1467.

26 Jin MS, Lee JO: Structures of TLR-ligand complexes. Curr Opin Immunol 2008;20:414–419.

27 Jin MS, Lee JO: Structures of the Toll-like receptor family and its ligand complexes. Immunity 2008;29:182–191.

28 Krieg AM: Therapeutic potential of Toll-like receptor 9 activation. Nat Rev Drug Discov 2006;5:471–484.

29 Mrabet-Dahbi S, Dalpke AH, Niebuhr M, Frey M, Draing C, Brand S, et al: The Toll-like receptor 2 R753Q mutation modifies cytokine production and Toll-like receptor expression in atopic dermatitis. J Allergy Clin Immunol 2008;121:1013–1019.

30 Niebuhr M, Lutat C, Sigel S, Werfel T: Impaired TLR-2 expression and TLR-2-mediated cytokine secretion in macrophages from patients with atopic dermatitis. Allergy 2009;64:1580–1587.

31 Niebuhr M, Langnickel J, Draing C, Renz H, Kapp A, Werfel T: Dysregulation of Toll-like receptor-2 (TLR-2)-induced effects in monocytes from patients with atopic dermatitis: impact of the TLR-2 R753Q polymorphism. Allergy 2008;63:728–734.

32 Niebuhr M, Langnickel J, Sigel S, Werfel T: Dysregulation of CD36 upon TLR-2 stimulation in monocytes from patients with atopic dermatitis and the TLR2 R753Q polymorphism. Exp Dermatol 2010;19:e296–e298.

33 Weidinger S, Novak N, Klopp N, Baurecht H, Wagenpfeil S, Rummler L, et al: Lack of association between Toll-like receptor 2 and Toll-like receptor 4 polymorphisms and atopic eczema. J Allergy Clin Immunol 2006;118:277–279.

34 Terhorst D, Kalali BN, Weidinger S, Illig T, Novak N, Ring J, et al: Monocyte-derived dendritic cells from highly atopic individuals are not impaired in their pro-inflammatory response to Toll-like receptor ligands. Clin Exp Allergy 2007;37:381–390.

35 Novak N, Yu CF, Bussmann C, Maintz L, Peng WM, Hart J, et al: Putative association of a TLR9 promoter polymorphism with atopic eczema. Allergy 2007;62:766–772.

36 Beygo J, Parwez Q, Petrasch-Parwez E, Epplen JT, Hoffjan S: No evidence of an association between polymorphisms in the IRAK-M gene and atopic dermatitis in a German cohort. Mol Cell Probes 2009;23:16–19.

37 Schimming TT, Parwez Q, Petrasch-Parwez E, Nothnagel M, Epplen JT, Hoffjan S: Association of Toll-interacting protein gene polymorphisms with atopic dermatitis. BMC Dermatol 2007;7:3.

38 Hasannejad H, Takahashi R, Kimishima M, Hayakawa K, Shiohara T: Selective impairment of Toll-like receptor 2-mediated proinflammatory cytokine production by monocytes from patients with atopic dermatitis. J Allergy Clin Immunol 2007; 120:69–75.

39 Novak N, Allam JP, Hagemann T, Jenneck C, Laffer S, Valenta R, et al: Characterization of FcepsilonRI-bearing CD123 blood dendritic cell antigen-2 plasmacytoid dendritic cells in atopic dermatitis. J Allergy Clin Immunol 2004;114:364–370.

40 Szabo G, Dolganiuc A: The role of plasmacytoid dendritic cell-derived IFNalpha in antiviral immunity. Crit Rev Immunol 2008;28:61–94.

41 Schroeder JT, Bieneman AP, Xiao H, Chichester KL, Vasagar K, Saini S, et al: TLR9- and FcepsilonRI-mediated responses oppose one another in plasmacytoid dendritic cells by down-regulating receptor expression. J Immunol 2005; 175:5724–5731.

42 Wollenberg A, Wagner M, Gunther S, Towarowski A, Tuma E, Moderer M, et al: Plasmacytoid dendritic cells: a new cutaneous dendritic cell subset with distinct role in inflammatory skin diseases. J Invest Dermatol 2002 119:1096–1102.

43 Peng WM, Jenneck C, Bussmann C, Bogdanow M, Hart J, Leung DY, et al. Risk factors of atopic dermatitis patients for eczema herpeticum. J Invest Dermatol 2007;127:1261–1263.

44 Wollenberg A, Zoch C, Wetzel S, Plewig G, Przybilla B: Predisposing factors and clinical features of eczema herpeticum: a retrospective analysis of 100 cases. J Am Acad Dermatol 2003;49:198–205.

45 Beck LA, Boguniewicz M, Hata T, Schneider LC, Hanifin J, Gallo R, et al: Phenotype of atopic dermatitis subjects with a history of eczema herpeticum. J Allergy Clin Immunol 2009;124:260–269.

Natalija Novak, MD
Department of Dermatology and Allergy
University of Bonn, Sigmund-Freud-Strasse 25
DE–53105 Bonn (Germany)
Tel. +49 228 287 15370, E-Mail Natalija.Novak@ukb.uni-bonn.de

Shiohara T (ed): Pathogenesis and Management of Atopic Dermatitis.
Curr Probl Dermatol. Basel, Karger, 2011, vol 41, pp 54–67

The Antimicrobial Skin Barrier in Patients with Atopic Dermatitis

Birgit Schittek

Department of Dermatology, University of Tübingen, Tübingen, Germany

Abstract

Keratinocytes represent the major cell population in the epithelial skin barrier and actively participate in innate immune responses by recognizing pathogenic microorganisms, followed by a fine-tuned production of cytokines, chemokines and antimicrobial peptides or proteins (AMPs). Patients with atopic dermatitis (AD) suffer from a defective permeability barrier which favors pathogen infection indicating that the permeability and antimicrobial barrier functions are interdependent. Several early studies showed that the inducible AMPs LL-37, HBD-2 and HBD-3 are expressed at lower levels in atopic skin compared to psoriatic skin. However, recent data indicate that AMP induction is not compromised in AD patients and that several AMPs are expressed at significantly higher amounts in AD compared to healthy skin. AD patients have an increased susceptibility to *Staphylococcus aureus* skin infection suggesting that AMP levels expressed by keratinocytes of AD patients might not be sufficient to combat pathogenic skin infection or that AMP function is disturbed. Increasing AMP expression in AD skin and repairing the skin barrier defect might have a therapeutic effect in AD patients enabling the skin to mount an enhanced response to pathogens.

Human skin, as the primary interface between the body and the environment, gets only rarely infected, although it is constantly exposed to a myriad of potential pathogens. At the same time it allows harmless, nonpathogenic microorganisms to survive and colonize the skin. Therefore, it seems that skin integrity is maintained by some kind of immune homeostasis in which the extent of skin immune response is controlled by active defense mechanisms and tolerogenic signals. In this respect, keratinocytes – as the main constituents of epithelial cells in skin and mucosa – sense signals from the environment and are able to initiate a differential immune response to harmless commensals and harmful pathogens, respectively. By this, keratinocytes actively participate in the skin innate immune response. Several inflammatory skin disorders, such as psoriasis, rosacea and atopic dermatitis (AD), are associated with a defective skin barrier and a dysregulation of immune responses in the skin. In this review we will highlight the role of keratinocytes as part of the antimicrobial barrier in the skin innate immune response in healthy individuals and in AD patients.

Innate Immune Responses in Healthy Human Skin

Keratinocytes as Skin-Resident Immune Sentinels

Human epidermis consists of a multilayered stratified epithelium in which keratinocytes represent the major cell population in the epithelial barrier. They are known to influence skin functions such as extracellular matrix composition, growth, differentiation, antimicrobial defense, inflammation and wound healing. Keratinocytes actively participate in the innate immune response by the production of cytokines, chemokines and antimicrobial peptides or proteins (AMPs) [1]. Therefore, they function not only as a physical barrier, but they can be considered as immune sentinels capable of recognizing pathogenic microorganisms and secreting a variety of defense effector molecules. By this, they orchestrate an immune inflammatory response [1–4].

Keratinocytes express several pattern recognition receptors such as the Toll-like receptors (TLRs), which recognize conserved microbial products like lipopolysaccharide, lipoteichoic acid, peptidoglycan, flagellin or nucleic acids. Epidermal keratinocytes express the cell-surface-associated TLRs 1, 2, 4, 5 and 6 and the endosomal TLRs 3 and 9 [4–8]. In addition, TLR7 expression is induced by triggering of TLR3 by double-stranded RNA [9]. Activation of TLR receptors on human keratinocytes leads to a predominant Th1-type immune response and to the production of type I interferons [10].

Keratinocytes are important producers of proinflammatory mediators such as interleukin (IL) 1 and tumor necrosis factor α. In addition, they can produce IL-6, IL-10 and IL-18 [4, 11]. The knowledge about the variety of mediators expressed by human keratinocytes is constantly growing. Keratinocytes are also able to attract different cell types into the skin by expression of several chemokines and chemokine receptors [12]. By expressing CC chemokine ligand 20 (CCL20), CXC chemokine ligand 9 (CXCL9), CXCL10- and CXCL11-activated keratinocytes attract effector T cells into the skin during inflammatory diseases [11]. By producing CXCL1 and CXCL8 (also known as IL-8) they can recruit neutrophils to the epidermis. Through the expression of CCL20 Langerhans cell precursors can traffic to the skin [13]. Keratinocytes are important cellular sources of the T-cell growth factor IL-15 in the skin. IL-15 has been implicated in the pathogenesis of different skin diseases by virtue of its action on the maintenance of T cells – possibly also on intraepithelial T cells. These interactions between keratinocytes and T cells have been extensively analyzed in the context of inflammatory skin diseases [14]. In summary, keratinocytes are proinflammatory effector cells producing AMPs, proinflammatory cytokines and chemokines. These are able to attract and activate members of the innate and adaptive immune system combatting harmful microbial infections.

AMPs, also called host defense peptides, are ancient players in innate immunity [3, 15]. AMPs show a broad spectrum of antimicrobial activity against a wide range of pathogens including bacteria, fungi and enveloped viruses, and therefore play an important role in the innate host defense [1, 16]. In human skin, keratinocytes are a major source of antimicrobial active peptides or larger proteins. In addition, cells present in skin like neutrophils [17], mast cells [18], T cells [19], eccrine sweat glands [20–22], hair bulb cells [23] and sebocytes [24, 25] are able to produce AMPs.

AMPs are either expressed constitutively at a basal level, or the expression is upregulated in response to microbial stimuli such as pathogen-associated molecular patterns or proinflammatory stimuli [1, 3, 26]. Dermcidin is constitutively expressed by eccrine sweat glands and secreted into sweat. In sweat several proteolytically processed dermcidin-derived antimicrobial peptides are found differing in charge and length. Dermcidin-derived peptides contribute to the first line of defense by building a constant barrier that overlies the epithelial skin [20–22]. The most abundant AMPs produced by human keratinocytes are the β-defensins HBD-1, HBD-2 and HBD-3, psoriasin, the cathelicidin LL-37 and the antimicrobial protein ribonuclease (RNase) 7 [3, 26, 27]. The AMPs HBD-1, RNase 7 and psoriasin are constitutively expressed by keratinocytes [26, 28]. Psoriasin is focally present at different levels in healthy skin [29]. Psoriasin, HBD-3 and RNase 7 are inducible upon skin inflammation or wounding [1, 26]. Others (HBD-2, LL-37) are found only in inflamed, but not in healthy skin [1, 16, 30, 31]. In healthy human skin, AMPs significantly contribute to the protection from infection by pathogenic microorganisms, and it has been shown that in some human skin diseases recurrent skin infections are associated with a dysregulation of AMP production (fig. 1) [1, 26, 30]. AMPs additionally play a crucial role as signaling molecules in linking innate and adaptive immune responses. They can mediate chemotaxis of dendritic cells and T cells and maturation and activation of dendritic cells and activate the acquired immune responses against infectious agents [32–34].

Regulation of Antimicrobial Protein Expression

AMP expression can be induced by proinflammatory cytokines including IL-1β, tumor necrosis factor α [35, 36], IL-17 and IL-22 [37, 38], after bacterial contact [35, 39], during epidermal differentiation [36] or wound healing [40]. Contact of cultured differentiated epidermal keratinocytes to *S. aureus* upregulates the expression of HBD-2, HBD-3 and LL-37 in keratinocytes [41, 42]. Proinflammatory cytokines as well as heat-killed bacteria induce RNase 7 expression which indicates that RNase 7 expression is increased under inflammatory conditions in human skin [3]. Psoriasin can be induced in vitro and in vivo in keratinocytes by contact with *Escherichia coli,* and it was shown that flagellin is responsible for the induction of psoriasin expression in

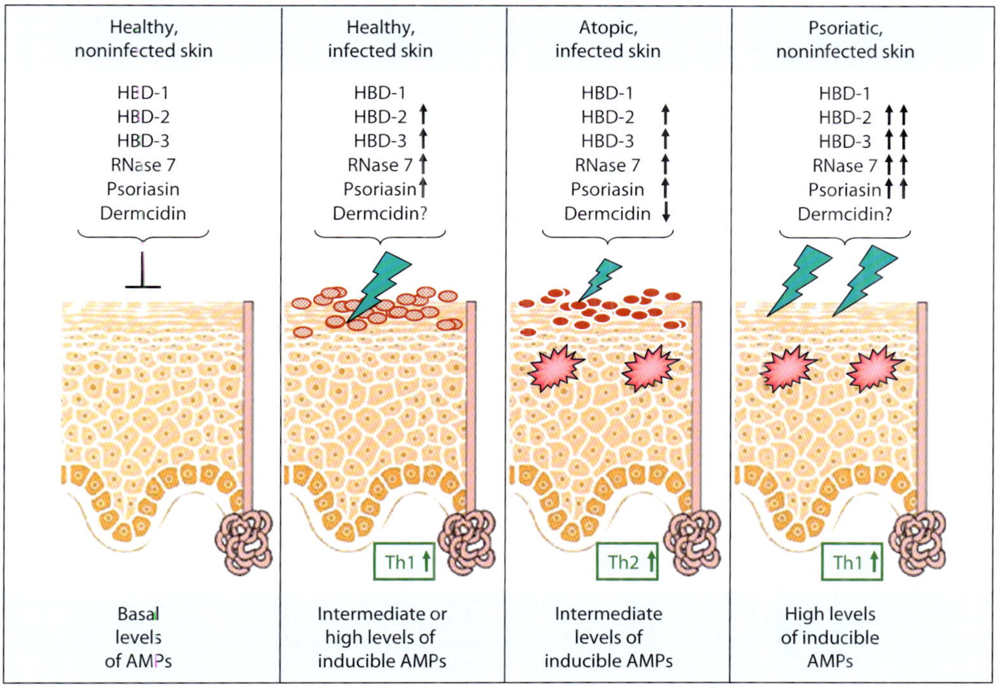

Fig. 1. AMP expression and function in healthy, AD and psoriatic skin. In healthy, noninfected skin, a basal expression level of the AMPs HBD1–3, RNase 7 and psoriasin expressed by keratinocytes and dermcidin expressed by eccrine sweat glands protects against pathogen infection. After infection of healthy skin with *S. aureus*, expressions of the inducible AMPs HBD-2, HBD-3, RNase 7 and psoriasin are increased to intermediate or high levels resulting in destruction of the pathogen. In atopic, inflamed skin, the AMPs HBD-2, HBD-3, RNase 7 and psoriasin are expressed at a higher, intermediate level compared to healthy skin, whereas dermcidin-derived peptides are found at reduced amounts in sweat. The expression level of the inducible AMPs in atopic skin seems not to solve pathogen infection with *S. aureus*. In contrast, in inflamed psoriatic skin, high expression levels of the inducible AMPs result in successful prevention of skin colonization of pathogens.

keratinocytes [28, 43]. During skin infections, the local production of AMPs by keratinocytes is increased by T-cell-derived cytokines. In particular, IL-17A and IL-22, which are produced by Th17 cells, increase AMP production by keratinocytes [4, 37, 44, 45]. Sorensen et al. [46, 47] have shown that wounding of skin stimulates HBD-3 expression via transactivation of the epidermal growth factor receptor. In addition, the expression of LL-37 in keratinocytes is induced by $1,25(OH)_2$ vitamin D_3 [48–51]. Recently, it was found that TLR3 and TLR2/6 ligands induce cyclooxygenase 2. Inhibiting cyclooxygenase 2 abrogates TLR ligand-induced HBD-2 and HBD-3 induction, but not cathelicidin expression, by abrogation of nuclear factor κB activation, which attenuates antistaphylococcal activity [52]. In general, it seems that HBD-3 and RNase 7 expression can be induced by multiple bacterial factors and several signaling pathways [6, 41, 53].

Requirements for Colonization of Human Skin by Staphylococcus aureus and Antimicrobial Protein Induction

It has been shown that HBD-3 is both necessary and sufficient to account for the constitutive ability of human keratinocytes to kill *S. aureus* within minutes of contact with the cell surface [39]. Gläser et al. [29] demonstrated that psoriasin is mainly responsible for preventing *E. coli* from colonizing the skin. Two recent studies showed that a high baseline expression level of RNase 7 confers protection against *S. aureus* infection of the skin, whereas there was no association with expression levels of HBD-2 and HBD-3 with skin infection [54, 55]. These studies emphasize the importance of RNase 7 in the control of *S. aureus* growth on the skin surface and in susceptibility to infection. Furthermore, a recent study showed that a higher inducibility of HBD-3, but not HBD-2, is associated with a more favorable clinical course and outcome of *S. aureus* skin infections [56]. The data suggest that limiting the extent of *S. aureus* skin colonization involves HBD-3 induction, while susceptibility to infection is substantially influenced by expression levels of RNase 7.

Recent work has revealed that skin commensals such as *S. epidermidis* may have a protective effect on skin infection in several ways. They can produce their own antimicrobial peptides that inhibit pathogenic organisms [57]. Lipoteichoic acid produced by *S. epidermidis* served to inhibit skin inflammation through a TLR crosstalk between TLR2 and TLR3 [58]. Furthermore commensal and pathogenic bacteria are able to activate different signaling pathways which act in a synergistic way to amplify immune responses in human skin by upregulation of AMP expression [6, 59–61]. Interestingly, several *S. aureus* isolates able to colonize human skin were not able to induce high-level expression of AMPs. This could facilitate their growth on human skin [6]. Furthermore, staphylococci have evolved mechanisms to resist the innate host defense. It has been nicely shown that *S. epidermidis* sense AMPs – as shown for HBD-3 – by a 3-component sensor/regulator system which upregulates resistance mechanisms to cationic AMPs. This seems to be of great importance for the efficient colonization of epithelia [62]. Interestingly, *S. aureus* has a similiar AMP sensing system which is, however, AMP selective [63]. For example, HBD-3 is a much weaker inducer of this resistance mechanism in *S. aureus* compared with *S. epidermidis*.

Innate Immune Responses in Atopic Dermatitis Skin

Skin Barrier Function in Patients with Atopic Dermatitis

AD is a chronic inflammatory skin disease that is frequently associated with recurrent bacterial and viral infections [64]. The microbial flora of atopic skin shows striking differences with more than 90% of inflammatory lesions and 76% of normal skin being colonized by *S. aureus* as compared to less than 10% in healthy individuals [65, 66]. AD has a complex etiology involving susceptibility genes, defects in skin barrier function and a dysregulation of immunological responses and inflammatory pathways which influence the differential colonization of atopic skin [67, 68].

Inherited defects either in serine protease activity or filaggrin production result in primary defects in stratum corneum structure and function. This compromises barrier function by accelerated degradation of stratum corneum lipid-processing enzymes resulting in the reduction of extracellular lipids and ceramide levels [69–71]. Consequently, low levels of sphingosine are found in the stratum corneum, an antimicrobial agent which is involved in the susceptibility of AD skin to colonization by *S. aureus*. Loss-of-function variants of the epidermal barrier protein filaggrin are a major predisposing factor for AD [72]. However, a significant number of AD patients do not have any of the known filaggrin mutations, and, conversely, approximately 40% of patients with a defective filaggrin gene do not suffer from AD [73–75]. In AD, a slight alcalinization in the average pH of the skin from pH 5.0 to pH 5.5 can be observed [76]. A recent study suggests that maintenance of an acidic stratum corneum pH prevents the emergence of AD induced in mice by attenuation of the development of a Th2-dominant inflammation [77].

Innate Immune Responses in Patients with Atopic Dermatitis

Several studies showed that impaired innate immune mechanisms in AD contribute to the propensity of atopic patients to skin infections [1, 26, 75, 78]. AD is characterized by abnormalities in the key effector cells in AD skin such as T cells and especially the cytokines that are produced by Th1 and Th2 cells, antigen-presenting cells and keratinocytes [67, 79]. Skin of AD patients has an increased number of Th2 cells which leads to an overexpression of the Th2 cytokines IL-4, IL-10 and IL-13 and low levels of proinflammatory cytokines (tumor necrosis factor α, γ-interferon, IL-1β) [80]. The expression of the innate immune response genes inducible nitric oxide synthetase and IL-8 was found to be decreased in AD, due to the overexpression of Th2 cytokines and low levels of proinflammatory cytokines [80]. Increased serine protease activity generates elevated levels of IL-1α and IL-1β by enhanced processing of the precursor forms which contribute to inflammation in AD skin [70, 81, 82]. The barrier defect enhances antigen penetration leading to a Th2 dominant infiltrate [83]. It is known that certain antigens such as those of mites trigger AD, particularly in filaggrin-deficient patients [84]. Accordingly, correction of the barrier abnormality alone should ameliorate both the cytokine cascade and allergen-induced inflammation in AD patients.

It has been demonstrated that keratinocytes as well as peripheral blood monocytes show an impaired TLR2-, but not TLR4-induced inflammatory cytokine production promoting a Th2-biased immune response [78, 85, 86]. Several studies suggest that the TLR2 pathway may be defective in AD patients due to TLR2 mutations or genetic TLR2 polymorphisms [75, 78, 87, 88]. In contrast, other studies did not find a correlation of TLR2 haplotypes and AD [89, 90]. Other pattern recognition receptors such as

TLR9, Nod1–2 and CD14 have also been described to be adequately expressed in AD patients [78]. Finally, several types of immune cells such as natural killer cells, plasmacytoid dendritic cells or polymorphonuclear neutrophil granulocytes are found in significantly lower amounts in AD patients compared to controls [75]. This might make AD patients more susceptible to a wide range of cutaneous microbes.

Data achieved in the last years point to the 'outside-inside' view of disease pathogenesis which claims that the permeability barrier abnormality in AD is the 'driver' of disease activity and antimicrobial barrier dysfunction [70]. Indeed, the extent of the permeability barrier abnormality seems to parallel the severity of the disease phenotype in AD [91–93]. Failure of the permeability barrier itself favors secondary infection, and, conversely, pathogen colonization/infection further aggravates the permeability abnormality indicating that these two functions are coregulated and interdependent [70, 94].

Antimicrobial Protein Expression in Patients with Atopic Dermatitis – Early Reports

Early reports showed that the inducible antimicrobial peptides LL-37, HBD-2 and HBD-3 are expressed at a significantly lower level in lesional atopic skin compared to lesional skin in psoriasis [80, 95]. Furthermore, our data showed that AD patients have a reduced amount of the constitutively produced antimicrobial peptide dermcidin in sweat which correlates with an impaired innate defense of human skin in vivo [96]. In healthy individuals, a significant reduction in viable bacteria on the skin surface occurs after sweating, but this does not occur in AD patients. These data indicate that reduced expression of dermcidin in AD patients contributes to the high susceptibility of these patients to skin infections and to altered skin colonization.

It has been shown that Th2 cytokines such as IL-4 and IL-13 suppress the cytokine-mediated induction of HBD-2 and HBD-3 in keratinocytes [80, 95]. Additionally, the lack of the major AMP inducers IL-1β or IL-22 could lead to a reduced expression of AMPs in AD skin [97]. It was demonstrated by microarray analysis that several other AMPs are expressed at lower amounts in AD skin compared to skin of patients with psoriasis [98]. Interestingly, neutralization of the Th2 cytokines augments LL-37, HBD-2 and HBD-3 expression in AD skin [99, 100]. These data indicate that the reduced expression of inducible AMPs in AD skin is not a constitutive but an acquired defect resulting from increased Th2 cytokine expression. This suggests that neutralizing the Th2 cytokine milieu in the skin of AD patients would augment the AMP response and reduce the susceptibility of these patients towards recurrent bacterial and viral skin infections. However, whereas acute lesions of AD are characterized by the overexpression of Th2 cytokines such as IL-4 and IL-13 [101, 102], Th1 cytokines appear to be more relevant in the chronic phase [103, 104].

Antimicrobial Protein Expression in Patients with Atopic Dermatitis – Recent Reports

The first studies analyzing the expression of AMPs in AD skin reported a reduced expression of several AMPs in lesional skin of AD patients, suggesting that an impaired induction of AMPs contributes to the increased susceptibility of atopic skin to infection [30, 80, 95, 100]. However, most of the studies analyzing AMP expression in AD compared the expression levels primarily with psoriatic but not with healthy skin [80, 95, 98].

Recent studies compared the expression level of several AMPs in the skin of AD patients not only to the expression level observed in psoriatic, but also in healthy skin [28, 105–108]. Gambichler et al. [105] showed mRNA induction of HBD-2, HBD-3, psoriasin and RNase 7 in psoriatic and AD skin when compared to controls. Asano et al. [106] found a significantly higher expression of HBD-2 in AD lesional skin compared with healthy control skin. Interestingly, HBD-2 levels in lesional skin of AD patients increase in proportion to the severity of AD. This correlates with higher systemic HBD-2 levels in the serum of AD patients compared to serum of healthy people. The HBD-2 levels found in the serum of AD patients are, however, reduced to the amounts found in patients with psoriasis [107]. Furthermore, there is an enhanced expression of LL-37 in lesional AD skin compared to healthy skin [109]. However, there was no correlation between LL-37 expression and severity of AD [109]. Interestingly, oral supplementation with vitamin D enhances the production of LL-37 in AD patients [75, 110]. Upregulation of LL-37 might be mediated by B-cell leukemia (Bcl) 3, an element of the nuclear factor κB signaling pathway [111]. It was shown that Bcl-3 is overexpressed in lesional skin from AD patients compared with normal skin and induced by Th2 cytokines IL-4 and IL-13. Bcl-3 modulates the expression of HBD-3 and cathelicidin, as well as the cytokines IL-8 and IL-6 [111]. Bcl-3 silencing enhanced vitamin-D_3-induced gene expression of cathelicidin AMP in keratinocytes, suggesting a negative regulatory function of Bcl-3 on cathelicidin expression. It might be that blocking signaling downstream of Bcl-3 in keratinocytes may be a potential therapeutic strategy in treating AD.

Two recent studies indicated that the expression and secretion of psoriasin, RNase 7, HBD-2 and HBD-3 are strongly induced in nonlesional and lesional skin of AD patients when compared with healthy skin, indicating that the expression of AMPs is not generally impaired in AD [28, 108]. However, the absolute levels of AMP expression and secretion were lower than levels detected in psoriasis [28, 108]. Interestingly, the secretion levels of RNase 7 and HBD-2 were higher in patients with acute exacerbation of AD when compared with patients suffering from chronic AD. This suggests that elevated Th2 cytokines, which have been associated with acute AD, are not sufficient enough to inhibit the induction of RNase 7, HBD-2 and HBD-3 in the acute AD lesions. Furthermore, superficial skin barrier disruption by tape-stripping of healthy skin induced the expression of HBD-2, HBD-3 and RNase 7, suggesting that the enhanced expression of AMPs in psoriatic and AD skin may be driven by the disrupted epidermal barrier [108]. Interestingly, there was no significant correlation between the presence and concentrations of the AMPs RNase 7, psoriasin and HBD-2 on AD skin and *S. aureus* colonization or disease severity [108]. This supports the hypothesis that the increased susceptibility of AD skin to *S. aureus* colonization and infection is not mainly caused by reduced amounts of these inducible AMPs, but by a disrupted skin barrier. It might be that the reduced amounts of the constitutively produced dermcidin-derived peptides in the sweat of AD patients have a greater influence on *S. aureus* colonization [96].

In summary, the expression and secretion of the AMPs RNase 7, psoriasin, HBD-2 and HBD-3 is induced in AD compared to healthy skin, but the expression levels are reduced when compared to the levels found in psoriatic skin. This points out that the induction of AMP expression is not generally impaired in AD patients. In addition, no correlation of AMP secretion and *S. aureus* colonization or severity of AD was observed. Clearly, the functional role of AMPs in AD needs further investigations.

Conclusions

Several defects in innate immune responses in AD patients contribute to the enhanced susceptibility of these patients towards microbial infections. Among the contributing factors are genetic polymorphisms in TLR expression, impaired recruitment or activation of innate immune cells to sites of inflammation, a Th2-based cytokine profile, skin barrier defects and a changed expression of AMPs. The antimicrobial barrier is intimately linked to the permeability barrier. Moreover, an impaired permeability barrier alone predisposes to pathogen colonization. The question remains whether a restoration of the permeability barrier alone can improve antimicrobial defense in AD patients. Since AD patients show an enhanced expression of several AMPs compared to healthy subjects, it has to be determined whether AMP function might be impaired in AD patients. Furthermore, the AMP levels expressed by keratinocytes of AD patients are possibly not sufficient to combat pathogenic skin infection. This situation could be similar to the AMP expression level induced by skin commensals which is too low to influence their survival, whereas the level induced by *S. aureus* is able to kill pathogenic, but not commensal staphylococci [6]. Recent data indicate that increasing the expression of HBD-3 and RNase 7 might be sufficient to increase the antimicrobial barrier function [39, 54, 56]. Furthermore, *S. aureus* able to colonize human skin have evolved resistance mechanisms to circumvent killing by AMPs as a failure to induce AMP expression [6] or an AMP-sensing system [63]. Interestingly, colonization of AD skin by *S. aureus* seems to successfully compete with skin colonization of the commensal *S. epidermidis* [112]. This indicates that the protective effect commensal bacteria have on pathogen infection of human skin by amplification of AMP expression might be disturbed in AD patients. Increasing AMP expression in AD skin by several possible options and simultaneous repair of the skin barrier defect could have a therapeutic effect in AD patients to increase the antimicrobial skin barrier function.

Acknowledgments

I thank Ines Wanke and Tobias Sinnberg for critically reading the manuscript. This work was supported by the Deutsche Forschungsgemeinschaft (SFB766).

References

1 Schittek B, Paulmann M, Senyurek I, Steffen H: The role of antimicrobial peptides in human skin and in skin infectious diseases. Infect Disord Drug Targets 2008;8:135–143.

2 Harder J, Schroder JM: Antimicrobial peptides in human skin. Chem Immunol Allergy 2005;86:22–41.

3 Schröder JM, Harder J: Antimicrobial skin peptides and proteins. Cell Mol Life Sci 2006;63:469–486.

4 Nestle FO, Di Meglio P, Qin JZ, Nickoloff BJ: Skin immune sentinels in health and disease. Nat Rev Immunol 2009;9:679–691.

5 Lebre MC, van der Aar AM, van Baarsen L, van Capel TM, Schuitemaker JH, Kapsenberg ML, de Jong EC: Human keratinocytes express functional Toll-like receptor 3, 4, 5, and 9. J Invest Dermatol 2007;127:331–341.

6 Wanke I, Steffen H, Christ C, Krismer B, Götz F, Peschel A, Schaller M, Schittek B: Skin commensals amplify the innate immune response to pathogens by activation of distinct signaling pathways. J Invest Dermatol 2010, E-pub ahead of print.

7 Kollisch G, Kalali BN, Voelcker V, Wallich R, Behrendt H, Ring J, Bauer S, Jakob T, Mempel M, Ollert M: Various members of the Toll-like receptor family contribute to the innate immune response of human epidermal keratinocytes. Immunology 2005;114:531–541.

8 Terhorst D, Kalali BN, Ollert M, Ring J, Mempel M: The role of Toll-like receptors in host defenses and their relevance to dermatologic diseases. Am J Clin Dermatol 2010;11:1–10.

9 Kalali BN, Kollisch G, Mages J, Muller T, Bauer S, Wagner H, Ring J, Lang R, Mempel M, Ollert M: Double-stranded RNA induces an antiviral defense status in epidermal keratinocytes through TLR3-, PKR-, and MDA5/RIG-I-mediated differential signaling. J Immunol 2008;181:2694–2704.

10 Miller LS, Modlin RL: Human keratinocyte Toll-like receptors promote distinct immune responses. J Invest Dermatol 2007;127:262–263.

11 Albanesi C, Scarponi C, Giustizieri ML, Girolomoni G: Keratinocytes in inflammatory skin diseases. Curr Drug Targets Inflamm Allergy 2005;4:329–334.

12 Homey B: Chemokines and inflammatory skin diseases. Adv Dermatol 2005;21:251–277.

13 Purwar R, Wittmann M, Zwirner J, Oppermann M, Kracht M, Dittrich-Breiholz O, Gutzmer R, Werfel T: Induction of C3 and CCL2 by C3a in keratinocytes: a novel autocrine amplification loop of inflammatory skin reactions. J Immunol 2006;177:4444–4450.

14 Wittmann M, Werfel T: Interaction of keratinocytes with infiltrating lymphocytes in allergic eczematous skin diseases. Curr Opin Allergy Clin Immunol 2006;6:329–334.

15 Boman HG: Peptide antibiotics and their role in innate immunity. Annu Rev Immunol 1995;13:61–92.

16 Zasloff M: Antimicrobial peptides in health and disease. N Engl J Med 2002;347:1199–1200.

17 Turner J, Cho Y, Dinh NN, Waring AJ, Lehrer RI: Activities of LL-37, a cathelin-associated antimicrobial peptide of human neutrophils. Antimicrob Agents Chemother 1998;42:2206–2214.

18 Di Nardo A, Vitiello A, Gallo RL: Cutting edge: mast cell antimicrobial activity is mediated by expression of cathelicidin antimicrobial peptide. J Immunol 2003;170:2274–2278.

19 Agerberth B, Charo J, Werr J, Olsson B, Idali F, Lindbom L, Kiessling R, Jornvall H, Wigzell H, Gudmundsson GH: The human antimicrobial and chemotactic peptides LL-37 and alpha-defensins are expressed by specific lymphocyte and monocyte populations. Blood 2000;96:3086–3093.

20 Schittek B, Hipfel R, Sauer B, Bauer J, Kalbacher H, Stevanovic S, Schirle M, Schroeder K, Blin N, Meier F, Rassner G, Garbe C: Dermcidin: a novel human antibiotic peptide secreted by sweat glands. Nat Immunol 2001;2:1133–1137.

21 Rieg S, Garbe C, Sauer B, Kalbacher H, Schittek B: Dermcidin is constitutively produced by eccrine sweat glands and is not induced in epidermal cells under inflammatory skin conditions. Br J Dermatol 2004;151:534–539.

22 Rieg S, Seeber S, Steffen H, Humeny A, Kalbacher H, Stevanovic S, Kimura A, Garbe C, Schittek B: Generation of multiple stable dermcidin-derived antimicrobial peptides in sweat of different body sites. J Invest Dermatol 2006;126:354–365.

23 Muller FB, Muller-Rover S, Korge BP, Kapas S, Hinson JP, Philpott MP: Adrenomedullin: expression and possible role in human skin and hair growth. Br J Dermatol 2003;148:30–38.
24 Lee DY, Yamasaki K, Rudsil J, Zouboulis CC, Park GT, Yang JM, Gallo RL: Sebocytes express functional cathelicidin antimicrobial peptides and can act to kill *Propionibacterium acnes.* J Invest Dermatol 2008;128:1863–1866.
25 Nagy I, Pivarcsi A, Kis K, Koreck A, Bodai L, McDowell A, Seltmann H, Patrick S, Zouboulis CC, Kemeny L: *Propionibacterium acnes* and lipopolysaccharide induce the expression of antimicrobial peptides and proinflammatory cytokines/chemokines in human sebocytes. Microbes Infect 2006;8: 2195–2205.
26 Harder J, Glaser R, Schroder JM: The role and potential therapeutical applications of antimicrobial proteins in infectious and inflammatory diseases. Endocr Metab Immune Disord Drug Targets 2007;7: 75–82.
27 Fulton C, Anderson GM, Zasloff M, Bull R, Quinn AG: Expression of natural peptide antibiotics in human skin. Lancet 1997;350:1750–1751.
28 Glaser R, Meyer-Hoffert U, Harder J, Cordes J, Wittersheim M, Kobliakova J, Folster-Holst R, Proksch E, Schroder JM, Schwarz T: The antimicrobial protein psoriasin (S100A7) is upregulated in atopic dermatitis and after experimental skin barrier disruption. J Invest Dermatol 2009;129: 641–649.
29 Gläser R, Harder J, Lange H, Bartels J, Christophers E, Schroder JM: Antimicrobial psoriasin (S100A7) protects human skin from *Escherichia coli* infection. Nat Immunol 2005;6:57–64.
30 Yamasaki K, Gallo RL: Antimicrobial peptides in human skin disease. Eur J Dermatol 2008;18: 11–21.
31 Bals R: Epithelial antimicrobial peptides in host defense against infection. Respir Res 2000;1: 141–150.
32 Medzhitov R, Janeway CJ: Innate immunity. N Engl J Med 2000;343:338–344.
33 Namjoshi S, Caccetta R, Benson HA: Skin peptides: biological activity and therapeutic opportunities. J Pharm Sci 2008;97:2524–2542.
34 Tosi MF: Innate immune responses to infection. J Allergy Clin Immunol 2005;116:241–249.
35 Harder J, Meyer-Hoffert U, Teran LM, Schwichtenberg L, Bartels J, Maune S, Schroder JM: Mucoid *Pseudomonas aeruginosa,* TNF-alpha, and IL-1beta, but not IL-6, induce human beta-defensin-2 in respiratory epithelia. Am J Respir Cell Mol Biol 2000;22:714–721.
36 Harder J, Meyer-Hoffert U, Wehkamp K, Schwichtenberg L, Schroder JM: Differential gene induction of human beta-defensins (hBD-1, -2, -3, and -4) in keratinocytes is inhibited by retinoic acid. J Invest Dermatol 2004;123:522–529.
37 Liang SC, Tan XY, Luxenberg DP, Karim R, Dunussi-Joannopoulos K, Collins M, Fouser LA: Interleukin (IL)-22 and IL-17 are coexpressed by Th17 cells and cooperatively enhance expression of antimicrobial peptides. J Exp Med 2006;203:2271–2279.
38 Wolk K, Witte E, Wallace E, Docke WD, Kunz S, Asadullah K, Volk HD, Sterry W, Sabat R: IL-22 regulates the expression of genes responsible for antimicrobial defense, cellular differentiation, and mobility in keratinocytes: a potential role in psoriasis. Eur J Immunol 2006;36:1309–1323.
39 Kisich KO, Howell MD, Boguniewicz M, Heizer HR, Watson NU, Leung DY: The constitutive capacity of human keratinocytes to kill *Staphylococcus aureus* is dependent on beta-defensin 3. J Invest Dermatol 2007;127:2368–2380.
40 Sorensen OE, Cowland JB, Theilgaard-Monch K, Liu L, Ganz T, Borregaard N: Wound healing and expression of antimicrobial peptides/polypeptides in human keratinocytes, a consequence of common growth factors. J Immunol 2003;170:5583–5589.
41 Menzies BE, Kenoyer A: *Staphylococcus aureus* infection of epidermal keratinocytes promotes expression of innate antimicrobial peptides. Infect Immun 2005;73:5241–5244.
42 Midorikawa K, Ouhara K, Komatsuzawa H, Kawai T, Yamada S, Fujiwara T, Yamazaki K, Sayama K, Taubman MA, Kurihara H, Hashimoto K, Sugai M: *Staphylococcus aureus* susceptibility to innate antimicrobial peptides, beta-defensins and CAP18, expressed by human keratinocytes. Infect Immun 2003;71:3730–3739.
43 Abtin A, Eckhart L, Mildner M, Gruber F, Schroder JM, Tschachler E: Flagellin is the principal inducer of the antimicrobial peptide S100A7c (psoriasin) in human epidermal keratinocytes exposed to *Escherichia coli.* FASEB J 2008;22:2168–2176.
44 Weaver CT, Hatton RD, Mangan PR, Harrington LE: IL-17 family cytokines and the expanding diversity of effector T cell lineages. Annu Rev Immunol 2007;25:821–852.
45 Kolls JK, McCray PB Jr, Chan YR: Cytokine-mediated regulation of antimicrobial proteins. Nat Rev Immunol 2008;8:829–835.
46 Sorensen OE, Thapa DR, Roupe KM, Valore EV, Sjobring U, Roberts AA, Schmidtchen A, Ganz T: Injury-induced innate immune response in human skin mediated by transactivation of the epidermal growth factor receptor. J Clin Invest 2006;116: 1878–1885.

47 Sorensen OE, Thapa DR, Rosenthal A, Liu L, Roberts AA, Ganz T: Differential regulation of beta-defensin expression in human skin by microbial stimuli. J Immunol 2005;174:4870–4879.
48 Wang TT, Nestel FP, Bourdeau V, Nagai Y, Wang Q, Liao J, Tavera-Mendoza L, Lin R, Hanrahan JW, Mader S, White JH: Cutting edge: 1,25-dihydroxyvitamin D_3 is a direct inducer of antimicrobial peptide gene expression. J Immunol 2004;173:2909–2912.
49 Weber G, Heilborn JD, Chamorro Jimenez CI, Hammarsjo A, Torma H, Stahle M: Vitamin D induces the antimicrobial protein hCAP18 in human skin. J Invest Dermatol 2005;124:1080–1082.
50 Schauber J, Dorschner RA, Coda AB, Buchau AS, Liu PT, Kiken D, Helfrich YR, Kang S, Elalieh HZ, Steinmeyer A, Zugel U, Bikle DD, Modlin RL, Gallo RL: Injury enhances TLR2 function and antimicrobial peptide expression through a vitamin D-dependent mechanism. J Clin Invest 2007;117:803–811.
51 Heilborn JD, Weber G, Gronberg A, Dieterich C, Stahle M: Topical treatment with the vitamin D analogue calcipotriol enhances the upregulation of the antimicrobial protein hCAP18/LL-37 during wounding in human skin in vivo. Exp Dermatol 2010;19:332–338.
52 Bernard JJ, Gallo RL: Cyclooxygenase-2 enhances antimicrobial peptide expression and killing of *Staphylococcus aureus*. J Immunol 2010;185:6535–6544.
53 Menzies BE, Kenoyer A: Signal transduction and nuclear responses in *Staphylococcus aureus*-induced expression of human beta-defensin 3 in skin keratinocytes. Infect Immun 2006;74:6847–6854.
54 Zanger P, Holzer J, Schleucher R, Steffen H, Schittek B, Gabrysch S: Constitutive expression of the antimicrobial peptide RNase 7 is associated with *Staphylococcus aureus* infection of the skin. J Infect Dis 2009;200:1907–1915.
55 Simanski M, Dressel S, Glaser R, Harder J: RNase 7 protects healthy skin from *Staphylococcus aureus* colonization. J Invest Dermatol 2010;130:2836–2838.
56 Zanger P, Holzer J, Schleucher R, Scherbaum H, Schittek B, Gabrysch S: Severity of *Staphylococcus aureus* infection of the skin is associated with inducibility of human beta-defensin 3 but not human beta-defensin 2. Infect Immun 2010;78:3112–3117.
57 Cogen AL, Yamasaki K, Muto J, Sanchez KM, Crotty AL, Tanios J, Lai Y, Kim JE, Nizet V, Gallo RL: *Staphylococcus epidermidis* antimicrobial delta-toxin (phenol-soluble modulin-gamma) cooperates with host antimicrobial peptides to kill group A *Streptococcus*. PLoS One 2010;5:e8557.
58 Lai Y, Di Nardo A, Nakatsuji T, Leichtle A, Yang Y, Cogen AL, Wu ZR, Hooper LV, Schmidt RR, von Aulock S, Radek KA, Huang CM, Ryan AF, Gallo RL: Commensal bacteria regulate Toll-like receptor 3-dependent inflammation after skin injury. Nat Med 2009;15:1377–1382.
59 Chung WO, Dale BA: Differential utilization of nuclear factor-kappaB signaling pathways for gingival epithelial cell responses to oral commensal and pathogenic bacteria. Oral Microbiol Immunol 2008;23:119–126.
60 Chung WO, Dale BA: Innate immune response of oral and foreskin keratinocytes: utilization of different signaling pathways by various bacterial species. Infect Immun 2004;72:352–358.
61 Lai Y, Cogen AL, Radek KA, Park HJ, Macleod DT, Leichtle A, Ryan AF, Di Nardo A, Gallo RL: Activation of TLR2 by a small molecule produced by *Staphylococcus epidermidis* increases antimicrobial defense against bacterial skin infections. J Invest Dermatol 2010;130:2211–2221.
62 Li M, Lai Y, Villaruz AE, Cha DJ, Sturdevant DE, Otto M: Gram-positive three-component antimicrobial peptide-sensing system. Proc Natl Acad Sci USA 2007;104:9469–9474.
63 Li M, Cha DJ, Lai Y, Villaruz AE, Sturdevant DE, Otto M: The antimicrobial peptide-sensing system aps of *Staphylococcus aureus*. Mol Microbiol 2007;66:1136–1147.
64 Biedermann T: Dissecting the role of infections in atopic dermatitis. Acta Derm Venereol 2006;86:99–109.
65 Aly R, Maibach HI, Shinefield HR: Microbial flora of atopic dermatitis. Arch Dermatol 1977;113:780–782.
66 Leyden JJ, Marples RR, Kligman AM: *Staphylococcus aureus* in the lesions of atopic dermatitis. Br J Dermatol 1974;90:525–530.
67 Leung DY, Boguniewicz M, Howell MD, Nomura I, Hamid QA: New insights into atopic dermatitis. J Clin Invest 2004;113:651–657.
68 Novak N, Bieber T, Leung DY: Immune mechanisms leading to atopic dermatitis. J Allergy Clin Immunol 2003;112:S128–S139.
69 Hachem JP, Crumrine D, Fluhr J, Brown BE, Feingold KR, Elias PM: pH directly regulates epidermal permeability barrier homeostasis, and stratum corneum integrity/cohesion. J Invest Dermatol 2003;121:345–353.
70 Elias PM, Schmuth M: Abnormal skin barrier in the etiopathogenesis of atopic dermatitis. Curr Opin Allergy Clin Immunol 2009;9:437–446.

71 Sator PG, Schmidt JB, Honigsmann H: Comparison of epidermal hydration and skin surface lipids in healthy individuals and in patients with atopic dermatitis. J Am Acad Dermatol 2003;48:352–358.
72 Palmer CN, Irvine AD, Terron-Kwiatkowski A, Zhao Y, Liao H, Lee SP, Goudie DR, Sandilands A, Campbell LE, Smith FJ, O'Regan GM, Watson RM, Cecil JE, Bale SJ, Compton JG, Di Giovanna JJ, Fleckman P, Lewis-Jones S, Arseculeratne G, Sergeant A, Munro CS, El Houate B, McElreavey K, Halkjaer LB, Bisgaard H, Mukhopadhyay S, McLean WH: Common loss-of-function variants of the epidermal barrier protein filaggrin are a major predisposing factor for atopic dermatitis. Nat Genet 2006; 38:441–446.
73 O'Regan GM, Sandilands A, McLean WH, Irvine AD: Filaggrin in atopic dermatitis. J Allergy Clin Immunol 2009;124:R2–R6.
74 Henderson J, Northstone K, Lee SP, Liao H, Zhao Y, Pembrey M, Mukhopadhyay S, Smith GD, Palmer CN, McLean WH, Irvine AD: The burden of disease associated with filaggrin mutations: a population-based, longitudinal birth cohort study. J Allergy Clin Immunol 2008;121:872–877.
75 Niebuhr M, Werfel T: Innate immunity, allergy and atopic dermatitis. Curr Opin Allergy Clin Immunol 2010;10:463–468.
76 Imokawa G: Skin moisturizers: development and clinical use of ceramides; in Loden M (ed): Dry Skin and Moisturizers. Boca Raton, CRC Press, 1999, pp 269–299.
77 Hatano Y, Man MQ, Uchida Y, Crumrine D, Scharschmidt TC, Kim EG, Mauro TM, Feingold KR, Elias PM, Holleran WM: Maintenance of an acidic stratum corneum prevents emergence of murine atopic dermatitis. J Invest Dermatol 2009; 129:1824–1835.
78 De Benedetto A, Agnihothri R, McGirt LY, Bankova LG, Beck LA: Atopic dermatitis: a disease caused by innate immune defects? J Invest Dermatol 2009; 129:14–30.
79 Baker BS: The role of microorganisms in atopic dermatitis. Clin Exp Immunol 2006;144:1–9.
80 Nomura I, Goleva E, Howell MD, Hamid QA, Ong PY, Hall CF, Darst MA, Gao B, Boguniewicz M, Travers JB, Leung DY: Cytokine milieu of atopic dermatitis, as compared to psoriasis, skin prevents induction of innate immune response genes. J Immunol 2003;171:3262–3269.
81 Elias PM, Feingold KR: Does the tail wag the dog? Role of the barrier in the pathogenesis of inflammatory dermatoses and therapeutic implications. Arch Dermatol 2001;137:1079–1081.
82 Elias PM, Wood LC, Feingold KR: Epidermal pathogenesis of inflammatory dermatoses. Am J Contact Dermat 1999;10:119–126.
83 Elias PM, Hatano Y, Williams ML: Basis for the barrier abnormality in atopic dermatitis: outside-inside-outside pathogenic mechanisms. J Allergy Clin Immunol 2008;121:1337–1343.
84 Lomholt H, Andersen KE, Kilian M: *Staphylococcus aureus* clonal dynamics and virulence factors in children with atopic dermatitis. J Invest Dermatol 2005;125:977–982.
85 Hasannejad H, Takahashi R, Kimishima M, Hayakawa K, Shiohara T: Selective impairment of Toll-like receptor 2-mediated proinflammatory cytokine production by monocytes from patients with atopic dermatitis. J Allergy Clin Immunol 2007;120:69–75.
86 McGirt LY, Beck LA: Innate immune defects in atopic dermatitis. J Allergy Clin Immunol 2006;118: 202–208.
87 Ahmad-Nejad P, Mrabet-Dahbi S, Breuer K, Klotz M, Werfel T, Herz U, Heeg K, Neumaier M, Renz H: The Toll-like receptor 2 R753Q polymorphism defines a subgroup of patients with atopic dermatitis having severe phenotype. J Allergy Clin Immunol 2004;113:565–567.
88 Mrabet-Dahbi S, Dalpke AH, Niebuhr M, Frey M, Draing C, Brand S, Heeg K, Werfel T, Renz H: The Toll-like receptor 2 R753Q mutation modifies cytokine production and Toll-like receptor expression in atopic dermatitis. J Allergy Clin Immunol 2008;121:1013–1019.
89 Akdis CA, Akdis M, Bieber T, Bindslev-Jensen C, Boguniewicz M, Eigenmann P, Hamid Q, Kapp A, Leung DY, Lipozencic J, Luger TA, Muraro A, Novak N, Platts-Mills TA, Rosenwasser L, Scheynius A, Simons FE, Spergel J, Turjanmaa K, Wahn U, Weidinger S, Werfel T, Zuberbier T: Diagnosis and treatment of atopic dermatitis in children and adults: European Academy of Allergology and Clinical Immunology/American Academy of Allergy, Asthma and Immunology/PRACTALL Consensus Report. Allergy 2006;61:969–987.
90 Schimming TT, Parwez Q, Petrasch-Parwez E, Nothnagel M, Epplen JT, Hoffjan S: Association of Toll-interacting protein gene polymorphisms with atopic dermatitis. BMC Dermatol 2007;7:3.
91 Sugarman JL, Fluhr JW, Fowler AJ, Bruckner T, Diepgen TL, Williams ML: The objective severity assessment of atopic dermatitis score: an objective measure using permeability barrier function and stratum corneum hydration with computer-assisted estimates for extent of disease. Arch Dermatol 2003; 139:1417–1422.
92 Seidenari S, Giusti G: Objective assessment of the skin of children affected by atopic dermatitis: a study of pH, capacitance and TEWL in eczematous and clinically uninvolved skin. Acta Derm Venereol 1995;75:429–433.

93 Chamlin SL, Kao J, Frieden IJ, Sheu MY, Fowler AJ, Fluhr JW, Williams ML, Elias PM: Ceramide-dominant barrier repair lipids alleviate childhood atopic dermatitis: changes in barrier function provide a sensitive indicator of disease activity. J Am Acad Dermatol 2002;47:198–208.
94 Elias PM: The skin barrier as an innate immune element. Semin Immunopathol 2007;29:3–14.
95 Ong PY, Ohtake T, Brandt C, Strickland I, Boguniewicz M, Ganz T, Gallo RL, Leung DY: Endogenous antimicrobial peptides and skin infections in atopic dermatitis. N Engl J Med 2002;347: 1151–1160.
96 Rieg S, Steffen H, Seeber S, Humeny A, Kalbacher H, Dietz K, Garbe C, Schittek B: Deficiency of dermcidin-derived antimicrobial peptides in sweat of patients with atopic dermatitis correlates with an impaired innate defense of human skin in vivo. J Immunol 2005;174:8003–8010.
97 Wolk K, Kunz S, Witte E, Friedrich M, Asadullah K, Sabat R: IL-22 increases the innate immunity of tissues. Immunity 2004;21:241–254.
98 De Jongh GJ, Zeeuwen PL, Kucharekova M, Pfundt R, van der Valk PG, Blokx W, Dogan A, Hiemstra PS, van de Kerkhof PC, Schalkwijk J: High expression levels of keratinocyte antimicrobial proteins in psoriasis compared with atopic dermatitis. J Invest Dermatol 2005;125:1163–1173.
99 Howell MD, Wollenberg A, Gallo RL, Flaig M, Streib JE, Wong C, Pavicic T, Boguniewicz M, Leung DY: Cathelicidin deficiency predisposes to eczema herpeticum. J Allergy Clin Immunol 2006;117: 836–841.
100 Howell MD, Novak N, Bieber T, Pastore S, Girolomoni G, Boguniewicz M, Streib J, Wong C, Gallo RL, Leung DY: Interleukin-10 downregulates anti-microbial peptide expression in atopic dermatitis. J Invest Dermatol 2005;125:738–745.
101 Jeong CW, Ahn KS, Rho NK, Park YD, Lee DY Lee JH, Lee ES, Yang JM: Differential in vivo cytokine mRNA expression in lesional skin of intrinsic vs extrinsic atopic dermatitis patients using semiquantitative RT-PCR. Clin Exp Allergy 2003;33: 1717–1724.
102 Homey B, Steinhoff M, Ruzicka T, Leung DY: Cytokines and chemokines orchestrate atopic skin inflammation. J Allergy Clin Immunol 2006;118: 178–189.
103 Grewe M, Gyufko K, Schopf E, Krutmann J: Lesional expression of interferon-gamma in atopic eczema. Lancet 1994;343:25–26.
104 Leung DY, Bieber T: Atopic dermatitis. Lancet 2003; 361:151–160.
105 Gambichler T, Skrygan M, Tomi NS, Othlinghaus N, Brockmeyer NH, Altmeyer P, Kreuter A: Differential mRNA expression of antimicrobial peptides and proteins in atopic dermatitis as compared to psoriasis vulgaris and healthy skin. Int Arch Allergy Immunol 2008;147:17–24.
106 Asano S, Ichikawa Y, Kumagai T, Kawashima M, Imokawa G: Microanalysis of an antimicrobial peptide, beta-defensin-2, in the stratum corneum from patients with atopic dermatitis. Br J Dermatol 2008;159:97–104.
107 Jansen PA, Rodijk-Olthuis D, Hollox EJ, Kamsteeg M, Tjabringa GS, de Jongh GJ, van Vlijmen-Willems IM, Bergboer JG, van Rossum MM, de Jong EM, den Heijer M, Evers AW, Bergers M, Armour JA, Zeeuwen PL, Schalkwijk J: Beta-defensin-2 protein is a serum biomarker for disease activity in psoriasis and reaches biologically relevant concentrations in lesional skin. PLoS One 2009;4:e4725.
108 Harder J, Dressel S, Wittersheim M, Cordes J, Meyer-Hoffert U, Mrowietz U, Folster-Holst R, Proksch E, Schroder JM, Schwarz T, Glaser R: Enhanced expression and secretion of antimicrobial peptides in atopic dermatitis and after superficial skin injury. J Invest Dermatol 2010;130:1355–1364.
109 Ballardini N, Johansson C, Lilja G, Lindh M, Linde Y, Scheynius A, Agerberth B: Enhanced expression of the antimicrobial peptide LL-37 in lesional skin of adults with atopic eczema. Br J Dermatol 2009; 161:40–47.
110 Hata TR, Kotol P, Jackson M, Nguyen M, Paik A, Udall D, Kanada K, Yamasaki K, Alexandrescu D, Gallo RL: Administration of oral vitamin D induces cathelicidin production in atopic individuals. J Allergy Clin Immunol 2008;122:829–831.
111 Buchau AS, Macleod DT, Morizane S, Kotol PF, Hata T, Gallo RL: Bcl-3 acts as an innate immune modulator by controlling antimicrobial responses in keratinocytes. J Invest Dermatol 2009;129:2148–2155.
112 Higaki S, Morohashi M, Yamagishi T, Hasegawa Y: Comparative study of staphylococci from the skin of atopic dermatitis patients and from healthy subjects. Int J Dermatol 1999;38:265–269.

Birgit Schittek
Department of Dermatology
University of Tübingen, Liebermeisterstrasse 25
DE–72076 Tübingen (Germany)
Tel. +49 7071 2980 832, Fax +49 7071 295 187, E-Mail birgit.schittek@med.uni-tuebingen.de

Shiohara T (ed): Pathogenesis and Management of Atopic Dermatitis.
Curr Probl Dermatol. Basel, Karger, 2011, vol 41, pp 68–79

Defective Sweating Responses in Atopic Dermatitis

Tetsuo Shiohara · Takaaki Doi · Jun Hayakawa

Department of Dermatology, Kyorin University School of Medicine, Tokyo, Japan

Abstract

While sweat is thought to be one of the important factors provoking exacerbations of clinical symptoms in atopic dermatitis (AD), little attention has been drawn to a beneficial role of sweat in the development of AD lesions. However, if the permeability barrier and antimicrobial barrier dysfunction represents the primary event in the development of AD, an evaluation of sweating responses in AD is a logical place to look for changes that predispose to the disease. In this regard, there have been conflicting data regarding whether sweating responses are impaired, normal or enhanced in AD patients. Consistent with the results of most recent studies, our recent study showed that most AD patients exhibit a defective ability to deliver sweat to the skin surface in response to thermal stress. Despite such defective sweating responses observed in the most part, a marked augmentation in the sweating response with delayed kinetics can be paradoxically detected in some sweating glands of these AD patients, indicating compensatory hyperhidrosis. Dermcidin, a new antimicrobial peptide exclusively produced by sweat glands, was abundantly detected not only in the sweat glands and ducts, and the lumen, but also in the dermal tissues adjacent to the sweat glands. These results indicate that the sweat may be retained in the lumen or pour into the dermal tissues, thereby causing inflammation. Thus, chronic inflammation in AD may be caused in part by a dysfunction of the sweat delivery system.

A marked rise in the prevalence of allergic diseases such as atopic dermatitis (AD) in the industrialized world has often been explained by an increase in ambient air pollution and robust allergic plants as the ecological consequences of global warming, together with a decline in infections during childhood [1]: apparently, genetic mutations alone cannot explain the marked rise in the prevalence. Because the epithelium serves as a first line of defense between the body and the environment, disturbance of the epidermal barrier is the most likely candidate that can favor the increased penetration of such allergens, thereby facilitating the occurrence of allergic inflammatory reactions: it has become clear that the epidermal barrier is an important site for gene-environment interactions in the development of AD [2, 3]. Thus, much attention has been focused on a genetic disturbance in epidermal barrier function as one of the primary events in the development of AD. In this regard, the convincing evidence for a primary defect of the stratum corneum underlying the pathogenesis of AD derives from the recent studies successfully linking loss-of-function mutations in the genes encoding the epidermal structure protein filaggrin (FLG) and AD [4–6]. After identification of *FLG* mutations as a major risk factor for AD, however, much less attention has been directed to the fact that sweating is one of the major mechanisms responsible for not only regulation of skin surface hydration, but also host defense against infections, both of which have been shown to be impaired in AD patients. If the permeability barrier and antimicrobial barrier dysfunction represents the primary event in the development of AD, sweating responses are a logical place to look for changes that predispose to the disease. In this review, we highlight these recent advances in our understanding of sweating disturbance in AD.

Clinical and Laboratory Aspects of Atopic Dermatitis Suggesting Sweating Disturbance

Sweat is well known to be one of the factors provoking exacerbations of clinical symptoms in AD. Indeed, AD patients often complain of aggravation of pruritus and eczematous skin lesions after severe sweating. Contrary to this widely held clinical opinion, however, there is mounting evidence for the protective role of sweat on the development of AD skin lesions. First, AD skin lesions, particularly in adult patients, often spare well-hydrated flexural areas, such as the axillae, and diaper areas. Second, AD patients characterized by dry itchy skin often experience a spontaneous remission in summer. Third, infants born in autumn show the highest prevalence of AD while those born in spring show the lowest [7]. Fourth, dermcidin (DCD), a new antimicrobial peptide exclusively produced by the eccrine sweat glands, contributes to the first line of defense against invading pathogens by building a constant barrier that overlies the epithelial skin [8]. Fifth, excreted sweat can serve to increase skin surface hydration. These findings suggest that sweat may play an essential role in mediating innate immune defenses and that sweating responses may be impaired in patients with AD as compared with healthy controls.

There has been conflicting data regarding whether sweating responses are impaired, normal or enhanced in patients with AD. Sulzberger et al. [9] initially reported that in AD skin there is sweat retention similar to that seen in miliaria. In 1953, Lobitz and Campbell [10] reported normal sweating responses to intradermally injected acetylcholine and epinephrine in AD patients, although these results were not compared with those in healthy controls. Subsequent quantitative studies performed on forearm skin in AD demonstrated increased sweating responses to cholinergic stimulation [11, 12], while others demonstrated normal sweating responses [13]. Varying results were also obtained when adrenergic stimulation was used [14, 15]. Later quantitative studies comparing the cholinergic and adrenergic sweat stimulation in AD again showed that the sweating responses to either cholinergic or adrenergic stimulation were significantly lowered in AD patients and that sweating disturbances were more obvious in dry-appearing AD skin than normal-appearing AD skin [16]. Sweating responses to moderate thermal stress were reported to be impaired in AD patients, although about half of the AD patients showed a normal sweating response [17]: a reduced sweating response was common in both the mildly involved, dry-appearing and uninvolved, normal-appearing skin. In addition, the sweating responses were also retarded as compared with those in healthy controls. Thus, a consensus has emerged from these and other studies that sweating responses are impaired in AD patients, particularly in dry-appearing skin, and retarded: the discrepancy in the results among previous studies could be attributable to a difference in the sensitivity of the method employed to quantify sweating responses.

Reduced Sweating Responses to Thermal Stress in Atopic Dermatitis-

We also investigated sweating responses to thermal stimulus by using an equipment for continuous recording of local sweating volumes, KenzPerspiro OSS-100® (Suzuken Technologies, Nagoya, Japan). In this study, the sweating response was induced by immersion of the trunk and extremities to neck level for 10 min in a water bath maintained at 43°C. Usually, 4 measurements were taken for each site, and 4 sites including involved areas and uninvolved areas were measured. Sweating responses thus measured were markedly decreased in either the involved areas or the uninvolved areas as compared with those in healthy controls [18], although sweating responses were rather lower in the uninvolved areas than those in the involved areas. These findings suggest that a reduced sweating response observed in AD is not a mere consequence of sweat pore closure by inflammation, tissue damage and nonspecific proteolysis, contrary to the previous suggestion that sweat may be prevented from reaching the skin surface due to sweat pore closure by obstructive materials.

A decrease in sweating responses in some areas may be compensated for by a significant increase in sweating responses at other sites [18, 19]. Such compensatory hyperhidrosis can be observed in some AD patients and may provide an explanation why some previous reports demonstrated a hyperhidrotic sweating response to cholinergic local stimulation in a typical lichenified skin area of a child with AD [11, 12]. Thus, hypohidrosis in one area may lead to compensatory hyperhidrosis in another, indicating that contradictory results in previous reports might have been explained by such regional differences.

To investigate whether such regional differences in sweating responses could exist as a function of time in patients with AD, we compared the time course of the sweating responses to thermal stress in involved areas and uninvolved areas of atopic subjects. The sweating response was induced by immersion of both legs to knee levels for 30 min in a water bath maintained at 43°C, a milder condition than our

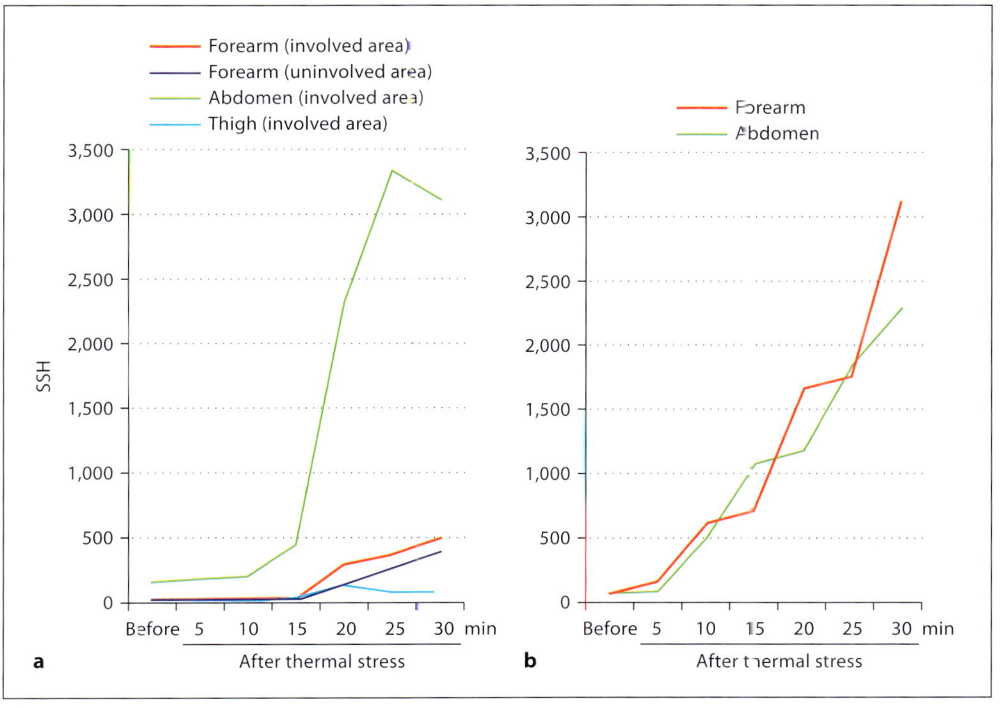

Fig. 1. Time course of sweating responses to thermal stress as measured by the skin surface hydration (SSH), expressed as μS, in different sites of a representative AD subject (**a**) and a normal subject (**b**). The difference in the mean SSH values before and at various time points after starting immersion of both legs to knee level in a water bath (43°C) can be regarded as sweating responses. Four measurements were taken for each site, and 2–4 sites including the involved area were measured.

previous studies. We also investigated how changes in the sweating responses can be related to changes in the local skin temperature. A representative result is shown in figure 1. In this experiment, the degree of sweating was determined by measuring the skin surface hydration (SSH) at different time points after starting thermal stress: before thermal stress and after every 5-min period of thermal stress, measurements of the SSH were performed in healthy controls and atopic subjects. In a representative healthy control, sweat secretion determined by measuring the SSH at each point increased gradually after starting thermal stress either in forearm or abdominal skin: no significant difference existed between the two sites examined. In contrast, sweat secretion in a representative atopic subject was severely impaired in the two sites, forearm and thigh, regardless of whether involved or uninvolved areas were measured. Unexpectedly however, dramatically increased sweat secretion was observed in the involved area of the abdomen in the 20- to 25-min period. These results indicate that a compensatory increase in sweating responses would occur in some areas of atopic subjects. Our results with many atopic subjects show that compensatory hyperhidrosis can be observed in limited areas of some, but not all, AD patients. Similar findings were also reported by Rovensky and Saxl [11]: they demonstrated that a more intense sweat response to thermal, effort and emotional stimuli occurred in lichenified areas while a reaction was absent in normal skin of the same AD patients. Because they did not observe impaired sweating responses in normal skin, they supposed that these increased sweating responses observed in the involved areas would be secondary to a decreased threshold in sudomotor nerves. However, this possibility is less likely to occur, because our ongoing studies showed that such hyperhidrosis can only be observed in limited areas regardless of whether the areas examined are involved or uninvolved. Thus, it is unlikely that sweating increased only in limited areas due to a decreased threshold in sudomotor nerves while it decreased in the majority of other areas. As suggested by Parkkinen et al. [20] and Hanifin [21], these increased sweating responses as determined by the increase in TEWL might have included nonsweat water originating from transudation of inflammatory tissue fluid.

In general, atopic subjects exhibit a lower skin temperature than that of normal subjects. Indeed, there was a difference in the mean skin temperature between atopic and normal subjects before thermal stress. Nevertheless, when the legs of the subjects were immersed in a water bath maintained at 43°C, a decrease in the mean skin temperature was much less apparent in atopic subjects than in control subjects (fig. 2): indeed, the body temperatures measured at any skin sites were not adequately decreased in patients with AD at the end of thermal stress, while those in healthy controls were sufficiently decreased owing to increased sweating responses. The mean skin temperature rather increased in the abdomen despite sweating during the 5- to 20-min period after starting thermal stress. Although the skin temperature in the abdomen eventually decreased at 25–30 min by a local effect of dramatically increased sweating, the levels of mean skin temperature were significantly higher at the end of thermal stress in atopic subjects than those in control subjects. Thus, impaired ability to sweat in response to heat in AD patients results in failure to increase the evaporative loss of heat from the skin and thus predispose to the development of heat tolerance. AD patients are generally unable to adapt physiologically to heat load and often develop symptoms of heat tolerance in hot and humid conditions. These results suggest that there is a disturbance in thermoregulatory responses in atopic subjects and that atopic subjects have greater difficulty in tolerating heat in a hot humid environment than normal subjects, because a reduced sweating response to thermal stress would result in a reduced ability to dissipate excessive heat in a hot environment.

Evaluation of Sweat Gland Activity with Imprint Techniques

Several methods are currently in use to identify the distribution and number of actively secreting sweat glands. The first introduced by Minor [22] is the method

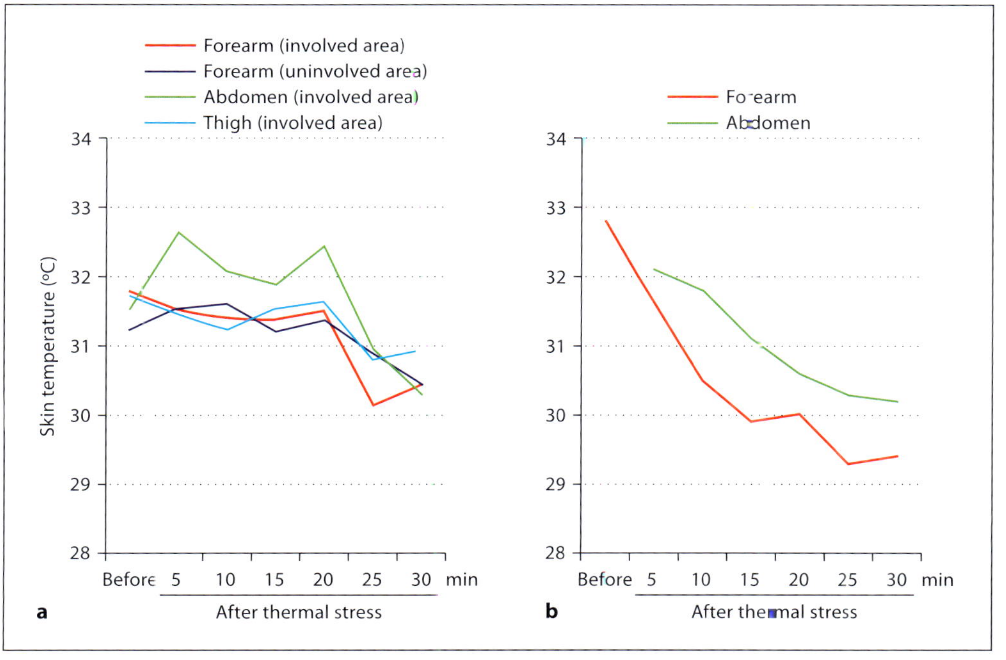

Fig. 2. Time course of skin temperature in the representative AD patient (**a**) and the normal subject (**b**) after exposure to thermal stress. Measurements were done in parallel to those shown in figure 1.

which utilizes the starch-iodine reaction. This starch-iodine reaction is also used for obtaining sweat imprint papers, but the imprint can be obtained only from flat body surfaces, such as the trunk, palms and soles, or small areas of skin. This method has also obvious disadvantages, such as inadequate sensitivity and consistency, and spotty definition of separate sweat gland openings [23].

Another useful method is plastic or silicone impression which allows an accurate quantification of sweat glands actively delivering sweat and the volume of sweat they produce, repeatedly over time. In this method, sweat droplets are visualized as small holes corresponding to the sweat pores. After stimulation, Silasoft, the silicone material of choice for the impression mold technique (IMT), was mixed and spread onto the sweating skin [24]. As the silicone hardened, it retained the impressions of the sweat droplets as they emerged from the sweat ducts and pushed up into the mold [25]. The number of sweat droplets was counted using a dissecting microscope. An estimate of the volume of sweat per square centimeter was obtained by measuring the mean diameter of the outline of each droplet. As described above, sweating was induced by immersing both legs to knee level for 30 min in a water bath (43°C). Usually, impression molds hardened in 3–4 min and they were then removed. Consecutive prints were taken every 15 min. Sweat droplets usually occupied each dermal crest, while they were rarely detected in the skin folds in normal subjects.

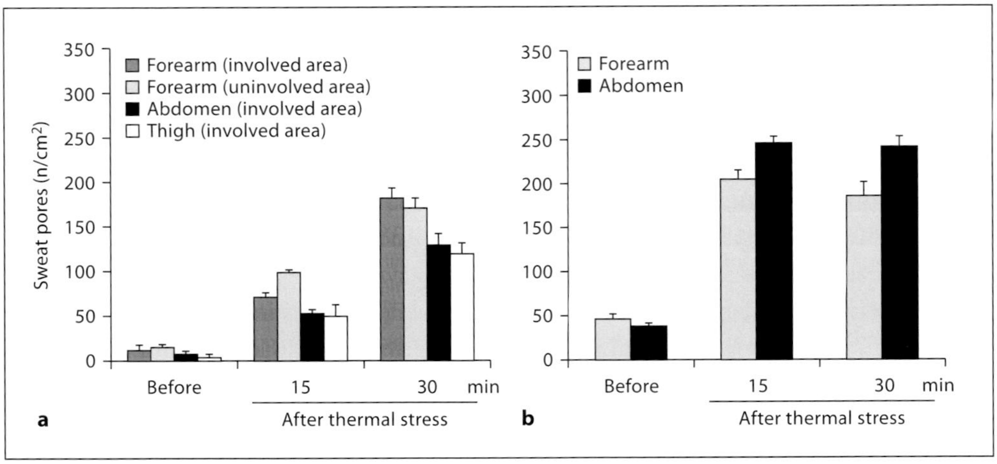

Fig. 3. Time course of the number of sweat gland droplets in the representative AD subject (**a**) and the normal subject (**b**) after exposure to thermal stress. Measurements were done in parallel to those in figures 1 and 2.

Sweat droplets were distributed evenly in healthy controls (data not shown). In contrast, the droplets shown from a representative AD patient were longer in diameter, less numerous and distributed much less evenly than those shown in a control subject. Because the starch-iodine technique yielded counts averaging 30–50/cm^2 in a normal subject, this IMT yielded significantly greater counts in comparison to the starch-iodine reaction.

Figure 3a and b summarizes the results of the number of sweat droplets taken from 3–4 different sites in a normal subject and a representative AD patient over the 15- to 30-min period after starting the thermal stimulus. The number of sweat droplets per square centimeter was apparently lower in an AD subject than that in a normal subject. The number of sweat droplets in a normal subject reached a plateau at 15 min and remained constant till 30 min while that in an AD patient remained low until 15 min and abruptly increased at 30 min in some sites, thus indicating a marked augmentation in the sweating response with delayed kinetics. Figure 4a, b and c shows the histograms of sweat droplet diameter and sweat droplet counts from a normal subject and a representative AD patient, respectively. Regardless of the sites tested, the diameter of sweat droplets ranged widely from 80 to >200 μm in the AD patient, while that in a normal subject remained relatively constant and ranged form 80 to 140 μm. This tendency was more apparent when the involved skin was tested. In many other AD patients, the numbers of sweat droplets counted per square centimeter were much lower than those in control subjects and the size was highly variable, although occasional patients with severe AD lesions only showed a decreased mean droplet count but retained a normal droplet volume. A good relationship existed between

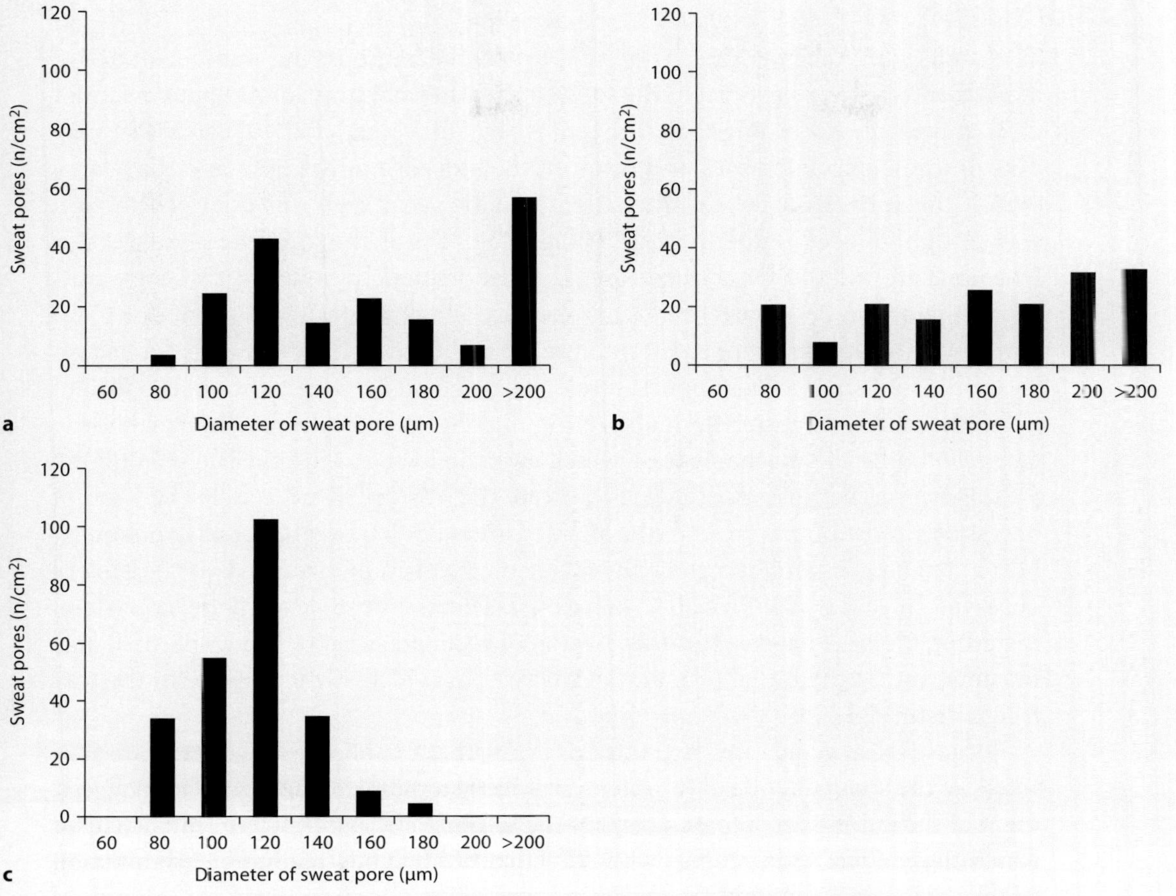

Fig. 4. Histograms of sweat droplet diameter and sweat droplet counts from the involved area (**a**) and uninvolved area (**b**) on the forearm of the representative AD subject and those from the forearm of the control subject (**c**) 30 min after starting thermal stress.

the number of sweat droplets and the volume in control subjects, while this relationship was not obvious in AD patients. Although there was a relationship between the results of the volume as determined by the difference in the mean SSH before and at different time points after starting immersion in a water bath and those of the volume as determined by the IMT, the latter was found to be more sensitive to detect a pinpoint of hypohidrosis and hyperhidrosis. The patients with severer and long-standing AD showed a marked decrease in the number of sweat droplets and a wide site-to-site variation in size. In contrast, our results using the IMT demonstrated that the number and size of the sweat droplets in control subjects were constant and there was a small subject-to-subject or site-to-site variation.

Mechanism of Sweating Disturbance in Atopic Dermatitis

The underlying mechanism responsible for the decrease in the number of active sweat glands delivering sweat to the surface after thermal stress in AD patients is not clear at present. According to earlier reports by Sulzberger et al. [9], the sweat may pour into the dermal tissues as a result of the blockage of the pore and thus carry with it the antigens to which the patient may be sensitized: this duct obstruction was thought to occur either by horny plugging of the openings of the sweat pore or by edema around the sweat duct pore [26]. Unfortunately, however, this early concept remained to be proved because of the lack of histological verification for plugging and the outpouring of sweat into the dermal tissues. In this regard, Rajka also suggested that some functional closure of sweat gland orifices, either in a transient nature or increased absorption/adsorption of secreted sweat by an abnormal horny layer, would be the mechanism by which sweat delivery to the surface is inhibited [27]. However, because our findings indicate that disturbed sweat delivery was not necessarily most pronounced in the affected areas of AD, sweat duct obstruction by horny plugging is not likely to be the major mechanism of disturbed sweat delivery observed in our study. Probably, functional defects in the sweat delivery system, including increased absorption/adsorption of secreted sweat by the epidermis, may in some way be the initial or main mechanism by which sweat delivery to the surface is disturbed.

Because sweat glands are innervated by sympathetic cholinergic fibers and are activated by the sympathetic nerve system, previous studies provided evidence suggesting that the autonomic nervous system, the sympathetic nerve system in particular, is negatively affected in patients with AD [16, 28–32]. Thus, autonomic dysfunction could also be an additional, important factor leading to a decrease in the amount of sweating in AD.

Deficiency of Dermcidin-Derived Peptides in Sweat of Atopic Patients

DCD is constitutively expressed in human eccrine sweat glands, secreted into sweat and transported to the epidermal surface [8, 33, 34]: it is not inducible by skin injury or inflammation. In eccrine sweat, different processed DCD-derived C-terminal peptides of 48-amino-acid residues (DCD-1L), 47-amino-acid residues (DCD-1) and shorter fragments can be detected [35]. DCD-1L and DCD-1 show antimicrobial activity against pathogenic microorganisms such as *Staphylococcus aureus*, *Escherichia coli* and *Candida albicans* under in vitro conditions resembling human sweat [32]. Rieg et al. [36] further demonstrated that DCD-derived peptides in sweat of AD patients are specifically reduced as compared with sweat of healthy individuals and that decreased DCD expression correlates with clinical infectious complications. Nevertheless, because sweat collected from AD patients by physical exercise on a bicycle ergometer was used for quantitative analyses of DCD peptides in this study, it is possible that the decreased DCD expression in sweat secreted from AD patients does not necessarily reflect the ability of the sweat gland to generate DCD peptides. We therefore investigated whether DCD antigen expression could be detected in the sweat glands of AD patients by immunohistochemical techniques. Surprisingly, the expression intensity of DCD antigen in both secretory and ductal cells of AD patients was significantly stronger than that in those of other inflammatory disease lesions, such as lichen planus and psoriasis: the secretory cells showed stronger labeling than the ductal cells. In some AD patients, positive staining was also seen in the lumen of the secretory and ductal portion and the dermis adjacent to the sweat glands, indicating that the sweat, instead of pouring out and being removed from the skin surface, may be retained in the lumen of the secretory and ductal portion or pour into the dermal tissues. In view of the fact that DCD peptides are sweat-specific components but not the components common to other body fluids, the detection of DCD antigen in the lumen of sweat glands and ducts and in the dermal tissues could be interpreted as an indication that the leading hypothesis formulated by Sulzberger et al. [9, 26] proves to be true, and that the sweat glands of AD patients have the potent ability to produce DCD peptides but fail to deliver them to the skin surface.

Conclusion

After a period of neglect in the eighties and nineties, sweating disturbance in AD has again attracted attention since a better understanding of sweat as the first element of the innate immune defense system is now thought to be the basis of improvements in the therapeutic intervention to correct these defects. Chronic inflammation in AD may not only be due to aberrant overwhelming Th2 and Th17 responses, but might also be caused in part by a dysfunction of the sweat delivery system, a long-standing hypothesis formulated by Sulzberger et al. [9, 26]. Accumulated evidence suggests an overall beneficial effect of sweat on host defense and anti-inflammatory mechanisms. We believe that the beneficial effects of sweat so far demonstrated are only the tip of the iceberg. Further investigations are warranted on the beneficial role of sweat in the pathogenesis of AD.

Acknowledgment

This work was supported in part by grants from the Ministry of Education, Culture, Sports, Science and Technology (to T.S.) and Health and Labour Sciences Research Grants (Research on Intractable Diseases) from the Ministry of Health, Labour and Welfare of Japan (to T.S.).

References

1 Yazdanbakhsh M, Kremsner RG, van Ree R: Allergy, parasites, and the hygiene hypothesis. Science 2002; 296:490–494.
2 Walley AJ, Chavanas S, Moffatt MF, Esnouf RM, Ubhi B, Lawrence R, Wong K, Abecasis GR, Jones EY, Harper JI, Hovnanian A, Cookson WO: Gene polymorphism in Netherton and common atopic disease. Nat Genet 2001;29:175–178.
3 Vasilopoulos Y, Cork MJ, Murphy R, Williams HC, Robinson DA, Duff GW, Ward SJ, Tazi-Ahnini R: Genetic association between an AACC insertion in the 3′-UTR of the stratum corneum chymotryptic enzyme gene and atopic dermatitis. J Invest Dermatol 2004;123:62–66.
4 Palmer CN, Irvine AD, Terron-Kwiatkowski A, Zhao Y, Liao H, Lee SP, Goudie DR, Sandilands A, Campbell LE, Smith FJ, O'Regan GW, Watson RM, Cecil JE, Bale SJ, Compton JG, Di Giovanna JJ, Fleckman P, Lewis-Jones S, Arseculeratne G, Sergeant A, Munro CS, EI Houate B, McElreavey K, Halkjaer LB, Bisgaard H, Mukhopadhyay S, McLean WH: Common loss-of-function variants of the epidermal barrier protein filaggrin are a major predisposing factor for atopic dermatitis. Nat Genet 2006;38:441–446.
5 Hudson TJ: Skin barrier function and allergic risk. Nat Genet 2006;38:399–400.
6 Weidinger S, Illig T, Baurecht H, Irvine AD, Rodriguez E, Diaz-Lacava A, Klopp N, Wagenpfeil S, Zhao Y, Liao H, Lee SP, Palmer CN, Jenneck C, Maintz L, Hagemann T, Behrendt H, Ring J, Nothen MM, McLean WH, Novak N: Loss-of-function variations within the filaggrin gene predispose for atopic dermatitis with allergic sensitizations. J Allergy Clin Immunol 2006;118:214–219.
7 Kusunoki T, Asai K, Harazaki M, Korematsu S, Hosoi S: Month of birth and prevalence of atopic dermatitis in schoolchildren: dry skin in early infancy as a possible etiologic factor. J Allergy Clin Immunol 1991;103:1148–1152.
8 Rieg S, Seeber S, Steffen H, Humeny A, Kalbacher H, Stevanovic S, Kimura A, Garbe C, Schittek B: Generation of multiple stable dermcidin-derived antimicrobial peptides in sweat of different body sites. J Invest Dermatol 2006;126:354–365.
9 Sulzberger MB, Herrmann F, Zak FG: Studies of sweating: preliminary report with particular emphasis of a sweat retention syndrome. J Invest Dermatol 1947;9:221–242.
10 Lobitz WC Jr, Campbell CJ: Physiologic studies in atopic dermatitis (disseminated neurodermatitis). I. The local cutaneous response to intradermally injected acetylcholine and epinephrine. Arch Dermatol Syphilol 1953;67:575–589.
11 Rovensky J, Saxl O: Differences in dynamics of sweat secretion in atopic children. J Invest Dermatol 1964;43:171–176.
12 Warndorff JA: The response of sweat gland to acetylcholine in atopic subjects. Br J Dermatol 1970;83:306–311.
13 Murphy GM, Smith SE, Smith SA, Greaves MW: Autonomic function in cholinergic urticaria and atopic eczema. Br J Dermatol 1984;110:581–586
14 Warndorff JA, Neefs J: Quantitative measurement of sweat production after local injection of adrenalin. J Invest Dermatol 1971;56:384–386.
15 Thune P, Kocsis M: Effects of adrenergic stimulating and blocking agents on eccrine sweat secretion in atopic dermatitis and psoriasis. Arch Dermatol Res 1975;253:97–103.
16 Kiistala R: Cholinergic and adrenergic sweating in atopic dermatitis. Acta Derm Venereol 1992;72: 106–108.
17 Candas V, Libert JP, Vogt JJ: Human skin wettedness and evaporative efficiency of sweating. J Appl Physiol 1979;46:522–528.
18 Hayakawa J, Shiohara T: Analysis of abnormal sweating responses in patients with atopic dermatitis (in Japanese). Jpn J Dermatol 2000;110: 1115–1119.
19 Sato K, Ohtsuyama M, Samman G: Eccrine sweat gland disorders. J Am Acad Dermatol 1991;24: 1010–1014.
20 Parkkinen MU, Kiistala R, Kiistala U: Sweating response to moderate thermal stress in atopic dermatitis. Br J Dermatol 1992;126:346–350.
21 Hanifin JM: Pharmacophysiology of atopic dermatitis. Clin Rev Allergy 1986;4:43–65.
22 Minor V: Ein neues Verfahren zu der klinischen Untersuchung der Schweissabsonderung. Zentralbl Ges Neurol Psychiatrie 1927;47:800–803.
23 Harris DR, Polk BF, Willis I: Evaluating sweat gland activity with imprint techniques. J Invest Dermatol 1972;58:78–84.
24 Vilches JJ, Navarro X: New silicones for the evaluation of sudomotor function with the impression mold technique. Clin Auton Res 2002;12:20–23.
25 Kennedy WR, Sakuta M: Collateral reinnervation of sweat glands. Ann Neurol 1984;15:73–78.
26 Sulzberger MB, Herrmann F: Hypohidrosis or anhidrosis attributable to structural changes of the sweat gland; in Sulzberger MB, Hermann F (eds): The Clinical Significance of Disturbances in the Delivery of Sweat. Springfield, Thomas, 1954, pp 62–118.
27 Rajka G: Sweat secretion; in: Essential aspects of atopic dermatitis. 1989, Springer, Berlin Heidelberg New York, pp 174–176.

28 Murphy GM, Smith SE, Smith SA, Greaves MW: Autonomic function in cholinergic urticaria and atopic dermatitis. Br J Dermatol 1984;110: 581–586.
29 Kaliner M: The cholinergic nervous system and immediate hypersensitivity. 1. Eccrine sweat responses in allergic patients. J Allergy Clin Immunol 1976;58:308–315.
30 Kiistala R: Adrenalin-induced local sweating and vasoconstructive response in atopic skin. Br J Dermatol 1992;126:246–249.
31 Kato F, Saga K, Morimoto Y, Kaneko R: Pilocarpine-induced cholinergic sweat secretion compared with emotional sweat secretion in atopic dermatitis. Br J Dermatol 1999;140:1110–1113.
32 Cicek D, Kandi B, Berilgen MS, Bulut S, Tekatas A, Dertlioglu SB, Ozel S, Saral Y: Does autonomic dysfunction play a role in atopic dermatitis? Br J Dermatol 2008;159:834–838.
33 Schittek B, Hipfel R, Sauer B, Bauer J, Kalbacher H, Stevanovic S, Schirle M, Schroeder K, Blin N, Meier F, Rassner G, Garbe C: Dermcidin: a novel human antibiotic peptide secreted by sweat glands. Nat Immunol 2001;2:1133–1137.
34 Rieg S, Garbe C, Sauer B, Kalbacher H, Schittek B: Dermcidin is constitutively produced by eccrine sweat glands and is not induced in epidermal cells under inflammatory skin conditions. Br J Dermatol 2004;151:534–539.
35 Flad T, Bogumil R, Tolson J, Schittek B, Garbe C, Deeg M, Mueller CA, Kalbacher H: Detection of dermcidin-derived peptides in sweat by ProteinChip technology. J Immunol Methods 2002;270:53–62.
36 Rieg S, Steffen H, Seeber S, Humeny A, Kalbacher H, Dietz K, Garbe C, Schittek B: Deficiency of dermcidin-derived antimicrobial peptides in sweat of patients with atopic dermatitis correlates with an impaired innate defense of human skin in vivo. J Immunol 2005;174:8003–8010.

Tetsuo Shiohara, MD, PhD
Department of Dermatology
Kyorin University School of Medicine
6-20-2 Shinkawa, Mitaka, Tokyo 181-8611 (Japan)
Tel. +81 422 47 5511, Fax +81 422 41 4741, E-Mail tpshio@ks.kyorin-u.ac.jp

Shiohara T (ed): Pathogenesis and Management of Atopic Dermatitis.
Curr Probl Dermatol. Basel, Karger, 2011, vol 41, pp 80–92

The Role of Cytokines/Chemokines in the Pathogenesis of Atopic Dermatitis

Kei-ichi Yamanaka · Hitoshi Mizutani

Department of Dermatology, Mie University Graduate School of Medicine, Tsu, Japan

Abstract

Atopic dermatitis (AD) is the most common and relapsing allergic disease of the skin. AD is characterized by a predominant expression of Th2-type cytokines associated with increased cellular infiltration in the skin, elevated circulating levels of IgE and eosinophilia. These findings are positively correlated with interleukin (IL)-4 and IL-13 expression in CD4+ T cells. In AD patients, Th2 cells, eosinophils, mast cells and dendritic cells are markedly increased in the skin lesions. However, Th1 cells are also involved in the development of AD lesions. In fact, Th1 cytokine mRNA expressions including γ-interferon and IL-12 are elevated in the chronic lesions as well as elevated Th2 cytokines in the acute AD lesions. The discovery of Th17 lineage and regulatory T (T_{reg}) cells shifted the simple Th1/Th2 balance concept into a 4-way balance system. Th17/22 cells, Foxp3+ T_{reg} and IL-10-producing T cells (Tr1) are involved in the mechanism of a local and systemic immunological milieu. In addition, super Th1 cells arranged from Th1 cells in high IL-18 milieu are also involved in the development of mouse AD lesions. Correction of Th2 cytokine predominance by Th1 inducers shows effectiveness in experimental models. However, fine-tuning of the delicate 4-way balance among Th1, Th2, Th17/22 and T_{reg} cells is required for the control of AD. Efficacy of some biological agents in AD has been reported. However, further investigations are required to make possible the therapeutic application of biologicals, antigen-specific immunotherapy, non-antigen-specific immunotherapy, antagonists and biological response modifiers in the clinic. These novel approaches may constitute a potential curative therapy for AD.

Atopic dermatitis (AD) is a common allergic skin disorder characterized by recurrent pruritic inflammatory skin lesions. The pathogenesis of AD is multifactorial including genetic, environmental, skin barrier, psychological and immunological factors. AD is a chronic dermatitis characterized by a predominant expression of Th2-type cytokines; that is associated with increased cellular infiltration of the skin and overproduction of IgE [1]. AD has been recognized as a Th2 disease for the abundant production of Th2 cytokines, interleukin (IL)-4, IL-5 and IL-13 associated with eosinophilia and elevated serum IgE level. There is a significant positive correlation between IL-4 and IL-13 expression in CD4+ T cells and also with peripheral blood eosinophil counts [2, 3]. In the AD skin lesions, CD4+ T cells, CD8+ T cells, eosinophils, mast cells and dendritic cells are markedly increased in the dermis; however, Th1 cells have also been involved. In fact, in addition to the high RNA expression of IL-5, IL-13 and IL-4 in the acute AD lesions, that of Th1 cytokines such as γ-interferon (IFN-γ) and IL-12 has also been found to be increased [4]. IL-17 is another important component of allergic and inflammatory diseases, and infiltration of IL-17-producing T cells (Th17) is known to be also abundant in the acute AD skin lesions [5]. Foxp3+ regulatory T cells (T_{reg}) and IL-10-producing T cells (Tr1) play critical roles locally and systemically in the control of AD symptoms. Super Th1 cells are also involved in AD formation in the mouse. Recently, AD has been categorized into 2 distinct types: extrinsic or intrinsic type. Patients with extrinsic AD show high levels of specific serum IgE against environmental or food allergens, whereas intrinsic or nonallergic AD exhibits absence of specific IgE and no association with respiratory diseases [6].

Th2 Cytokines

A generalized Th2-deviated immune response is closely linked to the condition of AD; however, the skin disease itself is a biphasic inflammation with an initial Th2 phase and a chronic Th1 phase [7]. The immune response in clinical AD lesions is a mixture of Th1 and Th2 features. A predominant systemic Th2 cytokine response with increased IgE levels and eosinophilia is widely accepted as part of the pathogenesis of atopic diseases. IL-4, IL-5 and IL-13 are major Th2 cytokines that participate in AD as well as in other allergic disorders. IL-4 and IL-13 have essential roles in the initial phase of tissue inflammation as well as in the increased expression of adhesion molecules on endothelial cells [7]. Both cytokines are also responsible for the differentiation of allergen-specific Th2 cells and the class switching of activated B cells to IgE-producing cells. IL-5 contributes to the increase and survival of eosinophils [7]. Recent studies have demonstrated high RNA expression of the cytokines described above, and low RNA expression of IFN-γ in the skin lesions and in peripheral blood of patients with extrinsic-type acute AD [2, 3, 8]. By contrast, IFN-γ expression is upregulated in the chronic phase. The epidermis with atopic inflammation contains 2 distinct types of dendritic cells including the classical Langerhans cells and the inflammatory dendritic epidermal cells [9]. The latter population induces Th1 cytokines, whereas the Langerhans cell population induces Th2-type reactions [10]. The balance of these populations may induce Th2/Th1 cytokine profile switching characteristic of the chronic phase of AD. Persistence of chronic dermatitis depends on both Th1 and Th2 responses. In contrast, in the intrinsic type of AD, there is a lack of specific IgE and it is associated with much lower levels of IL-4 and IL-13 and higher IFN-γ expression. Barrier dysfunction is

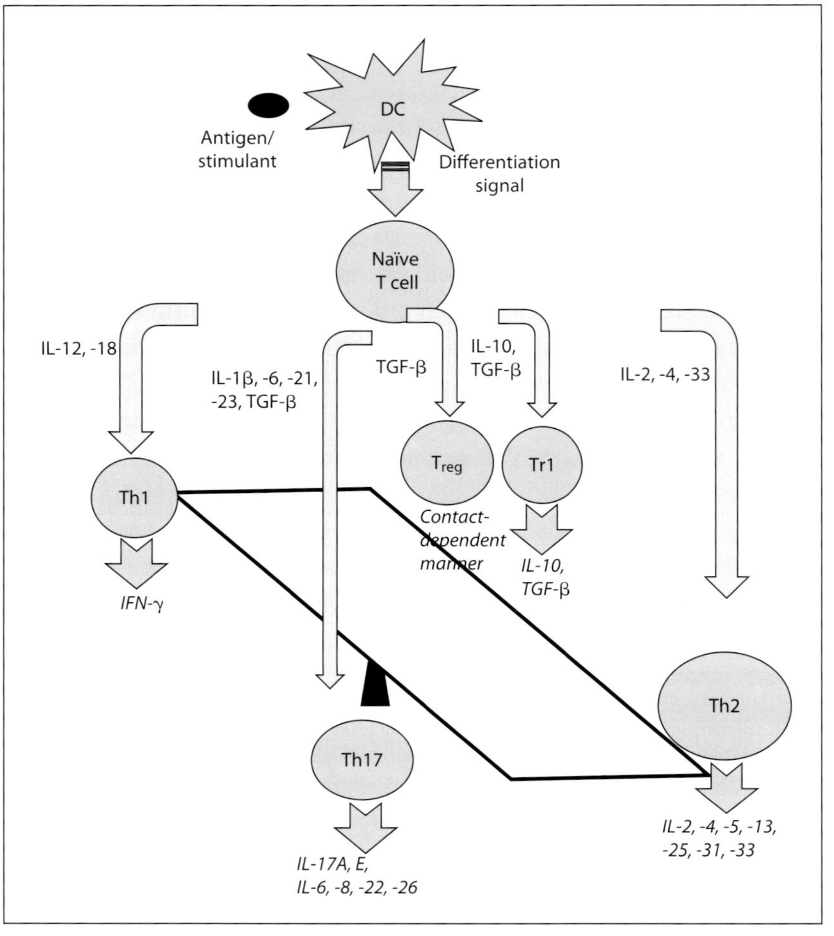

Fig. 1. Naïve T cells differentiate to effector T cells including Th1, Th2, Th17 and T_{reg} cells after the stimulation of allergens or antigens together with appropriate cytokines in the microenvironment. These components constitute a 4-way balance. DC = Dendritic cell; TGF = transforming growth factor.

apparent in extrinsic AD, suggesting that antigen exposure to the host immune system is enhanced in extrinsic AD. Therefore, patients with intrinsic AD are less sensitized to exogenous protein allergens that induce Th2 responses, or less sensitive to antibody production. Further investigation is required to clarify the mechanism of intrinsic AD.

GATA-3 is a transcription factor that is specifically expressed in Th2 cells and plays a critical role in the differentiation of naïve CD4 T cells to Th2 cells. In addition, GATA-3 is essential for the gene expression of the Th2 cytokines IL-4, IL-5 and IL-13 that mediate allergic inflammation. GATA-3 is inhibited by the Th1 master regulatory transcription T-bet, but in turn counteracts STAT4 and T-bet [11] (fig. 1).

Thymic Stromal Lymphopoietin

Thymic stromal lymphopoietin (TSLP) is an IL-7-like cytokine which promotes Th2 cytokine-associated inflammation by directly stimulating the effector functions of Th2 cells and basophils [12, 13]. TSLP is produced by epithelial, stromal and mast cells, and especially by keratinocytes in AD but not in other types of skin inflammation. TSLP binds to a heterodimer receptor consisting of IL-7 receptor α and TSLP receptor chains [14, 15]. TSLP promotes the activation and migration of dendritic cells within the dermis of AD, and TSLP-activated dendritic cells produce the Th2-attracting chemokines TARC (thymus- and activation-regulated chemokine; CC motif chemokine ligand 17, CCL17) and MDC (macrophage-derived chemokine; CCL22) [13], and prime differentiation of naïve CD4 T cells to effector Th2 cells. Thus, TSLP ultimately contributes to the induction of allergic inflammation by producing IL-4, IL-5 and IL-13. Additionally, TSLP inhibits IL-10 and IFN-γ production. On the other hand, microbial products, proinflammatory cytokines (tumor necrosis factor α and IL-1α) and Th2 cytokines (IL-4 or IL-13) induce the production of TSLP in human skin explants [16, 17]. Recent studies have shown evidence that eosinophil- and basophil-derived IL-25, a distinct member of the IL-17 cytokine family, enhances the expansion and functions of TSLP-activated Th2 memory cells, thus augmenting allergic tissue inflammation [18, 19]. TSLP has central roles for initiating the allergic responses [20, 21].

Interleukin 31

IL-31 is preferentially expressed by Th2 cells and is highly recognized in AD skin lesions [22]. IL-31 expression is significantly increased in pruritic AD skin compared with healthy skin [23, 24]. T cells are thought to be the main source of IL-31 in AD [23], and there is a correlation between serum IL-31 levels and the severity of AD [25]. IL-31 receptor is a heterodimer containing the IL-31 receptor A and oncostatin M receptor; those are expressed on human keratinocytes. IL-31 induces the expression of the inflammatory T cell attracting chemokines CCL17/TARC and CCL22/MDC in cultured keratinocytes [22, 24]. Thus, IL-31 has an essential role in the perpetuation of atopic skin inflammation.

Interleukin 33

IL-33, a newly described member of the IL-1 family, is expressed by many cell types including keratinocytes during inflammatory responses. Previous reports suggested the involvement of IL-33 in the development of Th2 type allergy. IL-33 receptor, which contains the ST2 and IL-1 receptor accessory protein, is also widely expressed in immunocytes, particularly in Th2 cells and mast cells. IL-33 promotes maturation of mast cells and induces cytokine and chemokine production in umbilical cord blood-derived mast cells [26]. IL-33 augmented IgE cross-linking-primed IL-8 and IL-13 production in human mast cells. Thus, IL-33 is involved in the pathogenesis of allergic disorders by promoting the expansion of Th2 cells and mast cell activation. Thus, IL-33 is a potent therapeutic target to control allergic diseases [27].

Th1 Cytokines

Chronic skin lesions are associated with a dominant Th1 response characterized by high levels of IFN-γ, IL-12 and granulocyte-macrophage colony-stimulating factor. For effective IFN-γ production during chronic AD lesions, a combined expression of IL-12 and IL-18 is required. In addition, remodeling-associated cytokines, i.e. IL-11 and transforming growth factor β_1, are expressed preferentially in chronic forms of the disease. The cause and mechanism of intrinsic AD remain unknown. The intrinsic type of the disease is characterized by IFN-γ-producing cells [28]. Acute AD skin lesions are characterized by T cells and eosinophils with deposition of eosinophil-derived products and increased skin expression of Th2 cytokines IL-4, IL-5, IL-13 and with only little IFN-γ expression. Increased expression of IFN-γ, IL-12 and granulocyte-macrophage colony-stimulating factor [29] is detected in chronic AD lesions. The characteristic findings of chronic AD lesions are dermal thickening caused by tissue remodeling and collagen deposition. IFN-γ is not only an initiator of inflammation. Recent studies have shown that IFN-γ is a strong stimulant of fibrosis [30]. The IFN-γ knockout mouse showed reduced dermal thickening in a mouse model of the dermatitis. The mechanism behind this switch from Th2 to Th1 type is not well understood. Some microbial products that activate TLR2 are believed to switch toward a Th1 response [31].

Th1 and Th2 Chemokines

Leukocyte trafficking into the skin is mainly regulated by adhesion molecules and the chemoattractive small protein chemokines [32, 33]. AD patients have high CCL17 and CCL22 levels [34] in their sera, and high CCL17 and CCL22 expressions on peripheral blood mononuclear cells compared to normal subjects [35]. These chemokines that recruit Th2 cells into inflammatory sites have been categorized as Th2 chemokines. CCL17 belongs to the CC chemokine family that is also known as TARC. CCL17 is expressed constitutively in the thymus and only transiently in stimulated peripheral blood mononuclear cells [36]. CCL17 binds and induces chemotaxis in T cells and elicits its effects by interacting with the chemokine receptor CCR4 [36, 37] that is selectively expressed on Th2 cells. CCL22 is also called MDC and is secreted by dendritic cells and macrophages. CCL22 also acts on its target cells through its CCR4 receptor [38]. CCL17/TARC and CCL22/MDC are high-affinity ligands for CCR4. Thus, they attract IL-4- and/or IL-13-producing Th2 lymphocytes, and their concentrations are strongly correlated with disease activity [39, 40]. Chemokines also control Th1 cell chemotaxis [41, 42]. CCL20/MIP-3a is an important Th1 chemokine responsible for the recruitment of CCR6-expressing immature dendritic cells and memory/effector T cells into the dermis of atopic skin through CCR6 [43, 44]. CCL20 is induced by IL-1 or tumor necrosis factor α [34]. CCL20 is constitutively but weakly expressed in the normal skin. However, CCL20 is abundantly identified in the basal layer of the lesional epidermis in AD patients [34, 45–47]. Thus, chemokines such as CCL11, CCL17 and CCL22 induce infiltration of cells with a Th2-dominated pattern. On the other hand, CXCL9, CXCL10 and CXCL11 recruit mainly Th1-type lymphocytes to the inflammatory sites [48].

The Pleiotropic Cytokine IL-18

In the presence of IL-12, 18-kDa mature IL-18 induces differentiation of naïve T cells into Th1 cells that secrete IFN-γ [49] and suppress IgE production from B cells. However, administration of IL-18 alone leads to increased IgE levels and enhanced production of IL-4 and IL-13 by basophils, mast cells and CD4+ T cells [50, 51]. Thus, in the absence of IL-12, IL-18 promotes a Th2 response in vivo. The levels of IL-18 in the serum and in the tape-stripped stratum corneum samples are also elevated in AD patients. As a member of the IL-1 family, IL-18 lacks the leader sequence. It is constitutively produced but stored as an inactive precursor form, pro-IL-18. Pro-IL-18 needs appropriate post-translational processing to become biologically active and to be extracellularly released. Caspase 1 is an authentic processing enzyme for IL-18 and IL-1β. Hematopoietic cells such as macrophages produce pro-IL-18 in the steady state and release IL-18 through endogenous caspase 1. Epithelial cells from the skin such as keratinocytes constitutively produce pro-IL-18 without converting into the mature form. Recently, as a novel function of mast cell chymase, an enzyme localized in the granules of mast cells, was found to cleave pro-IL-18 into the biologically active IL-18 [52]. Mast cells densely accumulate in the AD skin lesions [53]. Some immunological and physical stress (scratching) stimulates mast cells and keratinocytes to discharge mast cell granule chymase and keratinocyte contents (pro-IL-β and IL-18) to the surrounding microenvironment. Thus, an increased IL-18 level is directly associated with systemic Th2 dominance [51]. Therefore, the clinical effectiveness of antihistamine and antiallergic compounds on AD may be in part explained by the mast cell/keratinocyte cytokine paracrine network. More recently pro-IL-18 was found to be cleaved by granzyme B released from CD8+ T cells [54]. In AD skin lesions there are abundant skin-infiltrating cells including CD8+ T cells. It is conceivable that granzyme B from CD8+ T cells triggers inflammation activation of keratinocyte pro-IL-18 as well as silent apoptosis.

Super Th1 Cells

A recent study has revealed a second important role of IL-18 in the adaptive immunity. Upon simultaneous engagement of T-cell receptor and IL-18 receptor, Th1 cytokine-producing cells that have IL-18 receptor transform to produce Th2 cytokines including IL-3, IL-13 and IL-9, but not IL-4. They also produce larger amounts of chemokines that recruit inflammatory cells including granulocytes, macrophages and lymphocytes. These IL-13/IL-9/chemokine-producing Th1 cells were categorized as super Th1 cells [55]. Further studies to target super Th1 cells and associated cytokines are required to control long-lasting chronic skin lesions. Anti-human IL-18 monoclonal antibody is a potential candidate as a therapeutic agent for this disease [55, 56].

Staphylococcal Infection and Atopic Dermatitis

AD is frequently complicated with recurrent bacterial and viral infections [57]. Exacerbation of dermatitis after infection is a well-known phenomenon in AD. Keratinocytes defend themselves from bacterial infection by producing antimicrobial peptides; however, antimicrobial peptide production is suppressed in AD skin. *Staphylococcus aureus* is commonly cultivated from the skin lesions of AD patients and AD model animals. *S. aureus* has been ascribed to be one of the causative agents for AD. AD patients are sensitized to various *S. aureus*-derived toxins, and specific IgE is identified in their sera.

Epidermal keratinocytes produce the inflammatory cytokines IL-1α and IL-18. *S. aureus* infection augments production of IL-1α in the mouse skin [58]. Topical application of *S. aureus*-derived protein A (SpA) to the barrier-disrupted skin develops AD-like pruritic dermatitis in NC/Nga mice [59] inducing super Th1 cells. CD4+ T cells in the draining lymph nodes of the SpA-treated skin exhibit the features of super Th1 cells [55]. Keratinocytes freshly isolated from naïve mice release IL-18 in response to SpA in vitro [59], suggesting the involvement of *S. aureus* and keratinocyte-derived IL-18 in the development of super Th1 cells in vivo. SpA-positive *S. aureus* is commonly cultivated from AD lesions.

Th17 Cells

IL-17-producing CD4+ T cells (Th17) are distinct from Th1 and Th2 cells, and have roles in innate and acquired immunity. Differentiation of Th17 (IL-17A-producing and IL-17F-producing) cells is supported by IL-1β, IL-6, IL-21, IL-23, and transforming growth factor β [60]. Immunohistochemical analysis demonstrated the presence of IL-17-secreting cells in the dermis in acute AD lesions, but not in chronic lesions [5, 61, 62]. In the peripheral blood, the number of Th17 cells is increased in AD patients

[5]. Secreted IL-17 together with IL-22 in the skin lesions regulates the expression of antimicrobial proteins and proinflammatory cytokine granulocyte-macrophage colony-stimulating factor, tumor necrosis factor α and IL-8 in the epidermis. Thus, IL-17 induces and augments skin inflammation [5, 63]. Th17 cells are increased in psoriatic and AD lesions. In psoriatic lesions, the number of Th1 and Th17 cells is increased; however, Th2 cells are dominant in acute AD skin. IL-22 is a cytokine that promotes epidermal thickening. IL-22-producing T cells are significantly increased in AD skin [64] as well as in psoriatic lesions. Although lesions in AD and psoriasis have apparently different immunological backgrounds, similar IL-22 and IL-17 pathways are involved in the epidermal changes. Further studies should be carried out to clarify additional factors that induce the differentiation in both diseases.

Tr1 Cells

Allergen-specific immunotherapy for allergic diseases has been reevaluated for use as a curative therapy. In pollinosis, circulating IL-10-producing T regulatory type 1 (Tr1) is decreased compared to normal controls. After successful antigen-specific immunotherapy, the number of Tr1 cells was recovered to the levels of normal controls [65]. Effective and safety induction of Tr1 cells is a key for successful antigen-specific immunotherapy. In contrast to successful results in pollinosis, limited positive effects have recently been reported in AD. The number of Tr1 cells is elevated in the peripheral blood of patients with AD [66]. The role of Tr1 cells in AD is not fully understood. There may be differences in the property of Tr1 cells between AD and pollinosis. Tr1 cells in AD should be characterized. Systemic cyclosporine is indicated in severe cases. Cyclosporine suppresses the T_{reg} at high doses, but augments it at low doses. Control of Tr1 may be of general importance in AD therapy as well as in specific immunotherapy.

Experimental Immunotherapy for Atopic Dermatitis

The increase in AD and Th2-related diseases has been attributed in part to a decreased exposure to microorganisms ('hygiene theory'). The effect of bacille Calmette-Guérin vaccination in AD is still controversial. To correct the polarized Th2 immune imbalance in AD, *Propionibacterium acnes* was administered to AD model mice [67] to induce a Th1 response. Vaccination with low doses of *P. acnes* successfully prevented clinical manifestations of AD by increasing IFN-γ+ T cells, natural T_{reg} and Tr1 cells [68]. Avoiding granuloma formation of bacille Calmette-Guérin vaccination, a secretory protein, Ag85B, from acid-fast bacilli was selected as a Th1 inducer and was vaccinated as a DNA vaccine to a mouse AD model. This controlled AD skin lesions with elevation of IFN-γ expression and induction of natural T_{reg} cells [69]. Although these trials have been performed in mice, Th1 biological response modifiers are potent candidates for AD in the future.

Monoclonal Antibodies and Antagonists against Cytokines

Monoclonal antibodies and antagonists (biologicals) are hopeful therapeutic tools for allergic diseases [70]. Omalizumab is utilized for the treatment of asthma. Several successful results for AD have been reported. The involvement of IgE in AD pathogenesis is clear, and it was shown that it ameliorates AD manifestations directly or indirectly. Compared with asthma, serum IgE levels in AD patients are high and exceed 700 IU/ml. Therefore, higher doses of omalizumab are required to control AD than that used for asthma. The anti-IL-5 antibody mepolizumab decreased the peripheral blood eosinophil counts; however, it failed to improve clinical manifestations of AD [71–73]. Therapy using biologicals such as alefacept, an LFA-3/IgG1 fusion protein, and efalizumab, an anti-CD11a antibody, has been described by Jung and Stingl [18]. Alefacept ameliorates clinical manifestations in patients with AD [74, 75], and efalizumab significantly improved the clinical severity in patients with severe AD [76]. These biologicals improve AD interfering with antigen presentation and chemotaxis. The anti-CD20 antibody rituximab dramatically improves clinical severity, reduces the infiltration of B cells in the peripheral blood and skin, and decreases IL-5- and IL-13-producing skin cells [77]. Unexpected side effects are reported for biologicals together with these clinical improvements. A large-scale control study is needed to confirm the beneficial effects of biologicals.

An additional candidate is a receptor antagonist. Antagonistic IL-4 mutants are available to inhibit IL-4. Variants of human IL-4 that bind to the receptor subunit IL-4 receptor α are competitive antagonists of IL-4 [78, 79], and IL-13 is inhibited by similar variants [80, 81]. IL-4 and IL-13 double mutant is also reported as an effective antagonist for human IL-4 and IL-13 signaling [80, 82].

Conclusions

We are facing an era of transition in AD therapy. Recent findings of new T-cell subsets have changed the theory of Th1/Th2 2-way balance to a 4-way balance of Th1, Th2, Th17/22 and T_{reg}. Innate immunity plays an important role in AD manifestations and in the initiation of acquired immunity. There are still many unanswered questions. Fortunately, novel therapeutic tools are currently available for AD including biologicals, antagonists, specific and nonspecific immunomodulators, and immunosuppressants. Future research will clarify the remaining enigmas in the complex network of the AD immune system, and hopefully it will provide better therapeutic strategies for AD.

Acknowledgments

We thank Prof. Esteban C. Gabazza for his careful and critical reading and discussion of this manuscript. The authors are supported by funding from grants for scientific research from the Ministry of Education, Culture, Sports, Science and Technology, Japan, and by Maruho Co. Ltd.

References

1 Del Prete G: Human Th1 and Th2 lymphocytes: their role in the pathophysiology of atopy. Allergy 1992;47:450–455.
2 Kaminishi K, Soma Y, Kawa Y, Mizoguchi M: Flow cytometric analysis of IL-4, IL-13 and IFN-gamma expression in peripheral blood mononuclear cells and detection of circulating IL-13 in patients with atopic dermatitis provide evidence for the involvement of type 2 cytokines in the disease. J Dermatol Sci 2002;29:19–25.
3 Metwally SS, Mosaad YM, Abdel-Samee ER, El-Gayyar MA, Abdel-Aziz AM, El-Chennawi FA: IL-13 gene expression in patients with atopic dermatitis: relation to IgE level and to disease severity. Egypt J Immunol 2004;11:171–177.
4 Grewe M, Gyufko K, Schopf E, Krutmann J: Lesional expression of interferon-gamma in atopic eczema. Lancet 1994;343:25–26.
5 Koga C, Kabashima K, Shiraishi N, Kobayashi M, Tokura Y: Possible pathogenic role of Th17 cells for atopic dermatitis. J Invest Dermatol 2008;128: 2625–2630.
6 Wuthrich B, Schmid-Grendelmeier P: The atopic eczema/dermatitis syndrome: epidemiology, natural course, and immunology of the IgE-associated ('extrinsic') and the nonallergic ('intrinsic') AEDS. J Investig Allergol Clin Immunol 2003;13:1–5.
7 Bieber T: Atopic dermatitis. Ann Dermatol 2010;22: 125–137.
8 Miraglia del Giudice M, Decimo F, Leonardi S, et al: Immune dysregulation in atopic dermatitis. Allergy Asthma Proc 2006;27:451–455.
9 Wollenberg A, Kraft S, Hanau D, Bieber T: Immunomorphological and ultrastructural characterization of Langerhans cells and a novel, inflammatory dendritic epidermal cell (IDEC) population in lesional skin of atopic eczema. J Invest Dermatol 1996;106:446–453.
10 Novak N, Bieber T. The role of dendritic cell subtypes in the pathophysiology of atopic dermatitis. J Am Acad Dermatol 2005;53:S171–S176.
11 Barnes PJ: Role of GATA-3 in allergic diseases. Curr Mol Med 2008;8:330–334.
12 Ziegler SF, Artis D: Sensing the outside world: TSLP regulates barrier immunity. Nat Immunol 2010;11: 289–293.
13 Soumelis V, Reche PA, Kanzler H, et al: Human epithelial cells trigger dendritic cell mediated allergic inflammation by producing TSLP. Nat Immunol 2002;3:673–680.
14 Pandey A, Ozaki K, Baumann H, et al: Cloning of a receptor subunit required for signaling by thymic stromal lymphopoietin. Nat Immunol 2000;1:59–64.
15 Park LS, Martin U, Garka K, et al: Cloning of the murine thymic stromal lymphopoietin (TSLP) receptor: formation of a functional heteromeric complex requires interleukin 7 receptor. J Exp Med 2000;192:659–670.
16 Allakhverdi Z, Comeau MR, Jessup HK, et al: Thymic stromal lymphopoietin is released by human epithelial cells in response to microbes, trauma, or inflammation and potently activates mast cells. J Exp Med 2007;204:253–258.
17 Bogiatzi SI, Fernandez I, Bichet JC, et al: Cutting edge: proinflammatory and Th2 cytokines synergize to induce thymic stromal lymphopoietin production by human skin keratinocytes. J Immunol 2007; 178:3373–3377.
18 Jung T, Stingl G: Atopic dermatitis: therapeutic concepts evolving from new pathophysiologic insights. J Allergy Clin Immunol 2008;122:1074–1081.
19 Wang YH, Angkasekwinai P, Lu N, et al: IL-25 augments type 2 immune responses by enhancing the expansion and functions of TSLP-DC-activated Th2 memory cells. J Exp Med 2007;204:1837–1847.
20 Soumelis V, Liu YJ: Human thymic stromal lymphopoietin: a novel epithelial cell-derived cytokine and a potential key player in the induction of allergic inflammation. Springer Semin Immunopathol 2004;25:325–333.
21 Liu YJ: Thymic stromal lymphopoietin: master switch for allergic inflammation. J Exp Med 2006; 203:269–273.
22 Dillon SR, Sprecher C, Hammond A, et al: Interleukin 31, a cytokine produced by activated T cells, induces dermatitis in mice. Nat Immunol 2004;5:752–760.

23 Bilsborough J, Leung DY, Maurer M, et al: IL-31 is associated with cutaneous lymphocyte antigen-positive skin homing T cells in patients with atopic dermatitis. J Allergy Clin Immunol 2006;117: 418–425.
24 Sonkoly E, Muller A, Lauerma AI, et al: IL-31: a new link between T cells and pruritus in atopic skin inflammation. J Allergy Clin Immunol 2006;117: 411–417.
25 Raap U, Wichmann K, Bruder M, et al: Correlation of IL-31 serum levels with severity of atopic dermatitis. J Allergy Clin Immunol 2008;122:421–423.
26 Iikura M, Suto H, Kajiwara N, et al: IL-33 can promote survival, adhesion and cytokine production in human mast cells. Lab Invest 2007;87:971–978.
27 Liew FY, Pitman NI, McInnes IB: Disease-associated functions of IL-33: the new kid in the IL-1 family. Nat Rev Immunol 2010;10:103–110.
28 Simon D, von Gunten S, Borelli S, Braathen LR, Simon HU: The interleukin-13 production by peripheral blood T cells from atopic dermatitis patients does not require CD2 costimulation. Int Arch Allergy Immunol 2003;132:148–155.
29 Hamid Q, Boguniewicz M, Leung DY: Differential in situ cytokine gene expression in acute versus chronic atopic dermatitis. J Clin Invest 1994;94: 870–876.
30 Kosaka H, Yoshimoto T, Fujimoto J, Nakanishi K: Interferon-gamma is a therapeutic target molecule for prevention of postoperative adhesion formation. Nat Med 2008;14:437–441.
31 Jin H, Kumar L, Mathias C, et al: Toll-like receptor 2 is important for the T(H)1 response to cutaneous sensitization. J Allergy Clin Immunol 2009;123: 875–882.
32 Butcher EC, Picker LJ: Lymphocyte homing and homeostasis. Science 1996;272:60–66.
33 Campbell JJ, Butcher EC: Chemokines in tissue-specific and microenvironment-specific lymphocyte homing. Curr Opin Immunol 2000;12: 336–341.
34 Narbutt J, Lesiak A, Sysa-Jedrzeiowska A, et al: The imbalance in serum concentration of Th-1- and Th-2-derived chemokines as one of the factors involved in pathogenesis of atopic dermatitis. Mediators Inflamm 2009;2009:269541.
35 Park CO, Lee HJ, Lee JH, et al: Increased expression of CC chemokine ligand 18 in extrinsic atopic dermatitis patients. Exp Dermatol 2008;17:24–29.
36 Imai T, Yoshida T, Baba M, Nishimura M, Kakizaki M, Yoshie O: Molecular cloning of a novel T cell-directed CC chemokine expressed in thymus by signal sequence trap using Epstein-Barr virus vector. J Biol Chem 1996;271:21514–21521.
37 Imai T, Baba M, Nishimura M, Kakizaki M, Takagi S, Yoshie O: The T cell-directed CC chemokine TARC is a highly specific biological ligand for CC chemokine receptor 4. J Biol Chem 1997;272: 15036–15042.
38 Vulcano M, Albanesi C, Stoppacciaro A, et al: Dendritic cells as a major source of macrophage-derived chemokine/CCL22 in vitro and in vivo. Eur J Immunol 2001;31:812–822.
39 Kakinuma T, Nakamura K, Wakugawa M, et al: Thymus and activation-regulated chemokine in atopic dermatitis: serum thymus and activation-regulated chemokine level is closely related with disease activity. J Allergy Clin Immunol 2001;107: 535–541.
40 Kakinuma T, Nakamura K, Wakugawa M, et al: Serum macrophage-derived chemokine (MDC) levels are closely related with the disease activity of atopic dermatitis. Clin Exp Immunol 2002;127: 270–273.
41 Shimada Y, Takehara K, Sato S: Both Th2 and Th1 chemokines (TARC/CCL17, MDC/CCL22, and Mig/CXCL9) are elevated in sera from patients with atopic dermatitis. J Dermatol Sci 2004;34:201–208.
42 Nakazato J, Kishida M, Kuroiwa R, Fujiwara J, Shimoda M, Shinomiya N: Serum levels of Th2 chemokines, CCL17, CCL22, and CCL27, were the important markers of severity in infantile atopic dermatitis. Pediatr Allergy Immunol 2008;19: 605–613.
43 Nakayama T, Fujisawa R, Yamada H, et al: Inducible expression of a CC chemokine liver- and activation-regulated chemokine (LARC)/macrophage inflammatory protein (MIP)-3 alpha/CCL20 by epidermal keratinocytes and its role in atopic dermatitis. Int Immunol 2001;13:95–103.
44 Vanbervliet B, Homey B, Durand I, et al: Sequential involvement of CCR2 and CCR6 ligands for immature dendritic cell recruitment: possible role at inflamed epithelial surfaces. Eur J Immunol 2002;32: 231–242.
45 Oyama T, Miura S, Watanabe C, et al: CXCL12 and CCL20 play a significant role in mucosal T-lymphocyte adherence to intestinal microvessels in mice. Microcirculation 2007;14:753–766.
46 Nomura I, Gao B, Boguniewicz M, Darst MA, Travers JB, Leung DY: Distinct patterns of gene expression in the skin lesions of atopic dermatitis and psoriasis: a gene microarray analysis. J Allergy Clin Immunol 2003;112:1195–1202.
47 Schmuth M, Neyer S, Rainer C, et al: Expression of the C-C chemokine MIP-3 alpha/CCL20 in human epidermis with impaired permeability barrier function. Exp Dermatol 2002;11:135–142.

48 Schon MP, Zollner TM, Boehncke WH: The molecular basis of lymphocyte recruitment to the skin: clues for pathogenesis and selective therapies of inflammatory disorders. J Invest Dermatol 2003;121: 951–962.
49 Tsutsui H, Yoshimoto T, Hayashi N, Mizutani H, Nakanishi K: Induction of allergic inflammation by interleukin-18 in experimental animal models. Immunol Rev 2004;202:115–138.
50 Yoshimoto T, Tsutsui H, Tominaga K, et al: IL-18, although antiallergic when administered with IL-12, stimulates IL-4 and histamine release by basophils. Proc Natl Acad Sci USA 1999;96: 13962–13966.
51 Yoshimoto T, Mizutani H, Tsutsui H, et al: IL-18 induction of IgE: dependence on CD4+ T cells, IL-4 and STAT6. Nat Immunol 2000;1:132–137.
52 Omoto Y, Tokime K, Yamanaka K, et al: Human mast cell chymase cleaves pro-IL-18 and generates a novel and biologically active IL-18 fragment. J Immunol 2006;177:8315–8319.
53 Mihm MC Jr, Soter NA, Dvorak HF, Austen KF: The structure of normal skin and the morphology of atopic eczema. J Invest Dermatol 1976;67:305–312.
54 Omoto Y, Yamanaka K, Tokime K, et al: Granzyme B is a novel interleukin-18 converting enzyme. J Dermatol Sci 2010;59:129–135.
55 Nakanishi K, Tsutsui H, Yoshimoto T: Importance of IL-18-induced super Th1 cells for the development of allergic inflammation. Allergol Int 2010;59: 137–141.
56 Hamasaki T, Hashiguchi S, Ito Y, et al: Human anti-human IL-18 antibody recognizing the IL-18-binding site 3 with IL-18 signaling blocking activity. J Biochem 2005;138:433–442.
57 Howell MD, Boguniewicz M, Pastore S, et al: Mechanism of HBD-3 deficiency in atopic dermatitis. Clin Immunol 2006;121:332–338.
58 Miller LS, O'Connell RM, Gutierrez MA, et al: MyD88 mediates neutrophil recruitment initiated by IL-1R but not TLR2 activation in immunity against *Staphylococcus aureus*. Immunity 2006;24: 79–91.
59 Terada M, Tsutsui H, Imai Y, et al: Contribution of IL-18 to atopic-dermatitis-like skin inflammation induced by *Staphylococcus aureus* product in mice. Proc Natl Acad Sci USA 2006;103:8816–8821.
60 Akdis CA, Akdis M: Mechanisms and treatment of allergic disease in the big picture of regulatory T cells. J Allergy Clin Immunol 2009;123:735–746, quiz 47–48.
61 Toda M, Leung DY, Molet S, et al: Polarized in vivo expression of IL-11 and IL-17 between acute and chronic skin lesions. J Allergy Clin Immunol 2003; 111:875–881.
62 Guttman-Yassky E, Lowes MA, Fuentes-Duculan J, et al: Low expression of the IL-23/Th17 pathway in atopic dermatitis compared to psoriasis. J Immunol 2008;181:7420–7427.
63 Boniface K, Diveu C, Morel F, et al: Oncostatin M secreted by skin infiltrating T lymphocytes is a potent keratinocyte activator involved in skin inflammation. J Immunol 2007;178:4615–4622.
64 Nograles KE, Zaba LC, Shemer A, et al: IL-22-producing 'T22' T cells account for upregulated IL-22 in atopic dermatitis despite reduced IL-17-producing TH17 T cells. J Allergy Clin Immunol 2009;123:1244–1252.
65 Yamanaka K, Yuta A, Kakeda M, et al: Induction of IL-10-producing regulatory T cells with TCR diversity by epitope-specific immunotherapy in pollinosis. J Allergy Clin Immunol 2009;124: 842–845.
66 Szegedi A, Barath S, Nagy G, et al: Regulatory T cells in atopic dermatitis: epidermal dendritic cell clusters may contribute to their local expansion. Br J Dermatol 2009;160:984–993.
67 Yamanaka K, Tanaka M, Tsutsui H, et al: Skin-specific caspase-1-transgenic mice show cutaneous apoptosis and pre-endotoxin shock condition with a high serum level of IL-18. J Immunol 2000;165: 997–1003.
68 Kitagawa H, Yamanaka K, Kakeda M, et al: *Propionibacterium acnes* vaccination induces regulatory T cells and Th1 immune responses and improves mouse atopic dermatitis. Exp Dermatol, in press.
69 Mori H, Yamanaka K, Matsuo K, Kurokawa I, Yasutomi Y, Mizutani H: Administration of Ag85B showed therapeutic effects to Th2-type cytokine-mediated acute phase atopic dermatitis by inducing regulatory T cells. Arch Dermatol Res 2009;301: 151–157.
70 Tokura Y: Extrinsic and intrinsic types of atopic dermatitis. J Dermatol Sci 2010;58:1–7.
71 Phipps S, Flood-Page P, Menzies-Gow A, Ong YE, Kay AB: Intravenous anti-IL-5 monoclonal antibody reduces eosinophils and tenascin deposition in allergen-challenged human atopic skin. J Invest Dermatol 2004;122:1406–1412.
72 Oldhoff JM, Darsow U, Werfel T, et al: No effect of anti-interleukin-5 therapy (mepolizumab) on the atopy patch test in atopic dermatitis patients. Int Arch Allergy Immunol 2006;141:290–294.
73 Oldhoff JM, Darsow U, Werfel T, et al: Anti-IL-5 recombinant humanized monoclonal antibody (mepolizumab) for the treatment of atopic dermatitis. Allergy 2005;60:693–696

74 Simon D, Wittwer J, Kostylina G, Buettiker U, Simon HU, Yawalkar N: Alefacept (lymphocyte function-associated molecule 3/IgG fusion protein) treatment for atopic eczema. J Allergy Clin Immunol 2008;122:423–424.

75 Moul DK, Routhouska SB, Robinson MR, Korman NJ: Alefacept for moderate to severe atopic dermatitis: a pilot study in adults. J Am Acad Dermatol 2008;58:984–989.

76 Takiguchi R, Tofte S, Simpson B, et al: Efalizumab for severe atopic dermatitis: a pilot study in adults. J Am Acad Dermatol 2007;56:222–227.

77 Simon D, Hosli S, Kostylina G, Yawalkar N, Simon HU: Anti-CD20 (rituximab) treatment improves atopic eczema. J Allergy Clin Immunol 2008;121:122–128.

78 Kruse N, Tony HP, Sebald W: Conversion of human interleukin-4 into a high affinity antagonist by a single amino acid replacement. EMBO J 1992;11:3237–3244.

79 Kruse N, Shen BJ, Arnold S, Tony HP, Muller T, Sebald W. Two distinct functional sites of human interleukin 4 are identified by variants impaired in either receptor binding or receptor activation. EMBO J 1993;12:5121–5129.

80 Tony HP, Shen BJ, Reusch P, Sebald W: Design of human interleukin-4 antagonists inhibiting interleukin-4-dependent and interleukin-13-dependent responses in T-cells and B-cells with high efficiency. Eur J Biochem 1994;225:659–665.

81 Zurawski SM, Vega F Jr, Huyghe B, Zurawski G: Receptors for interleukin-13 and interleukin-4 are complex and share a novel component that functions in signal transduction. EMBO J 1993;12:2663–2670.

82 Schnarr B, Ezernieks J, Sebald W, Duschl A: IL-4 receptor complexes containing or lacking the gamma C chain are inhibited by an overlapping set of antagonistic IL-4 mutant proteins. Int Immunol 1997;9:861–868.

Kei-ichi Yamanaka
Department of Dermatology
Mie University Graduate School of Medicine
2-174 Edobashi, Tsu, Mie 514-8507 (Japan)
Tel. +81 59 231 5025, Fax +81 59 231 5206, E-Mail yamake@clin.medic.mie-u.ac.jp

Shiohara T (ed): Pathogenesis and Management of Atopic Dermatitis.
Curr Probl Dermatol. Basel, Karger, 2011, vol 41, pp 93–103

Contribution of Interleukin 18 to the Development of Infection-Associated Atopic Dermatitis

Hiroko Tsutsui[a] · Hitoshi Mizutani[c] · Kenji Nakanishi[b,d]

Departments of [a]Microbiology and [b]Immunology and Medical Zoology, Hyogo College of Medicine, Nishinomiya, [c]Department of Dermatology, Mie University Graduate School of Medicine, Tsu, and [d]Collaborative Development of Innovation Seeds, Japan Science and Technology Cooperation, Tokyo, Japan

Abstract

Atopic dermatitis (AD) has diverse etiologies. Some AD patients possess pathologically aberrant allergen-specific Th2 cells and resulting allergen-specific IgE, and exposure to the allergen exacerbates the skin lesions. This might be classified into the Th2-type AD. However, recent clinical studies revealed that the treatment with neutralizing anti-IgE monoclonal antibody does not always protect against AD, but rather has efficacy only in some variants of AD, perhaps Th2-type AD. This implicates that other factors might be involved. Interleukin (IL) 18 is a pleiotropic cytokine involved in both Th1- and Th2-type diseases. Many cell types including keratinocytes and dermal macrophages and dendritic cells are capable of producing IL-18. Our previous studies demonstrate that skin-specific overexpression of biologically active IL-18 causes AD-like skin lesions in mice. Loss of T cells and B cells cannot rescue these mice from AD-like lesions at all. Thus, aberrant IL-18 in the skin seems to be relevant to some types of AD. Furthermore, consecutive, topical application of *Staphylococcus aureus* product induces AD-like lesions in certain mice with a genetically impaired skin barrier. We found substantial efficacy of IL-18 blockade against this AD. Here, we review the recent finding that IL-18 is a possible therapeutic target of certain types of AD.

Atopic dermatitis (AD) was believed to be a single disease simply due to the pathological development of Th2 cells upon exposure to and challenge with allergens. In these decades, however, we found that AD is a syndrome developed by immunologically diverse situations [1]. Nonetheless, it is still to be accepted that both genetic backgrounds and environmental circumstances determine the development of AD. Twin studies have revealed the importance of genetic factors. A cotwin of an affected identical twin (monozygotic twin) has a significantly increased risk of AD compared to the cotwin of an affected fraternal twin (dizygotic twin). Thus, the genetic factors profoundly contribute to the susceptibility to AD [2, 3]. Environmental exposures are the other important factor. Exposure to allergens, such as house dust mite allergen that is a ubiquitous indoor allergen, and to lesional infection with microbes, exemplified by *Staphylococcus aureus*, is clinically well established to be important for induction and/or exacerbation of the disease [4–6]. In this section, we would like to review the molecular and cellular mechanisms underlying *S. aureus* product-induced AD-like skin inflammation in mice, particularly focusing on the involvement of interleukin (IL) 18 and IL-18-involving immune responses.

Preferential Production of Interleukin 18 in Atopic Patients

IL-18 is a proinflammatory cytokine in terms of its potential to induce robust γ-interferon (IFN-γ), particularly in collaboration with IL-12p70 [7]. IL-18 has the opposite feature as a proatopic cytokine as well [1]. IL-18 in combination with IL-2 or IL-3 induces CD4+ T cells, invariant natural killer (NK) T cells, NK cells, mast cells and basophils to produce substantial amounts of IL-13, a proasthmatic cytokine in terms of its potent induction of mucin production, airway hyperresponsiveness and respiratory remodeling [8–12]. Thus, IL-18 exerts biologically distinct actions under strict control of the cytokine milieu.

Serum IL-18 levels of AD patients are higher than those of healthy volunteers and well parallel to disease severity [13, 14]. Furthermore, single-nucleotide polymorphism studies on the promoters of *Il18* revealed that AD patients more frequently possess the polymorphism prone to express *Il18* upon stimulation as compared to healthy volunteers [15]. Thus, IL-18 seems to be involved in or associated with AD.

Innate Type of Atopic Dermatitis in Mice

IL-18 is intracellularly produced as biologically inactive precursor (pro). After being appropriately cleaved, pro-IL-18 becomes active and extracellularly released [16]. Many cell types including keratinocytes produce and store pro-IL-18 in the steady states. Caspase 1 (Casp1) is an authentic intracellular IL-18-processing enzyme [17, 18]. Plausibly, gene-manipulated mice that overexpress *Casp1* under control of a keratin promoter, keratin 14, have considerably high levels of serum IL-18 under specific pathogen-free conditions [19]. These keratinocyte-specific *Casp1* transgenic mice (K14Casp1Tg) are born healthy but show skin alterations with age [20] (table 1). Intriguingly, they frequently and seriously scratch the skin lesion, suggesting pruritus. As they fulfill the criteria of AD, we consider K14Casp1Tg as a mouse model of AD-like skin inflammation. Since the depletion of *Il18* profoundly inhibits the dermatitis in K14Casp1Tg and since K14IL-18Tg, which overexpress the gene encoding biologically active IL-18, display the phenotype similar to K14Casp1Tg, IL-18 is a relevant factor to this AD-like skin lesion [20] (table 1). Moreover, absence of the gene encoding STAT6 that is necessary

Table 1. Innate-type AD-like skin alterations in K14Casp1Tg mice

Genotype	AD score	Serum IL-18 levels ng/ml	Mast cells n/field	Serum IgE μg/ml
K14Casp1Tg	+++	+++	+++	+++
Il18$^{-/-}$K14Casp1Tg	–	–	<10	+
Rag2$^{-/-}$ K14Casp1Tg	+++	+++	+++	ND
WT	–	<0.1	<10	<0.5

The clinical AD score is determined as previously reported; +++ indicates that the AD score is more than 8. Serum IL-18 is measured by ELISA; +++ indicates that serum IL-18 levels are more than 5 ng/ml; + indicates that they are more than 0.1 ng/ml but less than 5 ng/ml. Mast cell numbers per field in the dermis are counted; +++ indicates that the mast cell number is more than 50/field at a magnification of ×50. Serum total IgE is measured by ELISA; +++ indicates that serum IgE levels are more than 5 μg/ml; + indicates that they are more than 0.5 μg/ml but less than 5 μg/ml. ND = Not determined; WT = wild type.

for signaling of IL-4 and IL-13 does not reduce the dermatitis of K14Casp1Tg [20]. Loss of T cells and B cells by the depletion of *Rag2* cannot protect against their dermatitis as well [20] (table 1). Thus, some type of human AD might develop without help from Th2 and IgE responses or even independently of acquired immune responses.

Topical Application of Staphylococcal Product Causes Atopic-Dermatitis-Like Skin Lesions in Mice

It is important to know which stimuli induce release of active IL-18 from keratinocytes. We incubated a murine keratinocyte cell line or primary cultured keratinocytes with various products of *S. aureus* and found that protein A (SpA) has the capacity to induce secretion of active IL-18 [21]. Therefore, we tried to generate a mouse AD model by using SpA.

We generated an SpA-associated AD-like dermatitis model in a limited strain of mouse. NC/Nga mice, which have a genetically impaired skin epithelial barrier, have healthy skin under specific pathogen-free conditions. However, upon exposure to house dust mites, NC/Nga mice, but not BALB/c or C57BL/6 (B6) mice, develop chronic dermatitis with frequent skin scratching [13]. After shaving, we painted the back of NC/Nga mice with a subclinical dose of sodium dodecyl sulfate (SDS) in order to destroy their skin barrier and subsequently with SpA. One week and later after daily application with SDS and subsequent SpA, we could find development of AD-like dermatitis in all the mice [22] (fig. 1e). Levels of IL-18 and histamine in the circulation were substantially increased with time. Eosinophils, neutrophils and mast

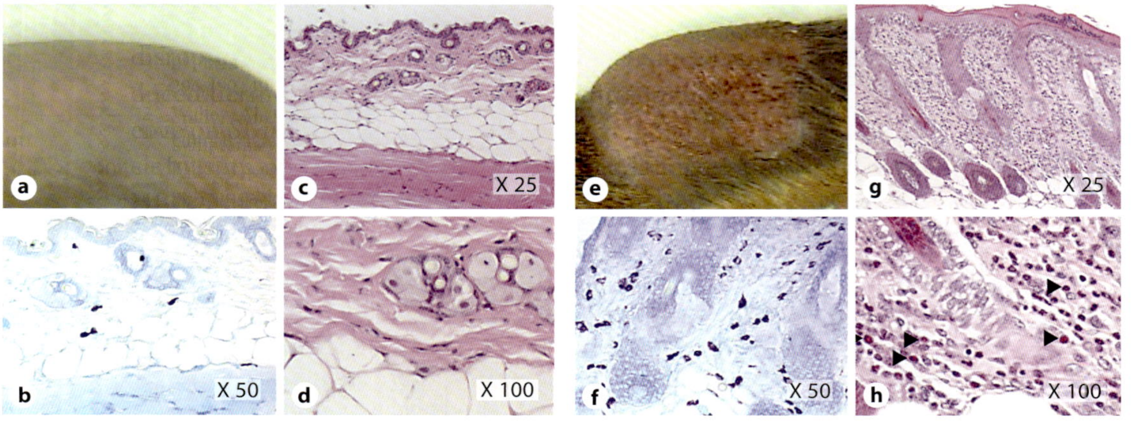

Fig. 1. SDS/SpA-induced AD-like cutaneous lesion. NC/Nga mice were treated with SDS alone (**a–d**) or with SDS and SpA (**e–h**) for 28 consecutive days. Skin sections were stained with hematoxylin and eosin (**c**, **d**, **g**, **h**) or with trypan blue (**b**, **e**). Eosinophils (arrowheads) are stained red, while mast cells are purple.

cells were numerically increased in the dermis of the lesion (fig. 1f, g, h). However, treatment with SDS alone or SpA alone caused little cutaneous alterations [22] (fig. 1a–d). It is intriguing to note that BALB/c mice are susceptible to SDS/SpA-induced dermatitis but with lesser severity than NC/Nga mice [22] (table 2a). B6 mice are completely resistant to SDS/SpA application [22] (table 2a). Thus, like human AD, this *S. aureus*-associated AD develops in hosts with limited genetic backgrounds.

Critical Role for Interleukin 18

As IL-18 is released from SpA-activated keratinocytes and as serum IL-18 levels are elevated in mice with SDS/SpA-induced AD, it is important to know whether and how IL-18 is involved in the development of AD. Treatment with neutralizing anti-IL-18 antibodies can rescue NC/Nga mice from SDS/SpA-induced AD [22] (table 2a). In contrast to $Il18^{+/+}$ BALB/c mice, $Il18^{-/-}$ BALB/c mice are resistant to SDS/SpA treatment [22]. Therefore, IL-18 is important for the development of SDS/SpA-induced AD-like dermatitis.

Super Th1 Cells in Atopic Dermatitis Induced by Sodium Dodecyl Sulfate/Protein A

As previously demonstrated, naïve CD4+ T cells or Th2 cells express little IL-18 receptor [9]. In contrast, Th1 cells express IL-18 receptor on their surface [23].

Table 2. Susceptibility to super Th1 cell differentiation and to SDS/SpA-induced dermatitis

a Susceptibility of different mouse strains

	Mouse strains		
	NC/Nga	BALB/c	B6
Susceptibility to SDS/SpA	++	+	–
IL-18 blockade	effective	effective	ND
Potential to differentiate into super Th1	++	+	–

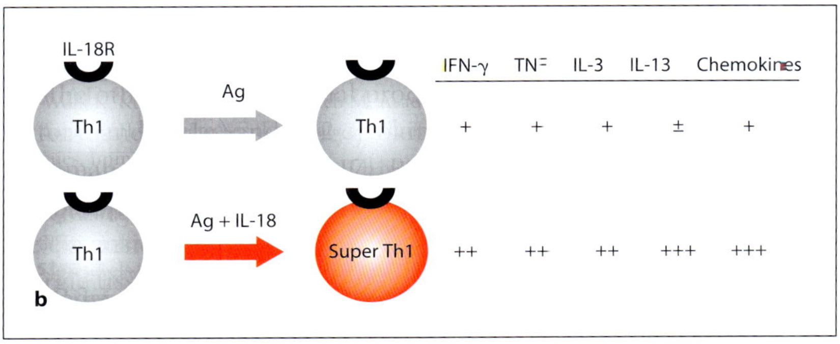

c SDS/SpA-induced dermatitis

Treatment (SDS + SpA)	CD4+ DLN cells
Control	super Th1
Anti-IL-18 antibodies	Th1

a CD4+ draining lymph node (DLN) cells from NC/Nga mice, BALB/c mice or B6 mice were incubated under the Th1 condition, and the cells were activated with immobilized anti-CD3 monoclonal antibody plus IL-18. Super Th1 cell differentiation was determined by the ability to produce the super Th1 cell cytokines. NC/Nga mice have potent ability to differentiate into super Th1 cells, while B6 mice lack this potential. BALB/c mice have intermediate potential. Potentials to differentiate toward super Th1 cells appear to reflect on the susceptibility to SDS/SpA-induced dermatitis. **b** When being activated with antigen (Ag) plus IL-18, Th1 cells produce twice and more (++) the amounts of IFN-γ, tumor necrosis factor (TNF) and IL-3 as compared to those in response to antigen alone. They also produce excessive amounts (+++) of IL-13 and chemokines, such as CCL5 (RANTES). **c** NC/Nga mice are topically applied with SDS + SpA and systemically treated with or without neutralizing anti-IL-18 antibodies (Abs). CD4+ DLN cells are incubated with plate-bound anti-CD3 monoclonal antibody (mAb), and differentiation into super Th1 cells or Th1 cells is determined by their cytokine production profile. Their AD scores are calculated as well. ND = Not determined; IL-18R = IL-18 receptor.

Th1 cells produce IFN-γ and tumor necrosis factor (TNF) in response to antigen (Ag). Expectedly, upon stimulation with Ag + IL-18, Th1 cells produce larger amounts of IFN-γ and TNF. Unexpectedly they begin to produce much larger amounts of IL-13, IL-3 and various chemokines for neutrophils and eosinophils [22, 24] (table 2b). Furthermore, once being stimulated with IL-18 + Ag, Th1 cells differentiate into the subpopulation that steadily produces these cytokines and chemokines in response to Ag alone [22]. As IL-13 and IFN-γ/TNF are powerful proatopic and proinflammatory cytokines, respectively, we designated this subpopulation as super Th1 cells. As super Th1 cells remain to express IL-18 receptor, IL-18 in combination with Ag facilitates their production of super Th1-associated cytokines and chemokines.

We investigated whether CD4+ T cells from draining lymph nodes (DLNs) of mice with SDS/SpA-induced AD have characteristics of super Th1 cells [22]. Two to 3 days after consecutive treatment with SDS/SpA, the skin appears intact. Their CD4+ DLN cells have the characteristics of Th1 cells. They produce IFN-γ and TNF but little IL-4 or IL-13 upon T-cell receptor engagement. Thus, Th1 cells are not harmful at least in the skin [22]. However, after 14 days and later, CD4+ DLN cells turn to produce larger amounts of IFN-γ, TNF, IL-3 and IL-13 [22]. Thus, repeated application of SDS/SpA causes further differentiation of Th1 cells into super Th1 cells. Notably, IL-18 blockade inhibits their development toward super Th1 cells and leave them to be Th1 cells [22] (table 2c), demonstrating IL-18 as an inducer of super Th1 cells. From these observations one can suppose that super Th1 cells, but not Th1 cells, are dangerous enough to trigger the inflammatory diseases and that SpA serves as an IL-18 inducer as well as Ag.

CD4+ DLN cells from NC/Nga mice are preferentially differentiated into super Th1 cells after incubation with Th1 followed by reactivation with T-cell receptor engagement + IL-18 in vitro. In contrast, cells from B6 mice remain Th1 cells under the same super Th1 cell-inducing condition. BALB/c mice have the intermediate potential. Thus, the susceptibility to SDS/SpA-induced dermatitis appears to be at least partly accounted for by the predisposition to super Th1 cells (table 2a).

How do super Th1 cells participate in the development of AD? To investigate this, we examined whether blockade of each super Th1 cytokine prevents AD. Administration of neutralizing anti-IFN-γ monoclonal antibody, anti-TNF antibodies or anti-IL-3 antibodies profoundly protects against AD [22] (table 3; fig. 2). As they are well-known potent proinflammatory cytokines, IFN-γ and TNF are accepted as the key. IL-3 is capable of activating mast cells and powerfully synergizes with IL-18 for mast cell activation. Thus, large amounts of IL-3 produced by super Th1 cells might contribute to the activation of effector mast cells perhaps in collaboration with endogenous IL-18. In contrast to the blockade of these cytokines, *Stat6*$^{-/-}$ NC/Nga mice, lacking signaling of IL-4 and IL-13, comparably suffer from the dermatitis as do STAT6-sufficient NC/Nga mice [22] (table 3; fig. 2). Thus, IL-3, IFN-γ and TNF, but not IL-13, principally participate in the SDS/SpA-induced chronic dermatitis.

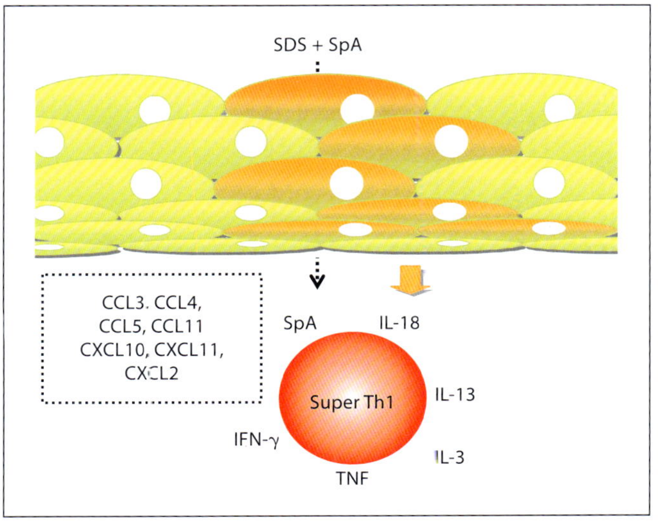

Fig. 2. Cellular and molecular mechanisms of SDS/SpA-induced AD-like skin lesions. After treatment with SDS, the skin barrier is destroyed. Applied SpA might activate keratinocytes to produce IL-18. Dermal dendritic cells might capture SpA and activate naïve T cells in the DLNs. CD4+ DLN cells promptly differentiate into Th1 cells and then super Th1 cells. These super Th1 cells are recruited in the lesional sites and are reactivated with SpA and IL-18 to release robust IFN-γ, TNF, IL-3, IL-13 and various chemokines. In collaboration with IL-18, these cytokines and chemokines, in turn, recruit and activate eosinophils, mast cells and neutrophils, leading to the development of itchy dermatitis. CCL = CC chemokine ligand; CXCL = CXC chemokine ligand.

Table 3. Requirement of IL-18 for super Th1 cell development and SDS/SpA-induced AD

Treatment	AD score
SDS + SpA	
Control	+++
Anti-IFN-γ mAb	–
Anti-TNF Abs	–
Anti-IL-3 Abs	–
Loss of *Stat6*	+++
SDS control	–

NC/Nga mice are treated with neutralizing anti-IFN-γ, anti-TNF or anti-IL-3 monoclonal antibodies, instead of anti-IL-18 antibodies, and their AD scores are calculated. *Stat6*$^{-/-}$ NC/Nga mice and their litter *Stat6*$^{+/-}$ NC/Nga mice are treated with SDS and SpA.

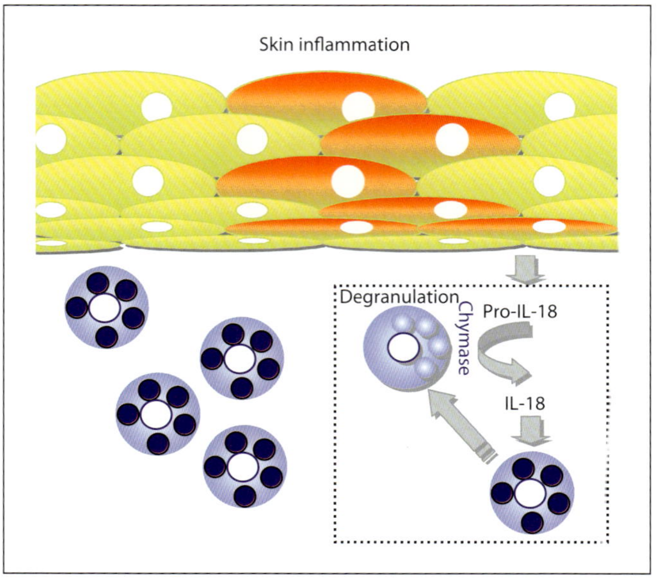

Fig. 3. Cutaneous IL-18 activation circuit between infiltrated mast cells and destroyed keratinocytes. IL-18 activates mast cells to produce IL-13 and degranulate for release of histamine and maybe chymase. Chymase can process pro-IL-18 possibly derived from destroyed keratinocytes of AD lesions. This IL-18-processing circuit might accelerate inflammatory responses in AD lesions.

Possible Acceleration Pathways for Production of Active Interleukin 18 in the Lesion

Recently, we demonstrated that human chymase is capable of cleaving pro-IL-18 into biologically active IL-18 [25]. As the resulting active fragment is different from that of Casp1, the cleavage site of chymase is different from that of Casp1. It is believed that mast cells principally exert their actions as effector cells in the development of AD. After microbial infection, pathogen-associated molecular patterns activate mast cells to produce various proinflammatory cytokines, such as TNF, for host defense. Upon exposure to allergen, allergen-specific IgE-loaded mast cells are strongly activated to release proatopic cytokines/chemokines and chemical mediators, shortly inducing type I allergic outcome. IL-18 can solely activate mast cells to release IL-13 and histamine [11]. Chymase, like histamine, might be released from the IL-18-activated mast cells. Thus, it is plausible that mast cells accumulated in the AD lesion release chymase, which in turn processes pro-IL-18 presumably derived from destroyed keratinocytes. This might serve as a positive circuit for IL-18 accumulation, which eventually results in the acceleration of SDS/SpA-induced AD (fig. 3).

Patients with AD sometimes suffer from reactivation of latent herpes viruses such as herpes simplex virus [5]. Upon recognition of virus-infected target cells, NK cells release perforin to make micropores on the target cells through which granzyme B is inserted into the cytosol. This is also the case for virus-specific cytotoxic T lymphocytes. Then, granzyme B cleaves DNA, eventually resulting in apoptotic death of the target cells. Very recently, we demonstrated that human granzyme B, a cysteine protease, has potential to process pro-IL-18 as well [26] (fig. 4). This may

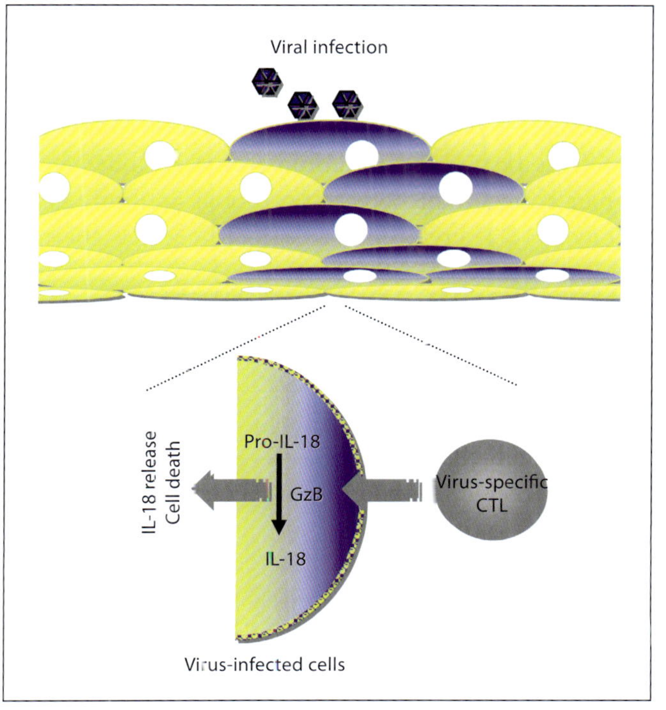

Fig. 4. Involvement of cytotoxic T lymphocytes (CTLs) for IL-18 release. After recognition of virus-infected keratinocytes, cytotoxic T lymphocytes release perforin to make a small pore in the keratinocytes, through which they insert granzyme B (GzB), eventually leading to apoptotic cell death. Granyzme B can process pro-IL-18 stored in the target keratinocytes, resulting in the accumulation of biologically active IL-18. IL-18 might upregulate the cutaneous inflammatory responses.

occur in the skin of AD patients. Keratinocytes infected with herpes simplex virus might be attacked by perforin/granzyme B of virus-specific cytotoxic T lymphocytes or perhaps of NK cells. In these keratinocytes, stored pro-IL-18 might be processed to biologically active IL-18, and simultaneously the death process progresses, which converges on the accumulation of IL-18 in the lesion. This IL-18 may accelerate AD (fig. 4).

Closing Remarks

We established an SpA-induced bronchial asthma model, in which IL-18 is important as well [27]. Mice are immunized with SpA in Freund's complete adjuvant and then with Freund's incomplete adjuvant, which gives rise to SpA-specific Th1 cells. After intranasal challenge with SpA, SpA-immunized mice, but not naïve mice, show asthmatic disorders in terms of airway hypersensitivity, peribronchial eosinophilic inflammation and numerical increase in eosinophils in bronchoalveolar lavage fluid. CD4+ DLN cells from mice immunized with SpA alone, and SpA-immunized and SpA-challenged asthma mice possess Th1 cells and super Th1 cells, respectively. IL-18 blockade prevents the individual signs of SpA-induced asthma. Naïve mice receiving CD4+ DLN cells from SpA-immunized mice suffer from asthma after intranasal challenge with SpA. Thus, SpA might be involved in microbial infection-associated allergic alterations.

Immunodeficient mice transfected with SpA-stimulated human peripheral blood mononuclear cells undergo bronchial inflammation after intranasal challenge with SpA. This respiratory inflammation is inhibited by pretreatment with neutralizing human anti-human IL-18 monoclonal antibody generated by a new immunotechnology [28]. Therefore, IL-18 might be a new therapeutic target for infectious-type atopic diseases.

References

1 Tsutsui H, Yoshimoto T, Hayashi N, Mizutani H, Nakanishi K: Induction of allergic inflammation by interleukin-18 in experimental animal models. Immunol Rev 2004;202:115–138.

2 Feijen M, Gerritsen J, Postma DS: Genetics of allergic disease. Br Med Bull 2000;56:894–907.

3 Van Beijsterveldt CEM, Boomsma DI: Genetics of parentally reported asthma, eczema and rhinitis in 5-year-old twins. Eur Respir J 2007;29:516–521.

4 Hammad H, Chieppa M, Perros F, Willart MA, Germain RN, lambrecht BN: House dust mite allergen induces asthma via Toll-like receptor 4 triggering of airway structural cells. Nat Med 2009;15: 410–416.

5 Leung DY, Bieber T: Atopic dermatitis. Lancet 2003; 361:151–160.

6 Leung DY, Boguniewicz M, Howell MD, Nomura I, Hamid QA: New insights into atopic dermatitis. J Clin Invest 2004;113:651–657.

7 Nakanishi K, Yoshimoto T, Tsutsui H, Okamura H: Interleukin-18 regulates both Th1 and Th2 responses. Annu Rev Immunol 2001;19:423–474.

8 Hoshino T, Wiltrout RH, Young HA: IL-18 is a potent coinducer of IL-13 in NK and T cells: a new potential role for IL-18 in modulating the immune response. J Immunol 1999;162:5070–5077.

9 Yoshimoto T, Min B, Sugimoto T, Hayashi N, Ishikawa Y, Sasaki Y, et al: Nonredundant roles for CD1d-restricted natural killer T cells and conventional CD4+ T cells in the induction of immunoglobulin E antibodies in response to interleukin 18 treatment of mice. J Exp Med 2003;197:997–1005.

10 Wynn TA: IL-13 effector functions. Annu Rev Immunol 2003;21:425–456.

11 Yoshimoto T, Tsutsui H, Tominaga K, Hoshino K, Okamura H, Akira S, et al: IL-18, although antiallergic when administered with IL-12, stimulates IL-4 and histamine release by basophils. Proc Natl Acad Sci USA 1999;96:13962–13966.

12 Sasaki Y, Yoshimoto T, Maruyama H, Tegoshi T, Ohta N, Arizono N, et al: IL-18 with IL-2 protects against *Strongyloides venezuelensis* infection by activating mucosal mast cell-dependent type 2 innate immunity. J Exp Med 2005;202:607–616.

13 Tanaka T, Tsutsui H, Yoshimoto T, Kotani M, Matsumoto M, Fujita A, et al: Interleukin-18 is elevated in the sera from patients with atopic dermatitis and from atopic dermatitis model mice, NC/Nga. Int Arch Allergy Immunol 2001;125: 236–240.

14 Ohnishi H, Kato Z, Watanabe M, Fukutomi O, Inoue R, Teramoto T, et al: Interleukin 18 is associated with the severity of atopic dermatitis. Allergol Int 2003;52:123–130.

15 Novak N, Kruse S, Potreck J, Maintz L, Jenneck C, Weidinger S, et al: Single nucleotide polymorphisms of the IL18 gene are associated with atopic eczema. J Allergy Clin Immunol 2005;115: 828–833.

16 Okamura H, Tsutsui H, Komatsu T, Yutsudo M, Hakura A, Tanimoto T, et al: Cloning of a new cytokine that induces IFN-gamma production by T cells. Nature 1995;378:88–91.

17 Gu Y, Kuida K, Tsutsui H, Ku G, Hsiao K, Fleming MA, et al: Activation of interferon-A inducing factor mediated by interleukin-1 converting enzyme. Science 1997;275:206–209.

18 Ghayur T, Banerjee S, Hugunin M, Butler D, Herzog L, Carter A, et al: Caspase-1 processes IFN-γ-inducing factor and regulates LPS-induced IFN-γ production. Nature 1997;386:619–623.

19 Yamanaka K, Tanaka M, Tsutsui H, Kupper TS, Asahi K, Okamura H, et al: Skin-specific caspase-1 transgenic mice show cutaneous apoptosis and pre-endotoxin shock condition with a high serum level of IL-18. J Immunol 2000;165:997–1003.

20 Konishi H, Tsutsui H, Murakami T, Yumikura-Futatsugi S, Yamanaka K, Tanaka M, et al: IL-18 contributes to the spontaneous development of atopic dermatitis-like inflammatory skin lesion independently of IgE/stat6 under specific pathogen-free conditions. Proc Natl Acad Sci USA 2002;99:11340–11345.
21 Nakano H, Tsutsui H, Terada M, Yasuda K, Matsui K, Yumikura-Futatsugi S, et al: Persistent secretion of IL-18 in the skin contributes to IgE response in mice. Int Immunol 2003;15:611–621.
22 Terada M, Tsutsui H, Imai Y, Yasuda K, Mizutani H, Yamanishi K, et al: Contribution of IL-18 to atopic-dermatitis-like skin inflammation induced by *Staphylococcus aureus* product in mice. Proc Natl Acad Sci USA 2006;103:8816–8821.
23 Yoshimoto T, Takeda K, Tanaka T, Ohkusu K, Kashiwamura S, Okamura H, et al: IL-12 up-regulates IL-18 receptor expression on T cells, Th1 cells, and B cells: synergism with IL-18 for IFN-gamma production. J Immunol 1998;161:3400–3407.
24 Sugimoto T, Ishikawa Y, Yoshimoto T, Hayashi N, Fujimoto J, Nakanishi K: Interleukin 18 acts on memory T helper cells type 1 to induce airway inflammation and hyperresponsiveness in a naive host mouse. J Exp Med 2004;199:535–545.
25 Omoto Y, Tokime K, Yamanaka K, Habe K, Morioka T, Kurokawa I, et al: Human mast cell chymase cleaves pro-IL-18 and generates a novel and biologically active IL-18 fragment. J Immunol 2006;177:8315–8319.
26 Omoto Y, Yamanaka K, Tokime K, Kitano S, Kakeda M, Akeda T, et al: Granzyme B is a novel interleukin-18 converting enzyme. J Dermatol Sci 2010;59:129–135.
27 Kuroda-Morimoto M, Tanaka H, Hayashi N, Nakahira M, Imai Y, Imamura M, et al: Contribution of IL-18 to eosinophilic airway inflammation induced by immunization and challenge with *Staphylococcus aureus* proteins. Int Immunol 2010;22:561–570.
28 Hamasaki T, Hashiguchi S, Ito Y, Kato Z, Nakanishi K, Nakashima T, et al: Human anti-human IL-18 antibody recognizing the IL-18-binding site 3 with IL-18 signaling blocking activity. J Biochem 2005;138:433–442.

Kenji Nakanishi
President Hyogo College of Medicine
1-1, Mukogawa-cho
Nishinomiya 663-8501 (Japan)
Tel. +81 798 45 6151, Fax +81 798 40 5423, E-Mail nakaken@hyo-med.ac.jp

Shiohara T (ed): Pathogenesis and Management of Atopic Dermatitis.
Curr Probl Dermatol. Basel, Karger, 2011, vol 41, pp 104–111

Innate Immunity in Atopic Dermatitis

S. Mrabet-Dahbi · M. Maurer

Department of Dermatology and Allergy, Allergiezentrum Charité/European Centre for Allergy Research Foundation, Charité-Universitätsmedizin, Berlin, Germany

Abstract

One of the most important functions of the skin is to provide protection from infectious pathogens. This is achieved by two complex and complementary powerful strategies, namely by preventing pathogen invasion and by raising innate and/or adaptive immune responses following infection. Most pathogens cannot penetrate healthy skin, and the vast majority of skin infections, thus, results from breaches of cutaneous integrity (skin wounds, arthropod bites, barrier function defects). Cutaneous infections, in turn, are controlled primarily by a functioning skin innate immune system and efficient host defence responses. Patients with atopic dermatitis (AD) exhibit both, impaired skin barrier function and defects in skin innate immunity. As a result, AD patients frequently develop skin infections which contribute to the pathogenesis and the course of their chronic inflammatory skin condition. Here, we discuss how skin innate immunity works in healthy individuals and how skin innate immunity is impaired in patients with AD.

How Does Cutaneous Innate Immunity Work?

The skin protects us from pathogens by providing physical/anatomical barriers and by activating its innate immune system, namely cellular sentinels with cognate receptors and chemical/secretory defence molecules.

The Physical/Anatomical Barrier

The physical/anatomical barriers of the skin include the stratum corneum of the epidermis with several layers of cornified keratinocytes embedded in a lipid matrix of water-retaining ceramides, cholesterol and sphingosines with direct antibacterial activities, thus preventing pathogen entry [1]. Historically, keratinocyte functions were believed to be limited to maintaining the structure of the epidermis and to providing a physical barrier to various exogenous micro-organisms. Today, it is well established that keratinocytes can also actively participate in bacterial clearance by sensing microbes and by subsequently releasing antimicrobial peptides [2]. Additional important cutaneous physical/anatomical barrier mechanisms include sweat and sebum production as well as body temperature and acidic pH [3].

Cellular Sentinels of the Cutaneous Innate Immune System

The cellular compartment of the cutaneous innate immune system, in addition to keratinocytes, consists of many rapidly mobilized cells such as neutrophils, dendritic cells, macrophages, mast cells and eosinophils [4]. All of them can recognize structurally conserved motifs of bacteria, viruses, parasites and fungi by so-called pattern recognition receptors (PRRs). These receptors allow the cutaneous innate immune system to rapidly detect potential danger and to raise protective responses. The recognition of pathogen-associated molecular patterns by PRRs initiates phagocytosis, and the secretion of antimicrobial peptides and inflammatory mediators, which finally results in the killing of the invading pathogen(s) [5].

Innate Immune Receptors

The best-known PRRs are the Toll-like receptors (TLRs), a family of currently 11 members in humans [6]. TLRs are located on the cell surface or in intracellular compartments [6]. Structurally, they are transmembrane proteins with an extracellular leucine-rich repeat domain needed for pathogen recognition and a cytoplasmic signaling part, which resembles the interleukin (IL) 1 receptor, called TIR [7]. Ligand binding induces a common signal transduction pathway mainly based on the interaction between the adaptor molecule MyD88 and TIR which in turn results in the activation of IRAK and subsequent oligomerization of TRAF6 [8]. Followed by activation of downstream kinases, this MyD88-IRAK-TRAF pathway leads to the activation of MAP kinases and the transcription factor NF-κB, finally culminating in the expression of pro-inflammatory mediators [9, 10]. Pathogen-associated molecular patterns originating from different pathogens can be distinguished by various TLR combinations, each of them providing a specific immune response [11].

Soon after the discovery of the TLRs it became clear that these PRRs could not account for full host protection due to their inability to sense intracellular pathogens. Indeed subsequent studies identified further cytosolic PRRs belonging to the Nod-like receptor (NLR) family, and bio-informatic analyses revealed the existence of more than 20 *NLR* genes in the human genome [12]. Based on the structure of the N-terminal domains, NLRs can be classified into 3 subgroups also referred to as CARD-containing NODs, PYD-containing NALPs, or BIR-containing NAIPs. While the leucine-rich repeat domain at the C terminus is responsible for pathogen recognition, exposition of the protein-protein interaction site at the N terminus mediates the recruitment and activation of CARD- and PYD-containing effector molecules [13]. This ends in the activation of the NF-κB and MAP kinase pathways which together upregulate the expression of pro-inflammatory molecules. Further innate immune receptors are the mannose receptors (CD206) [14] and the retinoid acid-inducible gene I-like receptors [15].

Secretory Effector Molecules of the Cutaneous Innate Immune System: Cytokines and Antimicrobial Peptides

TLR activation ends in the release of effector molecules, mainly pro-inflammatory cytokines and antimicrobial peptides. Two cytokines that are of special interest in this context are tumour necrosis factor (TNF) and IL-1, which trigger adhesion molecule expression on endothelial cells, thereby contributing to the recruitment of phagocytic cells to the sites of infection [16, 17]. In addition, the so-called novel cytokines IL-18 and IL-17 have recently been shown to be particularly relevant for pathogen clearance. Here, IL-18 is functionally similar to IL-12 in that it activates natural killer cells and induces IL-1 and TNF secretion [18]. In contrast, IL-17 potentiates neutrophilic cytotoxicity and phagocytosis [19]. Mice infected by extracellular bacterial pathogens, for example *Klebsiella pneumoniae* [19], mount a Th17 response, and disruption of IL-17 signalling increases susceptibility in this model.

Among the group of antimicrobial peptides, β-defensin 3 and the cathelicidin CAP18/LL-37, the only human antimicrobial peptide within the cathelicidin gene family, are potent, broad-spectrum antibiotics killing both Gram-positive and Gram-negative bacteria, and the yeast *Candida albicans* by pore formation and membrane permeabilization [20]. Also, antimicrobial peptides function as chemo-attractants for neutrophils, monocytes and mast cells, which at the same time are the source for these natural antibiotics next to the main producers, epithelial cells [20]. Their expression also involves NF-κB and can be further increased by the cytokines TNF, IL-1 or γ-interferon.

Regulatory Elements of the Cutaneous Innate Immune System

The skin innate immune system must discriminate pathogens from commensals, i.e. pathogens must be detected and controlled while commensal bacteria such as *Propionibacterium acnes*, *Staphylococcus epidermidis*, *Micrococcus luteus* and *Malassezia furfur* are tolerated and ignored. Factors that contribute to this include the anatomical localization of TLRs. Keratinocyte TLRs are expressed at the basal side which is not exposed to commensals living on the surface of the skin. Therefore, a pro-inflammatory response would only occur during destructive or invasive infections once the stratum corneum has been breached [4]. Unwanted responses against commensals are also avoided by simultaneous usage of multiple TLRs by the host to detect numerous features on a microbe [11]. As a consequence, effective immune responses occur only when specific combinations of antigens are identified and all of the involved receptors are present or functional. For example, keratinocyte activation by *Mycobacterium tuberculosis* can be suppressed by blocking of either TLR2 or TLR4 demonstrating the need of simultaneous TLR cooperation in this context [21]. In contrast to this, keratinocyte activation by *S. aureus*-derived peptidoglycan is restricted to TLR2 engagement, the principal receptor for Gram-positive bacteria, and remains unaffected by TLR4 blockage [22]. Host inactivity to commensals can also result from tolerance, a state of acquired functional unresponsiveness. Tolerance can be achieved by prolonged exposure to pathogen-associated molecular patterns which either results in decreased TLR expression or in activation of negative regulators within the TLR-signalling cascade such as TOLLIP, IRAK-M, SOCS or a truncated form of MyD88 (MyD88s) that control inflammatory cytokine production [23–25].

Defects of the Cutaneous Innate Immune System in Atopic Dermatitis

Why is it that atopic dermatitis (AD) patients are highly susceptible to recurrent and persistent bacterial infections? AD patients exhibit major defects in important skin barrier functions. In addition, cutaneous innate immunity in AD patients is impaired on several levels.

Impaired Function of the Physical/Anatomical Barrier

AD patients exhibit several changes in skin barrier functions that predispose them to cutaneous infections: (1) changes in skin pH values toward alkalinity increase transepidermal water loss, bacterial counts and microbial infections [26]; (2) lipid deficiencies (in ceramides and sphingosines) reduce antimicrobial activity and simultaneously increase transepidermal water loss contributing to dryness and cracked skin [27]; pruritus and extensive scratching may contribute to these effects as extracellular matrix molecules become exposed and serve as anchors for bacterial adherence; (3) AD is associated with loss-of-function mutations in the skin structural protein filaggrin [28–31], which leads to impaired aggregation of keratin filaments during the terminal differentiation of keratinocytes and consequently to improper formation of the physical barrier [32, 33]. Th2 cytokines were found to inhibit the S100 calcium-binding protein A11 (S100/A11) thereby downregulating skin filaggrin expression, which may be particularly relevant for AD patients who do not carry filaggrin mutations [34, 35].

Defects of the Cellular Compartment

Since patients with psoriasis, who also show skin barrier defects, are much more resistant to bacterial infections than AD patients, the increase in microbial infections in atopic patients must have other, additional reasons, which are likely to include abnormalities within the cellular compartment of the skin immune system. For example, natural killer cells and $\gamma\delta$+ T cells of atopic patients reportedly preferentially undergo apoptosis on cell-to-cell contact with activated monocytes [36], thereby affecting the recognition of malignant and virus-infected cells and increasing the susceptibility to viral infections. Moreover, AD skin has been shown to exhibit decreased levels of the neutrophil chemo-attractant IL-8 [37].

Consequences of Altered Expression or Mutations of the Major Innate Immune Receptor TLR2

Inadequate pathogen recognition, either because of marginal expression or aberrant signal transduction of PRRs, also contributes to impaired host defence in AD. TLR2, which is critical for the detection and control of Gram-positive bacteria and fungi [38], is constitutively expressed in healthy skin. In contrast, atopic individuals exhibit defective TLR2-mediated, but not TLR4-mediated, pro-inflammatory cytokine responses (TNF and IL-1) of monocytes and keratinocytes [39, 40].

Single-nucleotide polymorphisms of this receptor may additionally impair pathogen detection and control. The heterozygous TLR2 R753Q mutation, located in the TIR domain and initially linked to enhanced *S. aureus* infection [41], is frequently found in AD patients exhibiting severe disease, markedly elevated IgE and staphylococcal colonization in selected cases [42]. Monocytes from these subjects reportedly produce dramatically less IL-8 as compared to monocytes from patients lacking this mutation [43].

Defects within the Regulatory Compartment and the Secretory Effector Molecules

Recently, a mutation in the distal promoter region of the ST2 gene, which encodes an inhibitor of TLR activation, has been linked to AD severity [44]. The TOLLIP protein represents another negative regulator [45] which specifically controls the magnitude of TLR-induced inflammatory cytokine production upon endotoxin exposure [46]. Here, several mutations have been identified, 2 of them in the coding region (Pro139Pro in exon 4 and Ala222Ser in exon 6) and 4 non-coding mutations where only the promoter polymorphism (–526 C/G) showed a modest association with AD [47]. The precise role and relevance of these defects in the skin immune system of atopic individuals for innate immune responses to pathogens remains to be investigated.

AD is associated with an impaired expression of several effector molecules of antibacterial host defence responses. One of these mediators affected is IL-12, the key cytokine for Th1 differentiation, which is markedly reduced in AD, thus impairing the establishment of protective Th1 immunity [48]. More importantly, AD patients are deficient in the antimicrobial peptides β-defensin 2 and β-defensin 3 as compared to normal as well as psoriatic individuals, a finding which has been linked to Th2- but not Th1-driven skin disorders [49]. Indeed, the combination of IL-4 and IL-13 can significantly suppress antimicrobial peptide production by keratinocytes. Lack of these 'natural antibiotics' is not an acquired but rather a constitutive defect since neutralizing Th2 cytokines given to eczematous explants restored β-defensin 3 expression in AD [50]. In addition, neutralization of IL-4 and IL-13 in AD skin augmented LL-37 and thus limited viral infections [51].

References

1 Elias PM: Stratum corneum defensive functions: an integrated view. J Invest Dermatol 2005;125: 183–200.
2 Barker JN, Mitra RS, Griffiths CE, Dixit VM, Nickoloff BJ: Keratinocytes as initiators of inflammation. Lancet 1991;337:211–214.
3 Goodarzi H, Trowbridge J, Gallo RL: Innate immunity: a cutaneous perspective. Clin Rev Allergy Immunol 2007;33:15–26.
4 Pivarcsi A, Kemény L, Dobozy A: Innate immune functions of the keratinocytes: a review. Acta Microbiol Immunol Hung 2004;51:303–310.
5 Janeway CA Jr, Medzhitov R: Innate immune recognition. Annu Rev Immunol 2002;20:197–216.
6 Takeda K, Kaisho T, Akira S: Toll-like receptors. Annu Rev Immunol 2003;21:335–76.
7 Beutler B, Hoebe K, Du X, Ulevitch RJ: How we detect microbes and respond to them: the Toll-like receptors and their transducers. J Leukoc Biol 2003; 74:479–485.
8 Medzhitov R, Preston-Hurlburt P, Kopp E, Stadlen A, Chen C, Ghosh S, Janeway CA Jr: MyD88 is an adaptor protein in the hToll/IL-1 receptor family signalling pathways. Mol Cell 1998;2:253–258.
9 Muzio M, Natoli G, Saccani S, Levrero M, Mantovani A: The human Toll signaling pathway: divergence of nuclear factor kappaB and JNK/SAPK activation upstream of tumor necrosis factor receptor-associated factor 6 (TRAF6). J Exp Med 1998;187: 2097–2101.
10 Baud V, Liu ZG, Bennett B, Suzuki N, Xia Y, Karin M: Signaling by proinflammatory cytokines: oligomerization of TRAF2 and TRAF6 is sufficient for JNK and IKK activation and target gene induction via an amino-terminal effector domain. Genes Dev 1999;13:1297–1308.
11 Ozinsky A, Underhill DM, Fontenot JD, Hajjar AM, Smith KD, Wilson CB, Schroeder L, Aderem A: The repertoire for pattern recognition of pathogens by the innate immune system is defined by cooperation between Toll-like receptors. Proc Natl Acad Sci USA 2000;97:13766–13771.
12 Harton JA, Linhoff MW, Zhang J, Ting JP: Cutting edge: CATERPILLER – a large family of mammalian genes containing CARD, pyrin, nucleotide-binding, and leucine-rich repeat domains. J Immunol 2002;169:4088–4093.
13 Martinon F, Tschopp J: NLRs join TLRs as innate sensors of pathogens. Trends Immunol 2005;26: 447–454.
14 Wollenberg A, Mommaas M, Oppel T, Schottdorf EM, Günther S, Moderer M: Expression and function of the mannose receptor CD206 on epidermal dendritic cells in inflammatory skin diseases. J Invest Dermatol 2002;118:327–334.
15 Takeuchi O, Akira S: Recognition of viruses by innate immunity. Immunol Rev 2007;220: 214–224.
16 Lidington EA, McCormack AM, Yacoub MH, Rose ML: The effects of monocytes on the transendothelial migration of T lymphocytes. Immunology 1998;94:221–227.
17 Labow M, Shuster D, Zetterstrom M, Nunes P, Terry R, Cullinan EB, Bartfai T, Solorzano C, Moldawer LL, Chizzonite R, McIntyre KW: Absence of IL-1 signaling and reduced inflammatory response in IL-1 type I receptor-deficient mice. J Immunol 1997; 159:2452–2461.
18 Dinarello CA: IL-18: a Th1-inducing, proinflammatory cytokine and new member of the IL-1 family. J Allergy Clin Immunol 1999;103:11–24.

19 Ye P, Rodriguez FH, Kanaly S, Stocking KL, Schurr J, Schwarzenberger P, Oliver P, Huang W, Zhang P, Zhang J, Shellito JE, Bagby GJ, Nelson S, Charrier K, Peschon JJ, Kolls JK: Requirement of interleukin 17 receptor signaling for lung CXC chemokine and granulocyte colony-stimulating factor expression, neutrophil recruitment, and host defense. J Exp Med 2001;194:519–527.
20 Izadpanah A, Gallo RL: Antimicrobial peptides. J Am Acad Dermatol 2005;52:381–392.
21 Pivarcsi A, Bodai L, Réthi B, Kenderessy-Szabó A, Koreck A, Széll M, Beer Z, Bata-Csörgoo Z, Magócsi M, Rajnavölgyi E, Dobozy A, Kemény L: Expression and function of Toll-like receptors 2 and 4 in human keratinocytes. Int Immunol 2003;15:721–730.
22 Mempel M, Voelcker V, Köllisch G, Plank C, Rad R, Gerhard M, Schnopp C, Fraunberger P, Walli AK, Ring J, Abeck D, Ollert M: Toll-like receptor expression in human keratinocytes: nuclear factor kappaB controlled gene activation by *Staphylococcus aureus* is Toll-like receptor 2 but not Toll-like receptor 4 or platelet activating factor receptor dependent. J Invest Dermatol 2003;121:1389–1396.
23 Strober W: Epithelial cells pay a Toll for protection. Nat Med 2004;10:898–900.
24 Fukao T, Koyasu S: PI3K and negative regulation of TLR signaling. Trends Immunol 2003;24:358–363.
25 Otte JM, Cario E, Podolsky DK: Mechanisms of cross hyporesponsiveness to Toll-like receptor bacterial ligands in intestinal epithelial cells. Gastroenterology 2004;126:1054–1070.
26 Rippke F, Schreiner V, Doering T, Maibach HI: Stratum corneum pH in atopic dermatitis: impact on skin barrier function and colonization with *Staphylococcus aureus*. Am J Clin Dermatol 2004;5: 217–223.
27 Arikawa J, Ishibashi M, Kawashima M, Takagi Y, Ichikawa Y, Imokawa G: Decreased levels of sphingosine, a natural antimicrobial agent, may be associated with vulnerability of the stratum corneum from patients with atopic dermatitis to colonization by *Staphylococcus aureus*. J Invest Dermatol 2002; 119:433–439.
28 Palmer CN, Irvine AD, Terron-Kwiatkowski A, Zhao Y, Liao H, Lee SP, Goudie DR, Sandilands A, Campbell LE, Smith FJ, O'Regan GM, Watson RM, Cecil JE, Bale SJ, Compton JG, Di Giovanna JJ, Fleckman P, Lewis-Jones S, Arseculeratne G, Sergeant A, Munro CS, El Houate B, McElreavey K, Halkjaer LB, Bisgaard H, Mukhopadhyay S, McLean WH: Common loss-of-function variants of the epidermal barrier protein filaggrin are a major predisposing factor for atopic dermatitis. Nat Genet 2006;38:441–446.
29 Henderson J, Northstone K, Lee SP, Liao H, Zhao Y, Pembrey M, Mukhopadhyay S, Smith GD, Palmer CN, McLean WH, Irvine AD: The burden of disease associated with filaggrin mutations: a population-based, longitudinal birth cohort study. J Allergy Clin Immunol 2008;121:872–877.
30 Brown SJ, Relton CL, Liao H, Zhao Y, Sandilands A, Wilson IJ, Burn J, Reynolds NJ, McLean WH, Cordell HJ: Filaggrin null mutations and childhood atopic eczema: a population-based case-control study. J Allergy Clin Immunol 2008;121:940–946.
31 Rice NE, Patel BD, Lang IA, Kumari M, Frayling TM, Murray A, Melzer D: Filaggrin gene mutations are associated with asthma and eczema in later life. J Allergy Clin Immunol 2008;122:834–836.
32 Mischke D, Korge BP, Marenholz I, Volz A, Ziegler A: Genes encoding structural proteins of epidermal cornification and S100 calcium-binding proteins form a gene complex ('epidermal differentiation complex') on human chromosome 1q21. J Invest Dermatol 1996;106:989–992.
33 Candi E, Schmidt R, Molino G: The cornified envelope: a model of cell death in the skin. Nat Rev Mol Cell Biol 2005;6:328–340.
34 Howell MD, Kim BE, Gao P, Grant AV, Boguniewicz M, Debenedetto A, Schneider L, Beck LA, Barnes KC, Leung DY: Cytokine modulation of atopic dermatitis filaggrin skin expression. J Allergy Clin Immunol 2007;120:150–155.
35 Howell MD, Fairchild HR, Kim BE, Bin L, Boguniewicz M, Redzic JS, Hansen KC, Leung DY: Th2 cytokines act on S100/A11 to downregulate keratinocyte differentiation. J Invest Dermatol 2008; 128:1591–1594.
36 Katsuta M, Takigawa Y, Kimishima M, Inaoka M, Takahashi R, Shiohara T: NK cells and γδ+ T cells are phenotypically and functionally defective due to preferential apoptosis in patients with atopic dermatitis. J Immunol 2006;176:7736–7744.
37 Rogge JL, Hanifin JM: Immunodeficiencies in severe atopic dermatitis: depressed chemotaxis and lymphocyte transformation. Arch Dermatol 1976; 112:1391–1396.
38 Takeuchi O, Hoshino K, Kawai T, Sanjo H, Takada H, Ogawa T, Takeda K, Akira S: Differential roles of TLR2 and TLR4 in recognition of Gram-negative and Gram-positive bacterial cell wall components. Immunity 1999;11:443–451.
39 Hasannejad H, Takahashi R, Kimishima M, Hayakawa K, Shiohara T: Selective impairment of Toll-like receptor 2-mediated proinflammatory cytokine production by monocytes from patients with atopic dermatitis. J Allergy Clin Immunol 2007;120:69–75.

40 McGirt LY, Beck LA: Innate immune defects in atopic dermatitis. J Allergy Clin Immunol 2006;118: 202–208.
41 Lorenz E, Mira JP, Cornish KL, Arbour NC, Schwartz DA: A novel polymorphism in the Toll-like receptor 2 gene and its potential association with staphylococcal infection. Infect Immun 2000; 68:6398–6401.
42 Mrabet-Dahbi S, Ahmad-Nejad P, Breuer K, Klotz M, Werfel T, Herz U, et al: The Toll-like receptor 2 R753Q polymorphism defines a subgroup of patients with atopic dermatitis having severe phenotype. J Allergy Clin Immunol 2004;113:565–567.
43 Mrabet-Dahbi S, Dalpke AH, Niebuhr M, Frey M, Draing C, Brand S, et al: The Toll-like receptor 2 R753Q mutation modifies cytokine production and Toll-like receptor expression in atopic dermatitis. J Allergy Clin Immunol 2008;121:1013–1019.
44 Shimizu M, Matsuda A, Yanagisawa K, Hirota T, Akahoshi M, Inomata N, Ebe K, Tanaka K, Sugiura H, Nakashima K, Tamari M, Takahashi N, Obara K, Enomoto T, Okayama Y, Gao PS, Huang SK, Tominaga S, Ikezawa Z, Shirakawa T: Functional SNPs in the distal promoter of the ST2 gene are associated with atopic dermatitis. Hum Mol Genet 2005;14:2919–2927.
45 Zhang G, Ghosh S: Negative regulation of Toll-like receptor-mediated signaling by Tollip. J Biol Chem 2002;277:7059–7065.
46 Didierlaurent A, Brissoni B, Velin D, Aebi N, Tardivel A, Käslin E, Sirard JC, Angelov G, Tschopp J, Burns K: Tollip regulates proinflammatory responses to interleukin-1 and lipopolysaccharide. Mol Cell Biol 2006;26:735–742.
47 Schimming TT, Parwez Q, Petrasch-Parwez E, Nothnagel M, Epplen JT, Hoffjan S: Association of Toll-interacting protein gene polymorphisms with atopic dermatitis. BMC Dermatol 2007;7:3.
48 Matsui E, Kaneko H, Teramoto T, Fukao T, Inoue R, Kasahara K, et al: Reduced IFN-γ production in response to IL-12 stimulation and/or IL-12 production in atopic patients. Clin Exp Allergy 2000;30: 1250–1256.
49 Ong PY, Ohtake T, Brandt C, Strickland I, Boguniewicz M, Ganz T, et al: Endogenous antimicrobial peptides and skin infections in atopic dermatitis. N Engl J Med 2002;347:1151–1160.
50 Howell MD, Boguniewicz M, Pastore S, Novak N, Bieber T, Girolomoni G, et al: Mechanism of HBD-3 deficiency in atopic dermatitis. Clin Immunol 2006; 121:332–338.
51 Howell MD, Gallo RL, Boguniewicz M, Jones JF, Wong C, Streib JE, et al: Cytokine milieu of atopic dermatitis skin subverts the innate immune response to vaccinia virus. Immunity 2006;24: 341–348.

Marcus Maurer, MD
Professor of Dermatology and Allergy, Department of Dermatology and Allergy
Allergie-Centrum-Charité, Charité-Universitätsmedizin Berlin
Charitéplatz 1, DE–10117 Berlin (Germany)
Tel. +49 30 450 518 043, Fax +49 30 450 518 972, E-Mail marcus.maurer@charite.de

Shiohara T (ed): Pathogenesis and Management of Atopic Dermatitis.
Curr Probl Dermatol. Basel, Karger, 2011, vol 41, pp 112–124

The Role of Regulatory T Cells in Atopic Dermatitis

Rachana Agrawal · Julia A. Wisniewski · Judith A. Woodfolk

Asthma and Allergic Diseases Center, University of Virginia Health System, Charlottesville, Va., USA

Abstract

Regulatory T (T_{reg}) cells play a pivotal role in immune suppression and are integral to the control of allergic responses. The chronic inflammatory skin condition atopic dermatitis (AD) is severest in patients who are sensitized to allergens from diverse sources including foods, pollens and animal danders, as well as skin-colonizing organisms. These individuals typically present with eczematous skin eruptions in early childhood, and evolution of the disease is thought to reflect an underlying dysregulated T-cell response to allergens that manifests as a Th2 response. Studying T_{reg} cells in the context of AD from infancy into adulthood could yield insight into their role in disease pathogenesis and reveal new strategies for exploiting these cells for therapeutic purposes. Such studies are challenging in humans owing to the heterogeneous nature of T_{reg} cells, lack of a reliable surface marker, and the paucity of knowledge surrounding the emergence of specialized T cells in early life. Moreover, the blurred distinction between activated effector T cells and T_{reg} cells further complicates studies in the context of inflammatory disorders such as AD. There is emerging evidence to suggest that T_{reg} cells can convert to Th2 cells and that this pathway is bidirectional. This phenomenon may be a double-edged sword with important implications not only for subverting T_{reg} cells in disease, but also for potential treatments designed to amplify these cells in order to suppress the allergic inflammatory cascade in AD.

Atopic dermatitis (AD) is a chronic inflammatory skin condition that can be severe and debilitating. A cellular infiltrate comprising predominantly T cells is a key feature of AD skin lesions supporting the view that these cells play a role in disease pathogenesis, and possibly in resolution. As we learn more about the existence of specialized T cell types, the nature of these cells will likely continue to evolve. As is true for many inflammatory disorders, regulatory T (T_{reg}) cells play a pivotal role in AD. Many AD patients are highly allergic, and thus, much of what we can glean about T_{reg} cells in AD comes from studies on T cells in the context of allergens and allergic disease. This article provides an overview of key concepts related to T_{reg} cells and highlights their relevance to AD.

Regulatory T Cells in Humans

Molecular Signature of Regulatory T Cells

There is general consensus that T_{reg} cells play an important role in controlling or suppressing T-cell responses to allergens. Human T_{reg} cells comprise a highly heterogeneous population as judged by their molecular signature and functional properties [1]. While the characteristics of these cells continue to be the subject of much debate, those most frequently studied express CD25 [interleukin (IL)-2 receptor α-chain] and the transcription factor Foxp3 (Forkhead/winged-helix transcription factor box P3). In humans, the levels of CD25 expression appear to correlate with Foxp3 expression. Specifically, CD25hiCD4+ cells express higher levels of Foxp3, CD25intCD4+ cells express lower amounts, and those that are CD25– lack Foxp3 expression [1]. Importantly, only those cells that express the highest levels of CD25 (typically comprising approx. 1–3% of total CD4+ T cells) exhibit suppressive properties.

Verifying human T_{reg} cells in health and disease has proven problematic owing to the lack of a distinguishing molecular phenotype. While Foxp3 is a feature of these cells, this molecule can also be induced in resting human effector T cells (CD25–CD4+) through T-cell receptor activation; however, expression is transient and does not confer suppressive properties [2–4]. Similarly, CD25 is also induced on activated effector T cells. It has recently been suggested that demethylation in the Foxp3 locus provides an improved method for identifying T cells with suppressor function rather than expression of Foxp3 protein itself [5, 6]. Other markers that have been used to identify human T_{reg} cells include low expression of CD127 (IL-7 receptor α-chain), expression of lymphocyte activation gene 3 on activated T_{reg} cells, and expression of GITR (glucocorticoid-induced tumor necrosis factor receptor family-related protein) and CTLA4 (cytotoxic T lymphocyte-associated antigen 4) [7–10]. However, none of these are exclusive to T_{reg} cells.

Preferential expression of several surface molecules has recently been reported on activated human T_{reg} cells. One of these, named glycoprotein A repetitions predominant (GARP or LRRC32), is a leucine-rich transmembrane protein. This receptor selectively identifies activated human Foxp3+ T_{reg} cells [11, 12] and regulates *Foxp3* gene expression [13, 14]. Notably, overexpression in human effector cells leads to stable reprogramming towards a regulatory phenotype and function which includes suppression of effector cytokine production, expression of Foxp3 and acquisition of suppressive capacity [13, 15]. By contrast, downregulation of GARP in human T_{reg} cells by gene knockdown impairs suppressor function [16]. Other molecules that are expressed on activated Foxp3+ T_{reg} cells include latency-associated peptide and IL-1 receptor types 1 and 2 (CD121a/CD121b) [17]. However, latency-associated peptide is also expressed on a novel T_{reg} cell subset that lacks Foxp3 [18]. Nonetheless, GARP and latency-associated peptide may prove useful markers for isolating human CD25+Foxp3+ T_{reg} cells following expansion ex vivo [19].

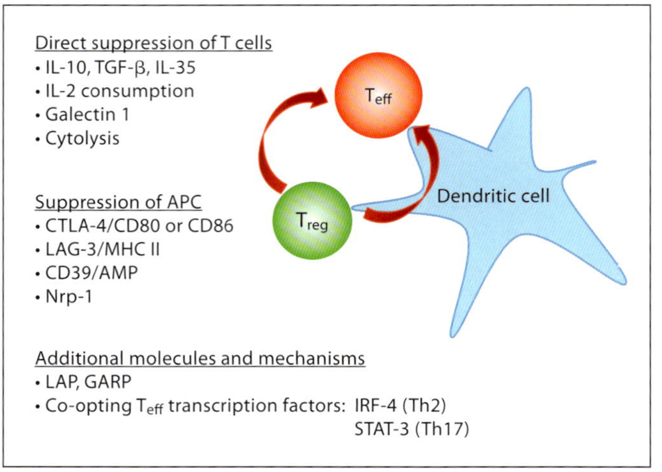

Fig. 1. Molecules and mechanisms implicated in suppression mediated by human T_{reg} cells. APC = Antigen-presenting cell; LAG-3 = lymphocyte activation gene 3; MHC II = major histocompatibility complex II; AMP = adenosine monophosphate; Nrp-1 = neuropilin-1; LAP = latency-associated peptide; STAT-3 = signal transducer and activator of transcription 3; T_{eff} = effector T cell.

Mechanisms of Suppression

T_{reg} cells that exhibit the CD25hiFoxp3+ phenotype may represent natural T_{reg} cells that constitutively express CD25 upon egress from the thymus. Another type of T_{reg} cell, the so-called 'adaptive T_{reg} cells' are induced by foreign antigens in the periphery. This T_{reg} cell type includes type-1-like regulatory T cells (Tr1) that secrete IL-10 and suppress antigen-specific responses in a cytokine-dependent manner [1]. In humans, the distinction between natural and adaptive T_{reg} cells is unclear, and the mechanism of suppression mediated by specific T_{reg} cell types continues to be debated. There is a broad array of molecules and pathways that have been implicated in suppressive pathways in vitro. The two primary modes include direct suppression of T cells and suppression through the antigen-presenting cell (fig. 1) [16–24]. Unfortunately, we still have a lot to learn about the relevance of these in vitro mechanisms to T_{reg} cell actions in vivo, and how these pathways may be impacted in disease [20, 21]. Pathways implicated in the control or suppression of allergic diseases such as AD include suppression via IL-10 or transforming growth factor (TGF) β, as well as contact-dependent mechanisms. Adding to the complex picture, it is increasingly apparent that specialized T cells, including T_{reg} cells, can exhibit plasticity and have the capacity to adapt in an inflammatory milieu [22]. For example, T_{reg} cells can 'co-opt' transcription factors of the corresponding target effector population in animal models [23, 24]. It has been proposed that this capability may equip T_{reg} cells to operate optimally at sites of inflammation.

Regulatory T Cells in Allergic Disease

Allergic diseases are driven by the development of Th2 cells which mastermind antibody isotype switching to IgE production and an inflammatory cascade involving recruitment and activation of diverse cell types including mast cells, basophils, eosinophils, dendritic cells and fibroblasts. The Th2 cytokines IL-4, IL-5, IL-9 and IL-13 initiate and perpetuate a chronic cycle of inflammation that results in the manifestation of different types of allergic diseases such as allergic rhinitis, asthma and AD. It is generally accepted that CD25+ T_{reg} cells have the capacity to suppress Th2 responses to allergen in vitro. Most experimental systems have used suppression assays that involve reconstituting CD25– responder cells with CD25+ T cells and monitoring the resulting dose-dependent suppression of proliferation or cytokine responses to allergen. One of the drawbacks of this approach is that CD25+ T cells may be contaminated with activated effectors, and strategies for isolating CD25hi T cells are not consistent between studies making these assays difficult to interpret. Moreover, some have argued that the diminished responses observed using this approach do not reflect suppression mediated by T_{reg} cells per se, but instead arise from sequestration of IL-2 by CD25+ T cells. Nevertheless, when considering the substantial body of data collected from allergic and nonallergic subjects, as well as from animal models of allergic disease, a role for T_{reg} cells in modulating T-cell responses to allergens is without doubt.

While multiple pathways have been implicated in controlling T-cell responses to allergen, perhaps the most abundant evidence in humans, as well as animal models, supports a role for IL-10. A decrease in the ratio of circulating allergen-specific IL-10- to IL-4-secreting T cells among allergic individuals as compared with healthy nonallergic subjects suggests that alterations in the 'balance' between T_{reg} cells and Th2 effectors may be a determinant in the development of allergy [25]. Consistent with this notion, a more recent study described decreased CD25hi T_{reg} cell numbers in asthmatic children in both the blood and the respiratory tract, as compared to children with cough or healthy children [26].

Studying T cells obtained from allergic patients during immunotherapy (IT) has yielded important clues regarding the role of T_{reg} cells in the induction of protective responses. While an extensive review of these studies is beyond the scope of this article, we will highlight several key findings. Allergen IT, which involves administration of incremental doses of allergen through subcutaneous or sublingual routes, has proven clinically efficacious for a variety of allergens including those derived from tree and grass pollens, animal sources and insects. In subjects who are monosensitized (i.e. sensitized to a single allergen), symptoms are improved for years after stopping treatment [27]. Induction of CD25+Foxp3+ T cells by IT has been widely reported and while not all studies have verified the functional properties of these cells, those that have generally report suppressive properties. Notably, IL-10 is often implicated in the suppressive mechanism, though other cytokines (TGF-β) and T-cell-associated inhibitory signaling molecules (e.g. CTLA4, PD-1) may also be involved [25, 28–31].

Early work linking IL-10 to successful IT in bee venom-allergic patients described increased IL-10 production by CD25+CD4+ T cells following in vitro activation by the major bee venom allergen phospholipase A_2 [32]. This phenomenon was associated with suppressed T-cell proliferation and Th2 cytokine responses to allergen as early as 7 days after initiating treatment. Notably, neutralization of IL-10 fully reconstituted allergen-induced proliferation and cytokine production. In the same study, IL-10 was shown to inhibit phospholipase-A_2-specific and total IgE while enhancing production of IgG4 antibodies. This latter observation suggested that IL-10 not only mediated allergen-specific T-cell anergy, but also skewed serum antibody profiles in favor of regulatory isotypes that can inhibit IgE-facilitated allergen presentation [33].

In more recent work on beekeepers exposed to high doses of phospholipase A_2 through natural stings, increases in allergen-specific IL-10-secreting T cells were observed soon after onset of the beekeeping season [31]. This corresponded with a decrease in both IL-4- and γ-interferon-secreting T cells that coincided with suppressed in vitro T-cell responses to allergen. Notably, it appeared that in vivo expansion of IL-10-secreting allergen-specific T cells arose from conversion of IL-4-secreting T cells through a mechanism involving histamine binding to the histamine receptor HR2 on Th2 cells. This supports the view that allergen-specific Th2 cells exhibit functional plasticity. Further elucidation of T_{reg} cells induced during IT is warranted in order to better understand their origins and functional properties.

It is not clear which T-cell-suppressive mechanisms are involved by administration of allergen using different dosing regimens (e.g. conventional IT vs. rush IT) and different routes (e.g. skin vs. sublingual). Nonetheless, it is widely held that the appearance of T_{reg} cells during IT reflects the development of allergen tolerance. In addition to their induction by therapeutic administration of allergen, T_{reg} cells may also be induced by high-dose natural exposure. Some individuals who are exposed to high levels of cat allergen in the environment develop a protective immune response that is characterized by the presence of high-titer IgG and IgG4 antibodies to the major cat allergen Fel d 1, in the absence of IgE antibodies and allergic symptoms [34]. Our group performed T-cell epitope mapping studies of Fel d 1 using cultures established from allergic and cat-tolerant individuals in order to analyze T-cell mechanisms involved in the development of this 'modified Th2' response. Those studies identified a region of the Fel d 1 molecule that preferentially induced IL-10, indicating that this allergen had intrinsic tolerogenic properties [35].

The abundant literature on the biological properties of allergens highlights the diversity of these molecules and the complex immune pathways that may be triggered by interactions with immune cells. Dendritic cells (DCs) play a key role in driving Th2 responses to allergen, and this professional antigen-presenting cell is also likely to be critical to the development of T_{reg} cells. These cells express an array of surface molecules that may bind allergen and condition DCs to induce specialized T-cell subsets. Perhaps the best described is the high-affinity IgE receptor FcεRI, which is expressed at increased levels on DCs from highly atopic individuals, including those with AD [36]. Facilitated allergen presentation through this receptor may augment Th2 responses during the effector phase. However, in the initiation phase, generation of Th2 responses likely reflects triggering and convergence of multiple pathways during a critical developmental window in the first years of life. A key role continues to emerge for innate signaling pathways, notably the Toll-like receptor 4 pathway, in modulating allergic responses at the T-cell level [37]. While much has been written about the ability for the Toll-like receptor 4 ligand, lipopolysaccharide, to dampen Th2 responses based on its Th1-promoting properties at high dose, less is known about the role of innate signaling pathways in the induction of T_{reg} cells. There is evidence in animal models to suggest that Toll-like receptor pathways are involved in modulating T_{reg} cells [38, 39]. However, a variety of different mechanisms have been reported to induce DC-mediated tolerance. These are reviewed elsewhere [40]. When considering allergic disease, it is important to note that the status of the host is also an important factor in determining immune outcome. Recent work by our group suggests that DCs from highly atopic subjects, including those with AD, exhibit intrinsic Th2-promoting properties [41]. Thus, studying these cells in the context of disease could provide new insight into pathways that skew the immune response away from T_{reg} cells in favor of Th2 responses.

Regulatory T Cells and Atopic Dermatitis

In humans, CD4+ T_{reg} cells are present in both the peripheral blood and lymphoid tissues [10, 42–44]. A notable feature of T_{reg} cells is that they express a variety of skin-homing addressins including CC chemokine receptor (CCR) 4, CCR6 and cutaneous lymphocyte-associated antigen (CLA) [45–47]. Indeed, it has been suggested that the majority of human T_{reg} cells actually reside in the skin where they may play a key role in immune surveillance [48]. While there is no doubt that T cells infiltrate the inflamed skin of patients with AD, there has been considerable debate surrounding the nature of these cells. Early work reported that Th2 cells are the predominant T-cell type in acute lesions, while those in chronic lesions represented a mixed T helper profile [49, 50]. Not surprisingly, increased knowledge of the existence of novel T-cell subsets provided the impetus for new observations indicating the presence of a variety of T-cell types, including Th17 cells, in eczematous skin [51]. Despite this, relatively little remains known about recruitment of T_{reg} cells to AD skin, and their function at this site remains enigmatic. IL-10-secreting Tr1 cells can be isolated from lesional AD skin; however, in that study, CD25+Foxp3+ T_{reg} cells were absent [52]. By contrast, other work has reported the presence of CD25+Foxp3+ 'T_{reg} cells' at lesional sites [53–55]. Given that activated effector T cells can express Foxp3, further elucidation of these cells is warranted.

Perhaps the most striking evidence of a role for T_{reg} cells in protecting against the development of AD comes from the clinical syndrome associated with mutations in the *Foxp3* gene. Immune dysregulation, polyendocrinopathy and enteropathy X-linked syndrome is a congenital disorder that is associated with a deficiency in CD25+ T_{reg} cells, resulting in severe immune dysregulation. This syndrome includes several manifestations that are characteristic of allergic disorders including spontaneous development of allergic airway inflammation, hyper-IgE, eosinophilia, food allergy and eczema [56–58]. This has led investigators to question whether a decrease in T_{reg} cells, or changes in their function, contribute to the pathogenesis of AD.

Studying how T_{reg} cells evolve in childhood could yield insight into the development and persistence of AD. Sensitization to food allergens in infancy and beyond may herald the onset of the 'atopic march' which culminates in sensitization to a broad array of allergens and progression of skin disease [59]. Patients with severe AD are often highly atopic, exhibiting sensitization to diverse allergens including inhalants (e.g. cat, mite, pollens) and bacterial sources (e.g. skin-colonizing bacteria and fungi). A key question is why some children outgrow their eczema while others do not. Increased CD25+ T_{reg} cells have been reported in children who outgrew cow's milk allergy [60]. In addition, increased numbers of allergen-specific CD25+Foxp3+ T_{reg} cells were reported in children who developed tolerance to milk, and higher T_{reg} cell numbers correlated with milder clinical symptoms to milk [61]. Collectively, these findings imply that increased T_{reg} cells in early life are protective.

In adults with established disease, the T-cell landscape may be more complex. Work by our group revealed an increase in the frequency of circulating CD25hiFoxp3+ T cells in patients with AD as compared with healthy controls, and a similar expansion of CD25+Foxp3+ T cells has been reported by others [45, 62]. These findings contrast with a report of elevated numbers of Tr1 cells with no variation in CD25+Foxp3+ T cells in the blood of patients with AD [54]. While at first glance, expansion of T cells that coexpress CD25 and Foxp3 in AD may seem paradoxical, this likely reflects a mixed population comprising activated effector T cells and T_{reg} cells. In order to further elucidate the properties of expanded CD25hi T cells in AD, we examined the expression of additional markers. The results showed that CD25hiFoxp3+ T cells exhibited skin-homing potential based on the expression of CLA and CCR4, the receptor for thymus- and activation-regulated chemokine (TARC)/CCL17. Notably, TARC is highly expressed in AD skin lesions, and we and others have shown that serum levels of this chemokine correlate with disease severity and IgE titers [63–65]. Thus, CCR4 likely plays a pivotal role in recruitment of T cells, including T_{reg} cells, to inflamed skin in AD. Despite possessing a molecular signature that comprises a characteristic array of molecules (i.e. CD25, CLA, CCR4 and Foxp3), 2 discrete subtypes of CD25hi T cells were discernable in AD patients based on differential expression of the chemokine receptor CCR6. Specifically, those cells lacking expression of this receptor exhibited Th2-like properties as judged by their cytokine secretion profile upon activation with the bacterial superantigen staphylococcal enterotoxin B. Moreover, these cells actually amplified secretion of Th2 cytokines when mixed with CD25– effectors [45]. Thus, this novel CD25hiCCR6– subtype exhibited Th2-like properties despite bearing the molecular signature of T_{reg} cells.

The presence of discrete T-cell subtypes within an expanded CD25hi compartment in AD is consistent with the theory of 'parallel amplification' whereby expansion of effector

T cells is counterregulated by an expansion of T_{reg} cells. In accordance with this, recent work using peripheral blood mononuclear leukocyte cultures established from subjects allergic to ryegrass pollen showed that allergen stimulation induced proliferation of both CD25+Foxp3hi T_{reg} cells and effector T cells. Interestingly, proliferation of T_{reg} cells was decreased in allergic patients, and the authors concluded that induction of T_{reg} cells may be impaired in these subjects, thereby evoking the notion of a T_{reg} cell deficiency [66].

An important alternate theory to consider is that T_{reg} cells are not reduced in numbers in AD, but instead are present, but fail to function in an optimal manner. Impaired T_{reg}-mediated suppression of Th2 cytokine responses to allergen has been observed in pollen-allergic subjects, possibly regulated by levels of pollen exposure [67, 68]. T_{reg} cells may also be influenced by 'proallergic' molecules expressed in AD skin. This could include allergens derived from environmental sources or skin-colonizing organisms, as well as a broad array of cytokines. As an example, thymic stromal lymphopoietin (TLSP) is a Th2-promoting cytokine that is expressed by keratinocytes in AD skin lesions [69]. This cytokine mediates its effects primarily at the DC level, but was recently shown to directly and selectively impair IL-10 production by pulmonary T_{reg} cells, thereby abrogating their suppressive capacity in patients with asthma [70]. This observation appears to contradict the role of TSLP in intrathymic generation of natural T_{reg} cells [71]. Other work supports a role for factors derived from skin-colonizing bacteria in altering T_{reg} cell function (fig. 2). Many patients with AD are colonized with *Staphylococcus aureus*, and IgE antibodies to staphylococcal enterotoxins are common among highly atopic patients [65]. Interestingly, CD25+ T_{reg} cells fail to suppress proliferation of autologous effector T cells in the presence of staphylococcal enterotoxin B, but effectively suppress proliferation induced by anti-CD3 [62]. The inhibitory GITR/GITR ligand pathway has been implicated in T_{reg} cell subversion mediated by staphylococcal enterotoxin B through upregulation of GITR ligand on monocytes [72].

The idea that T cells may be influenced by the inflammatory milieu is certainly not new. However, it is increasingly apparent that specific T-cell types can exhibit plasticity depending on the microenvironment, and this appears to hold true for T_{reg} cells. Notably, attenuation of Foxp3 expression results in conversion of T_{reg} cells to Th2 cells and this occurs even in a Th1-polarizing environment [73, 74]. Moreover, there is evidence to suggest that the conversion pathway is bidirectional. For example, antigen-specific Th2 cells can be redifferentiated into Foxp3+ T_{reg} cells by TGF-β in the presence of all-*trans*-retinoic acid and rapamycin [75]. Additionally, T_{reg} cells can also convert to other T-cell types including Th17 cells. This cell type is induced from naïve T cells by TGF-β and IL-6. However, T_{reg} cells producing TGF-β can differentiate into Th17 cells in the presence of IL-6 without the requirement for TGF-β [76]. These aspects of T-cell plasticity may be highly relevant to disease processes in the skin. Numerous studies have demonstrated expression of a broad array of inflammatory factors in AD skin [77]. These include IL-4, IL-5, IL-12, IL-13, IL-17, γ-interferon, granulocyte-macrophage colony-stimulating factor, IL-31, TSLP, and TNF-α. Thus, T_{reg} cells recruited to inflamed skin are exposed to a host of factors that

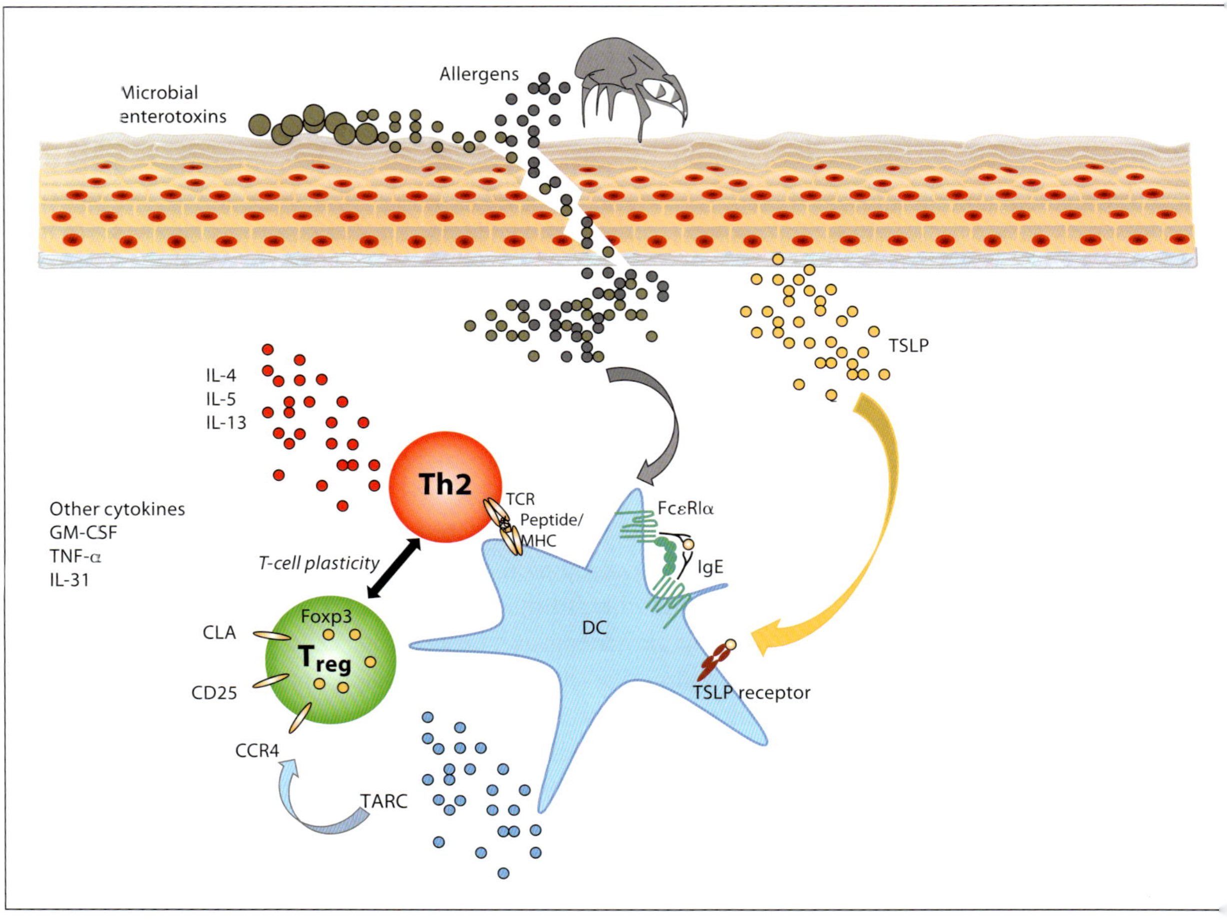

Fig. 2. Schematic depicting the 'proinflammatory milieu' in AD skin lesions that may influence T-cell function at this site. GM-CSF = Granulocyte-macrophage colony-stimulating factor; CLA = cutaneous lymphocyte-associated antigen; TCR = T-cell receptor; MHC = major histocompatibility complex.

could influence their ability to function. An intriguing question is whether CD25hi cells that exhibit Th2-like properties in the blood of AD patients constitute T_{reg} cells that have undergone conversion [45]. Such a phenomenon could exacerbate the inflammatory cascade in the skin.

Future Directions

We still have a lot to learn about human T_{reg} cells. Further studies on these cells in the context of diseases such as AD will prove valuable not only for understanding immune processes in the skin, but also for designing new therapies. Identification of new surface markers could facilitate improved methods of detection and isolation of T_{reg} cells for functional studies. While there is substantial evidence that T_{reg} cells can suppress T-cell responses to allergens, it remains unclear whether CD25+ T_{reg} cells in AD are allergen-specific. Techniques using peptide/major histocompatibility complex tetramers to test for T-cell receptor specificity could provide further insight in this regard. Until we learn more about T_{reg} cells in AD, it will be difficult to ascertain whether boosting T_{reg} cells is an appropriate therapeutic objective. While studies in animal models suggest that Th2 conversion to T_{reg} cells is feasible, it is not known whether this approach would translate successfully to humans. An important consideration is whether the Th2-promoting milieu in AD could hinder or subvert the types of T_{reg}-enhancing strategies used. In contrast to allergic patients without AD, conventional IT can exacerbate skin disease in AD patients. This may arise from uptake of allergen by skin DCs that have been primed with TSLP [69, 78]. We and others have shown that DCs from AD patients are equipped with the molecular machinery to induce robust Th2 responses [36, 41]. This includes the propensity to efficiently upregulate TSLP receptor upon Fc receptor ligation [41]. Thus, allergen-based treatments that target DCs may not be an appropriate mode for enhancing T_{reg} cells in AD. Despite this, there is substantial evidence to suggest that exploiting T_{reg} cells could prove a valuable strategy in the armory of treatments for this severe and often debilitating disease.

Acknowledgment

This work was supported by NIH grants AI-052196 and AI-070364.

References

1 Shevach EM: From vanilla to 28 flavors: multiple varieties of T regulatory cells. Immunity 2006;25: 195–201.

2 Gavin MA, Torgerson TR, Houston E, De Roos P, Ho WY, Stray-Pedersen A, et al: Single-cell analysis of normal and FOXP3-mutant human T cells: FOXP3 expression without regulatory T cell development. Proc Natl Acad Sci USA. 2006;103: 6659–6664.

3 Pillai V, Ortega SB, Wang CK, Karandikar NJ: Transient regulatory T-cells: a state attained by all activated human T-cells. Clin Immunol 2007;123: 18–29.

4 Allan SE, Crome SQ, Crellin NK, Passerini L, Steiner TS, Bacchetta R, et al: Activation-induced FOXP3 in human T effector cells does not suppress proliferation or cytokine production. Int Immunol 2007; 19:345–354.

5 Baron U, Floess S, Wieczorek G, Baumann K, Grutzkau A, Dong J, et al: DNA demethylation in the human FOXP3 locus discriminates regulatory T cells from activated FOXP3+ conventional T cells. Eur J Immunol 2007;37:2378–2389.

6 Janson PC, Winerdal ME, Marits P, Thorn M, Ohlsson R, Winqvist O: *FOXP3* promoter demethylation reveals the committed T_{reg} population in humans. PLoS One 2008;3:e1612.

7 Liu W, Putnam AL, Xu-Yu Z, Szot GL, Lee MR, Zhu S, et al: CD127 expression inversely correlates with FoxP3 and suppressive function of human CD4+ T reg cells. J Exp Med 2006;203:1701–1711.

8 Bayry J, Triebel F, Kaveri SV, Tough DF: Human dendritic cells acquire a semimature phenotype and lymph node homing potential through interaction with CD4+CD25+ regulatory T cells. J Immunol 2007;178:4184–4193.

9 Clark RA, Kupper TS: IL-15 and dermal fibroblasts induce proliferation of natural regulatory T cells isolated from human skin. Blood 2007;109: 194–202.
10 Jonuleit H, Schmitt E, Stassen M, Tuettenberg A, Knop J, Enk AH: Identification and functional characterization of human CD4+CD25+ T cells with regulatory properties isolated from peripheral blood. J Exp Med 2001;193:1285–1294.
11 Wang R, Kozhaya L, Mercer F, Khaitan A, Fujii H, Unutmaz D: Expression of GARP selectively identifies activated human FOXP3+ regulatory T cells. Proc Natl Acad Sci USA 2009;106:13439–13444.
12 Stockis J, Colau D, Coulie PG, Lucas S: Membrane protein GARP is a receptor for latent TGF-beta on the surface of activated human T_{reg}. Eur J Immunol 2009;39:3315–3322.
13 Probst-Kepper M, Geffers R, Kroger A, Viegas N, Erck C, Hecht HJ, et al: GARP: a key receptor controlling FOXP3 in human regulatory T cells. J Cell Mol Med 2009;13:3343–3357.
14 Wang R, Wan Q, Kozhaya L, Fujii H, Unutmaz D: Identification of a regulatory T cell specific cell surface molecule that mediates suppressive signals and induces Foxp3 expression. PLoS One 2008;3: e2705.
15 Probst-Kepper M, Balling R, Buer J: FOXP3: required but not sufficient – the role of GARP (LRRC32) as a safeguard of the regulatory phenotype. Curr Mol Med 2010;10:533–539.
16 Probst-Kepper M, Buer J: FOXP3 and GARP (LRRC32): the master and its minion. Biol Direct 2010;5:8.
17 Tran DQ, Andersson J, Hardwick D, Bebris L, Illei GG, Shevach EM: Selective expression of latency-associated peptide (LAP) and IL-1 receptor type I/II (CD121a/CD121b) on activated human FOXP3+ regulatory T cells allows for their purification from expansion cultures. Blood 2009;113:5125–5133.
18 Gandhi R, Farez MF, Wang Y, Kozoriz D, Quintana FJ, Weiner HL: Cutting edge: human latency-associated peptide+ T cells: a novel regulatory T cell subset. J Immunol 2010;184:4620–4624.
19 Tran DQ, Shevach EM: Therapeutic potential of FOXP3+ regulatory T cells and their interactions with dendritic cells. Hum Immunol 2009;70: 294–299.
20 Shevach EM: Mechanisms of Foxp3+ T regulatory cell-mediated suppression. Immunity 2009;30: 636–645.
21 Bettini M, Vignali DA: Regulatory T cells and inhibitory cytokines in autoimmunity. Curr Opin Immunol 2009;21:612–618.
22 Wan YY: Multi-tasking of helper T cells. Immunology 2010;130:166–171.
23 Chaudhry A, Rudra D, Treuting P, Samstein RM, Liang Y, Kas A, et al: CD4+ regulatory T cells control Th17 responses in a Stat3-dependent manner. Science 2009;326:986–991.
24 Zheng Y, Chaudhry A, Kas A, de Roos P, Kim JM, Chu TT, et al: Regulatory T-cell suppressor program co-opts transcription factor IRF4 to control Th2 responses. Nature 2009;458:351–356.
25 Akdis M, Verhagen J, Taylor A, Karamloo F, Karagiannidis C, Crameri R, et al. Immune responses in healthy and allergic individuals are characterized by a fine balance between allergen-specific T regulatory 1 and T helper 2 cells. J Exp Med 2004;199:1567–1575.
26 Hartl D, Koller B, Mehlhorn AT, Reinhardt D, Nicolai T, Schendel DJ, et al: Quantitative and functional impairment of pulmonary CD4+CD25hi regulatory T cells in pediatric asthma. J Allergy Clin Immunol 2007;119:1258–1266.
27 Durham SR, Walker SM, Varga EM, Jacobson MR, O'Brien F, Noble W, et al: Long-term clinical efficacy of grass-pollen immunotherapy. N Engl J Med 1999;341:468–475.
28 O'Hehir RE, Gardner LM, de Leon MP, Hales BJ, Biondo M, Douglass JA, et al: House dust mite sublingual immunotherapy: the role for transforming growth factor-beta and functional regulatory T cells. Am J Respir Crit Care Med 2009;180:936–947.
29 Jutel M, Akdis M, Budak F, Aebischer-Casaulta C, Wrzyszcz M, Blaser K, et al: IL-10 and TGF-beta cooperate in the regulatory T cell response to mucosal allergens in normal immunity and specific immunotherapy. Eur J Immunol 2003;33: 1205–1214.
30 Francis JN, Till SJ, Durham SR: Induction of IL-10+CD4+CD25+ T cells by grass pollen immunotherapy. J Allergy Clin Immunol 2003;111: 1255–1261.
31 Meiler F, Zumkehr J, Klunker S, Ruckert B, Akdis CA, Akdis M: In vivo switch to IL-10-secreting T regulatory cells in high dose allergen exposure. J Exp Med 2008;205:2887–2898.
32 Akdis CA, Blesken T, Akdis M, Wuthrich B, Blaser K: Role of interleukin 10 in specific immunotherapy. J Clin Invest 1998;102:98–106.
33 Nouri-Aria KT, Wachholz PA, Francis JN, Jacobson MR, Walker SM, Wilcock LK, et al: Grass pollen immunotherapy induces mucosal and peripheral IL-10 responses and blocking IgG activity. J Immunol 2004;172:3252–3259.
34 Platts-Mills T, Vaughan J, Squillace S, Woodfolk J, Sporik R: Sensitisation, asthma, and a modified Th2 response in children exposed to cat allergen: a population-based cross-sectional study. Lancet 2001;357:752–756.

35 Reefer AJ, Carneiro RM, Custis NJ, Platts-Mills TA, Sung SS, Hammer J, et al: A role for IL-10-mediated HLA-DR7-restricted T cell-dependent events in development of the modified Th2 response to cat allergen. J Immunol 2004;172:2763–2772.

36 Novak N, Tepel C, Koch S, Brix K, Bieber T, Kraft S: Evidence for a differential expression of the FcεRIγ chain in dendritic cells of atopic and nonatopic donors. J Clin Invest 2003;111: 1047–1056.

37 Trompette A, Divanovic S, Visintin A, Blanchard C, Hegde RS, Madan R, et al: Allergenicity resulting from functional mimicry of a Toll-like receptor complex protein. Nature 2009;457:585–588.

38 Aumeunier A, Grela F, Ramadan A, Pham Van L, Bardel E, Gomez Alcala A, et al: Systemic Toll-like receptor stimulation suppresses experimental allergic asthma and autoimmune diabetes in NOD mice. PLoS One 2010;5:e11484.

39 Abdollahi-Roodsaz S, Joosten LA, Koenders MI, Devesa I, Roelofs MF, Radstake TR, et al: Stimulation of TLR2 and TLR4 differentially skews the balance of T cells in a mouse model of arthritis. J Clin Invest 2008;118:205–216.

40 Pulendran B, Tang H, Manicassamy S: Programming dendritic cells to induce Th2 and tolerogenic responses. Nat Immunol 2010;11:647–655.

41 Hulse KE, Reefer AJ, Engelhard VH, Patrie JT, Ziegler SF, Chapman MD, et al: Targeting allergen to FcgammaRI reveals a novel Th2 regulatory pathway linked to thymic stromal lymphopoietin receptor. J Allergy Clin Immunol 2010;125:247–255.

42 Ng WF, Duggan PJ, Ponchel F, Matarese G, Lombardi G, Edwards AD, et al: Human CD4+CD25+ cells: a naturally occurring population of regulatory T cells. Blood 2001;98 2736–2744.

43 Dieckmann D, Plottner H, Berchtold S, Berger T, Schuler G: Ex vivo isolation and characterization of CD4+CD25+ T cells with regulatory properties from human blood. J Exp Med 2001;193:1303–1310.

44 Levings MK, Sangregorio R, Roncarolo MG: Human CD25+CD4+ T regulatory cells suppress naive and memory T cell proliferation and can be expanded in vitro without loss of function. J Exp Med 2001;193:1295–1302.

45 Reefer AJ, Satinover SM, Solga MD, Lannigan JA, Nguyen JT, Wilson BB, et al: Analysis of CD25hiCD4+ 'regulatory' T-cell subtypes in atopic dermatitis reveals a novel Th2-like population. J Allergy Clin Immunol 2008;121:415–422.

46 Clark RA, Chong B, Mirchandani N, Brinster NK, Yamanaka K, Dowgiert RK, et al: The vast majority of CLA+ T cells are resident in normal skin. J Immunol 2006;176:4431–4439.

47 Hirahara K, Liu L, Clark RA, Yamanaka K, Fuhlbrigge RC, Kupper TS: The majority of human peripheral blood CD4–CD25highFoxp3+ regulatory T cells bear functional skin-homing receptors. J Immunol 2006;177:4488–4494.

48 Kupper TS, Fuhlbrigge RC. Immune surveillance in the skin: mechanisms and clinical consequences. Nat Rev Immunol 2004;4:211–222.

49 Thepen T, Langeveld-Wildschut EG, Bihari IC, van Wichen DF, van Reijsen FC, Mudde GC, et al: Biphasic response against aeroallergen in atopic dermatitis showing a switch from an initial Th2 response to a Th1 response in situ: an immunocytochemical study. J Allergy Clin Immunol 1996;97: 828–837.

50 Grewe M, Bruijnzeel-Koomen CA, Schopf E, Thepen T, Langeveld-Wildschut AG, Ruzicka T, et al: A role for Th1 and Th2 cells in the immunopathogenesis of atopic dermatitis. Immunol Today 1998;19:359–361.

51 Eyerich K, Pennino D, Scarponi C, Foerster S, Nasorri F, Behrendt H, et al: IL-17 in atopic eczema: linking allergen-specific adaptive and microbial-triggered innate immune response. J Allergy Clin Immunol 2009;123:59–66.

52 Verhagen J, Akdis M, Traidl-Hoffmann C, Schmid-Grendelmeier P, Hijnen D, Knol EF, et al: Absence of T-regulatory cell expression and function in atopic dermatitis skin. J Allergy Clin Immunol 2006;117:176–183.

53 Caproni M, Antiga E, Torchia D, Volpi W, Barletta E, Gitti G, et al: Foxp3-expressing T regulatory cells in atopic dermatitis lesions. Allergy Asthma Proc 2007;28:525–528.

54 Szegedi A, Barath S, Nagy G, Szodoray P, Gal M, Sipka S, et al: Regulatory T cells in atopic dermatitis: epidermal dendritic cell clusters may contribute to their local expansion. Br J Dermatol 2009;160: 984–993.

55 Fujimura T, Okuyama R, Ito Y, Aiba S: Profiles of Foxp3+ regulatory T cells in eczematous dermatitis, psoriasis vulgaris and mycosis fungoides. Br J Dermatol 2008;158:1256–1263.

56 Bennett CL, Christie J, Ramsdell F, Brunkow ME, Ferguson PJ, Whitesell L, et al: The immune dysregulation, polyendocrinopathy, enteropathy, X-linked syndrome (IPEX) is caused by mutations of *FOXP3*. Nat Genet 2001;27:20–21.

57 Chatila TA, Blaeser F, Ho N, Lederman HM, Voulgaropoulos C, Helms C, et al: *JM2*, encoding a fork head-related protein, is mutated in X-linked autoimmunity-allergic disregulation syndrome. J Clin Invest 2000;106:R75–R81.

58 Wildin RS, Ramsdell F, Peake J, Faravelli F, Casanova JL, Buist N, et al: X-linked neonatal diabetes mellitus, enteropathy and endocrinopathy syndrome is the human equivalent of mouse scurfy. Nat Genet 2001;27:18–20.

59 Ker J, Hartert TV: The atopic march: what's the evidence? Ann Allergy Asthma Immunol 2009;103: 282–289.

60 Karlsson MR, Rugtveit J, Brandtzaeg P: Allergen-responsive CD4+CD25+ regulatory T cells in children who have outgrown cow's milk allergy. J Exp Med 2004;199:1679–1688.

61 Shreffler WG, Wanich N, Moloney M, Nowak-Wegrzyn A, Sampson HA: Association of allergen-specific regulatory T cells with the onset of clinical tolerance to milk protein. J Allergy Clin Immunol 2009;123:43–52.

62 Ou LS, Goleva E, Hall C, Leung DY: T regulatory cells in atopic dermatitis and subversion of their activity by superantigens. J Allergy Clin Immunol 2004;113:756–763.

63 Vestergaard C, Bang K, Gesser B, Yoneyama H, Matsushima K, Larsen CG: A Th2 chemokine, TARC, produced by keratinocytes may recruit CLA+CCR4+ lymphocytes into lesional atopic dermatitis skin. J Invest Dermatol 2000;115: 640–646.

64 Kakinuma T, Nakamura K, Wakugawa M, Mitsui H, Tada Y, Saeki H, et al: Thymus and activation-regulated chemokine in atopic dermatitis: serum thymus and activation-regulated chemokine level is closely related with disease activity. J Allergy Clin Immunol 2001;107:535–541.

65 Reefer AJ, Satinover SM, Wilson BB, Woodfolk JA: The relevance of microbial allergens to the IgE antibody repertoire in atopic and nonatopic eczema. J Allergy Clin Immunol 2007;120: 156–163.

66 Mittag D, Scholzen A, Varese N, Baxter L, Paukovics G, Harrison LC, et al: The effector T cell response to ryegrass pollen is counterregulated by simultaneous induction of regulatory T cells. J Immunol 2010;184: 4708–4716.

67 Grindebacke H, Wing K, Andersson AC, Suri-Payer E, Rak S, Rudin A: Defective suppression of Th2 cytokines by CD4+CD25+ regulatory T cells in birch allergics during birch pollen season. Clin Exp Allergy 2004;34:1364–1372.

68 Ling EM, Smith T, Nguyen XD, Pridgeon C, Dallman M, Arbery J, et al: Relation of CD4+CD25+ regulatory T-cell suppression of allergen-driven T-cell activation to atopic status and expression of allergic disease. Lancet 2004;363:608–615.

69 Soumelis V, Reche PA, Kanzler H, Yuan W, Edward G, Homey B, et al: Human epithelial cells trigger dendritic cell mediated allergic inflammation by producing TSLP. Nat Immunol 2002;3:673–680.

70 Nguyen KD, Vanichsarn C, Nadeau KC: TSLP directly impairs pulmonary T_{reg} function: association with aberrant tolerogenic immunity in asthmatic airway. Allergy Asthma Clin Immunol 2010;6:4.

71 Watanabe N, Wang YH, Lee HK, Ito T, Cao W, Liu YJ: Hassall's corpuscles instruct dendritic cells to induce CD4+CD25+ regulatory T cells in human thymus. Nature 2005;436:1181–1185.

72 Cardona ID, Goleva E, Ou LS, Leung DY: Staphylococcal enterotoxin B inhibits regulatory T cells by inducing glucocorticoid-induced TNF receptor-related protein ligand on monocytes. J Allergy Clin Immunol 2006;117:688–695.

73 Wan YY, Flavell RA: Regulatory T-cell functions are subverted and converted owing to attenuated Foxp3 expression. Nature 2007;445:766–770.

74 Joetham A, Matsubara S, Okamoto M, Takeda K, Miyahara N, Dakhama A, et al: Plasticity of regulatory T cells: subversion of suppressive function and conversion to enhancement of lung allergic responses. J Immunol 2008;180:7117–7124.

75 Kim BS, Kim IK, Park YJ, Kim YS, Kim YJ, Chang WS, et al: Conversion of Th2 memory cells into Foxp3+ regulatory T cells suppressing Th2-mediated allergic asthma. Proc Natl Acad Sci USA 2010;107:8742–8747.

76 Xu L, Kitani A, Fuss I, Strober W: Cutting edge: regulatory T cells induce CD4+CD25–Foxp3– T cells or are self-induced to become Th17 cells in the absence of exogenous TGF-beta. J Immunol 2007; 178:6725–6729.

77 Oyoshi MK, He R, Kumar L, Yoon J, Geha RS: Cellular and molecular mechanisms in atopic dermatitis. Adv Immunol 2009;102:135–226.

78 Ito T, Wang YH, Duramad O, Hori T, Delespesse GJ, Watanabe N, et al: TSLP-activated dendritic cells induce an inflammatory T helper type 2 cell response through OX40 ligand. J Exp Med 2005;202: 1213–1223.

Judith A. Woodfolk, MBChB, PhD
Allergy Division, PO Box 801355
University of Virginia Health System
Charlottesville, VA 22908-1355 (USA)
Tel. +1 434 924 1293, Fax +1 434 924 5779, E-Mail jaw4m@virginia.edu

Shiohara T (ed): Pathogenesis and Management of Atopic Dermatitis.
Curr Probl Dermatol. Basel, Karger, 2011, vol 41, pp 125–135

Increased Susceptibility to Cutaneous Viral Infections in Atopic Dermatitis: The Roles of Regulatory T Cells and Innate Immune Defects

Tetsuo Shiohara · Yohei Sato · Ryo Takahashi · Maiko Kurata · Yoshiko Mizukawa

Department of Dermatology, Kyorin University School of Medicine, Tokyo, Japan

Abstract

Much attention has been focused on the elucidation of mechanisms whereby atopic dermatitis (AD) skin lesions are especially susceptible to certain viral infections, such as herpes simplex virus (HSV). Although one of the most likely hypotheses is that the primary defect is in an impaired epidermal barrier function, alternative hypotheses include an imbalance between antiviral immune responses and regulatory T (T_{reg}) cells, and the defects in the innate immune system. Eczema herpeticum (EH) occurs almost exclusively in patients with AD, particularly in those who fail to control skin inflammation. According to our scenario, expansions of T_{reg} cells would be initially required for preventing such excessive inflammation resulting from the failure, and the expansions could in turn contribute to HSV reactivation, resulting in the initiation and progression of EH. A selective impairment of Toll-like-receptor-2-mediated proinflammatory cytokine production by monocytes could be the additional mechanism responsible for the increased susceptibility of AD subjects to curtain viral infections. Here we provide several potential explanations for why AD patients are at greater risk for eczema molluscatum.

Atopic dermatitis (AD) is a chronic inflammatory skin disease characterized by increased serum IgE levels, a predominance of a Th2 immune response, and increased susceptibility to cutaneous viral and bacterial infections [1, 2]. In recent years, much attention has been focused on the elucidation of the mechanisms whereby AD skin lesions are especially susceptible to certain bacterial and viral infections. One of the most likely hypotheses is that the primary defect is an impaired epidermal barrier function which results in increased protein antigen penetration through the epidermis and predisposes toward a Th2-dominated immune response [3], thereby facilitating bacterial and viral infections. An alternative hypothesis would be that the primary abnormality lies in the innate immune system that collectively affects the development and severity of AD [4]. In view of the clinical finding that there is no predisposition to any systemic infections in the majority of AD patients, we can postulate that there must be some intrinsic defects in innate defense mechanisms, particularly in the skin. Because regulatory T (T_{reg}) cells are shown to protect against the development of virus-induced inflammatory lesions [5], an imbalance between antiviral immune responses and T_{reg} cells is an alternative attractive candidate responsible for an increased susceptibility to certain viral infections in AD patients. In this review, we discuss recent advances in understanding viral infections associated with AD, with particular emphasis on T_{reg} cells and innate immune responses.

Clinical Aspects of Viral Complications in Atopic Dermatitis

AD patients run a higher risk of developing severe skin superinfections with a number of viruses including herpes simplex virus (HSV), molluscum contagiosum virus and vaccinia virus: after the causative virus they are named eczema herpeticum (EH), eczema molluscatum and eczema vaccinatum, respectively. EH caused by an extensive disseminated cutaneous infection with HSV 1 or 2 is the most commonly recognized viral complication in AD patients [6, 7]. EH was reported for the first time by Kaposi, who recognized similarities of this disease with varicella zoster virus (VZV) infection of the skin. Although the term 'Kaposi's varicelliform eruption' has still been widely used for complications of other skin diseases caused by a disseminated HSV infection, the term EH should be restricted to a disseminated HSV infection in AD or other types of dermatitis [7, 8]. EH can present in a primary form or a recurrent form, and the primary infection is generally considered to be severer with greater cutaneous involvement, lymphadenopathy and fever [9]. However, patients with recurrent HSV infections often develop disseminated vesicular lesions accompanied by systemic symptoms, such as fever, malaise and lymphadenopathy, findings indistinguishable from the primary infection. The eruption is most frequently located on the face, neck and the upper part of the chest, forearms and wrists while milder cases have lesions limited to the head and neck [9]. The vesicles rapidly evolve to pustules (fig. 1) or dry out, forming crusts. The vesiculopustular lesions tend to occur in areas where the skin has been most severely affected by the underlying skin disease in the primary form. Primary infections are thought to directly spread to a diseased cutaneous region by dissemination or autoinoculation. However, given that even recurrent EH lesions often occur in the previously affected site, the dissemination of vesiculopustular lesions is likely not true autoinoculation derived from the original infection site but may represent reactivation from viral latency at the site. Thus, it is difficult to distinguish between a primary infection and reactivation on clinical grounds alone without the aid of serological assays. These findings, together with the observation

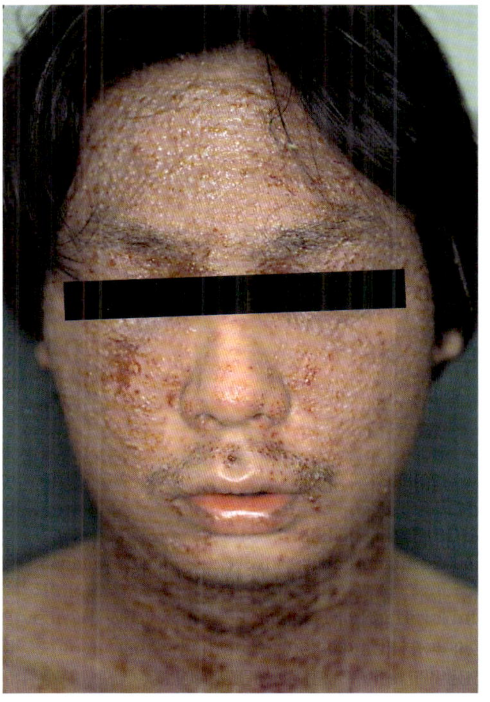

Fig. 1. Numerous, umbilicated pustules, erosions with purulent exudate and crusts cover the face and neck.

that severe, untreated AD lesions have EH develop more easily than patients with well-controlled disease [7], suggest that AD patients with uncontrolled eczematous lesions are at greater risk for the development of this viral complication. Consistently with this view, Wollenberg et al. [7] reported that the majority of the patients with EH had not received any corticosteroid therapy in the 4 weeks before the onset of EH, which suggests the possibility that EH may occur as a result of rebounding immune responses after withdrawal of topical corticosteroids. According to a retrospective study by Wollenberg et al. [7], risk factors for the development of EH are an early onset of AD and a high total serum IgE.

Although herpetic keratitis and herpetic meningitis are serious sequelae of EH, they are rare in the setting of EH [10]. Secondary bacterial infection is common and oral antibiotics are frequently given to treat bacterial superinfection. EH can often be associated with streptococcal impetigo, as a sequela of EH. Before the availability of acyclovir, the mortality rate of EH was approximately 75% [6]. The mainstay of therapy for EH is a nucleoside analog, such as acyclovir, valacyclovir and famciclovir. The use of topical or systemic corticosteroids is controversial, particularly in the acute phase of EH; however, most physicians suggest to avoid topical and systemic corticosteroids. Oral antibiotics are frequently given to prevent bacterial superinfection, because EH may be followed by group A β-hemolytic streptococcus or *Staphylococcus aureus* infections. If no response is seen upon these therapies, resistance to acyclovir or related drugs is a possibility: these patients should be treated with foscarnet, vidarabine or cidofovir [11]. Because severe recurrence of EH can take place in some AD patients who often interrupt topical treatment with corticosteroids, prophylactic acyclovir or valacyclovir can be a therapeutic option that may reduce recurrence.

Pathomechanisms of Eczema Herpeticum

EH occurs almost exclusively in patients with AD, particularly in those who fail to control the skin lesions. The reason why patients with AD or those with a history of AD are at great risk for the development of EH remains unknown. A dysfunctional epidermal barrier and decreased innate immune responses are possible predisposing factors, both of which will be described in detail in the next section. Another mechanism whereby this may exclusively occur in patients with AD is the involvement of CD4+ T_{reg} cells. The protective immunity to HSV in humans depends on CD4+ and CD8+ T effector (T_{eff}) cell populations that recognize viral antigens: on the other hand, damage to the skin is also initiated by these T_{eff} cell populations [12, 13], pointing to a critical role of HSV-specific T cells not only in the resolution, but also in the initiation of HSV lesions. Because T_{reg} cells are known to suppress such excessive T_{eff} cell responses to HSV, thereby limiting T_{eff}-mediated immunopathology, it has been tempting to speculate that an imbalance in the proportion of T_{eff} to T_{reg} cells may contribute to the development of EH. There are conflicting data with respect to T_{reg} cells in AD: many studies have reported an increase in the frequencies of circulating T_{reg} cells in patients with AD [14–16], while others demonstrated that AD patients with active lesions had a lower T_{reg} cell level than asymptomatic control subjects with similar levels of serum γ-interferon, total IgE and eosinophils and that T_{reg} cell frequencies correlated inversely with the severity of disease [17, 18]. However, no previous studies assessed alterations in their frequencies and functional properties depending on the clinical symptoms in patients with AD, particularly those associated with EH. Thus, it remains unknown how alterations of T_{reg} cell frequencies and functions could contribute to the initiation and resolution of EH lesions. Nevertheless, T_{reg} cells in AD with recurrent episodes of EH have not been extensively studied during the course of the illness.

Accordingly, we sequentially analyzed T_{reg} cell numbers and function at different stages of the illness. Nine patients with adult-type AD, who developed EH, were enrolled in this study. Eight patients out of the 9 were positive for HSV IgG and had recurrent HSV infection but with or without a history of EH: they were defined as recurrent EH. One patient was positive for HSV IgM without HSV IgG and had no history of EH: the patient was assumed to have primary HSV infection. AD patients who were positive for HSV IgG but had no EH at their presentation were selected as age-matched AD controls and defined as ADEH–. AD patients with EH had a significantly higher frequency of CD4+Foxp3+ T_{reg} cells in peripheral blood mononuclear cells at onset as compared with that after resolution and that in ADEH– cases. The increased T_{reg} cells at onset of EH exhibited phenotype characteristics similar to those in ADEH– patients and in healthy controls. After resolution of EH, the frequencies of Foxp3+ T_{reg} cells decreased to values similar to those in ADEH– and in healthy controls. These results suggest that expanded T_{reg} cells were contracted upon clinical resolution and that EH can be only aborted by a timely decrease in T_{reg} cell frequencies. We next analyzed T_{reg} cell frequencies in a single AD patient with primary EH over the ensuing 6-month period. In this patient, T_{reg} cells also increased at onset in the same range as what we observed in other AD patients with recurrent EH. Contrary to our expectation, however, after clinical resolution the frequency of T_{reg} cells remained elevated: the clinical improvement of EH was not associated with the decrease in T_{reg} cell frequency, a finding never observed in recurrent EH. However, the frequencies of T_{reg} cells eventually decreased. Since then, a flare of EH was no longer seen. These results indicate that a timely decrease in T_{reg} cell frequency may help prevent the further development of EH.

Because our recent study has demonstrated that the functional activity of T_{reg} cells was profoundly altered depending on the stage in severe drug eruptions [19], we next asked whether changes in T_{reg} cell frequency could be associated with alterations in T_{reg} cell function. Our functional assay showed that T_{reg} cells obtained from AD patients with EH retained the suppressive capacity to inhibit proliferation of T_{reg} cells, similar to that of healthy controls. In view of their increased frequency at onset, the net suppressive effects of T_{reg} cells could be maximal during the acute stage of EH. This was reflected in the impairment of γ-interferon production by CD8+ T cells and natural killer (NK) cells in these AD patients with EH. The impaired ability of these cells to produce γ-interferon was restored to levels comparable to those in healthy controls, upon a contraction of T_{reg} cells after clinical resolution. These findings suggest that an increase in T_{reg} cell frequencies would serve to attenuate anti-HSV immune responses necessary for elimination of HSV (fig. 2). This increase in T_{reg} cell frequency would contribute to HSV reactivation by prematurely limiting anti-HSV effector cell responses. Indeed, our immunohistochemical studies demonstrated that increased numbers of Foxp3+ T_{reg} cells occurred in the vicinity of HSV- and VZV-expressing cells in the EH lesions; interestingly, reactivations of VZV can also be seen in some EH lesions (fig. 3). Thus, an increase in the frequencies of T_{reg} cells observed at the onset of EH might be a cause of viral reactivation, but not a mere consequence.

If increased frequencies of T_{reg} cells are responsible at least in part for HSV reactivation in recurrent EH, then a question arises which factors are responsible for driving T_{reg} cell expansions that may induce HSV reactivations. In a recent retrospective analysis of 100 cases of EH, it has been described that 36% of the patients with EH had noted a severe exacerbation of their AD which had typically started 2 weeks before the onset of EH and that the majority of the patients had not received any corticosteroid therapy in the 4 weeks before the onset of EH [7]. A likely interpretation of these

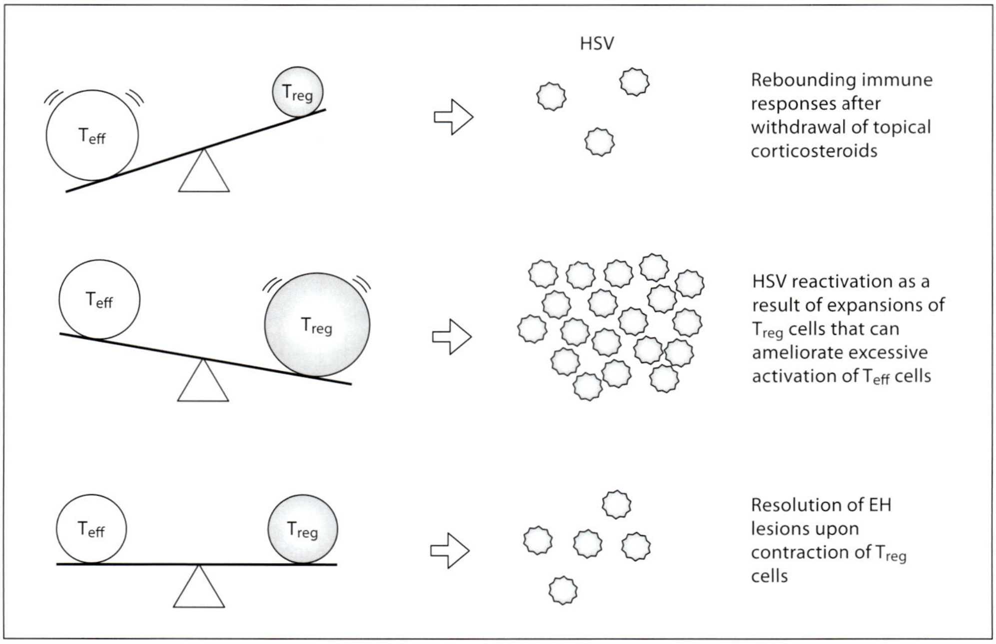

Fig. 2. The balance between T_{reg} cells and antiviral T_{eff} cells before the onset of EH and during the course of EH.

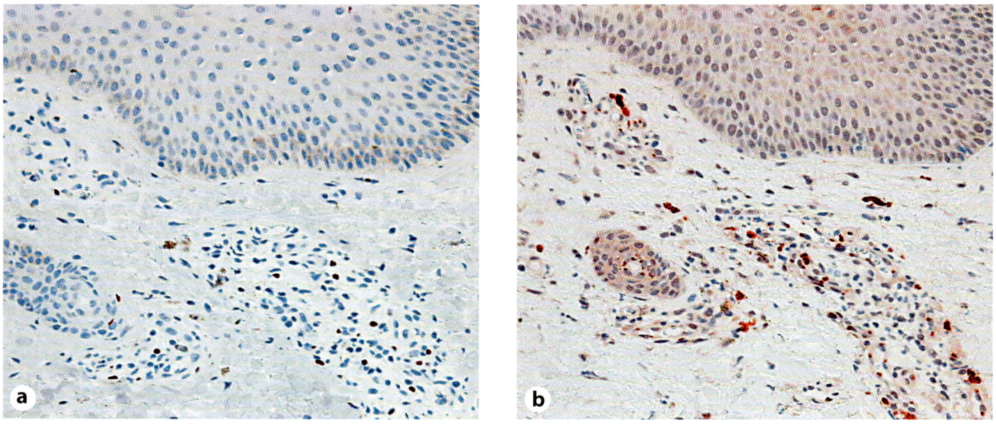

Fig. 3. Positive immunohistochemical staining for T_{reg} cells (**a**) and VZV antigen (**b**) in EH lesions.

observations is that an abrupt shift of host immune responses from a well-controlled state to a robust rebounding, pathogenic inflammatory state would occur upon withdrawal of immunosuppressive agents, such as corticosteroids in AD patients, which could be manifested as an exacerbation of clinical symptoms long before the onset of EH. Probably, this shift would allow latent HSV to be reactivated in an uncontrolled fashion. According to this scenario, expansions of T_{reg} cells initially required for preventing excessive pathogenic inflammation as a result of withdrawal of topical corticosteroids could in turn contribute to HSV reactivation, resulting in the initiation and progression of EH. These data propose a dual role of T_{reg} cells, either beneficial or harmful, by ameliorating the tissue-damaging effects of antiviral immune responses at the site of inflammation depending on how and when they are expanded. This scenario provides a potential explanation for why apparently disparate data on the role of T_{reg} cells in the pathogenesis of AD have been reported: this is due in part to a neglect in previous studies of evaluating the effects of T_{reg} cells on HSV reactivation.

Decreased Innate Immune Responses in Atopic Dermatitis

Decreased innate immune responses might also explain the susceptibility of AD patients to recurrent viral infections. An aberrant overwhelming Th2-dominated immune response in AD can also be caused by a dysfunction or failure of innate immune responses. In view of the fact that innate immune cells mediate a first line of defense against a wide variety of pathogens and determine the nature of subsequent acquired immune responses to these pathogens [20–22], one can imagine that innate immune cells are functionally defective in patients with AD. Indeed, we previously provided evidence to indicate that NK cells and γδ+ T cells from AD patients are prone to undergo apoptosis upon cell-to-cell contact with activated monocytes and that this preferential apoptosis is the major mechanism responsible for a sustained impairment of Th1 immune responses and increased susceptibility to cutaneous infections, both of which are the hallmarks of AD [23]. It remained unknown, however, whether the functional defect in AD resides fundamentally in the monocytes or the NK cells and γδ+ T cells. In view of recent observations that production of, or responsiveness to, IL-12 is clearly reduced in AD patients [24–26], prime candidates that are defective in AD patients would be a monocyte population rather than NK cells and γδ+ T cells. In support of this possibility, our previous study showed that the removal of monocytes from the culture restored the ability of NK cells and γδ+ T cells from AD patients to produce Th1 cytokines [23].

To determine which arms of innate immune responses are impaired in AD patients, attention should be focused on the fact that AD patients exhibit the increased susceptibility to limited pathogens, *S. aureus*, *Streptococcus pyogenes* and HSV [27–30], while preserving their capacity to mount innate immune responses to other pathogens. These findings suggest that the failure of AD patients to control these infections might result from either absence or inadequacy of innate immune responses to these pathogens, all of which are shown to stimulate Toll-like receptor (TLR) 2 [27, 31–33]. Thus, abnormalities in the TLR2 signaling pathway are likely potential targets in elucidating the pathomechanism of AD. In recent years, attention has been focused on TLR2 pathway defects.

TLR2 can recognize a remarkably broad range of pathogen-associated molecular patterns by homodimerizing as well as heterodimerizing with TLR1 and 6 [34]. Indeed, mice deficient in TLR2 and its downstream effector MyD88 were shown to be highly susceptible to an intravenous inoculation of *S. aureus* [35]. Ahmad-Nejad et al. [36] reported that a missense mutation in the *TLR2* gene R753Q is increased in AD patients with a severer phenotype characterized by markedly elevated IgE antibody levels and increased disease severity which renders these AD patients highly susceptible to *S. aureus* colonization.

We have recently demonstrated that TLR2-mediated proinflammatory cytokine (IL-1β and tumor necrosis factor α) production by monocytes was selectively impaired in AD patients when stimulated with the synthetic TLR2 ligand S-[2,3-bis(palmitoyloxy)-(2-RS)-propyl]-N-palmitoyl-R-Cys-S-Ser-S-Lys_4-OH trihydrochloride [37]: this impairment can be demonstrated with TLR2-mediated stimulation while phorbol-myristate-acetate- or TLR4-mediated proinflammatory cytokine production by the monocytes is not impaired [37]. This selective impairment cannot be explained by differences in cell surface TLR2 expression, because the levels of TLR2 and TLR4 expression on monocytes from AD patients were not significantly different from that in healthy controls [37]. Interestingly, the most remarkable reduction in TLR2-mediated proinflammatory cytokine production by monocytes was observed in the proinflammatory monocytes (CD14dimCD16+HLA-DR+ monocytes) expressing high FcεRI levels from AD patients, but not in those expressing low FcεRI levels [37]. These results suggest that cell surface FcεRI levels on monocytes regulate ongoing innate immune responses to invading pathogens. Therefore, it seems reasonable to speculate that the inhibitory effects FcεRI exerted on TLR2-mediated cytokine production by monocytes could be restored by reducing their FcεRI expression levels. In view of the notion that full activation of TLR2-mediated immune responses might require the assembly of receptor signaling complexes that influence signal transduction [38], the magnitude and consequences of TLR2-mediated immune responses could be influenced by coactivation through other transmembrane receptors. If so, the interplay between FcεRI and TLR2 might be essential in controlling cutaneous microbial infections and host skin inflammatory responses in AD patients. In support of this possibility, we have recently demonstrated that TLR2- and FcεRI-mediated responses counterregulate one another in mast cells [Mizukawa et al., manuscript submitted]. By analogy with our results, monocytes from AD patients heterozygous for the TLR2 R753Q mutation have been reported to produce dramatically less IL-8 than those from patients lacking this mutation [39]. In addition to monocytes, NK cells have been shown to play an important role in regulating ensuing acquired antiviral immune responses: they are shown to negatively regulate the duration and effectiveness of virus-specific CD4+ and CD8+ T cell responses by limiting exposure of T cells to infected antigen-presenting cells [40].

The production of antimicrobial peptides is also an important component of the cutaneous innate immune response. Antimicrobial peptides can directly kill not only a broad spectrum of microbes including Gram-positive and -negative bacteria, fungi and certain viruses, but also act as a link between innate and acquired immune responses [41, 42]. Human cathelicidin (LL-37) and some defensins have been shown to be chemoattractant for neutrophils, monocytes and T cells [42]. Because LL-37 possesses antiviral activity against HSV and skin from ADEH+ patients exhibits significantly lower levels of LL-37 expression than skin from ADEH– patients [43], a deficiency of LL-37 might render AD patients susceptible to the development of EH.

Conclusion

Viral clearance is a multifactorial process that involves a series of events mediated by T cells, monocytes, dendritic cells, NK cells and B cells, all of which work in combination and in sequence to resolve viral infections. Because each immune cell does not contribute equally to limit viral persistence, it is difficult to explain a special susceptibility to viral infections in atopic subjects solely by a functional defect in a single immune cell population. Possibly the variations in the functional level and/or impact of these immune cells between individuals may explain differences in the ability of each individual to control viral infections. Immune homeostasis in the skin immune system may rely on a delicate balance between the ability of immune cells to react to viral infections and the ability not to react with other harmless microbes, and if so, the imbalance may result in the loss of viral clearance and overwhelming Th2 responses to environmental allergens in AD.

Acknowledgment

This work was supported in part by grants from the Ministry of Education, Culture, Sports, Science and Technology (to T.S.) and Health and Labour Sciences Research Grants (Research on Intractable Diseases) from the Ministry of Health, Labour and Welfare of Japan (to T.S.).

References

1 Akdis CA, Akdis M, Bieber T, Bindslev-Jensen C, Boguniewicz M, Eigenmann P, Hamid Q, Kapp A, Leung DY, Lipozencic J, Luger TA, Muraro A, Novak N, Platts-Mills TA, Rosenwasser L, Scheynius A, Simons FE, Spergel J, Turjanmaa K, Wahn U, Weidinger S, Werfel T, Zuberbier T: Diagnosis and treatment of atopic dermatitis in children and adults: European Academy of Allergology and Clinical Immunology/American Academy of Allergy, Asthma and Immunology/PRACTALL Consensus Report. J Allergy Clin Immunol 2006; 118:152–169.

2 Homey B, Steinhoff M, Ruzicka T, Leung DY: Cytokines and chemokines orchestrate atopic skin inflammation. J Allergy Clin Immunol 2006;118: 178–189.

3 Kondo H, Ichikawa Y, Imokawa G: Percutaneous sensitization with allergens through barrier-disrupted skin elicits a Th2-dominant cytokine response. Eur J Immunol 1998;28:769–779.

4 De Benedetto A, Agnihothri R, McGirt LY, Barkova LG, Beck LA: Atopic dermatitis: a disease caused by innate immune defects? J Invest Dermatol 2009;129: 14–30.

5 Suvas S, Azkur AK, Kim BS, Kumaraguru U, Rouse BT: CD4+CD25+ regulatory T cells control the severity of viral immunoinflammatory lesions. J Immunol 2004;172:4123–4132.
6 Wollenberg A, Wetzel S, Burgdorf WH, Haas J: Viral infections in atopic dermatitis: pathogenic aspects and clinical management. J Allergy Clin Immunol 2003;112:667–674.
7 Wollenberg A, Zoch C, Wetzel S, Plewig G, Przybilla B: Predisposing factors and clinical features of eczema herpeticum: a retrospective analysis of 100 cases. J Am Acad Dermatol 2003;49:198–205.
8 Bussmann C, Peng WM, Bieber T, Novak N: Molecular pathogenesis and clinical implications of eczema herpeticum. Expert Rev Mol Med 2008;10: 1–8.
9 Wheeler CE Jr, Abele DC: Eczema herpeticum, primary and recurrent. Arch Dermatol 1966;93: 162–171.
10 Bork K, Brauninger W: Increasing incidence of eczema herpeticum: analysis of seventy-five cases. J Am Acad Dermatol 1988;19:1024–1029.
11 Chilukuri S, Rosen T: Management of acyclovir-resistant herpes simplex virus. Dermatol Clin 2003; 21:311–320.
12 Koelle DM, Posavad CM, Barnum GR, Johnson ML, Frank JM, Corey L: Clearance of HSV-2 from recurrent genital lesions correlates with infiltration of HSV-specific cytotoxic T lymphocytes. J Clin Invest 1998;101:1500–1508.
13 Banerjee K, Biswas PS, Kumaraguru U, Schoenberger SP, Rouse BT: Protective and pathological roles of virus-specific and bystander CD8+ T cells in herpetic stromal keratitis. J Immunol 2004;173:7575–7583.
14 Reefer AJ, Satinover SM, Solga MD, Lannigan JA, Nguyen JT, Wilson BB, Woodfolk JA: Analysis of CD25hiCD4+ 'regulatory' T-cell subtypes in atopic dermatitis reveals a novel Th2-like population. J Allergy Clin Immunol 2008;121:415–422.
15 Szegedi A, Baráth S, Nagy G, Szodoray P, Gál M, Sipka S, Bagdi E, Banham AH, Krenács L: Regulatory T cells in atopic dermatitis: epidermal dendritic cell clusters may contribute to their local expansion. Br J Dermatol 2009;160:984–993.
16 Ito Y, Adachi Y, Makino T, Higashiyama H, Fuchizawa T, Shimizu T, Miyawaki T: Expansion of FOXP3-positive CD4+CD25+ T cells associated with disease activity in atopic dermatitis. Ann Allergy Asthma Immunol 2009;103:160–165.
17 Verhagen J, Akdis M, Traidl-Hoffimann C, Schmid-Grendelmeier P, Hijnen D, Knol EF, Behrendt H, Blaser K, Akdis CA: Absence of T-regulatory cell expression and function in atopic dermatitis skin. J Allergy Clin Immunol 2006;117:176–183.
18 Orihara K, Narita M, Tobe T, Akasawa A, Ohya Y, Matsumoto K, Saito H: Circulating Foxp3+CD4+ cell numbers in atopic patients and healthy control subjects. J Allergy Clin Immunol 2007;120: 960–962.
19 Takahashi R, Kano Y, Yamazaki Y, Kimishima M, Mizukawa Y, Shiohara T. Defective regulatory T cells in patients with severe drug eruptions: timing of the dysfunction is associated with the pathological phenotype and outcome. J Immunol 2009;182: 8071–8079.
20 Janeway CA Jr, Medzhitov R: Innate immune recognition. Annu Rev Immunol 2002;20:197–216.
21 Goodarzi H, Trowbridge J, Gallo RL: Innate immunity: a cutaneous perspective. Clin Rev Allergy Immunol 2007;33:15–26.
22 Takeda K, Kaisho T, Akira S: Toll-like receptors. Annu Rev Immunol 2003;21:335–376.
23 Katsuta M, Takigawa Y, Kimishima M, Inaoka M, Takahashi R, Shiohara T: NK cells and gamma delta+ T cells are phenotypically and functionally defective due to preferential apoptosis in patients with atopic dermatitis. J Immunol 2006;176: 7736–7744.
24 Matsui E, Kaneko H, Teramoto T, Fukao T, Inoue R, Kasahara K, Takemura M, Seishima M, Kondo N: Reduced IFN gamma production in response to IL-12 stimulation and/or reduced IL-12 production in atopic patients. Clin Exp Allergy 2000;30: 1250–1256.
25 Kondo N, Matsui E, Kaneko H, Aoki M, Kato Z, Fukao T, Kasahara K, Morimoto N: RNA editing of interleukin-12 receptor beta2, 2451 C-to-U (Ala604Val) conversion, associated with atopy. Clin Exp Allergy 2004;34:363–368.
26 Reider N, Reider D, Ebner S, Holzmann S, Herold M, Fritsch P, Romani N: Dendritic cells contribute to the development of atopy by an insufficiency in IL-12 production. J Allergy Clin Immunol 2002;109: 89–95.
27 Kang SS, Kauls LS, Gaspari AA: Toll-like receptors: applications to dermatologic disease. J Am Acad Dermatol 2006;54:951–983.
28 Homey B, Steinhoff M, Ruzicka T, Leung DY: Cytokines and chemokines orchestrate atopic skin inflammation. J Allergy Clin Immunol 2006;118: 178–189.
29 McGirt LY, Beck LA: Innate immune defects in atopic dermatitis. J Allergy Clin Immunol 2006;118: 202–208.
30 De Benedetto A, Agnihothri R, McGirt LY, Bankova LG, Beck LA: Atopic dermatitis: a disease caused by innate immune defects? J Invest Dermatol 2009;129: 14–30.

31 Takeuchi O, Hoshino K, Kawai T, Sanjo H, Takada H, Ogawa T, Takeda K, Akira S: Differential roles of TLR2 and TLR4 in recognition of Gram-negative and Gram-positive bacterial cell wall components. Immunity 1999;11:443–451.
32 Miller LS, O'Connell RM, Gutierrez MA, Pietras EM, Shahangian A, Gross CE, Thirumala A, Cheung AL, Cheng G, Modlin RL: MyD88 mediates neutrophil recruitment initiated by IL-1R but not TLR2 activation in immunity against *Staphylococcus aureus*. Immunity 2006;24:79–91.
33 Kurt-Jones EA, Chan M, Zhou S, Wang J, Reed G, Bronson R, Amold MM, Knipe DM, Finberg RW: Herpes simplex virus 1 interaction with Toll-like receptor 2 contributes to lethal encephalitis. Proc Natl Acad Sci USA 2004;101:1315–1320.
34 Triantafilou M, Gamper FG, Haston RM, Mouratis MA, Morath S, Hartung T, Triantafilou K: Membrane sorting of Toll-like receptor (TLR)-2/6 and TLR2/1 heterodimers at the cell surface determines heterotypic associations with CD36 and intracellular targeting. J Biol Chem 2006;281: 31002–31011.
35 Takeuchi O, Hoshino K, Akira S: Cutting edge: TLR2-deficient and MyD88- deficient mice are highly susceptible to *Staphylococcus aureus* infection. J Immunol 2000;165:5392–5396.
36 Ahmad-Nejad P, Mrabet-Dahbi S, Breuer K, Klotz M, Werfel T, Herz U, Heeg K, Neumaier M, Renz H: The Toll-like receptor 2 R753Q polymorphism defines a subgroup of patients with atopic dermatitis having severe phenotype. J Allergy Clin Immunol 2004;113:565–567.
37 Hasannejad H, Takahashi R, Kimishima M, Hayakawa K, Shiohara T: Selective impairment of Toll-like receptor 2-mediated proinflammatory cytokine production by monocytes from patients with atopic dermatitis. J Allergy Clin Immunol 2007;120:69–75.
38 Underhill DM: Toll-like receptors: networking for success. Eur J Immunol 2003;33:1767–1775.
39 Mrabet-Dahbi S, Dalpke AH, Niebuhr M, Frey M, Draing C, Brand S, Heeg K, Werfel T, Renz H: The Toll-like receptor 2 R753Q mutation modifies cytokine production and Toll-like receptor expression in atopic dermatitis. J Allergy Clin Immunol 2008;121:1013–1019.
40 Andrews DM, Estcourt MJ, Andoniou CE, Wikstrom ME, Khong A, Voigt V, Fleming P, Tabarias H, Hill GR, van der Most RG, Scalzo AA, Smyth MJ, Degli-Esposti MA: Innate immunity defines the capacity of antiviral T cells to limit persistent infection. J Exp Med 2010;207: 1333–1343.
41 Izadpanah A, Gallo RL: Antimicrobial peptides. J Am Acad Dermatol 2005;52:381–390.
42 Yang D, Chertov O, Oppenheim JJ: Participation of mammalian defensins and cathelicidins in anti-microbial immunity: receptors and activities of human defensins and cathelicidin (LL-37). J Leukoc Biol 2001;69:691–697.
43 Howell MD, Wollenberg A, Gallo RL, Flaig M, Streib JE, Wong C, Pavicic T, Boguniewicz M, Leung DY: Cathelicidin deficiency predisposes to eczema herpeticum. J Allergy Clin Immunol 2006;117: 836–841.

Tetsuo Shiohara, MD, PhD
Department of Dermatology
Kyorin University School of Medicine
6-20-2 Shinkawa, Mitaka, Tokyo 181-8611 (Japan)
Tel. +81 422 47 5511, Fax +81 422 41 4741, E-Mail tpshio@ks.kyorin-u.ac.jp

Shiohara T (ed): Pathogenesis and Management of Atopic Dermatitis.
Curr Probl Dermatol. Basel, Karger, 2011, vol 41, pp 136–148

Biomarkers for Itch and Disease Severity in Atopic Dermatitis

Chih-Hung Lee[a,b] · Hsin-Su Yu[b]

[a]Department of Dermatology, Kaohsiung Municipal Hsiao-Kang Hospital, and [b]Department of Dermatology, Kaohsiung Medical University Hospital and Kaohsiung Medical University, Graduate Institute of Medicine, Kaohsiung, Taiwan, ROC

Abstract

Atopic dermatitis (AD) is a common allergic disease and constitutes a huge social and economic burden for the whole country. AD usually heralds other allergic diseases, such as asthma and allergic rhinitis. The pathogenesis of AD remains to be studied but generally includes abnormal skin barrier and aberrant cutaneous immune responses. Biomarkers are important in monitoring disease severity, prognosis and treatment responses. With the investigation and robust knowledge on AD pathophysiology, more and more biomarkers are being explored. Aberrant cutaneous inflammation is associated with Th2 polarization, chemokine upregulation in Langerhans cells and keratinocytes, IgE production by B cells, and degranulation of mast cells and eosinophils, subsequently leading to changes in the levels of cell-specific biomarkers in blood or urine. Furthermore, skin barrier abnormalities, including increased transepidermal water loss and decreased skin hydration, are biomarkers for severity and itch intensity in AD. Cross-talk between skin barrier abnormalities and aberrant immune responses is evidenced by epidermal abnormalities enhancing the release of keratinocyte-derived cytokines and chemokines, including CC chemokine ligand (CCL) 17, CCL27 and thymic stromal lymphopoietin, resulting in modulation of skin immune responses. The pathophysiology of itch in AD remains unclear. The subjective nature of itch makes biomarkers to estimate its intensity crucial in AD patients. Pruritus results from the activation of small nerve endings in the skin by noxious mediators, including neuropeptides, proinflammatory cytokines and prostaglandins, all of which might serve as potential biomarkers for itch. Recently, IL-31 and gastrin-releasing peptide have been reported to be involved in the development of itch, making the estimation of itch intensity a future reality. With the enormous amount of research in immunology, skin physiology and neurology in AD, more biomarkers in AD and its itch will be found in the near future.

Atopic dermatitis (AD) is a common allergic disease that is estimated to affect approximately 10% of the population. In recent years, there has been an increasing trend of AD prevalence in many developed countries. The chronic and relapsing course with intractable itch results in considerable suffering, impaired school and work performance, poor quality of life and substantial economic costs. It commonly heralds other allergic diseases, such as bronchial asthma, allergic rhinitis and allergic conjunctivitis, adding further to the health and economic burden [1]. Siblings and parents of AD patients are more likely to develop those allergic diseases [2]. AD can be classified based on its association with IgE, including an IgE-associated (extrinsic) and a non-IgE-associated (intrinsic) form. This implies they might be two distinct diseases [3]. However, in both AD types, dry skin due to abnormal barrier function is characteristic, and the absence of IgE sensitization is mostly only a transient factor [4]. The disease intensity in AD can be evaluated by several scoring systems, including the most commonly used SCORAD Index [5] and the Eczema Area and Severity Index [6].

Pathogenesis

There are many theories in AD pathogenesis. It is commonly believed that AD is a multifactorial disease with genetic and environmental components. To date, skin barrier abnormalities and immunological dysfunctions are usually indicated in the pathogenesis of AD. First, an impaired skin barrier is associated with the development of AD [7]. Profiles of ceramide, an intrinsic emollient, are altered in AD skin. Skin hydration is reduced even in grossly normal skin from AD patients [8]. Reconstitution of the skin barrier with emollients successfully alleviates AD severity and itch intensity. Filaggrin, a protein expressed in the upper epidermal layer, plays an important role in epidermal differentiation as well as intact barrier functions. Filaggrin mutations are found in 18–48% of patients with AD in the USA, Japan and Europe by several groups with case-control studies [9]. The two most common mutations (R501X and 2282del4) account for the majority of cases, while over 10 different other mutations have been reported. Patients with filaggrin-related AD have increased disease severity and defects in skin barrier function, as shown by poor transepidermal water loss (TEWL) and skin hydration [10], indicating a critical role of skin barrier abnormalities in AD pathogenesis. Second, AD patients are subject to various cutaneous infections, such as staphylococci and herpes simplex virus [11]. This susceptibility might result from both impaired innate and adaptive immunological responses [12]. In the acute Th2-predominant stage, macrophages and eosinophils are attracted by chemokines, while in the chronic mixed stage, interleukin (IL) 12 activates the Th1 response [13]. The immunological triggers in AD include aeroallergens, food allergens, microbes, autoallergens and contact allergens. In the Th2-predominant stage, degranulation of eosinophils [14] results in the release of several toxin proteins, such as eosinophil cationic protein (ECP) or major basic protein, that drive further inflammation [15]. In monocytes, prostaglandin E_2 production is enhanced, which in turn induces IL-4, IL-5 and IL-13 while it suppresses γ-interferon [16]

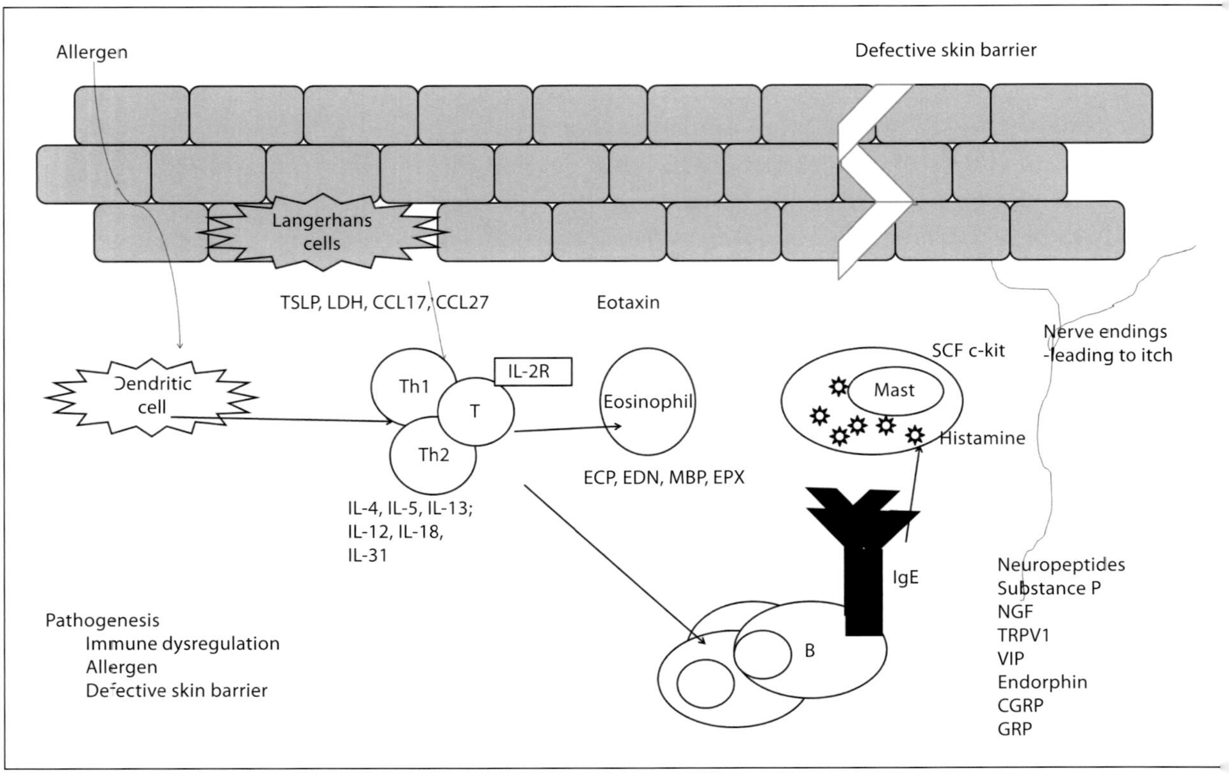

Fig. 1. Potential clinical biomarkers for AD and its itch. LDH = Lactate dehydrogenase; TSLP = thymic stromal lymphopoietin; CCL = CC chemokine ligand; MBP = major basic protein; EDN = eosinophil-derived neurotoxin; EPX = eosinophil protein X; SCF = stem cell factor; c-kit = cellular tyrosine kinase transmembrane receptor; NGF = nerve growth factor; TRPV1 = transient receptor potential V1; VIP = vasoactive intestinal peptide; CGRP = calcitonin gene-related peptide; GRP = gastrin-releasing peptide.

Biomarkers in Atopic Dermatitis

A biomarker is defined as a parameter that can be used to measure disease severity, disease progression or treatment effectiveness [17]. The parameter can be chemical, physical or biological. Effective and reliable biomarkers can help in many aspects of patient care and research, including early diagnosis, risk assessment, disease prevention and personalized treatment. Biomarkers are associated with the disease process and pathogenesis. Thus, understanding the pathophysiology of AD is of paramount importance to appreciate the translational significance of those biomarkers.

Depending on the clinical applications, biomarkers can be classified as severity markers, diagnostic markers, prognostic markers and drug-related markers. Biomarkers in AD are summarized in figure 1 and table 1. Most of the AD biomarkers belong to the severity markers. They may be further classified by their source:

Table 1. Severity biomarkers that have been reported in atopic dermatitis

Blood	Marker	Reference no.
Immunoglobulin	IgE	8
Cytokines	IL-31	84
	IL-12	27, 85, 86
	IL-18	27, 28, 85
Chemokines	Macrophage-derived cytokine (CCL28)	56, 87, 88
	Cutaneous T-cell-attracting chemokine (CCL10)	44, 46
	Thymus- and activation-regulated chemokine (CCL17)	47–49
	Eotaxin	89
	CCL22, CCL27	90
Eosinophil-related	Eosinophil cationic protein	2, 30, 38
	Major basic protein	35
Other soluble factors	E-selectin	39, 91, 92
	L-selectin	93
	Soluble IL-2 receptor	30, 31, 38
	Soluble CD30	41, 42
	Soluble stem cell factor and cellular tyrosine kinase transmembrane receptor	37
	Tissue inhibitor of metalloproteinase 1	94
	Lactate dehydrogenase	95
	Squamous cell carcinoma antigen	43
Neuropeptides	β-Endorphin	8, 96
	Brain-derived neurotrophic factor	97, 98
	Nerve growth factor	73, 74
	Substance P	73, 75
Urine	Eosinophil-derived neurotoxin	38, 99
	Eosinophil protein X	34
Skin barrier	TEWL	8, 100
	Hydration	2
	pH	2

CCL = CC chemokine ligand.

eosinophils, keratinocytes, mast cells and T cells. In contrast, there is no single reliable diagnostic biomarker for AD. IgE is increased in about 80% of AD patients. IgE is among the 20 minor criteria for AD in the diagnostic criteria of Hanifin and Rajka [18]. Increased blood IgE is helpful to confirm the AD diagnosis but not necessary. Further, IgE might serve as a predictive marker to some extent. The cord blood IgE levels might help in the early detection of infants at risk for atopic disorders [19]. Adult AD patients with high IgE values are expected to have ongoing dermatitis even after a decade [20]. Although blood IgE is not essential to diagnose AD, its elevation in AD defines the phenotype of extrinsic AD (elevated IgE) rather than intrinsic AD (normal IgE). For drug-related biomarkers, less is known; however, those might be explored after the application of advanced and high-throughput genomic profiling methods [21].

Recently a breakthrough in AD pathogenesis has resulted from abnormal expression or mutation of filaggrin, a critical component in epidermal differentiation and skin barrier function [22]. An impaired skin barrier enhances TEWL and decreases skin hydration. In AD, even in the clinically normal skin, those skin barrier parameters are abnormal [23]. In fact, increased TEWL is associated with itch intensity and disease severity in AD [8]. In AD skin, several inflammatory cell types are increased, including T cells, B cells, mast cells, Langerhans cells and eosinophils. There are increased numbers of IgE-bearing Langerhans cells, which are capable of binding allergens by their high-affinity IgE receptors. Langerhans cells are also crucial in the induction of Th2 responses by their antigen-presenting capacity in the skin.

Depending on coactivation signals and the communication between antigen-presenting cells and T cells, T cells can be activated to Th1, Th2, Th17 or regulatory T cell lineages [24]. In AD skin, there is a predominant Th2 activation, resulting in enhancement of Th2 cytokines, including IL-4 and IL-13, both of which are associated with AD disease severity [25]. In AD, there is usually a predominant Th2 cytokine milieu in the initiating stage of acute AD lesions, and a mixed Th1 and Th2 pattern in chronic lesions. Polarized Th2 responses [26] in AD usually result in provocation of allergic responses (increased IgE production by B cells and eosinophilia). As mentioned above, cytokines related to Th2 activation are increased in AD patients. In addition, IL-12 and IL-18 are also associated with disease severity in AD [23, 27]. The correlation between severity and IL-18 was confirmed by a subsequent study in children [28]. Of note, keratinocytes in AD skin can induce Th17 cytokine responses [29].

Th2 polarization further results in eosinophil recruitment and augments the production of IgE by B cells. Hence, eosinophils and their enzymes are increased in skin and blood from AD patients. ECP in blood has been reported to increase in AD patients [30, 31]. However, ECP as an indicator for AD severity is not settled. From a small set of AD patients, people reported that eosinophil-derived neurotoxin may reflect more strongly disease severity in AD patients than serum ECP [32]. A latter study measuring soluble E-selectin, soluble vascular cell adhesion molecule 1 and ECP showed that only soluble E-selectin is positively associated with disease severity [33]. Nevertheless, a recent study showed that ECP is highly associated with AD disease severity [34]. Major basic protein, derived from eosinophils, was also associated with the severity score [35]. Moreover, urinary eosinophil protein X was also reported to reflect AD disease severity [34].

Mast cells are increased in a majority of AD skin lesions [36]. Through IgE receptors in mast cells [36], they can release proinflammatory mediators and enzymes. One of the most important axes in mast cell chemotaxis and proliferation is the axis of stem cell factor and its receptor tyrosine kinase transmembrane receptor. Both soluble stem cell factor and tyrosine kinase transmembrane receptor levels were positively associated with disease severity and diminished after topical corticosteroid treatments [37].

Several soluble factors are also potential biomarkers for AD. L-selectin, which mediates leukocyte rolling in the endothelium, was also reported to be associated with disease severity. Some other reported severity biomarkers include E-selectin [38, 39], intercellular adhesion molecule 1 [40], CD30 [41, 42], IL-2 receptors [31, 38] and squamous cell carcinoma antigen [43].

CC chemokine ligand (CCL) 27 (cutaneous T-cell-attracting chemokine) is produced by basal keratinocytes. Its receptor CC chemokine receptor (CCR) 10 is expressed by circulating skin-homing T cells positive for cutaneous lymphocyte-associated antigen. Thus, keratinocytes in the skin initiate the inflammatory microenvironment through production and release of CCL27 [44]. The cutaneous T-cell-attracting chemokine level in the blood is associated with AD disease severity [45, 46]. Next, thymus- and activation-regulated chemokine (TARC/CCL17) is a chemokine that attracts CCR4+ or CCR8+ cells. Kakinuma et al. [47] reported an association of TARC and severity in 40 Japanese atopic patients. The association was later confirmed in 43 Polish AD patients [48]. In fact, from a population-based study on 1,359 children in Kyushu, Japan, blood TARC appears a very good indicator for biological monitoring of AD [49].

Thymic stromal lymphopoietin (TSLP), an IL-7-like cytokine, can promote the activation of B cells and dendritic cells. TSLP can promote a polarized Th2 response by directly promoting the effector functions of CD4+ Th2 cells. Epidermal-derived TSLP was sufficient to trigger atopy, sensitizing the lung airways to inhaled allergens in the absence of epicutaneous sensitization [50, 51] to develop subsequent airway hyperresponsiveness [50, 52]. Notably, TSLP from keratinocytes induced by double-stranded RNA is enhanced by the addition of IL-4 and IL-13 [52] and basophils while simultaneously inhibiting the expression of dendritic cell-derived proinflammatory cytokines and promoting regulatory T-cell responses in skin [53]. Thus, a complex interplay between adaptive and innate immunity networks coordinately contributes to AD pathogenesis [54].

Barrier defects and immune alterations can be linked by keratinocytes in the epidermis [55]. CCL28/mucosa-associated epithelial chemokine is involved in trafficking of Th2 cells in the skin. It may represent an objective prognostic marker for disease severity [56]. Of note, many of the cytokines and chemokines actually derive from keratinocytes, major cells in the epidermis. For example, CCL17, CCL27 and TSLP originate from keratinocytes. As chemokines, CCL17, CCL27 and TSLP selectively attract the cells with corresponding chemokine receptors. Further, TSLP is expressed by epidermal keratinocytes and polarizes Th2 allergic responses through dendritic cells in AD and asthma [57]. Filaggrin mutation is noticed in a substantial percentage of AD patients, and it explains the impaired epidermal barrier and the entrance of irritants and allergens [58]. Under Th2-dominant inflammation, keratinocytes produced less fillagrin [25].

The Physiological Biomarkers in Atopic Skin

The severity of AD was highly correlated with serum IgE and lactate dehydrogenase levels [59]. We also found that itch intensity in AD patients was closely related to IgE [8]. By assessing TEWL, pH and hydration, barrier impairment and a particular susceptibility to irritant substances have been documented in healthy skin of patients with AD [60, 61]. We also consistently observed increased TEWL, high pH value and decreased hydration of the stratum corneum in eczematous lesions of AD patients [8].

Patients with AD showed many physiological abnormalities of the skin, such as abnormal sweating, an altered vascular response to mechanical stimuli and an abnormal response to pharmacological agents [62, 63]. In contrast to the decreased microcirculation in normal controls, an aberrant increase in blood flow in AD patients was noted after delivery of the α_1-agonist phenylephrine by iontophoresis [unpubl. data]. The dermal blood vessels and sweat glands are regulated by sympathetic fibers. It is proposed that dysfunction of the sympathetic nerve system exists in AD patients, resulting in perspiration-induced flare-up in AD. The involvement of the sympathetic nerve system in itch needs further exploration.

Biomarkers of Itch Intensity

Itch is defined as an unpleasant sensation to external stimuli. Many diseases can result in itch through different mechanisms. Commonly encountered diseases with intense itch in clinical practice include chronic renal failure, lymphomas, cholestasis, HIV infection and other forms of dermatitis. Itch can be categorized as pruritoceptive, neurogenic, neuropathic and psychogenic [64]. Unmyelinated C fibers transmit itch and thermal changes in the skin [65]. The contralateral spinothalamic tract conveys itch to the thalamus and then projects to the cortex [66]. Mast cells release histamine that binds H_1 receptors in C fibers. Tryptase from mast cells activates protease-activated receptor 2 on afferent C nerve endings, which in turn enhances the release of substance P and ultimately contributes to the initiation of pruritus [67]. Neurotrophins such as nerve growth factor (NGF) are also important itch mediators. NGF causes the proliferation of C fibers and enhances the release of other neuropeptides. Keratinocytes from AD skin express high levels of NGF and its receptor [68]. Further, transient receptor potential V1 channels are expressed on nociceptor-sensory neurons. Capsaicin, depleting substance P in nociceptors via binding to transient receptor potential V1, can inhibit itch sensation [69]. Transient receptor potential V1 activation in keratinocytes leads to release of proinflammatory and pruritic mediators from these cells [70].

There are several very good reviews about the neurophysiology of itch [64, 65, 71, 72]. However, the discussion of mechanisms and biomarkers in diseases other than AD is outside the scope of this article. Herein we focus on the biomarkers of itch in AD. Due to the inflammatory nature of AD and the close association of disease severity and itch intensity in AD patients, it is difficult to define itch intensity alone without taking disease severity and status of inflammation into consideration. Nevertheless, some of the biomarkers in AD seem to be rather specific for itch because they are not present in other nonpruritic inflammatory skin diseases.

Among those, neuropeptides and neurotransmitters deserve further discussion. NGFs and substance P are associated with disease severity and itch in AD [73]. Vasoactive intestinal peptide was also reported to be associated with AD severity and itch [74]. Further, blood β-endorphin is an independent factor to determine itch intensity in AD [8]. Calcitonin gene-related peptide is also implicated in itch pathogenesis [75]. Of note, skin barrier and TEWL also serve as good biomarkers for itch intensity in AD patients [8]. Recently, gastrin-releasing peptide (GRP) and its receptor have been proven to be very important in itch perception and transmission [76, 77]. GRP is increased in the nerve endings of itchy NC/Nga mice [78]. How GRP can be used as a biomarker in AD remains to be determined.

Next, transgenic overexpression of IL-31, a T cell-derived cytokine, in lymphocytes induces severe pruritus and dermatitis in mice. IL-31 receptor subunits are heterodimeric and composed of IL-31 receptor A and oncostatin M receptor, which is expressed on epithelial cells and keratinocytes [79, 80]. Bilsborough et al. [81] first reported that IL-31 receptor A protein was expressed by keratinocytes and infiltrating macrophages in skin biopsy specimens from patients with AD. Comparisons between skin from patients with AD and healthy skin showed IL-31 receptor A expression at higher levels on epidermal keratinocytes in AD samples [81]. Moreover, IL-31 was significantly overexpressed in pruritic atopic skin compared with nonpruritic psoriatic inflamed skin, suggesting that IL-31 plays an important part in pruritus development beyond its proinflammatory action [82]. Using NC/Nga mice which spontaneously develop an eczematous AD-like skin lesion, there was a good association of scratching behavior and expression of IL-31 mRNA in conventional NC/Nga mice [83]. Hence, IL-31 is a potential cytokine that links the cutaneous immunity and pruritus of AD.

Conclusion

Many biomarkers in AD belong to the class of disease severity markers, and they can be used to objectively monitor disease progression and to assess treatment responses. The clinical use of those biomarkers depends on the facility, the costs and the individual biomarkers to reflect true disease biomarkers. IgE remains the most useful biomarker for AD. With more exploration on AD pathophysiology, further developments of disease biomarkers are anticipated in the future.

Acknowledgments

This work is supported by grants from the National Science Council (NSC95-2314-B-037-024, NSC96-2314-B-037-043), National Health Research Institutes (NHRI-EO-096-PP-11; NHRI CN-PD-9611P), Kaohsiung Medical University (KMU-QA096005) and Kaohsiung Medical University Center of Excellence for Environmental Medicine (98.2b). We thank Dr. Peihying (Peggy) Lu for her help in the English editing.

References

1 Kapoor R, Menon C, Hoffstad O, Bilker W, Leclerc P, Margolis DJ: The prevalence of atopic triad in children with physician-confirmed atopic dermatitis. J Am Acad Dermatol 2008;58:68–73.
2 Lee CH, Chuang HY, Shih CC, Jee SH, Wang LF, Chiu HC, Chang CH, Wu CS, Yu HS: Correlation of serum total IgE, eosinophil granule cationic proteins, sensitized allergens and family aggregation in atopic dermatitis patients with or without rhinitis. J Dermatol 2004;31:784–793.
3 Johansson SG, Bieber T, Dahl R, Friedmann PS, Lanier BQ, Lockey RF, Motala C, Ortega Martell JA, Platts-Mills TA, Ring J, Thien F, Van Cauwenberge P, Williams HC: Revised nomenclature for allergy for global use: report of the Nomenclature Review Committee of the World Allergy Organization, October 2003. J Allergy Clin Immunol 2004;113: 832–836.
4 Terui T: Analysis of the mechanism for the development of allergic skin inflammation and the application for its treatment: overview of the pathophysiology of atopic dermatitis. J Pharmacol Sci 2009;110:232–236.
5 Severity scoring of atopic dermatitis: the SCORAD index. Consensus report of the European Task Force on Atopic Dermatitis. Dermatology 1993;186:23–31.
6 Hanifin JM, Thurston M, Omoto M, Cherill R, Tofte SJ, Graeber M: The eczema area and severity index (EASI): assessment of reliability in atopic dermatitis. EASI Evaluator Group. Exp Dermatol 2001;10: 11–18.
7 Jungersted JM, Scheer H, Mempel M, Baurecht H, Cifuentes L, Hogh JK, Hellgren LI, Jemec GB, Agner T, Weidinger S: Stratum corneum lipids, skin barrier function and filaggrin mutations in patients with atopic eczema. Allergy 2010;65:911–918.
8 Lee CH, Chuang HY, Shih CC, Jong SB, Chang CH, Yu HS: Transepidermal water loss, serum IgE and beta-endorphin as important and independent biological markers for development of itch intensity in atopic dermatitis. Br J Dermatol 2006;154: 1100–1107.
9 Brown SJ, Irvine AD: Atopic eczema and the filaggrin story. Semin Cutan Med Surg 2008;27:128–137.
10 Nemoto-Hasebe I, Akiyama M, Nomura T, Sandilands A, McLean WH, Shimizu H: Clinical severity correlates with impaired barrier in filaggrin-related eczema. J Invest Dermatol 2009;129: 682–689.
11 Boguniewicz M, Leung DY: Recent insights into atopic dermatitis and implications for management of infectious complications. J Allergy Clin Immunol 2010;125:4–13, quiz 4–5.
12 De Benedetto A, Agnihothri R, McGirt LY, Bankova LG, Beck LA: Atopic dermatitis: a disease caused by innate immune defects? J Invest Dermatol 2009;129: 14–30.
13 Elias PM, Steinhoff M: 'Outside-to-inside' (and now back to 'outside') pathogenic mechanisms in atopic dermatitis. J Invest Dermatol 2008;128:1067–1070.
14 Leiferman KM: Eosinophils in atopic dermatitis. J Allergy Clin Immunol 1994;94:1310–1317.
15 Homey B, Steinhoff M, Ruzicka T, Leung DY: Cytokines and chemokines orchestrate atopic skin inflammation. J Allergy Clin Immunol 2006;118: 178–189.
16 Snijders A, Van der Pouw Kraan TC, Engel M, Wormmeester J, Widjaja P, Zonneveld IM, Bos JD, Kapsenberg ML: Enhanced prostaglandin E_2 production by monocytes in atopic dermatitis (AD) is not accompanied by enhanced production of IL-6, IL-10 or IL-12. Clin Exp Immunol 1998;111:472–476.

17 Puntmann VO: How-to guide on biomarkers: biomarker definitions, validation and applications with examples from cardiovascular disease. Postgrad Med J 2009;85:538–545.
18 Hanifin J, Rajka G: Diagnostic features of atopic dermatitis. Acta Dermatol Venereol (Stockh) 1980; 92:44–47.
19 Scirica CV, Gold DR, Ryan L, Abulkerim H, Celedon JC, Platts-Mills TA, Naccara LM, Weiss ST, Litonjua AA: Predictors of cord blood IgE levels in children at risk for asthma and atopy. J Allergy Clin Immunol 2007;119:81–88.
20 Katoh N, Hirano S, Kishimoto S: Prognostic factor of adult patients with atopic dermatitis. J Dermatol 2008;35:477–483.
21 Holloway JW, Yang IA, Holgate ST: Genetics of allergic disease. J Allergy Clin Immunol 2010;125: S81–S94.
22 Palmer CN, Irvine AD, Terron-Kwiatkowski A, Zhao Y, Liao H, Lee SP, Goudie DR, Sandilands A, Campbell LE, Smith FJ, O'Regan GM, Watson RM, Cecil JE, Bale SJ, Compton JG, Di Giovanna JJ, Fleckman P, Lewis-Jones S, Arseculeratne G, Sergeant A, Munro CS, El Houate B, McElreavey K, Halkjaer LB, Bisgaard H, Mukhopadhyay S, McLean WH: Common loss-of-function variants of the epidermal barrier protein filaggrin are a major predisposing factor for atopic dermatitis. Nat Genet 2006; 38:441–446.
23 Werner Y, Lindberg M: Transepidermal water loss in dry and clinically normal skin in patients with atopic dermatitis. Acta Derm Venereol 1985;65: 102–105.
24 Weaver CT, Harrington LE, Mangan PR, Gavrieli M, Murphy KM: Th17: an effector CD4 T cell lineage with regulatory T cell ties. Immunity 2006;24: 677–688.
25 Howell MD, Kim BE, Gao P, Grant AV, Boguniewicz M, De Benedetto A, Schneider L, Beck LA, Barnes KC, Leung DY: Cytokine modulation of atopic dermatitis filaggrin skin expression. J Allergy Clin Immunol 2009;124:R7–R12.
26 Coffman RL: Immunology: the origin of TH2 responses. Science 2010;328:1116–1117.
27 Aral M, Arican O, Gul M, Sasmaz S, Kocturk SA, Kastal U, Ekerbicer HC: The relationship between serum levels of total IgE, IL-18, IL-12, IFN-gamma and disease severity in children with atopic dermatitis. Mediators Inflamm 2006 2006: 73098.
28 Hon KL, Leung TF, Ma KC, Wong CK, Wan H, Lam CW: Serum concentration of IL-18 correlates with disease extent in young children with atopic dermatitis. Pediatr Dermatol 2004;21:619–622.
29 Nograles KE, Suarez-Farinas M, Shemer A, Fuentes-Duculan J, Chiricozzi A, Cardinale I, Zaba LC, Kikuchi T, Ramon M, Bergman R, Krueger JG, Guttman-Yassky E: Atopic dermatitis keratinocytes exhibit normal Th17 cytokine responses. J Allergy Clin Immunol 2010;125:744–746.
30 Czech W, Krutmann J, Schopf E, Kapp A: Serum eosinophil cationic protein (ECP) is a sensitive measure for disease activity in atopic dermatitis. Br J Dermatol 1992;126:351–355.
31 Furue M, Sugiyama H, Tsukamoto K, Ohtake N, Tamaki K: Serum soluble IL-2 receptor (sIL-2R) and eosinophil cationic protein (ECP) levels in atopic dermatitis. J Dermatol Sci 1994;7:89–95.
32 Taniuchi S, Chihara J, Kojima T, Yamamoto A, Sasai M, Kobayashi Y: Serum eosinophil derived neurotoxin may reflect more strongly disease severity in childhood atopic dermatitis than eosinophil cationic protein. J Dermatol Sci 2001;26:79–82.
33 Gutgesell C, Heise S, Seubert A, Stichtenoth DO, Frolich JC, Neumann C: Comparison of different activity parameters in atopic dermatitis: correlation with clinical scores. Br J Dermatol 2002;147: 914–919.
34 Pucci N, Novembre E, Cammarata MG, Bernardini R, Monaco MG, Calogero C, Vierucci A: Scoring atopic dermatitis in infants and young children: distinctive features of the SCORAD index. Allergy 2005;60:113–116.
35 Morita H, Yamamoto K, Kitano Y: Elevation of serum major basic protein in patients with atopic dermatitis. J Dermatol Sci 1995;9:165–168.
36 Kawakami T, Ando T, Kimura M, Wilson BS, Kawakami Y: Mast cells in atopic dermatitis. Curr Opin Immunol 2009;21:666–678.
37 Kanbe T, Soma Y, Kawa Y, Kashima M, Mizoguchi M: Serum levels of soluble stem cell factor and soluble KIT are elevated in patients with atopic dermatitis and correlate with the disease severity. Br J Dermatol 2001;144:1148–1153.
38 Halmerbauer G, Frischer T, Koller DY: Monitoring of disease activity by measurement of inflammatory markers in atopic dermatitis in childhood. Allergy 1997;52:765–769.
39 Laan MP, Koning H, Baert MR, Oranje AP, Buurman WA, Savelkoul HF, Neijens HJ: Levels of soluble intercellular adhesion molecule-1, soluble E-selectin, tumor necrosis factor-alpha, and soluble tumor necrosis factor receptor p55 and p75 in atopic children. Allergy 1998;53:51–58.
40 Hirai S, Kageshita T, Kimura T, Tsujisaki M, Okajima K, Imai K, Ono T: Soluble intercellular adhesion molecule-1 and soluble E-selectin levels in patients with atopic dermatitis. Br J Dermatol 1996;134: 657–661.

41 Katoh N, Hirano S, Suehiro M, Ikenaga K, Yamashita T, Sugawara N, Yasuno H: Soluble CD30 is more relevant to disease activity of atopic dermatitis than soluble CD26. Clin Exp Immunol 2000;121:187–192.
42 Heshmat NM, El-Hadidi ES: Soluble CD30 serum levels in atopic dermatitis and bronchial asthma and its relationship with disease severity in pediatric age. Pediatr Allergy Immunol 2006;17:297–303.
43 Mitsuishi K, Nakamura T, Sakata Y, Yuyama N, Arima K, Sugita Y, Suto H, Izuhara K, Ogawa H: The squamous cell carcinoma antigens as relevant biomarkers of atopic dermatitis. Clin Exp Allergy 2005;35:1327–1333.
44 Homey B, Alenius H, Muller A, Soto H, Bowman EP, Yuan W, McEvoy L, Lauerma AI, Assmann T, Bunemann E, Lehto M, Wolff H, Yen D, Marxhausen H, To W, Sedgwick J, Ruzicka T, Lehmann P, Zlotnik A: CCL27-CCR10 interactions regulate T cell-mediated skin inflammation. Nat Med 2002;8:157–165.
45 Hon KL, Lam MC, Leung TF, Wong KY, Chow CM, Fok TF, Ng PC: Are age-specific high serum IgE levels associated with worse symptomatology in children with atopic dermatitis? Int J Dermatol 2007;46:1258–1262.
46 Hon KL, Leung TF, Ma KC, Li AM, Wong Y, Fok TF: Serum levels of cutaneous T-cell attracting chemokine (CTACK) as a laboratory marker of the severity of atopic dermatitis in children. Clin Exp Dermatol 2004;29:293–296.
47 Kakinuma T, Nakamura K, Wakugawa M, Mitsui H, Tada Y, Saeki H, Torii H, Asahina A, Onai N, Matsushima K, Tamaki K: Thymus and activation-regulated chemokine in atopic dermatitis: serum thymus and activation-regulated chemokine level is closely related with disease activity. J Allergy Clin Immunol 2001;107:535–541.
48 Jahnz-Rozyk K, Targowski T, Paluchowska E, Owczarek W, Kucharczyk A: Serum thymus and activation-regulated chemokine, macrophage-derived chemokine and eotaxin as markers of severity of atopic dermatitis. Allergy 2005;60:685–688.
49 Furusyo N, Takeoka H, Toyoda K, Murata M, Maeda S, Ohnishi H, Fukiwake N, Uchi H, Furue M, Hayashi J: Thymus and activation regulated chemokines in children with atopic dermatitis: Kyushu University Ishigaki Atopic Dermatitis Study (KIDS). Eur J Dermatol 2007;17:397–404.
50 Zhang Z, Hener P, Frossard N, Kato S, Metzger D, Li M, Chambon P: Thymic stromal lymphopoietin overproduced by keratinocytes in mouse skin aggravates experimental asthma. Proc Natl Acad Sci USA 2009;106:1536–1541.
51 Demehri S, Morimoto M, Holtzman MJ, Kopan R: Skin-derived TSLP triggers progression from epidermal-barrier defects to asthma. PLoS Biol 2009;7:e1000067.
52 Kinoshita H, Takai T, Le TA, Kamijo S, Wang XL, Ushio H, Hara M, Kawasaki J, Vu AT, Ogawa T, Gunawan H, Ikeda S, Okumura K, Ogawa H: Cytokine milieu modulates release of thymic stromal lymphopoietin from human keratinocytes stimulated with double-stranded RNA. J Allergy Clin Immunol 2009;123:179–186.
53 Ziegler SF, Artis D: Sensing the outside world: TSLP regulates barrier immunity. Nat Immunol 2010;11:289–293.
54 Lee EB, Kim KW, Hong JY, Jee HM, Sohn MH, Kim KE: Increased serum thymic stromal lymphopoietin in children with atopic dermatitis. Pediatr Allergy Immunol 2010;21:e457–e460.
55 Komine M: Analysis of the mechanism for the development of allergic skin inflammation and the application for its treatment: keratinocytes in atopic dermatitis – their pathogenic involvement. J Pharmacol Sci 2009;110:260–264.
56 Ezzat MH, Sallam MA, Shaheen KY: Serum mucosa-associated epithelial chemokine (MEC/CCL28) in atopic dermatitis: a specific marker for severity. Int J Dermatol 2009;48:822–829.
57 He R, Geha RS: Thymic stromal lymphopoietin. Ann NY Acad Sci 2010;1183:13–24.
58 O'Regan GM, Sandilands A, McLean WH, Irvine AD: Filaggrin in atopic dermatitis. J Allergy Clin Immunol 2009;124:R2–R6.
59 Ogawa M, Berger PA, McIntyre OR, Clendenning WE, Ishizaka K: IgE in atopic dermatitis. Arch Dermatol 1971;103:575–580.
60 Seidenari S, Giusti G: Objective assessment of the skin of children affected by atopic dermatitis: a study of pH, capacitance and TEWL in eczematous and clinically uninvolved skin. Acta Derm Venereol 1995;75:429–433.
61 Seidenari S: Reactivity to nickel sulfate at sodium lauryl sulfate pretreated skin sites is higher in atopics: an echographic evaluation by means of image analysis performed on 20 MHz B-scan recordings. Acta Derm Venereol 1994;74:245–249.
62 Hanifin JM: Pharmacophysiology of atopic dermatitis. Clin Rev Allergy 1986;4:43–65.
63 Kato F, Saga K, Morimoto Y, Kaneko R: Pilocarpine-induced cholinergic sweat secretion compared with emotional sweat secretion in atopic dermatitis. Br J Dermatol 1999;140:1110–1113.
64 Yosipovitch G, Greaves MW, Schmelz M: Itch. Lancet 2003;361:690–694.

65 Stander S, Steinhoff M, Schmelz M, Weisshaar E, Metze D, Luger T: Neurophysiology of pruritus: cutaneous elicitation of itch. Arch Dermatol 2003; 139:1463–1470.
66 Davidson S, Zhang X, Yoon CH, Khasabov SG, Simone DA, Giesler GJ Jr: The itch-producing agents histamine and cowhage activate separate populations of primate spinothalamic tract neurons. J Neurosci 2007;27:10007–10014.
67 Handwerker HO: Microneurography of pruritus. Neurosci Lett 2010;470:193–196.
68 Grewe M, Vogelsang K, Ruzicka T, Stege H, Krutmann J: Neurotrophin-4 production by human epidermal keratinocytes: increased expression in atopic dermatitis. J Invest Dermatol 2000;114:1108–1112.
69 Stander S, Moormann C, Schumacher M, Buddenkotte J, Artuc M, Shpacovitch V, Brzoska T, Lippert U, Henz BM, Luger TA, Metze D, Steinhoff M: Expression of vanilloid receptor subtype 1 in cutaneous sensory nerve fibers, mast cells, and epithelial cells of appendage structures. Exp Dermatol 2004;13:129–139.
70 Imamachi N, Park GH, Lee H, Anderson DJ, Simon MI, Basbaum AI, Han SK: TRPV1-expressing primary afferents generate behavioral responses to pruritogens via multiple mechanisms. Proc Natl Acad Sci USA 2009;106:11330–11335.
71 Steinhoff M, Bienenstock J, Schmelz M, Maurer M, Wei E, Biro T: Neurophysiological, neuroimmunological, and neuroendocrine basis of pruritus. J Invest Dermatol 2006;126:1705–1718.
72 Ikoma A, Rukwied R, Stander S, Steinhoff M, Miyachi Y, Schmelz M: Neurophysiology of pruritus: interaction of itch and pain. Arch Dermatol 2003;139:1475–1478.
73 Toyoda M, Nakamura M, Makino T, Hino T, Kagoura M, Morohashi M: Nerve growth factor and substance P are useful plasma markers of disease activity in atopic dermatitis. Br J Dermatol 2002; 147:71–79.
74 Wang IJ, Hsieh WS, Guo YL, Jee SH, Hsieh CJ, Hwang YH, Chen PC: Neuro-mediators as predictors of paediatric atopic dermatitis. Clin Exp Allergy 2008;38:1302–1308.
75 Scholzen T, Armstrong CA, Bunnett NW, Luger TA, Olerud JE, Ansel JC: Neuropeptides in the skin: interactions between the neuroendocrine and the skin immune systems. Exp Dermatol 1998;7: 81–96.
76 Sun YG, Zhao ZQ, Meng XL, Yin J, Liu XY, Chen ZF: Cellular basis of itch sensation. Science 2009; 325:1531–1534.
77 Sun YG, Chen ZF: A gastrin-releasing peptide receptor mediates the itch sensation in the spinal cord. Nature 2007;448:700–703.
78 Tominaga M, Ogawa H, Takamori K: Histological characterization of cutaneous nerve fibers containing gastrin-releasing peptide in NC/Nga mice: an atopic dermatitis model. J Invest Dermatol 2009;129: 2901–2905.
79 Dillon SR, Sprecher C, Hammond A, Bilsborough J, Rosenfeld-Franklin M, Presnell SR, Haugen HS, Maurer M, Harder B, Johnston J, Bort S, Mudri S, Kuijper JL, Bukowski T, Shea P, Dong DL, Dasovich M, Grant FJ, Lockwood L, Levin SD, LeCiel C, Waggie K, Day H, Topouzis S, Kramer J, Kuestner R, Chen Z, Foster D, Parrish-Novak J, Gross JA: Interleukin 31, a cytokine produced by activated T cells, induces dermatitis in mice. Nat Immunol 2004;5:752–760.
80 Diveu C, Lak-Hal AH, Froger J, Ravon E, Grimaud L, Barbier F, Hermann J, Gascan H, Chevalier S: Predominant expression of the long isoform of GP130-like (GPL) receptor is required for interleukin-31 signaling. Eur Cytokine Netw 2004;15: 291–302.
81 Bilsborough J, Leung DY, Maurer M, Howell M, Boguniewicz M, Yao L, Storey H, Le Ciel C, Harder B, Gross JA: IL-31 is associated with cutaneous lymphocyte antigen-positive skin homing T cells in patients with atopic dermatitis. J Allergy Clin Immunol 2006;117:418–425.
82 Sonkoly E, Muller A, Lauerma AI, Pivarcsi A, Soto H, Kemeny L, Alenius H, Dieu-Nosjean MC, Meller S, Rieker J, Steinhoff M, Hoffmann TK, Ruzicka T, Zlotnik A, Homey B: IL-31: a new link between T cells and pruritus in atopic skin inflammation. J Allergy Clin Immunol 2006;117:411–417.
83 Takaoka A, Arai I, Sugimoto M, Honma Y, Futaki N, Nakamura A, Nakaike S: Involvement of IL-31 on scratching behavior in NC/Nga mice with atopic-like dermatitis. Exp Dermatol 2006;15:161–167.
84 Raap U, Wichmann K, Bruder M, Stander S, Wedi B, Kapp A, Werfel T: Correlation of IL-31 serum levels with severity of atopic dermatitis. J Allergy Clin Immunol 2008;122:421–423.
85 Yoshizawa Y, Nomaguchi H, Izaki S, Kitamura K: Serum cytokine levels in atopic dermatitis. Clin Exp Dermatol 2002;27:225–229.
86 Piancatelli D, Bellotta L, Del Beato T, Duse M, Della Penna MR: Total IL-12 levels are increased in paediatric atopic dermatitis: correlations with age and disease severity. Int J Immunopathol Pharmacol 2008;21:359–365.
87 Kagami S, Kakinuma T, Saeki H, Tsunemi Y, Fujita H, Sasaki K, Nakamura K, Takekoshi T, Kishimoto M, Mitsui H, Komine M, Asahina A, Tamaki K: Increased serum CCL28 levels in patients with atopic dermatitis, psoriasis vulgaris and bullous pemphigoid. J Invest Dermatol 2005;124:1088–1090.

88 Kakinuma T, Nakamura K, Wakugawa M, Mitsui H, Tada Y, Saeki H, Torii H, Komine M, Asahina A, Tamaki K: Serum macrophage-derived chemokine (MDC) levels are closely related with the disease activity of atopic dermatitis. Clin Exp Immunol 2002;127:270–273.
89 Kagami S, Kakinuma T, Saeki H, Tsunemi Y, Fujita H, Nakamura K, Takekoshi T, Kishimoto M, Mitsui H, Torii H, Komine M, Asahina A, Tamaki K: Significant elevation of serum levels of eotaxin-3/CCL26, but not of eotaxin-2/CCL24, in patients with atopic dermatitis: serum eotaxin-3/CCL26 levels reflect the disease activity of atopic dermatitis. Clin Exp Immunol 2003;134:309–313.
90 Nakazato J, Kishida M, Kuroiwa R, Fujiwara J, Shimoda M, Shinomiya N: Serum levels of Th2 chemokines, CCL17, CCL22, and CCL27, were the important markers of severity in infantile atopic dermatitis. Pediatr Allergy Immunol 2008;19:605–613.
91 Yamashita N, Kaneko S, Kouro O, Furue M, Yamamoto S, Sakane T: Soluble E-selectin as a marker of disease activity in atopic dermatitis. J Allergy Clin Immunol 1997;99:410–416.
92 Wolkerstorfer A, Laan MP, Savelkoul HF, Neijens HJ, Mulder PG, Oudesluys-Murphy AM, Sukhai RN, Oranje AP: Soluble E-selectin, other markers of inflammation and disease severity in children with atopic dermatitis. Br J Dermatol 1998;138:431–435.
93 Shimada Y, Sato S, Hasegawa M, Tedder TF, Takehara K: Elevated serum L-selectin levels and abnormal regulation of L-selectin expression on leukocytes in atopic dermatitis: soluble L-selectin levels indicate disease severity. J Allergy Clin Immunol 1999;104:163–168.
94 Katoh N, Hirano S, Suehiro M, Ikenaga K, Yasuno H: Increased levels of serum tissue inhibitor of metalloproteinase-1 but not metalloproteinase-3 in atopic dermatitis. Clin Exp Immunol 2002;127:283–288.
95 Mukai H, Noguchi T, Kamimura K, Nishioka K, Nishiyama S: Significance of elevated serum LDH (lactate dehydrogenase) activity in atopic dermatitis. J Dermatol 1990;17:477–481.
96 Glinski W, Brodecka H, Glinska-Ferenz M, Kowalski D: Increased concentration of beta-endorphin in the sera of patients with severe atopic dermatitis. Acta Derm Venereol 1995;75:9–11.
97 Raap U, Werfel T, Goltz C, Deneka N, Langer K, Bruder M, Kapp A, Schmid-Ott G, Wedi B: Circulating levels of brain-derived neurotrophic factor correlate with disease severity in the intrinsic type of atopic dermatitis. Allergy 2006;61:1416–1418.
98 Namura K, Hasegawa G, Egawa M, Matsumoto T, Kobayashi R, Yano T, Katoh N, Kishimoto S, Ohta M, Obayashi H, Ose H, Fukui M, Nakamura N, Yoshikawa T: Relationship of serum brain-derived neurotrophic factor level with other markers of disease severity in patients with atopic dermatitis. Clin Immunol 2007;122:181–186.
99 Goto T, Morioka J, Inamura H, Yano M, Kodaira K, Igarashi Y, Abe S, Kurosawa M: Urinary eosinophil-derived neurotoxin concentrations in patients with atopic dermatitis: a useful clinical marker for disease activity. Allergol Int 2007;56:433–438.
100 Ostlere LS, Taylor C, Baillod R, Wright S: Relationship between pruritus, transepidermal water loss, and biochemical markers of renal itch in haemodialysis patients. Nephrol Dial Transplant 1994;9:1302–1304.

Hsin-Su Yu, MD, PhD
Kaohsiung Medical University College of Medicine
100 Shih-Chuan 1st Road
Kaohsiung 807, Taiwan (ROC)
Tel. +886 7 3121 101, ext. 2101, Fax +886 7 3118 901, E-Mail dermyu@kmu.edu.tw

Shiohara T (ed): Pathogenesis and Management of Atopic Dermatitis.
Curr Probl Dermatol. Basel, Karger, 2011, vol 41, pp 149–155

Practical Issues on Interpretation of Scoring Atopic Dermatitis: SCORAD Index, Objective SCORAD, Patient-Oriented SCORAD and Three-Item Severity Score

Arnold P. Oranje

Department of Paediatrics, Paediatric Dermatology, Erasmus Medical Centre, Rotterdam, The Netherlands

Abstract

The SCORAD (Index) is the best validated scoring system in atopic dermatitis (AD). Modification of the SCORAD Index has led several times to incorrect use of the system. To measure the extent of AD, the rule of nines is applied on a front/back drawing of the patient's inflammatory lesions. The extent can be graded from 0 to 100. The intensity part of the SCORAD consists of 6 items: erythema, oedema/papulation, excoriations, lichenification, oozing/crusts and dryness. Each item can be graded on a scale from 0 to 3. The subjective items include daily pruritus and sleeplessness. The SCORAD Index formula is: A/5 + 7B/2 + C. In this formula A is defined as the extent (0–100), B is defined as the intensity (0–18) and C is defined as the subjective symptoms (0–20). The maximal score of the SCORAD Index is 103. The objective SCORAD consist of the extent and the intensity items; the formula is A/5 + 7B/2. The maximal objective SCORAD score is 83 (with 10 additional points for severe disfiguring eczema of the face and hands). Patients should also evaluate their dermatitis, because their well-being is the most important aspect of treating AD. Therefore different self-assessment scores for AD patients, including the patient-oriented SCORAD, were developed. The patient-oriented SCORAD correlates well with the SCORAD Index. The Three-Item Severity (TIS) score involves the scoring of erythema (redness), oedema and excoriations (scratches) in one representative lesion. The TIS score corresponds well with the objective SCORAD and can be used as prescreening system or as a quick system in studies and is excellent for epidemiological studies.

Atopic dermatitis (AD) is a multifactorial genetically based disease [1, 2]. Assessment of the severity of AD is necessary to evaluate the disease process and to measure intervention by therapy or elimination. Therefore it should be performed as objectively as possible. This is extremely important in clinical practice and for research purposes.

The text is an updated version of a previous publication [Br J Dermatol 2007;157:645–648].

The SCORAD system has been developed based on consensus by the European Task Force Group on Atopic Dermatitis (ETFAD). The ETFAD consists of a group of more than 20 dermatologists with much expertise in paediatric dermatology. The acronym SCORAD was proposed by Arnold Oranje and stands for 'scoring atopic dermatitis' [1]. Establishing the diagnosis of AD should be seen as separate from evaluating the well-being of the involved patient and the severity of the disorder [3–5].

Patient involvement in the evaluation and treatment process is of the utmost importance. There are very few validated patient self-assessment tools for AD. Recently the patient-oriented SCORAD was developed and investigated in a multicentre international study [Stalder et al., in preparation].

This report describes items of the SCORAD Index, objective SCORAD, patient-oriented SCORAD and TIS score (Three-Item Severity score).

SCORAD Index

The SCORAD Index was developed by the ETFAD in 1993. This initiative was undertaken by Alain Taïeb from Bordeaux and Jean-François Stalder from Nantes (France). The system was developed on the basis of the consensus of more than 20 dermatologists, almost each of whom had their own system. The SCORAD Index consists of the interpretation of the extent of the disorder (A: according to the rule of nines – 20% of the score), the intensity composed of 6 items (B: erythema, oedema/papules, effect of scratching, oozing/crust formation, lichenification and dryness – 60% of the score; each item has 4 grades: 0, 1, 2, 3) and subjective symptoms (C: itch, sleeplessness – 20% of the score).

In the SCORAD Index, the 'visual analogue scale' ruler is used for the evaluation of subjective symptoms. The distribution of the score is achieved using the formula $A/5 + 7B/2 + C$. The maximum achievable score is 103 (see SCORAD Index, fig. 1) [1, 6]. The evaluation form can be completed within 7–10 min depending upon the experience of the investigators. The end results of the SCORAD Index were too much influenced by unreliable and widely divergent gradings of the subjective items by the parents/caregivers or the patient.

Objective SCORAD

Two interesting studies have been conducted with actual patients and with a pictorial atlas [7]. In the period 1993–1994 three training sessions in Bordeaux, Rotterdam and Hamburg were performed (organized by Taïeb, Oranje and Ring, respectively) by the ETFAD. The scores completed by 12 dermatologists present at 2 sessions at least were analysed. Twenty-two patients were included; there were 3 drop-outs because of the use of tar ointment (in 1 case), use of eosin (in 1 case) and because of extremely

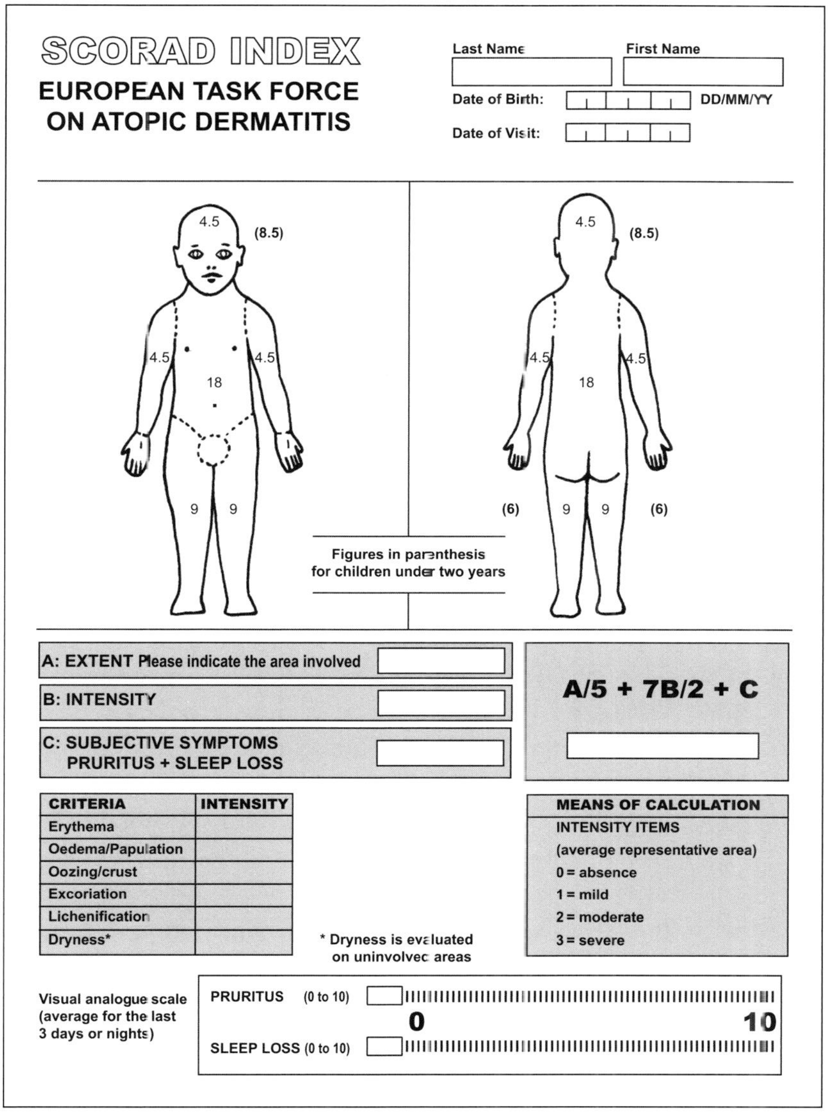

Fig. 1. SCORAD Index (derived from the report of the ETFAD [1]).

hard crying (red baby in another case). It appeared that there was 20–60% variability between various investigators from the combined sessions with actual patients. Moreover, there were 'high scorers and low scorers'. It is important that each item is chosen in the most representative lesion. Lesions involving less than 3% of the body surface are not included in the evaluation.

The subjective scores provide an overall assessment of disease severity, but in view of the complexity of scoring clinical signs with patient symptoms it was decided to concentrate on objective scores only for monitoring changes in disease severity.

Table 1. Formula of the SCORAD Index, the objective SCORAD and the TIS score

System	Formula
SCORAD Index (0–103) (= SCORAD composite index)	A/5 (20) + 7B/2 (0–63) + C (0–20); the maximal score is 103
Objective SCORAD (0–83)	A/5 (20) + 7B/2 (0–63); additional points for disfiguring lesions or functionally limiting lesions = 10 extra; in worst cases, the maximal score can reach 93
TIS (0–9)	erythema (redness) 0–3, oedema 0–3, excoriations (scratches) 0–3 = R-O-S; the maximal score is 9

A = Extent of eczema according to the rule of nines; B = intensity items; C = subjective items (pruritus, sleep loss during the last 3 days).

That subjective part scored by the patients or the parents had an unpredictable impact on the final score of the initial design of the scoring system. Therefore, the maximum score in the objective SCORAD was now set at 83 [7]. An additional 10 points were given in cases with severe disfiguring visible lesions (table 1) [7].

These additional points were chosen by Kunz and others of the ETFAD as a compensation for terribly disfiguring lesions of the face or hands [7].

In the other study, investigators of a multicentre trial were trained using the pictorial atlas for the trial Early Treatment of the Atopic Child, a double-blind placebo-controlled study on the effect of cetirizine in children with AD. It appeared that the interobserver agreement was high for oedema but low for lichenification. Erythema and excoriations were statistically significantly better scored by dermatologically trained physicians (t test, $p = 0.042$, $p = 0.063$). Also the extent was better scored by them ($p = 0.006$). Lichenification was better scored by dermatologically non-trained physicians ($p = 0.013$).

It appeared that such a training programme was useful for standardizing the evaluation of AD. It also appeared that non-dermatologists could be trained for this purpose [8].

Patient-Oriented SCORAD

The patient-oriented SCORAD is based on the SCORAD Index and is structurally the same as the latter. It consists of 3 parts: an assessment of the extent of disease, items evaluating severity and an evaluation of subjective symptoms. The extent of disease is assessed using 2 methods: patients are asked to shade a drawing and to describe the area affected in terms of the size of their hand (fingers included). Severity assessment was clearly divided into 2 subparts: dryness of non-inflamed skin and the characteristics of inflamed skin. With simplified questions, the patient is able to answer the items. The subjective items pruritus and sleep disturbance were assessed as in the SCORAD Index, using a visual analogue scale from 0 to 10.

Three-Item Severity Score

The TIS is a simple scoring system using 3 of the intensity items of the SCORAD. It evaluates the intensity of erythema (redness), oedema and excoriations (scratches). It can be regarded as a global scoring system [8]. For each item, the most representative lesion is selected and written down as R-O-S, for example as 1-0-1, total score 2.

The 3 items in the TIS can all be scored in different representative areas, as in the SCORAD system, rather than in 1 representative area.

We use this system for routine orientation within our daily practice. The TIS, ranging from 0 to 9, is a system with a much smaller grey area than the objective SCORAD, ranging from 0 to 83.

A good correlation between the TIS and objective SCORAD is obvious and not surprising as the TIS is a component of the SCORAD Index and they are bound to correlate.

A TIS examination can be completed within 1 min.

Discussion

The SCORAD Index is influenced by subjective ratings that may interfere by social and cultural factors. Therefore I and others recommend the objective SCORAD. The advantage of using the objective SCORAD system is that it is based on a European consensus. The system is representative and well evaluated but shows as all other systems intra- and interobserver disagreements. The variation of the scores is estimated to be about 20%. By using this instrument, different studies are better comparable, in routine as well as in observational or double-blind randomized clinical trials [9]. Other systems to be mentioned are the Six-Area, Six-Sign Atopic Dermatitis severity score and the Eczema Area and Severity Index (EASI) as well as the TIS. The first has also been shown to be an effective system for recording and monitoring disease activity in AD, but validity studies are limited. The score is obtained by grading 6 signs (erythema, exudation, excoriation, dryness, cracking and lichenification), each on a scale of 0 (absent), 1 (mild), 2 (moderate) or 3 (severe), at each of 6 sites: arms, hands, legs, feet, head and neck, trunk. The maximum score is 108 [10]. The EASI showed good validity, reliability and sensitivity to change and correlated well with other measures of severity [11]. Training and interobserver appointments are advisable to diminish unnecessary differences in interpretation [12]. The SCORAD system

Table 2. SCORAD Index, objective SCORAD and TIS: classification of severity of eczema

	Mild	Moderate	Severe
SCORAD Index	<25	25–50	≥50
Objective SCORAD	<15	15–40	≥40
TIS	<3	3–6	≥6

takes time, and even experienced dermatologists will require 7 min in total. An inexperienced physician will need 10 min. Most comparable with the SCORAD is the EASI method, which was also validated in a large multinational patient population with AD.

However, the EASI places a significant emphasis on body surface area assessments and incorporates them into the total score in a very complex way. Given the potential difficulties assessing body surface area accurately, this may certainly lead to problems.

A major problem, relevant for all scoring systems developed for AD, raised by different dermatologists, is that pigmented skin could be a problem for the evaluation of erythema. However, if experienced in using scoring systems for pigmented skin, the investigator can recognize redness as darkening of the skin depending upon the individual skin type.

The TIS is less sensitive than the objective SCORAD. The objective SCORAD gives more information about extent (not included in the TIS) and intensity of eczema (table 2). The TIS contains only (sub)acute items. Therefore the objective SCORAD should be used in clinical comparative trials, while the TIS score is to be preferred in epidemiological studies and in daily practice. The TIS has a great advantage, because it is simple, quick and easy to perform in routine settings with less experienced physicians. It takes only 1 min.

Researchers are still widely using untested and unstandardized severity indices. This was demonstrated in the paper by Charman et al. [13], showing that in randomized controlled trials of AD treatment published between 1994 and 2001 (93 trials) only 27% of trials used a published scoring system, of which the SCORAD was the most widely used.

More widespread use of the objective SCORAD is needed, while the TIS, as a simplified component of the objective SCORAD, is an excellent system for evaluation in epidemiological studies [14]. Recently, Cosickic et al. [15] did perform a comparative study in 261 children with AD of the SCORAD Index and TIS and found a significant correlation ($r = 0.531$; $p < 0.0001$).

Also Willemsen et al. [16] found in a study in the general practice a moderate-to-good agreement between the observers for the TIS ($\kappa = 0.604$ or 0.464) or objective

SCORAD (κ = 0.695 or 0.700). Most important was the finding of an excellent correlation between TIS and objective SCORAD (r_s = 0.755–0.839). Because of the moderate-to-good interobserver agreement and the high correlation with the objective SCORAD, the authors (including myself) recommend the TIS to determine the severity of AD in general practice. This proposal by Dirven (general physician) was accepted in the Netherlands in the consensus for AD 2009.

References

1 European Task Force on Atopic Dermatitis: Severity scoring of atopic dermatitis: the SCORAD index – consensus report of the European Task Force on Atopic Dermatitis. Dermatology 1993; 186:23–31.

2 Harper JI, Prose NP, Oranje AP: Textbook of Pediatric Dermatology. London, Blackwell Science, 2006.

3 Sampson H: Pathogenesis of eczema. Clin Exp Allergy 1990;20:459–467.

4 Oranje AP, Glazenburg EJ, Wolkerstorfer A, de Waard-van der Spek FB: Practical issues on interpretation of scoring atopic dermatitis: the SCORAD index, objective SCORAD and the three-item severity score. Br J Dermatol 2007;157:645–648.

5 Vourc'h-Jourdain M, Barbarot S, Taieb A, Diepgen T, Ambonati M, Durosier V, Sibaud V, Stalder JF: Patient-oriented SCORAD: a self-assessment score in atopic dermatitis. A preliminary feasibility study. Dermatology. 2009;218:246–251.

6 Kunz B, Oranje AP, Labrèze L, et al: Clinical validation and guidelines for the SCORAD index: consensus report of the European Task Force on Atopic Dermatitis. Dermatology 1997;195:10–19.

7 Oranje AP, Stalder JF, Taïeb A, et al: Scoring of atopic dermatitis by SCORAD using a training atlas by investigators from different disciplines. Pediatr Allergy Immunol 1997;8:28–34.

8 Wolkerstorfer A, de Waard-van der Spek FB, Glazenburg EJ, Mulder PGH, Oranje AP: Scoring the severity of atopic dermatitis: three item severity (TIS) score as a rough system for daily practice and as a prescreening tool for studies. Acta Derm Venereol 1999;79:356–359.

9 Gelmetti C, Colonna C: The value of SCORAD and beyond: towards a standardized evaluation of severity? Allergy 2004;59(suppl 78):61–65.

10 Berth-Jones J: Six area, six sign atopic dermatitis (SASSAD) severity score: a simple system for monitoring disease activity in atopic dermatitis. Br J Dermatol 1996;135(suppl 48):25–30.

11 Barbier N, Paul C, Luger T, et al: Validation of the Eczema Area and Severity Index for atopic dermatitis in a cohort of 1,550 patients from the pimecrolimus cream 1% randomized controlled clinical trials programme. Br J Dermatol 2004;150: 96–102.

12 Charman CR, Venn AJ, Williams HC: Reliability testing of the Six Area, Six Sign Atopic Dermatitis severity score. Br J Dermatol 2002;146:1057–1060.

13 Charman CR, Chambers C, Williams HC: Measuring atopic dermatitis severity in randomized controlled clinical trials: what exactly are we measuring? J Invest Dermatol 2003;120:932–941.

14 Charman CR, Williams HC: Measuring atopic eczema severity visually: which variables are most important to patients. Arch Dermatol 2005;141: 1146–1151.

15 Cosickic A, Skokic F, Colic-Hadzic B, Jahic M: Clinical characteristics and estimation severity of the atopic dermatitis in children. Med Arh 2010;64: 178–182.

16 Willemsen MG, van Valburg WC, Dirven-Meijer PC, Oranje AP, van der Wouden JC, Moed H: Determining the severity of atopic dermatitis in children presenting in general practice: an easy and fast method. Dermatol Res Pract DOI: 10.1155/2009/357046.

Prof. Arnold P. Oranje
Department of Paediatrics, Paediatric Dermatology Unit
Erasmus Medical Centre Rotterdam, Postbus 2040, NL–3000 CA Rotterdam
Dr. Molewaterplein 60, NL–3015 GD Rotterdam (The Netherlands)
Tel. +31 10 703 6653, Fax +31 10 202 1274, E-Mail arnold.p.oranje@inter.nl.net

Shiohara T (ed): Pathogenesis and Management of Atopic Dermatitis.
Curr Probl Dermatol. Basel, Karger, 2011, vol 41, pp 156–164

Systemic Therapy of Atopic Dermatitis in Children and Adults

Dagmar Simon

Department of Dermatology, Inselspital, Bern University Hospital, University of Bern, Bern, Switzerland

Abstract

Systemic therapy is required in patients with severe atopic dermatitis (AD) refractory to adequate topical therapy. The aim of a systemic therapy is the rapid and efficient improvement of skin symptoms and pruritus in acute exacerbation and/or the long-term control of severe chronic disease. A number of immunosuppressive and immunomodulating substances are available that may efficiently reduce skin inflammation and thus lead to a relief of symptoms including pruritus. The excellent effects of cyclosporine as short-term as well as maintenance therapy have been documented in several studies in children and adults. Furthermore, other immunosuppressive substances such as azathioprine, mycophenolate mofetil and methotrexate are effective in patients with moderate to severe AD. Intravenous immunoglobulins and γ-interferon exert immunomodulatory effects and thus may improve severe AD. Biological agents are a new approach in AD therapy since they may specifically target cells, cytokines or mediators involved in the pathogenesis of AD.

Systemic therapy is required in patients with severe atopic dermatitis (AD) not responding to topical therapy. Just in cases, in which the combination of topical treatment modalities such as anti-inflammatory therapy including topical corticosteroids and calcineurin inhibitors, antimicrobial therapy with disinfectants, and skin care with emollients has been applied adequately and sufficiently without satisfactory effect, should systemic therapy be considered. The aim of any systemic therapy is a drastic inhibition of skin inflammation resulting in a reduction of skin symptoms and pruritus as well as improvement of the quality of life. For all available systemic therapies, drug-specific side effects and interactions as well as interference with the immune system have to be taken into account. In order to do so, periodical examinations of the patients including clinical checkups and laboratory tests are required. Usually, in severe AD systemic therapy is limited in time and applied for several weeks to months.

Systemic Corticosteroids

Because of their mode of action, corticosteroids affect the gene expression of several cytokines, adhesion molecules, growth factors, mediators, extracellular matrix proteins and enzymes by inflammatory cells involved in the pathogenesis of AD as well as resident cells resulting in an inhibition of inflammation, cell proliferation and vasoconstriction. Based on clinical experiences, systemic corticosteroids are widely used in the treatment of AD. However, controlled trials of short-term or long-term therapy in adults are lacking. In children, methylprednisolone bolus (20 mg/day for 3 days) and flunisolide therapy over 2 weeks have been reported to improve severe AD for several weeks [1, 2]. Short-term therapy with systemic corticosteroids may be helpful in severe exacerbations of AD to stop acute symptoms and pruritus [3]. As a clinical rule, the dose of initially 0.75–1 mg/kg body weight per day should be tapered quickly within 7–10 days. Long-term treatment with systemic corticosteroids is not recommended because of potential side effects, e.g. diabetes, hypertension, gastric ulcers, osteoporosis, skin atrophy, glaucoma, Cushing syndrome and growth retardation in children [3, 4].

Cyclosporine

Cyclosporine inhibits T-cell activation and proliferation [5]. After binding to its cytoplasmic receptor, cyclosporine blocks the calcium-dependent phosphatase calcineurin. Thus, the dephosphorylation of the transcription factor nuclear factor of activated T cells is blocked resulting in an interruption of the signal transduction pathway between T-cell receptor activation and cytokine production. The efficacy and safety of cyclosporine therapy in adults and children with AD is well documented by randomized controlled studies [6, 7]. A meta-analysis of 15 studies including over 600 patients revealed a dose-dependent decrease in AD severity after 2 weeks of therapy with a further improvement and a relative effectiveness of 55% after 6–8 weeks [7]. Cyclosporine is recommended for severe AD. It is administered in doses between 2.5 and 5 mg/kg body weight. Although a therapy with higher doses (300 mg/day) of cyclosporine was shown to be more effective after 2 weeks, an initial dose of 150 mg/day was recommended because of better renal tolerability [8]. Continuous therapy with cyclosporine led to a more consistent disease control compared to intermittent short-course therapy [9]. However, since short-term courses were adequate in some patients, an individually tailored therapy was recommended [9]. After discontinuing cyclosporine therapy, the rate of relapse was 50% after 2 weeks and 80% after 6 weeks in patients continuously treated for 6 weeks [10]. Long-term therapy with low-dose cyclosporine was reported to lead to a significant decrease in AD severity after 6 months starting 1 month after initiating therapy [11]. Furthermore, long-term oral cyclosporine therapy given at doses of 3–5 mg/kg daily was shown to improve severe atopic keratoconjunctivitis associated with AD [12]. Currently, 2 therapy schemes are recommended: (1) a short-term interval therapy, in which immediately after achieving a marked improvement of AD, the cyclosporine dose is tapered to 0 – in case of flare-up, cyclosporine therapy is initiated again; (2) a long-term therapy for patients with chronic severe AD and frequent exacerbations, with an individually adjusted maintenance dose at lowest levels controlling the disease for a maximum of 2 years [13]. Due to potential side effects, in particular renal toxicity and hypertension, renal function parameters and blood pressure have to be monitored regularly [13]. Adverse events appeared more likely in patients treated with higher doses [7]. Because of an increased risk for skin cancer, cyclosporine therapy should not be combined with phototherapy.

Azathioprine

The prodrug azathioprine is converted to 6-mercaptopurine, an atypical nucleoside which blocks the synthesis of RNA and DNA and thus inhibits the proliferation of T and B cells. Upon azathioprine therapy, a clearance or marked improvement of AD could be achieved in up to 80% of patients [14, 15]. After 2 years of treatment with azathioprine, a significant decrease in total IgE levels was noted [15]. However, despite initial good responses to azathioprine, in approximately 25% of patients a remission of symptoms allowing a stop of therapy could not be achieved, or flare-ups occurred during therapy [16]. A double-blind, placebo-controlled, crossover trial of 2.5 mg/kg azathioprine per day in patients with severe AD revealed a significant effect of azathioprine by reducing symptoms including pruritus and sleep loss compared to placebo [17]. A significant reduction of disease severity, pruritus, antihistamine usage and staphylococcal colonization was observed in children and young adults after 3 months [18]. However, azathioprine may cause severe side effects including gastrointestinal disturbances, liver dysfunction and leukopenia [17]. The underlying cause for myelosuppressive effects of azathioprine is a partial or total deficiency in thiopurine methyltransferase (TPMT) activity due to gene polymorphisms. Patients at risk can be identified by determining TPMT activity and/or genotyping. Adult AD patients, in whom the azathioprine dose was adapted to TPMT activity, showed a similar disease improvement compared with patients with normal TPMT activity receiving 2.5 mg/kg azathioprine [19]. In 48 children screened for normal TPMT levels before therapy, no myelosuppression was observed under treatment with 2.5–3.5 mg/kg azathioprine for severe AD [20]. Out of these patients, 28 had an excellent and 13 a good response to azathioprine [20].

Mycophenolate Mofetil

Mycophenolate mofetil (MMF) is a prodrug that is metabolized to mycophenolic acid in the gut. It selectively and reversibly inhibits the enzyme inosine monophosphate dehydrogenase required for the synthesis of guanosine nucleotides, components of DNA and RNA. Since the de novo synthesis of purines is essential for T- and B-cell proliferation, MMF preferentially targets these lymphocytes. Successful treatment with MMF was first reported in 2 patients refractory to topical and systemic therapy including prednisone and PUVA [21]. Monotherapy with MMF with initial doses of 1 g twice daily over 4 weeks, followed by 4 weeks with 0.5 g twice daily, led to a significant reduction in disease severity with a sustained improvement during the follow-up until week 20 [22]. The percentage of patients responding to MMF therapy can be estimated to be 70–80% [22, 23]. Whereas remission allowing a stop of MMF can be achieved in some patients, others require maintenance therapy with MMF to control AD. Successful long-term treatment in 3 patients with MMF 1–2 g daily over 12–29 months has been reported [24]. A retrospective analysis of 14 children and adolescents with AD treated with MMF revealed an improvement in 13 patients, of whom 4 achieved complete remission, 4 a >90% and 5 a 60–90% reduction of symptoms [25]. MMF was given at daily doses of 40–50 mg/kg in younger children and 30–40 mg/kg in adolescents. Initial responses were seen after 4–8 weeks, the maximum effect after 8–12 weeks [25]. In parallel with the reduction of disease severity after MMF treatment for 12 weeks in 10 patients with severe AD, an increase in the blood γ-interferon (IFN-γ) level and a significant decrease in total IgE levels have been observed [26]. Main adverse events reported under MMF therapy in AD patients were nausea, liver enzyme abnormalities and infections such as herpes zoster, herpes simplex and staphylococcal infection [22, 23, 27].

Methotrexate

Methotrexate is an immunosuppressant and widely used in dermatology to treat chronic inflammatory diseases. As an analog of folic acid, it interferes with the folic acid metabolism, resulting in a reduced production of pyrimidine and purine nucleotides required for DNA and RNA synthesis. Thus, methotrexate may reduce chemotaxis of and cytokine production by lymphocytes or induce cell death. Methotrexate was shown to be effective in moderate to severe AD. In an open-label, dose-ranging study involving 12 patients, a decrease in disease activity by 52% from baseline was observed after 24 weeks [28]. The median dose was 15 mg/week. Eight patients experienced a persistent improvement over 12 weeks after stopping therapy. A retrospective study reported an improvement of >70% as assessed by the physician in 75% of patients treated intramuscularly with weekly doses of 7.5–25 mg methotrexate after 3 months [29]. These results were confirmed by another retrospective study on low-dose methotrexate therapy with 10–25 mg weekly for 8–12 weeks [30]. 80% of patients with moderate to severe AD responded with a mean decrease in the SCORAD by 44% [30]. Symptoms started to improve 2 weeks to 3 months after initiating therapy [28–30]. Patients not responding to 15 mg methotrexate per week after 3 months failed to improve with further dose escalation [28]. Before starting methotrexate therapy, liver toxicity and teratogenicity have to be considered. Nausea and increase in liver enzymes were the main adverse events observed that eventually caused transient or total discontinuation of methotrexate therapy [29, 30].

Alitretinoin

Alitretinoin, 9-*cis*-retinoic acid, is an antagonist vitamin A derivate which binds to both retinoic acid and retinoid X receptors. Alitretinoin has been shown to be effective in the treatment of severe hand eczema [31]. Recently is has been reported that alitretinoin at a standard dose of 30 mg daily significantly improved extrapalmar AD lesions in 6 patients treated for severe atopic hand eczema [32].

Intravenous Immunoglobulins

Intravenous immunoglobulins (IVIgs), thought to exert immunomodulating effects in inflammatory diseases, have been used for treatment of severe refractory AD. Interesting observations on an improvement of AD skin symptoms were made in patients treated with intravenous gammaglobulins for Kawasaki disease or idiopathic thrombocytopenic purpura, who had AD in addition [33]. Six cycles with high-dose IVIg (2 g/kg per month) given as adjunctive therapy were shown to be effective in 4 out of 6 patients and to significantly improve skin scores [34]. Moreover, IVIg therapy allowed the reduction of concomitant systemic drugs in patients under long-term corticosteroid therapy [35]. A significant decrease in the SCORAD as well as in inflammatory markers including eosinophil cationic protein in the peripheral blood was observed in 5 children treated with 3 cycles of 2 g/kg IVIg per month [36]. However, the results of the effect of IVIgs in patients with severe AD are controversial, as some reports reveal no or just slight improvement [37, 38].

γ-Interferon

Based on findings that patients with AD have an increased interleukin (IL) 4 but a decreased IFN-γ production, clinical trials with recombinant IFN-γ (rIFN-γ) in patients with severe AD have been performed. Treatment with rIFN-γ at increasing dose levels (0.01, 0.05, 0.1 mg/m^2, each for 5 days) showed an improvement at each level, but worsening 3 days after stopping therapy [39]. Better results and a sustained effect were achieved upon 6 weeks of therapy with 0.05 mg/m^2 rIFN-γ daily and a maintenance therapy 3 times per week over 14 weeks [39]. In a double-blind placebo-controlled study, therapy with 0.05 mg/m^2 IFN-γ daily over 12 weeks was shown to be superior to placebo [40]. By continuing rIFN-γ therapy, the initial efficacy was maintained over 2 years in these patients [41]. Long-term IFN-γ therapy has also been administered to children [42]. All studies reported that rIFN-γ was safe and well tolerated. Flu-like symptoms, which occurred in 30–60% of the patients treated with rIFN-γ, could effectively be prevented by dosing at bedtime and pretreatment with nonsteroidal anti-inflammatory drugs [40].

Monoclonal Antibodies and Fusion Proteins

Biological agents present a new group of therapeutics that include monoclonal antibodies and fusion proteins. Biologicals specifically target inflammatory cells and mediators, respectively. In AD, biologicals can be used in order to reduce inflammation by modulating the number, activation and function of immune cells or the action of cytokines or disease-relevant antibodies. A number of case reports and small studies on the effect of biologicals in patients with moderate to severe AD have been published. However, representative, randomized, placebo-controlled studies evaluating the efficacy and safety of biologicals in AD are still not available.

Alefacept is a fusion protein of lymphocyte function-associated antigen 3 (CD58) and IgG that inhibits costimulation and induces apoptosis of T cells. A 12-week course of alefacept 15 mg weekly was reported to significantly reduce skin symptoms, pruritus and concomitant topical steroid therapy [43]. Another study on alefacept demonstrated a clinical improvement in 6 of 9 patients [44]. The anti-CD11a antibody efalizumab shown to be effective in AD [45, 46] is no longer available because of the high risk of infections including progressive multifocal leukoencephalopathy. The depletion of B cells with rituximab, an anti-CD20 antibody, resulted in a rapid reduction of skin inflammation in all patients with a sustained effect over 5 months in 5 of 6 patients, although specific IgE levels were not affected [47]. However, a report on 2 cases of severe AD receiving rituximab could not confirm these findings [48]. Upon short-term therapy with the anti-IL-5 antibody mepolizumab (2 × 750 mg), a moderate improvement of clinical symptoms was observed, although a rapid depletion of eosinophils in the peripheral blood was noted [49]. Upon low-dose anti-IgE therapy (omalizumab, 10 cycles of 150 mg), 6 of 11 AD patients with serum IgE levels >1,000 kU/l before therapy responded as shown by a decrease in the SCORAD over 50% in 2 and between 25 and 50% in 4 patients [50]. Recent studies reported that accompanying AD significantly improved in patients receiving omalizumab because of severe bronchial asthma [51–53]. Anti-tumor-necrosis-factor (TNF)-α antibody (infliximab) has been shown to significantly decrease skin symptoms and pruritus in patients with severe AD during induction therapy [54]. However, a sustained improvement was seen only in 2 of 9 patients during maintenance therapy [54]. A patient with severe AD and concomitant contact allergy responded well to anti-TNF-α [55]. To note, some authors observed atopic eczema-like skin eruptions in patients treated with anti-TNF-α [56, 57], while others did not [58].

Currently, efficacy and safety of cyclosporine and azathioprine for systemic therapy of AD are best documented. There are numerous efforts to develop new drugs that might specifically target cells or cytokines involved in the pathogenesis of AD, e.g. IL-4, IL-13, eotaxin, CC chemokine receptors 3 and 5, histamine H_4 receptor and thymic stromal lymphopoietin.

References

1 Galli E, Chini L, Moschese V, Paone F, Menichelli A, Fraioli G, Rossi P: Methylprednisolone bolus: a novel therapy for severe atopic dermatitis. Acta Paediatr 1994;83:315–317.

2 La Rosa M, Musarra I, Ranno C, Maiello N, Negri L, Del Giudice MM: A randomized, double-blind, placebo-controlled crossover trial of systemic flunisolode in the treatment of children with severe atopic dermatitis. Curr Ther Res 1995;56:720–726.

3 Akdis CA, Akdis M, Bieber T, Bindslev-Jensen C, Boguniewicz M, Eigenmann P, Hamid Q, Kapp A, Leung DY, Lipozencic J, Luger TA, Muraro A, Novak N, Platts-Mills TA, Rosenwasser L, Scheynius A, Simons FE, Spergel J, Turjanmaa K, Wahn U, Weidinger S, Werfel T, Zuberbier T, European Academy of Allergology and Clinical Immunology/American Academy of Allergy, Asthma and Immunology: Diagnosis and treatment of atopic dermatitis in children and adults: European Academy of Allergology and Clinical Immunology/American Academy of Allergy, Asthma and Immunology/PRACTALL Consensus Report. J Allergy Clin Immunol 2006;118: 152–169.

4 Aylett SE, Atherton DJ, Preece MA: The treatment of difficult atopic dermatitis in childhood with oral beclomethasone dipropionate. Acta Derm Venereol Suppl (Stockh) 1992;176:123–125.

5 Liu J: FK506 and cyclosporin, molecular probes for studying intracellular signal transduction. Immunol Today 1993;14:290–295.

6 Hoare C, Li Wan Po A, Williams H: Systematic review of treatments for atopic eczema. Health Technol Assess 2000;4:1–191.

7 Schmitt J, Schmitt N, Meurer M: Cyclosporin in the treatment of patients with atopic eczema – a systematic review and meta-analysis. J Eur Acad Dermatol Venereol 2007;21:606–619.

8 Czech W, Bräutigam M, Weidinger G, Schöpf E: A body-weight-independent dosing regimen of cyclosporine microemulsion is effective in severe atopic dermatitis and improves the quality of life. J Am Acad Dermatol 2000;42:653–659.

9 Harper JI, Ahmed I, Barclay G, Lacour M, Hoeger P, Cork MJ, Finlay AY, Wilson NJ, Graham-Brown RA, Sowden JM, Beard AL, Sumner MJ, Berth-Jones J: Cyclosporin for severe childhood atopic dermatitis: short course versus continuous therapy. Br J Dermatol 2000;142:52–58.

10 Granlund H, Erkko P, Sinisalo M, Reitamo S: Cyclosporin in atopic dermatitis: time to relapse and effect of intermittent therapy. Br J Dermatol 1995;132:106–112.

11 Haw S, Shin MK, Haw CR: The efficacy and safety of long-term oral cyclosporine treatment for patients with atopic dermatitis. Ann Dermatol 2010; 22:9–15.

12 Hoang-Xuan T, Prisant O, Hannouche D, Robin H: Systemic cyclosporine A in severe atopic keratoconjunctivitis. Ophthalmology 1997;104:1300–1305.

13 Mrowietz U, Klein CE, Reich K, Rosenbach T, Ruzicka T, Sebastian M, Werfel T: Cyclosporine therapy in dermatology. J Dtsch Dermatol Ges 2009; 7:474–479.

14 Buckley DA, Baldwin P, Rogers S. The use of azathioprine in severe adult atopic eczema. J Eur Acad Dermatol Venereol 1998;11:137–140.

15 Kuanprasert N, Herbert O, Barnetson RS: Clinical improvement and significant reduction of total serum IgE in patients suffering from severe atopic dermatitis treated with oral azathioprine. Austral J Dermatol 2002;43:125–127.

16 Hughes R, Collins P, Rogers S: Further experience of using azathioprine in the treatment of severe atopic dermatitis. Clin Exp Dermatol 2008;33: 710–711.

17 Berth-Jones J, Takwale A, Tan E, Barclay G, Agarwal S, Ahmed I, Hotchkiss K, Graham-Brown RA: Azathioprine in severe adult atopic dermatitis: a double-blind, placebo-controlled, crossover trial. Br J Dermatol 2002;147:324–330.

18 Hon KL, Ching GK, Leung TF, Chow CM, Lee KK, Ng PC: Efficacy and tolerability at 3 and 6 months following use of azathioprine for recalcitrant atopic dermatitis in children and young adults. J Dermatol Treat 2009;20:141–145.

19 Meggitt SJ, Gray JC, Reynolds NJ: Azathioprine dosed by thiopurine methyltransferase activity for moderate-to-severe atopic eczema: a double-blind, randomised controlled trial. Lancet 2006;367:839–846.

20 Murphy LA, Atherton DJ: Azathioprine as a treatment for severe atopic eczema in children with a partial thiopurine methyl transferase (TPMT) deficiency. Pediatr Dermatol 2003;20:531–534.

21 Grundmann-Kollmann M, Korting HC, Behrens S, Leiter U, Krähn G, Kaufmann R, Peter RU, Kerscher M: Successful treatment of severe refractory atopic dermatitis with mycophenolate mofetil. Br J Dermatol 1999;141:175–176.

22 Grundmann-Kollmann M, Podda M, Ochsendorf F, Boehncke WH, Kaufmann R, Zollner TM: Mycophenolate mofetil is effective in the treatment of atopic dermatitis. Arch Dermatol 2001;137:870–873.

23 Murray ML, Cohen JB: Mycophenolate mofetil therapy for moderate to severe atopic dermatitis. Clin Exp Dermatol 2007;32:23–27.

24 Benez A, Fierlbeck G: Successful long-term treatment of severe atopic dermatitis with mycophenolate mofetil. Br J Dermatol 2001;144:638–639.

25 Heller M, Shin HT, Orlow SJ, Schaffer JV: Mycophenolate mofetil for severe childhood atopic dermatitis: experience in 14 patients. Br J Dermatol 2007;157:127–132.

26 Neuber K, Schwartz I, Itschert G, Dieck AT: Treatment of atopic eczema with oral mycophenolate mofetil. Br J Dermatol 2000;143:385–391.

27 Hantash B, Fiorentino D: Liver enzyme abnormalities in patients with atopic dermatitis treated with mycophenolate mofetil. Arch Dermatol 2006; 142: 109–110.

28 Weatherhead SC, Wahie S, Reynolds NJ, Meggitt SJ: An open-label, dose-ranging study of methotrexate for moderate-to-severe adult atopic eczema. Br J Dermatol 2007;156:346–351.

29 Goujon C, Bérard F, Dahel K, Guillot I, Hennino A, Nosbaum A, Saad N, Nicolas JF: Methotrexate for the treatment of adult atopic dermatitis. Eur J Dermatol 2006;16:155–158.

30 Lyakhovitsky A, Barzilai A, Heyman R Baum S, Amichai B, Solomon M, Shpiro D, Trau H: Low-dose methotrexate treatment for moderate-to-severe atopic dermatitis in adults. J Eur Acad Dermatol Venereol 2010;24:43–49.

31 Ruzicka T, Lynde CW, Jemec GB, Diepgen T, Berth-Jones J, Coenraads PJ, Kaszuba A, Bissonnette R, Varjonen E, Holló P, Cambazard F, Lahfa M, Elsner P, Nyberg F, Svensson A, Brown TC, Harsch M, Maares J: Efficacy and safety of oral alitretinoin (9-*cis*-retinoic acid) in patients with severe chronic hand eczema refractory to topical corticosteroids: results of a randomized, double-blind, placebo-controlled, multicentre trial. Br J Dermatol 2008;158:808–817.

32 Grahovac M, Molin S, Prinz JC, Ruzicka T, Wollenberg A: Treatment of atopic eczema with oral alitretinoin. Br J Dermatol. 2010;162:217–218.

33 Kimata H: High dose gammaglobulin treatment for atopic dermatitis. Arch Dis Child 1994;70:335–336.

34 Jolles S, Sewell C, Webster D, Ryan A, Heelan B, Waite A, Rustin M: Adjunctive high-dose intravenous immunoglobulin treatment for resistant atopic dermatitis: efficacy and effects on intracellular cytokine levels and CD4 counts. Acta Derm Venereol 2003;83:433–437.

35 Jolles S, Hughes J, Rustin M: The treatment of atopic dermatitis with adjunctive high-dose intravenous immunoglobulin: a report of three patients and review of the literature. Br J Dermatol 2000;142: 551–554.

36 Huang JL, Lee WY, Chen LC, Kuo ML, Hsieh KH: Changes of serum levels of interleukin-2, intercellular adhesion molecule-1, endothelial leukocyte adhesion molecule-1 and Th1 and Th2 cell in severe atopic dermatitis after intravenous immunoglobulin therapy. Ann Allergy Asthma Immunol 2000;84: 345–352.

37 Wakim M, Alazard M, Yajima A, Speights D, Saxon A, Stiehm ER: High dose intravenous immunoglobulin in atopic dermatitis and hyper-IgE syndrome. Ann Allergy Asthma Immunol 1998;81:153–158.

38 Paul C, Lahfa M, Bachelez H, Chevret S, Dubertret L: A randomized controlled evaluator-blinded trial of intravenous immunoglobulin in adults with severe atopic dermatitis. Br J Dermatol 2002;147: 518–522.

39 Boguniewicz M, Jaffe HS, Izu A, Sullivan MJ, York D, Geha RS, Leung DY: Recombinant gamma interferon in treatment of patients with atopic dermatitis and elevated IgE levels. Am J Med 1990;88: 365–370.

40 Hanifin JM, Schneider LC, Leung DY, Ellis CN, Jaffe HS, Izu AE, Bucalo LR, Hirabayashi SE, Tofte SJ, Cantu-Gonzales G, et al: Recombinant interferon gamma therapy for atopic dermatitis. J Am Acad Dermatol 1993;28:189–197.

41 Stevens SR, Hanifin JM, Hamilton T, Tofte SJ, Cooper KD: Long-term effectiveness and safety of recombinant human interferon gamma therapy for atopic dermatitis despite unchanged serum IgE levels. Arch Dermatol 1998;134:799–804.

42 Schneider LC, Baz Z, Zarcone C, Zurakowski D: Long-term therapy with recombinant interferon-gamma (rIFN-gamma) for atopic dermatitis. Ann Allergy Asthma Immunol 1998;80:263–268.

43 Simon D, Wittwer J, Kostylina G, Buettiker U, Simon HU, Yawalkar N: Alefacept (lymphocyte function-associated molecule 3/IgG fusion protein) treatment for atopic eczema. J Allergy Clin Immunol 2008;122:423–424.

44 Moul DK, Routhouska SB, Robinson MR, Korman NJ: Alefacept for moderate to severe atopic dermatitis: a pilot study in adults. J Am Acad Dermatol 2008;58:984–989.
45 Takiguchi R, Tofte S, Simpson B, Harper E, Blauvelt A, Hanifin J, Simpson E: Efalizumab for severe atopic dermatitis: a pilot study in adults. J Am Acad Dermatol 2007;56:222–227.
46 Ibler K, Dam TN, Gniadecki R, Kragballe K, Jemec GB, Agner T: Efalizumab for severe refractory atopic eczema: retrospective study on 11 cases. J Eur Acad Dermatol Venereol 2010;24:837–839.
47 Simon D, Hösli S, Kostylina G, Yawalkar N, Simon HU: Anti-CD20 (rituximab) treatment improves atopic eczema. J Allergy Clin Immunol 2008;121: 122–128.
48 Sedivá A, Kayserová J, Vernerová E, Polouckova A, Capková S, Spísek R, Bartůnková J: Anti-CD20 (rituximab) treatment for atopic eczema. J Allergy Clin Immunol 2008;121:1515–1516.
49 Oldhoff JM, Darsow U, Werfel T, Katzer K, Wulf A, Laifaoui J, Hijnen DJ, Plötz S, Knol EF, Kapp A, Bruijnzeel-Koomen CA, Ring J, de Bruin-Weller MS: Anti-IL-5 recombinant humanized monoclonal antibody (mepolizumab) for the treatment of atopic dermatitis. Allergy 2005;60:693–696.
50 Belloni B, Ziai M, Lim A, Lemercier B, Sbornik M, Weidinger S, Andres C, Schnopp C, Ring J, Hein R, Ollert M, Mempel M: Low-dose anti-IgE therapy in patients with atopic eczema with high serum IgE levels. J Allergy Clin Immunol 2007;120:1223–1225.
51 Sheinkopf LE, Rafi AW, Do LT, Katz RM, Klaustermeyer WB: Efficacy of omalizumab in the treatment of atopic dermatitis: a pilot study. Allergy Asthma Proc 2008;29:530–537.
52 Vigo PG, Girgis KR, Pfuetze BL, Critchlow ME, Fisher J, Hussain I: Efficacy of anti-IgE therapy in patients with atopic dermatitis. J Am Acad Dermatol 2006;55:168–170.
53 Incorvaia C, Pravettoni C, Mauro M, Yacoub MR, Tarantini F, Riario-Sforza GG: Effectiveness of omalizumab in a patient with severe asthma and atopic dermatitis. Monaldi Arch Chest Dis 2008;69: 78–80.
54 Jacobi A, Antoni C, Manger B, Schuler G, Hertl M: Infliximab in the treatment of moderate to severe atopic dermatitis. J Am Acad Dermatol 2005;52: 522–526.
55 Cassano N, Loconsole F, Coviello C, Vena GA: Infliximab in recalcitrant severe atopic eczema associated with contact allergy. Int J Immunopathol Pharmacol 2006;19:237–240.
56 Lee HH, Song IH, Friedrich M, Gauliard A, Detert J, Röwert J, Audring H, Kary S, Burmester GR, Sterry W, Worm M: Cutaneous side-effects in patients with rheumatic diseases during application of tumour necrosis factor-alpha antagonists. Br J Dermatol 2007;156:486–491.
57 Vestergaard C, Deleuran M, Kragballe K: Two cases of atopic dermatitis-like conditions induced in psoriasis patients treated with infliximab. J Eur Acad Dermatol Venereol 2007;21:1272–1274.
58 Davaine AC, Saraux A, Prigent S, Kupfer-Bessaguet I, Roswag D, Plantin P, Schoenlaub P, Talarmin F, Zagnoli A, Misery L: Cutaneous events during treatment of chronic inflammatory joint disorders with anti-tumour necrosis factor alpha: a cross-sectional study. J Eur Acad Dermatol Venereol 2008;22:1471–1477.

Dagmar Simon, MD
Department of Dermatology
Inselspital
CH–3010 Bern (Switzerland)
Tel. +41 31 632 2278, Fax +41 31 632 2233, E-Mail dagmar.simon@insel.ch

Author Index

Subject Index

PRINCIPLES OF

Environmental Science

INQUIRY AND APPLICATIONS

Third Edition

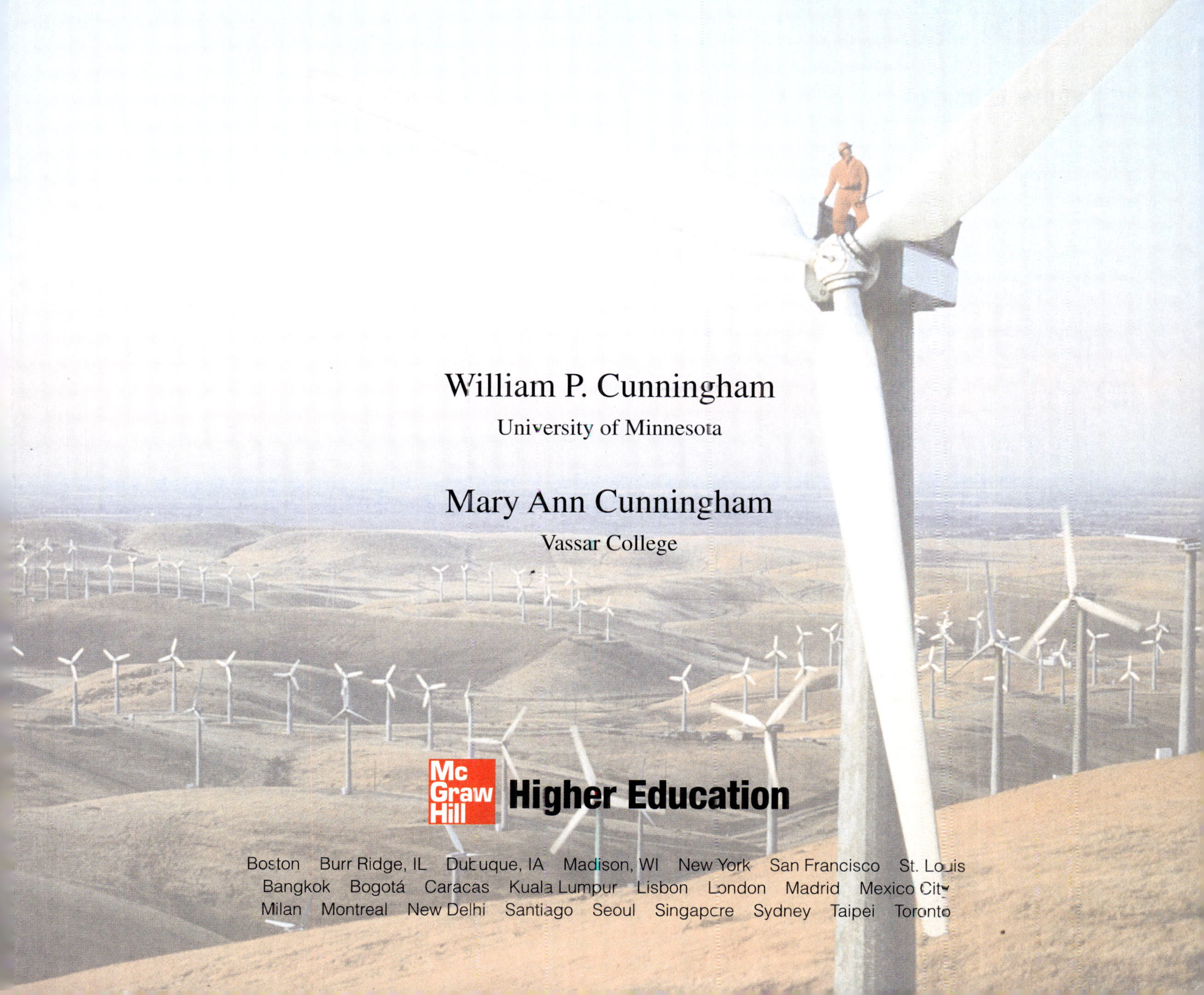

William P. Cunningham
University of Minnesota

Mary Ann Cunningham
Vassar College

McGraw Hill Higher Education

Boston Burr Ridge, IL Dubuque, IA Madison, WI New York San Francisco St. Louis
Bangkok Bogotá Caracas Kuala Lumpur Lisbon London Madrid Mexico City
Milan Montreal New Delhi Santiago Seoul Singapore Sydney Taipei Toronto

The McGraw-Hill Companies

Higher Education

PRINCIPLES OF ENVIRONMENTAL SCIENCE: INQUIRY AND APPLICATIONS
THIRD EDITION

Published by McGraw-Hill, a business unit of The McGraw-Hill Companies, Inc., 1221 Avenue of the Americas, New York, NY 10020.

This book is printed on recycled, acid-free paper containing 10% postconsumer waste.

1 2 3 4 5 6 7 8 9 0 QPD/QPD 0 9 8 7 6 5

ISBN 0–07–111574–9

www.mhhe.com

PRINCIPLES OF

Environmental Science

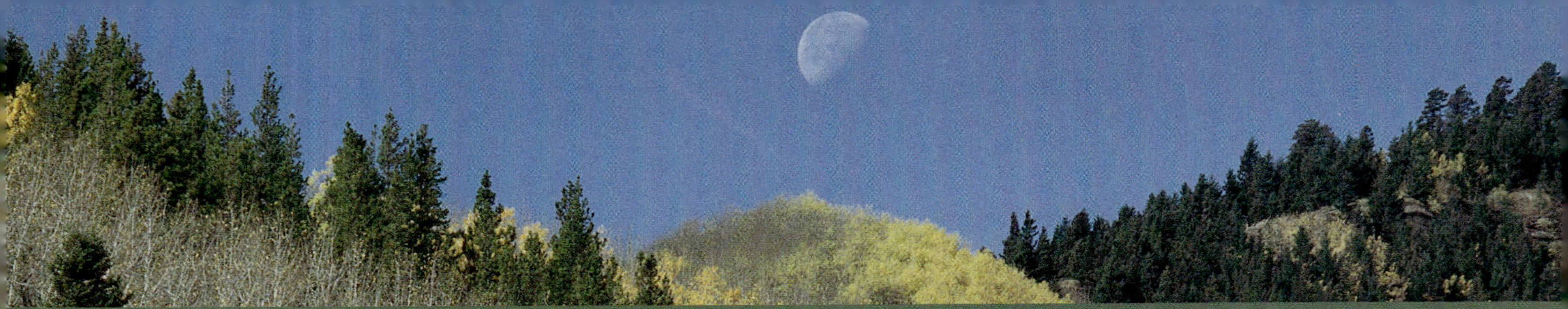

CONTENTS IN BRIEF

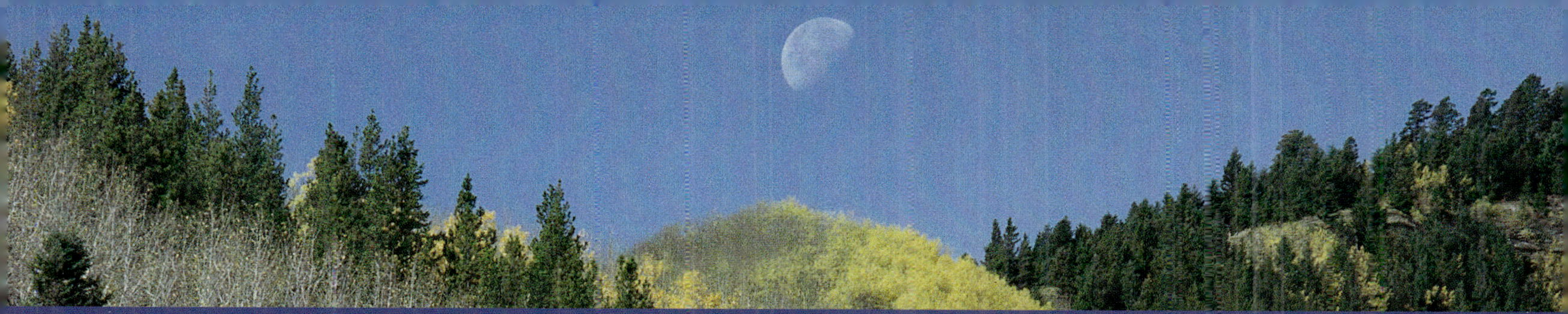

CONTENTS

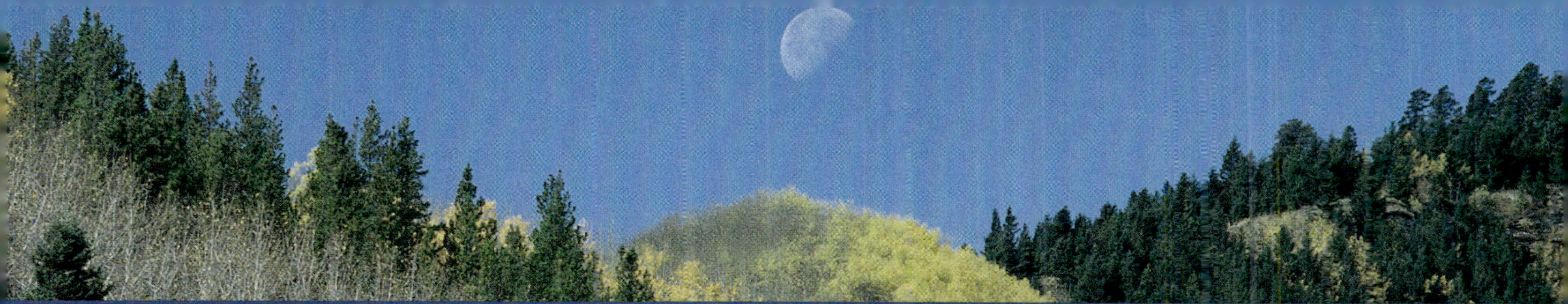

PREFACE

Can we learn to live sustainably on this planet, drawing only on nature's surplus and protecting the ecological processes on which life depends, while still providing a healthy, fulfilling life for everyone? This dilemma lies at the heart of environmental science.

Recent progress in environmental protection and improved human welfare gives us hope for reaching the goal of meeting urgent human needs while still preserving the earth's fragile life-support systems. Chlorofluorocarbon (CFC) releases into the atmosphere have decreased dramatically since the passage of the 1987 Montreal Protocol, for example, and destruction of UV-absorbing stratospheric ozone appears to be slowing. Similarly, clean air regulations have reduced sulfur dioxide emissions over North America by 31 percent over the past two decades. In many areas, acid precipitation, which threatened forests, crops, and aquatic ecosystems, has lessened. Currently, some 16.3 million km^2 (about 11 percent of the world land area) is protected in parks and nature preserves. Over the past 20 years, the average number of children born per woman worldwide has dropped nearly by half, and demographers predict that world population will stabilize by the middle of this century.

Still, many problems remain. Increasingly, we see evidence that human-caused global climate change is already underway. Biodiversity losses appear to be occurring at rates unmatched since the demise of the dinosaurs 65 million years ago. Hydrologists predict that, in a few decades, three-quarters of all humans will live in countries where freshwater supplies are inadequate to meet demand. Water wars could become a major source of conflict in the future. Bioconcentration of mercury and other toxins in food webs is a growing concern, not only in industrialized countries but even in remote areas where long-range transport of air pollutants can result in contamination problems. Currently, more than 800 million people are chronically undernourished, and more than 1.2 billion don't have enough money to provide the clean drinking water, shelter, medicine, sanitation, and education needed for a healthy, productive life.

Good science is needed to provide answers for solving these problems, but we also need an educated public that understands how science works and how to evaluate the difficult trade-offs we face. A broad-based environmental science course is an excellent way to teach a wide range of students about both scientific and social issues. It can show how valid information is gathered and analyzed as well as how to think critically and creatively about complex issues. Many instructors have asked for a textbook that gives students a strong foundation in the basic principles of environmental science. We understand and agree with that goal.

This book provides a solid foundation in scientific approaches to environmental problems and solutions. We integrate information from a wide range of disciplines from both the natural and social sciences. And we attempt to present a **balanced, objective perspective** that presents both sides of controversial issues. While much current environmental news is discouraging, we also present positive examples in which progress toward sustainability is being made. We also suggest ways that individuals can contribute to environmental protection and resource conservation. Although this book is suitable for nonscience majors, you will find that it isn't simplistic or condescending. The presentation, while condensed, remains sophisticated and discerning.

CONCISE AND AFFORDABLE

In recent years, environmental science textbooks have gotten bigger, more encyclopedic, and increasingly expensive. Both instructors and students call for a concise and affordable text. This book was written to fill that need. Rather than the 25 to 30 chapters found in most environmental science textbooks, we've limited this book to 15 chapters, or about 1 chapter per week for a typical semester course. The more concise presentation focuses on key principles, on scientific methods and ideas, and on life-long learning skills for students. We have also included enough case studies and current events to provide the real-world context for the themes discussed here. Additional case studies and current issues are also available on the book's website to help enrich your course's content. At the same time, the moderate size and price of this book should allow you to add supplementary materials to meet your individual teaching/learning objectives.

The outline of this book follows a topic sequence widely used in many environmental science textbooks and courses, but we know that many instructors choose to organize their courses around their own outlines. We've written each chapter in a way that doesn't assume that students have already read other chapters in any particular order. If instructors prefer a different organization of course topics, chapters can be presented in any order that suits their course's needs.

ACTIVE LEARNING AND CRITICAL THINKING

Learning how scientists approach problems can help students develop habits of independent, orderly, and objective thought. But it takes active involvement to master these skills. Throughout this book, we encourage students to practice thinking for themselves. Data and interpretations aren't presented as immutable truths but, rather, as evidence to be examined and tested. We try to give a balanced view of controversial topics. Orderly, critical assessment of complex problems is a key part of **scientific literacy,** which is essential for understanding current environmental science. In every chapter, students are invited to practice **critical thinking** and to apply new ideas. We also include case studies demonstrating how scientists have thought about important environmental questions.

Because we think a discouraged student is unlikely to take positive action toward sustainability, we also strive to avoid "gloom and doom" or "shame and blame" attitudes. Instead, we adopt a thoughtful but cautiously optimistic view that will encourage readers to look for ways that we can solve problems and make our world a better place in which to live. In nearly every chapter, we include "What Can You Do?" boxes that give practical suggestions for things individuals can do to make a difference. Most chapters also have short applications boxes that invite readers to stop for a moment and practice using the principles they've learned.

An introductory story at the beginning of each chapter illustrates an important current issue and relates it to practical environmental concerns. These stories also start the process of exploring how scientists study complex issues. In addition to these introductory stories, case studies and examples of how scientists investigate our environment appear periodically throughout the book to remind readers about the practical importance of these issues.

INTEGRATION AND SUSTAINABILITY

Environmental problems and their solutions occur at the intersection of natural systems and the human systems that manipulate the natural world. In this book, we present an **integrated approach** to physical sciences—biology, ecology, geology, air and water resources—and to human systems that affect nature—food and agriculture, population growth, urbanization, environmental health, resource economics, and policy. Although it is tempting to emphasize purely natural systems, we feel that students can never understand why coral reefs are threatened or why tropical forests are being cut down if they don't know something about the cultural, economic, and political forces that shape our decisions.

This integrated approach is essential if we are to work toward sustainable solutions in our environment. Throughout the book, we present **sustainability** as an ultimate goal for both preserving nature and improving the lives of people everywhere. Sustainability implies that human well-being and environmental health need to be complementary, not contradictory, efforts. The goal of sustainability also requires a global view. We take a **global perspective** in this book because we believe that the most important and difficult environmental problems we now face involve worldwide resources and international institutions. To help students gain geographical literacy, we have included many maps and international case studies in this book, including a valuable set of world maps in the appendices.

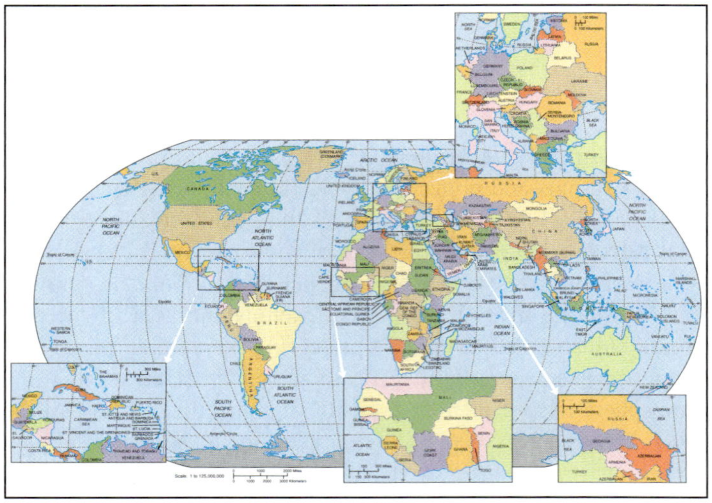

CURRENCY

Throughout this book, we present up-to-date tables and graphs with the most current available data. We hope these data will give students an appreciation of the kinds of information available in environmental science. Among the sources we have called upon here are geographic information systems (GIS) data and maps, current census and population data, international news and data sources, and federal data-collection agencies.

This text has had the benefit of input from more than 400 researchers, professionals, and instructors who have reviewed this book or our larger text, *Environmental Science: A Global Concern*. These reviewers have helped us keep the text current and focused. We deeply appreciate their many helpful suggestions and comments.

WEB-ENHANCEMENT

The World Wide Web has become a vast and valuable resource for students. You can find a wealth of information there to update or supplement topics in environmental science. We incorporate this resource more fully in this text than in any other environmental science book currently available. Every chapter opens with a list of **web-based resources** that relate to and enrich the chapter contents. We have also placed further readings and extra case studies on the Web and have referenced these readings in the text. We encourage instructors to make use of these additional resources. At the end of each chapter, a **web-based exercise** invites students to visit specific webpages and use the data found there to create graphs, make comparisons, or do some other practical analysis of real data. These aren't simplistic exercises that just ask the reader to look at a site and report on what it contains. Rather, we ask the student to explore these resources and use the information they find in pragmatic ways. Note that these exercises are just a beginning: instructors and students can modify or add to these exercises if they wish. One of our objectives in these exercises is simply to expose students to important data sources. Another objective in these exercises is to make students work with data, create graphs, map data, and experience some of the ways that scientists create and share information today.

LEARNING TOOLS

This book is intentionally written in a **lively, accessible style** and illustrated with nearly 400 full-color photographs and figures that help explain important concepts. We have also integrated a number of learning tools to help students gain an informed, thoughtful view of our environment:

- *"Investigating Our Environment" essays.* These examples give students some experience with tools and approaches scientists use to solve contemporary environmental problems. Each boxed essay shows how scientists work to solve complex environmental questions.

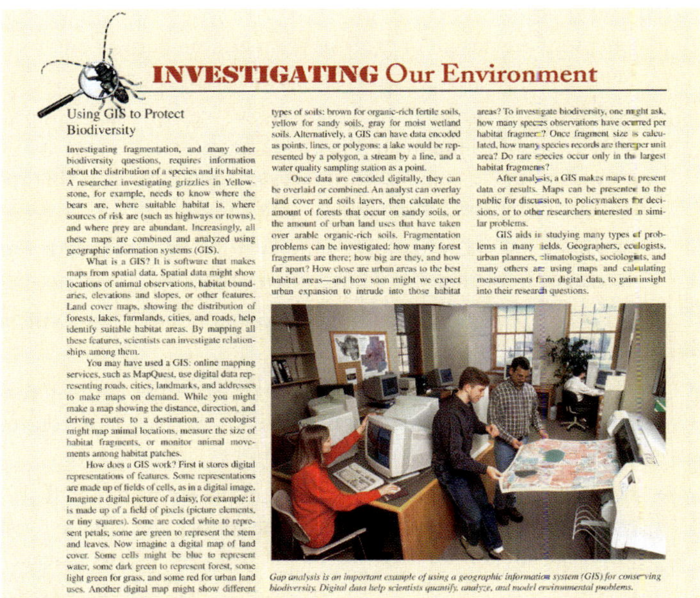

INVESTIGATING Our Environment

Using GIS to Protect Biodiversity

Investigating fragmentation, and many other biodiversity questions, requires information about the distribution of a species and its habitat. A researcher investigating grizzlies in Yellowstone, for example, needs to know where the bears are, where suitable habitat is, where sources of risk are (such as highways or towns), and where prey are abundant. Increasingly, all these maps are combined and analyzed using geographic information systems (GIS).

What is a GIS? It is software that makes maps from spatial data. Spatial data might show locations of animal observations, habitat boundaries, elevations and slopes, or other features. Land cover maps, showing the distribution of forests, lakes, farmlands, cities, and roads, help identify suitable habitat areas. By mapping all these features, scientists can investigate relationships among them.

You may have used a GIS: online mapping services, such as MapQuest, use digital data representing roads, cities, landmarks, and addresses to make maps on demand. While you might make a map showing the distance, direction, and driving routes to a destination, an ecologist might map animal locations, measure the size of habitat fragments, or monitor animal movements among habitat patches.

How does a GIS work? First it stores digital representations of features. Some representations are made up of fields of cells, as in a digital image. Imagine a digital picture of a daisy, for example: it is made up of a field of pixels (picture elements, or tiny squares). Some are coded white to represent petals; some are green to represent the stem and leaves. Now imagine a digital map of land cover. Some cells might be blue to represent water, some dark green to represent forest, some light green for grass, and some red for urban land uses. Another digital map might show different types of soils: brown for organic-rich fertile soils, yellow for sandy soils, gray for moist wetland soils. Alternatively, a GIS can have data encoded as points, lines, or polygons: a lake would be represented by a polygon, a stream by a line, and a water quality sampling station as a point.

Once data are encoded digitally, they can be overlaid or combined. An analyst can overlay land cover and soils layers, then calculate the amount of forests that occur on sandy soils, or the amount of urban land uses that have taken over arable organic-rich soils. Fragmentation problems can be investigated: how many forest fragments are there; how big are they, and how far apart? How close are urban areas to the best habitat areas—and how soon might we expect urban expansion to intrude into those habitat areas? To investigate biodiversity, one might ask, how many species observations have occurred per habitat fragment? Once fragment size is calculated, how many species records are there per unit area? Do rare species occur only in the largest habitat fragments?

After analysis, a GIS makes maps to present data or results. Maps can be presented to the public for discussion, to policymakers for decisions, or to other researchers interested in similar problems.

GIS aids in studying many types of problems in many fields. Geographers, ecologists, urban planners, climatologists, sociologists, and many others are using maps and calculating measurements from digital data, to gain insight into their research questions.

Gap analysis is an important example of using a geographic information system (GIS) for conserving biodiversity. Digital data help scientists quantify, analyze, and model environmental problems.

- *Study aids.* Each chapter opens with a list of objectives that summarize the main points of the chapter. These objectives are written in active terms that suggest to the student that it requires active involvement on their part to learn environmental science. Notice that, while some objectives call for simple, concrete thinking skills, others are deliberately aimed at higher cognitive levels to encourage students to think reflectively, analytically, and critically. Although asking students to analyze, understand, explore, or question don't have simple, clear endpoints that can be measured objectively, we believe it's important to point out the need for higher-level thinking about complex issues. Every chapter ends with a summary of main points, a list of key terms, and review questions that help the student review material and prepare for tests.
- *Scientific thinking.* A more challenging, open-ended set of questions titled "Thinking Scientifically" encourages students to think more deeply and independently about issues and principles presented in the chapter. These questions make excellent starting points for discussion sections. They also could be used to practice for essay exams or might even serve as an essay exam themselves.
- *Statistics, graphs, and data.* Knowing that many students have little background in math, we've included special features on statistical methods and how they apply to environmental science, as well as discussion of how graphs can be used to present data. To give students practice in graphing, several end-of-chapter web exercises include graphing exercises.
- *Applications.* Because few of us learn effectively without an opportunity to actively apply new ideas, we have included application boxes. These boxes provide a break in reading the text and invite students to practice or apply skills they have just learned. In addition, "What Can You Do?" boxes in nearly every chapter suggest practical things that individuals can do to help improve environmental quality and resource conservation.

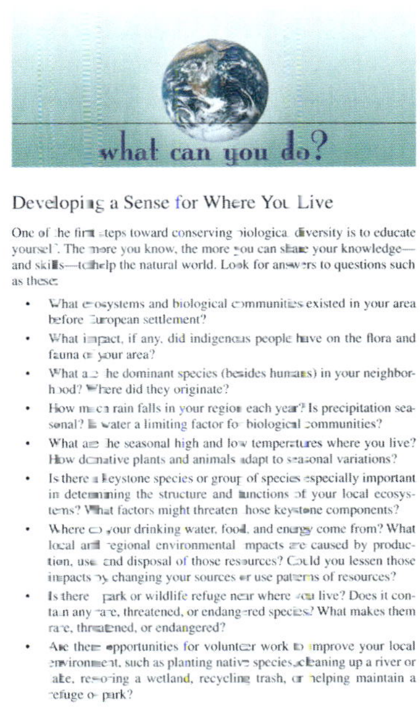

what can you do?

Developing a Sense for Where You Live

One of the first steps toward conserving biological diversity is to educate yourself. The more you know, the more you can share your knowledge—and skills—to help the natural world. Look for answers to questions such as these:

- What ecosystems and biological communities existed in your area before European settlement?
- What impact, if any, did indigenous people have on the flora and fauna of your area?
- What are the dominant species (besides humans) in your neighborhood? Where did they originate?
- How much rain falls in your region each year? Is precipitation seasonal? Is water a limiting factor for biological communities?
- What are the seasonal high and low temperatures where you live? How do native plants and animals adapt to seasonal variations?
- Is there a keystone species or group of species especially important in determining the structure and functions of your local ecosystems? What factors might threaten those keystone components?
- Where do your drinking water, food, and energy come from? What local and regional environmental impacts are caused by production, use, and disposal of those resources? Could you lessen those impacts by changing your sources or use patterns of resources?
- Is there a park or wildlife refuge near where you live? Does it contain any rare, threatened, or endangered species? What makes them rare, threatened, or endangered?
- Are there opportunities for volunteer work to improve your local environment, such as planting native species, cleaning up a river or lake, restoring a wetland, recycling trash, or helping maintain a refuge or park?

- *Web exercises.* The World Wide Web has become an extremely important source of current data, but many students know little about the kinds of information available or the agencies and organizations that produce it. Our web exercises make use of current data and ask students to perform activities such as graphing data, comparing maps, and using live GIS sources to learn about environmental issues and information sources.

- *Maps and appendices*. The appendices include conversion factors for weights and measures in an easy-to-locate position on the inside back cover. A new and expanded set of maps serves as a reference for the whole book and should help students expand their geographical knowledge and global perspective. The glossary defines all key terms as well as other important vocabulary words. A list of further readings will be posted on the webpage, where it can be updated periodically.

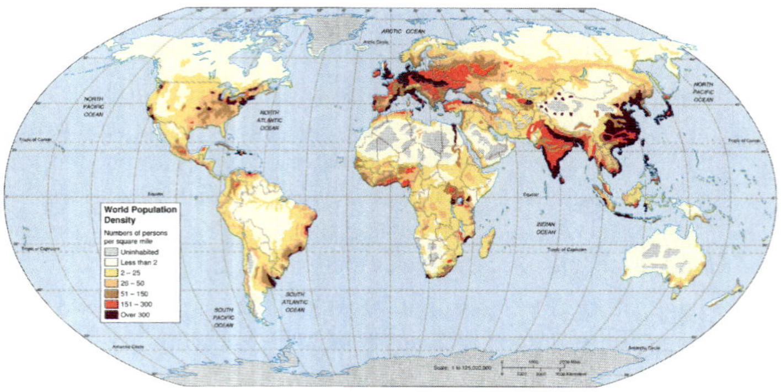

NEW FEATURES IN THIS EDITION

Updated Art Program

We are fortunate to have a collection of beautiful, three-dimensional, photo-realistic drawings by Kandis Elliott, of the University of Wisconsin, that illustrate ecological cycles and relationships in a more realistic and recognizable style to help students understand important environmental principles. More than 50 new or revised graphs, drawings, and other graphics (about 200 in total) provide valuable information as well as making the text attractive and highly readable. Additional maps have been added to give students an understanding of geography, including small place maps to locate major world biomes. In addition, 10 new tables allow readers to compare and understand data in greater depth than provided by straight text. A fold-out world map is included at the end of the book as additional reference for political and physical world regions.

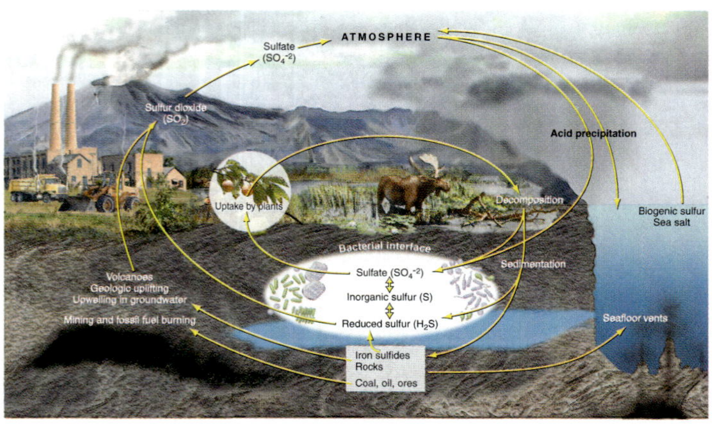

New Photographs

We believe that students benefit from seeing photographs of people and nature in actual settings. For students who may rarely get outdoors and whose primary contact with the world around them is the computer screen or TV, photographs can add interest and authenticity to their study of environmental science. While other textbooks in this area have reduced or eliminated photographs from their texts, we continue to use high-quality photographs. Roughly half of our 406 figures are photographs, and approximately half of those are new for this edition. We are fortunate to have access to the outstanding photography of Dr. Barry Barker of Nova Southeastern University and David L. Hansen of the University of Minnesota Agricultural Experiment Station, whose works are prominently featured in this edition.

Updated Information

Much has happened in environmental science since the second edition of this text. Every chapter has been updated with new information.

- Chapter One has an entirely new section on current environmental conditions.
- Following reviewers' suggestions, we've moved the Periodic Table of Elements to the appendix, where it's still available for those who are interested but doesn't disrupt information flow for those who don't use it.
- In chapter 4, new data on human populations and recent advances in birth control have been added.
- Chapter 5 has undergone extensive reorganization, with a new section on marine ecosystems.
- The discussion of threats to biodiversity in chapter 5 also has been reorganized around E. O. Wilson's acronym HIPPO.
- In one of the most dramatic changes in environmental science in recent years, the WHO documents a shift in the most important health threats worldwide from infectious diseases to chronic conditions such as obesity, depression, trauma, and cardiovascular diseases once thought to be limited to the richest countries. As Western lifestyles spread to developing countries, however, the diseases of affluence have become the leading causes of death and morbidity nearly everywhere. Chapter 8 has been rewritten to reflect this new reality.
- Chapter 9 contains a wealth of new information on global climate change together with a discussion of clean air controversies in the United States.

- Chapter 10 incorporates updated data on water quality, water shortages, and water pollution, including the terrible problem of arsenic poisoning of groundwater in South Asia.
- The expert advice of Dr. John Pratt has guided revisions to chapters 11 and 12, and these chapters are strengthened and improved by his suggestions.

Many other chapters also have new data and features that we don't have room to detail here. Altogether, we believe you'll find this edition the most up-to-date of any textbook currently on the market.

GIS and Remote Sensing

Drawing on Mary Ann Cunningham's expertise in the areas of GIS, remote sensing, and biogeography, we have added several boxed readings to explain these important techniques and to show how they can be used in environmental science.

New Case Studies, Opening Stories, and Other Special Readings

Every chapter starts with an opening vignette, which presents a fascinating current environmental problem that illustrates the principles to be presented in the text. Interspersed throughout each chapter are other special features that show concrete application of theoretical knowledge. Ranging from controversy over dredging PCBs from the Hudson River to the threat of bioterrorism, these special readings also provide an opportunity to bring up current events and to make connections to real-life issues. Of the 30 special readings in the book, 16 are new to this edition, making the text thoroughly up-to-date and relevant.

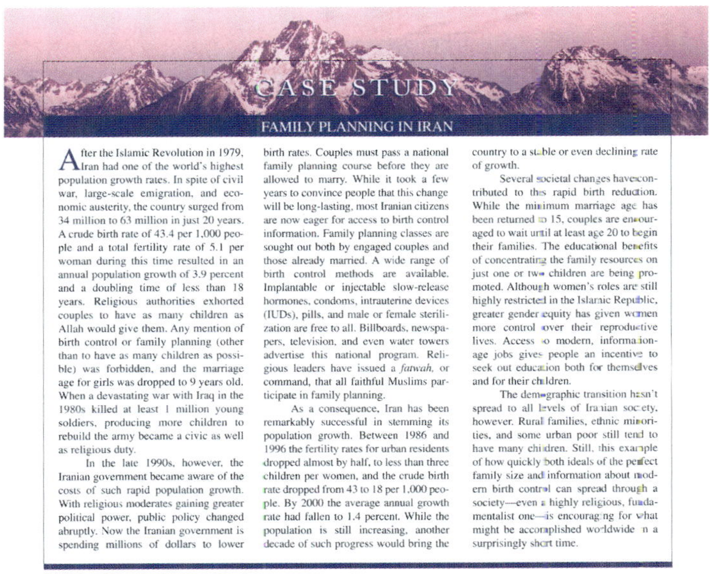

CASE STUDY

FAMILY PLANNING IN IRAN

After the Islamic Revolution in 1979, Iran had one of the world's highest population growth rates. In spite of civil war, large-scale emigration, and economic austerity, the country surged from 34 million to 63 million in just 20 years. A crude birth rate of 43.4 per 1,000 people and a total fertility rate of 5.1 per woman during this time resulted in an annual population growth of 3.9 percent and a doubling time of less than 18 years. Religious authorities exhorted couples to have as many children as Allah would give them. Any mention of birth control or family planning (other than to have as many children as possible) was forbidden, and the marriage age for girls was dropped to 9 years old. When a devastating war with Iraq in the 1980s killed at least 1 million young soldiers, producing more children to rebuild the army became a civic as well as religious duty.

In the late 1990s, however, the Iranian government became aware of the costs of such rapid population growth. With religious moderates gaining greater political power, public policy changed abruptly. Now the Iranian government is spending millions of dollars to lower birth rates. Couples must pass a national family planning course before they are allowed to marry. While it took a few years to convince people that this change will be long-lasting, most Iranian citizens are now eager for access to birth control information. Family planning classes are sought out both by engaged couples and those already married. A wide range of birth control methods are available. Implantable or injectable slow-release hormones, condoms, intrauterine devices (IUDs), pills, and male or female sterilization are free to all. Billboards, newspapers, television, and even water towers advertise this national program. Religious leaders have issued a *fatwah*, or command, that all faithful Muslims participate in family planning.

As a consequence, Iran has been remarkably successful in stemming its population growth. Between 1986 and 1996 the fertility rates for urban residents dropped almost by half, to less than three children per women, and the crude birth rate dropped from 43 to 18 per 1,000 people. By 2000 the average annual growth rate had fallen to 1.4 percent. While the population is still increasing, another decade of such progress would bring the country to a stable or even declining rate of growth.

Several societal changes have contributed to this rapid birth reduction. While the minimum marriage age has been returned to 15, couples are encouraged to wait until at least age 20 to begin their families. The educational benefits of concentrating the family resources on just one or two children are being promoted. Although women's roles are still highly restricted in the Islamic Republic, greater gender equity has given women more control over their reproductive lives. Access to modern, information-age jobs gives people an incentive to seek out education both for themselves and for their children.

The demographic transition hasn't spread to all levels of Iranian society, however. Rural families, ethnic minorities, and some urban poor still tend to have many children. Still, this example of how quickly both ideals of the perfect family size and information about modern birth control can spread through a society—even a highly religious, fundamentalist one—is encouraging for what might be accomplished worldwide in a surprisingly short time.

Suggested Readings

Our Online Learning Center website has an extensive list of more than 2,500 annotated citations to important environmental articles. We know, however, that few students take the time to investigate this database, so we've added a short list of suggested readings to each chapter to show important data sources and current directions in science.

LET US KNOW WHAT YOU THINK

We'd appreciate hearing from both students and instructors about where—and how—we could improve this text. You, the users, are the real test of whether we have accomplished our goal of presenting the principles of environmental science in an engaging and understandable way. Please let us know what you think. We value your comments and suggestions. Please send your recommendations to the Integrative Biology Division of McGraw-Hill, 2460 Kerper Blvd., Dubuque, IA, 52001.

USEFUL SUPPLEMENTS

- **Digital Content Manager (DCM) CD-ROM.** This multimedia collection of visual resources allows instructors to utilize artwork from the text in multiple formats to create customized classroom presentations, visually based tests and/or quizzes, dynamic course website content, and attractive printed support materials. The digital assets on this cross-platform CD-ROM are grouped within the following easy-to-use folders:
    - *Illustrations and photos.* All of the line drawings from the text and hundreds of photos are in ready-to-use digital files.
    - *PowerPoint lecture outline.* Ready-made presentations combine art from the text with customized, instructor-written lecture notes, covering all 15 chapters.
    - *Tables.* Every table that appears in the text is provided in electronic form.
    - *Active art.* These special art pieces consist of key images from the text that are converted to a format that allows instructors to break the art down into core elements and then group the various pieces and create customized

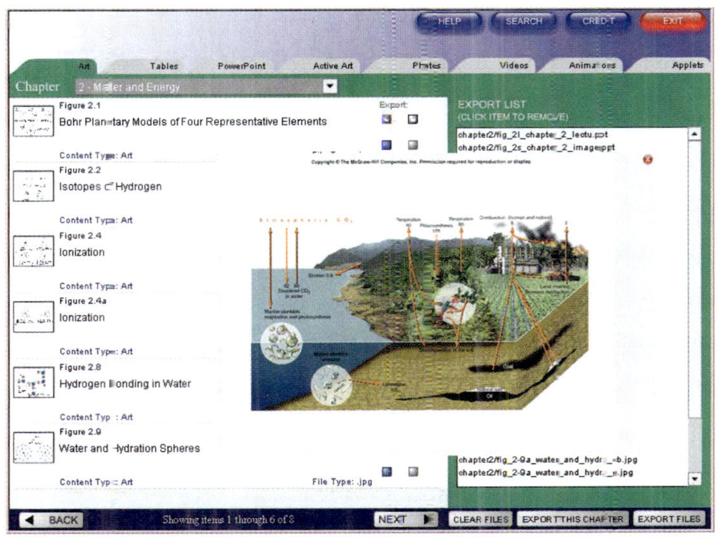

images. This is especially helpful with difficult concepts; they can be presented step-by-step.

- *Animations.* Numerous full-color animations illustrating many different concepts covered in the study of environmental science are provided. The visual impact of motion will enhance classroom presentations and increase comprehension.

- *Additional photo library.* Over 400 full-color photographs *additional* to those already in the textbook are included in the Digital Content Manager. These photos are specific to environmental science topics, and are searchable by content.

• **Instructor's Testing and Resource CD-ROM.** This cross-platform CD-ROM provides a wealth of resources for the instructor. Supplements featured on this CD-ROM include lab activities, and a computerized test bank to quickly create customized exams. This user-friendly program allows instructors to search for questions by format, edit existing questions or add new ones, and scramble questions and answer keys for multiple versions of the same test. Other assets on the Instructor's Testing and Resource CD-ROM are grouped within easy-to-use folders.

• **Transparencies.** A set of 100 transparencies is available to users of the text. These acetates include key figures from the text, including new art from this edition.

• **Interactive World Issues CD-ROM.** This CD explores environmental issues that affect various geographic regions. For example, you'll visit Oregon and investigate water rights of the Columbia River. Listen to Native Americans whose living depends on salmon fishing and then to the farmers who need water to irrigate their crops. Additional case studies discuss migration in Mexico, apartheid in South Africa, population issues in China, and farming in urban Chicago.

• **Online Learning Center.** (http://www.mhhe.com/cunningham3e). This comprehensive website offers numerous resources for both students and instructors.

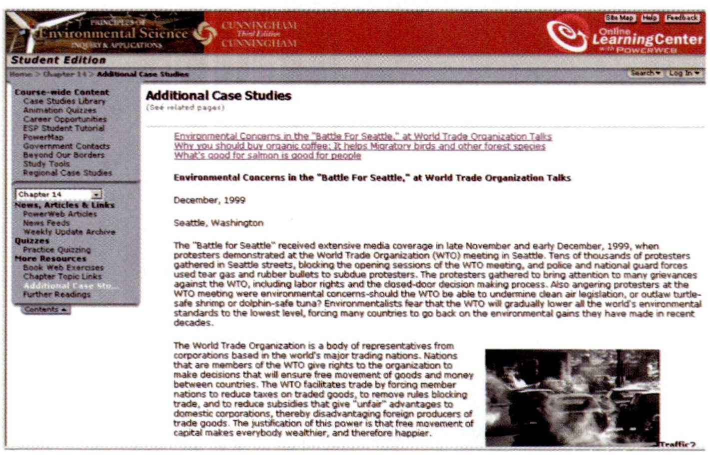

Student Resources—Everything you need in one place

- Practice quizzing
- How-to study tips
- Web links to related topics
- Web exercises
- Guide to electronic research
- Regional perspectives (case studies)
- Environmental issues world map
- Key term flashcards
- How to write a paper
- How to contact your elected officials
- Further readings
- Metric equivalents and conversion tables
- Career information
- Access Science offering the advantage of an online, interactive encyclopedia

Instructor Resources—in addition to all of the above, you'll receive:

- Supplements resource chart for each chapter
- Answers to web exercises
- Additional case studies
- Answers to critical thinking questions
- PageOut (create your own course website)

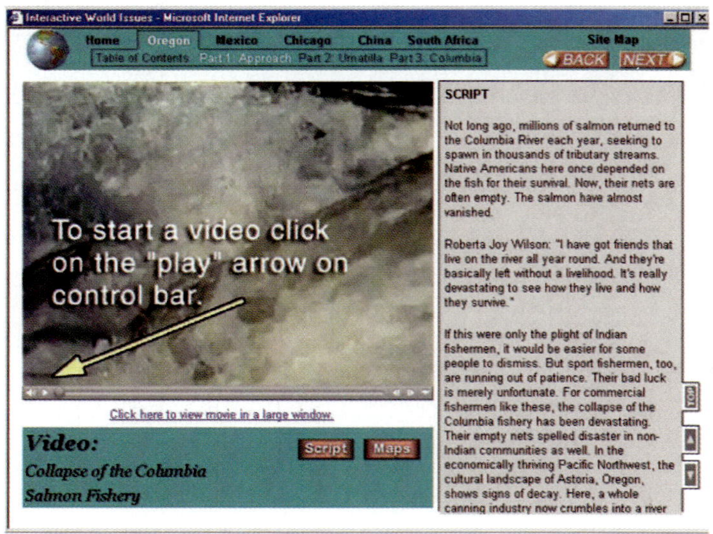

• **New!! Exploring Environmental Solutions with GIS.** This short book provides exercises for students and instructors who are new to GIS but are familiar with the Windows operating system. The exercises focus on improving analytical skills, understanding spatial relationships, and understanding the nature and structure of environmental data. Because the software used is distributed free of charge, this text is appropriate for courses and schools that are not yet ready to commit to the expense and time involved in acquiring other GIS packages.

RELATED TITLES OF INTEREST

1. *Exploring Environmental Solutions with GIS* (includes CD-ROM) (0-07-297744-2) by Stewart, Schneiderman, Cunningham, and Gold.
2. *Field and Laboratory Activities Manual,* 7th ed. (0-07-290913-7) by Enger and Smith.
3. *Interactive World Issues: Of Place and Planet CD-ROM* (0-07-255648-X), Cambridge Studios.
4. *Annual Editions: Environment 04/05* (0-07-286147-9). Editor: John L. Allen.
5. *Taking Sides: Clashing Views on Controversial Environmental Issues,* revised 10th ed. (0-07-293317-8). Editors: Thomas Easton, Theodore D. Goldfarb.
6. *Sources: Notable Selections in Environmental Studies,* 2nd ed. (0-07-303186-0). Editor: Theodore D. Goldfarb.
7. The Dushkin *Student Atlas of Environmental Issues* (0-697-36520-4). Editor: John Allen. University of Connecticut.

ACKNOWLEDGMENTS

We're indebted to all the instructors who have reviewed the manuscript and made helpful suggestions, corrections, and recommendations for improving this book. Space does not permit inclusion of all the excellent ideas that were provided, but we will continue to do our best to incorporate the ideas that reviewers have given us. In addition, all of us owe a big debt to the many scholars whose work forms the basis of our understanding of environmental science. We stand on the shoulders of giants. If errors persist in spite of our best efforts to root them out, we accept responsibility.

We express our gratitude to the entire McGraw-Hill book team for their wonderful work in putting together this edition. Donna Nemmers and Brian Loehr oversaw the developmental stages and have made many creative contributions to this book. April Southwood, production project manager, kept everything running smoothly. Lori Hancock found excellent photographs. The folks at Precision Graphics did an excellent job of composition and page layout. Tami Petsche and Marge Kemp have supported this project with their enthusiasm and creative ideas.

The following individuals provided reviews for this book. We thank them for their suggestions.

Shannon A. Bliss
Cerro Coso Community College

Robert Buschbacher
University of Florida

Catherine W. Carter
Georgia Perimeter College

Richard Clements
Chattanooga State Technical Community College

Michael L. Denniston
Georgia Perimeter College

Laurie S. Eberhardt
Valparaiso University

Brad C. Fiero
Pima Community College

Steven P. Frysinger
James Madison University, Harrisonburg

Zofia E. Gagnon
Marist College

Carey A. Gazis
Central Washington University

Marcia L. Gillette
Indiana University, Kokomo

Daniel F. Gleason
Georgia Southern University

Lawrence J. Gray
Utah Valley State College

Mark F. Hammer
Wayne State College

Charles Kaminski
Middlesex Community College

Paul Kimball
Northeast Iowa Community College

Ned J. Knight
Linfield College

Jeff Kushner
James Madison University

Matthew Laposata
Kennesaw State University

Kurt M. Leuschner
College of the Desert

Edward M. Lignowski
Holy Family College

Les M. Lynn
Bergen Community College

Timothy F. Lyon
Ball State University

Janet S. MacFall
Elon University

Nancy Jean Mann
Cuesta College

Ken R. Marion
University of Alabama, Birmingham

Thomas C. Moon
California University of Pennsylvania

Michele Morek
Brescia University

Michael J. Neilson
The University of Alabama, Birmingham

Pamela Pape-Lindstrom
Everett Community College

David R. Perault
Lynchburg College

Ervand M. Peterson
Sonoma State University

Julie Phillips
De Anza College

Mark D. Plunkett
Bellevue Community College

John M. Pratte
Kennesaw State University

Carlton Lee Rockett
Bowling Green State University

Robert J. Sager
Pierce College

Ronald L. Sass
Rice University

Jeffry A. Schneider
SUNY-Oswego

Bruce A. Schulte
Georgia Southern University

Julie A. Seiter
Oakland Community College

Jill Singer
Buffalo State College

Denise L. Stetson
Johnson and Wales University

L. Harold Stevenson
McNeese State University

Ronald C. Sundell
Northern Michigan University

John A. Tiedemann
Monmouth University

Michael Toscano
San Joaquin Delta College

Edward R. Wells
Wilson College

Arlene A. Westhoven
Ferris State University

Ray E. Williams
Rio Hondo College

Thomas B. Wilson
University of Arizona

Bruce C. Wyman
McNeese State University

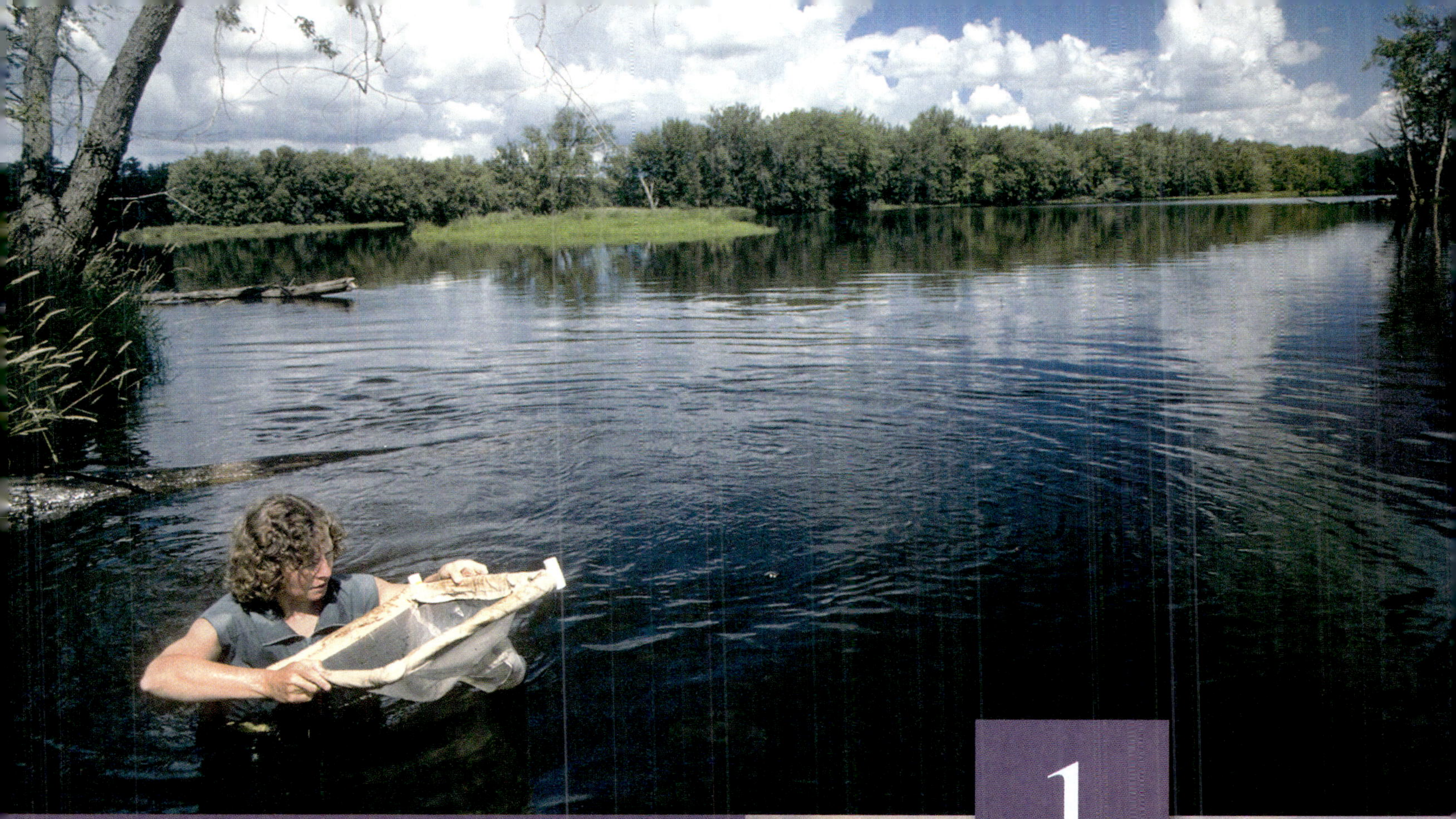

A limnologist studies freshwater organisms as indicators of water quality.

1

Understanding Our Environment

We travel together, passengers on a little spaceship, dependent upon its vulnerable reserves of air and soil, all committed for our safety to its security and peace; preserved from annihilation only by the care, the work, and I will say, the love that we give to our fragile craft.

–Adlai Stevenson

Welcome to McGraw-Hill's Online Learning Center
http://www.mhhe.com/cunningham3e

LEARNING ONLINE

Visit our webpage at www.mhhe.com/cunningham3e for data sources, further readings, additional case studies, current environmental news, and regional examples within the Online Learning Center to help you understand the material in this chapter. You'll also find active links to information pertaining to this chapter, including

Conservation history
Environmental justice
Environmental philosophy
State of the world
Human development
Sustainable development
Indigenous rights
Science

OBJECTIVES

After studying this chapter, you should be able to

- define the term *environment* and identify some important environmental concerns that we face today.
- explain the scientific method and why it refutes or supports theories but never proves them beyond any doubt.
- apply the scientific method to problem solving.
- explain how statistics can help evaluate the accuracy and significance of results.
- summarize four stages in the history of conservation.
- distinguish among analytical, creative, logical, critical, and reflective thinking.
- summarize some major environmental dilemmas and issues that shape our current environmental agenda.
- discuss the implications of sustainability and sustainable development.

Dredging the Hudson River

In February 2002 the U.S. Environmental Protection Agency (EPA) signed a decision to begin the most expensive river cleanup in U.S. history. Over the next decade, a $460 million dredging project will remove some 2 million m^3 of contaminated sediment from a 40-mile stretch of the Hudson River north of Albany, New York. The main target of this expensive operation is polychlorinated biphenyls (PCBs)—oily, persistent organic compounds once widely used as electrical insulators in capacitors and transformers.

Between 1946 and 1977, General Electric Company (GE) legally discharged an estimated 500,000 kg (1.1 million lbs) of PCBs into the river from its factories in Hudson Falls and Fort Edward. Production, processing, and distribution of PCBs were banned in the United States in 1976 after these chemicals were shown to cause cancer in laboratory animals. GE stopped releasing PCBs in 1977, but seepage from the river bottom still continues. In addition to being classified as potential carcinogens in humans, PCBs also are suspected of triggering other serious health problems, including low birth weight, thyroid disease, and mental, reproductive, and immunological abnormalities. Because of these health concerns, a $40 million per year Hudson River fishing industry was shut down in 1976. Although PCB concentrations in the Hudson have dropped significantly in recent years, women of childbearing age and children under age 15 still are warned not to eat fish from the river, and no one should eat fish caught between Troy and Hudson Falls. In 1983 a 200-mile stretch of the Hudson south of Hudson Falls was declared the largest Superfund site in the United States.

Despite decades of research and debate, what to do about polluted sediment from the river bottom remains highly controversial. Although environmentalists and most residents farther south support dredging, many who live along affected sections of the river remain strongly opposed. Local residents fear the noise, lights, and commotion of the 19-hour per day operation will disrupt fish and wildlife populations, drive away tourists, and spoil the quiet beauty of their neighborhoods. They argue that dredging the river will stir up sediments and contaminate the water even more.

These fears were magnified by GE's multimillion-dollar advertising campaign showing giant clamshell dredges dumping dripping loads of muck into barges. A much better plan, according to GE—which will have to pay most of the dredging costs—would be to leave the PCBs in the sediment, where bacteria would eventually metabolize and deactivate them. The EPA replies that the environmental dredges to be used on the Hudson are not much larger than the average recreational fishing boat (fig. 1.1). Operating as large vacuum cleaners, they suck up sediment inside silt curtains that keep contaminants from escaping into nearby water. The EPA claims residents will hardly notice that the operation is underway and that it will be completely open and transparent in reporting water quality data and cooperating with affected communities.

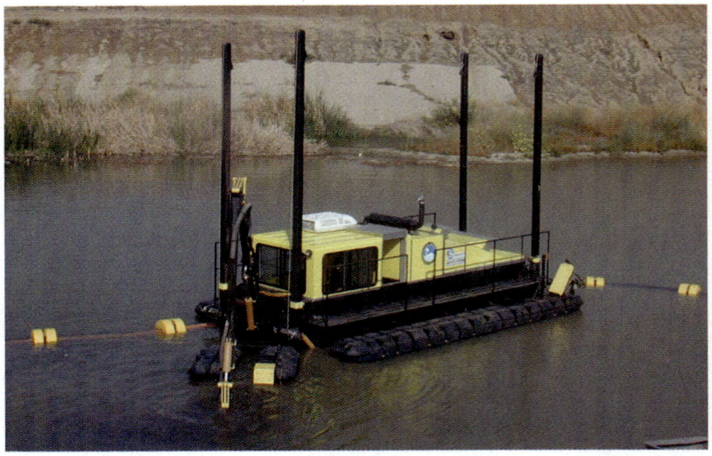

FIGURE 1.1 *An environmental dredge removes contaminants from the river bottom.*

EPA scientists agree that bacterial action would eventually destroy PCBs in the river sediment, but they point out that this process would take centuries. Meanwhile, according to EPA estimates, about 500 lbs (227 kg) of PCBs seep from the river mud and from fractured bedrock beneath the Hudson Falls factory every year. The total amount of PCBs released in six years of dredging, according to the EPA, will be about 200 lbs (91 kg). We can't be sure if these estimates are correct until the dredging has been carried out, but EPA scientists argue that the benefits of dredging far outweigh its potential risks. Many local residents distrust these calculations and doubt the benefits are as large as promised. Meanwhile, GE has challenged the entire Superfund program as an unconstitutional constraint on business.

The dilemma over what to do about contamination of the Hudson River shares aspects of many issues we will discuss in this book. We are changing our environment in ways that we suspect are hazardous, both to us and to other living things. It often is uncertain, however, exactly how dangerous these threats are or what we ought to do about them. Science can't predict what will happen in the future, or offer absolute certainty about how safe, or unsafe, particular options may be. Scientists can only give reasoned judgments about potential benefits and risks. Both policymakers and ordinary citizens need training and experience to understand the advantages and limits of scientific information.

Often, as in the case of dredging the Hudson, seemingly equal authorities give exactly opposite opinions about what we should do. It takes careful, critical thinking to fashion an independent, rational position when the evidence presented is confusing or contradictory. Studying environmental science will help you find answers to some important questions we all face. It's the first step in becoming an informed environmental citizen. Welcome to an important and, we hope, engaging voyage of discovery.

UNDERSTANDING OUR ENVIRONMENT

The debate about dredging the Hudson River illustrates some of the complexity and importance of contemporary environmental issues. Human actions are having widespread impacts on our world and the other organisms with which we share it. Science and technology have become pervasive forces, both to explain how things work and to reveal how we can make our environment safer, more comfortable, and more enduring. The knowledge being gained by scientists is fundamental to our ability to manage the earth's resources in a sustainable manner and to improve the quality of our lives and those of our children. Environmental scientists work on many problems that critically affect our well-being in many ways. Because of the significance of its findings, an understanding of environmental science is becoming increasingly necessary for any educated person.

As you study environmental science, you will learn about many serious problems. But environmental science can also be exciting and highly gratifying. As they study the world around us, environmental scientists explore coral reefs, live with great apes, collect ice samples from deep within glaciers, study exotic plant species, and listen to whales. They also examine the social institutions and built environment that we create for ourselves using science, technology, and political organization. There is room for many different kinds of interests and abilities within this broad discipline. Whether you are a professional scientist or a concerned citizen, you can apply your knowledge of environmental science in enjoyable and useful ways.

A Marvelous Planet

Before proceeding in our discussion of current dilemmas and how scientists are trying to understand them, we should pause for a moment to consider the extraordinary natural world that we inherited and that we hope to pass on to future generations in as good—or perhaps even better—condition than we found it.

Imagine that you are an astronaut returning to the earth after a long trip to the moon or Mars. What a relief it would be, after experiencing the hostile environment of outer space, to come back to this beautiful, bountiful planet (fig. 1.2). Although there are dangers and difficulties here, we live in a remarkably prolific and hospitable world that is, as far as we know, unique in the universe. Compared with the conditions on other planets in our solar system, temperatures on the earth are mild and relatively constant. Plentiful supplies of clean air, fresh water, and fertile soil are regenerated endlessly and spontaneously by biogeochemical cycles and biological communities (discussed in chapters 2 and 3).

Perhaps the most amazing feature of our planet is its rich diversity of life. Millions of beautiful and intriguing species populate the earth and help sustain a habitable environment (fig. 1.3). This vast multitude of life creates complex, interrelated communities where towering trees and huge animals live together with, and depend upon, such tiny life-forms as viruses, bacteria, and fungi. Together, all these organisms make up delightfully diverse, self-sustaining ecosystems, including dense, moist forests; vast, sunny savannas; and richly colorful coral reefs.

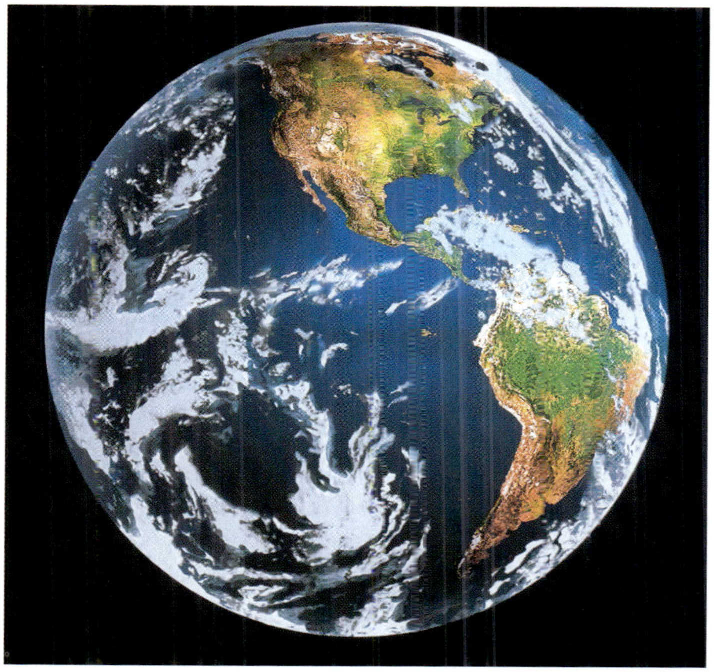

FIGURE 1.2 *The life-sustaining ecosystems on which we all depend are unique in the universe, as far as we know.*

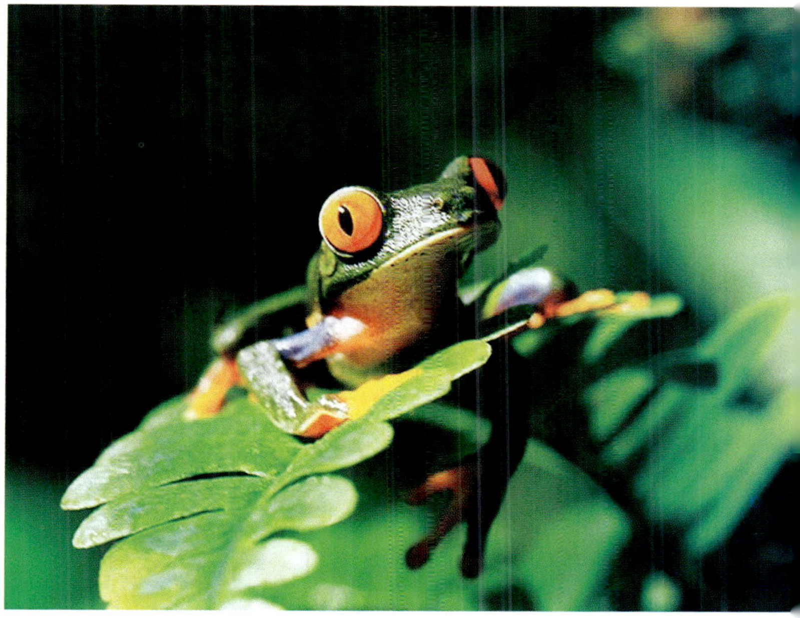

FIGURE 1.3 *Perhaps the most amazing feature of our planet is its rich diversity of life.*

From time to time, we should pause to remember that, in spite of the challenges and complications of life on earth, we are incredibly lucky to be here. We should ask ourselves: what is our proper place in nature? What *ought* we do and what *can* we do to protect the irreplaceable habitat that produced and supports us? These are some of the central questions of environmental science.

What Is Environmental Science?

We inhabit two worlds. One is the natural world of plants, animals, soils, air, and water that preceded us by billions of years and of which we are a part. The other is the world of social institutions and artifacts that we create for ourselves using science, technology, and political organization. Both worlds are essential to our lives, but integrating them successfully causes enduring tensions.

Environment (from the French *environner:* to encircle or surround) can be defined as (1) the circumstances and conditions that surround an organism or a group of organisms or (2) the social and cultural conditions that affect an individual or a community. Since humans inhabit the natural world as well as the "built" or technological, social, and cultural world, all constitute important parts of our environment (fig. 1.4).

Environmental science is the systematic study of our environment and our place in it. A relatively new field, environmental science is highly interdisciplinary. It integrates information from biology, chemistry, geography, agriculture, and many other fields. To apply this information to improve the ways we treat our world, environmental scientists also incorporate knowledge of social organization, politics, and the humanities. In other words, environmental science is inclusive and holistic. Environmental science is also mission-oriented: it implies that we all have a responsibility to get involved and try to do something about the problems we have created.

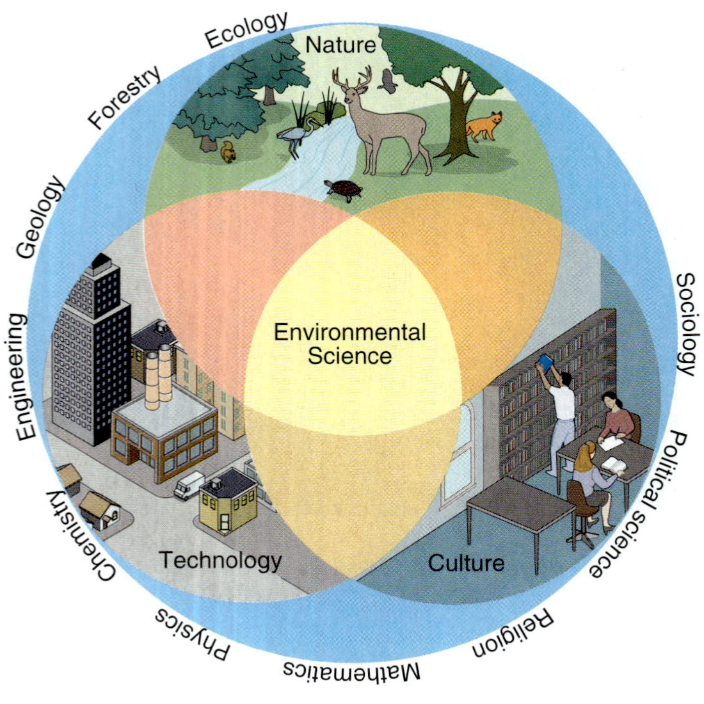

FIGURE 1.4 *The intersections of the natural, cultural, and technological worlds outline the province of environmental science. Many disciplines contribute to our understanding and management of our environment.*

As distinguished economist Barbara Ward pointed out, for an increasing number of environmental issues, the difficulty is not to identify remedies. Remedies are now well understood; the problem is to make them socially, economically, and politically acceptable. Foresters know how to plant trees, but not how to establish conditions under which villagers in developing countries can manage plantations for themselves. Engineers know how to control pollution, but not how to persuade factories to install the necessary equipment. City planners know how to design urban areas, but not how to make them affordable for the poorest members of society. The solutions to these problems increasingly involve human social systems as well as natural science.

Criteria for environmental literacy have been suggested by the National Environmental Education Advancement Project in Wisconsin. These criteria include awareness and appreciation of the natural and built environment, knowledge of natural systems and ecological concepts, understanding of current environmental issues, and ability to use analytical and problem-solving skills on environmental issues. These are good goals to keep in mind as you study this book.

SCIENCE AS A WAY OF KNOWING

Science, derived from "knowing" in Latin, is a process for producing knowledge. It depends on making precise observations of natural phenomena and on formulating reasonable theories to make sense out of those observations. Science rests on the assumptions that the world is knowable and that we can learn about how things work through careful empirical study and logical analysis. Moreover, because science provides information about both materials and mechanisms in the world around us, it can help us find practical solutions for many problems (table 1.1).

An important value of scientific thinking is that it reduces our tendency to rely on emotional reactions and unexamined assumptions. In the Middle Ages, the ultimate source of knowledge about matters such as how crops grow or how diseases spread was religious authorities or cultural traditions. While these sources may have provided useful insights in many cases, there was no way to test their explanations independently and objectively. They were right because custom, politics, or theology said so. The benefit of scientific thinking is that it searches for testable evidence: if you suspect that a disease spreads through contaminated water, you can close off access to that water source and see if the disease stops spreading.

Ideally, scientists are skeptical. They don't accept proposed explanations until there is substantial evidence to support them. Even then, every explanation is considered only provisionally true because there is always a possibility that some additional evidence may appear to disprove it. Scientists also try to be methodical, rigorous, and unbiased. Because bias and methodical errors are hard to avoid, scientific tests are subject to review by informed peers, who can help evaluate results and conclusions.

Modern science has its roots in antiquity. Greek philosophers such as Pythagoras (about 520 B.C.), Socrates (464–399 B.C.), and Aristotle (380–320 B.C.) laid the foundations for inquiry and logic

TABLE 1.1 Some Scientific Assumptions

1. The world is knowable. With careful, impartial observation and logical analysis, we can make sense of the fundamental processes and laws that shape our environment.
2. Basic patterns that describe events in the natural world are uniform throughout time and space. The forces at work now are the same as those that shaped the world in the past and will continue to do so in the future.
3. Where two equally plausible explanations for a phenomenon are possible, we should choose the simpler one (also known as the law of **parsimony,** or Ockham's razor after the English philosopher who first proposed this rule).
4. Change in knowledge is inevitable because new evidence may challenge prevailing theories. No matter how well one theory explains a set of observations, another theory may fit just as well or better, or it may fit a still wider range of data.
5. Although new facts can disprove existing theories, science can never provide absolute proof that a theory is correct. Every theory should be considered only conditionally or provisionally correct until contrary evidence is found.
6. Even if there is no way to secure complete and absolute truth, increasingly accurate approximations can be made to account for the world and how it works.
7. Because science provides information about both mechanisms and processes in the world around us, it can help find practical solutions for many problems.

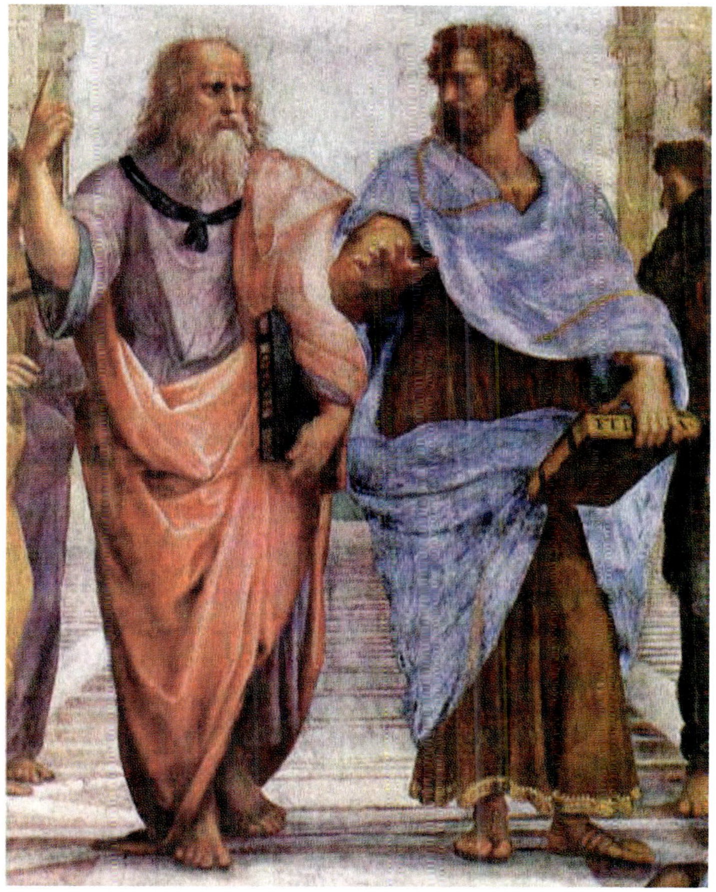

FIGURE 1.5 *Plato and Aristotle debate moral philosophy in a painting by Raphael. Plato* (left) *motions upward, indicating a transcendent, universal moral truth, while Aristotle* (right) *motions downward to suggest grounded, contingent knowledge.*

(fig. 1.5). Arabic mathematicians and astronomers added to this store of knowledge and reintroduced it to the Western world at the end of the Middle Ages. Much of what we now know as the scientific worldview and scientific method, however, originated in seventeenth- and eighteenth-century Europe. Among the scholars who pioneered empirical, experimental approaches to science were Galileo Galilei (1564–1642), a pioneer in physics and astronomy; philosophers such as René Descartes (1596–1650) and Francis Bacon (1561–1626), who emphasized the use of objective observation and inductive reasoning; and Isaac Newton (1642–1727), who invented calculus and studied optics and gravitation. The insights and methods introduced by these scientific pioneers laid the foundation for much of the material progress that we now enjoy.

Cooperation and Insight in Science

Good science rarely is carried out by a single individual working in isolation. Instead, a community of scientists collaborates in a cumulative, self-correcting process. Ideas and information are freely exchanged, debated, and tested to find the most correct ones. Ideally, scientists compare results and challenge interpretations in a democratic, impartial way. You often hear about big breakthroughs and dramatic discoveries that change our understanding overnight, but these are rare in ordinary science. Instead, many people work on different aspects of a common problem, each adding small insights into how a system works.

Confusing or erroneous results often misdirect researchers temporarily until mistakes are recognized and the search for truth gets back on the right track. One of the main benefits of research work is the realization it gives you of how contradictory science often is. If you're working at the cutting edge of either your theories or your instruments, you may well get wrong answers as often as you get right ones. Making sense of a baffling mass of information is one of the greatest challenges that scientists face (fig. 1.6).

Many people—even scientists—fail to recognize the role that creativity, insight, aesthetics, and luck play in research. Often our most important discoveries were made not through superior scientific method or equipment, but because the investigators were passionate and tenacious in their pursuit of knowledge. Some great physicists such as Albert Einstein, Richard Feynman, and Murray Gell-Mann have been attracted to certain theories as much by their elegance and beauty as by their scientific importance.

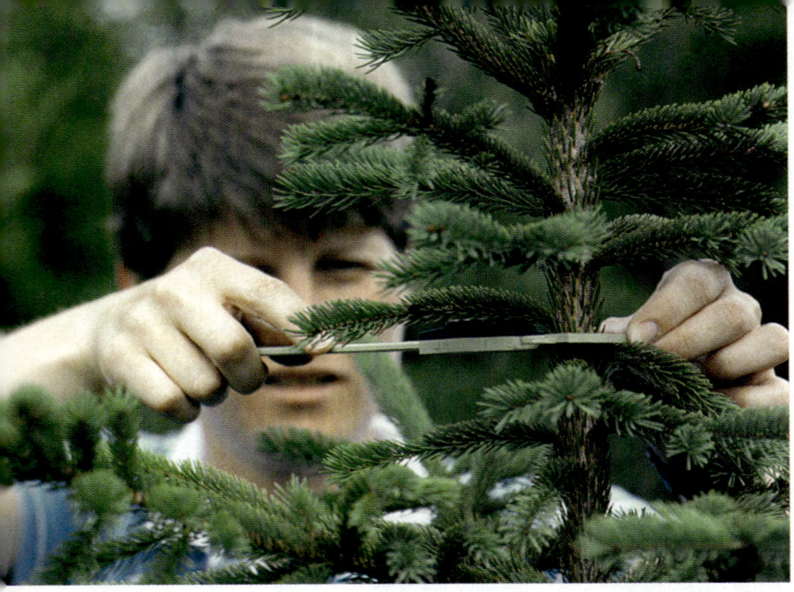

FIGURE 1.6 *Making careful, accurate measurements and keeping good records are essential in scientific research.*

Scientific Design

Scientists demand lots of evidence before they are willing to accept the accuracy of any data or the usefulness of a particular interpretation. One of the most important tests of any data is their **reproducibility.** Making an observation or obtaining a particular result just once doesn't count for much. You have to produce the same result consistently to be sure that your first outcome wasn't a fluke. Even more important, you ought to be able to describe in sufficient detail the conditions under which you made the observation or obtained the result so that someone else can reproduce your findings.

It's often difficult to study natural systems because so many important factors vary simultaneously. To avoid this problem, scientists design **controlled studies** in which comparisons are made between experimental and control populations that are identical (as far as possible) in every factor except the one being studied. Studies must be designed very carefully so that experimenters don't inadvertently treat the experimental and control groups differently or that data coders don't unconsciously let bias creep into their scoring. To avoid investigator bias, **blind experiments** are designed in which those carrying out the experiment don't know which treatment the subjects received until after data have been gathered and analyzed. In medical research involving human subjects you have to be careful that expectations of the subjects and the experimenters don't bias results (the placebo effect). In a **double-blind design,** neither the subject (participant) nor the experimenter knows which participants are receiving the experimental or the control treatments. Analysis of the results is done by a third party who does know which participants are allocated to which group.

Researchers try very hard to be accurate, but it's important to avoid unnecessary or meaningless precision. Suppose you've had a fresh snowfall in your area, and you want to know its depth. You have a ruler marked in millimeters. The first measurement you make is 24 mm, but the surface of the snow isn't even. By moving your ruler slightly, you can get measurements of 21 mm and 25 mm. What's the true depth of the snowfall? If you average these three measurements, you get 23.3333 mm, but this gives a false notion of precision. The last three digits aren't **significant numbers.** Your ruler isn't accurate to tenths of a millimeter, let alone thousandths or ten-thousandths, nor is the surface of the snow even enough to make such a precise measurement. The most accurate answer is an approximation of about 23 mm.

Deductive and Inductive Reasoning

In 1919 Sir Arthur Eddington led an expedition to Principe Island off the coast of West Africa to photograph stars during a solar eclipse. These photographs were a landmark in modern science because they were the first successful empirical test of Einstein's theory of general relativity. Einstein's calculations predicted that photons of light are affected by gravity. Thus, light coming from distant stars should be deflected if it passes close to our sun's surface. These stars should appear shifted slightly in position during the day, when the sun is present, compared with the night, when it is not. Normally, you can't make such an observation because the stars close to the sun are invisible in the daytime. During an eclipse, however, it is possible to photograph stars and compare their apparent day and night locations. This is what Eddington did, and his corroboration of Einstein's prediction was a triumphant moment in modern physics, one that helped Einstein's theory of relativity become widely accepted.

This series of logical steps is **deductive reasoning.** Starting with a general principle (the theory of general relativity), a testable prediction is derived about a specific case: that certain stars should appear closer together in the daytime than at night. You might think of this as "top-down" reasoning—proceeding from the general to the specific. Although deduction is often regarded as a scientific ideal, in many cases we don't have a general theory to explain certain phenomena in nature. Instead, we depend on "bottom-up" **inductive reasoning,** in which we study specific examples and try to discover patterns and derive general explanations from collected observations.

An example of inductive reasoning is seen in the brilliant work of Austrian zoologist Karl Von Frisch, who discovered how honeybees communicate. Although people had noticed for many years that bees seem to have an uncanny ability to find their way to nectar-bearing flowers, no theoretical explanation gave any insight into this phenomenon. Through meticulous, methodical observations, Von Frisch discovered and described the dances by which foraging honeybees (*Apis mellifera*) indicate the direction and distance of food sources to their hive mates. In 1973 Von Frisch shared the Nobel Prize in Medicine with Konrad Lorenz and Nikolaas Tinbergen, who had made similar discoveries in animal behavior through equally detailed and painstaking observations. While we still don't have many widely accepted laws of animal behavior or communication, these studies have given us fascinating insights into the lives of other organisms.

Hypotheses and Theories

You may already be using scientific technique without being aware of it. Suppose your flashlight doesn't work. The problem could be in the batteries, the bulb, or the switch—or all of them could be faulty. How can you distinguish among these possibilities? If you change all the components at once, you may have a working flashlight, but you won't know which was the faulty part. A series of methodical steps to test each component can be helpful.

Starting with the observation that your flashlight doesn't work, you make inferences about the component you think most likely to be defective. Perhaps that's the batteries. You propose a **hypothesis,** or a conditional explanation that can be tested by further observation or experiment. In this case, the hypothesis might be "The batteries are dead." From this tentative assumption, you make a prediction: "If I replace the dead batteries with fresh ones, the flashlight should work." If your hypothesis is correct, then when you perform the experiment (replacing the batteries), you will see the predicted result. If not, you reject your first hypothesis and form a new one: for example, "The bulb is burned out." By formulating testable hypotheses and evaluating each component in turn, you should eventually be able to isolate the problem and find a way to solve it.

What you have just employed in this example is the scientific method of observations, systematic testing, and interpretation of results shown in figure 1.7. As mentioned earlier, the results of one experiment may give us information that leads to further hypotheses and additional experiments. In each case, prior knowledge and experience help us design experiments and interpret results. Eventually, with evidence from a group of related investigations, we may be able to formulate a theory to explain a set of general principles.

Logically, you can show a hypothesis based on inductive reasoning to be wrong, but you can almost never show it to be unquestionably true. The philosopher Ludwig Wittgenstein gave the following example to illustrate this principle. Suppose all the swans you have ever seen are white. You might assume that *all* swans are white. This hypothesis could be tested by examining a large number of swans. If you never find a black one, you might tentatively conclude that your hypothesis is right. But even if you look at a million white swans, there could still be a black one somewhere (actually, there are black swans in Australia) that would refute your conjecture. Thus, you could show your hypothesis is wrong, but you could never be absolutely sure that it is correct, no matter how much evidence you collect.

As a result of this uncertainty, we should always regard evidence in science as provisional. Additional information might come along to undermine the observations we have made thus far. When a large number of tests supports an explanation, however, and a majority of experts in a given field have reached a general consensus that it is the best description or explanation available, we call it a **scientific theory.** Note that scientists' use of this term is very different from that of the general public. To many people, a theory is speculative and unsupported by facts. To a scientist, it means just the opposite; while all explanations are tentative and open to revision and correction, one that counts as a scientific theory is supported by an overwhelming body of data and experience, and it is generally accepted in the scientific community, at least for the present.

Modeling and Natural Experiments

Not every area that we might want to study scientifically is open to simple, direct experiments like those described earlier. A geologist, for instance, might want to study mountain building, or an

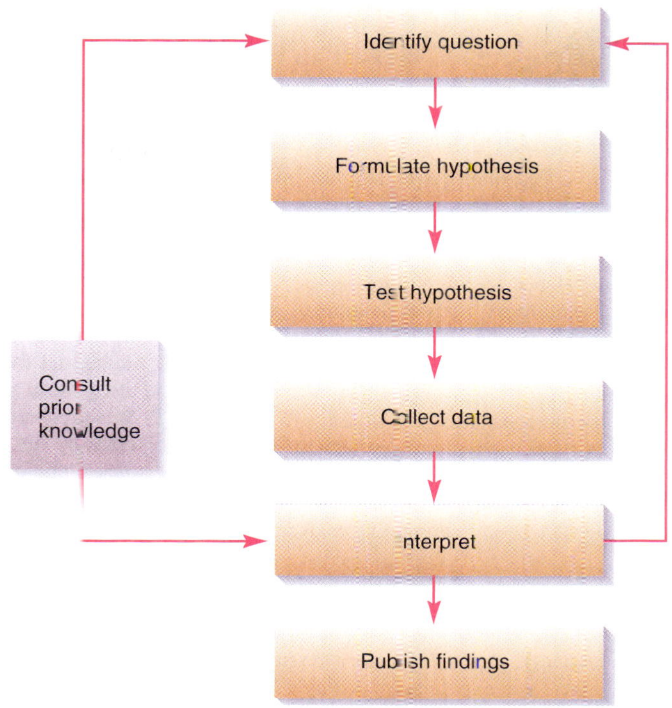

FIGURE 1.7 *Ideally, scientific investigation follows a series of logical, orderly steps to formulate and test hypotheses.*

ecologist might like to know how species coevolve, but neither scientist would be able to re-create the millions of years and complex environmental conditions required for these processes to occur. Similarly, a toxicologist might want to know about the effects of toxins but couldn't deliberately poison people, no matter how useful that information might be.

One way to gather information in fields such as these is to look for historic evidence, or what might be called "natural experiments," for support or contradiction of an idea. Can you find examples that would support or refute a given hypothesis from what has already happened? The geologist, for example, might propose the hypothesis that mountain building always involves folding and uplifting of surface strata. If she can find counterexamples, this hypothesis could be discarded.

Another way to gather information about environmental systems is to use models. A model could be a substitute organism or a physical mock-up that simulates a real system, or it could be a set of mathematical equations, often calculated in a computer program, that represents the phenomenon you want to study. For instance, the toxicologist might feed the toxin in question to rats and then attempt to extrapolate or infer how the rats' reaction is related to humans. The geologist might build a scale model of a mountain range to see what forces affect it. Mathematical models are especially useful when there are simultaneous variables. Input conditions (initial population size, population growth rate, and so on) can be manipulated to test their effect on resulting conditions.

Models, however, represent researchers' assumptions about how a system works, so models run by different people can produce contradictory results. Global warming models, for example,

INVESTIGATING Our Environment

What Are Statistics, and Why Are They Important?

Statistics are numbers that let you evaluate and compare things. "Statistics" is also a field of study that has developed meaningful methods of comparing those numbers. By both definitions, statistics are widely used in environmental sciences, partly because they can give us a useful way to assess patterns in a large population, and partly because the numbers can give us a measure of confidence in our research or observations. Understanding the details of statistical tests can take years of study, but a few basic ideas will give you a good start toward interpreting statistics.

1. *Descriptive statistics help you assess the general state of a group.* In many towns and cities, the air contains a dust, or particulate matter, as well as other pollutants. From personal experience you might know your air isn't as clean as you'd like, but you may not know how clean or dirty it is. You could start by collecting daily particulate measurements to find average levels. An averaged value is more useful than a single day's values, because daily values may vary a great deal, but general, long-term conditions affect your general health. Collect a sample every day for a year; then divide the sum by the number of days, to get a **mean** (average) dust level. Suppose you found a mean particulate level of 30 micrograms per cubic meter ($\mu g/m^3$) of air. Is this level high or low? In 1997 the EPA set a standard of 50 $\mu g/m^3$ as a limit for allowable levels of coarse particulates (2.5–10 micrometers in diameter). Higher levels tend to be associated with elevated rates of asthma and other respiratory diseases. Now you know that your town, with an annual average of 30 $\mu g/m^3$, has relatively clean air, after all.
2. *Statistical samples.* Although your town is clean by EPA standards, how does it compare with the rest of the cities in the country? Testing the air in *every* city is probably not possible. You could compare your town's air quality with a **sample,** or subset of cities, however. A large, random sample of cities should represent the general "population" of cities reasonably well. Taking a large sample reduces the effects of outliers (unusually high or low values) that might be included. A random sample minimizes the chance that you're getting only the worst sites, or only a collection of sites that are close together, which might all have similar conditions. Suppose you get average annual particulate levels from a sample of 50 randomly selected cities. You can draw a frequency distribution, or histogram, to display your results (fig. 1). The mean value of this group is 36.8 $\mu g/m^3$, so by comparison your town (at 30 $\mu g/m^3$) is relatively clean.

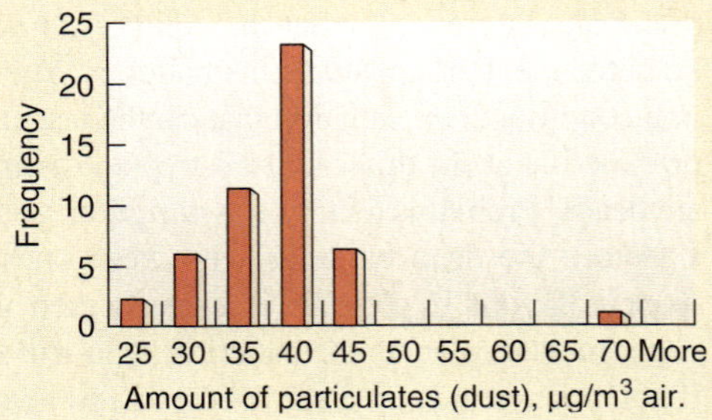

FIGURE 1 *Average annual airborne dust levels for 50 hypothetical cities in 2001.*
Source: Data from U.S. Environmental Protection Agency.

Many statistical tests assume that the sample has a normal, or Gaussian, frequency distribution, often described as a bell-shaped curve (fig. 2). In this distribution, the mean is near the center of the range of values, and most values are fairly close to the mean. Large and random samples are more likely to fit this shape than are small and nonrandom samples.

3. *Confidence.* How do you know that the 50 cities you sampled really represent all the cities in the country? You can't ever be completely certain, but you can use estimates, such as confidence limits, to express the reliability of your mean statistic. Depending on the size of your sample (not 10, not 100, but 50) and the amount of variability in the

disagree on the amount of climate change expected, as well as the rate of change. However, models do provide heuristic information—suggestions of how things might be—and they allow us to test our understanding of the relationships in a system. Even though climate models disagree on the degree of change, nearly all agree that temperatures will increase. Models have become an important scientific tool for exploring complex systems. In chapter 3 we will look at a few simple population models and at how these models help us understand population dynamics.

Statistics and Probability

You will encounter a lot of numbers in this book. It is important to think carefully about what they mean and what they don't mean. Quantitative data can be precise and easily compared, and they provide good benchmarks for measuring change. Suppose that you read—as you will in chapter 6—that 2.7 million ha (6.7 million acres) of forest burned in the United States in 2002. Is that a lot or a little? Is it an ominous change from previous years, or is it within the range that we might expect? It happens that 2000 was an exceptionally hot, dry year and that the number and sizes of forest fires were much greater than anytime in the previous 90 years. The total area of the fires was slightly larger than Maryland or Vermont, but some of the forests were probably only lightly burned, while other sections were more severely affected. You have to look carefully at what numbers mean, not just take them at face value. It also helps to try to develop some benchmarks to which you can compare statistics. How big is a hectare? How many people live in Canada? What is a gigaton? A useful conversion table can be found inside the back cover of this book.

Probability is another important concept in science. Probability, risk, and chance are all ideas that try to measure how likely something is. They never tell what *will* happen, only what might happen. If you have a 20 percent chance of catching a cold this month, that means that about 20 out of every 100 people will probably get a cold. You are relatively unlikely to get one, but you might. We rarely can be 100 percent sure of anything, but scientists consider a 95 percent probability—or confidence level—that

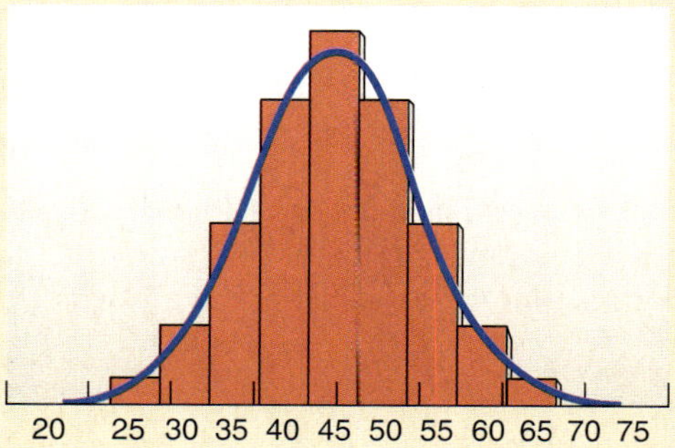

FIGURE 2 *A normal distribution.*

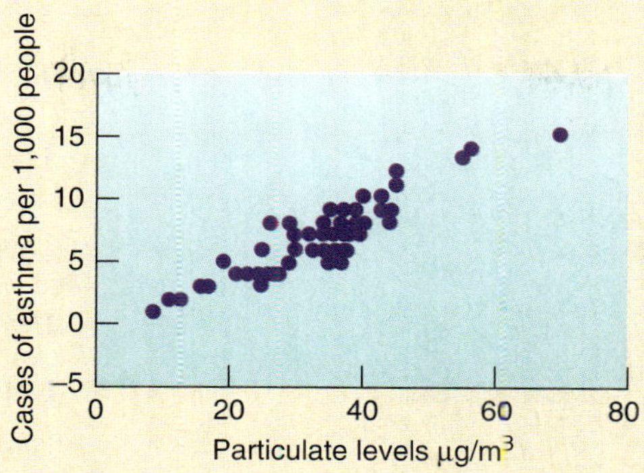

FIGURE 3 *A plot showing relationships between variables.*

sample data, you can calculate a confidence interval that the mean represents the whole population (all cities). Confidence levels, or confidence intervals, represent the likelihood that your statistics represent the entire population correctly. For the mean of your sample, a confidence interval tells you the probability that your sample is similar to other random samples of the population. A common convention is to compare values with a 95 percent confidence level, or a probability of 5 percent or less that your conclusions are misleading. Using statistical software, we can calculate that, for our 50 cities, the mean is 36.8 $\mu g/m^3$, and the confidence interval is 35.0 to 38.6. This suggests that, if you take 1,000 samples from the entire population of cities, 95 percent of those samples ought to be within 2 $\mu g/m^3$ of your mean. This indicates that your mean is reliable and representative.

4. *Is your group unusual?* Once you have described your group of cities, you can compare it with other groups. For example, you might believe that Canadian cities have cleaner air than U.S. cities. You can compare mean air quality levels for the two groups. Then you can calculate confidence intervals for the difference between the means, to see if the difference is meaningful.
5. *Evaluating relationships between variables.* Are respiratory diseases correlated with air pollution? For each city in your sample, you could graph pollution and asthma rates (fig. 3). If the graph looks like a loose cloud of dots, there is no clear relationship. A tight, linear pattern of dots trending upward to the right indicates a strong and positive relationship. You can also use a statistical package to calculate an equation to describe the relationship and, again, confidence intervals for the equation. This is known as a regression equation.
6. *Lies, damned lies, and statistics.* Can you trust a number to represent a complex or large phenomenon? One of the devilish details of representing the world with numbers is that those numbers can be tabulated in many ways. If we want to assess the greatest change in air quality statistics, do we report rates of change or the total amount of change? Do we look at change over five years? Twenty-five years? Do we accept numbers selected by the EPA, by the cities themselves, by industries, or by environmental groups? Do we trust that all the data were collected with a level of accuracy and precision that we would accept if we knew the hidden details in the data-gathering process? Like all information, statistics need to be interpreted in terms of who produced them, when, and why. Awareness of some of the standard assumptions behind statistics, such as sampling, confidence, and probability, will help you interpret statistics that you see and hear.

an event is not random a high degree of certainty (see Investigating Our Environment, p. 8).

A related question concerns appropriate sample size. How many individuals would you need to examine to have a reliable representation of a population? Is it better to sample small areas in many different places or one larger area? How many times do you need to replicate your investigation to ensure a reliable result (fig. 1.8)? The answers to these questions depend on the variables that you intend to study, as well as the accuracy level you hope to attain. These aspects of research design are the domain of statistics. Statistics is an important tool in both planning and evaluating scientific studies.

Paradigms and Scientific Consensus

The notion of paradigm shifts has been important since science historian Thomas Kuhn introduced it in the 1960s. **Paradigms,** according to Kuhn, are overarching models of the world that guide our interpretation of events. Two centuries ago, Noah's flood was considered one of the principal events that shaped our world. Geologic evidence was interpreted in terms of the flood and its impacts. Today geologists interpret the world's history in terms of tectonic plates that have rearranged themselves repeatedly over billions of years. Biogeographers and ecologists also now have entirely different explanations for the same physical evidence (such as distribution of fossils on different continents). Paradigms are also important because they guide the sorts of questions we ask. Today few people would search for evidence that Noah's flood redistributed fish species, but they might be interested in how mountain building separated species into different watersheds.

The shift from one guiding paradigm to another occurs when a majority of scientists accept that the old explanation no longer explains new observations very well. This shift can be contentious and political because a new model can undermine whole careers that are based on one sort of research and explanation. Sometimes this revolution is accomplished rather quickly. Quantum mechanics and Einstein's theory of relativity, for example, overturned classical physics in only about 30 years. In other

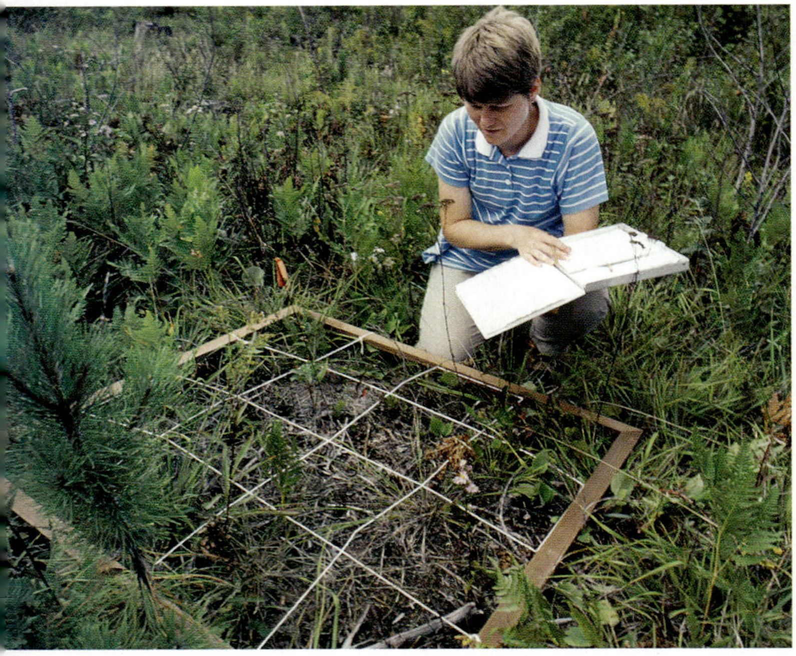

FIGURE 1.8 *What is an appropriate sample size for an investigation? How many individuals would you need to examine to have a representative sample of a population? These are statistical questions of variability, probability, and accuracy.*

APPLICATION: Calculating Probability

An understanding of statistical analysis and probability is fundamental in most areas of modern science. Working with these concepts is critical to your ability to comprehend scientific information.

Every time you flip a coin, the chance that heads will end up on top is 1 in 2 (50 percent, assuming you have a normal coin). The odds of getting heads two times in a row is $1/2 \times 1/2$, or 1/4.

1. What are the odds of getting heads five times in a row?
2. As you start the fifth flip, what are the odds of getting heads?
3. If there are 100 students in your class and everybody flips a coin five times, how many people are likely to get five heads in a row?

Answers: ***1.*** (1 in 2 to the 5th) = 1/32; ***2.*** 1 in 2; ***3.*** 100 students × 1/32 = about 3.

cases, it may take a century or more for new ideas to supplant old ones. Often a paradigm shifts as a new generation replaces an older generation.

As you study this book and think about environmental science, try to identify some of the paradigms that guide our investigations and explanations today. This is one of the skills involved in critical thinking, which we will discuss in further detail later in the chapter.

Pseudoscience and Baloney Detection

In every controversial topic, a few contrarian scientists champion a view diametrically opposed to the majority position of the scientific community. There are several reasons to adopt a contradictory view. One might be sincerely convinced, for instance, that the majority opinion is wrong. Often the most brilliant and original thinkers are regarded as hopelessly off track by conventional scientists. Others may be motivated simply by a desire to consider all possibilities in case unexpected evidence comes up.

Some people also may be tempted to take an opposing viewpoint because they know it will generate publicity and even, perhaps, generous payments from those who benefit from countertestimony. In many court cases, for example, opposing sides are able to produce paid "experts" who are willing to present a partisan agenda rather than objective science. A common tactic is to use scientific uncertainty as an excuse to postpone or reverse an action or a policy that a vast majority of the scientific community believes to be prudent. Opponents will claim that the evidence doesn't constitute conclusive proof that the action needs to be taken, or that the policy is based only on a scientific "theory" and therefore has no validity. As we've discussed earlier, theory describes an entirely different level of certainty in science than it does in common usage. In addition, while scientists usually avoid claims that a theory is unquestionably true, an overwhelming body of evidence is usually required before a consensus is reached on the provisional validity of a particular position.

Harvard's Edward O. Wilson writes, "We will always have contrarians whose sallies are characterized by willful ignorance, selective quotations, disregard for communications with genuine experts, and destructive campaigns to attract the attention of the media rather than scientists. They are the parasite load on scholars who earn success through the slow process of peer review and approval." How can we identify junk science that presents bogus analysis dressed up in quasi-scientific jargon but that really represents a perversion of objective inquiry? The astronomer Carl Sagan proposed a "Baloney Detection Kit" containing the questions in table 1.2. An example of a current scientific controversy is presented in Investigating Our Environment (p. 12).

THINKING ABOUT THINKING

Perhaps the most valuable skill you can learn in any of your classes is the ability to think clearly, creatively, and purposefully. Much of the most important information in environmental science is highly contested. As previous sections of this chapter show, facts can vary, depending on when and by whom they were gathered. How can you make sense out of a welter of conflicting information? Developing your ability to learn new skills, examine new facts, evaluate new theories, and formulate your own interpretations is essential for keeping up in a changing world.

TABLE 1.2 Questions for Baloney Detection

1. How reliable are the sources of this claim? Is there reason to believe that they might have an agenda to pursue in this case?
2. Have the claims been verified by other sources? What data are presented in support of this opinion?
3. What position does the majority of the scientific community hold in this issue?
4. How does this claim fit with what we know about how the world works? Is this a reasonable assertion or does it contradict established theories?
5. Are the arguments balanced and logical? Have proponents of a particular position considered alternate points of view or only selected supportive evidence for their particular beliefs?
6. What do you know about the sources of funding for a particular position? Are they financed by groups with partisan goals?
7. Where was evidence for competing theories published? Has it undergone impartial peer review or is it only in proprietary publication?

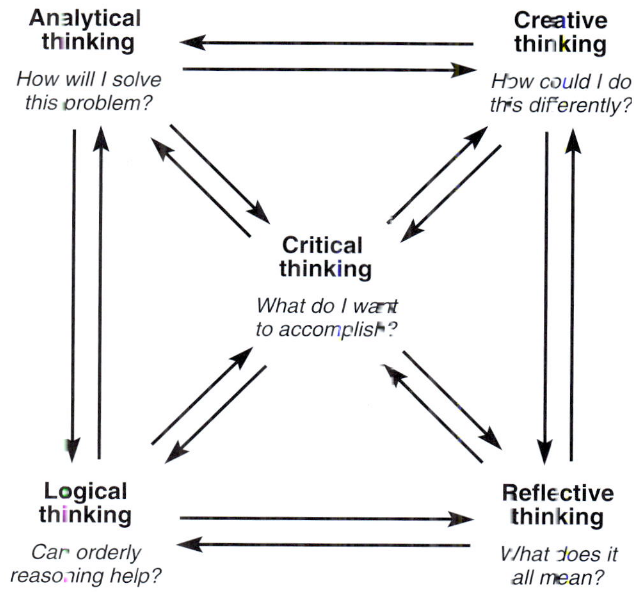

FIGURE 1.9 *Different approaches to thinking are used to solve different kinds of problems or to study alternate aspects of a single issue.*

A flood of information and misinformation inundates us every day. Competing explanations and contradictory ideas battle for our attention. The rapidly growing complexity of our world and our lives intensifies the difficulties of knowing what to believe or how to act. Consider how the communications revolution has brought us computers, email, cell phones, mobile faxes, pagers, the World Wide Web, hundreds of channels of satellite TV, and direct mail or electronic marketing that overwhelm us with conflicting information. We have more choices than we can possibly manage, and we know more about the world around us than ever before but, perhaps, understand less.

An additional complication is that distinguished authorities vehemently disagree about many important topics. Some cynics say that, for any expert, there is always an equal and opposite expert. How can you decide what is true and meaningful? Is it simply a matter of what feels good at the moment or what supports our preconceived notions? Or can we use logical, orderly, creative thinking procedures to reach decisions?

Approaches to Knowledge and Meaning

A number of skills, attitudes, and approaches can help us evaluate information and make decisions. **Analytical thinking** asks, "How can I break this problem down into its constituent parts?" **Creative thinking** asks, "How might I approach this problem in new and inventive ways?" **Logical thinking** asks, "How can orderly, deductive reasoning help me think clearly?" **Critical thinking** asks, "What am I trying to accomplish here, and how will I know when I've succeeded?" **Reflective thinking** asks, "What does it all mean?" (See fig. 1.9.)

While much of science is based on analytical and logical thinking, critical thinking adds elements of contextual sensitivity and empathy that can be very helpful in your study of environmental science. It challenges us to examine theories, facts, and options in a systematic, purposeful, and responsible manner. It shares many methods and approaches with other methods of reasoning but adds some important skills, attitudes, and dispositions. Furthermore, it challenges us to plan methodically and to assess the process of thinking as well as the implications of our decisions. Thinking critically can help us discover hidden ideas and meanings, develop strategies for evaluating reasons and conclusions in arguments, recognize the differences between facts and values, and avoid jumping to conclusions. Richard Paul, chair of the National Council for Critical Thinking, identifies ten steps in critical thinking (table 1.3).

TABLE 1.3 Steps in Critical Thinking

1. What is the purpose of my thinking?
2. What precise question am I trying to answer?
3. Within what point of view am I thinking?
4. What information am I using?
5. How am I interpreting that information?
6. What concepts or ideas are central to my thinking?
7. What conclusions am I aiming toward?
8. What am I taking for granted; what assumptions am I making?
9. If I accept the conclusions, what are the implications?
10. What would the consequences be if I put my thoughts into action?

Notice that many critical thinking processes are self-reflective and self-correcting. This form of thinking is sometimes called "thinking about thinking." It is an attempt to plan rationally how to analyze a problem, to monitor your progress while you are doing it, and to evaluate how your strategy worked and what you

INVESTIGATING Our Environment

A Skeptical Environmentalist?

In 2001 Cambridge University Press published *The Skeptical Environmentalist: Measuring the Real State of the World* by the Danish statistician Bjørn Lomborg. The book triggered a firestorm of criticism as natural scientists argued that Lomborg's book was serving to "confuse legislators and regulators, and poison the well of public environmental information."[1] In January 2002 *Scientific American* published a series of articles by five distinguished environmental scientists contesting Lomborg's claims. To some observers, the ferocity of the attack was surprising. Why was *The Skeptical Environmentalist* so controversial, and how can we judge the relative correctness of the claims and counterclaims in this debate?

Lomborg begins by saying that, although he is an "old left-wing Greenpeace member," he is worried about the unrelenting "doom and gloom" of mainstream environmentalism. He describes what he regards as an all-pervasive litany that says, among other things, "Our resources are running out. The population is ever growing, leaving less and less to eat. The air and water are becoming ever more polluted. The planet's species are becoming extinct in vast numbers. . . . The forests are disappearing, fish stocks are collapsing and coral reefs are dying."

Lomborg, however, says these claims about the collapse of ecosystems are "simply not in keeping with reality. We are not running out of energy or natural resources. There will be more and more food per head of the world's population. Fewer and fewer people are starving. In 1900 we lived for an average of 30 years; today we live for 67. According to the UN we have reduced poverty more in the last 50 years than we did in the preceding 500, and it has been reduced in practically every country." He goes on to challenge conventional scientific assessment of global warming, forest losses, freshwater scarcity, energy shortages, and a host of other environmental problems. Is Lomborg being deliberately (and some would say, hypocritically) optimistic, or are others being unreasonably pessimistic? Is this simply a case of regarding the glass as half full or half empty?

Part of the discrepancy is that Lomborg is unabashedly anthropocentric. He dismisses the value of biodiversity, for example. As long as there are plants and animals to supply human needs, what does it matter if a few nonessential species go extinct? Furthermore, he is intentionally positive. He cheerfully predicts that progress in population control, use of renewable energy, and extension of water supplies through desalination technology will spread to the whole world, thus avoiding crises in resource supplies and human impacts on our environment. Others, particularly Lester Brown of the Worldwatch Institute, according to Lomborg, seem to deliberately adopt worst-case scenarios. Are they merely being realistic or might they be attempting to scare us into supporting their agenda?

Perhaps the most effective criticism of Lomborg comes from his reporting of statistics and research results. Stephen Schneider, a distinguished climate scientist from Stanford University, for instance, writes in *Scientific American,* "Most of [Lomborg's] nearly 3,000 citations are to secondary literature and media articles. Moreover, even when cited, the peer-reviewed articles come elliptically from those studies that support his rosy view that only the low end of the uncertainty ranges [of climate change] will be plausible. IPCC authors, in contrast, were subjected to three rounds of review by hundreds of outside experts. They didn't have the luxury of reporting primarily from the part of the community that agrees with their individual views."[2]

Lomborg also criticizes extinction rate estimates as much too large, citing evidence from places like Brazil's Atlantic forest, where about 90 percent of the trees have been cleared without large numbers of recorded extinctions. Thomas Lovejoy, chief biodiversity adviser to the World Bank, responds, "First, this is a region with very few field biologists to record either species or their extinction. Second, there is abundant evidence that if the Atlantic forest remains as reduced and fragmented as it is, it will lose a sizable fraction of the species that at the moment are able to hang on."

How would you evaluate the claims and counterclaims in this debate? What questions from the Baloney Detection Kit in table 1.2 might be most appropriate here? Based on these limited quotes from Lomborg and his critics, what hidden agendas might you look for in the original articles, and what further evidence would you want to gather by examining the primary sources?

Although Lomborg has been rather thoroughly discredited by a majority of environmental scientists, others are bound to give similarly optimistic analyses in the future. Having examined this case may help you understand similar controversies when you encounter them.

[1]Richard C. Bell. 2002. Media sheep: How did *The Skeptical Environmentalist* pull the wool over the eyes of so many editors? Worldwatch 15(2):11–13.

[2]Stephen Schneider. 2002. Global warming: Neglecting the complexities. *Scientific American* 286(1):62–65.

have learned when you are finished. It is not critical in the sense of finding fault, but it makes a conscious, active, disciplined effort to be aware of hidden motives and assumptions; to uncover bias; and to recognize the reliability or unreliability of sources.

While critical thinking shares many of the orderly, systematic approaches of formal logic, it also invokes traits such as empathy, sensitivity, courage, and humility. Formulating intelligent opinions about some of the complex issues you will encounter in environmental science requires more than simple logic. Developing these attitudes and skills is not easy or simple. It takes practice. You have to develop your mental faculties just as you need to train for a sport. Intellectual integrity, modesty, fairness, compassion, and fortitude are not traits you use only occasionally. They must be cultivated until they become a part of your normal way of thinking.

Applying Critical Thinking

We all use critical or reflective thinking at times. Suppose a television commercial tells you that a new breakfast cereal is tasty and good for you. You may be suspicious and ask yourself a few questions: What do they mean by *good*? Good for whom or what? Does *tasty* simply mean more sugar and salt? Might the sources of this information have other motives besides your health and happiness? Although you may not have been aware of it, you already have used some of the techniques of critical analysis. Working to expand these skills helps you recognize how information and analysis can be distorted, misleading, prejudiced, superficial, unfair, or otherwise defective. Often, discussing complex ideas with others is a good way to clarify your own thoughts (fig. 1.10).

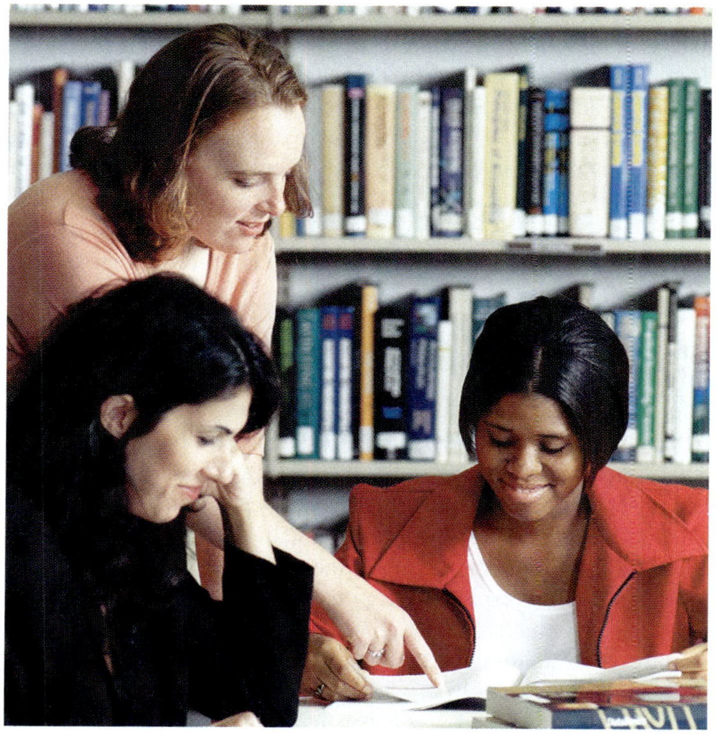

FIGURE 1.10 *Explaining ideas to others, debating points, or simply verbalizing your understanding of something is an excellent way to clarify your thoughts.*

Here are some steps in critical thinking:

1. *Identify and evaluate premises and conclusions in an argument.* What is the basis for the claims made here? What evidence is presented to support these claims, and what conclusions are drawn from this evidence? If the premises and evidence are correct, does it follow that the conclusions are necessarily true?

2. *Acknowledge and clarify uncertainties, vagueness, equivocation, and contradictions.* Do the terms used have more than one meaning? If so, are all participants in the argument using the same meanings? Is ambiguity or equivocation deliberate? Can all the claims be true simultaneously?
3. *Distinguish between facts and values.* Can claims be tested? (If so, these are statements of fact and should be verifiable by gathering evidence.) Are claims made about the worth or lack of worth of something? (If so, these are value statements or opinions and probably cannot be verified objectively.) For example, claims of what we ought to do to be moral or righteous or to respect nature are generally value statements.
4. *Recognize and assess assumptions.* Given the backgrounds and views of the protagonists, what underlying reasons might there be for the premises, evidence, or conclusions presented? Does anyone have an "axe to grind" or a personal agenda in this issue? What does s/he think you know, need, want, or believe? Is there a subtext based on race, gender, ethnicity, economics, or some belief system that distorts this discussion?
5. *Distinguish source reliability or unreliability.* What qualifies the experts on this issue? What special knowledge or information do they have? What evidence do they present? How can we determine whether the information offered is accurate, true, or even plausible?
6. *Recognize and understand conceptual frameworks.* What are the basic beliefs, attitudes, and values that this person, group, or society holds? What dominating philosophy or ethics control their outlooks and actions? How do these beliefs and values affect the way people view themselves and the world around them? If there are conflicting or contradictory beliefs and values, how can these differences be resolved?

Some Clues for "Unpacking" an Argument

A logical argument is made up of one or more introductory statements (called premises) and a conclusion that supposedly follows logically from the premises. In ordinary conversation, different kinds of statements often are mixed together, so distinguishing among them or deciphering hidden or implied meanings is difficult. Social theorists call the process of separating and analyzing textual components "unpacking." Applying this type of analysis to an argument can be useful.

An argument's premises are usually claimed to be based on facts; conclusions are usually opinions and values drawn from, or used to interpret, those facts. Words that often introduce a premise include *as, because, assume that, given that, since, whereas,* and *we all know that.* Words that generally indicate a conclusion or statement of opinion or values include *and, so, thus, therefore, it follows that, consequently, the evidence shows,* and *we can conclude that.*

For instance, in the example we used earlier, the television cereal ad might have said, "Since we all need vitamins, and since this cereal contains vitamins, the cereal must be good for you." Which are the premises, and which is the conclusion? Does one necessarily follow from the other? Remember that, even if the facts in a premise are correct, the conclusions drawn from those facts may not be. Information may be withheld from the argument, such as the fact that the cereal is also loaded with unhealthy amounts of sugar.

Using Critical Thinking

In this book, you will have many opportunities to practice critical thinking skills. Every chapter includes many facts, figures, opinions, and theories. Are all of them true? No, probably not. They were the best information available when this text was written, but much in environmental science is in a state of flux. Data change constantly, as does our interpretation of data. Do the ideas presented here give a complete picture of the state of our environment? Unfortunately, they probably don't. No matter how comprehensive our discussion is of this complex, diverse subject, it can never capture everything worth knowing, nor can it reveal all possible points of view.

When reading this text, try to distinguish between statements of fact and opinion. Ask yourself if the premises support the conclusions drawn from them. Although we have tried to be fair and even-handed in presenting controversies, our personal biases and values—some of which we may not even recognize—affect how we see issues and present arguments. Watch for cases in which you need to think for yourself, and use your critical and reflective thinking skills to uncover the truth.

A BRIEF HISTORY OF CONSERVATION AND ENVIRONMENTALISM

Although some early societies had negative impacts on their surroundings, others lived in relative harmony with nature. In modern times, however, growing human populations and the power of our technology have heightened concern about what we are doing to our environment. We can divide conservation history and environmental activism into at least four distinct stages: (1) pragmatic resource conservation, (2) moral and aesthetic nature preservation, (3) a growing concern about health and ecological damage caused by pollution, and (4) global environmental citizenship. These stages aren't necessarily mutually exclusive, however; parts of each persist today in the environmental movement, and one person may embrace them all simultaneously.

Historic Roots of Nature Protection

Recognizing human misuse of nature is not unique to modern times. Plato complained in the fourth century B.C. that Greece once was blessed with fertile soil and clothed with abundant forests of fine trees. After the trees were cut to build houses and ships, however, heavy rains washed the soil into the sea, leaving only a rocky "skeleton of a body wasted by disease." Springs and rivers dried up, while farming became all but impossible. Many classical authors regarded earth as a living being, vulnerable to aging, illness, and even mortality. Periodic threats about the impending death of nature from human misuse have persisted to our own times. As Mostafa K. Tolba, former director of the United Nations Environment Programme said, "The problems that overwhelm us today are precisely those we failed to solve decades ago."

Some of the earliest scientific studies of environmental damage were carried out in the eighteenth century by French or British colonial administrators, many of whom were trained scientists and who considered responsible environmental stewardship as an aesthetic and moral priority, as well as an economic necessity. These early conservationists observed and understood the connections between deforestation, soil erosion, and local climate change. The pioneering British plant physiologist Stephen Hales, for instance, suggested that conserving green plants preserves rainfall. His ideas were put into practice in 1764 on the Caribbean island of Tobago, where about 20 percent of the land was marked as "reserved in wood for rains."

Pierre Poivre, an early French governor of Mauritius, an island in the Indian Ocean, was appalled at the environmental and social devastation caused by destruction of wildlife (such as the flightless dodo) and the felling of ebony forests on the island by early European settlers. In 1769 Poivre ordered that one-quarter of the island be preserved in forests, particularly on steep mountain slopes and along waterways. Mauritius remains a model for balancing nature and human needs. Its forest reserves shelter a larger percentage of its original flora and fauna than most other human-occupied islands.

Pragmatic Resource Conservation

Many historians consider the publication of *Man and Nature* in 1864 by geographer George Perkins Marsh as the wellspring of environmental protection in North America. Marsh, who also was a lawyer, politician, and diplomat, traveled widely around the Mediterranean as part of his diplomatic duties in Turkey and Italy. He read widely in the classics (including Plato) and personally observed the damage caused by excessive grazing by goats and sheep and by the deforestation of steep hillsides. Alarmed by the wanton destruction and profligate waste of resources still occurring on the American frontier in his lifetime, he warned of its ecological consequences. Largely because of his book, national forest reserves were established in the United States in 1873 to protect dwindling timber supplies and endangered watersheds.

Among those influenced by Marsh's warnings were U.S. President Theodore Roosevelt and his chief conservation adviser, Gifford Pinchot. In 1905 Roosevelt, who was the leader of the populist, progressive movement, moved forest management out of the corruption-filled Interior Department into the Department of Agriculture. Pinchot, who was the first American-born professional forester, became the first chief of the new Forest Service (fig. 1.11). He put resource management on an honest, rational, and scientific basis for the first time in American history. Together with naturalists and activists such as John Muir, William Brewster, and George Bird Grinnell, Roosevelt and Pinchot established the framework of the national forest, park, and wildlife refuge system. They passed game protection laws and tried to stop some of the most flagrant abuses of the public domain. In 1908 Pinchot organized and chaired the White House Conference on Natural Resources, perhaps the most prestigious and influential environmental meeting ever held in the United States. Pinchot also was governor of Pennsylvania and founding head of the Tennessee Valley Authority, which provided inexpensive power to the southeastern United States.

The basis of Roosevelt's and Pinchot's policies was pragmatic **utilitarian conservation.** They argued that the forests should be saved "not because they are beautiful or because they shelter wild creatures of the wilderness, but only to provide homes and jobs for people." Resources should be used "for the greatest good, for the greatest number, for the longest time." "There has been a fundamental misconception," Pinchot wrote, "that conservation means nothing but husbanding of resources for future generations. Nothing could be further from the truth. The first principle of conservation is development and use of the natural

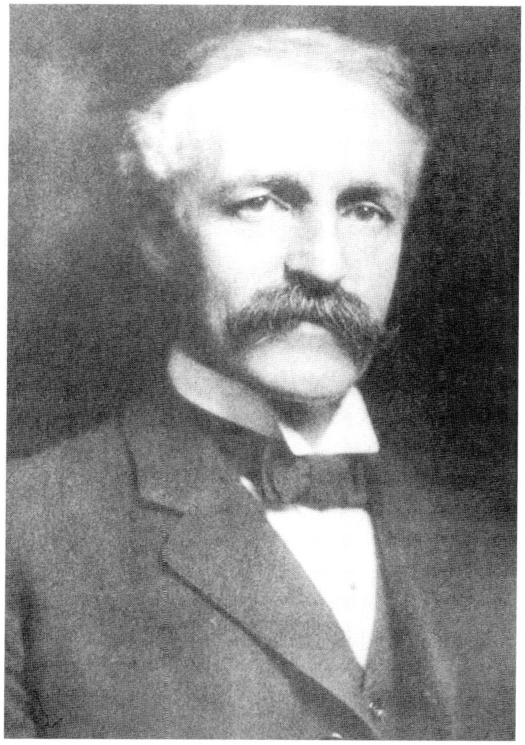

FIGURE 1.11 *Gifford Pinchot, first chief of the U.S. Forest Service and founder of the utilitarian conservation movement.*

resources now existing on this continent for the benefit of the people who live here now. There may be just as much waste in neglecting the development and use of certain natural resources as there is in their destruction." This pragmatic approach still can be seen in the multiple-use policies of the U.S. Forest Service.

Moral and Aesthetic Nature Preservation

John Muir (fig. 1.12), amateur geologist, popular author, and first president of the Sierra Club, strenuously opposed Pinchot's utilitarian policies. Muir argued that nature deserves to exist for its own sake, regardless of its usefulness to us. Aesthetic and spiritual values formed the core of his philosophy of nature protection. This outlook has been called **biocentric preservation** because it emphasizes the fundamental right of other organisms to exist and to pursue their own interests. Muir wrote: "The world, we are told, was made for man. A presumption that is totally unsupported by the facts. . . . Nature's object in making animals and plants might possibly be first of all the happiness of each one of them. . . . Why ought man to value himself as more than an infinitely small unit of the one great unit of creation?"

Muir, who was an early explorer and interpreter of California's Sierra Nevada range, fought long and hard for establishment of Yosemite and Kings Canyon National Parks. The National Park Service, established in 1916, was first headed by Muir's disciple, Stephen Mather, and has always been oriented toward preservation of nature in its purest state. It has often been at odds with Pinchot's utilitarian Forest Service. One of Muir and Pinchot's

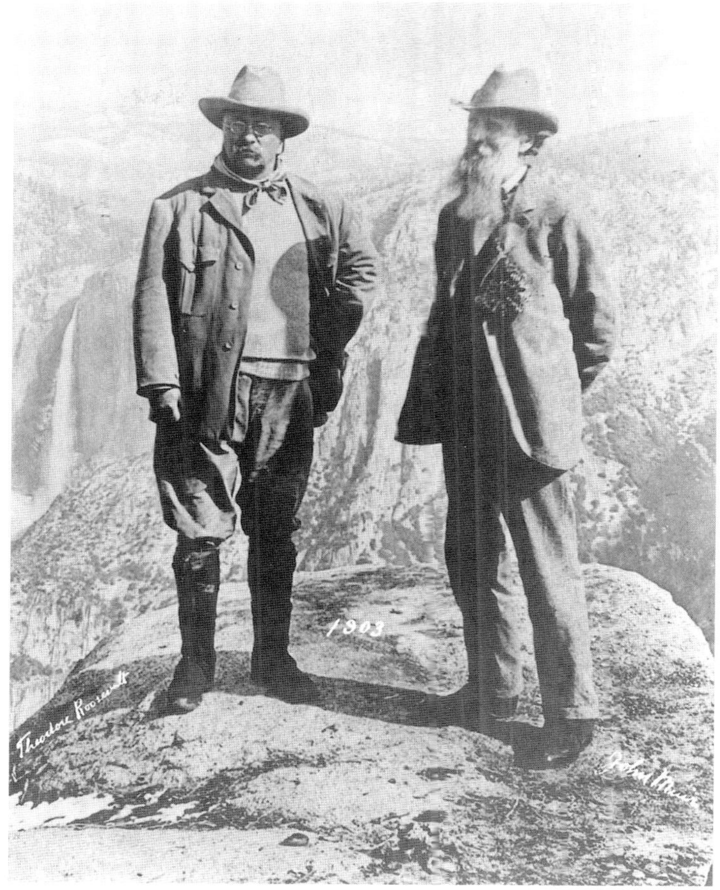

FIGURE 1.12 *Teddy Roosevelt and John Muir.*

biggest battles was over the damming of Hetch Hetchy Valley in Yosemite. Muir regarded flooding the valley a sacrilege against nature. Pinchot, who championed publicly owned utilities, viewed the dam as a way to free San Francisco residents from the clutches of greedy water and power monopolies.

Modern Environmentalism

The undesirable effects of pollution probably have been recognized as long as people have been building smoky fires. In 1273 King Edward I of England threatened to hang anyone burning coal in London because of the acrid smoke it produced. In 1661 the English diarist John Evelyn complained about the noxious air pollution caused by coal fires and factories and suggested that sweet-smelling trees be planted to purify city air. Increasingly dangerous smog attacks in Britain led, in 1880, to formation of a national Fog and Smoke Committee to combat this problem.

The tremendous expansion of chemical industries during and after World War II added a new set of concerns to the environmental agenda. *Silent Spring*, written by Rachel Carson (fig. 1.13) and published in 1962, awakened the public to the threats of pollution and toxic chemicals to humans as well as other species. The movement she engendered might be called **modern environmentalism** because its concerns extended to include both natural

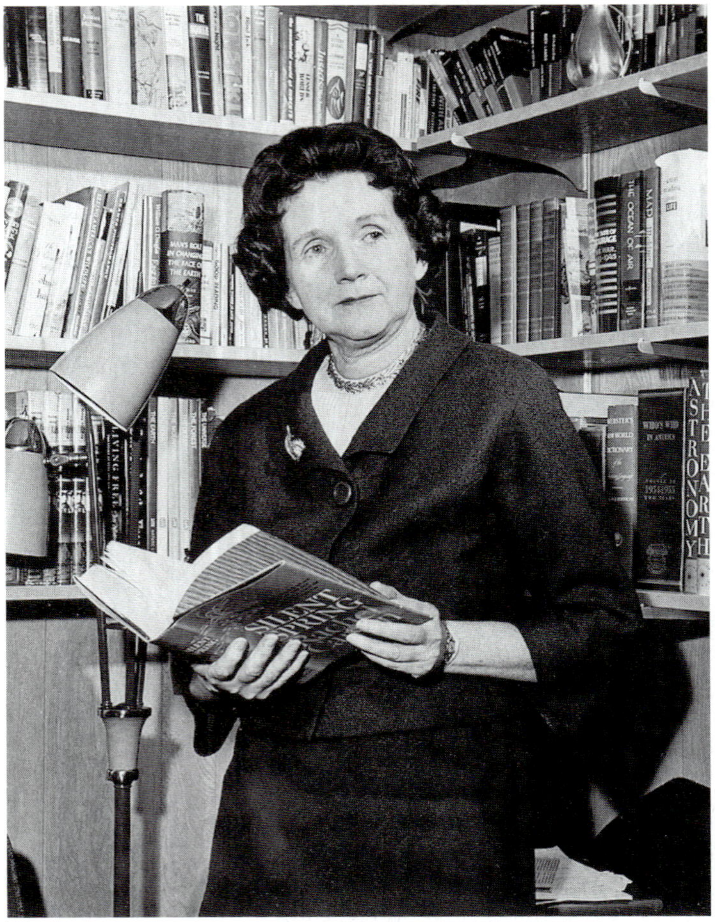

FIGURE 1.13 *Rachel Carson's book* Silent Spring *was a landmark in modern environmental history. She alerted readers to the dangers of indiscriminate pesticide use.*

resources and environmental pollution. Among some other pioneers of this movement were activist David Brower and scientist Barry Commoner. Brower, as executive director of the Sierra Club, Friends of the Earth, and Earth Island Institute, introduced many of the techniques of environmental lobbying and activism, including litigation, intervention in regulatory hearings, book and calendar publishing, and use of mass media for publicity campaigns. Commoner, who was trained as a molecular biologist, has been a leader in analyzing the links between science, technology, and society. Both activism and research remain hallmarks of the modern environmental movement.

Under the leadership of a number of other brilliant and dedicated activists and scientists, the environmental agenda was expanded in the 1960s and 1970s to most of the issues addressed in this textbook, such as human population growth, atomic weapons testing and atomic power, fossil fuel extraction and use, recycling, air and water pollution, and wilderness protection. Environmentalism has become well established in the public agenda since the first national Earth Day in 1970. A majority of Americans now consider themselves environmentalists, although there is considerable variation in what that term means.

Global Concerns

Increased opportunities to travel and expanded international communications now enable us to know about daily events in places unknown to our parents or grandparents. We have become, as Marshal McLuhan famously announced in the 1960s, a global village. As in a village, we are all interconnected in various ways. Events that occur on the other side of the globe have profound and immediate effects on our lives.

Photographs of the earth from space (see fig. 1.2) provide a powerful icon for the fourth wave of ecological concern, which might be called **global environmentalism.** Such photos remind us how small, fragile, beautiful, and rare our home planet is. We all share an environment at this global scale. As Ambassador Adlai Stevenson noted, in his 1965 farewell address to the United Nations (quoted at the beginning of this chapter), we now need to worry about the life-support systems of the planet as a whole. He went on to say in this speech, "We cannot maintain it half fortunate, half miserable, half confident, half despairing, half slave to the ancient enemies of mankind and half free in a liberation of resources undreamed of until this day. No craft, no crew, can travel with such vast contradictions. On their resolution depends the security of us all."

Among the leaders of the worldwide movement combining environmental protection with social justice have been British economist Barbara Ward, French/American scientist René Dubois, Norwegian prime minister Gro Harlem Brundtland, and Canadian diplomat Maurice Strong. All have been central in major international environmental conventions, such as the 1972 UN Conference on the Human Environment in Stockholm or the 1992 UN Earth Summit in Rio de Janeiro. Once again, new issues have become part of the agenda as our field of vision widens. We have begun to appreciate the links between poverty, injustice, oppression, and exploitation of humans and our environment. A concern about the human dimensions of environmental science is an important focus of this textbook.

CURRENT ENVIRONMENTAL CONDITIONS

Every year the World Resources Institute, the United Nations Environment Program, and the World Bank issue Earth Trends, a comprehensive assessment of current world environmental conditions. The most recent version describes many serious environmental and social challenges. With more than 6 billion humans currently, we're adding about 85 million more to the world every year. While demographers report a transition to slower growth rates in most countries, present trends project a population between 8 and 10 billion by 2050. The impacts of that many people on our natural resources and ecological systems is a serious concern.

Water may well be the most critical resource in the twenty-first century. Already at least 1.2 billion people lack access to safe drinking water, and twice that many don't have adequate sanitation. Polluted water contributes to the death of more than 5 million people every year, including 2.2 million children under age 5. About 40

APPLICATION: Making Sense of Data

You will see many numbers in this book. Instead of simply glossing over them, think about what they mean relative to some benchmark numbers.

1. For example, you just read that we are adding 85 million people to the world's population each year. How does that compare with the number of people in the United States? In Canada? In Mexico? (If you can't know, where can you find those numbers?)
2. What proportion of the current global population of about 6 billion is the 85 million people added each year?

Answers: *1.* The United States has about 270 million people, Canada has about 25 million, and Mexico has about 100 million. *2.* About 1.4 percent.

percent of the world population lives in countries where water demands now exceed supplies, and the UN projects that by 2025 as many as three-fourths of us could live under similar conditions.

Over the past century, global food production has more than kept pace with human population growth, but there are worries about whether we will be able to maintain this pace. Soil scientists report that about two-thirds of all agricultural lands show signs of degradation. The biotechnology and intensive farming techniques responsible for much of our recent production gains are too expensive for many poor farmers. Can we find ways to produce the food we need without further environmental degradation? And will that food be distributed equitably? In a world of food surpluses, currently more than 800 million people are chronically undernourished, and at least 20 million face acute food shortages due to bad weather or politics (fig. 1.14).

How we obtain and use energy is likely to play a crucial role in our environmental future. Fossil fuels (oil, coal, and natural gas) presently provide around 80 percent of the energy used in industrialized countries. Supplies of these fuels are diminishing, however, and problems associated with their acquisition and use—air and water pollution, mining damage, shipping accidents, and geopolitics—may limit what we do with remaining reserves. Cleaner, renewable energy resources—solar, wind, geothermal, and biomass power—together with conservation could give us cleaner, less destructive options if we invest in appropriate technology.

Burning fossil fuels, making cement, cultivating rice paddies, clearing forests, and other human activities release carbon dioxide and other so-called greenhouse gases, which trap heat in the atmosphere. Over the past 200 years, atmospheric CO_2 concentrations have increased about 30 percent. Climatologists warn that by 2100, if current trends continue, mean global temperatures will probably warm between 1.5° and 6°C (2.7° and 11°F). Global climate change already is affecting a wide variety of biological species (fig. 1.15). Further warming is likely to cause increasingly severe weather events, including droughts in some areas and floods in others. Melting alpine glaciers and snowfields could threaten

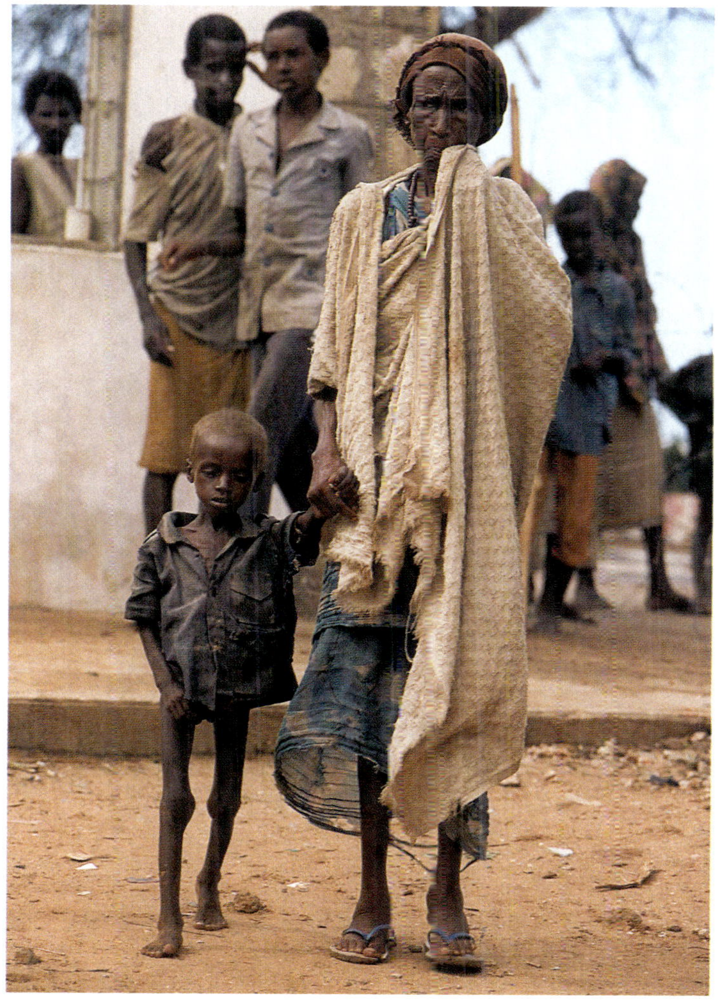

FIGURE 1.14 *More than 800 million people are chronically undernourished, and at least 20 million face life-threatening food shortages.*

water supplies on which millions of people depend. Rising sea levels already are flooding low-lying islands and coastal regions, while habitat losses and climate changes are affecting many biological species. Canadian Environment Minister David Anderson said, in 2004, that global climate change is a greater threat than terrorism because it could force hundreds of millions of people from their homes and trigger an economic and social catastrophe.

Air quality has worsened dramatically in many areas. Over southern Asia, for example, satellite images recently revealed a 3-km (2-mile)-thick toxic haze of ash, acids, aerosols, dust, and photochemical products, which regularly covers the entire Indian subcontinent for much of the year. Nobel laureate Paul Crutzen estimates that at least 3 million people die each year from diseases triggered by air pollution. Worldwide, the United Nations estimates, more than 2 billion metric tons of air pollutants (not including carbon dioxide or wind-blown soil) are released each year. Air pollution no longer is merely a local problem. Mercury, polychlorinated biphenyls (PCB), DDT, and other long-lasting pollutants accumulate in arctic ecosystems and native people after being transported by air currents from

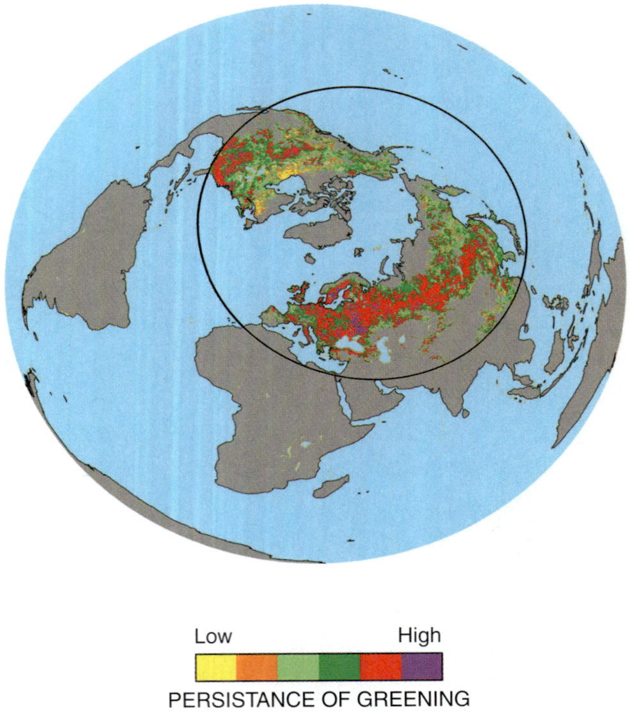

FIGURE 1.15 *Satellite images and surface temperature data show that polar regions, especially in Eurasia, are becoming green earlier and staying green longer than ever in recorded history. This appears to be evidence of a changing global climate.*
Source: NASA, 2002.

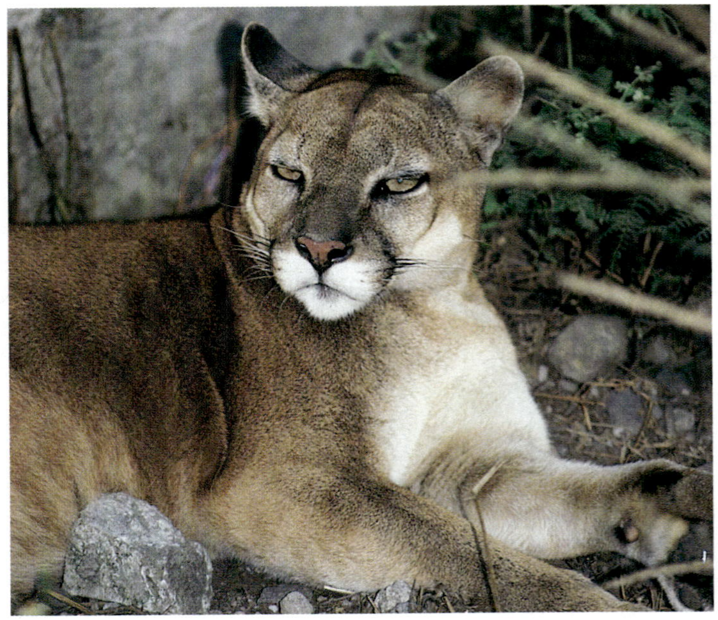

FIGURE 1.16 *Fewer than 80 Florida panthers remain in the wild. They have been crossbred with Texas cougars in an attempt to save the population.*

industrial regions thousands of kilometers to the south. And during certain days, as much as 75 percent of the smog and particulate pollution recorded on the west coast of North America can be traced to Asia.

Biologists report that habitat destruction, overexploitation, pollution, and introduction of exotic organisms are eliminating species at a rate comparable to the great extinction that marked the end of the age of dinosaurs. The UN Environment Programme reports that, over the past century, more than 800 species have disappeared and at least 10,000 species are now considered threatened. This includes about half of all primates and freshwater fish, together with around 10 percent of all plant species. Top predators, including nearly all the big cats in the world, are particularly rare and endangered (fig. 1.16). A nationwide survey of the United Kingdom in 2004 found that most bird and butterfly populations had declined between 50 and 75 percent over the previous 20 years. More than three-quarters of all global fisheries are overfished or harvested at their biological limit. At least half of the forests existing before the introduction of agriculture have been cleared, and much of the diverse "old growth" on which many species depend for habitat is rapidly being cut and replaced by secondary growth or monoculture.

Signs of Hope

The dismal litany of problems facing us seems overwhelming, doesn't it? Is there hope that we can find solutions to these dilemmas? We think so. As you will see in subsequent chapters in this book, progress has been made in many areas in reducing pollution and curbing wasteful resource use. Many cities in Europe and North America, for example, are cleaner and much more livable now than they were a century ago. Population has stabilized in most industrialized countries and even in some very poor countries where social security and democracy have been established. Over the past 20 years, the average number of children born per woman worldwide has decreased from 6.1 to 3.4. By 2050, the UN Population Division predicts, all developed countries and 75 percent of the developing world will experience a below-replacement fertility rate of 2.1 children per woman. This suggests that the world population will stabilize at about 8.9 billion, rather than the 9.3 billion previously estimated.

The incidence of life-threatening infectious diseases has been reduced sharply in most countries during the past century, while life expectancies have nearly doubled, on average. In 2004 the World Health Organization proposed a plan to rid the world of polio. Since 1990 more than 800 million people have gained access to improved water supplies and modern sanitation. In spite of population growth that added nearly a billion people to the world during the 1990s, the number facing food insecurity and chronic hunger during this period actually declined by about 40 million.

Deforestation has slowed in Asia, from more than 8 percent during the 1980s to less than 1 percent in the 1990s. Nature preserves and protected areas have increased nearly five-fold over the past 20 years, from about 2.6 million square km (1 million square mi) to about 12.2 million square km (4.7 million square mi). This represents only 8.2 percent of all land area—less than the 12 percent thought necessary to protect a viable sample of the world's biodiversity—but is a dramatic expansion, nonetheless.

Dramatic progress is being made in a transition to renewable energy sources. The European Union has announced a goal of obtaining 22 percent of its electricity and 12 percent of all energy from renewable sources by 2010. British Prime Minister Tony Blair has laid out ambitious plans to fight global warming by cutting carbon dioxide emissions in Britain by 60 percent through energy conservation and a switch to renewables. If nonpolluting, sustainable energy technology is made available to the world's poorer countries, it may be possible to enhance human development while simultaneously reducing environmental damage.

The increased speed at which information and technology now flow around the world holds promise that we can continue to find solutions to our environmental dilemmas. Although we continue to face many challenges, collectively we may be able to implement sustainable development that raises living standards for everyone while also reducing our negative environmental impacts.

HUMAN DIMENSIONS OF ENVIRONMENTAL SCIENCE

Because we live in both the natural and social worlds, and because we and our technology have become such dominant forces on the planet, environmental science must take human institutions and the human condition into account. We live in a world of haves and have-nots; a few of us live in increasing luxury, while many others lack the basic necessities for a decent, healthy, productive life. The World Bank estimates that more than 1.4 billion people—about one-fifth of the world's population—live in acute poverty with an income of less than $1 (U.S.) per day. These poorest of the poor generally lack access to an adequate diet, decent housing, basic sanitation, clean water, education, medical care, and other essentials for a humane existence. Seventy percent of those people are women and children. In fact, four out of five people in the world live in what would be considered poverty in the United States or Canada (see the related story "Getting to Know the Neighbors" at www.mhhe.com/cases).

Policymakers are becoming aware that eliminating poverty and protecting our common environment are inextricably interlinked because the world's poorest people are both the victims and the agents of environmental degradation. The poorest people are often forced to meet short-term survival needs at the cost of long-term sustainability. Desperate for croplands to feed themselves and their families, many move into virgin forests or cultivate steep, erosion-prone hillsides, where soil nutrients are exhausted after only a few years. Others migrate to the grimy, crowded slums and ramshackle shantytowns that now surround most major cities in the developing world. With no way to dispose of wastes, the residents often foul their environment further and contaminate the air they breathe and the water on which they depend for washing and drinking (fig. 1.17).

The cycle of poverty, illness, and limited opportunities can become a self-sustaining process that passes from one generation to another. People who are malnourished and ill can't work productively to obtain food, shelter, or medicine for themselves or their children, who also are malnourished and ill. About 250 million children—mostly in Asia and Africa and some as young as 4 years old—are forced to work under appalling conditions weaving carpets, making ceramics and jewelry, or working in the sex trade. Growing up in these conditions leads to educational, psychological, and developmental deficits that condemn these children to perpetuate this cycle.

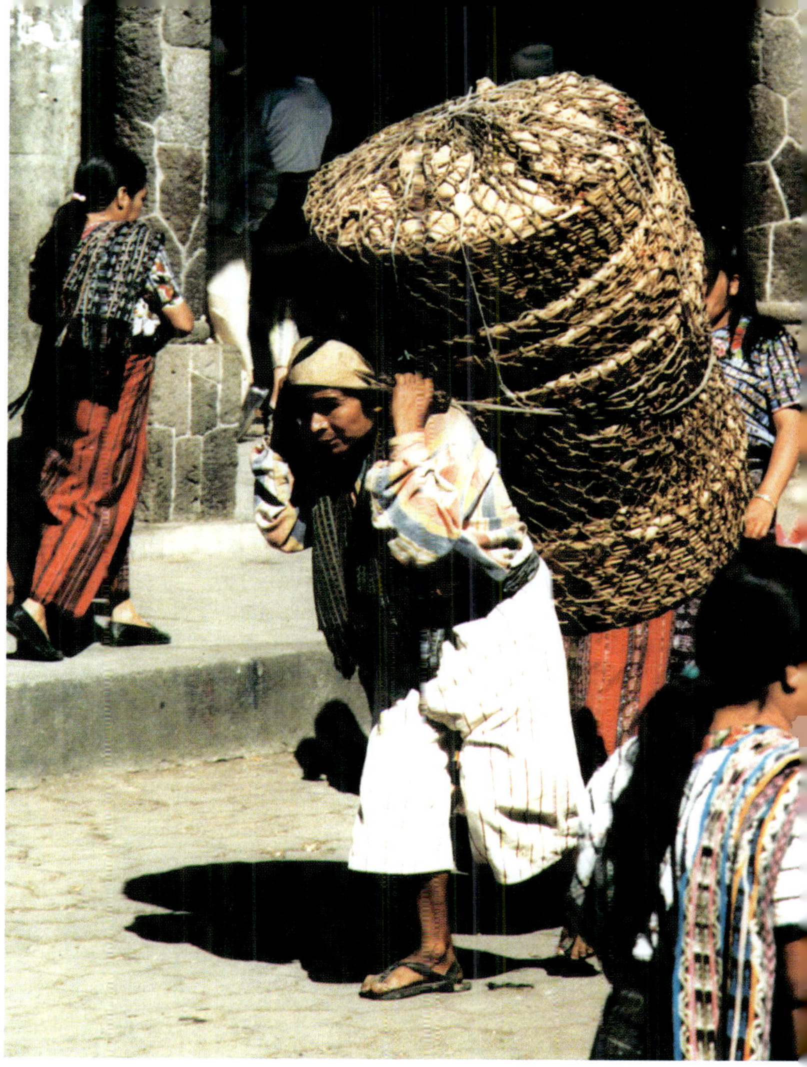

FIGURE 1.17 *While many of us live in luxury, more than a billion people lack access to resources for a healthy, productive life. Often the poorest people are both the victims and agents of environmental degradation as they struggle to survive.*

Faced with immediate survival needs and few options, these unfortunate people often have no choice but to overharvest resources; in doing so, however, they diminish not only their own options but also those of future generations. And in an increasingly interconnected world, the environments and resource bases damaged by poverty and ignorance are directly linked to those on which we depend.

Rich and Poor Countries

Where do the rich and poor live? About one-fifth of the world's population lives in the 20 richest countries, where the average per capita income is above $25,000 (U.S.) per year. Most of these countries are in North America or Western Europe, but Japan, Singapore, Australia, New Zealand, the United Arab Emirates, and Israel also fall into this group. Almost every country, however, even the richest, such as the United States and Canada, has poor people. No doubt everyone reading this book knows about homeless people or other individuals who lack resources for a safe, productive life. According to Bread for the World, 35 million Americans—one-third of them children—live in households without sufficient food.

The other four-fifths of the world's population lives in middle- or low-income countries, where nearly everyone is poor by North American standards (fig. 1.18). More than 3 billion people live in the poorest nations, where the average per capita income is below $620 (U.S.) per year. China and India are the largest of these countries, with a combined population of about 2.3 billion people. Among the 41 other nations in this category, 33 are in sub-Saharan Africa. All the other lowest-income nations, except Haiti, are in Asia. Although poverty levels in countries such as China and Indonesia have fallen in recent years, most countries in sub-Saharan Africa and much of Latin America have made little progress. The destabilizing and impoverishing effects of earlier colonialism continue to play important roles in the ongoing problems of these unfortunate countries. Meanwhile, the relative gap between rich and poor has increased dramatically (fig. 1.19).

As table 1.4 shows, the gulf between the richest and poorest nations affects many quality-of-life indicators. The average individual in the highest income countries has an annual income more than 100 times that of those in the lowest-income nations. Because of high infant mortality rates, the average family in the poorest countries has more than four times as many children as those in richer countries. If it were not for immigration, the population in most of the richer countries now would be declining; that in the poorer countries continues to grow at 2.6 percent per year.

The gulf between rich and poor is even greater at the individual level. The richest 200 people in the world have a combined wealth of $1 trillion. This is more than the total owned by the 3 billion people who make up the poorest half of the world's population.

A Fair Share of Resources?

The affluent lifestyle that many of us in the richer countries enjoy consumes an inordinate share of the world's natural resources and produces a shockingly high proportion of pollutants and wastes. The United States, for instance, with less than 5 percent of the total population, consumes about one-quarter of most commercially traded commodities and produces a quarter to half of most industrial wastes (table 1.5).

To get an average American through the day takes about 450 kg (nearly 1,000 lbs) of raw materials, including 18 kg (40 lbs) of fossil fuels, 13 kg (29 lbs) of other minerals, 12 kg (26 lbs) of farm products, 10 kg (22 lbs) of wood and paper, and 450 liters (119 gal) of water. Every year, Americans throw away some 160 million tons of garbage, including 50 million tons of paper, 67 billion cans and bottles, 25 billion styrofoam cups, 18 billion disposable diapers, and 2 billion disposable razors (fig. 1.20).

This profligate resource consumption and waste disposal strains the planet's life-support systems. If everyone in the world tried to live at consumption levels approaching ours, the results

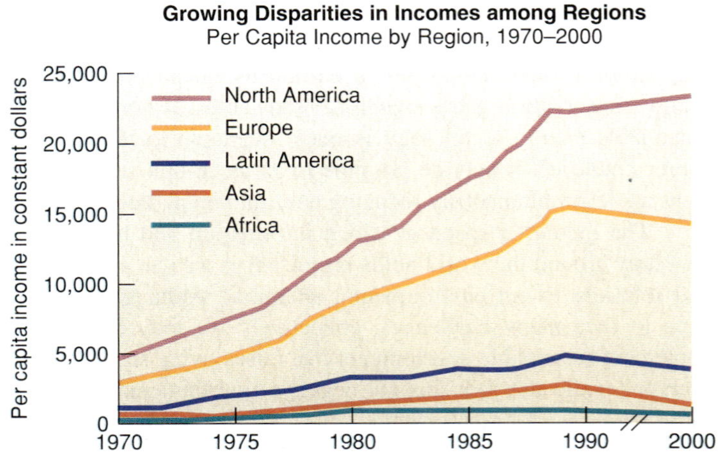

FIGURE 1.19 *Although the percentage of the world's population living in poverty has decreased slightly over the past 30 years, the relative gap between the rich and poor nations has increased sharply.* *Source:* United Nations, 2001.

TABLE 1.4 Average Indicators of Quality of Life for the 20 Richest and Poorest Countries

INDICATOR	POOR COUNTRIES	RICH COUNTRIES
GDP/capita[1]	$230 (U.S.)	$27,460 (U.S.)
Total fertility[2]	6.3	1.5
Life expectancy	49.3 years	77.8 years
Infant mortality[3]	100	5
Safe drinking water	44%	99%
Adult literacy	38%	99%
Annual population growth	2.6%	0.3%

Source: Data from UNDP Human Development Indicators, 2004.
[1]Annual gross domestic product.
[2]Average number of children per woman.
[3]Per 1,000 live births.

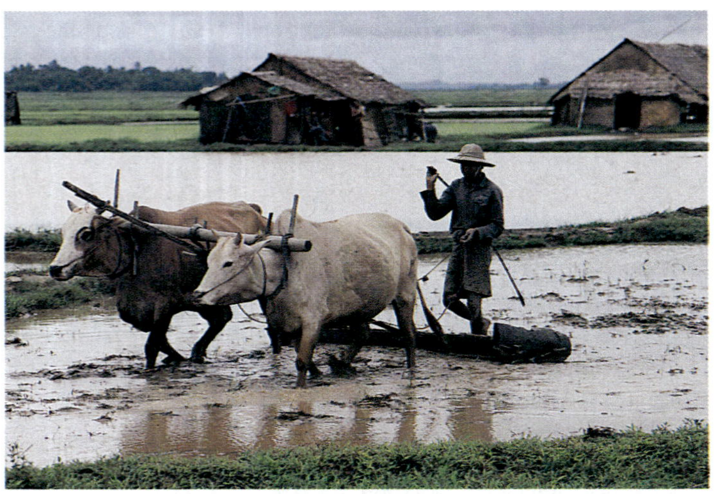

FIGURE 1.18 *About four-fifths of the world's population lives in countries where nearly everyone is poor by American standards.*

TABLE 1.5 The United States, with 4.5 Percent of the World's Population . . .

CONSUMES	PRODUCES
26 percent of all oil	50 percent of all toxic wastes
24 percent of aluminum	26 percent of nitrogen oxides
20 percent of copper	25 percent of sulfur oxides
19 percent of nickel	22 percent of chlorofluorocarbons
13 percent of steel	26 percent of carbon dioxide

Source: Data from World Resources Institute, 1998–99.

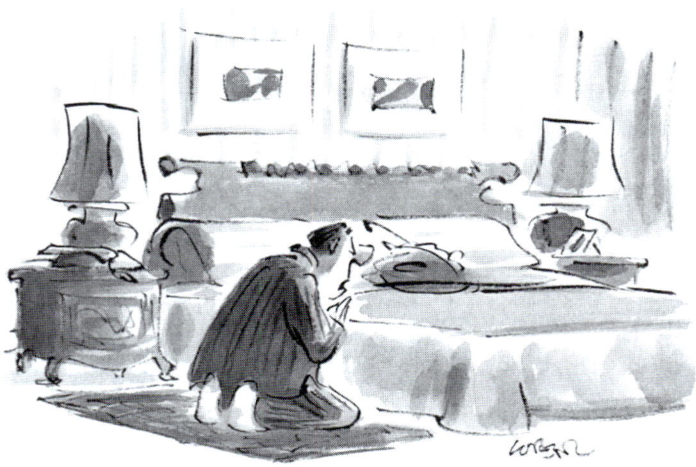

FIGURE 1.20 *"And may we continue to be worthy of consuming a disproportionate share of this planet's resources."*

would be disastrous. Unless we find ways to curb our desires and produce the things we truly need in less destructive ways, the sustainability of human life on our planet is questionable.

Sustainability

An overarching theme of this book is **sustainability:** a search for ecological stability and human progress that can last over the long term. Of course, neither ecological systems nor human institutions can continue forever. We can work, however, to protect the best aspects of both realms, and to encourage resiliency and adaptability in both of them. World Health Organization Director Gro Harlem Brundtland has defined **sustainable development** as "meeting the needs of the present without compromising the ability of future generations to meet their own needs." In these terms, development means bettering people's lives. Sustainable development, then, means progress in human well-being that we can extend or prolong over many generations, rather than just a few years. To be truly enduring, the benefits of sustainable development must be available to all humans and not just to the members of a privileged group. We will discuss this topic further in chapter 14.

Indigenous Peoples

In both rich and poor countries, indigenous, or native, peoples are generally the least powerful, most neglected groups in the world. Typically descendants of the original inhabitants of an area taken over by more powerful outsiders, they are distinct from their country's dominant language, culture, religion, and racial communities. Of the world's nearly 6,000 recognized cultures, 5,000 are indigenous ones that account for only about 10 percent of the total world population. In many countries, traditional caste systems, discriminatory laws, economics, or prejudice repress indigenous peoples. Their unique cultures are disappearing, along with biological diversity as natural habitats are destroyed to satisfy industrialized world appetites for resources. Traditional ways of life are disrupted further by dominant Western culture sweeping around the globe.

At least half of the world's 6,000 distinct languages are dying because they are no longer taught to children. When the last few elders who still speak the language die, so will the culture that was its origin. Lost with those cultures will be a rich repertoire of knowledge about nature and a keen understanding of a particular environment and way of life (fig. 1.21).

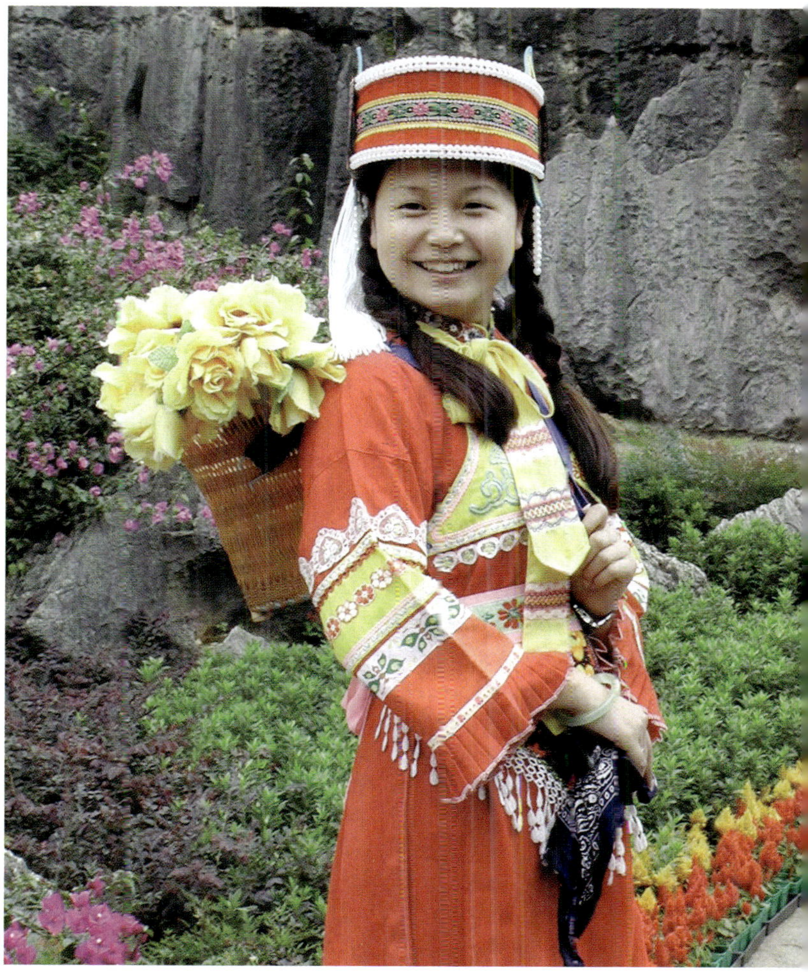

FIGURE 1.21 *Do indigenous people have unique knowledge about nature and inalienable rights to traditional territories?*

Nonetheless, in many places, the 500 million indigenous people who remain in traditional homelands still possess valuable ecological wisdom and remain the guardians of little-disturbed habitats that are refuges for rare and endangered species and undamaged ecosystems. In his book *The Future of Life,* the eminent ecologist E. O. Wilson argues that the cheapest and most effective way to preserve species is to protect the natural ecosystems in which they now live. Interestingly, just 12 countries account for 60 percent of all human languages (fig. 1.22). Seven of these are also among the "megadiversity" countries that contain more than half of all unique plant and animal species. Conditions that support evolution of many unique species seem to favor development of equally diverse human cultures as well.

Recognizing native land rights and promoting political pluralism can be among the best ways to safeguard ecological processes and endangered species. As the Kuna Indians of Panama say, "Where there are forests, there are native people, and where there are native people, there are forests." A few countries, such as Papua New Guinea, Fiji, Ecuador, Canada, and Australia, acknowledge indigenous title to extensive land areas.

Other countries, unfortunately, ignore the rights of native people. Indonesia, for instance, claims ownership of nearly three-quarters of its forestland and all waters and offshore fishing rights, ignoring the interests of indigenous inhabitants. Similarly, the Philippine government claims possession of all uncultivated land in its territory, while Cameroon and Tanzania recognize no rights at all for forest-dwelling pygmies who represent one of the world's oldest cultures.

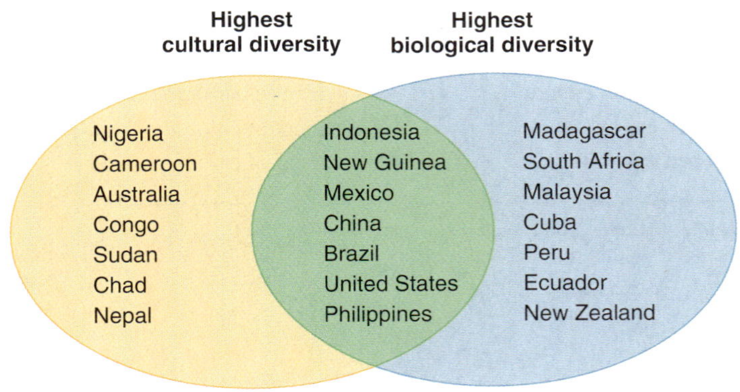

FIGURE 1.22 *Cultural diversity and biodiversity often go hand in hand. Seven of the countries with the highest cultural diversity in the world are also on the list of "megadiversity" countries with the highest number of unique biological organisms (listed in decreasing order of importance).*
Source: Norman Myers, Conservation International and Cultural Survival Inc., 2002.

SUMMARY

- Humans inhabit two worlds: one of nature and another of human society and technology. Environmental science is the systematic study of the intersection of these worlds. An interdisciplinary field, environmental science draws from many areas of inquiry to help us understand the worlds in which we live and how we might improve both of them.
- The most amazing features of our planet may be the self-sustaining ecological systems that make life possible and the rich diversity of life that is part of, and dependent upon, those ecological processes. In spite of the many problems that beset us, the earth is wonderfully bountiful and beautiful.
- Science is a way of exploring and understanding the world around us. It depends on making careful observations of natural phenomena and on formulating reasonable theories to explain those observations. Science rests on certain assumptions such as that the world is understandable and that we can learn about how things work through careful empirical study and rational analysis.
- Scientists strive to be methodical, rigorous, and unbiased. They also are skeptical, reserve judgment, and generally consider conclusions and interpretations to be conditional because new information can always overturn what is thought to be true. Scientists can use either deductive reasoning (arguing from laws or general theories to specific detail) or inductive reasoning (using individual observations to derive general rules).
- Scientists formulate testable hypotheses (provisional explanations) based on their inferences and attempt to test them through experimenting or looking for evidence in nature. Once a substantial body of evidence has been accumulated and a consensus emerges within the scientific community, an explanation is considered a theory.
- Statistics and probability are important concepts in environmental science. Descriptive statistics help us assess the general state of a group. Using a large, random sample helps prevent errors that arise from variations within the study group. Confidence levels represent the likelihood that your results are in error. Scientists usually compare values with a 95 percent confidence level, or a probability of 5 percent or less that the conclusions are misleading.
- Critical thinking shares many of the aspects of logical, analytical thinking but also includes empathy, context, and justice in its search for truth and meaning.

- Unprecedented population growth, food shortages, scarce energy supplies, air and water pollution, and destruction of habitats and biological resources are all serious threats to our environment and our way of life.
- There is good news. Pollution has been reduced and population growth has slowed in many places. Perhaps we can extend these advances to other areas as well.
- The 20 percent of us in the world's richest countries consume an inordinate amount of resources and produce a shocking amount of waste and pollution. Meanwhile, at least 1.4 billion people live in acute poverty and lack access to an adequate diet, decent housing, basic sanitation, clean water, education, medical care, and other essentials for a humane existence.
- Faced with immediate survival needs, the poorest poor often have little choice but to overharvest resources and reduce long-term sustainability for themselves and their children. Development means a real increase in standard of living for the average person. Sustainable development attempts to meet the needs of present generations without reducing the ability of future generations to meet their own needs.
- Indigenous, or native, people are generally among the poorest and most oppressed of any group. Nevertheless, they possess valuable ecological knowledge and remain the guardians of nature in many places. Recognizing the rights of indigenous people and minority communities is an important way to protect natural resources and environmental quality.

QUESTIONS FOR REVIEW

1. Define the terms *environment* and *environmental science.*
2. What is parsimony, and why is it important to scientists?
3. Describe how deductive and inductive reasoning differ.
4. Diagram the scientific method, and give one example of how you might apply it.
5. What are statistics and probability? How are they useful in science?
6. How do analytical, creative, critical, logical, and reflective thinking differ?
7. List six environmental dilemmas that we now face, and describe how each concerns us.
8. Compare some indicators of quality of life between the richest and poorest nations.
9. Define the terms *sustainability* and *sustainable development.*
10. What role might indigenous or tribal land rights have in protecting biodiversity?

THINKING SCIENTIFICALLY

1. If you were voting on whether to dredge PCBs out of the Hudson River, what information would you need, and what sources would you trust to supply it?
2. Do you believe the world is ultimately knowable? What values or evidence shape your views on this question? Why might some people have an attitude different from your own?
3. Why can we falsify a hypothesis but never prove it to be true?
4. Suppose you wanted to investigate the prevalence of a trait among your classmates (say, the percentage who are left-handed). How many out of a class of 100 would you need to question to get a sufficiently accurate result? How would you define *sufficiently accurate*?
5. Some field biologists claim that mathematical models and laboratory simulations can never capture the complexity and variability of the real world. Experimental scientists retort that complex systems have too many simultaneous variables to allow meaningful analysis. Where would you stand in this debate?
6. Identify and explain a paradigm that you and your friends use to help explain how things work.
7. Many social theorists argue that there is no such thing as objective truth or an impartial observer. If you were researching a controversial topic—perhaps whether grizzly bears can be safely restored to the Northern Rockies—what steps would you take to try to maintain objectivity and impartiality?
8. Does the world have enough resources for 8 or 10 billion people to live decent, secure, happy, fulfilling lives? What do those terms mean to you? Try to imagine what they mean to others in our global village.
9. Suppose you wanted to study the environmental impacts of a rich versus a poor country. What factors would you examine, and how would you compare them?

KEY TERMS

analytical thinking 11
biocentric preservation 15
blind experiments 6
controlled studies 6
creative thinking 11
critical thinking 11
deductive reasoning 6
double-blind design 6
environment 4
environmental science 4
global environmentalism 16
hypothesis 7
inductive reasoning 6
logical thinking 11
mean 8
modern environmentalism 15
paradigms 9
parsimony 5
probability 8
reflective thinking 11
reproducibility 6
sample 8
scientific theory 7
significant numbers 6
statistics 8
sustainability 21
sustainable development 21
utilitarian conservation 14

SUGGESTED READINGS

Blair, Tony. 2003. "Meeting the Sustainable Development Challenge." *Environment* 45(4):20–28.

Carson, Rachael. 1962. *Silent Spring*. Riverside Press.

Folke, Carl, et al. 2002. *Resilience and Sustainable Development: Building Adaptive Capacity in a World of Transformations.* International Council for Science.

Fox, Stephen. 1986. *The American Conservation Movement: John Muir and His Legacy.* University of Wisconsin Press.

Gardner, Gary, et al. 2004. *State of the World.* W.W. Norton/Worldwatch Institute.

Gruen, Lori, and Dale Jamieson, eds. 1994. *Reflecting on Nature: Readings in Environmental Philosophy.* Oxford University Press.

Halweil, Brian, et al. 2004. *State of the World.* W.W. Norton/Worldwatch Institute.

Mabogunje, Akin L. 2002. "Poverty and Environmental Degradation: Challenges Within the Global Economy." *Environment* January-February, 8–18.

Orr, David. 2003. "Walking North on a Southbound Train." *Conservation Biology* 17(2):348–51.

Sachs, Jeffery, Andrew D. Mellinger, and John L. Gallup. 2001. "The Geography of Poverty and Wealth." *Scientific American* 284(3):70–73.

Steffen, Will, et al. 2004. Global Change and the Earth System: A Planet Under Pressure. Springer Verlag.

World Resources Institute. 2003. *World Resources 2002–2004: Decisions for the Earth: Balance, voice, and power.* Oxford University Press.

For a far more extensive list of suggested readings, visit our website at www.mhhe.com/cunningham3e.

Welcome to McGraw-Hill's Online Learning Center

http://www.mhhe.com/cunningham3e

WEB EXERCISE

Satellites in Environmental Science

Satellite data are an important source of environmental information and monitoring. Satellite imagery is available from the National Atmospheric and Space Agency (NASA) at http://seawifs.gsfc.nasa.gov/SEAWIFS.html. What are some of the current topics shown in images on this page? Have you heard or read about these topics in the news?

Go to the big maps if you have a fast Internet connection: http://seawifs.gsfc.nasa.gov/cgi/level3.pl.

Click on the NDVI (normalized difference vegetation index) option in the table of themes. NDVI is a measure of how green the vegetation is. Then click on the current month in the table of months and years. (Click on a map to see a larger version.) Compare the view of the current month with the views at several different times of year. Find your location on the map. Can you identify local features that should (or should not) be green in the various months? How does the amount of vegetation in your area affect local environmental conditions? If satellites had existed 100 years ago, how might the view they would have shown differed from what we see today?

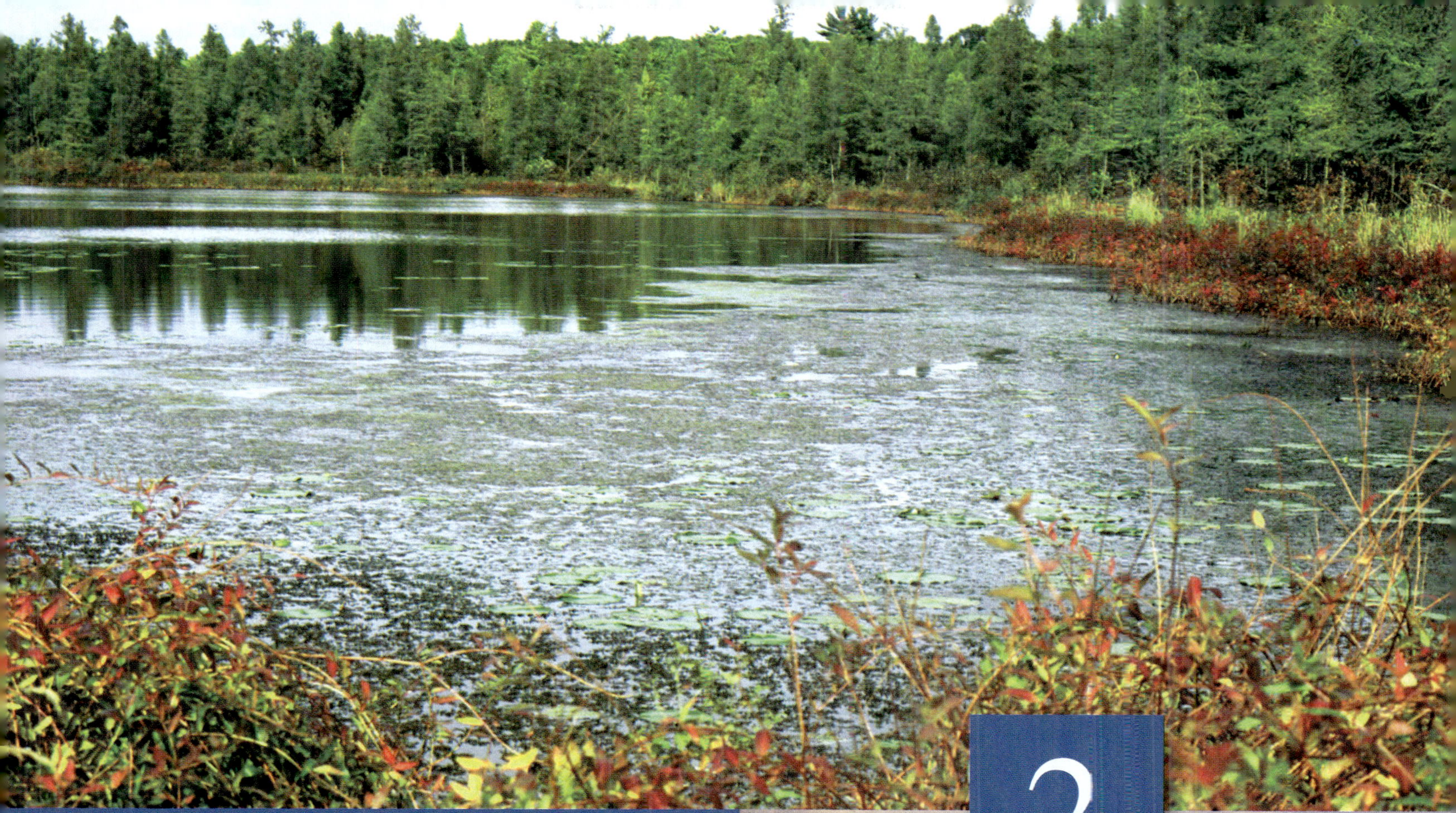

Cedar Bog Lake, the focus of the first detailed, quantitative study of matter and energy cycling in an ecosystem.

2

Principles of Ecology: Matter, Energy, and Life

When one tugs at a single thing in nature,
he finds it attached to the rest of the world.

—*John Muir*

Welcome to McGraw-Hill's Online Learning Center

http://www.mhhe.com/cunningham3e

LEARNING ONLINE

Visit our webpage at www.mhhe.com/cunningham3e for data sources, further readings, additional case studies, current environmental news, and regional examples within the Online Learning Center to help you understand the material in this chapter. You'll also find active links to information pertaining to this chapter, including

Chemistry primer
Cell biology and cell structure
Ecosystems
Thermodynamics
Photosynthesis
Nutrient cycles

OBJECTIVES

After studying this chapter, you should be able to

- describe matter, atoms and molecules, and give simple examples of the roles of four major kinds of organic compounds in living cells.
- define *energy,* and explain the difference between kinetic and potential energy.
- understand the principles of conservation of matter and energy, and appreciate how the laws of thermodynamics affect living systems.
- explain how photosynthesis captures energy for life and how cellular respiration releases that energy to do useful work.
- define *species, populations, biological communities,* and *ecosystems,* and understand the ecological significance of these levels of organization.
- discuss food chains, food webs, and trophic levels in biological communities, and explain why there are pyramids of energy, biomass, and numbers of individuals in the trophic levels of an ecosystem.
- explain the importance of material cycles, such as carbon and nitrogen cycles, in ecosystems.

Measuring Energy Flows in Cedar Bog Lake

In 1936 a young graduate student named Ray Lindeman began his Ph.D. research on a small, marshy pond in Minnesota called Cedar Bog Lake. His pioneering work helped reshape the way ecologists think about the systems they study. At the time, most ecologists were concerned primarily with descriptive histories and classifications of biological communities. A typical lake study might classify the taxonomy and life histories of resident species and describe the lake's stage in development from open water to marsh and then to forest. Blind in one eye, Lindeman couldn't do the microscopy necessary to identify the many species of algae, protozoans, and other aquatic organisms in the lake. Instead, following the ideas of two contemporary English ecologists, Charles Elton and A. G. Tansley, he concentrated on biological communities as systems and looked at broad categories of feeding relationships, for which he coined the term *trophic levels* (from the Greek word for eating) (fig. 2.1). Aided by his wife, Eleanor, Lindeman spent many hours collecting samples of aquatic plants and algae, grazing and predatory zooplankton and fish, and the benthic (bottom-dwelling) worms, insect larvae, crustaceans, and sediment. Back in the laboratory, he measured the plants' photosynthetic rates, the animals' respiration rates, and the total energy content of organic compounds in each of the different trophic levels.

Describing the system in terms of energy flows was a radical departure from ecological methods at the time. Lindeman made a careful balance sheet of the total energy content in the biomass at each trophic level, the energy used in respiration, and the energy content of organic matter deposited in the sediment. To his surprise, he found that each successive feeding level contained only about 10 percent of the energy captured by the level below it. The remainder is lost as heat or deposited in sediments, he argued, because of the work that organisms perform and the inefficiency of biological energy transformations. In his dissertation, Lindeman showed that energy represents a common denominator that allows us to sum up all the processes of production and consumption by the myriad organisms in a biological community.

Lindeman also broke from standard procedure by representing the relationships in his study lake as a mathematical model: he used a series of equations to describe thermodynamic relationships and the efficiency of energy capture and transfer. Ironically,

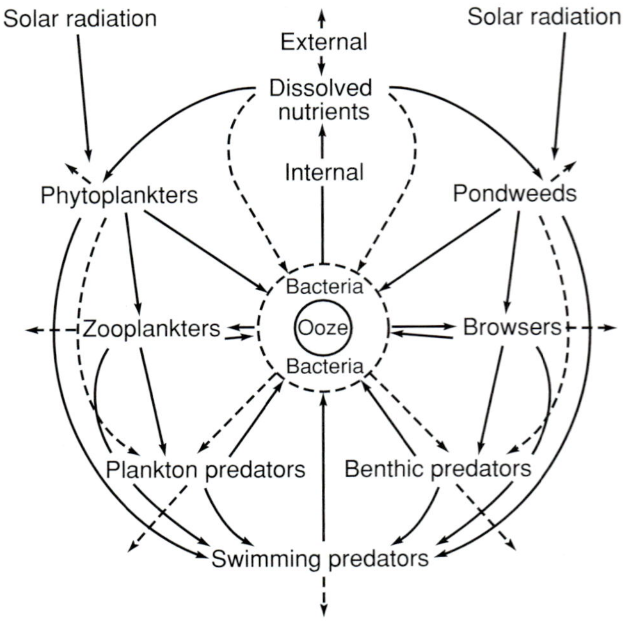

FIGURE 2.1 *Feeding relationships in Cedar Bog Lake.*
Source: After R. Lindeman, 1942. The trophic-dynamic aspect of ecology. *Ecology* 23(4):399–417.

Lindeman's most important paper was rejected by the journal *Ecology* as being too theoretical and too quantitative. It was only after the intercession of G. Evelyn Hutchinson from Yale, with whom Lindeman had a postdoctoral fellowship after finishing his studies at Minnesota, that his mathematical model and energy analysis of Cedar Bog Lake was finally published. Unfortunately, Ray Lindeman died of liver failure before his article appeared. It has since become a landmark in ecological history.

In the years since Lindeman's work, the idea of taking a systemic view of a biological community together with its physical and inorganic environment has become standard in ecology. Energy flows and nutrient cycles are central to the way we understand the workings of ecological systems. Constructing quantitative models to describe, explain, and explore ecological processes has become routine. In this chapter, we will investigate the ways living things use energy and matter and the ways these flows create relationships in ecosystems. (See R. L. Lindeman. 1942. The trophic-dynamic aspect of ecology. *Ecology* 23:399–418.)

PRINCIPLES OF MATTER AND ENERGY

How and why materials are cycled between the living and nonliving parts of our environment are the domain of **ecology,** the scientific study of relationships between organisms and their environment. Modern biology covers a wide range of scales and themes, from molecules to ecosystems to global systems. Ecology examines the life histories, distribution, and behavior of individual species, as well as the structure and function of natural systems at the level of populations, communities, ecosystems, and landscapes. The systems approach of ecology encourages us to think holistically about interconnections that make whole systems more than just the sum of their individual parts.

In a sense, every organism is a chemical factory that captures matter and energy from its environment and transforms them into structures and processes that make life possible. Therefore, to understand how ecosystems function, it is important first to know something of how energy and matter behave—both in the universe and in living things. In this chapter, we will survey some fundamental aspects of energy flow and material recycling within ecosystems.

What Is Matter?

Everything that takes up space and has mass is matter. All matter has three interchangeable physical forms, or phases: gas, liquid, and solid. Water, for example, can exist as a gas (water vapor), a liquid (water), or a solid (ice). Under ordinary circumstances, matter is neither created nor destroyed but is recycled over and over again. The elements in your body have been recycled through many other organisms, over millions of years. Matter is transformed and combined in different ways, but it doesn't disappear; everything goes somewhere. These statements paraphrase the physical principle of **conservation of matter.**

How does this principle apply to human relationships with the biosphere? It implies that, as we use more resources to produce more "disposable" goods, we should pay attention to where our waste products go. What happens to the garbage the truck hauls away? Where does the exhaust from your car go? Ultimately, we need to answer these questions because there is no "away" where we can throw things we don't want anymore.

What Is Energy?

Energy and matter are essential constituents of both the universe and living organisms. If **matter** is the material of which things are made, **energy** is the capacity to do work, such as moving matter over a distance. Energy can take many different forms. Heat, light, electricity, and chemical energy are common forms. The energy contained in moving objects is called **kinetic energy.** A rock rolling down a hill, the wind blowing through the trees, water flowing over a dam (fig. 2.2), and electrons speeding around the nucleus of an atom are all examples of kinetic energy. **Potential energy** is stored energy that is latent but available for use. A rock poised at the top of a hill contains potential energy, which is converted to kinetic energy when the rock starts rolling down the hill. Chemical energy, stored in the food you eat and the gasoline you put into your car, is also potential energy that can be released to do useful work. Energy is often measured in units of heat (calories) or work (joules). One joule (J) is the work done when 1 kg is accelerated 1 m per second per second ($1 \text{ J} = 1 \text{ kg} \cdot \text{m}^2/\text{s}^2$). One calorie is the amount of energy needed to heat 1 gram of pure water 1 degree Celsius. A calorie can also be measured as 4.184 J.

Heat describes the energy that can be transferred between objects of different temperature. When two objects of different temperature are placed in contact, heat transfers to the cooler one until the two reach the same temperature. When a substance absorbs heat, its internal energy increases; the kinetic energy (motion) of its molecules increases, or it may change state: a solid may become a liquid or a liquid become a gas. When you heat a tea kettle on a stove, for example, energy is transferred to the water. We sense the change in heat content as a change in temperature. Some of the water may change state from liquid to vapor. After the stove is turned off, heat gradually dissipates from the water into the surrounding air. Water requires a relatively large exchange of heat in order to warm or change to steam. One kilogram of iron, for example, would warm much faster than 1 kilogram of water on the same stove. We measure this difference in terms of *specific heat,* the amount of heat required to warm 1 gram of a substance 1 degree C. Water requires 4.18 J to warm 1 degree C; a gram of wood takes less than half as much energy (1.7 J), and iron just over one-tenth as much energy (0.45 J) to warm 1 degree C.

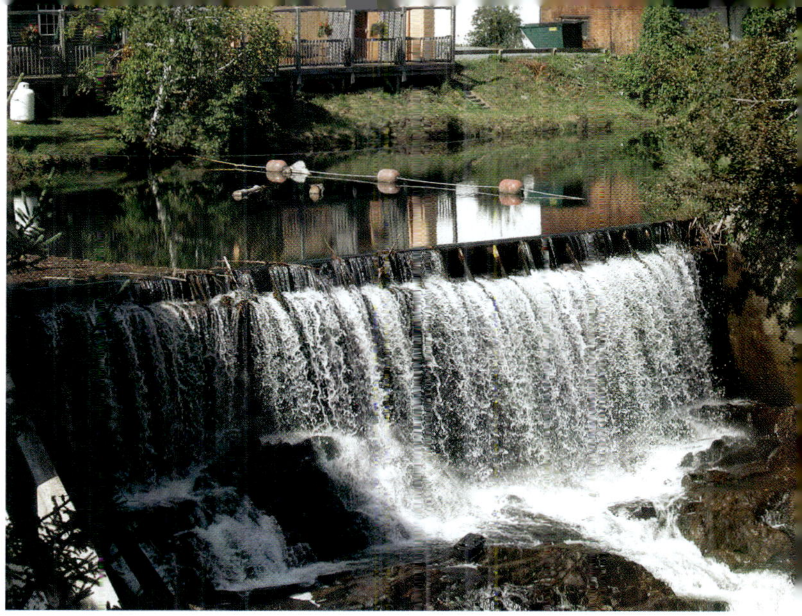

FIGURE 2.2 *Water stored behind this dam represents potential energy. Water flowing over the dam has kinetic energy, some of which is converted to heat.*

A substance can have a low temperature but a high heat content, as in the case of a lake that freezes slowly in the fall. Other objects, such as a burning match, have a high temperature but little heat content. Low-quality energy is diffused, dispersed, or low in temperature, so it is difficult to gather and use for productive purposes. Oceans store vast amounts of heat, but converting that heat to useful purposes is difficult. High-quality energy is intense, concentrated, or high in temperature, and it is useful in carrying out work. The intense flames of a very hot fire or high-voltage electrical energy are useful for many purposes. This distinction is important because many of our most common energy sources are low-quality and must be concentrated or transformed into high-quality before they are useful to us.

Why is understanding heat and energy important to understanding environmental science? Because physical characteristics of substances, and their ability to absorb and release energy, control environmental systems. Consider the properties of water, for example. Water's high specific heat keeps lakeshores and seashores relatively cool in the summer and warm in the winter (see "The Miracle of Water," p. 32). Because water absorbs so much heat as it evaporates, atmospheric water vapor redistributes heat around the globe, as well as contributing to the formation of thunderstorms and hurricanes (chapter 9). In addition, the concepts that energy can be converted from work to heat, or from potential to kinetic energy, help explain the ways we store and use energy, both in our bodies and in our electrical utility systems. Further, a common problem in alternative energy production is that alternative energy sources are often more diffuse and difficult to capture than conventional sources, such as oil or coal (chapter 12).

Thermodynamics and Energy Transfers

Matter is recycled endlessly through living things, but this recycling is made possible by something that cannot be recycled: energy. Most energy used in ecosystems originates as sunlight. Green plants capture and convert some of this energy to chemical energy, which can be used or stored. Animals consume plants and convert some of the stored chemical energy to kinetic energy and heat. Eventually the energy dissipates and becomes no longer useful. Thus, energy is reused, but it is degraded from higher quality to lower quality forms as it moves through living systems.

Thermodynamics is the study of how energy is transferred, its rates of flow and transformation from one form or quality to another. Thermodynamics is a complex, quantitative discipline, but you don't need a great deal of math to understand some of the broad principles that shape our world and our lives.

The **first law of thermodynamics** states that energy is conserved: it is neither created nor destroyed under normal conditions. It may be transferred or transformed, but the total amount of energy remains the same.

The **second law of thermodynamics** states that, with each successive energy transfer or transformation in a system, less energy is available to do work. Even though the total amount of energy remains the same, its intensity and usefulness deteriorate. The second law recognizes the principle known as *entropy,* the tendency of all natural systems to go from a state of order (for example, high-quality energy, such as chemical energy) toward a state of increasing disorder (for example, low-quality energy, such as heat or kinetic energy). Because of this law, all mechanical systems degrade and disperse energy as they operate. The need for an external source of high-quality energy is an important limitation on all human activities.

How does the second law of thermodynamics apply to organisms and biological systems? Organisms are highly organized, both structurally and metabolically. Constant care and maintenance are required to keep up this organization, and a constant supply of energy is required to maintain these processes. Every time some energy is used by a cell to do work, some of that energy is dissipated, or lost, as heat and movement. If cellular energy supplies are interrupted or depleted, the result—sooner or later—is death.

THE BUILDING BLOCKS OF EARTH AND LIFE

Matter consists of elements, which are combined to form molecules and compounds. Each of the 112 known elements has distinct chemical characteristics (see periodic table, Appendix 4 p.384). Among the more common elements in biology are carbon (C), hydrogen (H), oxygen (O), nitrogen (N), and phosphorus (P) (table 2.1).

TABLE 2.1 Important Elements in Environmental Science

Living things	C, H, O, N
Atmosphere	N, O, Ar, C, Ne, He
Earth, rocks	Fe, O, Si, Mg, Ni, Ca, Al, Na
Economic metals	Al, Cr, Cu, Fe, Pb, Mn, Ni
Primary toxins	Hg, Pb, Se, Br, Cd, Be, Rn, Ni, As

Atoms, Molecules, and Compounds

An **atom** is the smallest particle that exhibits the characteristics of an element. Atoms are tiny units of matter composed of positively charged *protons,* negatively charged *electrons,* and electrically neutral *neutrons.* Protons and neutrons, which have approximately the same mass, are clustered in the nucleus at the center of the atom (fig. 2.3). Electrons, which are tiny in comparison with protons and neutrons, orbit the nucleus in a rapidly moving cloud. Atoms that have equal numbers of electrons and protons are electrically neutral. Atoms frequently lose or gain electrons, acquiring a positive or negative electrical charge. Charged atoms are called **ions.** A *cation* has a positive charge (the atom has lost one or more electrons); an *anion* has a negative charge (the original atom has gained one or more extra electrons).

We identify atoms by their atomic number, the number of protons in their nuclei. A hydrogen (H) atom has one proton in its nucleus, while a carbon (C) atom has six. The number of neutrons in atoms of the same element can vary, producing slight variations in atomic mass (the sum of protons and neutrons). Atoms of a single element that differ in atomic mass are *isotopes.* For example, the nuclei of most hydrogen atoms contain only one proton. A small percentage of hydrogen nuclei in nature contain one proton *and* one neutron. We call this isotope deuterium (^2H). An even smaller percentage of hydrogen atoms have one proton and two neutrons in their nuclei. This isotope is known as tritium (^3H).

Tritium is an example of a radioactive isotope, an unstable form that spontaneously decays by emitting high-energy electromagnetic radiation, subatomic particles, or both. The rate of radioactive decay is indicated by the half-life of an isotope, or the time it takes for half of the atoms to decay. Tritium decays to helium-3 (^3He), with a half-life of 12.5 years. If we started with 1,000 ^3H nuclei, 500 of them would have decayed to ^3He after 12.5 years. Some isotopes of iodine have half-lives measured in seconds, while plutonium, a waste product of nuclear power reactions, has a half-life of 24,000 years. The radioactive emissions from these atoms may be neutrons, beta particles (high-energy electrons), alpha particles (helium nuclei consisting of two protons and two neutrons), positrons (high-energy, positively charged particles), or gamma rays (very short-wavelength radiation). These high-energy emissions can badly damage living cells and tissues. The decades-long debate about storing nuclear waste at Yucca Mountain, Nevada (chapter 12), reflects the danger of radioactive emissions and the long half-life of plutonium.

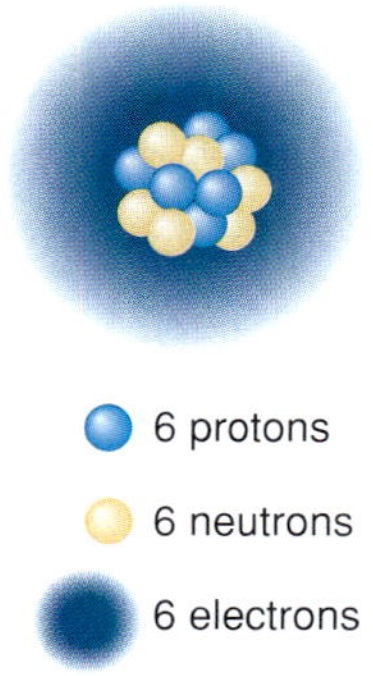

FIGURE 2.3 *As difficult as it may be to imagine when you look at a solid object, all matter is composed of tiny, moving particles, separated by space and held together by energy. This model represents a carbon-12 atom, with a nucleus containing six protons and six neutrons; the six electrons are represented as a fuzzy cloud of potential locations, rather than as individual particles.*

Two or more atoms can combine chemically to form units called **molecules** (fig. 2.4). For example, when two atoms of oxygen combine chemically, a molecule of oxygen is created. A molecule composed of atoms of the same type is called an elemental molecule. When atoms of two or more different elements combine, we call the resulting molecules **chemical compounds.** For example, water (H_2O) is a chemical compound made up of hydrogen and oxygen in a ratio of 2:1. The properties of a chemical compound can be quite different from those of its constituent elements: at room temperature, water is usually a liquid, while hydrogen and oxygen are gases.

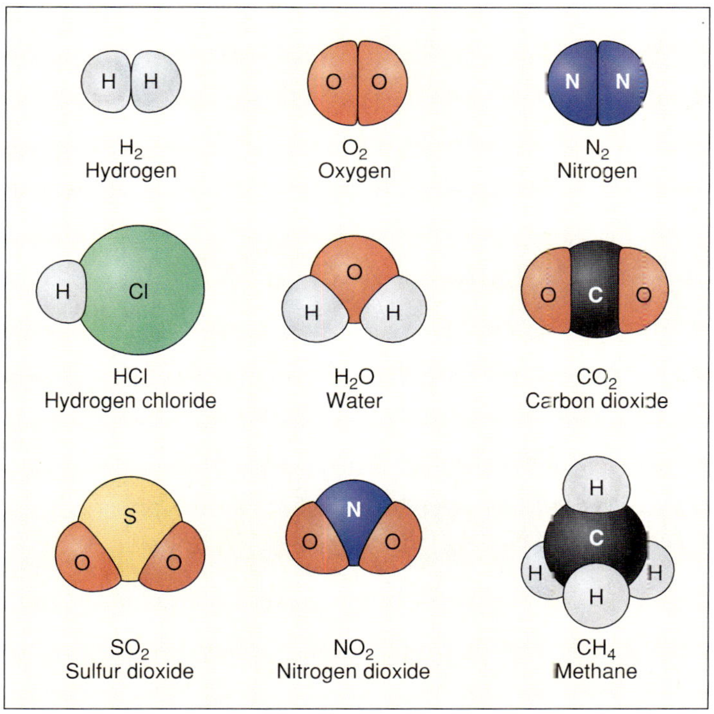

FIGURE 2.4 *These common molecules, with atoms held together by covalent bonds, are important components of the atmosphere or important pollutants.*

The atoms of a molecule or compound are held together by forces of attraction called chemical bonds. Each bond represents a certain amount of chemical energy. In covalent bonds, an electron or a pair of electrons is shared between adjacent atoms. A simple example is the joining of two hydrogen atoms in a molecule of hydrogen gas, H_2. Each hydrogen atom has only a single electron. Both atoms share their electrons so that both electrons spin around both atomic nuclei, thus joining the two atoms. Oxygen atoms, which are much larger than hydrogen and have more electrons, share a pair of electrons, forming an oxygen molecule (O_2). It takes a considerable amount of energy to break these covalent bonds.

Some atoms and molecules are not electrically neutral. When an atom or a molecule loses or gains one or more electrons, it becomes an ion. The loss of electrons creates positively charged cations. Atoms or molecules that have gained extra electrons become negatively charged anions. The attraction between the positive charge of a cation and the negative charge of an anion is called an ionic bond. An example is the attraction between sodium and chloride ions in ordinary table salt (NaCl). The sodium atom gives up an electron to become positively charged (Na^+), while the chlorine atom gains an electron to become negatively charged (Cl^-) These ions are attracted to each other as a result of their opposite charges.

When sodium chloride is in its solid crystal state, no discrete molecules of NaCl exist. Sodium and chloride ions are present in a 1:1 ratio, but each ion is surrounded by six ions of opposite charge. Compounds joined by ionic bonds have a tendency to dissociate (separate) into their individual ions when placed in water. Thus,

NaCl	$\longrightarrow$	Na^+	+	Cl^-
sodium chloride	in H_20	sodium ion		chloride ion

Because atoms are more stable when bonded ionically or covalently than when they stand alone, energy is needed to break chemical bonds, and energy is released when bonds are formed. Some bonds are stronger than others, so that more energy is needed to break them, and more energy is released when they are broken. For example, plants require energy from the sun to disrupt the very strong covalent bonds in carbon dioxide (CO_2) and water. Plants use atoms from these compounds to form complex molecules, such as sugars and cellulose. An animal that eats a plant breaks the relatively weak bonds of carbohydrates (sugars and starches), and the resulting atoms recombine to form much stronger bonds of CO_2 and H_2O. The net effect is a release of energy, which powers muscles and allows cells to perform functions such as transferring nutrients and synthesizing proteins.

Chemical Reactions

Chemical reactions occur when bonds are broken and re-formed among atoms and compounds. These reactions form the basic compounds on which life depends, and they underlie many of the processes (and problems) in environmental science. Some reactions, such as the breakdown of sugar molecules, can be very complex, but all chemical reactions follow the basic principles of physics: matter (atoms) can be neither created nor destroyed, and energy is transformed or dissipated as reactions occur.

Here is a reaction that occurs when you light a gas stove or furnace:

$$CH_4 + 2\ O_2 \rightarrow CO_2 + 2\ H_2O$$

This reaction shows how atoms are rearranged into new compounds when you burn natural gas, or methane. The reaction starts with two input components, or *reactants:* one methane (CH_4) molecule and two oxygen (O_2) molecules. The methane molecule is broken apart and recombined with oxygen. Two new compounds, or *products,* are formed: carbon dioxide and water. Energy (heat) is released as the methane bonds are broken. Note that the same number of each kind of atom appears on both sides of the reaction (one carbon, four hydrogen, and four oxygen atoms). This balance demonstrates the conservation of matter in chemical reactions.

Some reactions occur in a sequence, as in the breakdown of ozone (O_3) to molecular oxygen (O_2) by highly reactive chlorine atoms released from chlorofluorocarbons (CFCs) (see the related story, "Ozone Hole Continues to Grow," at www.mhhe.com/cases).

Step 1: CF_2Cl_2 + high energy sunlight $\rightarrow CF_2Cl + Cl$

Step 2: $Cl + O_3 \rightarrow ClO + O_2$

Step 3: $ClO + O_3 \rightarrow Cl + 2\ O_2$

When a molecule or an atom loses electrons it is said to be *oxidized.* For example, when iron in the steel body of your car is exposed to oxygen in the air, each iron atom gives up three electrons to the oxygen (O_2) molecules. The formerly blue-black iron becomes a red iron oxide compound commonly known as rust. In this process, we say that the iron, which lost electrons, was oxidized, while the oxygen, which gained electrons, was *reduced.* Not all oxidation-reduction reactions involve oxygen, but many do. Can you think of any other such reactions? What happens when a candle burns?

APPLICATION: Balance a Chemical Equation

In any chemical reaction the same number of atoms of each element must appear on both sides of the arrow. The following reaction represents the net reaction when two reactants, iron and water, combine to produce one product, iron oxide (rust). To balance the equation, first count the number of Fe atoms and O atoms on each side of the arrow. Then fill in the coefficients to make the number of Fe atoms balance. Then fill in the coefficient to make O atoms balance.

___ Fe + ___ $O_2 \rightarrow$ ___ Fe_2O_3

Here is a harder example, representing photosynthesis (see fig. 2.11). The reactants water and carbon dioxide are broken apart (with the aid of solar energy) and recombined to produce oxygen molecules, glucose ($C_6H_{12}O_6$), and water. Again, first count the number of H, C, and O atoms on each side of the equation. Fill in the blanks to balance C, then H, and finally O atoms.

___ H_2O + ___ CO_2 + light energy $\rightarrow$
___ O_2 + ___ $C_6H_{12}O_6$ + ___ H_2O

Answers: $4\ Fe + 3\ O_2 \rightarrow 2\ Fe_2O_3$; $12\ H_2O + 6\ CO_2$ + light energy $\rightarrow 6\ O_2 + C_6H_{12}O_6 + 6\ H_2O$.

Acids and Bases

You are probably familiar with **acids,** such as vinegar or battery acid. Mild acids add a sour flavor to foods; strong acids can burn your skin. Chemically, acids are compounds that readily release hydrogen ions (H^+) in water. Familiar alkaline substances, or **bases,** are also common, especially as cleaning agents: these include baking soda, ammonia, bleach, and drain cleaners. Concentrated bases are extremely caustic to your skin. Chemically, bases are substances that readily take up H^+ ions and release hydroxide ions (OH^-) in solution. The strength of an acid or a base solution can be described by its concentration of H^+ ions, or **pH** (fig. 2.5). Acids have pH values less than 7; they have more H^+ than OH^- ions. Bases have a pH greater than 7; they have more OH^- than H^+ ions. Substances with a pH of exactly 7 are neutral. The pH scale is logarithmic, which means it increases by factors of ten. A substance with pH 5, therefore, has ten times as many hydrogen ions as one with pH 6. In 2002 a train car filled with

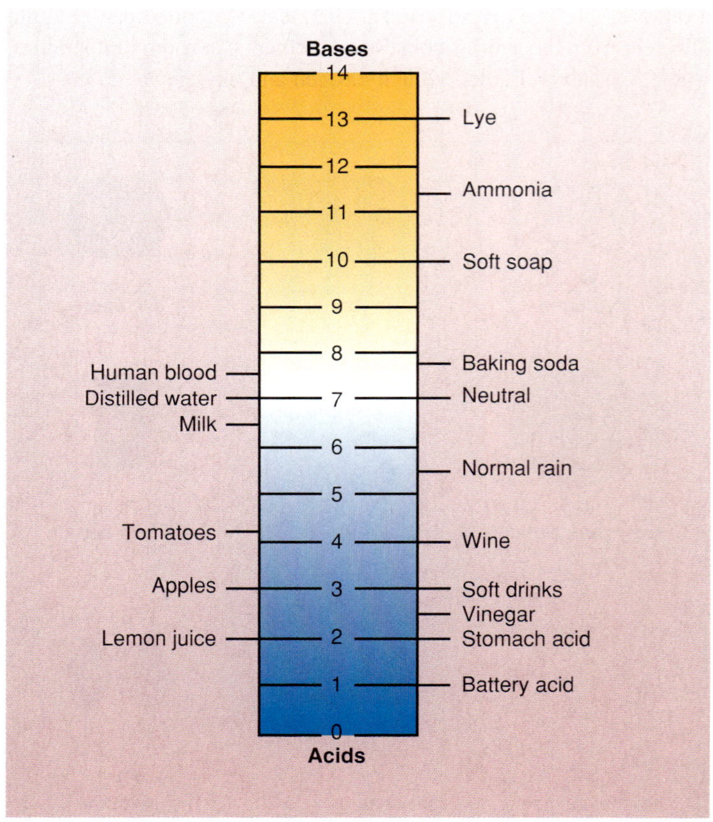

FIGURE 2.5 *The pH scale. The numbers represent the negative logarithm of the hydrogen ion concentration in water. Alkaline (basic) solutions have a pH greater than 7. Acids (pH less than 7) have high concentrations of reactive H^+ ions.*

ammonia (NH_3), the most common nitrogen fertilizer on midwestern farms, overturned in North Dakota. Nearby residents had to be evacuated because, in contact with moisture, ammonia is a strong basic compound that is extremely caustic to living tissue.

Organic Compounds

Organic compounds, the compounds that make up living things, are large, often complex molecules built on structures of carbon atoms. The carbon atoms can be arranged in chains, rings, or complex arrangements of many rings and chains. Aside from carbon, some of the most common elements in organic compounds are hydrogen, oxygen, nitrogen, phosphorus, and potassium. There are many types of bioorganic compounds, but they can be grouped into four major categories: lipids, carbohydrates, proteins, and nucleic acids (fig. 2.6, table 2.2). Together these form the structural and functional characteristics of cells.

Cells: The Fundamental Units of Life

All living organisms are composed of cells, minute compartments within which the processes of life are carried out (fig. 2.7). Microscopic organisms, such as bacteria, some algae, and protozoa, are composed of single cells. By contrast, your body contains several trillion cells of about 200 distinct types. Surrounding every cell is a thin membrane of lipid and protein, which receives information and regulates the flow of materials between the cell and its environment. Inside, cells are subdivided into tiny organelles and subcellular particles, which provide the machinery for life. Some of these organelles store and release energy. Others manage and distribute information. Still others create the internal structure that gives the cell its shape and allows it to fulfill its functions.

A special class of proteins, called enzymes, facilitates all the chemical reactions in cells—providing energy, disposing of wastes, building proteins, and creating new cells. Enzymes are molecular catalysts: they initiate chemical reactions without being used up or inactivated in the process. Think of them as tools. Like hammers or wrenches, they do their jobs without being consumed or damaged as they work. There are generally thousands of different kinds of enzymes in every cell, all designed to carry out the many individual processes on which life depends. Most enzymes work by temporarily binding molecules in a unique cavity, or slot, much as a key fits a lock. The multitude of enzymatic reactions an organism performs is called its **metabolism.**

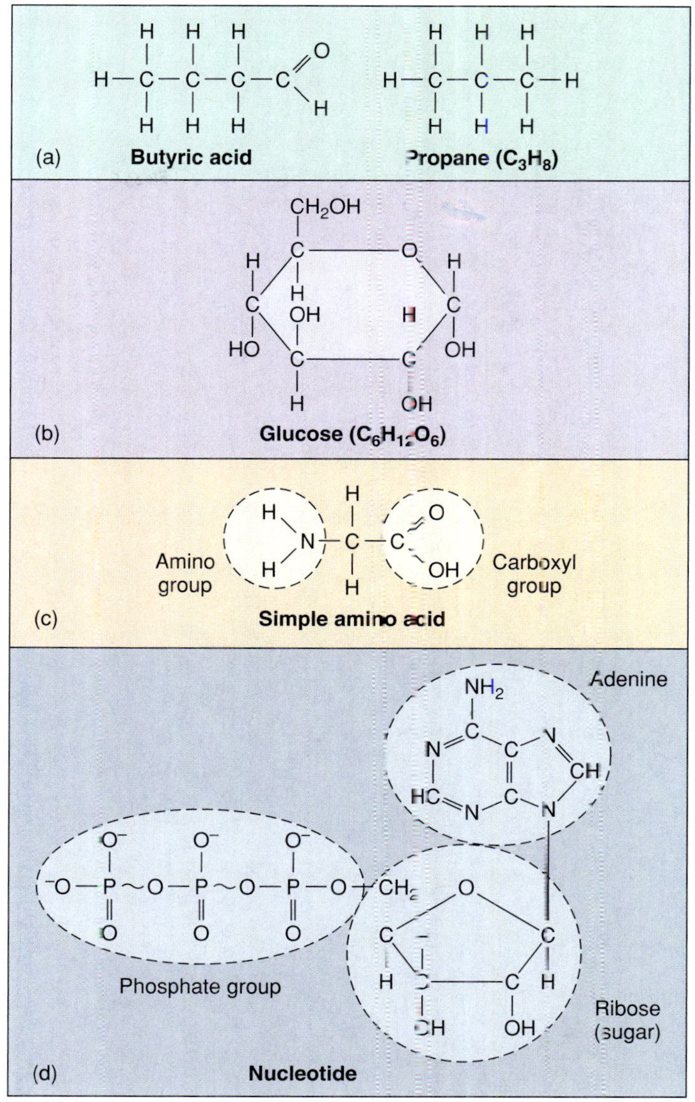

FIGURE 2.6 *The four major groups of organic molecules are based on repeating subunits of these carbon-based structures. Basic structures are shown for* (a) *butyric acid (a building block of lipids) and a hydrocarbon,* (b) *a simple carbohydrate,* (c) *a protein, and* (d) *a nucleic acid.*

TABLE 2.2 Major Classes of Organic Compounds

SUBSTANCE	EXAMPLES	SOME USES	BASIC STRUCTURES
Lipids and hydrocarbons	Fats, oils	Cell membranes, internal cell organelles	Chains of C with attached H
Carbohydrates	Sugars, starches, cellulose	Cell structure, energy storage	Rings or chains of C with attached H and O
Proteins	Muscles, enzymes	Cell structure, function	Chains of amino acids
Nucleic acids	DNA, RNA	Genetic information, protein synthesis	Chains of nucleotides linked by phosphate-sugar bonds

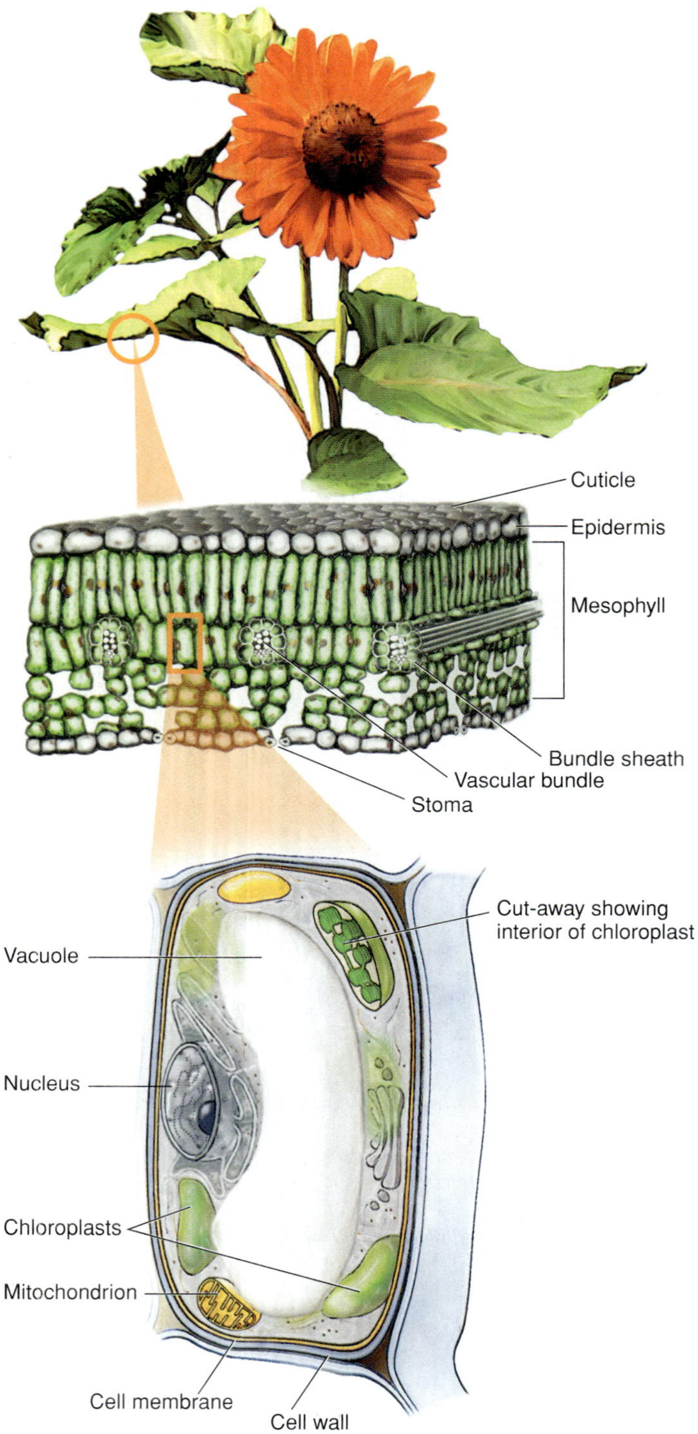

FIGURE 2.7 *Plant tissues and a single cell's interior. Cell components include a cellulose cell wall; a nucleus; a large, empty vacuole; and several chloroplasts, which carry out photosynthesis.*

The Miracle of Water

If travelers from other solar systems were to visit our lovely, cool, blue planet, they might call it Aqua rather than Terra because of its most outstanding feature: an abundance of streams, rivers, lakes, and oceans of liquid water. Without liquid water we would not exist. Water is the (nearly) universal solvent that carries nutrients and wastes to and from our cells. It participates in many organic functions and reactions that allow life as we know it to exist. The earth is the only place that we know of where water exists in liquid form in any appreciable quantity. Liquid water covers nearly three-fourths of the earth's surface, and during the winter, snow and ice cover a good deal of the rest. Not only is water essential for cell structure and metabolism, but water's unique physical and chemical properties directly affect the earth's surface temperatures, its atmosphere, and the interactions of life-forms with their environments. Water has many unique, almost magical, qualities, including the following:

1. Water makes up 60 to 70 percent (on average) of the weight of living organisms. It fills cells, thereby giving form and support to many tissues. Water is the medium in which all of life's chemical reactions occur, and it is an active participant in many of these reactions. Water is a solvent that dissolves the nutrients that cells need for life, as well as the wastes that cells produce. Thus, water is essential in delivering materials to and from cells.
2. Water dissolves salts and other compounds, producing solutions that conduct electricity. These solutions, called electrolytes, are essential in many physiological reactions, such as muscle contraction and nerve conduction.
3. Water molecules are cohesive, tending to stick together tenaciously. You have experienced this property if you have ever done a belly flop off a diving board. Water has the highest surface tension of any common natural liquid (fig. 2.8). As a result, water is subject to *capillary action;* that is, it can be drawn into small channels. Without capillary action, movement of water and nutrients into groundwater reservoirs and through living organisms might not be possible.
4. Water exists as a liquid over a wide temperature range that, for most of the world (at least during summer months), corresponds to the ambient temperature range. Most substances exist as either a solid or a gas, with only a very narrow liquid temperature range. Organisms synthesize important organic compounds, such as oils and alcohols, that remain liquid at ambient temperatures, but the original and predominant liquid in nature is water.
5. Water is unique in that it expands when it crystallizes. Most substances shrink as they change from liquid to solid. Ice floats because it is less dense than liquid water. When temperatures fall below freezing, the surface layers of lakes, rivers, and oceans cool faster and freeze before deeper water. Floating ice then insulates underlying layers, keeping most water bodies liquid (and aquatic organisms alive) throughout the winter. Without this feature, lakes, rivers, and even oceans in high latitudes would freeze solid and never melt.
6. Water has a high heat of vaporization: a great deal of energy is needed to convert it from liquid to vapor. Consequently, evaporating water is an effective way for organisms to shed excess heat. Many animals pant or sweat to moisten evaporative cooling surfaces. Why do you feel less comfortable on

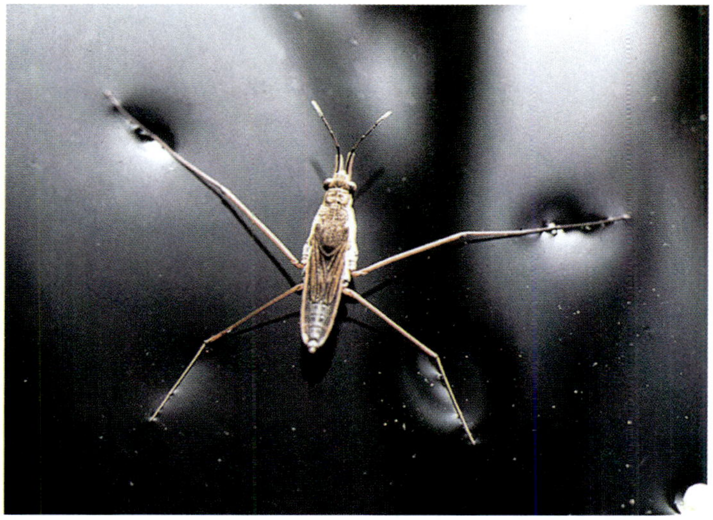

FIGURE 2.8 *Surface tension (cohesiveness of water molecules) prevents this water strider from breaking through as it walks on water.*

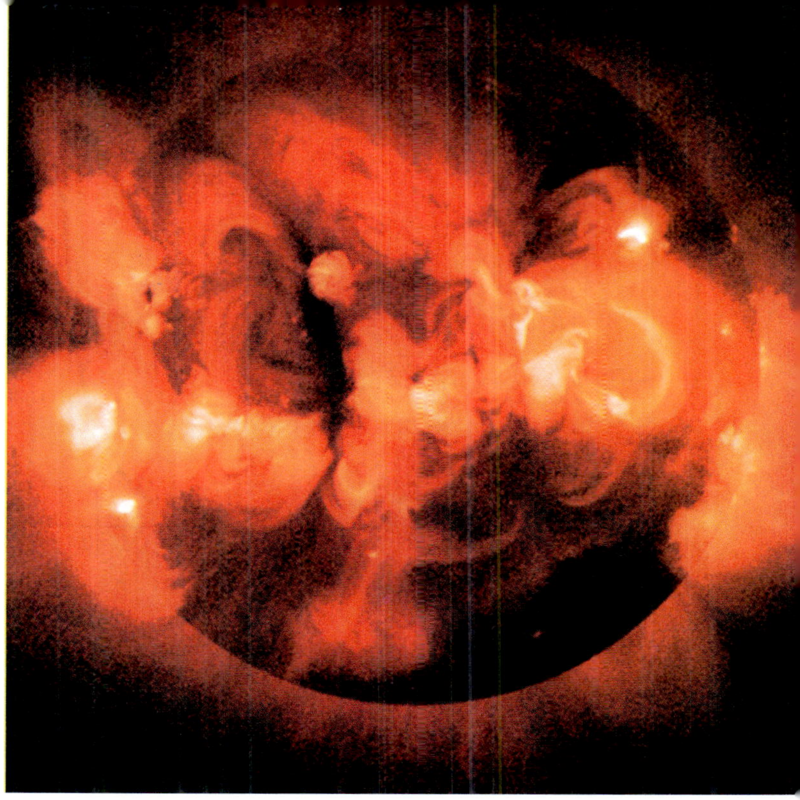

FIGURE 2.9 *Thermonuclear reactions in the sun provide the energy for life on earth.*

a hot, humid day than on a hot, dry day? The water vapor-laden air inhibits the rate of evaporation from your skin, thereby impairing your ability to shed heat.

7. Water also has a high specific heat; that is, water absorbs or loses a great deal of energy as it changes temperature. Water bodies such as lakes and oceans warm and cool slowly as seasons change. This temperature lag helps moderate global temperatures, keeping the environment warm in winter and cool in summer. This effect is especially noticeable near the ocean, but it is important globally.

Altogether, these unique properties of water not only shape life at the molecular and cellular level but also determine many of the features of both the biotic (living) and abiotic (nonliving) components of our world.

SUNLIGHT: ENERGY FOR LIFE

Although some organisms are able to live on chemical reactions in the earth's crust or around deep-sea thermal vents, most organisms depend directly or indirectly on the sun for the energy needed to create structures and carry out life processes. Our sun is a star, a fiery ball of exploding hydrogen gas (fig. 2.9). Its thermonuclear reactions emit powerful forms of radiation, including potentially deadly ultraviolet and nuclear radiation (fig. 2.10). Radiant energy is classified by its wavelengths. Intense energy, such as X rays or gamma rays, has short wavelengths. Lower-energy, longer wavelengths include heat (infrared) and radio wavelengths. By the time solar energy reaches the earth's surface, our atmosphere has filtered out most of the dangerous shortwave radiation. The remaining energy provides two critical factors for life: warmth and light.

Warmth is essential because most organisms survive within a relatively narrow temperature range. At very high temperatures, biomolecules break down or become distorted and nonfunctional. At very low temperatures, the chemical reactions of metabolism occur too slowly to enable organisms to grow and reproduce. Other planets in our solar system are either too hot or too cold to support life as we know it.

The dominant form of solar energy that reaches the earth's surface is in and near the wavelengths of visible light. Not coincidentally, these are the wavelengths that drive **photosynthesis** in green plants. Photosynthesis converts radiant energy into useful, high-quality chemical energy in the bonds that hold together organic molecules. Energy captured by photosynthesis supports nearly all life on earth.

How much incoming solar energy do organisms actually use? The amount of incoming solar radiation is enormous, about 1,372 watts/m^2 at the top of the atmosphere (1 watt = 1 J per second). However, more than half of the incoming sunlight may be reflected or absorbed by atmospheric clouds, dust, and gases. In particular, harmful, short wavelengths are filtered out by gases (especially ozone) in the upper atmosphere. Of the solar radiation that reaches the earth's surface, about 10 percent is ultraviolet, 45 percent is visible, and 45 percent is infrared. Photosynthesizing plants use light energy, especially the blue and red wavelengths, to power photosynthesis. Because most plants reflect, rather than absorb, green wavelengths, they appear green to our eyes. We can use the absorption of different wavelengths of light to measure photosynthetic activity. See Investigating our Environment, p. 35.

How Does Photosynthesis Capture Energy?

Photosynthesis occurs in tiny, membranous organelles called chloroplasts that reside within plant cells (see fig. 2.7). The key to this process is chlorophyll, a unique green molecule that captures

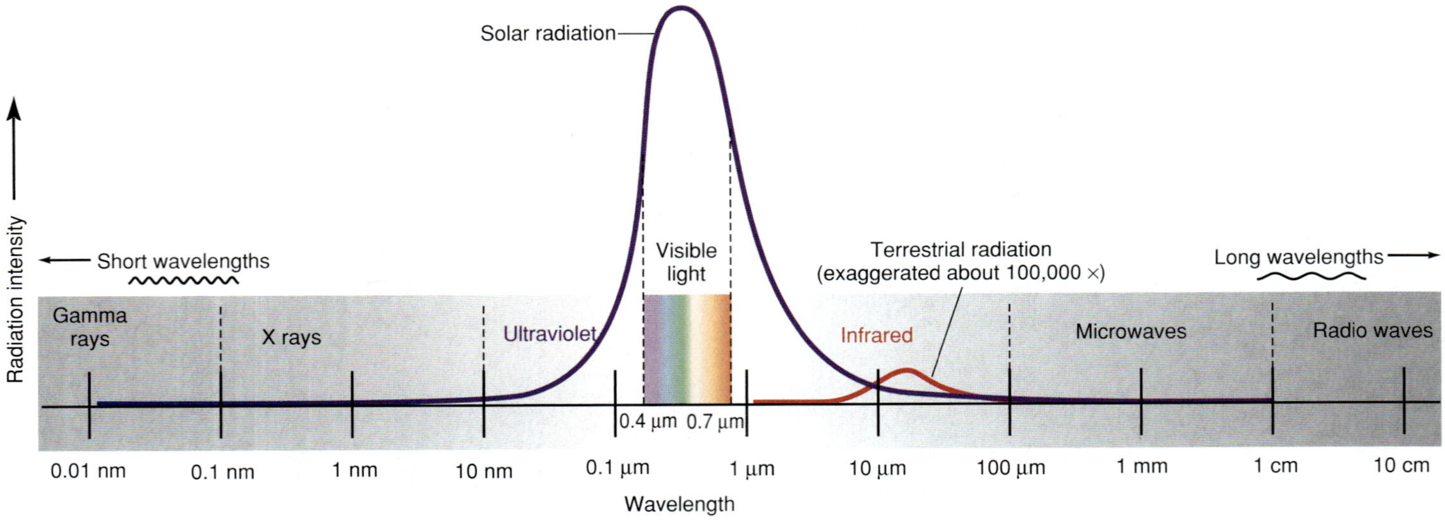

FIGURE 2.10 *The electromagnetic spectrum. Our eyes are sensitive to light wavelengths, which make up nearly half the energy that reaches the earth's surface (represented by the area under the "solar radiation" curve). Photosynthesizing plants use the most abundant solar wavelengths (light and infrared). The earth reemits lower-energy, longer wavelengths (shown by the "terrestrial radiation" curve), mainly the infrared part of the spectrum.*

light energy and uses it to do useful work. Chlorophyll doesn't do this important job alone, however. Many molecules within the chloroplast membranes participate in a series of oxidation-reduction steps called the light-dependent reactions (because they occur only when light strikes the chloroplast) (fig. 2.11). In these reactions, high-energy electrons pass from one intermediate to another. The electrons from this process are drawn from water. The oxygen released when water is split is the source of all the atmospheric oxygen on which all higher animals, including us, depend for life.

Ultimately, some of the energy captured in the light-dependent reactions is stored in two more stable compounds called adenosine triphosphate (ATP) and reduced nicotinamide adenine dinucleoside phosphate (NADPH). ATP and NADPH provide the energy for a series of steps called the light-independent reactions (they can take place after light is no longer present), which fix carbon; that is, they create complex organic molecules, such as sugars, out of atmospheric carbon dioxide (CO_2). The following equation summarizes the overall set of reactions in photosynthesis:

$$6\ H_2O + 6\ CO_2 + \text{solar energy} \xrightarrow[\text{chlorophyll}]{} C_6H_{12}O_6\ (\text{sugar}) + 6\ O_2$$

We read this as "water plus carbon dioxide plus energy (in the presence of chlorophyll) produces sugar plus oxygen." The sugar shown here is glucose, a simple six-carbon molecule that is one of the main products of photosynthesis in most plants. Glucose and other simple sugars are the building blocks for all the organic molecules that make up cells and provide the energy that drives cell physiology. The process of releasing chemical energy, called **cellular respiration,** essentially reverses photosynthesis by splitting

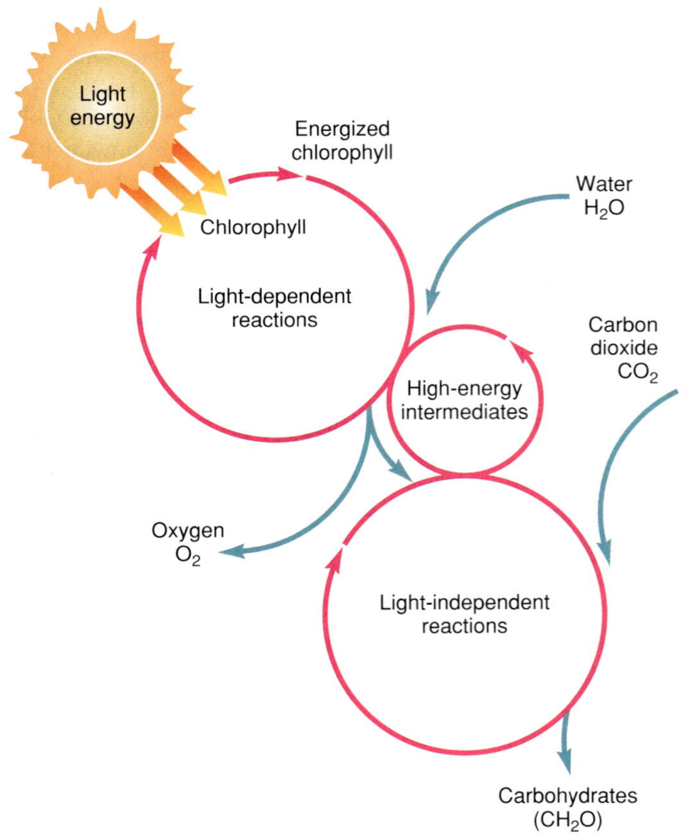

FIGURE 2.11 *During photosynthesis, chlorophyll molecules capture light energy and use it to synthesize energy-rich chemical compounds that cells can use to drive life processes. These reactions consume carbon dioxide and water, and they produce oxygen and carbohydrates.*

INVESTIGATING Our Environment

Remote Sensing, Photosynthesis, and Material Cycles

Measuring primary productivity is important for understanding individual plants and local environments. Understanding the rates of primary productivity is also key to understanding global processes, such as material cycling and biological activity:

- In global carbon cycles, how much carbon is stored by plants, how quickly is it stored, and how does carbon storage compare in contrasting environments, such as the Arctic and the tropics?
- How does this carbon storage affect global climates (chapter 9)?
- In global nutrient cycles, how much nitrogen and phosphorus wash offshore, and where?

How can environmental scientists measure primary production (photosynthesis) at a global scale? In the opening story of this chapter, you read that Ray Lindeman collected and weighed samples of all trophic levels in a small lake ecosystem. But that method is impossible for large ecosystems, especially for oceans, which cover 70 percent of the earth's surface. One of the newest methods of quantifying biological productivity involves remote sensing, or using data collected from satellite sensors that observe the energy reflected from the earth's surface.

As you have read in this chapter, chlorophyll in green plants *absorbs* red and blue wavelengths of light and *reflects* green wavelengths. Your eye receives, or senses, these green wavelengths. A white-sand beach, on the other hand, reflects approximately equal amounts of all light wavelengths that reach it from the sun, so it looks white (and bright!) to your eye. In a similar way, different surfaces of the earth reflect characteristic wavelengths. Snow-covered surfaces reflect light wavelengths; dark green forests with abundant chlorophyll-rich leaves—and ocean surfaces rich in photosynthetic algae and plants—reflect greens and near-infrared wavelengths. Dry, brown forests with little active chlorophyll reflect more red and less infrared energy than do dark green forests.

To detect land cover patterns on the earth's surface, we can put a sensor on a satellite that orbits the earth. As the satellite travels, the sensor receives and transmits to earth a series of "snapshots." One of the best known earth-imaging satellites, *Landsat 7,* produces images that cover an area 185 km (115 mi) wide, and each pixel represents an area of just 30 × 30 m on the ground. *Landsat* orbits approximately from pole to pole, so as the earth spins below the satellite it captures images of the entire surface every 16 days. Another satellite, *SeaWiFS,* was designed mainly for monitoring biological activity in oceans. *SeaWiFS* follows a path similar to *Landsat*'s, but it revisits each point on the earth every day and produces images with a pixel resolution of just over 1 km.

Since satellites detect a much greater range of wavelengths than our eyes can, they are able to monitor and map chlorophyll abundance. In oceans, this is a useful measure of ecosystem health, as well as carbon dioxide uptake. By quantifying and mapping primary production in oceans, climatologists are working to estimate the role of ocean ecosystems in moderating climate change: for example, they can estimate the extent of biomass production in the cold, oxygen-rich waters of the North Atlantic. Oceanographers can also detect nearshore areas where nutrients washing off the land surface fertilize marine ecosystems and stimulate high productivity, such as near the mouth of the Amazon or Mississippi River. Monitoring and mapping these patterns helps us estimate human impacts on nutrient flows from land to sea.

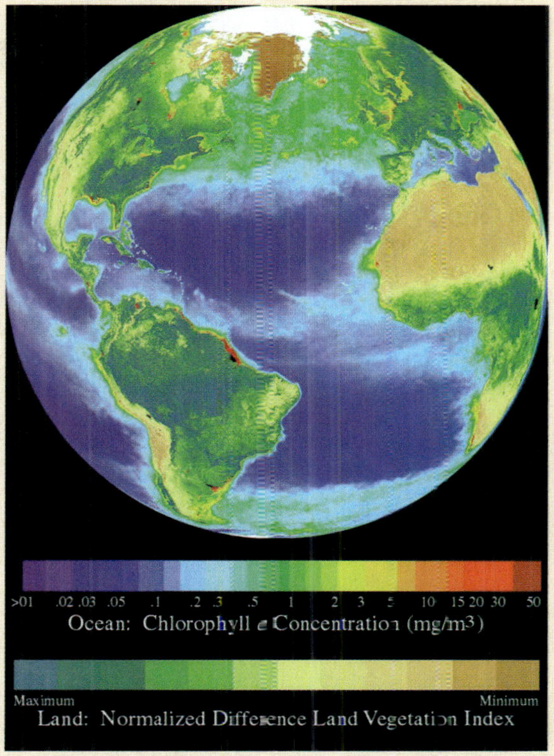

SeaWiFS *image showing chlorophyll abundance in oceans and plant growth on land (normalized difference vegetation index).*

carbon and hydrogen atoms from sugar molecules and recombining them with oxygen to re-create carbon dioxide and water. The net chemical reaction, then, is

$$C_6H_{12}O_6 + 6\ O_2 \rightarrow 6\ H_2O + 6\ CO_2 + \text{released energy}$$

Note that in photosynthesis energy is captured, while in respiration energy is released. Similarly, photosynthesis consumes water and carbon dioxide to produce sugar and oxygen, while respiration does the opposite. In both sets of reactions, energy is stored temporarily in chemical bonds, which constitute a kind of energy currency for the cell.

Organisms that cannot photosynthesize, such as ourselves, must get energy for cellular respiration by consuming plants or animals that eat plants (fig. 2.12). In the process, we also consume oxygen and release carbon dioxide, thus completing the cycle of photosynthesis and respiration. Later in this chapter, we will see more of how these feeding relationships work.

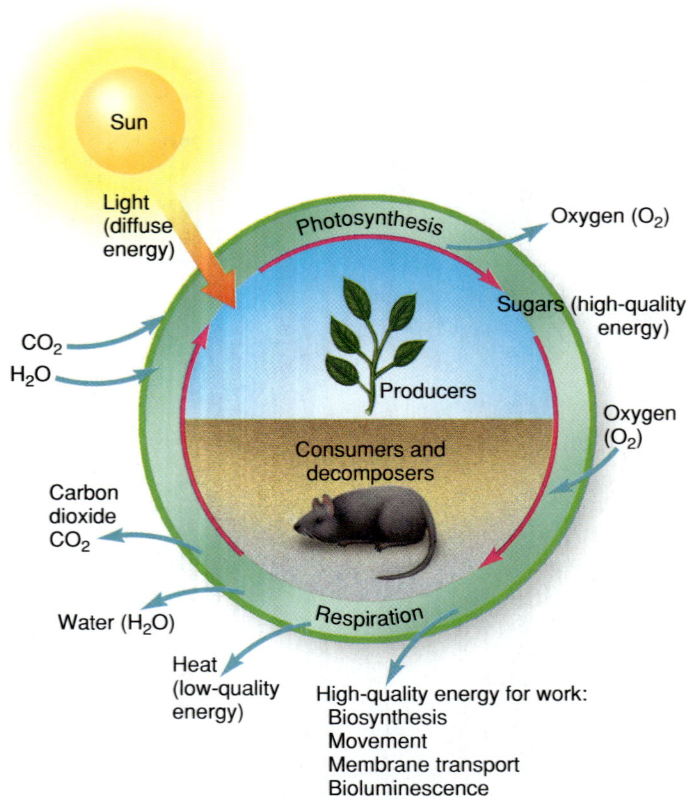

FIGURE 2.12 *Energy exchange in an ecosystem. Plants take water and carbon dioxide from the environment and use the energy from sunlight to convert them into energy-rich sugars and other organic chemicals, releasing oxygen in the process. Consumers and decomposers take up oxygen and break down sugars during cellular respiration to release useful energy for living. In this process, water, carbon dioxide, and low-quality heat are released to the environment.*

ENERGY AND MATTER IN THE ENVIRONMENT

Living systems are maintained by processes that capture energy from external sources and use it to carry out essential functions. Materials are used and recycled in these processes. Conceptually, we organize living systems in terms of species, populations, biological communities, and ecosystems. A **species** ("kind" in Latin) is most often defined as all organisms that are genetically similar enough to breed and produce live, fertile offspring in nature. A **population** consists of all members of a species that live in the same area at the same time. We might refer to the population of elk in Yellowstone National Park, for example: this group is genetically similar to an elk population in Oregon, but the two are considered separate populations because they are geographically separate. A **biological community** consists of all the populations living and interacting in an area. A biological community and its physical environment (water, mineral resources, air, sunlight) make up an ecological system, or **ecosystem.** Much of ecology is concerned with understanding the ways energy and matter move through ecosystems.

For the sake of simplicity, we often think of ecosystems and communities as fixed ecological units with distinct boundaries. A patch of woods surrounded by farm fields, for instance, has relatively sharp boundaries that separate the two environments. Contrasting levels of light, moisture, and wind occur in the fields and the woods, as well as different kinds of birds, rodents, and insects. Such contrasts differentiate ecosystems. On the other hand, the fields and forest are also interconnected: some animals cross the boundary, carrying nutrients and water from one to the other. Permeable boundaries, across which resources move, make most ecosystems *open systems.* In contrast, a *closed system* is one that does not exchange materials with its surroundings. In fact, few such closed systems exist in nature.

Ecosystems can also be delimited in terms of their dominant, or most visible, components. The Greater Yellowstone Ecosystem, which has been defined as an area reaching from southwestern Wyoming to southern Montana and Idaho, is often outlined as the area that would support a viable population of grizzly bears. A coral reef ecosystem is defined in terms of the extent and composition of the community of coral polyps (organisms) that give it structure and the myriad organisms that depend on the primary productivity of coral for sustenance.

Regardless of how we define the extent of an ecosystem, we understand its structure and organization largely in terms of the storage and movement of energy through organisms and their environment.

Food Chains, Food Webs, and Trophic Levels

Photosynthesis provides all the energy for nearly all ecosystems. (The chief exception is deep-sea ecosystems supported by geothermal heat and minerals.) One of the major properties of ecosystems is **productivity,** the amount of **biomass** (biological material) produced in a given area during a given period of time. Photosynthesis is often called primary productivity because it is the basis for almost all other growth in an ecosystem. Photosynthesizing organisms are called **primary producers.** Organisms that do not photosynthesize are **consumers,** and they get their nutrients and energy by eating other things. Net productivity is the amount of primary production that accumulates in a system. An ecosystem may have very high total productivity, but if decomposers break down organic material as rapidly as it is formed, the net productivity will be low.

Think about what you have eaten today, and trace it back to its photosynthetic source. If you have eaten an egg, you can trace it back to a chicken, which ate corn. This is an example of a food chain, a linked feeding series. Now think about a more complex food chain involving you, a chicken, a corn plant, and a grasshopper. The chicken could eat grasshoppers that had eaten leaves of the corn plant. You also could eat the grasshopper directly—some humans do. Or you could eat corn yourself, making the shortest possible food chain. Humans have several options of where we fit into food chains.

In ecosystems, some consumers feed on a single species, but most consumers have multiple food sources. Similarly, some species are prey to a single kind of predator, but many species in an ecosystem are beset by several types of predators and parasites.

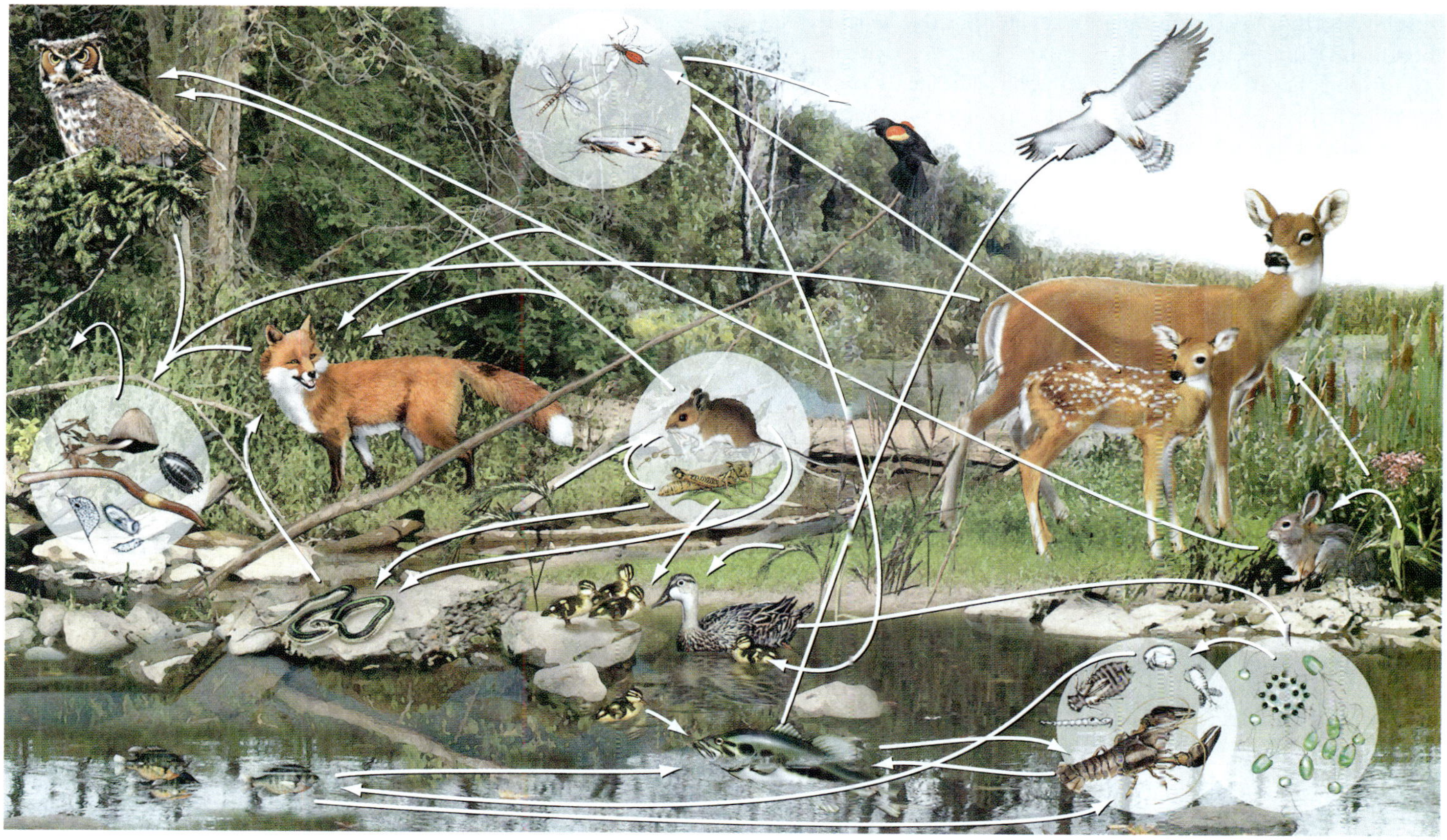

FIGURE 2.13 *Each time an organism feeds, it becomes a link in a food chain. In an ecosystem, food chains become interconnected when predators feed on more than one kind of prey, thus forming a food web. The arrows in this diagram indicate the direction in which matter and energy are transferred through feeding relationships.*

In this way, individual food chains interconnect to form a **food web.** Figure 2.13 shows feeding relationships among some of the larger organisms in a woodland and lake community. If we were to add all the insects, worms, and microscopic organisms that belong in this picture, however, it would be overwhelmingly complex.

An organism's feeding position in an ecosystem is its **trophic level.** A corn plant, for example, is at the primary producer level: it produces chemical energy from sunlight, water, and carbon dioxide. A grasshopper that eats the corn is a primary consumer. A chicken that eats the grasshopper is a secondary consumer, and if you eat the chicken, you are a tertiary consumer (sometimes called a "top carnivore").

Most terrestrial food chains are relatively short (seeds → mouse → owl), but aquatic food chains can be quite long (microscopic algae → copepod → minnow → crayfish → bass → osprey). The length of a food chain also may reflect the physical characteristics of a particular ecosystem. A harsh arctic landscape may have a much shorter food chain than a temperate or tropical one.

Organisms also can be identified by the kinds of food they eat (fig. 2.14). **Herbivores** eat plants, **carnivores** eat flesh, and **omnivores** eat both plant and animal matter. Humans are natural omnivores, something you can tell by looking at our teeth. Our teeth are suited for an omnivorous diet, with a combination of cutting and

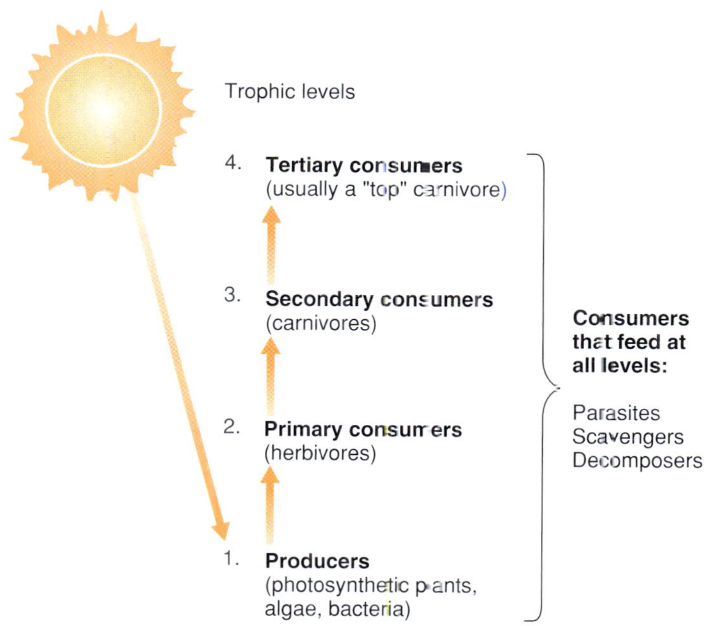

FIGURE 2.14 *Organisms in an ecosystem can be identified by how they obtain food for their life processes (producer, herbivore, carnivore, omnivore, scavenger, decomposer, reducer) or by consumer level (producer; primary, secondary, or tertiary consumer) or by trophic level (first, second, third, fourth).*

crushing surfaces that are not highly adapted for one specific kind of food, as are the teeth of a wolf (carnivore) or a horse (herbivore).

In the end, everything is consumed by the many organisms that recycle the dead bodies and waste products of others. Scavengers, such as crows, jackals, and vultures, clean up dead carcasses of larger animals. Detritivores, such as ants and beetles, consume detritus (litter, debris, and dung), while **decomposer** organisms, such as fungi and bacteria, complete the final breakdown and return nutrients to the soil to fertilize the primary producers. Without the activity of these microorganisms, nutrients would remain locked up in the organic compounds of dead organisms and discarded body wastes, rather than being made available to successive generations of organisms. Think for a moment about the food web that supports you. How many organisms, in how many places, does it include?

Ecological Pyramids

Most ecosystems have a huge number of primary producers supporting a smaller number of herbivores, which in turn support an even smaller number of secondary consumers. This relationship can be described in terms of a trophic pyramid, which represents the amount of energy stored in the bodies of living things. Most energy in most ecosystems is stored in the bodies of primary producers (fig. 2.15). The second law of thermodynamics (energy dissipates as it is used) explains this relationship.

This loss of energy occurs in several ways. First, some consumed energy is not used efficiently: a prairie dog that eats grass does not digest all the plant efficiently. Second, a great deal of energy dissipates as kinetic energy and heat. Prairie dogs spend a lot of energy running, playing, hiding, and simply living. When a coyote catches a prairie dog, only a small part of the energy the prairie dog has eaten is available to the coyote.

Furthermore, ecosystems don't operate at 100 percent efficiency. Some surplus usually exists at the lower levels. If there were enough foxes to catch all the rabbits available in the summer, when the rabbit supply is abundant, there would be too many foxes in the middle of the winter, when rabbits are scarce. A popular rule of thumb is that only about 10 percent of the energy at one consumer level is represented at the next higher level. The amount of energy available is often expressed in terms of biomass. For example, we could say that it takes about 100 kg of clover to make 10 kg of rabbit, as well as 10 kg of rabbit to make 1 kg of fox (fig. 2.16). The energy efficiency of real ecosystems varies a great deal, however, and may be considerably less than 10 percent captured in each successive trophic level.

The amount of biomass at each trophic level may also form a pyramid. A large population of rabbits, for example, is needed to support one fox. The total mass of those rabbits is much greater than the mass of the fox. Rapid fluctuations in producer and consumer populations can invert this pyramid, however: in lakes, winter populations of producers (plants and algae) can fall well below that of consumers. In some cases, the number of individuals in a community can also be described as a pyramid (fig. 2.17). However, the numbers pyramid is highly variable and can be inverted. For example, one fox can support numerous tapeworms.

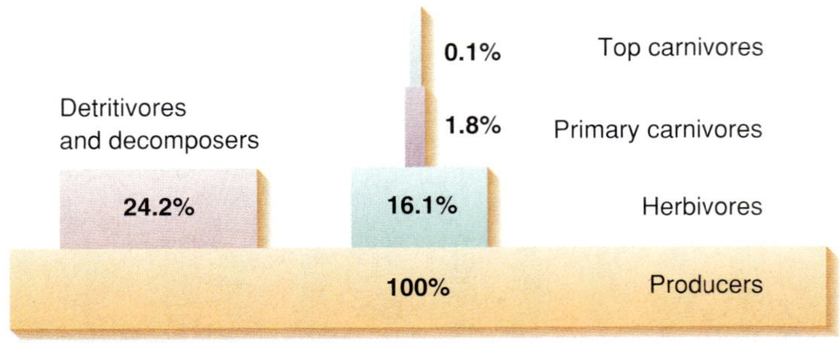

FIGURE 2.15 *A classic example of an energy pyramid from Silver Springs, Florida. The numbers in each bar show the percentage of the energy captured at the primary producer level that is incorporated in the biomass at each succeeding level. Detritivores and decomposers feed at every level but are shown attached to the producer bar because this level provides most of their energy.*

Source: Data from Howard T. Odum, "Trophic Structure and Productivity of Silver Springs, Florida" in *Ecological Monographs,* 27:55–112, 1957, Ecological Society of America.

BIOGEOCHEMICAL CYCLES AND LIFE PROCESSES

The elements and compounds that sustain us are cycled endlessly through living things and through the environment. On a global scale, this movement is referred to as biogeochemical cycling. Substances can move quickly or slowly: you might store carbon for hours or days, while carbon is stored in the earth for millions of years. When human activity alters flow rates or storage times in these natural cycles, overwhelming the environment's ability to process them, these materials can become pollutants. Sulfur, nitrogen, carbon dioxide, and phosphorus are some of the more serious examples of these. Global-scale movement of energy is discussed in detail in chapter 9. Here we will explore some of the paths involved in cycling several important elements: water, carbon, nitrogen, sulfur, and phosphorus.

The Hydrologic Cycle

The path of water through our environment is perhaps the most familiar material cycle, and it is discussed in greater detail in chapter 10 (fig. 2.18). Most of the earth's water is stored in the oceans, but solar energy continually evaporates this water, and winds distribute water vapor around the globe. Water that condenses over land surfaces, in the form of rain, snow, or fog, supports all terrestrial (land-based) ecosystems. Living organisms emit the moisture they have consumed through respiration and perspiration. Eventually this moisture reenters the atmosphere or enters lakes and streams, from which it ultimately returns to the ocean again.

As it moves through living things and through the atmosphere, water is responsible for metabolic processes within cells, for maintaining the flows of key nutrients through ecosystems, and for global-scale distribution of heat and energy (chapter 9). Water performs countless services because of its unusual properties (see "The Miracle of Water," p. 32). Water is so important that, when astronomers look for signs of life on distant planets, traces of water are the key evidence they seek.

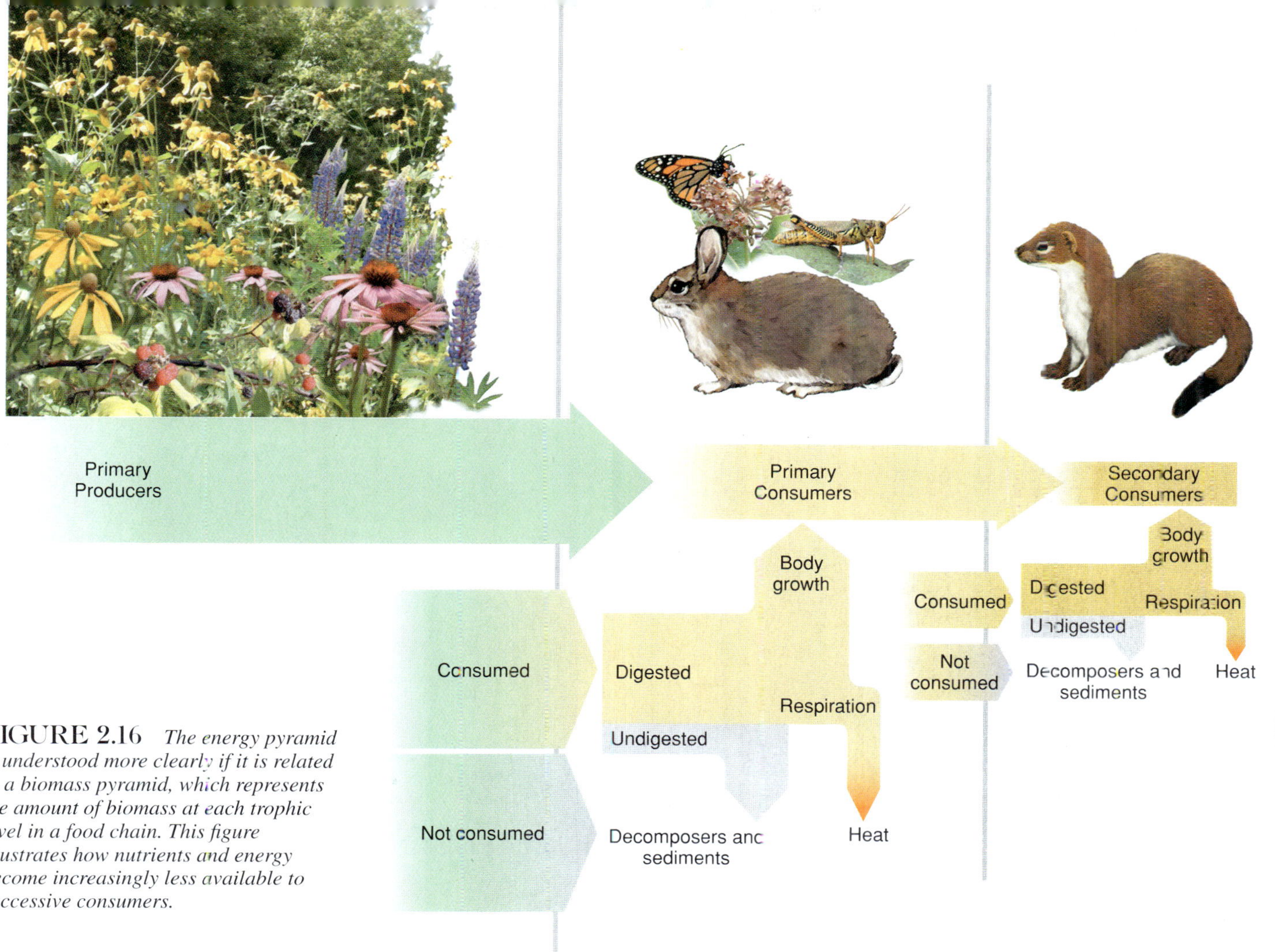

FIGURE 2.16 *The energy pyramid is understood more clearly if it is related to a biomass pyramid, which represents the amount of biomass at each trophic level in a food chain. This figure illustrates how nutrients and energy become increasingly less available to successive consumers.*

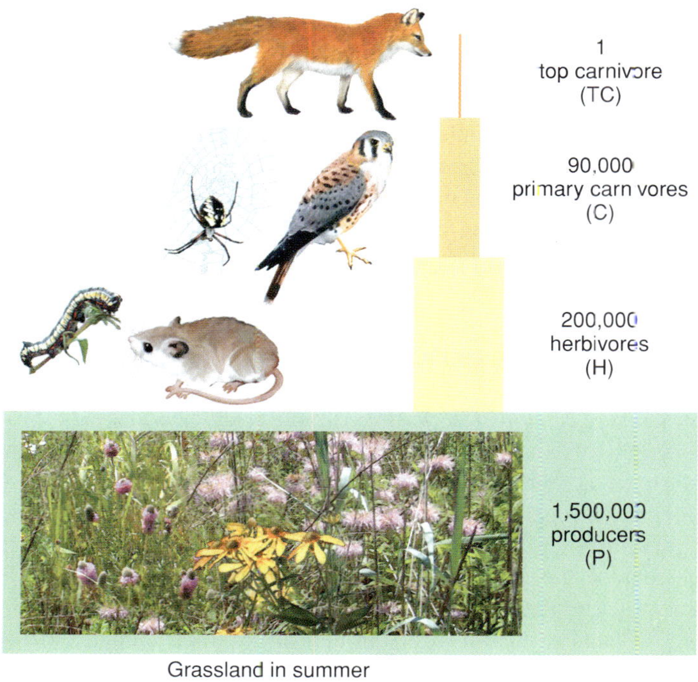

FIGURE 2.17 *Usually, smaller organisms are eaten by larger organisms, and it takes numerous small organisms to feed one large organism. The classic study represented in this pyramid shows numbers of individuals at each trophic level per 1,000 m² of grassland and reads like this: to support 1 individual at the top carnivore level, there were 90,000 primary carnivores feeding upon 200,000 herbivores, which in turn fed upon 1,500,000 producers.*

The Carbon Cycle

Carbon serves a dual purpose for organisms: (1) it is a structural component of organic molecules, and (2) chemical bonds in carbon compounds provide metabolic energy. The **carbon cycle** begins with photosynthetic organisms taking up carbon dioxide (CO_2) (fig. 2.19). This is called carbon fixation because carbon is changed from gaseous CO_2 to less mobile organic molecules. Once a carbon atom is incorporated into organic compounds, its path to recycling may be very quick or extremely slow. Imagine for a moment what happens to a simple sugar molecule you swallow in a glass of fruit juice. The sugar molecule is absorbed into

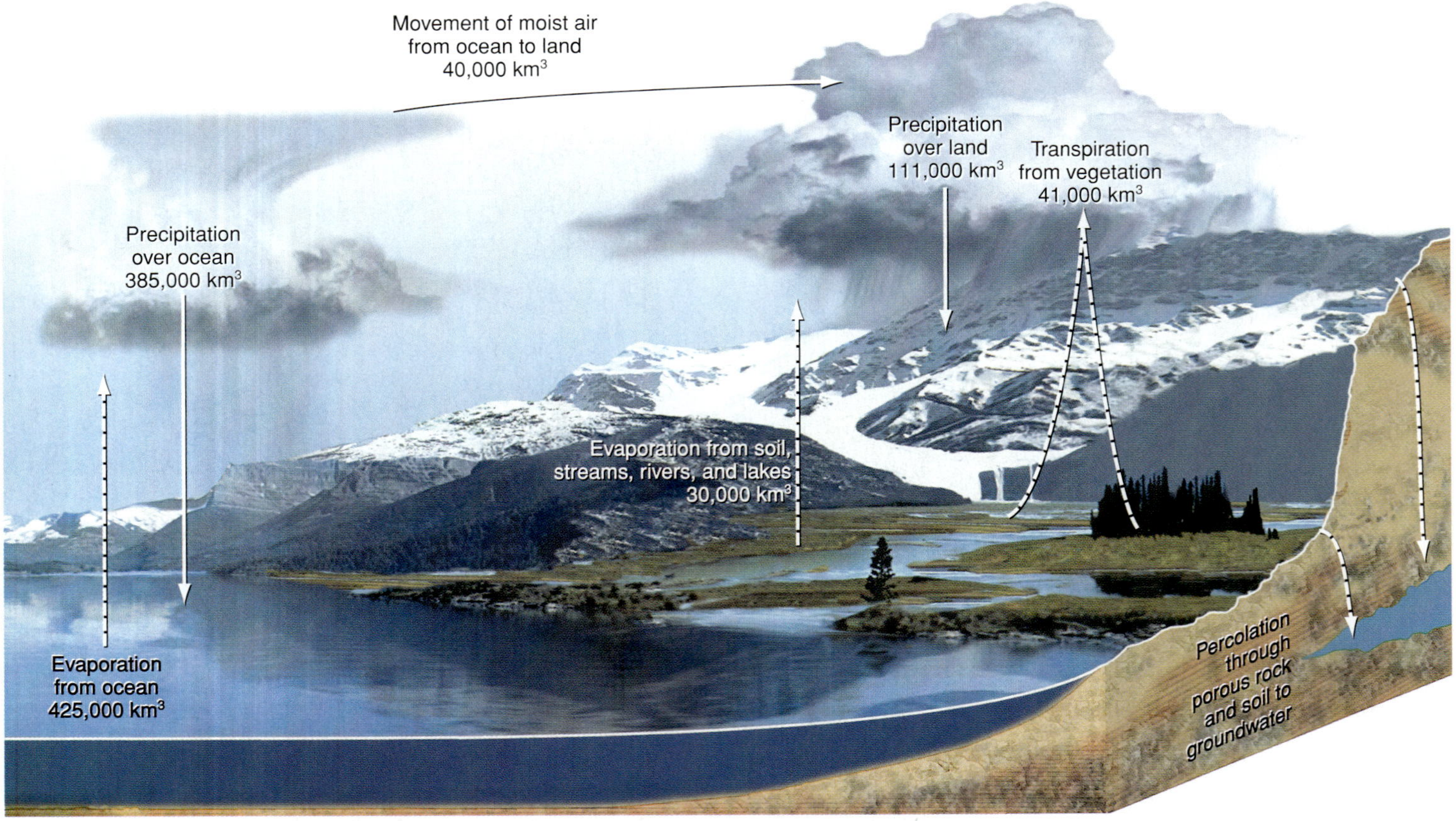
Movement of moist air
from ocean to land
40,000 km³
Precipitation
over land
111,000 km³
Transpiration
from vegetation
41,000 km³
Precipitation
over ocean
385,000 km³
Evaporation from soil,
streams, rivers, and lakes
30,000 km³
Evaporation
from ocean
425,000 km³
Percolation
through
porous rock
and soil to
groundwater

FIGURE 2.18 *The hydrologic cycle. Most exchange occurs with evaporation from oceans and precipitation back to oceans. About one-tenth of the water evaporated from oceans falls over land, is recycled through terrestrial systems, and eventually drains back to oceans in rivers.*

your bloodstream, where it is made available to your cells for cellular respiration or the production of more complex biomolecules. If it is used in respiration, you may exhale the same carbon atom as CO_2 in an hour or less, and a plant could take up that exhaled CO_2 the same afternoon.

Alternatively, your body may use that sugar molecule to make larger organic molecules that become part of your cellular structure. The carbon atoms in the sugar molecule could remain a part of your body until it decays after death. Similarly, carbon in the wood of a thousand-year-old tree will be released only when fungi and bacteria digest the wood and release carbon dioxide as a by-product of their respiration.

Sometimes recycling takes a very long time. Coal and oil are the compressed, chemically altered remains of plants and microorganisms that lived millions of years ago. Their carbon atoms (and hydrogen, oxygen, nitrogen, sulfur, etc.) are not released until the coal and oil are burned. Enormous amounts of carbon also are locked up as calcium carbonate ($CaCO_3$), used to build shells and skeletons of marine organisms from tiny protozoans to corals. The world's extensive surface limestone deposits are biologically formed calcium carbonate from ancient oceans, exposed by geological events. The carbon in limestone has been locked away for millennia, which is probably the fate of carbon currently being deposited in ocean sediments. Eventually, even the deep ocean deposits are recycled as they are drawn into deep molten layers and released via volcanic activity. Geologists estimate that every carbon atom on the earth has made about 30 such round trips over the past 4 billion years.

Materials that store carbon, including geologic formations and standing forests, are known as carbon sinks. When carbon is released from these sinks, as when we burn fossil fuels and inject CO_2 into the atmosphere, or when we clear extensive forests, natural recycling systems may not be able to keep up. This is the root of the global warming problem, discussed in chapter 9. Alternatively, extra atmospheric CO_2 could support faster plant growth, speeding some of the recycling processes.

The Nitrogen Cycle

Organisms cannot exist without amino acids, peptides, and proteins, all of which are organic molecules that contain nitrogen. Nitrogen is therefore an extremely important nutrient for living things. (Nitrogen is a primary component of many household and agricultural fertilizers.) Even though nitrogen makes up about 78 percent of the air around us, plants cannot use N_2, the stable diatomic (two-atom) molecule in the air.

Plants acquire nitrogen through an extremely complex **nitrogen cycle** (fig. 2.20). The key to this cycle is nitrogen-fixing bacte-

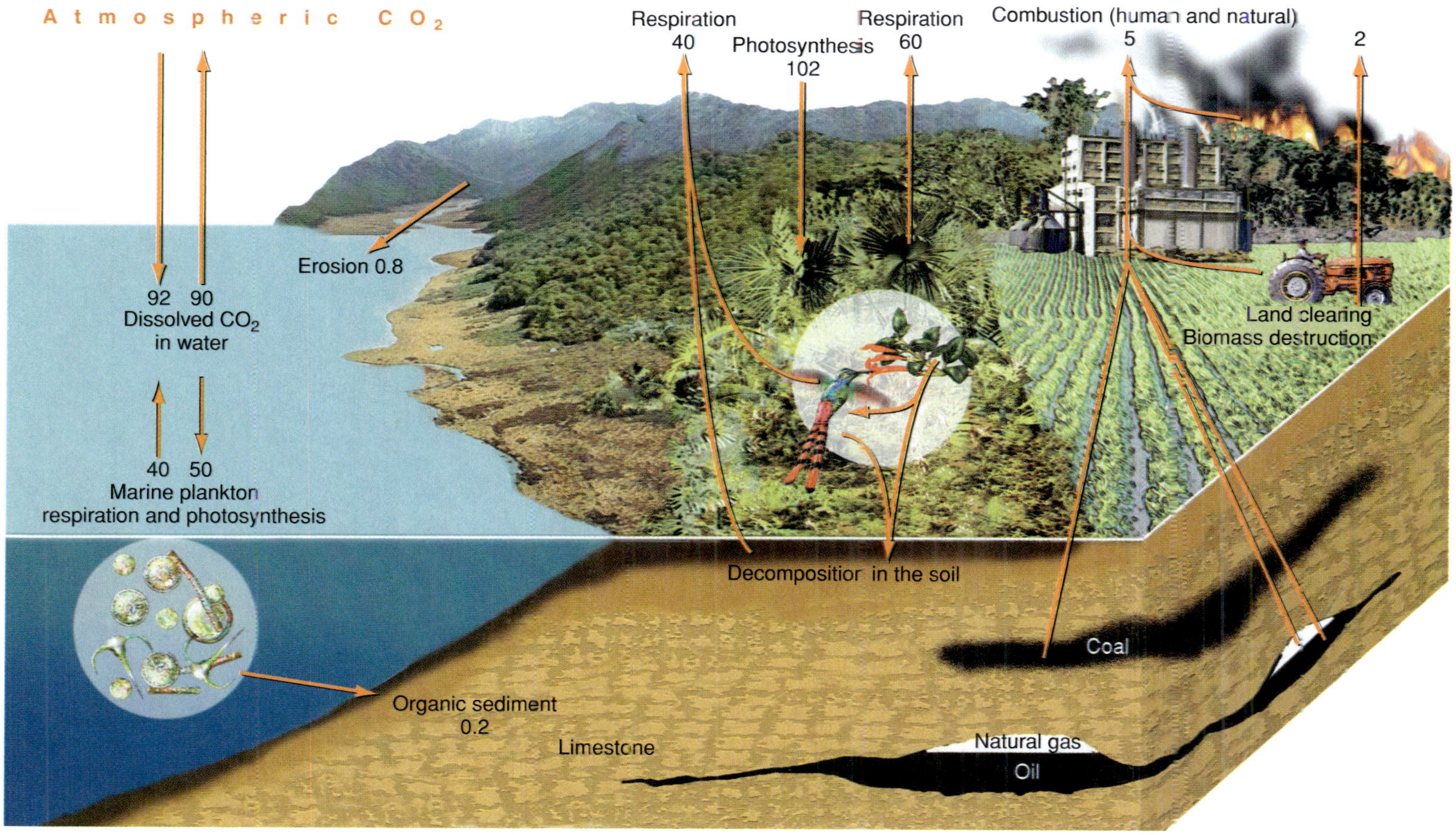

FIGURE 2.19 *The carbon cycle. Numbers indicate approximate exchange of carbon in gigatons (Gt) per year. Natural exchanges are balanced, but human sources produce a net increase of CO_2 in the atmosphere.*

ria (including some blue-green algae or cyanobacteria). These organisms have a highly specialized ability to "fix" nitrogen, or combine gaseous N_2 with hydrogen to make ammonia (NH_3).

Other bacteria then combine ammonia with oxygen to form nitrites (NO_2^-). Another group of bacteria converts nitrites to nitrates (NO_3^-), which green plants can absorb and use. After plant cells absorb nitrates, the nitrates are reduced to ammonium (NH_4^+), which cells use to build amino acids that become the building blocks for peptides and proteins.

Members of the bean family (legumes) and a few other kinds of plants are especially useful in agriculture because nitrogen-fixing bacteria actually live in their root tissues (fig. 2.21). Legumes and their associated bacteria add nitrogen to the soil, so interplanting and rotating legumes with crops, such as corn, that use but cannot replace soil nitrates are beneficial farming practices that take practical advantage of this relationship.

Nitrogen reenters the environment in several ways. The most obvious path is through the death of organisms. Fungi and bacteria decompose dead organisms, releasing ammonia and ammonium ions, which then are available for nitrate formation. Organisms don't have to die to donate proteins to the environment, however. Plants shed their leaves, needles, flowers, fruits, and cones; animals shed hair, feathers, skin, exoskeletons, pupal cases, and silk. Animals also produce excrement and urinary wastes that contain nitrogenous compounds. Urine is especially high in nitrogen because it contains the detoxified wastes of protein metabolism. All of these by-products of living organisms decompose, replenishing soil fertility.

How does nitrogen reenter the atmosphere, completing the cycle? Denitrifying bacteria break down nitrates into N_2 and nitrous oxide (N_2O), gases that return to the atmosphere; thus, denitrifying bacteria compete with plant roots for available nitrates. However, denitrification occurs mainly in waterlogged soils that have low oxygen availability and a large amount of decomposable organic matter. These are suitable growing conditions for many wild plant species in swamps and marshes, but not for most cultivated crop species, except for rice, a domesticated wetland grass.

In recent years, humans have profoundly altered the nitrogen cycle. By using synthetic fertilizers, cultivating nitrogen-fixing crops, and burning fossil fuels, we now convert more nitrogen to ammonia and nitrates than all natural land processes combined. This excess nitrogen input causes algal blooms and excess plant growth in water bodies, called eutrophication, which we will discuss in more detail in chapter 10. Excess nitrogen also causes serious loss of soil nutrients such as calcium and potassium; acidification of rivers and lakes; and rising atmospheric concentrations of nitrous oxide, a greenhouse gas. It also encourages the spread of weeds into areas such as prairies, where native plants are adapted to nitrogen-poor environments.

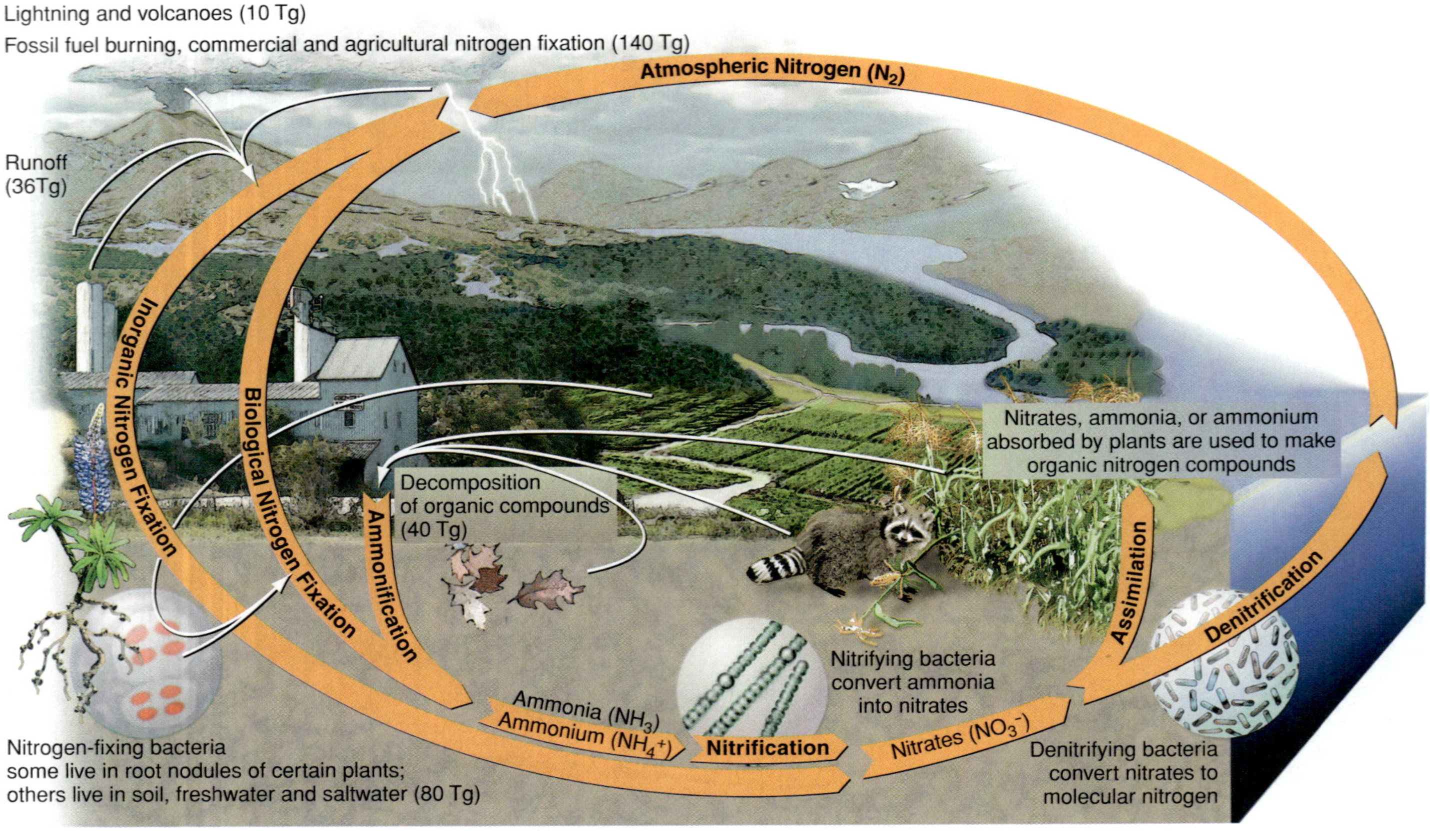

FIGURE 2.20 *The nitrogen cycle. Human sources of nitrogen fixation (conversion of molecular nitrogen to ammonia or ammonium) are now about 50 percent greater than natural sources. Bacteria convert ammonia to nitrates, which plants use to create organic nitrogen. Eventually, nitrogen is stored in sediments or converted back to molecular nitrogen (1 Tg = 10^{12} g).*

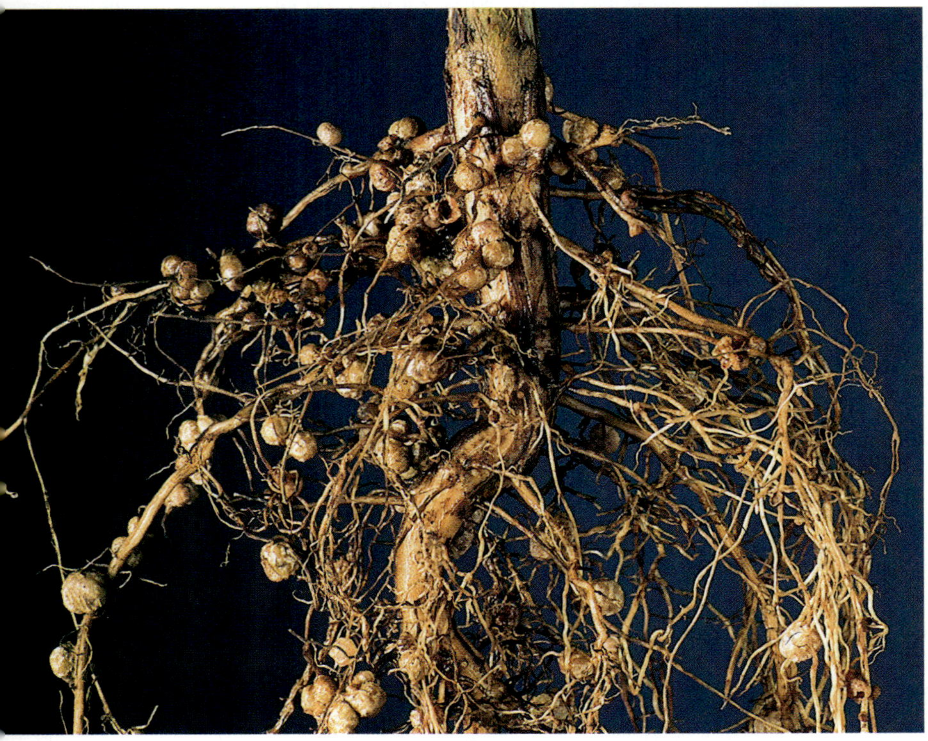

FIGURE 2.21 *Bumps called nodules cover the roots of this adzuki bean plant. Each nodule is a mass of root tissue containing many bacteria that help convert nitrogen in the soil to a form that the bean plant can assimilate and use to manufacture amino acids.*

The Phosphorus Cycle

Minerals become available to organisms after they are released from rocks. Two mineral cycles of particular significance to organisms are phosphorus and sulfur. Why do you suppose phosphorus is a primary ingredient in fertilizers? At the cellular level, energy-rich phosphorus-containing compounds are primary participants in energy-transfer reactions, as discussed earlier.

The amount of available phosphorus in an environment, therefore, can dramatically affect productivity. Abundant phosphorus stimulates lush plant and algal growth, making phosphorus a major contributor to water pollution.

The phosphorus cycle begins when phosphorus compounds leach from rocks and minerals over long periods of time (fig. 2.22). Because phosphorous has no atmospheric form, it is usually transported in water. Producer organisms take in inorganic phosphorus, incorporate it into organic molecules, and then pass it on to consumers. Phosphorus returns to the environment by decomposition. An important aspect of the phosphorus cycle is the very long time it takes for phosphorus atoms to pass through it. Deep ocean sediments are significant phosphorus sinks of extreme longevity. Phosphate ores that now are mined to make detergents and inorganic fertilizers represent exposed ocean sediments that are millennia old. You could think of our present use of phosphates, which are washed out into the river systems and eventually the oceans, as an accelerated mobilization of phosphorus from source to sink. Aquatic ecosystems often are dramatically affected in the process because excess phosphates can stimulate explosive growth of algae and photosynthetic bacteria populations (algae blooms), upsetting ecosystem stability (see "Investigating Our Environment," p. 44). Can you think of ways we could reduce the amount of phosphorus we put into our environment?

The Sulfur Cycle

Sulfur plays a vital role in organisms, especially as a minor but essential component of proteins. Sulfur compounds are important determinants of the acidity of rainfall, surface water, and soil. In addition, sulfur in particles and tiny airborne droplets may act as critical regulators of global climate. Most of the earth's sulfur is tied up underground in rocks and minerals, such as iron disulfide (pyrite) and calcium sulfate (gypsum). Weathering, emissions from deep seafloor vents, and volcanic eruptions release this inorganic sulfur into the air and water (fig. 2.23).

The sulfur cycle is complicated by the large number of oxidation states the element can assume, producing hydrogen sulfide (H_2S), sulfur dioxide (SO_2), sulfate ion (SO_4^{2-}), and others.

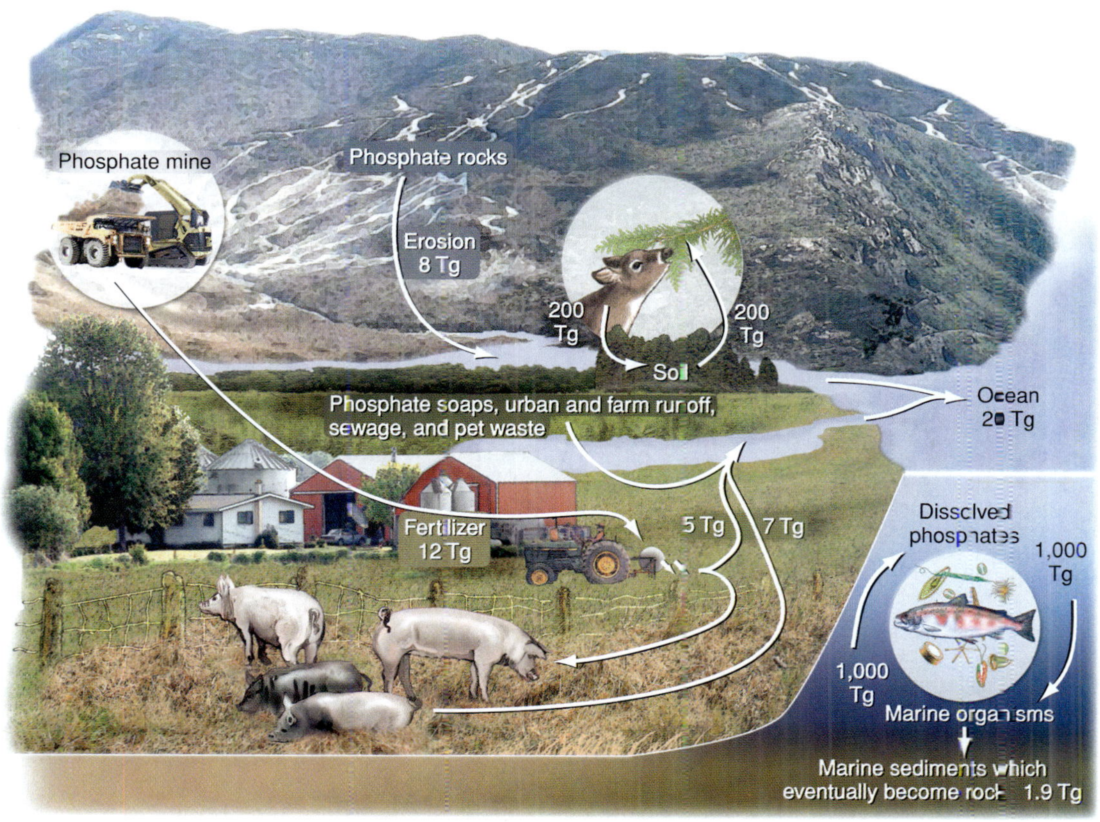

FIGURE 2.22 *The phosphorus cycle. Natural movement of phosphorus is slight, involving recycling within ecosystems and some erosion and sedimentation of phosphorus-bearing rock. Use of phosphate (PO_4^{-3}) fertilizers and cleaning agents increases phosphorus in aquatic systems, causing eutrophication. Units are teragrams (Tg) phosphorus per year.*

INVESTIGATING Our Environment

Environmental Chemistry of Phosphorus

In the 1950s and 1960s people across Canada, the United States, and Europe began to notice increasing rates of smelly algae growth in lakes and wetlands. Increased nutrient loading was accepted as the cause, but which nutrient? Nitrogen, phosphorus, potassium, calcium, and other elements are all known to increase plant growth. To find an answer, ecologist David Schindler decided to do a large-scale experiment. Schindler and his colleagues divided an Ontario lake into two parts. They enriched one-half of it with nitrogen and the other half with phosphorus. The phosphorus-enriched half of the lake rapidly became eutrophic: algae and plants grew in such profusion that they choked out the sunlight, died, and decayed, producing a warm, smelly chemically and biologically altered ecosystem. The other half showed little change. With this classic study, Schindler and his colleagues demonstrated that phosphorus is the key limiting factor for plant growth in aquatic ecosystems. Add abundant phosphorus, and eutrophication results. This discovery led to drastic reduction in phosphates in household detergents and other products.

Phosphorus is a natural and essential component of all living systems. Released by weathered rocks into soil and water, it is taken up by bacteria and algae, then incorporated into the food web. Our cells use it to produce countless essential compounds, including DNA and the energy-releasing molecule ATP. By weight, your bones are 7 percent phosphorus, and your body contains about 700 grams of the element.

But since the 1950s the use of phosphorus fertilizers on farms has increased dramatically, and their distribution has expanded globally. At the same time, agricultural intensification has increased erosion rates, sending fertilizer-laden soils into streams and lakes at an accelerating rate. Limnologists Elena Bennett and Steve Carpenter estimate that recent expansion in phosphorus mining and trading have more than quadrupled natural rates of phosphorus inputs into freshwater ecosystems around the world, from 3.5 terragrams (trillion grams) per year normally to 13 terragrams now. Eutrophication is increasingly evident in developing countries, where phosphorus-rich fertilizers have become common in recent years. Further, our past activities will affect our water bodies for decades or centuries to come. Fertilizers will continue to wash off of farm fields, and the phosphorus currently in aquatic ecosystems may be recycled for centuries.

As this case shows, understanding the chemistry of ecosystems is essential to minimizing damage to our environment, or to restoring already damaged ecosystems. Environmental chemistry is therefore a growing discipline that needs dedicated students to ensure that our environment stays healthy—or returns to health.

This case also demonstrates the broad, multidisciplinary nature of environmental science. Understanding global phosphorus imbalances requires the expertise of hydrologists (who study water sources and the geography of water movement), climatologists (who study atmospheric distribution of moisture and airborne compounds), ecologists (who study ecosystem structure and functions), and toxicologists (who study organically harmful compounds), in addition to environmental chemists. As you read this book, we hope you will discover the ways different scientific disciplines help us identify, and hopefully solve, emerging threats to our environment and our health.

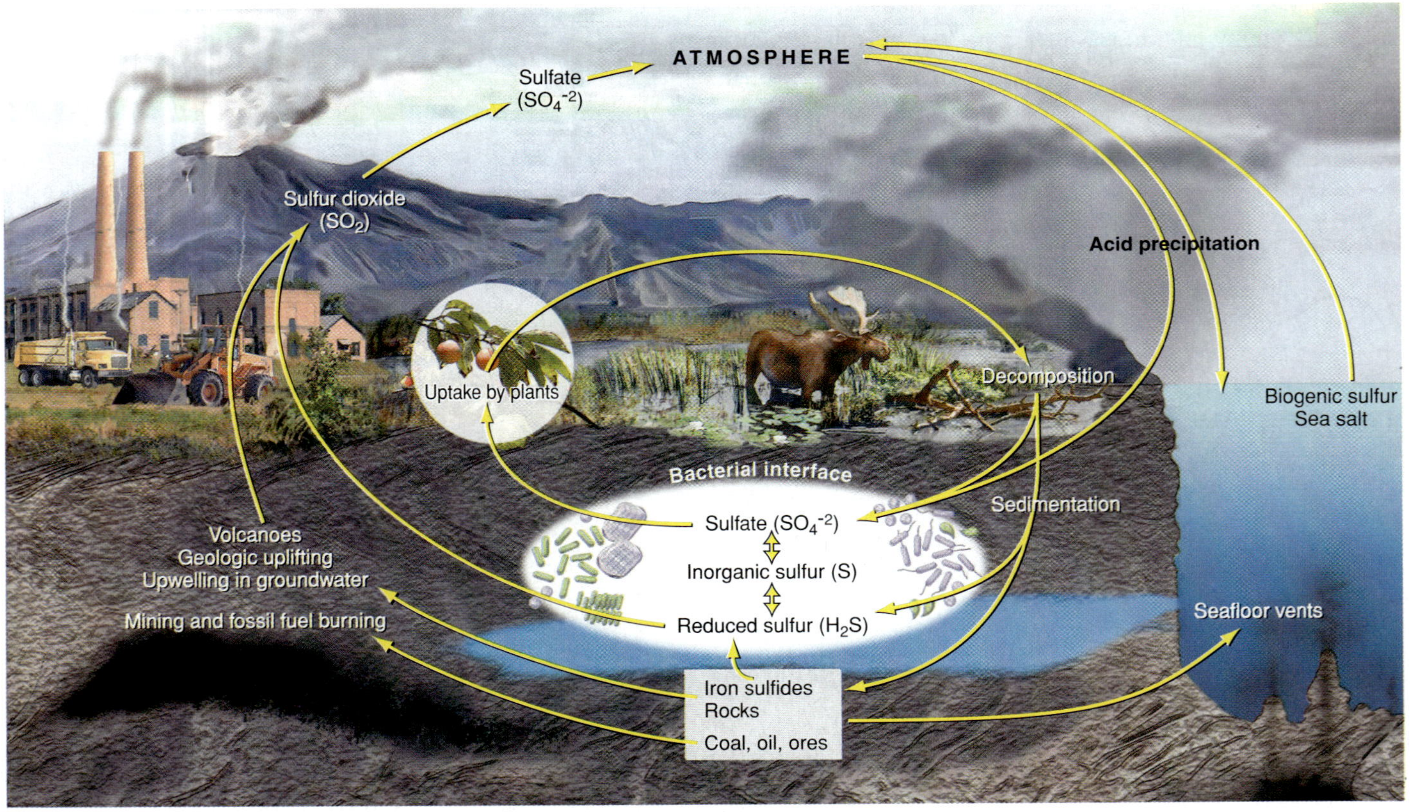

FIGURE 2.23 *The sulfur cycle. Sulfur is present mainly in rocks, soil, and water. It cycles through ecosystems when it is taken in by organisms. Combustion of fossil fuels causes increased levels of atmospheric sulfur compounds, which create problems related to acid precipitation.*

Inorganic processes are responsible for many of these transformations, but living organisms, especially bacteria, also sequester sulfur in biogenic deposits or release it into the environment. Which of the several kinds of sulfur bacteria prevails in any given situation depends on oxygen concentrations, pH level, and light level.

Human activities also release large quantities of sulfur, primarily through burning fossil fuels. Total yearly anthropogenic sulfur emissions rival those of natural processes, and acid rain (caused by sulfuric acid produced as a result of fossil fuel use) is a serious problem in many areas (see chapter 9). Sulfur dioxide and sulfate aerosols cause human health problems, damage buildings and vegetation, and reduce visibility. They also absorb ultraviolet (UV) radiation and create cloud cover that cools cities and may be offsetting greenhouse effects of rising CO_2 concentrations.

Interestingly, the biogenic sulfur emissions of oceanic phytoplankton may play a role in global climate regulation. When ocean water is warm, tiny, single-celled organisms release dimethylsulfide (DMS), which is oxidized to SO_2 and then SO_4^{2-} in the atmosphere. Acting as cloud droplet condensation nuclei, these sulfate aerosols increase the earth's albedo (reflectivity) and cool the earth. As ocean temperatures drop because less sunlight gets through, phytoplankton activity decreases, DMS production falls, and clouds disappear. Thus, DMS, which may account for half of all biogenic sulfur emissions, could be a feedback mechanism that keeps temperature within a suitable range for all life.

SUMMARY

- Ecology, the study of relationships between organisms and their environment, involves investigating how organisms acquire and use energy, nutrients, and water from their environment. Required conditions for life include chemical elements, availability of liquid water, and moderate temperatures.
- Matter—the substance of which things are made—is not created or destroyed under normal circumstances. It is recycled endlessly through organisms and their environment. This principle is known as the conservation of matter.
- Elements are identified by their atomic number, the number of protons in their nuclei. Atoms can have variable numbers of neutrons (isotopes) or electrons (ions). Four elements, oxygen, carbon, hydrogen, and nitrogen, make up more than 96 percent of most living organisms.
- Acids are substances that readily release hydrogen ions in solution; bases are substances that readily bond with hydrogen atoms. Acids and bases play important roles in life processes, and they are common sources of environmental problems, such as acid mine drainage. Buffers, substances that absorb or release hydrogen ions, neutralize acids and bases.
- Ionic or covalent bonds join atoms to produce compounds or molecules. Breaking bonds releases energy, including that used by living cells.
- Water's remarkable properties make it both the medium for life processes and a key factor in our global climate.
- Four major classes of organic compounds, hydrocarbons, carbohydrates, proteins, and nucleic acids, provide structure, function, and energy for cells.
- Energy cannot be created or destroyed (the first law of thermodynamics) but it is constantly degraded to less useful forms—entropy increases—as it is used (the second law of thermodynamics).
- Photosynthesis is the conversion of solar energy to chemical bonds in organic molecules, using carbon dioxide (from air) and water. Chlorophyll, the green pigment in plants, provides the energy for nearly all living things on earth. Photosynthesis involves a complex series of reactions, some light-dependent and others not dependent on light. Cellular respiration is the process of breaking down organic molecules to release energy.
- Species are often (but not always) defined as all organisms that can breed and produce fertile offspring in nature. A population is all the members of a species that live in an area, and a biological community comprises all the populations in an area. An ecosystem is a biological community and its physical environment. Ecosystems are generally open systems: they exchange materials and energy with their surroundings.
- Energy and nutrients flow through food webs and trophic levels in an ecosystem. Productivity is a measure of how rapidly an ecosystem accumulates biomass, or biological material. Organisms in a food web can be identified as primary producers or consumers; they can also be identified as herbivores, carnivores, omnivores, scavengers, detritivores, or decomposers. The concept of ecological pyramids is that there are many more individuals, and more biomass, at lower trophic levels than at higher trophic levels.
- Materials such as water, carbon, nitrogen, sulfur, and phosphorus also cycle through organisms and their environment. Substances are stored in rocks, air, water, and living things for varying lengths of time. One of the major impacts of humans on our environment has been to alter the rates of material cycling.

QUESTIONS FOR REVIEW

1. Define the terms *atom* and *element.* Are these terms interchangeable?
2. Your body contains vast numbers of carbon atoms. How is it possible that some of these carbon atoms may have been part of the body of a prehistoric creature?
3. In the biosphere, matter follows a circular pathway while energy follows a linear pathway. Explain.
4. The oceans store a vast amount of heat, but this huge reservoir of energy is of little use to humans (except for climate moderation). Explain the difference between high-quality and low-quality energy.
5. Ecosystems require energy to function. From where does this energy come? Where does it go? How does the flow of energy conform to the laws of thermodynamics?
6. Heat is released during metabolism. How is this heat useful to a cell and to a multicellular organism? How might it be detrimental, especially in a large, complex organism?
7. Photosynthesis and cellular respiration are complementary processes. Explain how they exemplify the laws of conservation of matter and thermodynamics.
8. What do we mean by carbon fixation or nitrogen fixation? Why is it important to humans that carbon and nitrogen be "fixed"?
9. The population density of large carnivores is always very small, compared with the population density of herbivores occupying the same ecosystem. Explain this in relation to the concept of an ecological pyramid.
10. A species is a specific kind of organism. What general characteristics do individuals of a particular species share? Why is it important for ecologists to differentiate among the various species in a biological community?

THINKING SCIENTIFICALLY

1. How does the principle of entropy (or the second law of thermodynamics) explain the idea of trophic pyramids?
2. Which wavelengths do our eyes respond to, and why (refer to fig. 2.10)? What is the ratio of short ultraviolet wavelengths to microwave wavelengths (used in a microwave oven)?
3. Ecosystems are often defined as a matter of convenience, because we can't study everything at once. How would you describe the character and extent of the natural ecosystem in which you live? What characteristics make your ecosystem an open system?
4. How would you delimit the human ecosystem (including food and energy production) in which you live?
5. If you had to define a research project to evaluate the relative biomass of producers and consumers in an ecosystem, what would you measure? (Note: This could be a natural ecosystem or an enclosed system, such as a terrarium.)
6. Understanding storage compartments is essential to understanding material cycles, such as the carbon cycle. If you look around your backyard, how many carbon storage compartments are there? Which ones are biggest? Which ones are longest-lasting?

KEY TERMS

acids 30
atom 28
bases 30
biological community 36
biomass 36
carbon cycle 39
carnivores 37
cellular respiration 34
chemical compounds 29
conservation of matter 27
consumers 36
decomposer 38
ecology 26
ecosystem 36
energy 27
first law of thermodynamics 28
food web 37
herbivores 37
ions 28
kinetic energy 27
matter 27
metabolism 31
molecules 29
nitrogen cycle 40
omnivores 37
organic compounds 31
pH 30
photosynthesis 33
population 36
potential energy 27
primary producers 36
productivity 36
second law of thermodynamics 28
species 36
trophic level 37

SUGGESTED READINGS

Beardsley, Tim. 1997. When nutrients turn noxious: A little nitrogen is nice, but too much is toxic. *Scientific American* 276(6): 24–25.

Daily, Gretchen, ed. 2002. *The New Economy of Nature.* Island Press.

Emsley, John. 2001. *Nature's Building Blocks: A–Z Guide to the Elements.* Oxford University Press.

Galloway, James N., and Ellis B. Cowling. 2002. Reactive nitrogen and the world: 200 years of change. *AMBIO* 31(7):501.

Lindeman, Ray L. 1942. The trophic-dynamic aspect of ecology. *Ecology* 23:399–418.

Smith, Stephen V., et al. 2003. Humans, hydrology, and the distribution of inorganic nutrient loading to the ocean. *BioScience* 53(3):235–45.

Welcome to McGraw-Hill's Online Learning Center

http://www.mhhe.com/cunningham3e

WEB EXERCISES

Calculating Your Carbon Budget

How much do *you* contribute to global carbon cycling? Possibly more than you think. Go to www.lpb.org/programs/forest/calculator.html (a site provided by the Public Broadcasting Service [PBS] of Louisiana) and calculate your personal carbon budget. How many trees would be needed to offset your yearly production of CO_2? Try modifying your lifestyle: suppose you drove half as much or recycled more. What are the most effective strategies for reducing your carbon budget?

Once you have figured your personal carbon budget, first multiply your carbon emissions by the number of people in your class, then by the number of people in your state. This multiplication should give you an idea of how individual actions contribute to global-scale processes. If everyone in your state reduced his or her carbon emissions by 10 percent, how many tons of carbon would be kept out of circulation?

Investigating Current Research Problems

Scientists exchange ideas and information through scientific journals. Thousands of journals exist, many in very specialized fields. *Conservation Ecology* is an important example of a new variety of scientific journals: e-journals, which you can access on the World Wide Web. This journal includes research articles, debates, discussions, and comments from a variety of well-respected and active ecologists, and it covers topics that are very current. Go to *Conservation Ecology* at www.consecol.org/Journal and look at the most recent issue.

1. Review the table of contents. What topics are ecologists concerned about today?
2. Look at one of the articles in detail. How does the tone of the article reflect some of the ideal approaches to science outlined in chapter 1 (hypothesis testing, cautious inspection of evidence, objectivity)?
3. What kinds of data (or other evidence) does the author present in support of his or her arguments?
4. Some of the articles are debates about a particular topic. Find one of these, and identify the positions on both sides of the debate. What is the question being debated? Describe two (or more) opposing views on the question.

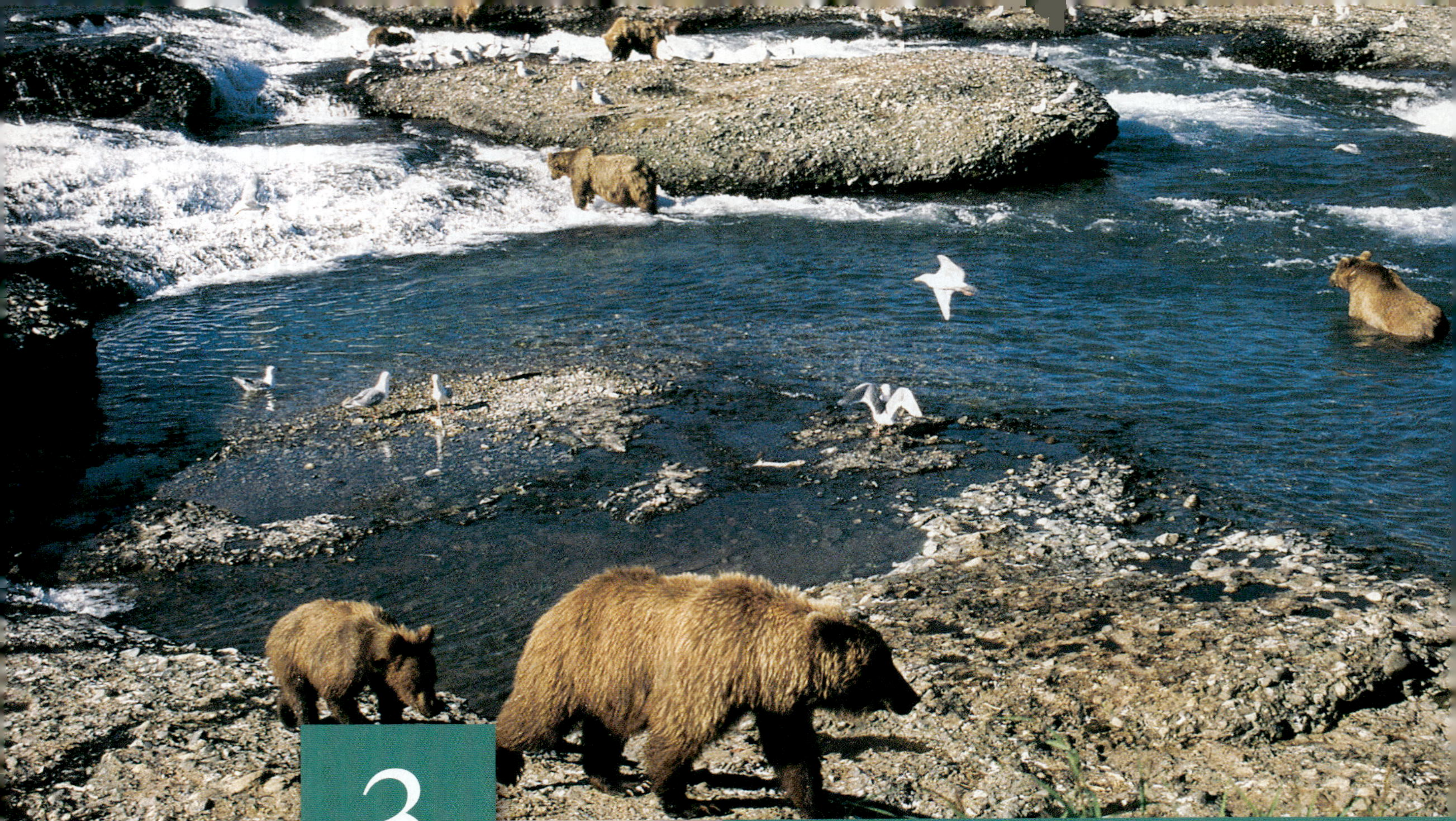

3

Populations, Communities, and Species Interaction

Conservation is a state of harmony between men and land.
–*Aldo Leopold*

The bears, birds, and fish of the McNeil River, Alaska, form an interconnected biological community together with terrestrial and aquatic plants and invertebrates.

Welcome to McGraw-Hill's Online Learning Center

http://www.mhhe.com/cunningham3e

LEARNING ONLINE

Visit our webpage at www.mhhe.com/cunningham3e for data sources, further readings, additional case studies, current environmental news, and regional examples within the Online Learning Center to help you understand the material in this chapter. You'll also find active links to information pertaining to this chapter, including

Community ecology
Cornell Lab of Ornithology
Biological Resources Division, USGS
National biological information
U.S. Long Term Ecological Research Network, Home
Quantitative Population Ecology
Chaos and complexity
Population dynamics models

OBJECTIVES

After studying this chapter, you should be able to

- describe how environmental factors determine which species live in a given ecosystem and where or how they live.
- understand how random genetic variation and natural selection lead to evolution, adaptation, niche specialization, and partitioning of resources in biological communities.
- compare and contrast interspecific predation, competition, symbiosis, commensalism, mutualism, and coevolution.
- explain population growth rates, carrying capacity, and factors that limit population growth.
- discuss productivity, diversity, complexity, and structure of biological communities and how these characteristics might be connected to resilience and stability.
- explain how ecological succession results in ecosystem development and allows one species to replace another.
- list some examples of exotic species introduced into biological communities, and describe the effects such introductions can have on indigenous species.

Darwin and the Theory of Evolution

Why do living things vary so much, and how is it that they fit so neatly into their environments and their biological communities? These questions, at the core of environmental science today, inspired Charles Darwin to explore the origin of species a century and a half ago. Darwin's work demonstrates the importance of careful observation, cautious explanation, and a willingness to consider new ideas, even controversial ones.

Darwin was only 22 years old when he set out on his epic five-year voyage aboard the ship *Beagle,* which left England in 1831 to map sailing routes around South America (fig. 3.1). Initially an indifferent student, Darwin had found inspiring professors in his last years in college. One of these helped him get a position as an unpaid naturalist on board the *Beagle.* Darwin turned out to be an inquisitive thinker, an avid collector of specimens, and a careful reader of explorers, natural historians, and geologists.

After four years of exploring and collecting, Darwin reached the Galápagos Islands. Six hundred miles from the coast of Ecuador, these islands are isolated from the mainland and from each other by strong, cold currents and high winds. By then, Darwin had read and seen enough to recognize that numerous species on each island occurred nowhere else in the world, yet their features suggested common ancestors on the South American mainland. The finches were especially interesting: each island had its own species, marked by distinct bill shapes, which graded from large and parrot-like to small and warbler-like. Each bird's beak type was suited to an available food source on its island. It seemed obvious that, somehow, these birds had been modified to survive in their distinct environments.

To convince others that species can adapt to their environments, and to make a useful contribution to scientific understanding, Darwin had to come up with an *explanation* of *how* they did so. Shortly after his return to England, he read an essay by the Reverend Thomas Malthus, proposing that humans invariably reproduce beyond the carrying capacity of their resources, after which famine, disease, and competition eliminate the surplus population. Here Darwin found a plausible explanation for evolution: species produce many offspring, but only the fittest survive to reproduce again; poorer competitors do not reproduce and pass on their traits.

It's important to note that Darwin wasn't the first to think about biological evolution. Many people in his time understood that organisms can have common ancestors but drift apart over time. Darwin spent a great deal of time, for example, interviewing animal and plant breeders about how traits change from generation to generation. What was missing—and what Darwin supplied with his brilliant insights about natural selection—was how this process works in nature. Darwin didn't know, however, how characteristics are passed from generation to generation. Only after many years of further research were Ernst Mayer and others able to put together a modern synthesis that explains the genetic basis of evolution.

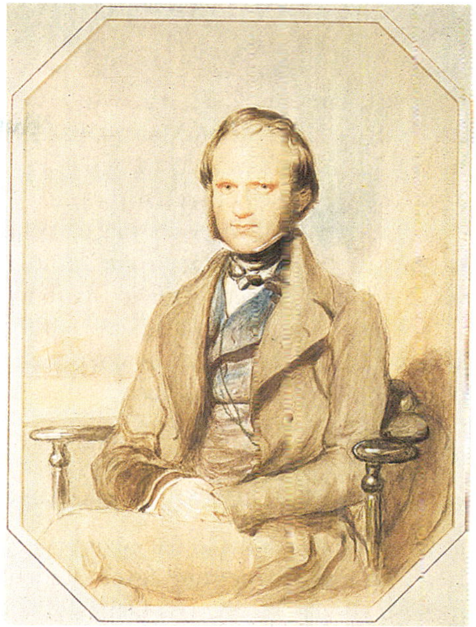

FIGURE 3.1 *Charles Darwin, in a portrait painted shortly after the voyage on the* Beagle.

An overwhelming majority of biologists now consider the theory of evolution through natural selection to be the cornerstone of their science. A huge body of evidence from both laboratory and field studies supports this theory. Neither Darwin nor his ideas are above scrutiny, however. Darwin believed, for example, that evolution probably proceeds very slowly and gradually. In 1972 the Harvard paleontologist Stephen Jay Gould challenged this idea of gradualism, suggesting instead that species and biological communities go through long periods of relatively little change but then have brief episodes of very rapid evolutionary development. Gould called this punctuated equilibrium. Darwin's work remains one of our foremost examples of bold, creative thinking and meticulous observation. A good theory is able to explain new evidence as it accumulates; it is also a springboard for further exploration and debate. How species multiply and how they interact, the subjects of this chapter, are aspects of evolution that scientists continue to explore and debate almost 150 years after Darwin's theory was first published.

For further reading, see Charles Darwin, *The Voyage of the Beagle* (1837) and *On the Origin of Species by Means of Natural Selection* (1859).

WHO LIVES WHERE, AND WHY?

"Why" questions often stimulate scientific research, but the research itself centers on "how" questions. Why, we wonder, does a particular species live where it does? More to the point, how does it deal with the physical resources and stresses of its environment? How does it interact with the other species present? And what gives one species an edge over another species in a particular habitat?

In this chapter, we will examine some specific ways organisms respond to physical aspects of their environment. We then will discuss how members of a biological community interact, pointing out a few of the difficulties ecologists encounter when they attempt to discern patterns and make generalizations about community interactions and organization.

Critical Factors and Tolerance Limits

Every living organism has limits to the environmental conditions it can endure. Temperature, moisture level, nutrient supply, soil and water chemistry, living space, and other environmental factors must be within appropriate levels for organisms to persist. In 1840 Justus von Liebig proposed that the single factor in shortest supply relative to demand is the critical determinant in species distribution. Ecologist Victor Shelford later expanded this principle of limiting factors by stating that each environmental factor has both minimum and maximum levels, called **tolerance limits,** beyond which a particular species cannot survive or is unable to reproduce (fig. 3.2). The single factor closest to these survival limits, Shelford postulated, is the critical limiting factor that determines where a particular organism can live.

At one time, ecologists accepted the critical limiting factor concept so completely that they called it Liebig's or Shelford's Law and tried to identify unique factors limiting the growth of every plant and animal population. For many species, however, we find that the interaction of several factors working together, rather than a single limiting factor, determines biogeographical distribution. If you have ever explored the rocky coasts of New England or the Pacific Northwest, for instance, you have probably noticed that mussels and barnacles endure extremely harsh conditions but generally are sharply limited to an intertidal zone, where they grow so thickly that they often completely cover the substrate. No single factor determines this distribution. Instead, a combination of temperature extremes, drying time between tides, salt concentrations, competitors, and food availability limits the number and location of these animals.

For other organisms, there may be a specific critical factor that, more than any other, determines the abundance and distribution of that species in a given area. A striking example of cold intolerance as a critical factor is found in the giant saguaro cactus (*Carnegiea gigantea*), which grows in the dry, hot Sonoran desert of southern Arizona and northern Mexico (fig. 3.3). Saguaros are extremely sensitive to low temperatures. A single exceptionally cold winter night with temperatures below freezing for 12 hours or more kills growing tips on the branches.

Animal species, too, exhibit tolerance limits, which often are more critical for the young than for the adults. The desert pupfish (*Cyprinodon*), for instance, occurs in small, isolated populations in warm springs in the northern Sonoran desert. Adult pupfish can survive temperatures between 0° and 42°C (a remarkably high temperature for a fish) and are tolerant to an equally wide range of salt concentrations. Eggs and juvenile fish, however, can live only between 20° and 36°C and are killed by high salt levels. Reproduction, therefore, is limited to a small part of the range of adult fish.

Sometimes the requirements and tolerances of species are useful indicators of specific environmental characteristics. The presence or absence of such species can tell us something about the community and the ecosystem as a whole. Lichens and eastern

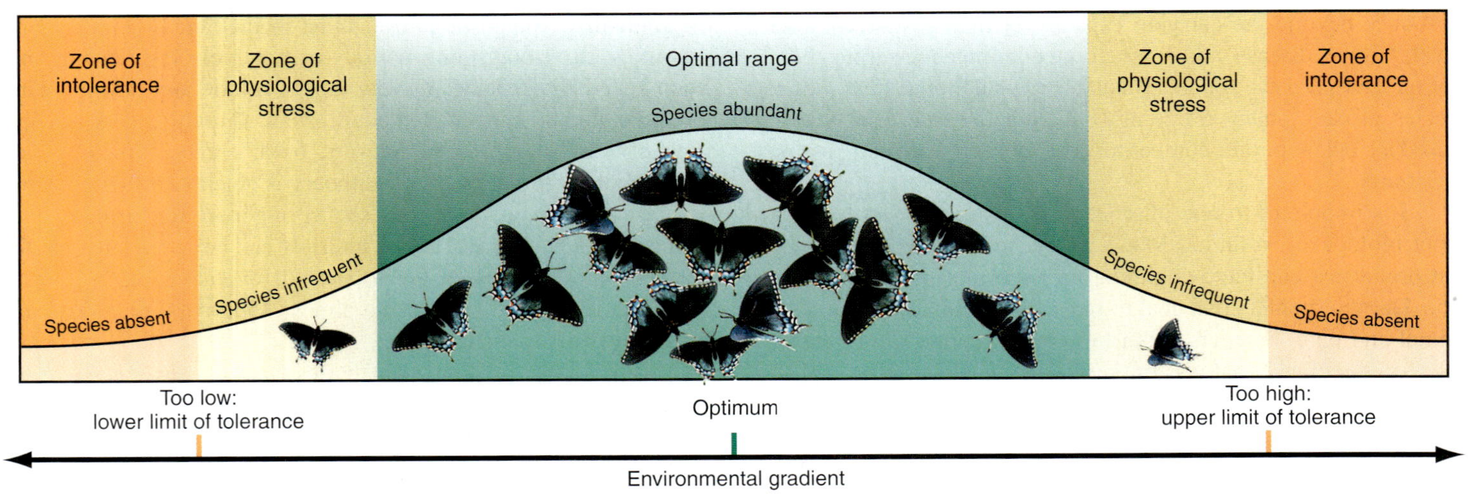

FIGURE 3.2 *The principle of tolerance limits states that, for every environmental factor, an organism has both maximum and minimum levels beyond which it cannot survive. The greatest abundance of any species along an environmental gradient is around the optimum level of the critical factor most important for that species. Near the tolerance limits, abundance decreases because fewer individuals are able to survive the stresses imposed by limiting factors.*

white pine, for example, are indicators of air pollution because they are extremely sensitive to sulfur dioxide and acid precipitation. Bull thistle is a weed that grows on disturbed soil but is not eaten by cattle; therefore, an abundant population of bull thistle in a pasture is a good indicator of overgrazing. Similarly, anglers know that trout species require clean, well-oxygenated water, so the presence or absence of trout can be an indicator of water quality.

Evolution: Natural Selection and Adaptation

How is it that mussels have developed the ability to endure pounding waves, daily exposure to drying sun and wind, and seasonal threats of extreme cold or hot temperature? How does the saguaro survive in the harsh temperatures and extreme dryness of the desert? We commonly say that each of these species is "adapted" to its special set of conditions, but what does that mean? **Adaptation,** when species acquire traits that allow them to survive in their environments, is one of the most important concepts in biology.

We use the term *adapt* in two ways. One is a limited range of physiological modifications (called acclimation) available to individual organisms. If you keep houseplants inside all winter, for example, and then put them out in full sunlight in the spring, they get sunburned. If the damage isn't too severe, your plants will probably grow new leaves with a thicker cuticle and denser pigments to protect them from the sun. They can adapt to some degree, but the change isn't permanent. Another winter inside will make them just as sensitive to the sun as before. Furthermore, the changes they acquire are not passed on to their offspring. Although the potential to acclimate is inherited, each generation must develop its own protective epidermis.

Another type of adaptation operates at the population level and is brought about by inheritance of specific genetic traits that allow a species to live in a particular environment. This process is explained by the theory of **evolution.** This theory is mainly attributed to Charles Darwin (see "Darwin and the Theory of Evolution" at the beginning of this chapter), but it was also developed independently and simultaneously by Alfred Russel Wallace, who documented species differentiation in Indonesia. According to this theory, species change gradually through competition for scarce resources. **Natural selection** describes the process in which better competitors survive and reproduce more successfully. Poorer competitors are more likely to die or to fail to reproduce. Note that "better competitors" can have any trait that provides individuals with some advantage over their peers. Bigger bills, better camouflage, or more attractive plumage or songs each can provide advantages in different circumstances. Individuals carrying advantageous traits are most likely to reproduce successfully, thus passing on those traits.

Natural selection occurs because small, random mutations (changes in genetic material) occur spontaneously in every population. These random differences create genetic diversity (natural variability in traits) in a population. Depending on environmental conditions, some traits may be more advantageous than others. Limited resources or environmental conditions may exert **selective pressure** on a population, reducing the chance that less fit

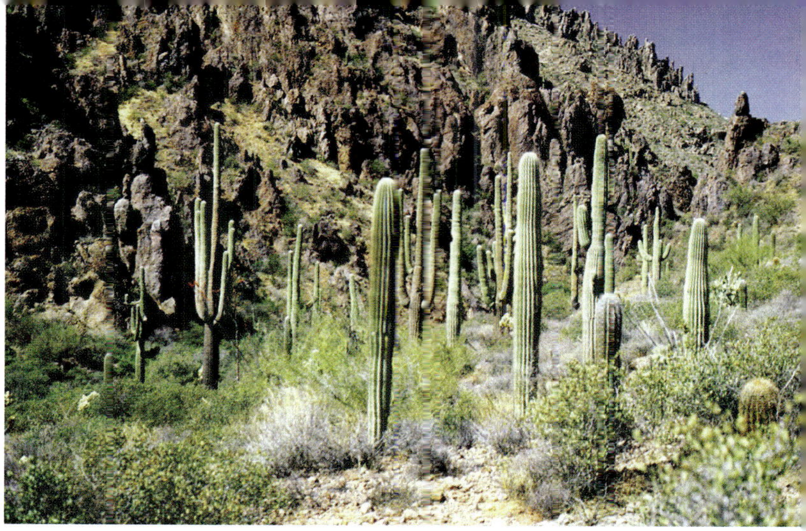

FIGURE 3.3 *Saguaro cacti, symbolic of the Sonoran desert, are an excellent example of distribution controlled by a critical environmental factor. Extremely sensitive to low temperatures, saguaros are found only where minimum temperatures never dip below freezing for more than a few hours at a time.*

individuals will reproduce successfully. In such cases, individuals with advantageous traits become relatively more abundant in the population.

It is important to remember that mutations can be negative as well as positive. That is, the characteristics created by a particular genetic change can be either harmful or beneficial. Natural selection tends to discard the negative traits and preserve the helpful ones.

What environmental factors cause selective pressure and influence fertility or survivorship in nature? Some important factors include (1) physiological stress due to inappropriate levels of some critical environmental factor, such as moisture, light, temperature, pH, or specific nutrients; (2) predation, including parasitism and disease; (3) competition; and (4) luck. In some cases, the organisms that survive environmental catastrophes or find their way to a new habitat, where they start a new population, may simply be lucky rather than more fit or better suited to subsequent environmental conditions than their less fortunate contemporaries.

Speciation

Given enough time, many small changes (mutations) may collectively allow a species to become better suited to new environmental conditions. Sometimes evolution creates entirely new species, physically, genetically, and/or behaviorally distinct from their ancestors. The development of new species is known as speciation. Speciation can result from the development of new opportunities (the appearance of a new food source or other resource) or risks (climate change or new predators or competitors). Isolation can also produce new species: if a small group is separated from the rest of the population (called geographic isolation), its genetic characteristics can diverge from those of the main group. Similarly, if a small population colonizes a new environment, island, or habitat, it might encounter new environmental conditions that produce selective pressure. The barriers that divide subpopulations are not always physical. In some cases, behaviors such as when and where population members feed, sleep, or mate, or even how they communicate, may separate them sufficiently for **divergent evolution** (separation into new types) to occur even though they occupy the same territory. This is called behavioral isolation. Although each genetic change may be very slight, many mutations over a long time have produced the incredible variety of life-forms that we observe in nature.

Cheetahs are remarkable examples of evolutionary adaptation (fig. 3.4). The fastest-running of any mammal, these big cats have a flexible skeleton, a sleek shape, and musculature that allows them to catch even the fleetest prey. Think about the adaptations of house cats. Which features might have been useful to their ancestors but are no longer so important?

The variety of finches observed by Charles Darwin on the Galápagos Islands is another classic example of speciation driven by availability of different environmental opportunities (fig. 3.5). Originally derived from a single seed-eating species that was perhaps carried over 1,000 km from the mainland in a storm, the finches have evolved into 13 distinct species that differ markedly in appearance, food preferences, and habitat. Fruit eaters have thick, parrot-like bills; seed eaters have heavy, crushing bills; insect eaters have thin, probing beaks to catch their prey. One of the most unusual species is the woodpecker finch, which pecks at tree bark for hidden insects. Lacking the woodpecker's long tongue, however, the finch uses a cactus spine as a tool to extract bugs.

The amazing variety of colors, shapes, and sizes of dogs, cats, rabbits, fish, flowers, vegetables, and other domestic species shows the effects of deliberate selective breeding. The various characteristics of these organisms arose through mutations. We have simply kept the ones we liked.

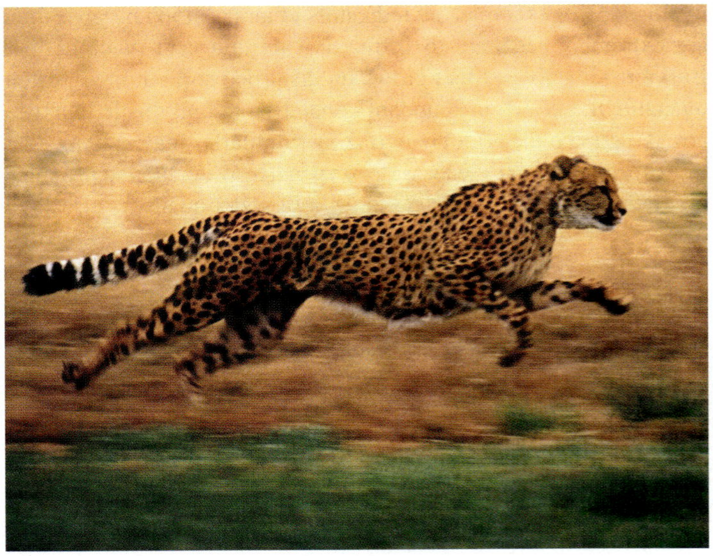

FIGURE 3.4 *Cheetahs are adapted by natural selection to run extremely fast.*

Natural selection and adaptation can produce very different organisms from a common origin, but it can also cause unrelated organisms to look and act very much alike. We call this latter

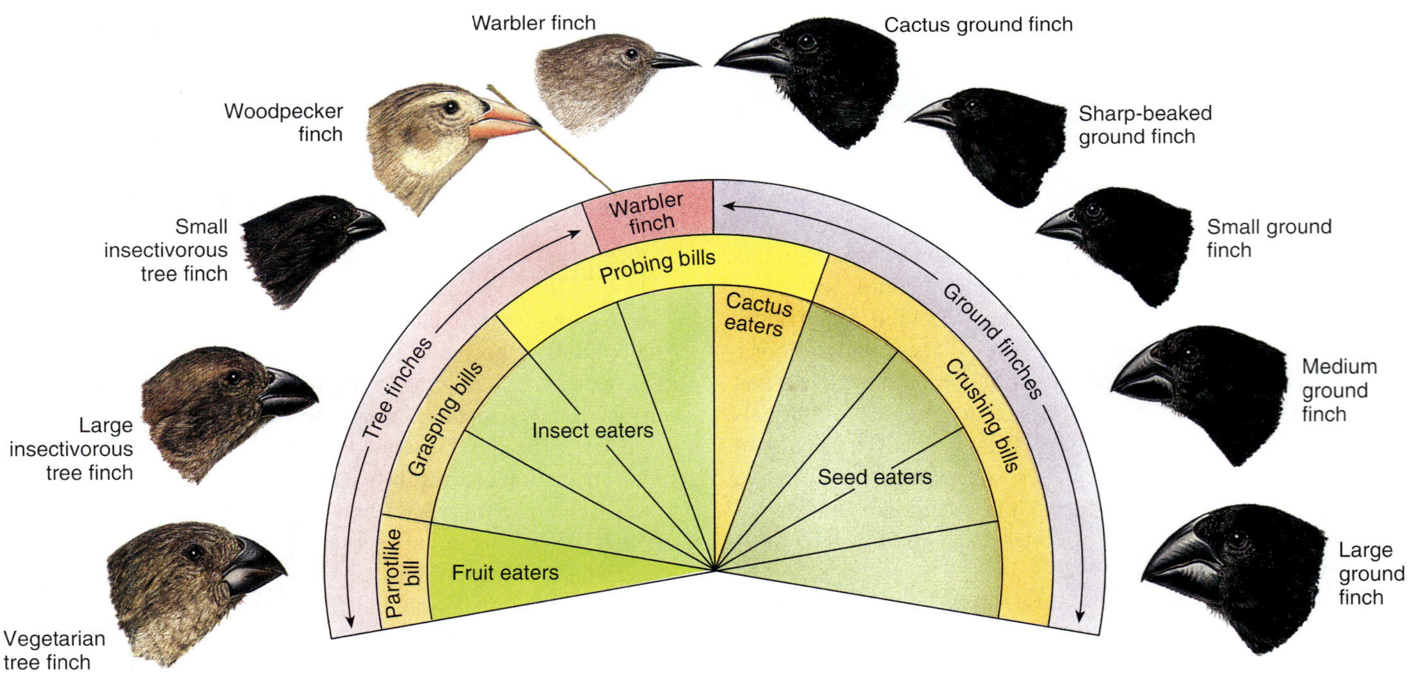

FIGURE 3.5 *Some species of Galápagos Island finches. Although all are descendents of a common ancestor, they now differ markedly in appearance, habitat, and feeding behavior. Ground finches* (lower right) *eat cactus leaves; warbler finches* (upper left) *eat insects; others eat seeds or have mixed diets. The woodpecker finch* (upper left) *pecks tree bark, as do woodpeckers, but lacks a long tongue. Instead, it uses cactus spines as tools to extract insects.*

process **convergent evolution.** The fruit-eating Galápagos finches, for example, look and act very much like parrots even though they are genetically very dissimilar. The features that enable parrots to eat fruit successfully work well for these finches also.

Be sure you understand that, while selection affects individuals, evolution and adaptation work at the population level. Individuals don't evolve; species do. Each individual is locked in by genetics to a particular way of life. Most plants, animals, and microbes have relatively limited ability to modify their physical makeup or behavior to better suit a particular environment. Over time, however, random genetic changes and natural selection can change an entire population.

Another common mistake is to believe that organisms develop certain characteristics because they want or need them. This is incorrect. A duck doesn't have webbed feet because it *wants* to swim or *needs* to swim in order to eat; it has webbed feet because some ancestor happened to have a gene for webbed feet that gave it some advantage over other ducks in acquiring food or evading predators. That successful duck produced more offspring than other ducks, and its webbed feet were passed on. A variety of genetic types is always present in any population, and natural selection simply favors those types best suited for particular conditions. Whether this process has a purpose or direction is a philosophical question rather than a scientific one and is beyond the scope of this book.

The Taxonomic Naming System

Taxonomy, or the study of types of organisms and their relationships, traces how organisms have evolved from common ancestors. Like a family tree, taxonomic relationships can be displayed in a tree-like arrangement. The most widely used part of this tree are the final levels, the genus and species, which make up the binomial name (or scientific name or Latin name) that identifies a species. These names follow a Latin-like naming style, although species are often named with non-Latin words or with names of people. These names help scientists communicate with each other, because they provide an international language to refer to organisms. Common names such as buttercup or bluebird might refer to a wide variety of organisms in different locations, and multiple names are often used for a single species. A scientific name such as *Pinus resinosa,* on the other hand, always means the same kind of pine tree, regardless of whether you think of it as a red pine or a Norway pine.

In general, taxonomic organization uses the following levels:

Kingdom
Phylum (or division)
Class
Order
Family
Genus
Species

For example, you are a *Homo sapiens,* and corn (maize) is *Zea mays* (table 3.1). These two species represent the two best-known kingdoms: animals and plants. Scientists recognize six kingdoms, however: animals, plants, fungi (molds and mushrooms), protists (algae, protozoans), eubacteria (ordinary bacteria), and archaebacteria (ancient, single-celled organisms that live in harsh environments, such as hot springs). Within these kingdoms are millions of different species (see chapter 5).

TABLE 3.1 Taxonomy of Two Common Species

TAXONOMIC LEVEL	HUMANS	CORN
Kingdom	Animalia	Plantae
Phylum	Chordata	Anthophyta
Class	Mammalia	Monocotyledons
Order	Primates	Commenales
Family	Hominidae	Poaceae
Genus	*Homo*	*Zea*
Species	*Homo sapiens*	*Zea mays*

The Ecological Niche

Habitat describes the place or set of environmental conditions in which a particular organism lives. A more functional term, **ecological niche,** is a description of either the role played by a species in a biological community or the total set of environmental factors that determine species distribution. The concept of niches, as community roles, describing how a species obtains food, what relationships it has with other species, and the services it provides its community, was first defined by the British ecologist Charles Elton in 1927. Thirty years later, the American limnologist G. E. Hutchinson proposed a more biophysical definition of this concept. Every species, he pointed out, has a range of physical and chemical conditions (temperature, light levels, acidity, humidity, salinity, etc.) as well as biological interactions (predators and prey present, defenses, nutritional resources available, etc.) within which it can exist. Figure 3.2, for example, shows the abundance of a hypothetical species along a single factor gradient. If it were possible to graph simultaneously all of the factors that affect a particular species, a multidimensional space would result that describes the ecological niche available to that species.

Some species, such as raccoons and coyotes, are generalists that eat a wide variety of food and live in a broad range of habitats (including urban areas). Others, such as the panda, are specialists that occupy a very narrow niche (fig. 3.6). Specialists often tend to be rarer than generalists and less resilient to disturbance or change.

A few species, such as elephants, chimpanzees, and baboons, learn how to behave from their social group and can invent new ways of doing things when presented with new opportunities or challenges. Most organisms, however, are limited by genetically determined physical structure and instinctive behavior to established niches.

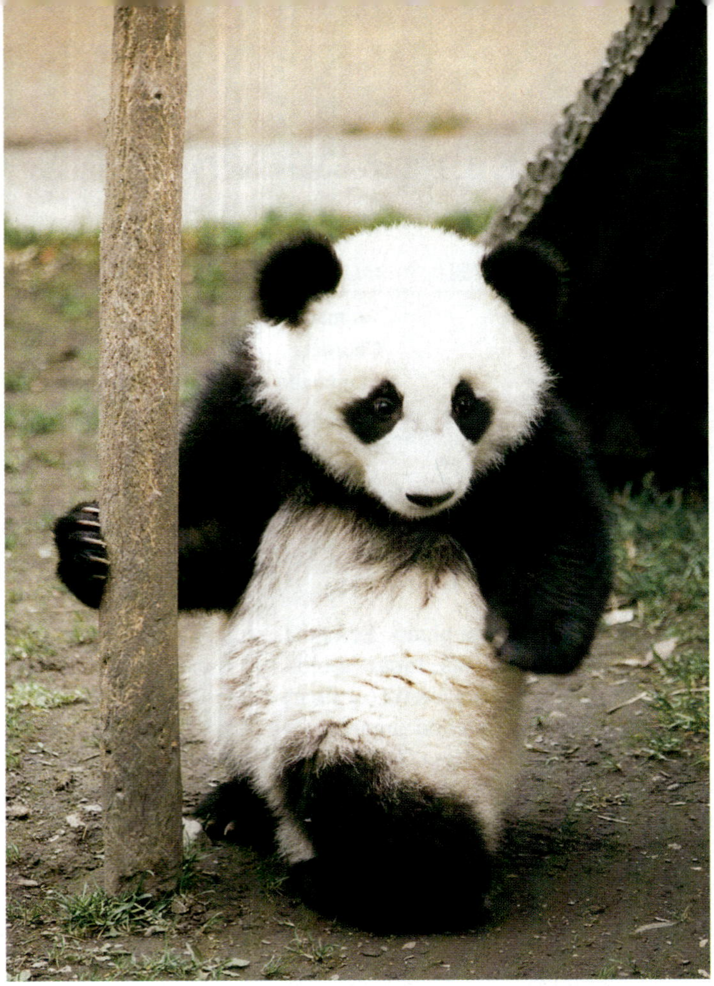

FIGURE 3.6 *The giant panda feeds exclusively on bamboo. Although its teeth and digestive system are those of a carnivore, it is not a good hunter and has adapted to a vegetarian diet. In the 1970s, huge acreages of bamboo flowered and died, and many pandas starved.*

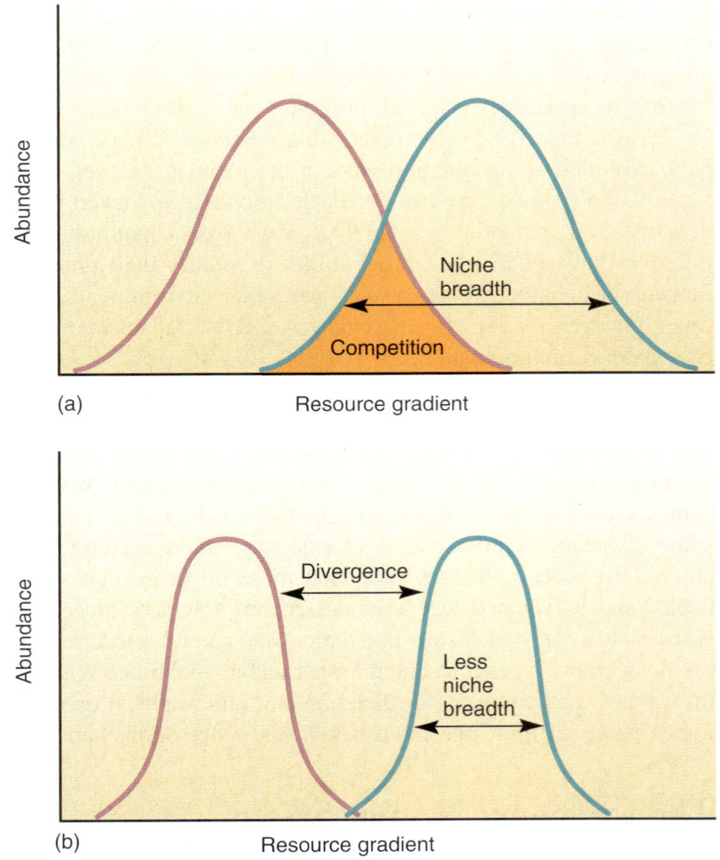

FIGURE 3.7 *Resource partitioning and niche specialization caused by competition.* (a) *Where niches of two species overlap along a resource gradient, competition occurs* (shaded area). (b) *Individuals occupying this part of the niche are less successful in reproduction. Characteristics of the population then diverge to produce more specialization, narrower niche breadth, and less competition between species.*

Over time, niches can change as species develop new strategies to exploit resources. The law of competitive exclusion states that no two species will occupy the same niche and compete for exactly the same resources in the same habitat for very long. Eventually, one group will gain a larger share of resources, while the other will either migrate to a new area, become extinct, or change its behavior or physiology in ways that minimize competition. We call this third process of niche evolution **resource partitioning** (fig. 3.7). Partitioning can allow several species to utilize different parts of the same resource and coexist within a single habitat (fig. 3.8). Species can specialize in time, too. Swallows and insectivorous bats both catch insects, but some insect species are active during the day and others at night, providing noncompetitive feeding opportunities for day-active swallows and night-active bats.

What Are Weedy Species?

Most of us have spent time trying to control weeds, but have you ever thought about what weeds are, ecologically? In your yard or garden, weeds are species that grow rapidly where you don't want them. They are *opportunistic,* quickly appearing wherever an opportunity arises. Weeds such as dandelions, crabgrass, and creeping Charlie can reproduce quickly, easily spreading many seeds long distances (fig. 3.9). Many weeds are generalist species, able to tolerate a wide variety of environmental conditions (hot, cold, sunny, shady, dry, wet) and to endure environmental change. Ecologically, these attributes make such species excellent competitors in the environmental conditions of your yard. Many weeds are also *pioneer species,* able to quickly colonize open, disturbed, or bare ground. Such species can play important ecological roles, covering bare soil and reducing erosion, for example. If they have no natural predators, they can also quickly overwhelm other vegetation, causing significant environmental change.

Many animals can be considered "weedy" species as well. Generalist, opportunistic species, such as starlings and English sparrows, raccoons, and rats, all spread readily and can tolerate a wide range of climate and environmental conditions. Ecologically, these traits are advantageous to these species. Their aggressiveness can quickly alter environments in which they arrive, however.

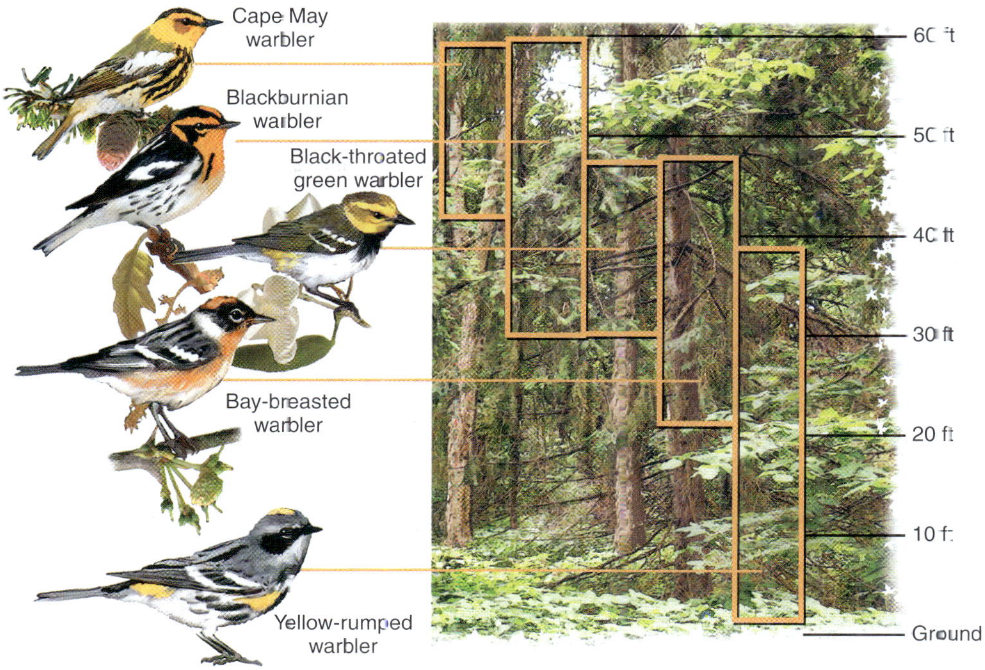

FIGURE 3.8 *Resource partitioning and the concept of the ecological niche are demonstrated by several species of wood warblers that use different strata of the same forest. This is a classic example of the principle of competitive exclusion.*
Source: Original observation by R. H. MacArthur.

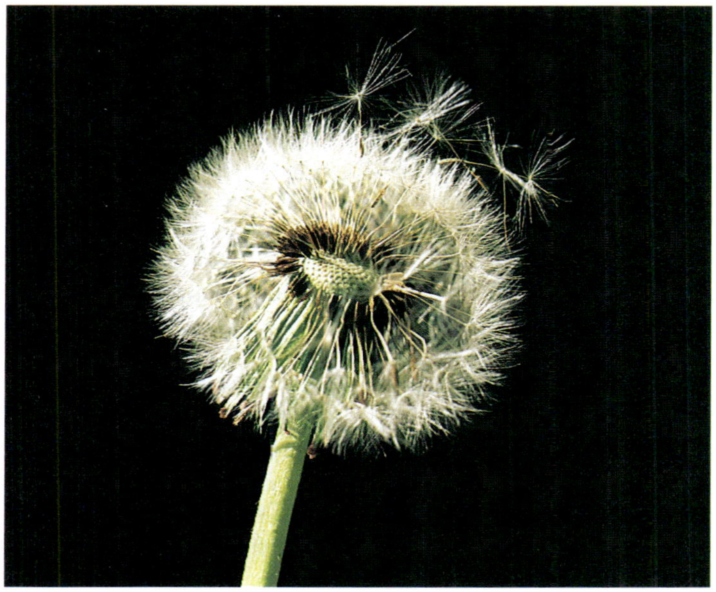

FIGURE 3.9 *Dandelions and other opportunistic species generally produce many highly mobile offspring.*

SPECIES INTERACTIONS

Predation and competition for scarce resources are major factors in evolution and adaptation. Not all biological interactions are competitive, however. Organisms also cooperate with, or at least tolerate, members of their own species as well as individuals of other species in order to survive and reproduce. In some cases, different organisms depend on each other to help acquire resources. In this section, we will look more closely at the different interactions within and between species that shape biological communities.

Predation

All organisms need food to live. Producers make their own food, and consumers eat organic matter created by other organisms. In most communities, as we saw in chapter 2, photosynthetic plants and algae are the producers. Consumers include herbivores, carnivores, omnivores, scavengers, detritivores, and decomposers. With which of these categories do you associate the term *predator?* Ecologically, a **predator** is any organism that feeds directly upon another living organism, whether or not it kills its prey to do so (fig. 3.10). By this definition, herbivores, carnivores, and omnivores that feed on live prey are predators, but scavengers, detritivores, and decomposers that feed on dead things are not. In this broad sense, parasites (organisms that feed on a host organism or steal resources from it without necessarily killing it) and even pathogens (disease-causing organisms) might also be considered predator organisms.

Predation is a potent and complex influence on the population balance of communities involving (1) all stages of the life cycles of predator and prey species, (2) many specialized food-obtaining mechanisms, and (3) specific prey-predator adaptations that either resist or encourage predation.

Predatory relationships can change dramatically with life stages. In marine intertidal ecosystems, many crustaceans, mollusks, and worms release eggs directly into the water, and the eggs and free-living larval and juvenile stages are part of the floating

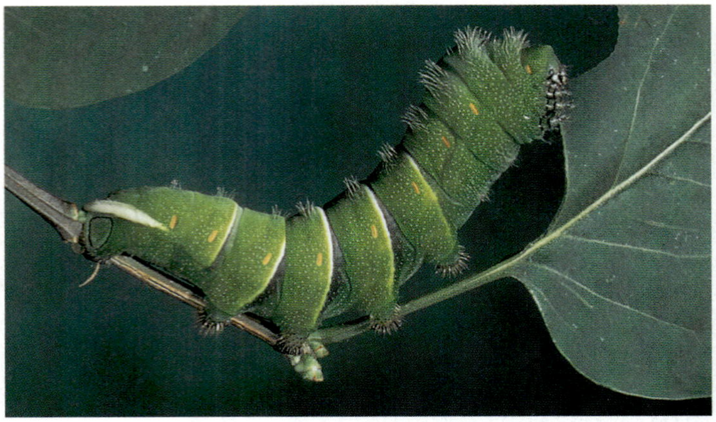

FIGURE 3.10 *Insect herbivores are predators as much as lions and tigers are. In fact, insects consume the vast majority of biomass in the world. Complex patterns of predation and defense have often evolved between insect predators and their plant prey.*

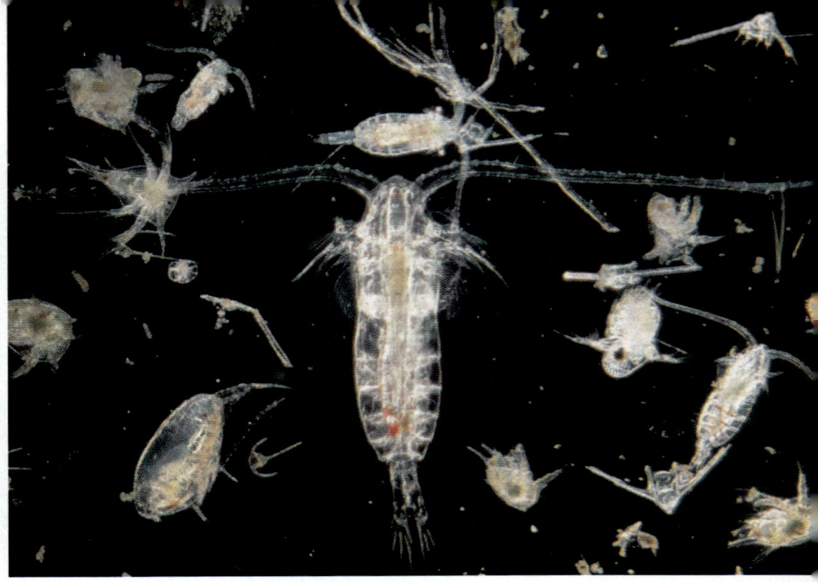

FIGURE 3.11 *Microscopic plants and animals form the basic levels of many aquatic food chains and account for a large percentage of total world biomass. Many oceanic plankton are larval forms that have habitats and feeding relationships very different from their adult forms.*

community, or plankton (fig. 3.11). Planktonic animals feed upon each other and are food for successively larger carnivores, including small fish. As prey species mature, their predators change. Barnacle larvae are planktonic and are eaten by fish. Adult barnacles, on the other hand, build hard shells that protect them from fish but can be crushed by limpets and other mollusks. Predators also may change their feeding targets. Adult frogs, for instance, are carnivores, but the tadpoles of most species are grazing herbivores. Sorting out the trophic levels in these communities can be very difficult.

Predation can be an important factor in controlling populations of both prey organisms and their consumers. The cyclamen mite (*Tarsonemus sp.*), for example, is a pest of strawberry crops in California. It is kept in check by a predatory mite in the genus *Typhlodromus.* When predators are removed, cyclamen mite populations explode and can severely damage a crop. If predators are reintroduced, they quickly reduce the cyclamen mite populations and bring them under control.

Given enough time, these trophic relationships can exert selective pressure that favors evolutionary adaptation. The predator becomes more efficient at finding and feeding, and the prey becomes more effective at escape or avoidance. In plants, predator avoidance is often accomplished with thick bark, spines, thorns, or chemical defenses. Animal prey may become very adept at hiding, fleeing, or fighting back against predators. Predators, in turn, evolve mechanisms to overcome the defenses of their prey. This process in which species exert selective pressure on each other is called **coevolution.** Coevolution can also be mutually beneficial: many plants and pollinators have evolved together, each aiding the other.

Competition

Competition is another kind of antagonistic relationship within a community. For what do organisms compete? To answer this question, think again about what all organisms need to survive: energy and matter in usable forms, space, and specific sites for life activities. Plants compete for growing space for root and shoot systems so they can absorb and process sunlight, water, and nutrients. Animals compete for living, nesting, and feeding sites, as well as for food, water, and mates. Competition among members of the same species is called intraspecific competition, whereas competition between members of different species is called interspecific competition.

If you look closely at a patch of weeds growing on good soil early in the summer, you likely will see several types of interspecific competition. First of all, many weedy species attempt to crowd out their rivals by producing prodigious numbers of seeds. After the seeds germinate, the plants race to grow the tallest, cover the most ground, and get the most sun. You may observe several strategies to do this. For example, vines don't build heavy stems of their own; they simply climb up over their neighbors to get to the light.

We often think of competition among animals as a bloody battle for resources, "nature red in tooth and claw." In fact, many animals tend to avoid fighting if possible. It's not worth getting injured. Most confrontations are more noise and show than actual fighting. Often competition is a matter of getting to food or habitat first or being able to use it more efficiently. As we discussed earlier, each species has a tolerance range for abiotic factors. Repeated studies have shown that, when two species compete, the one closest to its optimum range of abiotic conditions has an advantage and, more often than not, prevails.

Intraspecific (within species) competition can be just as intense as interspecific (between species) competition. Members of the same species have the same space and nutritional requirements; therefore, they compete directly for these environmental resources. How do organisms cope with intraspecific competition? One way is by dispersing: plants use wind, water, and passing animals to disperse seeds away from the parent plant. Young animals are forced to leave the parents' territory as soon as they are independent. Territoriality, vigorously defending territory, is a way of minimizing competition within a species. From grizzly bears to songbirds, many species vigorously defend territories—and food and water sources—from others of their own kind. Another way to reduce intraspecific competition is resource partitioning. Often the young of a species use resources differently than mature individuals. A leaf-munching caterpillar uses different food sources than a nectar-sipping adult butterfly. Crabs start out as floating planktonic larvae, which do not compete with bottom-crawling adult forms. In these examples, the adults and juveniles of each species do not compete because they occupy different ecological niches.

Symbiosis

In contrast to predation and competition, symbiotic interactions between organisms can be nonantagonistic. **Symbiosis** is the intimate living together of members of two or more species. Symbiotic relationships often enhance the survival of one or both partners. **Commensalism** is a type of symbiosis in which one member clearly benefits and the other apparently is neither benefited nor harmed. Cattle, for example, are often accompanied by cattle egrets and cowbirds, both of which catch insects kicked up as the cattle graze through a field. The birds benefit, while the cattle seem indifferent. Many of the mosses, bromeliads, and other plants growing on trees in the moist tropics are also considered to be commensals (fig. 3.12). These epiphytes get water from rain and nutrients from leaf litter and dust fall, and often they neither help nor hurt the trees on which they grow. In a way, the robins and sparrows that inhabit suburban yards are commensals with humans.

Lichens are a combination of a fungus and a photosynthetic partner, either an alga or a cyanobacteria. Their association is a type of symbiosis called **mutualism,** in which both members of the partnership benefit (fig. 3.13). Some ecologists believe that cooperative, mutualistic relationships may be more important in evolution than commonly thought. Aggressive interactions often are dangerous and destructive, while cooperation and compromise may have advantages that we tend to overlook. Survival of the fittest often may mean survival of those organisms that can live best with one another.

Parasitism, described earlier as a form of predation, also can be considered a type of symbiosis, where one species benefits and the other is harmed. All of these relationships have a bearing on such ecological issues as resource utilization, niche specialization, diversity, predation, and competition.

Symbiotic relationships often entail some degree of coadaptation or coevolution of the partners, shaping—at least in part—their structural and behavioral characteristics. An interesting case of mutualistic coadaptation is seen in Central and South American swollen thorn acacias and their symbiotic ants. Acacia ant colonies live within the swollen thorns on the acacia tree branches and feed on two kinds of food provided by the trees: nectar produced in glands at the leaf bases and special protein-rich structures produced on leaflet tips. The acacias thus provide shelter and food for the ants. Although they spend energy to provide these services, the trees are not physically harmed by ant feeding.

What do the acacias get in return? Ants defend their colonies and territories aggressively, and they drive off herbivorous insects that attempt to feed on their home acacia, thus reducing predation on the tree. Ants also trim away vegetation that grows around the tree, thereby reducing competition for water and nutrients. This is a fascinating example of how a symbiotic relationship fits into community interactions. It is also an example of coevolution based on mutualism rather than competition or predation.

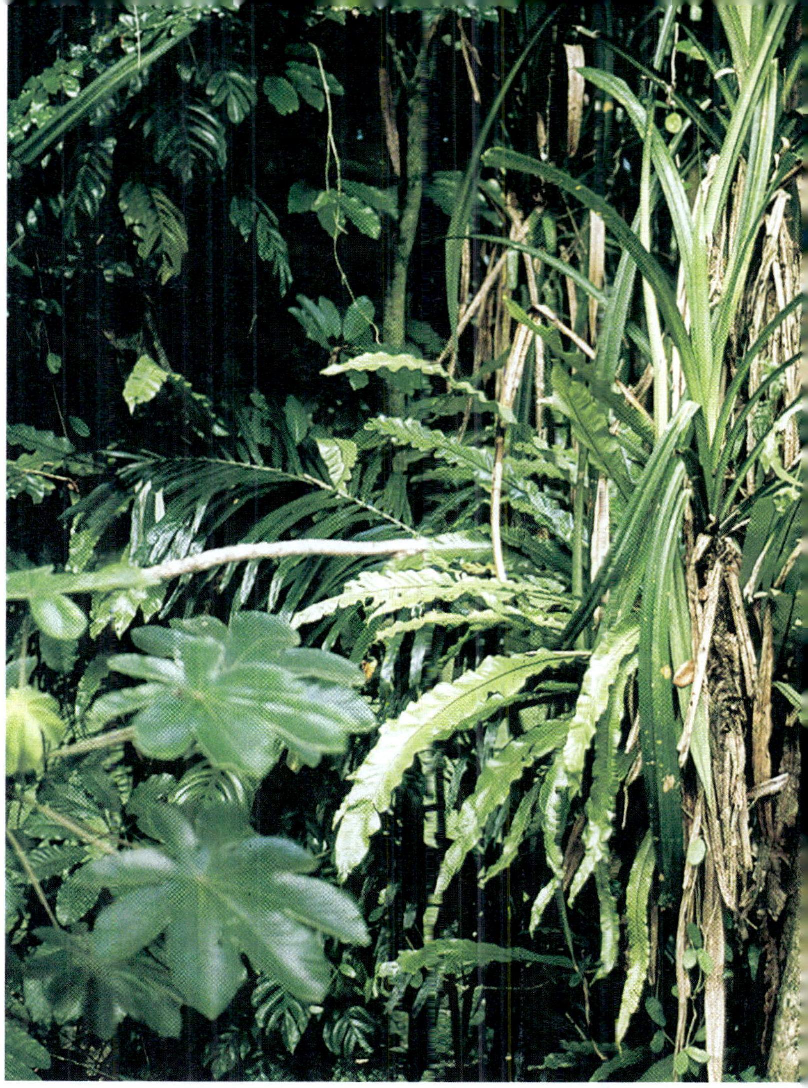

FIGURE 3.12 *Plants compete for light and growing space in this Indonesian rainforest. Epiphytes, such as the ferns and bromeliads shown here, find a place to grow in the forest canopy by perching on the limbs of large trees. This may be a commensal relationship if the epiphytes don't hurt their hosts. Sometimes, however, the weight of the epiphytes breaks off branches and even topples whole trees.*

Defensive Mechanisms

Evolution has produced a bewildering array of ingenious defensive adaptations. Toxic chemicals, body armor, extraordinary speed, and the ability to hide are a few strategies organisms use to protect themselves from competitors or predators. Arthropods, amphibians, snakes, and some mammals, for instance, produce noxious odors or poisonous secretions to induce other species to leave them alone. Poison ivy and stinging nettles use chemicals to discourage you from disturbing them. Often, species possessing these chemical defenses evolve distinctive colors or patterns to warn potential enemies (fig. 3.14).

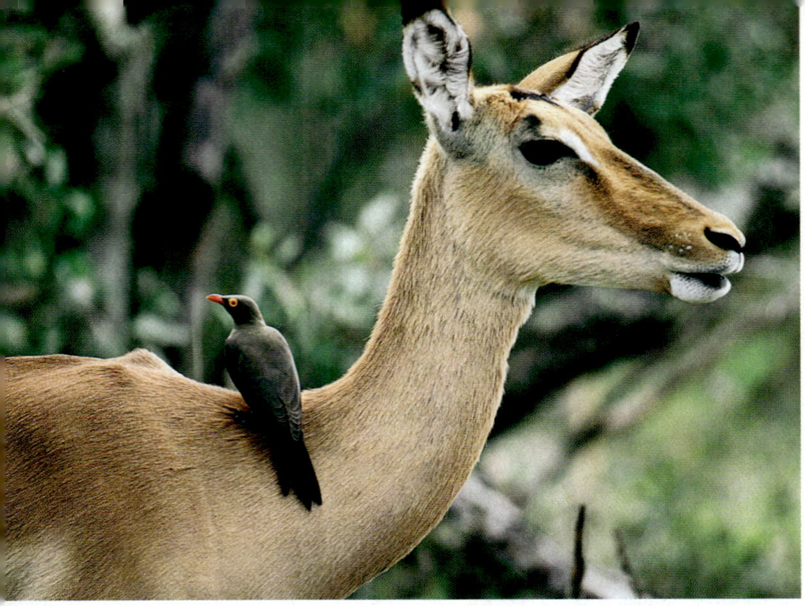

FIGURE 3.13 *A commensal relationship. The red-billed oxpecker benefits by eating parasites, while the impala benefits by being parasite-free.*

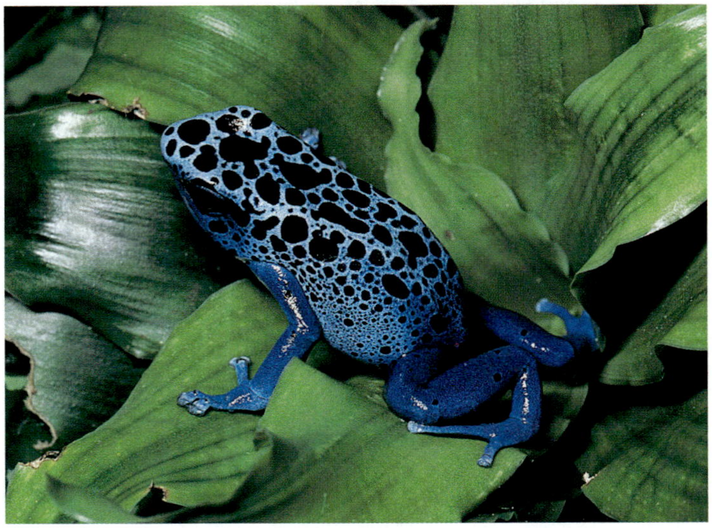

FIGURE 3.14 *Poison arrow frogs of the family* Dendrobatidae *use brilliant colors to warn potential predators of the extremely toxic secretions from their skin. Native people in Latin America use the toxin on blowgun darts.*

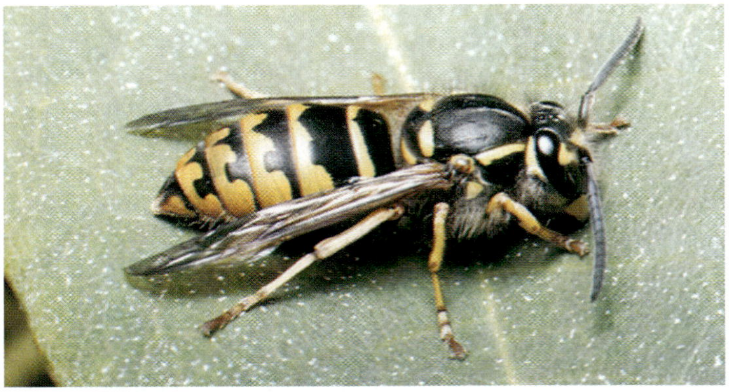

(a)

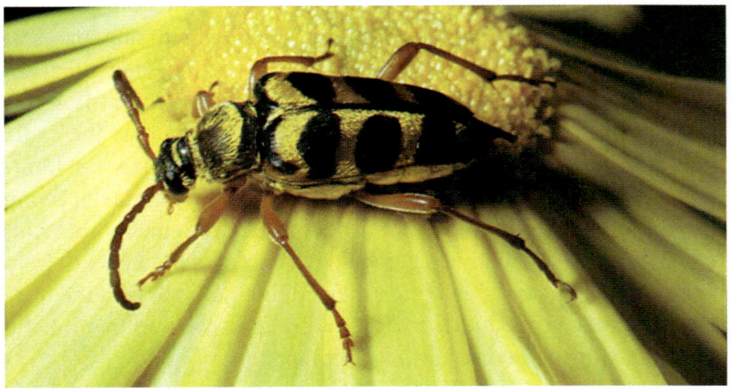

(b)

FIGURE 3.15 *An example of Batesian mimicry.* (a) *This dangerous wasp has bold yellow and black bands to warn away predators.* (b) *The much rarer longhorn beetle has no poisonous stinger but looks and acts like a wasp and thus avoids predators as well.*

Sometimes species that actually are harmless evolve colors, patterns, or body shapes that mimic unpalatable or poisonous species. This is called **Batesian mimicry,** after the English naturalist H. W. Bates, who described the strategy in 1857. Many wasps, for example, have bold patterns of black and yellow stripes to warn off potential predators (fig. 3.15a). The much rarer longhorn beetle has no stinger but looks and acts much like a wasp, tricking predators into avoiding it (fig. 3.15b). Another form of mimicry, called **Müllerian mimicry,** named for the German biologist Fritz Müller, who described it in 1878, involves two species, both of which are unpalatable or dangerous and have evolved to look alike. When predators learn to avoid either species, both benefit.

Species also evolve amazing abilities to avoid being discovered. You may have seen examples of insects that look exactly like dead leaves or twigs to hide from predators. Predators also use camouflage to hide as they lie in wait for their prey. Not all cases of mimicry are to avoid or carry out predation, however. Some tropical orchids have evolved flower structures that look exactly like female flies. Males attempting to mate unwittingly carry away pollen.

Keystone Species

A **keystone species** is a species or group of species whose impact on its community or ecosystem is much larger and more influential than would be expected from mere abundance. Originally, keystone species were thought to be top predators, such as wolves, whose presence limits the abundance of herbivores and thereby reduces their grazing or browsing on plants. Recently, scientists have recognized that less conspicuous species also play essential community roles. Certain tropical figs, for example, bear during seasons when no other fruit is available for frugivores (fruit-eating animals). If these figs were removed, many animals would starve to death during periods of fruit scarcity. With those animals gone, many other plant species that depend on them at other times of the year for pollination and seed dispersal would disappear as well.

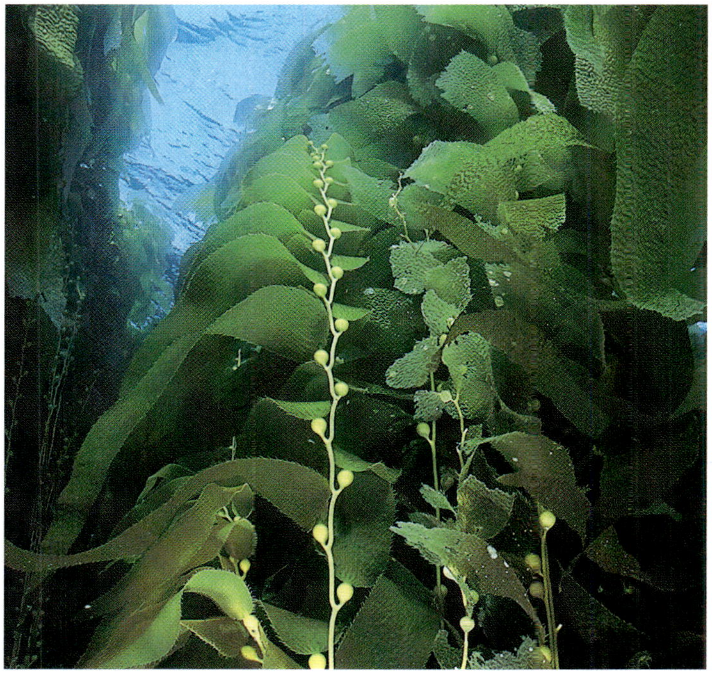

FIGURE 3.16 *Giant kelp is a massive alga that forms dense "forests" off the Pacific coast of California. It is a keystone species in that it provides food, shelter, and structure essential for a whole community. Removal of sea otters allows sea urchin populations to explode. When the urchins destroy the kelp, many other species suffer as well.*

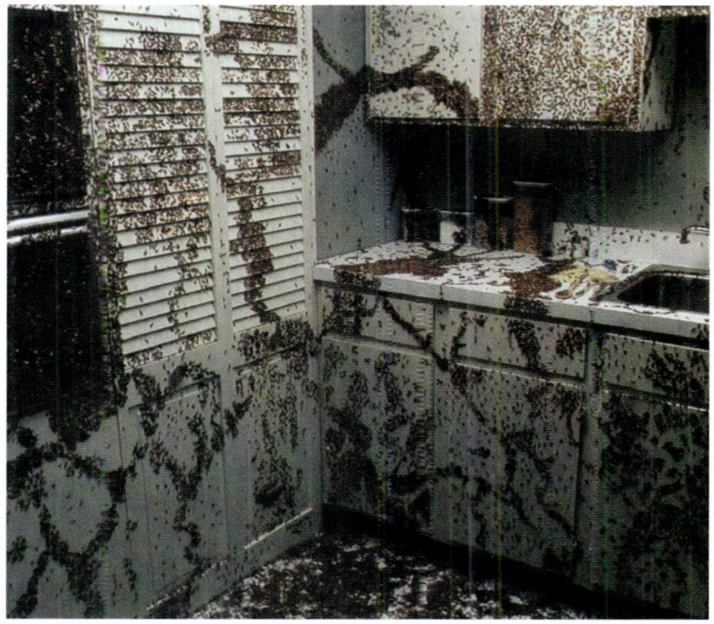

FIGURE 3.17 *High reproductive rates give many organisms the potential to expand populations explosively. The cockroaches in this kitchen could have been produced in only a few generations. A single female cockroach can produce up to 80 eggs every six months. This exhibit is in the Smithsonian Institution's National Museum of Natural History.*

Even microorganisms can play vital roles. In some forest ecosystems, mycorrhizae (fungi associated with tree roots) are essential for mineral mobilization and absorption. If the fungi die, so do the trees and many other species that depend on a healthy forest community. Rather than being a single species, mycorrhizae are actually a group of species that together fulfill a keystone function.

Often a number of species are intricately interconnected in biological communities so that it is difficult to tell which is the essential key. In the kelp "forests" off the California coast, the giant kelp (a kind of algae) provides shelter for many fish and shellfish species and so could be regarded as the key to community structure (fig. 3.16). However, kelp depends on sea otters, which eat the sea urchins that graze on the kelp. Are kelp or otters most important? Each depends on and affects the other. Perhaps we should think in terms of a "keystone set" of organisms in some ecosystems. Some ecological communities are functionally redundant in the sense that, if one important species disappears, another will replace it, and essential ecological functions will continue without much change. Such a community might be said to have no keystone species. We'll discuss the role of keystone species in preserving biodiversity in chapter 5.

POPULATION DYNAMICS

Many biological organisms can produce amazing numbers of offspring, given optimum environmental resources (fig. 3.17). Consider the example of the common fruitfly (*Drosophila melanogaster*). Under ideal conditions, 24 fly generations can be produced in a year. Typically, each female lays 50 to 100 eggs per generation. If one female fly were to lay 100 eggs and if all her offspring lived long enough to reproduce at the same rate with the same survival success, in a single year she would have about 6×10^{40} offspring. That's 60 billion trillion quadrillion insects! If this rate of reproduction continued for a decade, the whole earth would be covered several meters deep in fruitflies. Fortunately for us, fruitfly reproduction, like that of most organisms, is limited by a variety of environmental factors. This example demonstrates, however, the remarkable potential amplification of biological reproduction. Population dynamics describes the changes in number of organisms in a population.

Population Growth

As you learned in chapter 2, a population consists of all the members of a single species living in a specific area at the same time. We call the unrestricted increase in populations **exponential growth** because its rate can be expressed as a constant fraction, or exponent, by which the existing population is multiplied. The mathematical formula for exponential growth is

$$\frac{dN}{dt} = rN$$

That is, the change in numbers of individuals *(dN)* per change in time *(dt)* equals the rate of growth *(r)* times the number of individuals in the population *(N)*. The *r* term is a fraction representing the average individual contribution to population growth. If *r* is positive, the population is increasing. If r is negative, the population is shrinking. If r is zero, there is no change, and $dN / dt = 0$.

This equation for population growth is also referred to as **biotic potential,** the potential of a population to grow if nothing is limiting its expansion. Note that the equation is a very simple *model* (an idealized, simple description of the real world). In reality, many factors prevent most populations from growing at their biotic potential. (The same equation is used to calculate growth in your bank account due to interest rates; unfortunately, many factors also may keep your savings from growing at their potential rate.)

Boom and Bust Population Cycles

A graph of exponential population growth is described as a **J curve** (left portion of fig. 3.18) because of its shape. As you can see in this graph, the number of individuals added to a population at the beginning of an exponential growth curve can be rather small. But within a very short time, the numbers begin to increase quickly because a fixed percentage becomes a much larger amount as the population increases.

In the real world, however, there are limits to growth. We call the maximum number of individuals of any species that can be supported by a particular ecosystem on a sustainable basis the **carrying capacity.** When a population **overshoots,** or surpasses the carrying capacity of its environment, death rates begin to surpass birth rates. The growth curve becomes negative rather than positive, and the population may decrease as fast as, or faster than, it grew. We call this dieback a population crash. Populations may go through repeated oscillating cycles of population growth and decline as shown in fig. 3.18. These cycles may be very regular if they depend on a few simple factors, such as the seasonal light- and temperature-dependent bloom of algae in a lake. They also may be very irregular if they depend on complex environmental and biotic relationships that control cycles, such as the outbreaks of migratory locusts in the desert or tent caterpillars in northern forests. We call long periods of low population size followed by a sudden population explosion irruptive growth.

Sometimes predator and prey populations oscillate in a sort of synchrony with each other, as shown in fig. 3.19. This is a classic study of the number of furs taken into Hudson Bay Company trading posts in Canada between 1840 and 1930. As you can see, the numbers of Canada lynx fluctuate on about a ten-year cycle that is similar to, but slightly out of phase with, the population peaks of snowshoe hares. When the hare population is high and food is plentiful, lynx reproduction is very successful, and lynx populations grow rapidly. Eventually, declining food supplies limit hare populations. For a while lynx populations continue to grow because starving hares are easier to catch than healthy ones. As hares become more scarce, however, so do the lynx. When hares are at their lowest levels, food supplies recover and population growth of both prey and predator begins again. This predator-prey oscillation is known as the Lotka-Volterra model, after the scientists who first described it mathematically.

Growth to a Stable Population

Not all biological populations go through cycles of exponential overshoot and catastrophic diebacks. Many species are regulated by both internal and external factors, so that they come into equilibrium with their environmental resources and maintain relatively stable population sizes. These species may grow exponentially when resources are unlimited, but their growth slows as they approach the carrying capacity of the environment. This pattern is called **logistic growth** because of its constantly changing rate.

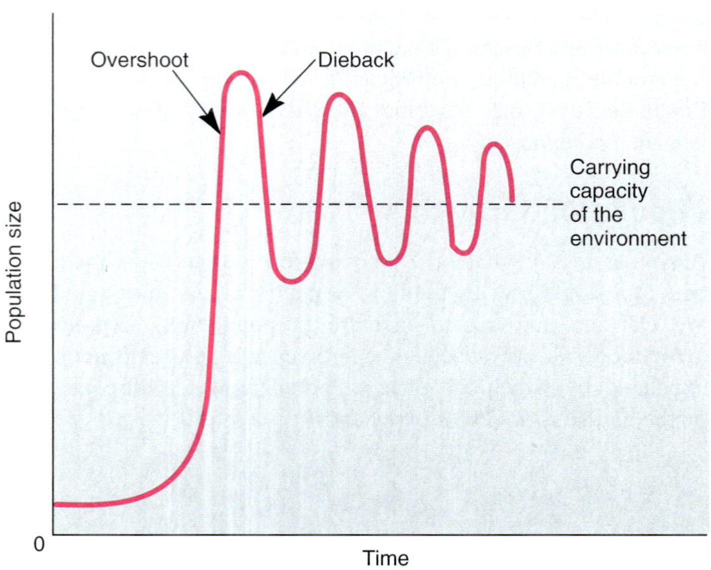

FIGURE 3.18 *Population oscillations. Some species demonstrate a pattern of cyclic overshoot and dieback.*

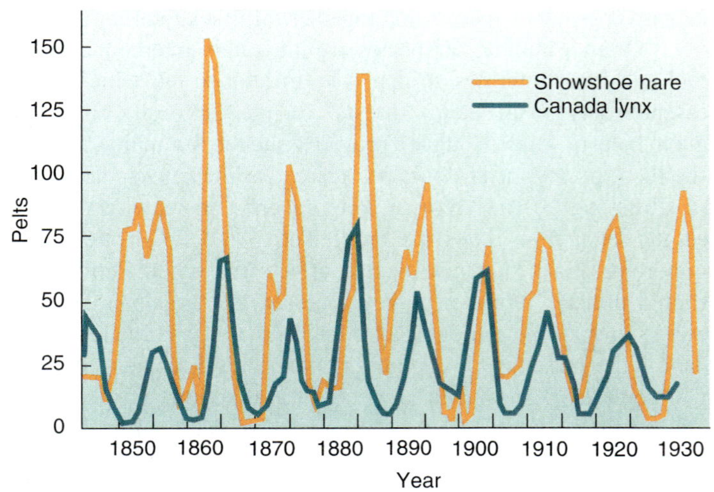

FIGURE 3.19 *Oscillations in the population of snowshoe hare and lynx in Canada suggest the close interdependency of this prey-predator relationship. These data are based on the number of pelts received by the Hudson Bay Company. Both predator and prey show a ten-year cycle in population growth and decline.*

Source: Data from D. A. MacLulich. *Fluctuations in the Numbers of the Varying Hare (Lepus americus).* Toronto: University of Toronto Press, 1937, reprinted 1974.

Mathematically, this growth pattern is described by the following equation, which adds a term for carrying capacity (K) to the biotic potential growth equation:

$$\frac{dN}{dt} = rN\left(1 - \frac{N}{K}\right)$$

This equation says that the change in numbers over time (dN/dt) equals the exponential growth rate (r times N) times the portion of the carrying capacity (K) represented by the population size (N). The term $(1 - N/K)$ represents the relationship between N at any given time step and K, the number of individuals the environment can support. If N is less than K—say, 100, compared with 120—then $(1 - N/K)$ is a positive number $(1 - 100/120 = 0.17)$, and population growth, dN/dt, is slow but positive. If N is greater than K; that is, if the population is greater than the environment can support, then $(1 - N/K)$ is a negative number. For example, if N is 150 and K is 120, then $(1 - N/K)$ is $(1 - 150/120)$, which is equal to $(1 - 1.25)$, or -0.25. In this case, the growth rate is negative. The logistic growth model, then, describes a population that decreases if its numbers exceed carrying capacity.

How does the growth curve of a stable population differ from the J curve of an exploding population? Figure 3.20 shows an idealized comparison between exponential and logistic growth.

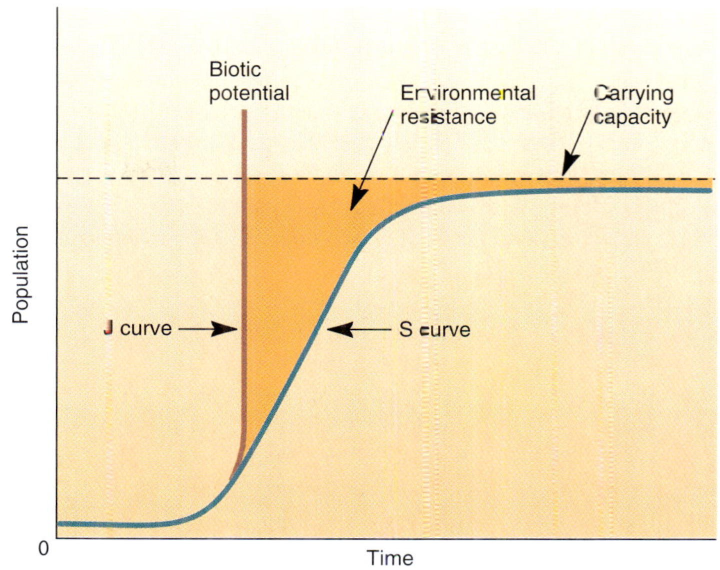

FIGURE 3.20 *J and S population curves. The J curve represents theoretical unlimited growth. The S curve represents population growth and stabilization in response to environmental resistance.*

APPLICATION:	Calculate Population Growth

Think of exponential growth as occurring in time steps. Start with ten cockroaches that can produce enough young to increase at a rate of 150 percent per month ($r = 1.5$). Calculate the number of roaches after seven time steps: for each t, multiply r times the N of the previous time step (round N to the nearest whole number). Then graph the results.

$t = 0$ (start): $N = 10$

$t = 1$: $N = 1.5 \times 10 = 15$

$t = 2$: $N = 1.5 \times 15 = 22$

$t = 3$: $N = 1.5 \times 22 =$ ____

$t = 4$: $N = 1.5 \times$ ____ $=$ ____

$t = 5$: $N = 1.5 \times$ ____ $=$ ____

$t = 6$: $N = 1.5 \times$ ____ $=$ ____

$t = 7$: $N = 1.5 \times$ ____ $=$ ____

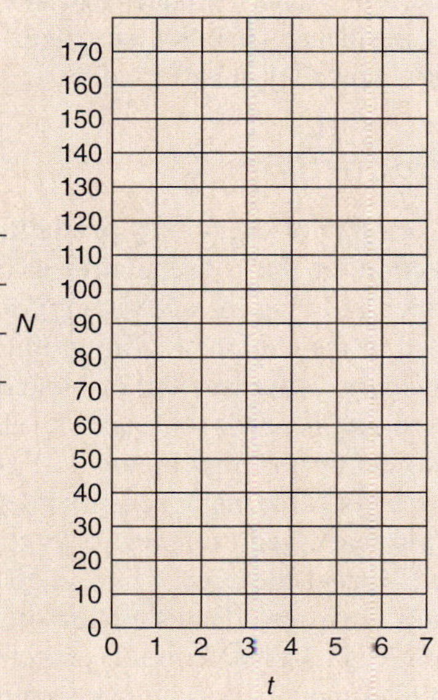

Answer: The final graph should be a J-shaped curve.

The J curve on the left in this figure represents the growth without restraint toward the biotic potential, or the maximum number a species might possibly attain. The curve to the right represents logistic growth. We call this later pattern an **S curve** or a sigmoidal curve (for the Greek letter sigma).

Limiting Factors

In many species, population growth is regulated by both internal and external factors. Maturity, body size, and hormonal status are examples of internal factors. Habitat and food availability and interactions with other organisms are examples of external factors. Some of these limits are dependent on population density. Food and water, for example, become more limited as populations grow. Disease, stress, and exposure to predators or parasites can all increase mortality rates as populations increase. These factors are called *density-dependent.*

Other limits to growth are *density-independent.* Many of these factors are abiotic: drought or early frost can reduce populations of mosquitoes drastically, regardless of how many mosquitoes there were to start with. Habitat destruction—because of floods, landslides, or human activities—can also limit population growth.

Together, factors that tend to reduce population growth rates are called **environmental resistance.** The area between the two curves in figure 3.20 is the cumulative effect of environmental resistance. Note that the resistance becomes larger and the rate of logistic growth becomes smaller as the population approaches the carrying capacity of the environment.

K-adapted and *r*-adapted Species

Some organisms, such as dandelions, persist by depending on a high rate of reproduction and growth (rN). These organisms are described as **r-adapted species.** They tend to have rapid reproduction and high mortality of offspring, and they may frequently overshoot carrying capacity and die back. Other organisms tend to reproduce more slowly as they approach the carrying capacity (*K*) of their environment. These species are referred to as ***K*-adapted species.**

Many species don't fit neatly into either exponential (*r*-adapted) or logistic (*K*-adapted) growth patterns. Still, it's useful to contrast the advantages and disadvantages of some organisms at the extremes of a continuum of growth patterns. Although we should avoid implying intention in natural systems, it sometimes helps us see these differences in terms of "strategies" of adaptation and "logic" in different modes of reproduction.

Organisms with *r*-adapted, or exponential, growth patterns tend to occupy low trophic levels in their ecosystems (see chapter 2) or to be successional pioneers. As generalists or opportunists, they move quickly into disturbed environments, grow rapidly, mature early, and produce many offspring. They usually do little to care for their offspring or protect them from predation. They depend on sheer numbers and dispersal mechanisms to ensure that some offspring survive to adulthood. They have little investment in individual offspring, using their energy to produce vast numbers instead (table 3.2).

A female clam, for example, can release up to 1 million eggs over her lifetime. As the eggs drift away on water currents, they are entirely on their own. The mother clam can neither protect them from predators nor help them find food or a place to live. The vast majority of all young clams die before reaching maturity, but if even a few survive, the species will continue. Many marine invertebrates, parasites, insects, rodents, and annual plants follow this reproductive strategy. Predators and other external factors generally limit their numbers. Also included in this group are the weeds, pests, and other species we consider nuisances that reproduce profusely, adapt quickly to environmental change, and survive under a broad range of conditions.

So-called *K*-adapted organisms are usually larger, live longer, mature more slowly, produce fewer offspring in each generation, and have fewer natural predators than the species below them in the ecological hierarchy. Elephants, for example, are not reproductively mature until they are 18 to 20 years old. During youth and adolescence, a young elephant is part of a complex extended family that cares for it, protects it, and teaches it how to behave. A female elephant normally conceives only once every 4 or 5 years after she matures. The gestation period is about 18 months; thus, an elephant herd doesn't produce many babies in a given year. Since elephants have few enemies and live a long life (often 60 or 70 years), however, this low reproductive rate usually produces enough elephants to keep the population stable, given appropriate environmental conditions.

Think of how you would categorize some other familiar animals in terms of reproductive strategies. Are ants, bald eagles, cheetahs, clams, squirrels, and sharks *K*- or *r*-adapted?

An important underlying question to much of the discussion in this book is which of these strategies humans follow. Do we more closely resemble wolves and elephants in our population growth, or does our population growth pattern more closely resemble that of moose and rabbits? Will we overshoot our environment's carrying capacity (or are we already doing so), or will our population growth come into balance with our resources?

TABLE 3.2 Reproductive Strategies

r-ADAPTED SPECIES	*K*-ADAPTED SPECIES
1. Short life	1. Long life
2. Rapid growth	2. Slower growth
3. Early maturity	3. Late maturity
4. Many, small offspring	4. Few, large offspring
5. Little parental care and protection	5. High parental care or protection
6. Little investment in individual offspring	6. High investment in individual offspring
7. Adapted to unstable environment	7. Adapted to stable environment
8. Pioneers, colonizers	8. Later stages of succession
9. Niche generalists	9. Niche specialists
10. Prey	10. Predators
11. Regulated mainly by intrinsic factors	11. Regulated mainly by extrinsic factors
12. Low trophic level	12. High trophic level

COMMUNITY PROPERTIES

The processes and principles that we have studied thus far in this chapter—tolerance limits, species interactions, resource partitioning, evolution, and adaptation—play important roles in determining the characteristics of populations and species. In this section, we will look at some fundamental properties of biological communities and ecosystems—productivity, abundance and diversity, complexity, resilience, stability, structure, and edges and boundaries—to learn how they are affected by these factors.

Productivity

A community's **primary productivity** is the rate of biomass production, or the conversion of solar energy into chemical energy stored in living (or once-living) organisms. Since much energy is used in respiration, a more useful term is often *net primary productivity,* or the amount of biomass stored after respiration. Productivity depends on light levels, temperature, moisture, and nutrient availability. Figure 3.21 shows approximate productivity levels for some major ecosystems. As you can see, tropical forests, coral reefs, and estuaries (bays or inundated river valleys where rivers meet the ocean) have high levels of productivity because they have abundant supplies of all the required resources. In deserts, lack of water limits photosynthesis. On the arctic tundra or in high mountains, low temperatures inhibit plant growth. In the open ocean, a lack of nutrients reduces the ability of algae to make use of plentiful sunshine and water.

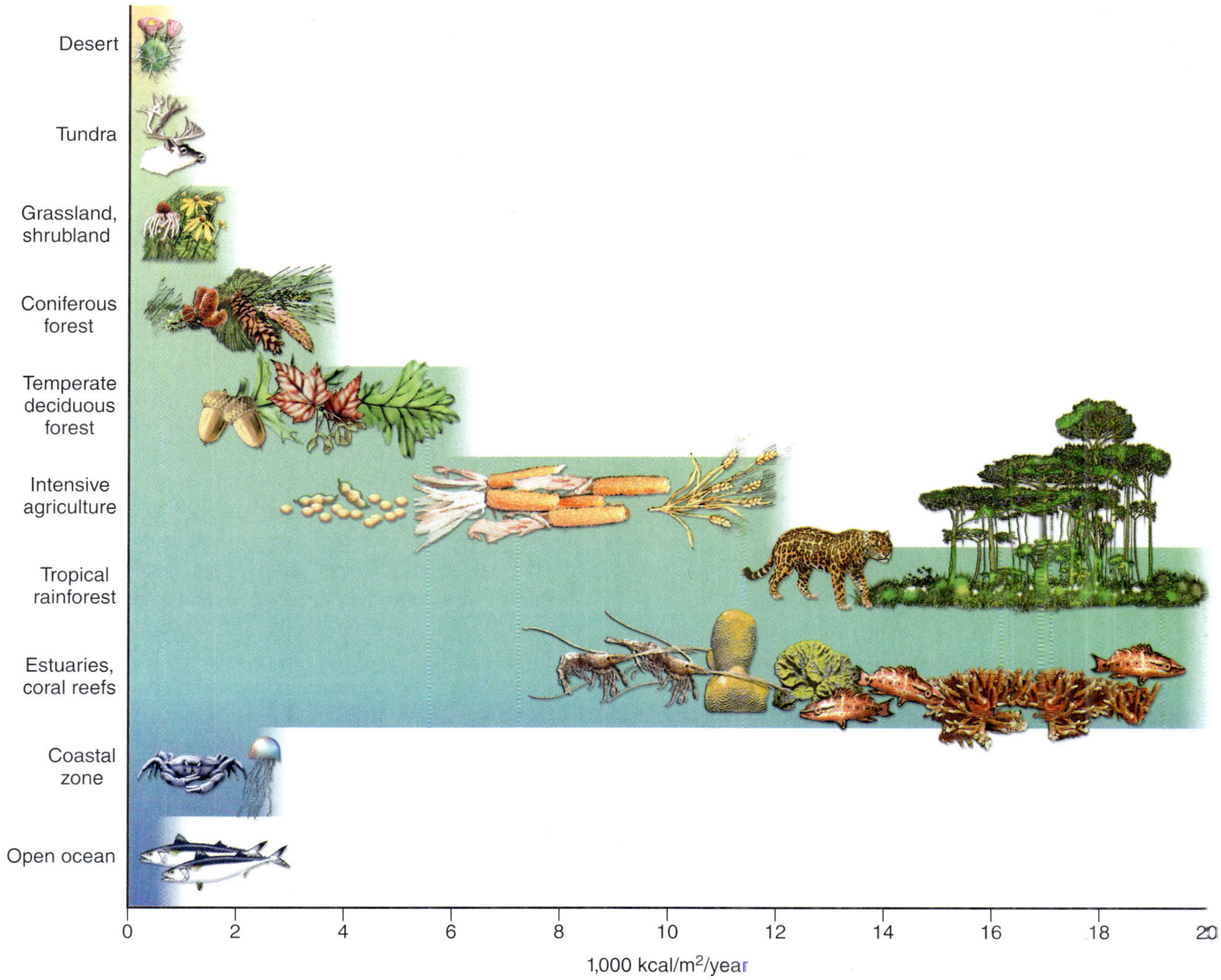

FIGURE 3.21 *Relative biomass accumulation of major world ecosystems. Only plants and some bacteria capture solar energy. Animals consume biomass to build their own bodies.*

Even the most photosynthetically active ecosystems capture only a small percentage of the available sunlight and use it to make energy-rich compounds. In a temperate-climate oak forest, leaves absorb only about half the available light on a midsummer day. Of this absorbed energy, 99 percent is used to evaporate water in respiration and cooling. A large oak tree can transpire (evaporate) several thousand liters of water on a warm, dry, sunny day, while making only a few kilograms of sugars and other energy-rich organic compounds.

Abundance and Diversity

Abundance is an expression of the number of individuals of a species in an area. **Diversity** is the number of different species in an area. Diversity is also a useful measure of the variety of ecological niches or genetic variation in a community. Communities with high diversity often have low abundance of most species. As a general rule, diversity decreases as we go from the equator toward the poles, but abundance of a smaller number of species increases. The Arctic has a vast abundance of mosquitoes, for example, but relatively few other insect species. The tropics, on the other hand, have vast numbers of insect species—some of which have incredibly bizarre forms and habits—but often only a few individuals of any particular species in a given area.

Bird populations also vary dramatically with latitude. Greenland is home to 56 species of breeding birds, while Colombia, which is only one-fifth the size of Greenland, has 1,395. Why are there so many species in Colombia and so few in Greenland? Climate and history are important factors. Greenland has such a harsh climate that the need to survive through the winter or escape to milder climates becomes the single most important critical factor that overwhelms all other considerations and severely limits the ability of species to specialize or differentiate into new forms. Furthermore, because glaciers covered Greenland until about 10,000 years ago, new species have had little time to develop.

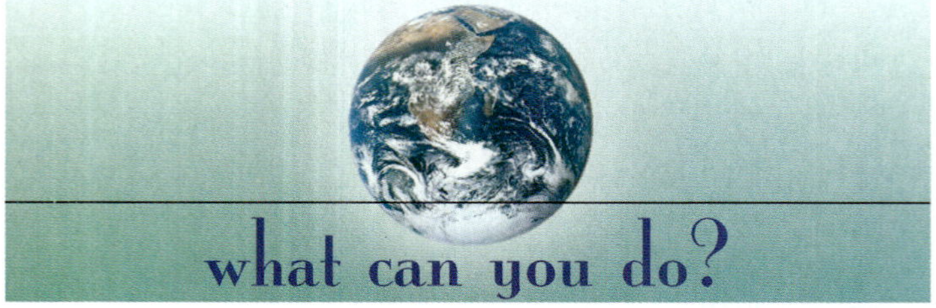

what can you do?

Developing a Sense for Where You Live

One of the first steps toward conserving biological diversity is to educate yourself. The more you know, the more you can share your knowledge—and skills—to help the natural world. Look for answers to questions such as these:

- What ecosystems and biological communities existed in your area before European settlement?
- What impact, if any, did indigenous people have on the flora and fauna of your area?
- What are the dominant species (besides humans) in your neighborhood? Where did they originate?
- How much rain falls in your region each year? Is precipitation seasonal? Is water a limiting factor for biological communities?
- What are the seasonal high and low temperatures where you live? How do native plants and animals adapt to seasonal variations?
- Is there a keystone species or group of species especially important in determining the structure and functions of your local ecosystems? What factors might threaten those keystone components?
- Where do your drinking water, food, and energy come from? What local and regional environmental impacts are caused by production, use, and disposal of those resources? Could you lessen those impacts by changing your sources or use patterns of resources?
- Is there a park or wildlife refuge near where you live? Does it contain any rare, threatened, or endangered species? What makes them rare, threatened, or endangered?
- Are there opportunities for volunteer work to improve your local environment, such as planting native species, cleaning up a river or lake, restoring a wetland, recycling trash, or helping maintain a refuge or park?

Many areas in the tropics, by contrast, have relatively abundant rainfall and warm temperatures year-round, so that ecosystems there are highly productive. The year-round availability of food, moisture, and warmth supports a great exuberance of life and allows a high degree of specialization in physical shape and behavior. Coral reefs are similarly stable, productive, and conducive to proliferation of diverse and exotic life-forms. The enormous abundance of brightly colored and fantastically shaped fish, corals, sponges, and arthropods in the reef community is one of the best examples we have of community diversity.

Productivity is related to abundance and diversity (both of which depend on total resource availability in an ecosystem), as well as the reliability of resources, the adaptations of the member species, and the interactions between species. You shouldn't assume that all communities are perfectly suited to their environment. A relatively new community that hasn't had time for niche specialization, or a disturbed one where roles such as top predators are missing, may not achieve maximum efficiency of resource use or reach its maximum level of either abundance or diversity. We will discuss the importance of biodiversity and abundance further in chapter 5.

Complexity, Resilience, and Stability

Community complexity involves diversity and community functions. **Complexity** in ecological terms refers to the number of species at each trophic level and the number of trophic levels in a community. A diverse community may not be very complex if all of its species are clustered in only a few trophic levels and form a relatively simple food chain.

A complex, highly interconnected community might have many trophic levels, some of which can be compartmentalized into subdivisions (fig. 3.22). In tropical rainforests, for instance, herbivores can be grouped into "guilds," based on the specialized ways they feed on plants. There may be fruit-eaters, leaf-nibblers, root-borers, seed-gnawers, and sap-suckers—each composed of species of very different size, shape, and even biological kingdom but that feed in related ways. A highly interconnected community such as this can form a very elaborate food web.

How is complexity related to stability in an ecosystem and to resilience (the ability to recover from disturbance)? Ecologists have debated this question for many years. We can identify three kinds of stability or resiliency in ecosystems: (1) constancy (lack of fluctuations in composition or functions), (2) inertia (resistance to perturbations), and (3) renewal (ability to repair damage after disturbance).

In 1955 Robert MacArthur, who was then a graduate student at Yale, proposed that, the more complex and interconnected a community is, the more stable and resilient it is in the face of disturbance. If many different species occupy each trophic level, some can fill in if others are stressed or eliminated by external forces, making the whole community resistant to perturbations and able to recover relatively easily from disruptions. On the other hand, in a diverse and highly specialized ecosystem, removal of a few keystone members can eliminate many other associated species. Eliminating a major tree species from a tropical forest, for example, may destroy pollinators and fruit distributors as well. We might replant the trees, but could we replace the whole web of relationships on which they depend? In this case, diversity makes the forest less resilient, rather than more. This relationship between diversity and stability remains controversial (see Case Study, p. 66).

Community Structure

Ecological structure refers to patterns of spatial distribution of individuals and populations within a community, as well as the relation of a particular community to its surroundings. At the local level, even in a relatively homogeneous environment, individuals in a single population can be distributed randomly, clumped together, or in highly regular patterns (fig. 3.23). In randomly arranged populations, individuals live wherever resources are

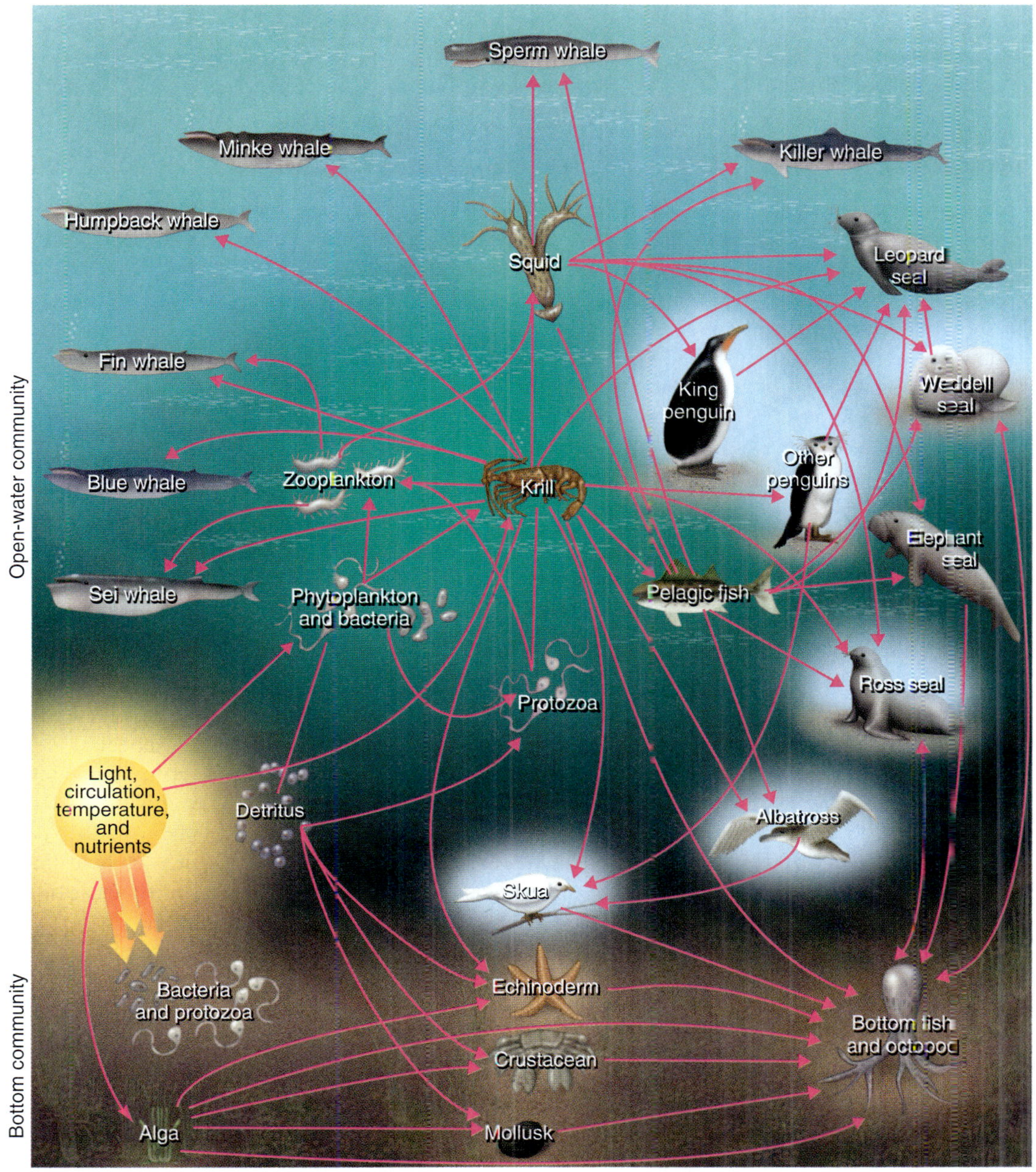

FIGURE 3.22 *A complex and highly interconnected community can have many species at each trophic level and many relationships, as this Antarctic marine food web illustrates.*

available. Ordered patterns may be determined by the physical environment but are more often the result of biological competition. For example, competition for nesting space in a penguin colony is often fierce. Each nest tends to be just out of reach of the neighbors sitting on their own nests. Constant squabbling produces a highly regular pattern. Similarly, sagebrush releases toxins from roots and fallen leaves, which inhibit the growth of competitors and create a circle of bare ground around each bush. As neighbors fill in empty spaces up to the limit of this chemical barrier, a regular spacing results.

Some other species cluster together for protection, mutual assistance, reproduction, or access to a particular environmental resource (fig. 3.23c). Dense schools of fish, for instance, cluster closely together in the ocean, increasing their chances of detecting and escaping predators (fig. 3.24). Similarly, predators, whether sharks, wolves, or humans, often hunt in packs to catch their prey. A flock of blackbirds descending on a cornfield or a troop of baboons traveling across the African savanna band together both to avoid predators and to find food more efficiently.

Plants can cluster for protection, as well. A grove of wind-sheared evergreen trees is often found packed tightly together at the crest of a high mountain or along the seashore. They offer mutual protection from the wind not only to each other but also to other creatures that find shelter in or under their branches.

CASE STUDY

BIODIVERSITY AND STABILITY

Is a more diverse community more stable and resilient in the face of environmental stress? This has been an ongoing debate among ecologists. One of the important contributors to the debate has been experimental ecologist David Tilman. Since 1982 Tilman and his colleagues have been studying the effects of nitrogen fertilization on grassland plots. Initially, Tilman's goal was to study the effect of fertilizer on regenerating grass on abandoned farm fields and natural oak savannas in central Minnesota. The experimental design was to randomly assign different fertilizer treatments to a set of sample plots on old fields and natural savannas. Study plots varied considerably in species diversity: some contained only 1 species, some had as many as 26. Using the same set of sample plots for over two decades, Tilman and his colleagues—and platoons of student assistants—carefully gathered, counted, and weighed all the plants growing on the plots. The result has been a long record of highly detailed data.

In a fortuitous turn of events, an extreme case of environmental stress occurred 6 years into the experiment. The summer of 1988 was the hottest, driest summer in 50 years. When researchers tallied up the total plant productivity on the study plots that year, they found that the plots with the most species suffered much less than those with few species. On species-rich plots, drought-tolerant plants still grew, while more sensitive species languished. By contrast, the most species-poor plots had only about one-eighth their predrought productivity.

In subsequent years, the species-poor plots also took longer to recover from the drought. Ability to recover from stress—resilience—is an important factor in ecosystem stability.

The idea that biodiversity increases ecosystem stability is one that ecologists have long believed was true but that they have had difficulty proving. Many field researchers have concluded that complex communities are more stable, but their evidence has been ambiguous because natural environments have so many simultaneously changing variables. Other field ecologists have found simple systems to be very stable and resilient, depending on the types of organisms present. Mathematical models have suggested that simple communities of a few generalist species can be more stable than more complex assemblages of specialists. Experiments such as Tilman's, with long-term data gathering on a set of controlled sample plots, provide an important type of evidence to the debate. Experimental data are relatively controlled—reducing the number of simultaneously changing variables of a natural system—but they are more realistic (and often more convincing) than computer models.

Ecologists continue to dispute whether it is the variety of organisms in a community, the particular type of organisms, or both that control ecosystem stability and resilience, but experiments such as Tilman's provide important contributions to the discussion. This work also shows the value of careful, long-term record keeping in science. This work was carried out on one of 18 Long-Term Ecological Research sites, funded by the National Science Foundation precisely to allow long-term monitoring of ecological systems. Tilman's work also shows the importance of attention to unexpected implications of your research. As Louis Pasteur said, "Chance favors the prepared mind." In this case, the 1988 drought provided an unexpected opportunity to explore critical questions about stability and resilience.

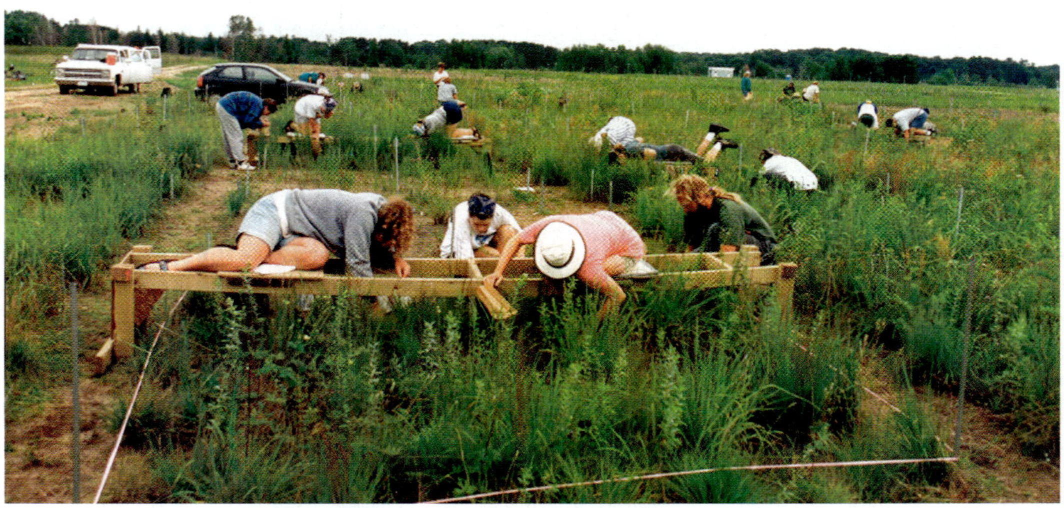

Student interns weed experimental biodiversity plots at Cedar Creek Natural History Area in Minnesota.

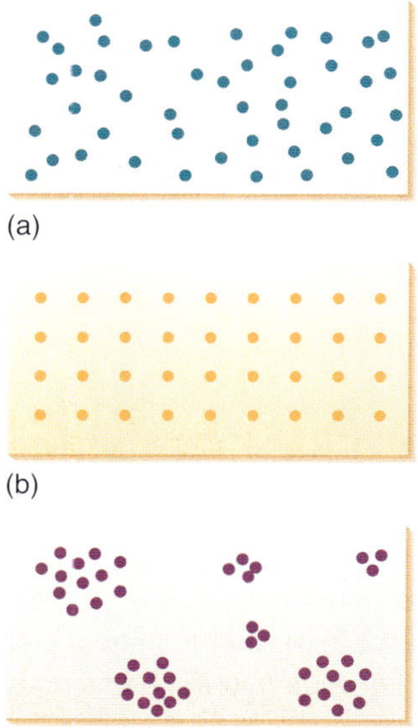

FIGURE 3.23 *Distribution of members of a population in a given space can be* (a) *random,* (b) *ordered, or* (c) *clustered. The physical environment and biological interactions determine these patterns. The patterns may produce a graininess or patchiness in community structure.*

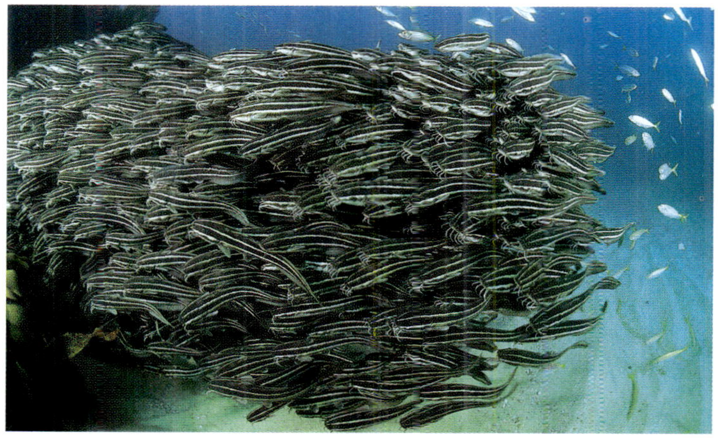

FIGURE 3.24 *Fish and birds often flock in dense groups for protection or mutual feeding.*

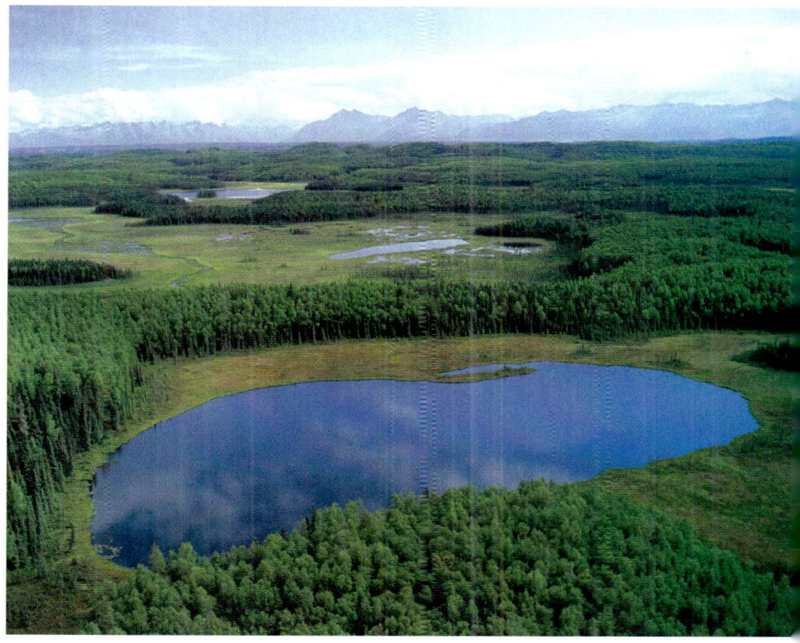

FIGURE 3.25 *Ecological edges are known as ecotones, as seen here between lake/wetland and wetland/forest. Temperature, wind, and humidity differ at the edges in a landscape. Edge conditions do extend into patches of habitat. Small or linear fragments may be mostly edge.*

Most environments are patchy at some scale. Organisms cluster or disperse according to patchy availability of water, nutrients, or other resources. Distribution in a community can be vertical as well as horizontal. The tropical forest, for instance, has many layers, each with different environmental conditions and combinations of species. Distinct communities of smaller plants, animals, and microbes live at different levels. Similarly, aquatic communities are often stratified into layers based on light penetration in the water, temperature, salinity, pressure, or other factors.

Edges and Boundaries

An important aspect of community structure is the boundary between one habitat and its neighbors. We call these relationships edge effects. Sometimes the edge of a patch of habitat is relatively sharp and distinct. In moving from a woodland patch into a grassland or cultivated field, you sense a dramatic change from the cool, dark, quiet forest interior to the windy, sunny, warmer, open space of the field or pasture. In other cases, one habitat type may intergrade very gradually into another, so that there is no distinct border.

Ecologists call the boundaries between adjacent communities **ecotones** (fig. 3.25). Ecotones are often rich in species diversity because individuals from both environments occupy the boundary area. In addition, many species actively occupy an ecotone, taking advantage of resources in both environments. White-tailed deer, for example, browse in open fields but hide in forest cover.

Other species avoid edges and ecotones and prefer interior environments. Spotted owls of the Pacific Northwest, for example, nest only in the forest "core," relatively deep, cool rainforest. **Edge effects**, the environmental and biotic conditions on the edges, may extend hundreds of meters into a forest fragment. In a rainforest, edges are sunnier, drier, hotter, and more susceptible to storm damage than the interior. Edges also have a different set of predators and competitors than does the forest core. These conditions discourage spotted owls from nesting near edges.

Depending on how far edge effects extend from the boundary, differently shaped habitat patches may have very dissimilar amounts of interior area (fig. 3.26). If edge effects extended 200 m into a forest, a 40-acre square block (400 m^2) surrounded by clearcut would have no true core habitat at all.

Many popular game animals, such as white-tailed deer and pheasants that are adapted to human disturbance, are most plentiful

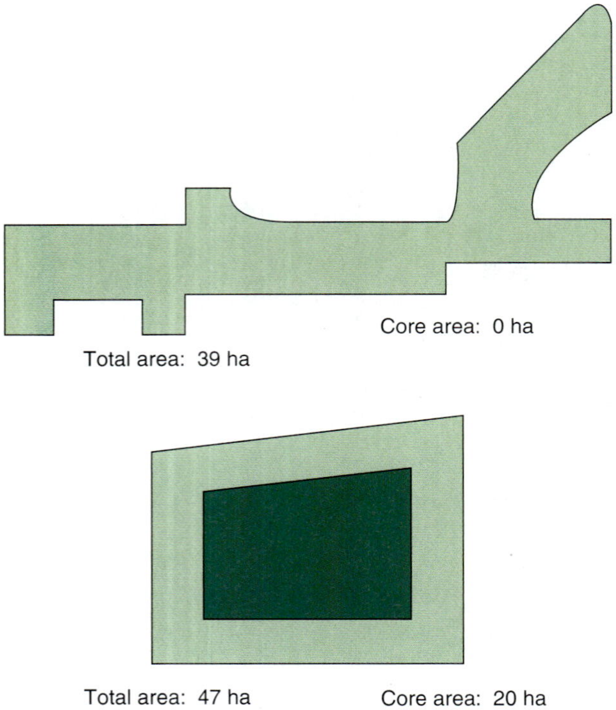

FIGURE 3.26 *Shape can be as important as size in small preserves. While these areas are similar in size, no place in the top figure is far enough from the edge to have characteristics of core habitat, while the bottom patch has a significant core.*

in boundary zones between different types of habitat. Game managers once were urged to develop as much edge as possible to promote large game populations. Today, however, most wildlife conservationists recognize that the edge effects associated with habitat fragmentation are generally detrimental to biodiversity. Preserving large habitat blocks and linking smaller blocks with migration corridors may be a good way to protect some rare and endangered species. (See chapter 6; see also related story, "Where Have All the Songbirds Gone?" at www.mhhe.com/cases.)

COMMUNITIES IN TRANSITION

So far, our view of communities has focused on the day-to-day interactions of organisms with their environments, set in a context of survival and selection. In this section, we'll step back to look at some transitional aspects of communities, including where communities meet and how communities change over time.

Ecological Succession

Biological communities have a history in a given landscape. The process by which organisms occupy a site and gradually change environmental conditions by creating soil, shade, or shelter or by increasing humidity is called ecological succession or development. **Primary succession** occurs when a community begins to develop on a site previously unoccupied by living organisms, such as an island, a sand or silt bed, a body of water, or a new volcanic flow (fig. 3.27). **Secondary succession** occurs when an existing community is disrupted and a new one subsequently develops at the site. The disruption may be caused by a natural catastrophe, such as fire or flooding, or by a human activity, such as deforesta-

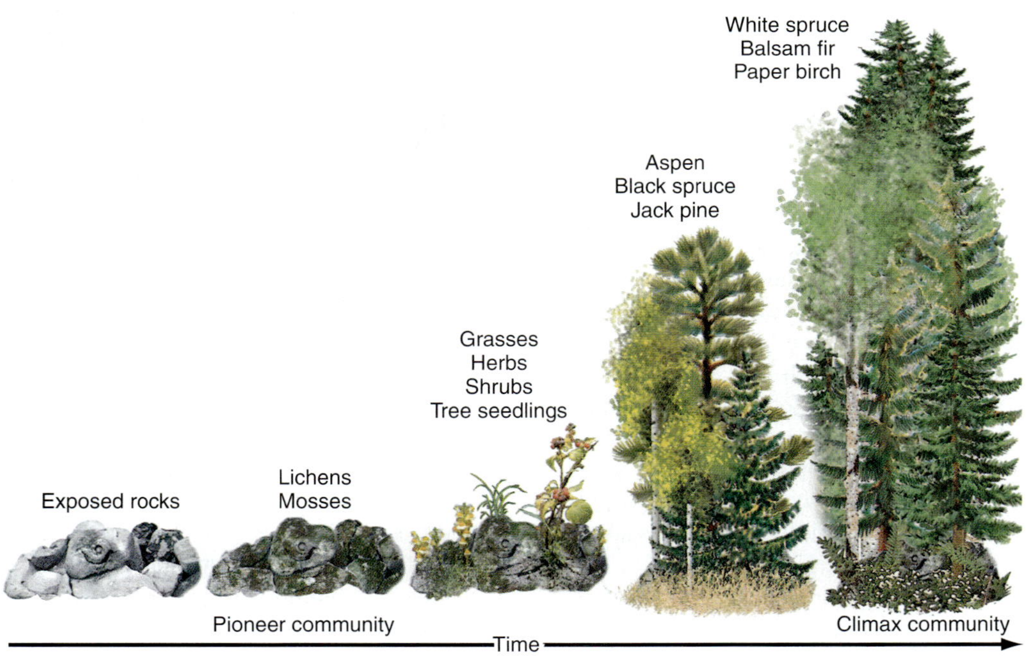

FIGURE 3.27 *One example of primary succession, shown in five stages* (left to right). *Here, bare rocks are colonized by lichens and mosses, which trap moisture and build soil for grasses, shrubs, and eventually trees.*

tion, plowing, or mining. In each case, organisms modify the environment in ways that allow one species to replace another.

In primary succession on a terrestrial site, the new site first is colonized by a few hardy **pioneer species,** often microbes, mosses, and lichens that can withstand harsh conditions and lack of resources. Their bodies create patches of organic matter. Debris accumulates in pockets and crevices, providing soil in which seeds can become lodged and grow. We call this process of environmental modification by organisms **ecological development** or facilitation. The community of organisms often becomes more diverse and increasingly competitive as development continues and new niche opportunities appear. The pioneer species gradually disappear as the environment changes and new species combinations replace the preceding community.

Examples of secondary succession are easy to find. Observe an abandoned farm field or a clear-cut forest (fig. 3.28) in a temperate climate. The bare soil first is colonized by rapidly growing annual plants (those that grow, flower, and die the same year) that have light, wind-blown seeds and can tolerate full sunlight and exposed soil. They are followed and replaced by perennial plants (those that live for several to many years), including grasses, flowering plants, shrubs, and trees. As in primary succession, plant species progressively change the environmental conditions. Biomass accumulates and the site becomes richer, better able to capture and store moisture, more sheltered from wind and climate change, and biologically more complex. Species that cannot survive in a bare, dry, sunny, open area find shelter and food as the field turns to prairie or forest.

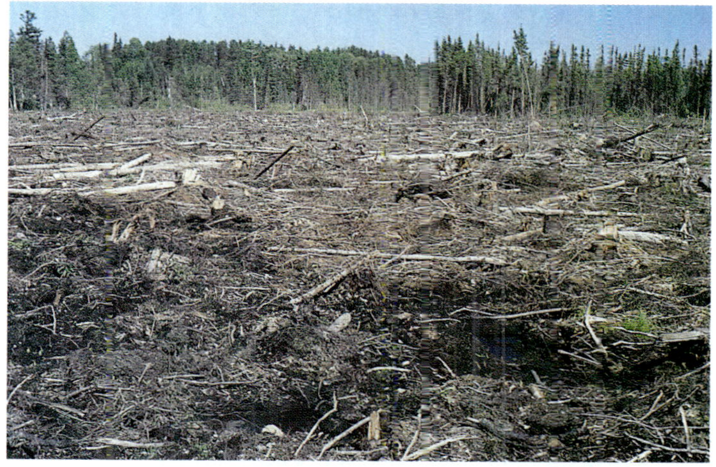

FIGURE 3.28 *Clear-cutting and burning have turned what was once a cool, shady black spruce bog into a dry, sunny, barren opening in which few of the former residents can survive. Secondary succession may eventually restore conditions, given enough time.*

Climax Communities or Individualistic Succession?

Eventually, in either primary or secondary succession, many communities reach a state that resists further change. Fifty years ago, ecologists called this a mature or climax community because it appeared to be the culmination of the successional process. An analogy was made between community succession and organism maturation. Beginning with a primitive, or juvenile, state and going through a complex developmental process, both individual organisms and communities progress until complex, stable, and mature forms are reached. It's dangerous to carry this analogy too far, however, because no mechanism is known to regulate communities in the same way that genetics and physiology regulate development of the body.

The concept of succession to a climax community was first championed by the pioneer biogeographer F. E. Clements. He viewed this process as being like a parade or relay, in which species replace each other in predictable groups and in a fixed, regular order. Clements argued that every landscape has a characteristic climax community, determined mainly by climate conditions. If left undisturbed, this community would mature to a characteristic set of organisms, each performing its optimal functions. The climax community would represent the maximum possible state of complexity and stability.

This community-unit theory was opposed by Clements' contemporary, H. A. Gleason, who saw community history as a much more unpredictable process. He argued that species are individualistic, each getting established according to its ability to colonize and reproduce in an area. Myriad temporary associations of plants and animals might form, according to the conditions prevailing at a particular time and the species available to colonize a given area. You might think of the Gleasonian model as a time-lapse movie of a busy railroad station. Passengers come and go; groups form and then dissipate. Patterns and assemblages that seem significant to us may not mean much in the long run. Gleason suggested that we see ecosystems as stable and uniform only because our lifetimes are so short and our view so limited.

The process of succession may not be as deterministic as we once thought, yet steady-state or highly developed ecological communities do often tend to be resilient and stable over long periods. Complex, mature communities, characterized by high species diversity, narrow niche specialization, well-organized community structure, good nutrient conservation, and recycling, can be highly resistant to disturbance. Community functions, such as productivity and nutrient cycling, tend to be self-stabilizing or self-perpetuating. What we once regarded as "final" climax communities, however, may still be changing. It's probably more accurate to say that the rate of succession is so slow in some mature communities that, from the perspective of a single human lifetime, it appears to be unchanging.

Some landscapes never reach a stable climax in the traditional sense because they are characterized by, and adapted to, periodic disruption. Grasslands, the chaparral scrubland of California, and some kinds of coniferous forests, for instance, are shaped and maintained by the periodic fires that have long been a part of their history (fig. 3.29). Plants in these communities are adapted to resist fires, reseed quickly after fires, or both. In fact, many of the plant species we recognize as dominants in these communities require fire to eliminate competition, to prepare seedbeds for germination of seedlings, or to open cones or thick seed coats. Without fire, community structure may be quite different.

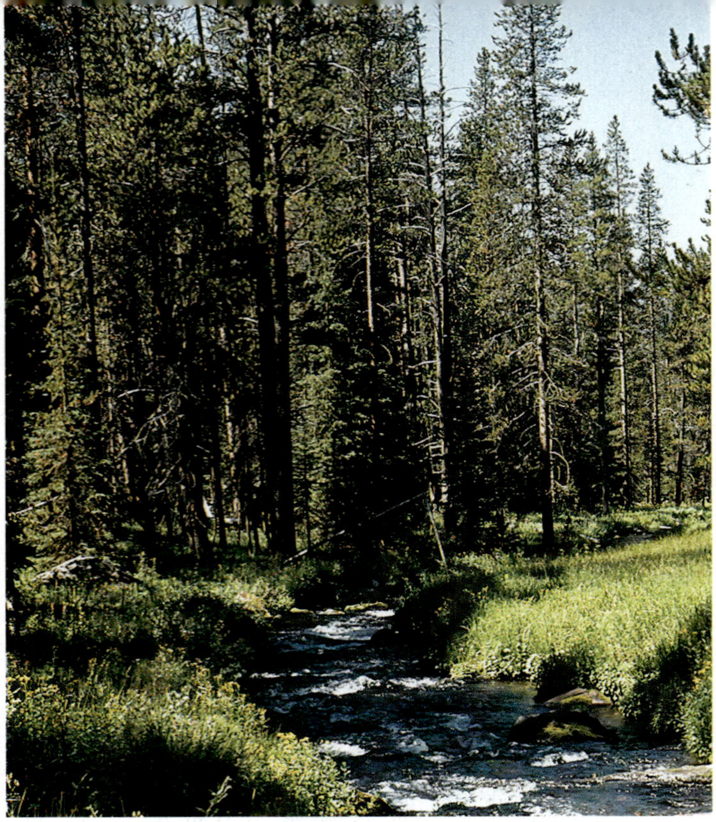

FIGURE 3.29 *This lodgepole pine forest in Yellowstone National Park was once thought to be a climax forest, but we now know that this forest exists only when renewed by periodic fire.*

The differences in these points of view influence how we manage ecosystems. Disturbance in ecosystems was long seen as disrupting climax conditions and, thus, inherently bad. Accordingly, fire suppression and flood control have been central policies in the United States and elsewhere for most of the twentieth century. In recent years, more conservationists have come to see disturbance as a natural part of ecosystems. Grasslands and some forests are now described as "fire-adapted," for example, and many fires are allowed to burn naturally. Similarly, floods are increasingly considered healthy for floodplains and river corridors, and policymakers are more cautious about funding dams and levees than they once were. (See further discussion in chapter 6 and related stories "Prescribed Fires in New Mexico" and "Fires in the Boundary Waters Canoe Area Wilderness" at www.mhhe.com/cases.)

Introduced Species and Community Change

Succession requires the continual introduction of new community members and the disappearance of previously existing species. Sometimes communities can be completely altered, however, by the introduction of non-native, **invasive species,** organisms not normally occurring in a particular location that invade and disrupt the local community. Usually we think of invasive species as introduced by humans from different continents. Because these organisms arrive without their natural predators, they can invade aggressively, drastically altering local environments. European rats in Polynesia, for example, have decimated breeding birds on many islands, and kudzu, a Japanese vine, has run rampant in much of the southern United States. Many ecologists consider invasive species the most pressing hazard for biological communities in the 21st century (see chapter 5).

Successful invasives tend to be prolific, opportunistic species. Sailing ships visiting oceanic islands, for example, took rats, goats, cats, and pigs. All these animals are prolific, quickly developing large populations. Goats are efficient, nonspecific herbivores; they eat nearly any vegetation, from grasses and herbs to seedlings and shrubs. In addition, their sharp hooves are hard on plants rooted in thin island soils. Rats and pigs are opportunistic omnivores, eating the eggs and nestlings of seabirds that tend to nest in large, densely packed colonies and digging up sea turtle eggs. Cats prey upon nestlings of both ground- and tree-nesting birds. Native species, those that originate in an area or have occupied the area for a very long time, are particularly vulnerable to invasive species because they did not evolve under circumstances that required them to have defensive adaptations to these predators.

Sometimes we introduce new species in an attempt to solve problems created by previous introductions but end up making the situation worse. In Hawaii and on several Caribbean islands, for instance, mongooses were imported to help control rats that had escaped from ships and were destroying indigenous birds and devastating pineapple plantations (fig. 3.30). Since the mongooses are diurnal (active in the day), however, and rats are nocturnal, they tended to ignore each other. Instead, the mongooses killed native birds and further threatened endangered species. Our lessons from this and similar introductions have a new technological twist. Some of the ethical questions currently surrounding the release of genetically engineered organisms are based on concerns that they are novel organisms, and we might not be able to predict how they will interact with other species in natural ecosystems—let alone how they might respond to natural selective forces. It is argued that we can't predict either their behavior or their evolution.

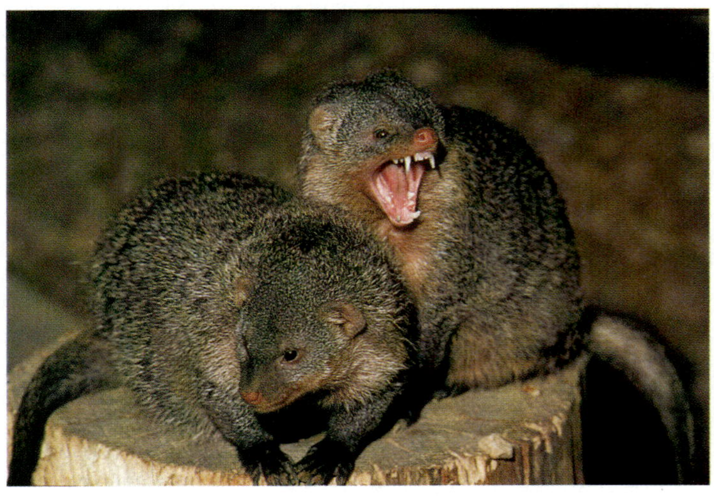

FIGURE 3.30 *Mongooses were released in Hawaii in an effort to control rats. The mongooses are active during the day, however, while the rats are night creatures, so they ignored each other. Instead, the mongooses attacked defenseless native birds and became as great a problem as the rats.*

SUMMARY

- Organisms are adapted to live within certain ranges of environmental conditions. Tolerance limits are the maximum or minimum conditions, such as temperature or moisture, that an organism can survive. Since many environmental factors affect survival, it is useful to consider critical factors that limit a species' growth or expansion.
- Evolution is gradual change of organisms by natural selection. Natural selection refers to a higher rate of survival and reproduction among individuals that happen to have advantageous traits. Environmental conditions can exert *selective pressure* by making some traits more advantageous than others.
- An ecological niche is usually described as its ecological role in a community; a niche can also be the place or set of environmental conditions in which an organism lives. Generalist species can occupy a range of habitats and ecological roles or environmental conditions. Highly specialized species occupy narrower niches.
- Resource partitioning occurs when species adapt to use a single resource differently.
- Species interact in many ways. Some general classes of interaction include predation, parasitism, symbiosis, and competition. All of these interactions can exert selective pressure, as organisms develop defenses against predators or parasites, as they develop traits that improve competitiveness, or as they develop mutually beneficial interactions. Both interspecific (between species) and intraspecific (within a species) competition can lead to changes in traits or behavior.
- Defensive mechanisms include Batesian mimicry, in which a harmless species looks like a dangerous one, and Müllerian mimicry, in which two dangerous species look like each other and thus both discourage predation.
- Primary productivity, or the rate of biomass accumulation, is a basic characteristic of communities. Abundance and species diversity are also important characteristics.
- Complexity refers to the number of species at each trophic level and the number of trophic levels in a community. Many ecologists believe that complexity contributes to stability in an ecosystem or resilience to abrupt change, such as fire, flood, or drought. Others believe that complex communities can be less resilient than simple ones.
- Edges, where contrasting conditions meet, are important features in biological communities. Ecotones, or zones of transition, have great diversity. Edges also reduce habitat quality for interior species.
- Primary succession occurs when pioneer species occupy areas previously lacking living things. Secondary succession occurs when an existing community is disrupted and a new, different community develops.
- The idea of a climax community is a stable community that appears to be the culmination of successional processes. A contrasting idea is that species occur individualistically, each according to its ability to colonize an area.
- Introduced species are one of the greatest modern threats to biological diversity and ecosystem complexity. When introduced species are free of predators, they can become abundant and cause significant damage to ecosystems.

QUESTIONS FOR REVIEW

1. Explain how tolerance limits to environmental factors determine distribution of a highly specialized species, such as the desert pupfish. Compare this with the distribution of a generalist species, such as cowbirds or starlings.
2. Productivity, diversity, complexity, resilience, and structure are exhibited to some extent by all communities and ecosystems. Describe how these characteristics apply to the ecosystem in which you live.
3. Describe the general niche occupied by a bird of prey, such as a hawk or an owl. How can hawks and owls exist in the same ecosystem and not adversely affect each other?
4. Define *keystone species* and explain their importance in community structure and function.
5. Relationships between predators and prey play an important role in the energy transfers that occur in ecosystems. They also influence the process of natural selection. Explain how predators affect the adaptations of their prey. How do prey species affect the adaptations of their predators?
6. Competition for a limited quantity of resources occurs in all ecosystems. This competition can be interspecific or intraspecific. Explain some of the ways an organism might deal with these different types of competition.
7. Explain the difference between exponential and logistic population growth. In the exponential growth model, $dN/dt = rN$, what do r, N, and dN represent?
8. What are some factors that prevent exponential growth in a population? What are some density-dependent and density-independent limiting factors?

9. Explain the concept of climax community. Why do mature, late-stage communities often exhibit a higher level of stability than that found in other successional stages?
10. Discuss the dangers posed to existing community members when new species are introduced into ecosystems. What type of organism would be most likely to survive and cause problems in a new habitat?

THINKING SCIENTIFICALLY

1. Ecologists debate whether biological communities have self-sustaining, self-regulating characteristics or are highly variable, accidental assemblages of individually acting species. What outlook or worldview might lead scientists to favor one or the other of these theories?
2. The concepts of natural selection and evolution are central to how most biologists understand and interpret the world, yet the theory of evolution is contrary to the beliefs of many religious groups. Why do you think this theory is so important to science and so strongly opposed by others? What evidence would be required to convince opponents of evolution?
3. What is the difference between saying that a duck has webbed feet because it needs them to swim and saying that a duck is able to swim because it has webbed feet?
4. The concept of keystone species is controversial among ecologists because most organisms are highly interdependent. If each of the trophic levels is dependent on all the others, how can we say one is most important? Choose an ecosystem with which you are familiar and decide whether it has a keystone species or keystone set.
5. Some scientists look at the boundary between two biological communities and see a sharp dividing line. Others looking at the same boundary see a gradual transition with much intermixing of species and many interactions between communities. Why are there such different interpretations of the same landscape?

KEY TERMS

adaptation 51
Batesian mimicry 58
biotic potential 60
carrying capacity 60
coevolution 56
commensalism 57
complexity 64
convergent evolution 53
divergent evolution 52
diversity 63
ecological development 69
ecological niche 53
ecotones 67
edge effects 67
environmental resistance 61
evolution 51
exponential growth 59
habitat 53
invasive species 70
J curve 60
K-adapted species 62
keystone species 58
logistic growth 60
Müllerian mimicry 58
mutualism 57
natural selection 51
overshoots 60
pioneer species 69
predator 55
primary productivity 62
primary succession 68
r-adapted species 62
resource partitioning 54
S curve 61
secondary succession 68
selective pressure 51
symbiosis 57
tolerance limits 50

SUGGESTED READINGS

Botkin, Daniel B. 1989. *Discordant harmonies: A New Ecology for the Twenty-First Century.* Oxford University Press.

Ehrlich, Paul R., and Peter H. Raven. 1967. Butterflies and plants: A study in coevolution. *Evolution* 18:586–608.

Gleason, Henry A. 1926. The individualistic concept of the plant association. *Bulletin of the Torrey Botanical Club* 53:7–26.

MacArthur, R. H. 1958. Population ecology of some warblers of northeastern coniferous forests. *Ecology* 39:599–619.

Paracer, S., and V. Ahmadjian. 2000. *Symbiosis: An Introduction to Biological Associations.* Oxford University Press.

Simberloff, D. 1997. Flagships, umbrellas, and keystones: Is single-species management passé in the landscape era? *Biological Conservation* 83:247–57.

Tilman, David, et al. 1997. The influence of functional diversity and composition on ecosystem processes. *Science* 277(5330): 1300–02.

Welcome to McGraw-Hill's Online Learning Center

http://www.mhhe.com/cunningham3e

WEB EXERCISES

Environments and Species Distributions

The Breeding Bird Survey (BBS) is one of the most comprehensive, current population databases available. This database, maintained by the Biological Resources Division of the U.S. Geological Survey, documents population fluctuations and geographic ranges of birds across the United States and southern Canada. Go to the BBS website at www.mbr-pwrc.usgs.gov/bbs/bbs.html.

Clicking on the "Distribution Maps" option on this page will produce a list of the birds in North America. You can see species distribution and breeding density maps by clicking on the name of any species. Find these species in the list and look at the map for each in order to answer the questions below:

Double crested cormorant

Great blue heron

Wood stork

American robin

1. Assuming that generalist/opportunistic species are widespread *and* more or less uniformly distributed, which of these species would you guess are generalists, and which might be specialists, with narrow niche preferences or environmental tolerance ranges? As you look at the range maps, consider especially each species' climate range, presence in densely populated areas, and evenness of distribution throughout the species' range. If you are unsure of environmental conditions across the continent, refer to the precipitation, biome, and climate maps.
2. Also look at the map for the bald eagle. Would you guess that temperature, water, forest cover, or mountainous terrain best explains its distribution? Why might this be so?
3. Now look at the range of the American dipper. Which of the four variables in question 2 best explains its distribution?

Diversity in Taxonomic Groups

Go to the Breeding Bird Survey (BBS) taxonomic list at www.mbr-pwrc.usgs.gov/bbs/htm96/map617/all.html.

Count the number of heron species. Now count the number of warbler species. What traits or ecological adaptations can you think of to describe these two groups? (For information and photos for each species, go to the Bird Information page on the BBS home page at www.mbr-pwrc.usgs.gov/id/framlst/framlst.html.

How might the different lifestyles, environments, or suites of competitive species help explain differences in diversity in these two groups?

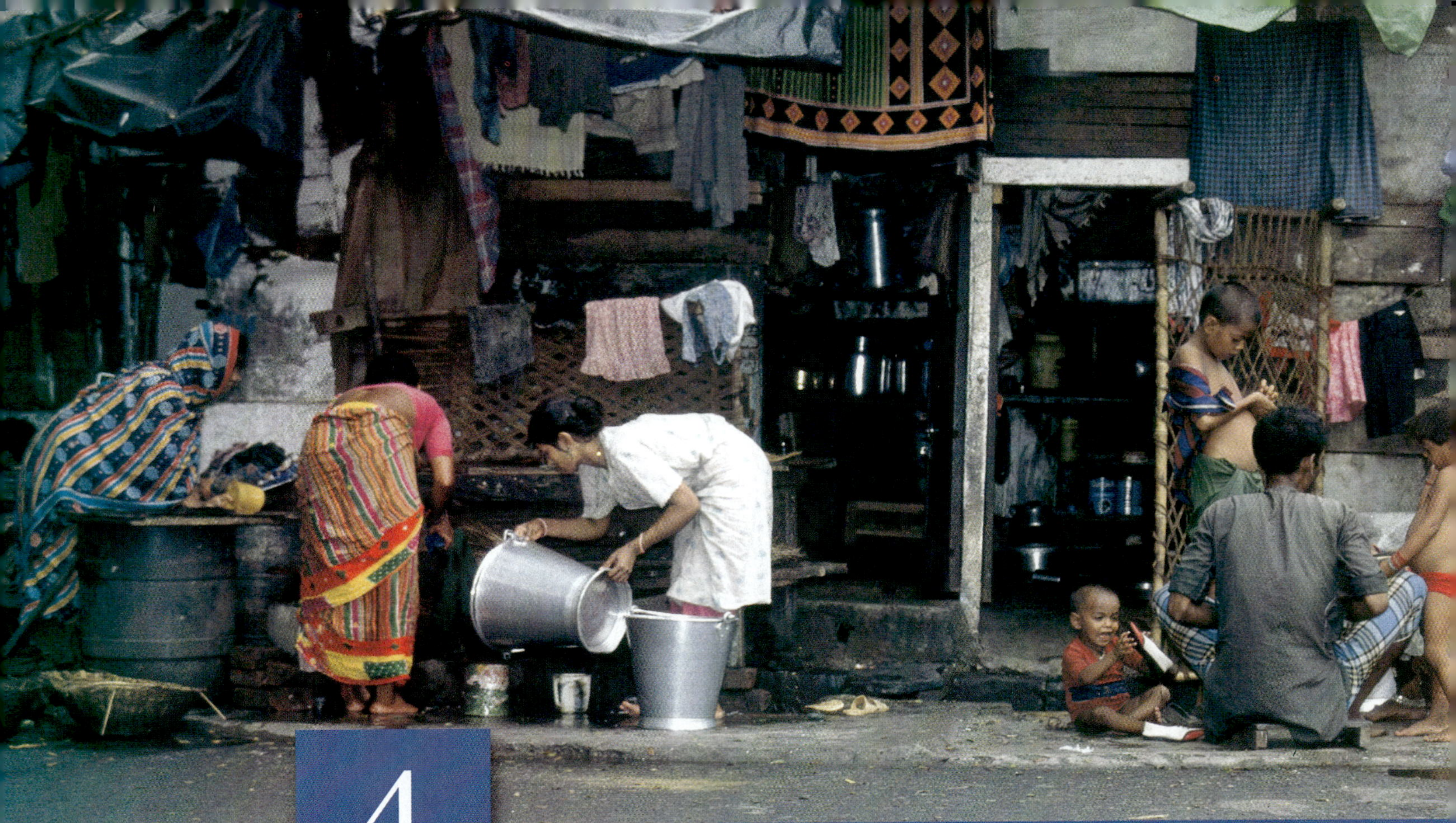

More than a billion people now live in India.

4 Human Populations

Live simply so that others may simply live.
–Mahatma Gandhi

Welcome to McGraw-Hill's Online Learning Center
http://www.mhhe.com/cunningham3e

LEARNING ONLINE

Visit our webpage at www.mhhe.com/cunningham3e for data sources, further readings, additional case studies, current environmental news, and regional examples within the Online Learning Center to help you understand the material in this chapter. You'll also find active links to information pertaining to this chapter, including

World population information
Census and demographic data
Population groups
Population models
Demographic transition

OBJECTIVES

After studying this chapter, you should be able to

- summarize historic factors that have contributed to human population growth.
- calculate doubling times for different annual growth rates.
- describe Malthusian and Marxian theories of limits to population growth, and explain why technological optimists and supporters of social justice oppose these theories.
- explain the process of demographic transition and why it produces a temporary population surge.
- understand how changes in life expectancy, infant mortality, women's literacy, standards of living, and democracy affect population changes.
- evaluate pressures for and against family planning in traditional and modern societies.
- compare modern birth control methods and think about a personal family planning agenda.

A Billion People and Growing

In 1999, having added more than 180 million people in just a decade, India reached a population of 1 billion humans. If current growth rates persist, India will have 1.63 billion residents in 2050 and will surpass China as the world's most populous country. How will the country, which already has more than a quarter of its population living in abject poverty, feed, house, educate, and employ all those being added each year? And what's the best way to slow this rapid growth? The fierce debate now taking place about how to control India's population has ramifications for the rest of the world as well.

On one side of this issue are those who believe that the best way to reduce the number of children born is poverty eradication and progress for women. Drawing on social justice principles established at the 1994 UN Conference on Population and Development in Cairo, some argue that responsible economic development, a broad-based social welfare system, education and empowerment of women, and high-quality health care—including family planning services—are essential components of population control. Without progress in these areas, they believe, efforts to provide contraceptives or encourage sterilization are futile.

On the other side of this debate are those who contend that, while social progress is an admirable goal, India doesn't have the time or resources to wait for an indirect approach to population control. The government must push aggressively, they argue, to reduce births now or the population will be so huge and its use of resources so great that only mass starvation, class war, crime, and disease will be able to bring it down to a manageable size.

Unable to reach a consensus on population policy, the Indian government decided in 2000 to let each state approach the problem in its own way. Some states have chosen to focus on social justice, while others have adopted more direct, interventionist policies.

The model for the social justice approach is the southern state of Kerala, which achieved population stabilization in the mid-1980s, the first Indian state to do so. Although still one of the poorest places in the world economically, Kerala's fertility rate is comparable to that of many industrialized nations, including the United States. Both women and men have a nearly 100 percent literacy rate and share affordable and accessible health care, family planning, and educational opportunities; therefore, women have only the number of children they want, usually two. The Kerala experience suggests that increased wealth isn't a prerequisite for zero population growth.

Taking a far different path to birth reduction is the neighboring state of Andra Pradesh, which reached a stable growth rate in 2001. Boasting the most dramatic fertility decline of any large Indian state, Andra Pradesh has focused on targeted, strongly enforced sterilization programs. The poor are encouraged—some would say compelled—to be sterilized after having only one or two children. The incentives include cash payments. You might receive 500 rupees—equivalent to $11 (U.S.) or a month's wages for an illiterate farm worker—if you agree to have "the operation." In addition, participants are eligible for better housing, land, wells, and subsidized loans.

The pressure to be sterilized is overwhelmingly directed at women, for whom the procedure is major abdominal surgery. Sterilizations often are done by animal husbandry staff and carried out in government sterilization camps. This practice raises troubling memories of the 1970s for many people, when then-Prime Minister Indira Gandhi suspended democracy and instituted a program of forced sterilization of poor people. There were reports at the time of people being rounded up like livestock and castrated or neutered against their will.

While many feminists and academics regard Andra Pradesh's policies as appallingly intrusive and coercive to women and the poor, the state has successfully reduced population growth. By contrast, the hugely populous northern states of Uttar Pradesh and Bihar have increased their growth rates slightly over the past two decades to a current rate above 2.5 percent per year. How will they slow this exponential growth, and what might be the social and environmental costs of not doing so?

India's population problems introduce several of the important themes of this chapter. What are the trends in human populations around the world, what do those trends mean for our resources and environment, and what is the best way to approach population planning? Keep in mind, as you read this chapter, that resource limits aren't simply a matter of total number of people; they also depend on consumption levels and the types of technology used to produce the things we use and consume.

POPULATION GROWTH

Every second, on average, four or five children are born, somewhere on the earth. In that same second, two other people die. This difference between births and deaths means a net gain of roughly 2.3 more humans per second in the world's population. At midyear 2004 the U.S. Census Bureau estimated that the total world population stood at roughly 6.4 billion people and was growing at 1.14 percent per year. This means we are adding nearly 73 million more people per year. Humans are now probably the most numerous vertebrate species on the earth. We also are more widely distributed and manifestly have a greater global environmental impact than any other species. For the families to whom these children are born, this may well be a joyous and long-awaited event (fig. 4.1). But is a continuing increase in humans good for the planet in the long run?

Many people worry that overpopulation will cause—or perhaps already is causing—resource depletion and environmental degradation that threaten the ecological life-support systems on which we all depend. These fears often lead to demands for

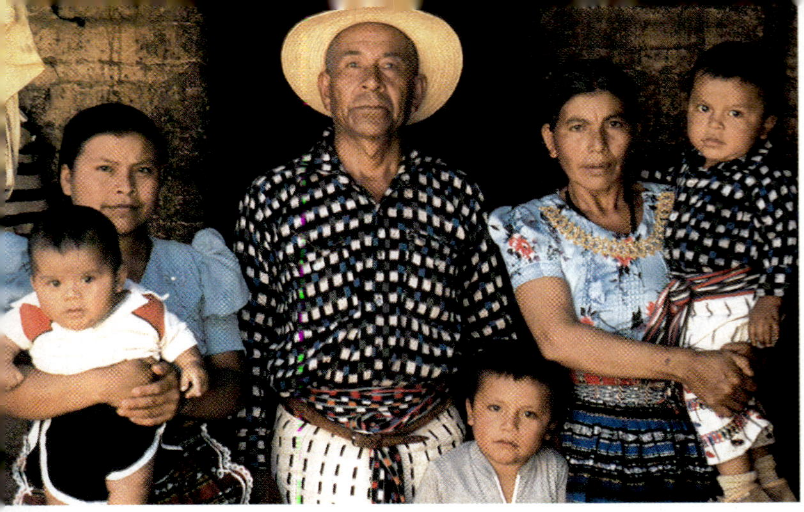

FIGURE 4.1 *A Mayan family in Guatemala with four of their six living children. Decisions on how many children to have are influenced by many factors, including culture, religion, need for old-age security for parents, immediate family finances, household help, child survival rates, and power relationships within the family.*

immediate, worldwide birth-control programs to reduce fertility rates and to eventually stabilize or even shrink the total number of humans.

Others believe that human ingenuity, technology, and enterprise can extend the world's carrying capacity and allow us to overcome any problems we encounter. From this perspective, more people may be beneficial, rather than disastrous. A larger population means a larger workforce, more geniuses, more ideas about what to do. Along with every new mouth comes a pair of hands. Proponents of this worldview argue that continued economic and technological growth can both feed the world's billions and enrich everyone enough to end the population explosion voluntarily.

Yet another perspective on this subject derives from social justice concerns. According to this worldview, resources are sufficient for everyone. Current shortages are only signs of greed, waste, and oppression. The root cause of environmental degradation, in this view, is inequitable distribution of wealth and power rather than merely population size. Fostering democracy, empowering women and minorities, and improving the standard of living of the world's poorest people are what are really needed. A narrow focus on population growth only fosters racism and an attitude that blames the poor for their problems, while ignoring the deeper social and economic forces at work.

Whether human populations will continue to grow at present rates and what that growth would imply for environmental quality and human life are among the most central and pressing questions in environmental science. In this chapter, we will look at some causes of population growth, as well as at how populations are measured and described. Family planning and birth control are essential for stabilizing populations. The number of children a couple decides to have and the methods they use to regulate fertility, however, are strongly influenced by culture, religion, politics, and economics, as well as basic biological and medical considerations. We will examine how some of these factors influence human demographics.

Human Population History

For most of our history, humans have not been very numerous, compared with other species. Studies of hunting and gathering societies suggest that the total world population was probably only a few million people before the invention of agriculture and the domestication of animals around 10,000 years ago. The agricultural revolution produced a larger and more secure food supply and allowed the human population to grow, reaching perhaps 50 million people by 5000 B.C. For thousands of years, the number of humans increased very slowly. Archaeological evidence and historical descriptions suggest that only about 300 million people were living at the time of Christ (table 4.1).

As you can see in figure 4.2, human populations began to increase rapidly after about A.D. 1600. Many factors contributed to this rapid growth. Increased sailing and navigating skills stimulated commerce and communication among nations. Agricultural developments, better sources of power, and better health care and hygiene also played a role. We are now in an exponential, or J curve, pattern of growth, described in chapter 3.

It took all of human history to reach 1 billion people in 1804 but little more than 150 years to reach 3 billion in 1960. It took us only 12 years—from 1987 to 1999—to add the sixth billion. Another way to look at population growth is that the number of humans tripled during the twentieth century. Will it do so again in the twenty-first century? If it does, will we overshoot our environment's carrying capacity and experience a catastrophic dieback similar to those described in chapter 3? As you will see later in this chapter, there is some evidence that population growth already is slowing, but whether we will reach equilibrium soon enough and at a size that can be sustained over the long term remains a difficult but important question.

Population Doubling Times

If the current world population is growing at approximately 1.14 percent per year, how long will it take to double the population if

TABLE 4.1 World Population Growth and Doubling Times

DATE	POPULATION	DOUBLING TIME
5000 B.C.	50 million	?
800 B.C.	100 million	4,200 years
200 B.C.	200 million	600 years
A.D. 1200	400 million	1,400 years
A.D. 1700	800 million	500 years
A.D. 1900	1,600 million	200 years
A.D. 1965	3,200 million	65 years
A.D. 2000	6,100 million	51 years
A.D. 2050 (estimate)	9,300 million	140 years

Source: Data from Population Reference Bureau and United Nations Population Division.

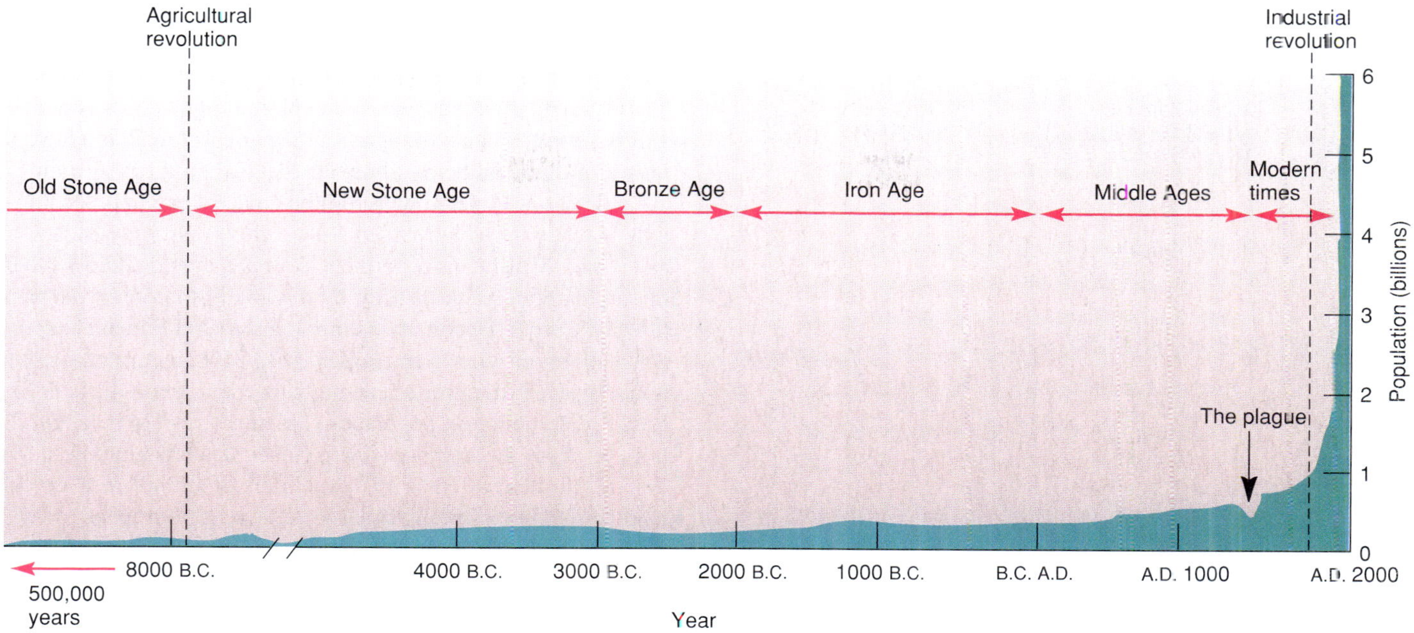

FIGURE 4.2 *Human population levels throughout history. Since about* A.D. *1000, our population curve has assumed a J shape. Are we on the upward slope of a population overshoot? Will we be able to adjust our population growth to an S curve? Or can we just continue the present trend indefinitely?*

APPLICATION: Population Doubling Times

Using the "rule of 70," calculate the doubling time of populations growing at the following annual percentage growth rates: 0.1 percent, 1.0 percent, 5 percent.

Example: $\frac{\text{70 years}}{\text{(percent growth)}}$ = doubling time in years

Answers: 0.1 = 700 years; 1.0 = 70 years; 5.0 = 14 years.

that rate persists? A useful rule of thumb is that, if you divide 70 by the annual percentage growth, you get the approximate doubling time in years for anything growing exponentially. For example, a savings account or a biological population growing at a compound interest rate of 1 percent per year will double in about 70 years. By the same measure, a population growing at 35 percent doubles every 2 years. Countries growing at 4 percent per year will double their populations in 17.5 years. A country growing at a rate of 0.1 percent annually will double its population in 700 years.

LIMITS TO GROWTH: SOME OPPOSING VIEWS

As with many topics in environmental science, people have widely differing opinions about population and resources. Some believe that population growth is the ultimate cause of poverty and environmental degradation. Others argue that poverty, environmental degradation, and overpopulation are all merely symptoms of deeper social and political factors. Which of these opposing worldviews we accept as most correct will have a great impact on our population policies. In this section, we will examine some of the major figures and their arguments in this debate.

Malthusian Checks on Population

In 1798 the Reverend Thomas Malthus wrote *An Essay on the Principle of Population* to refute the views of progressives and optimists—including his father—who, inspired by the egalitarian principles of the French Revolution, predicted a coming utopia. The younger Malthus argued that human populations tend to increase at an exponential, or compound, rate, while food production either remains stable or increases only slowly. The result, according to Malthus, is that human populations inevitably outstrip their food supply and eventually collapse into starvation, crime, and misery. Figure 4.3a summarizes his theory.

According to Malthus, the only ways to stabilize human populations are "positive checks," such as diseases or famines that kill people, or "preventative checks," including all the factors that prevent human birth. Among the preventative checks he advocated were "moral restraint," including late marriage and celibacy until a couple could afford to support children. Malthus himself, however, had several illegitimate children and didn't have much faith in moral restraint. Many social scientists and biologists have been influenced by Malthus. Charles Darwin, for instance, derived his theories about the struggle for scarce resources and survival of the fittest after reading Malthus' essay.

If Malthus' views of the consequences of exponential population growth were dismal, the corollary he drew was even more

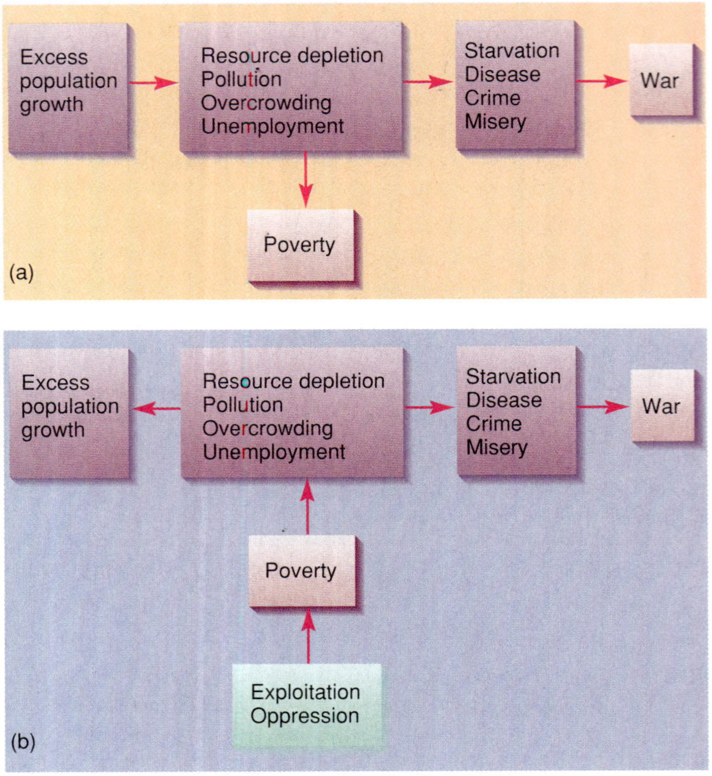

FIGURE 4.3 (a) *Thomas Malthus argued that excess population growth is the ultimate cause of many other social and environmental problems.* (b) *Karl Marx argued that oppression and exploitation are the real causes of poverty and environmental degradation. In his view, population growth is a symptom or result of other problems, not the source.*

bleak. He believed that most people are too lazy and immoral to regulate birth rates voluntarily. Consequently, he opposed efforts to feed and assist the poor in England because he feared that more food would simply increase their fertility and thereby perpetuate the problems of starvation and misery. (See the related story "The Saga of Easter Island" at www.mhhe.com/cases.)

Not surprisingly, Malthus' ideas provoked a great social and economic debate. Karl Marx was one of his most vehement critics, claiming that Malthus was a "shameless sycophant of the ruling classes." According to Marx, population growth is a symptom rather than a root cause of poverty, resource depletion, pollution, and other social ills. The real causes of these problems, he believed, are exploitation and oppression (fig. 4.3b). Marx argued that workers always provide for their own sustenance, given access to means of production and a fair share of the fruits of their labor. According to Marxians, the way to slow population growth and to alleviate crime, disease, starvation, misery, and environmental degradation is through social justice.

Malthus and Marx Today

Both Marx and Malthus developed their theories about human population growth in the nineteenth century, when understanding of the world, technology, and society were much different than they are now. Still, as the opening story in this chapter shows, the questions they raised are relevant today. While the evils of racism, classism, and the other forms of exploitation that Marx denounced still beset us, it is also true that at some point available resources must limit the numbers of humans that the earth can sustain.

Those who agree with Malthus that we are approaching—or may already have surpassed—the earth's carrying capacity are called **neo-Malthusians.** In their view, we should address the issue of surplus population directly by making birth control our highest priority. Cornell University entomologist David Pimentel expressed a version of this view when he said, "By 2100, if current trends continue, twelve billion miserable humans will suffer a difficult life on Earth." The optimum population, he argues, would be about 2 billion, or about the number on the planet at the beginning of World War II. He believes that this population would allow everyone to enjoy a standard of living equal to the average European today.

Neo-Marxians, on the other hand, believe that only eliminating oppression and poverty through technological development and social justice will solve population problems. Claims of resource scarcity, they argue, are only an excuse for inequity and exclusion. They believe that, if distribution of wealth and resources were more fair, there would be plenty for everyone. As Mohandas Gandhi said, "There is enough for everyone's need, but not enough for anyone's greed."

Perhaps a compromise position between these opposing views is that population growth, poverty, and environmental degradation are all interrelated. No factor exclusively causes any other, but each influences and, in turn, is influenced by the others.

Can Technology Make the World More Habitable?

Technological optimists argue that Malthus was wrong in his predictions of famine and disaster 200 years ago because he failed to account for scientific progress. In fact, food supplies have increased faster than population growth since Malthus' time. There have been terrible famines in the past two centuries, but they were caused more by politics and economics than lack of resources or sheer population size. Whether this progress will continue remains to be seen, but technological advances have vastly increased human carrying capacity so far.

The burst of world population growth that began 200 years ago was stimulated by scientific and industrial revolutions. Progress in agricultural productivity, engineering, information technology, commerce, medicine, sanitation, and other achievements of modern life have made it possible to support approximately 1,000 times as many people per unit area as was possible 10,000 years ago. Economist Stephen Moore of the Cato Institute in Washington, D.C. regards this achievement as "a real tribute to human ingenuity and our ability to innovate." There is no reason, he argues, to think that our ability to find technological solutions to our problems will diminish in the future.

Much of our growth in the past 200 years, however, has been based on availability of easily acquired natural resources, especially cheap, abundant fossil fuels. Whether we can develop alternative, renewable energy sources in time to avert disaster when current fossil fuels run out is a matter of great concern.

Could More People Be Beneficial?

Larger populations can have benefits as well as disadvantages. More people mean larger markets, more workers, and efficiencies of scale in mass production of goods. Greater numbers also provide more intelligence and enterprise to overcome such problems as underdevelopment, pollution, and resource limitations. Human ingenuity and intelligence can create new resources through substitution of new materials and can discover new ways of doing things for old materials and old ways. For instance, utility companies are finding it cheaper and more environmentally sound to finance insulation and energy-efficient appliances for their customers rather than build new power plants. The effect of saving energy that was formerly wasted is comparable to creating a new fuel supply.

Economist Julian Simon was one of the most outspoken champions of this rosy view of human history. He argued that people are the "ultimate resource" and that no evidence suggests that pollution, crime, unemployment, crowding, the loss of species, or any other resource limitations will worsen with population growth. Leaders of many developing countries share this outlook and insist that, instead of being obsessed with population growth, we should focus on the inordinate consumption of the world's resources by people in richer countries.

HUMAN DEMOGRAPHY

Demography (derived from the Greek words *demos* [people] and *graphein* [to write or to measure]) encompasses vital statistics about people, such as births, deaths, and where they live, as well as total population size. In this section, we will survey ways to measure and describe human populations and discuss demographic factors that contribute to population growth.

How Many of Us Are There?

The U.S. Census Bureau estimate of 6.4 billion people in the world in mid-2004 quoted at the beginning of this chapter is only an educated guess. Even in this age of information technology and communication, counting the number of people in the world is like shooting at a moving target. People continue to be born and die. Furthermore, some countries have never even taken a census, and those that have been done may not be accurate. Governments may overstate or understate their populations to make their countries appear larger and more important or smaller and more stable than they really are. Individuals, especially if they are homeless, refugees, or illegal aliens, may not want to be counted or identified.

We really live in two very different demographic worlds. One of these worlds is poor, young, and growing rapidly. It is occupied by the vast majority of people who live in the less-developed countries of Africa, Asia, and Latin America. These countries represent 80 percent of the world population but more than 90 percent of all projected growth (fig. 4.4). (See Investigating Our Environment, p. 80.)

The highest population growth rates occur in a few "hot spots," such as sub-Saharan Africa and the Middle East, where economics, politics, religion, and civil unrest keep birth rates high and contraceptive use low. In Chad and the Democratic Republic of Congo, for example, annual population growth is above 3.2 percent. Less than 10 percent of all couples use any form of birth control, women average more than seven children each, and nearly half the population is less than 15 years old. Even faster growth rates occur in Oman and Palestine, where the population doubling time is only 18 years.

Some countries in the developing world have experienced amazing growth rates and are expected to reach extraordinary population sizes by the middle of the twenty-first century. Table 4.2 shows the 15 largest countries in the world, arranged by their estimated size in 2002 and projected size in 2050. Note that, while China was the most populous country throughout the twentieth century, as the opening of this chapter shows, India is expected to pass China in the twenty-first century. Nigeria, which had only 33 million residents in 1950, is forecast to have more than 300 million in 2050. Ethiopia, with about 18 million people 50 years ago, is likely to grow at least ten-fold over a century. In many of these countries, rapid population growth is a serious problem. Bangladesh, about the size of Iowa, is already overcrowded at 128 million people. Another 83 million people by 2050 will only add to current problems.

The other demographic world is made up of the richer countries of North America, Western Europe, Japan, Australia, and New Zealand. This world is wealthy, old, and shrinking. Italy, Germany, Hungary, and Japan, for example, all have negative growth rates. The average age in these countries is now 40, and life expectancy of their residents is expected to exceed 90 by 2050. With many couples choosing to have either one or no children, the populations of these countries are expected to decline

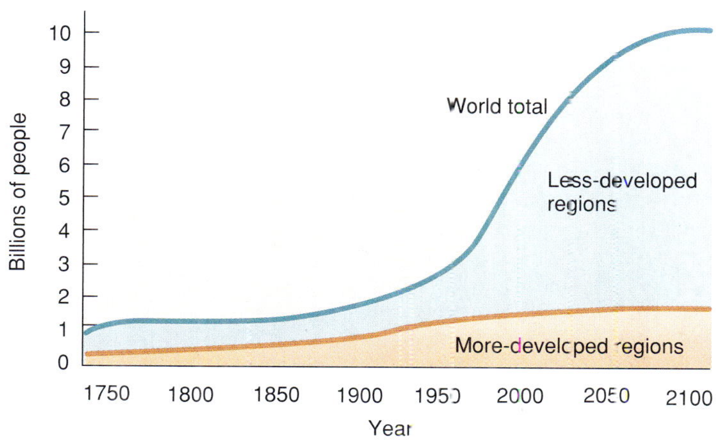

FIGURE 4.4 *Estimated human population growth, 1750–2100, in less-developed and more-developed regions. More than 90 percent of all growth in the twentieth century and projected for the twenty-first century is in the less-developed countries.*

INVESTIGATING Our Environment

Interpreting Graphs

An important part of any scientific investigation is presenting the data. Graphs and other pictorial representations of information are particularly good for helping others to understand what we have to say. It is one thing to read that "the human population is rising explosively," but it is considerably more compelling to see the J curve along with concrete numbers as evidence. The combination of picture and numbers often conveys powerful impressions beyond the numbers themselves. But it is important to recognize that graphs can be as truthful or misleading as the person who creates them intends to be.

Central questions addressed in this chapter are how serious is the worldwide population problem and does it demand action. The graphs in figures 1 and 2 present information relevant to human population studies, yet the impressions these figures convey vary considerably, depending on the type of data used and the design of the graph.

Reexamine figure 4.2, which presents a historical perspective on the growth in human numbers. What conclusions do you draw from it? Does it suggest that we are experiencing an explosive rise in human numbers? Does it indicate that the current increase is unprecedented in our species history? Does it also imply, perhaps more indirectly, that the earth's population problem is serious and urgent? In light of the concepts of environmental resistance, carrying capacity, and overshoot and dieback, many people would conclude that the current population growth, highlighted by the graph, is unsustainable.

Now examine figure 1. It plots the same variables as figure 4.2 but suggests that population is rising at a modest rate. It does not produce the same sense of explosiveness and urgency as figure 4.2. How can the impressions be so different?

Notice that the graph in figure 1 covers a much shorter time period. This greatly changes the time interval lengths on the horizontal scale. In figure 4.2, 1 mm represents about 50 years, but in figure 1, it represents less than 1 year. This changes the line's slope from nearly vertical in figure 4.2 to a modest incline in figure 1. Slope impacts the visual impression created by a graph and, therefore, its interpretation. How could you change the time axis in figure 1 to flatten the slope even more?

Next examine figure 2. This graph plots the stabilization ratio, rather than population size over time. The graph reveals that the growth rate for most regions except Africa has been declining since about 1970. Do the graph's downward-trending lines suggest that there really isn't much of a population problem, or at least not much reason for concern?

All three graphs present information relevant to a discussion of worldwide population growth, yet each gives a different impression of the seriousness of the problem. So, how can we analyze graphs and their messages in a thoughtful way? Certainly, no single formula is applicable to all situations, but the following questions are worth keeping in mind:

1. Is the graph's time frame of reference appropriate, or is it too restricted to allow a valid, comprehensive assessment of the issue?
2. Are the unit intervals on the graph appropriately sized?
3. Is the impression the graph creates real or simply an artifact of the graph's format?
4. Do the data the graph presents provide only a partial, perhaps misleading, view of the whole?

Because graphs can create powerful impressions, we need to use and interpret them with care.

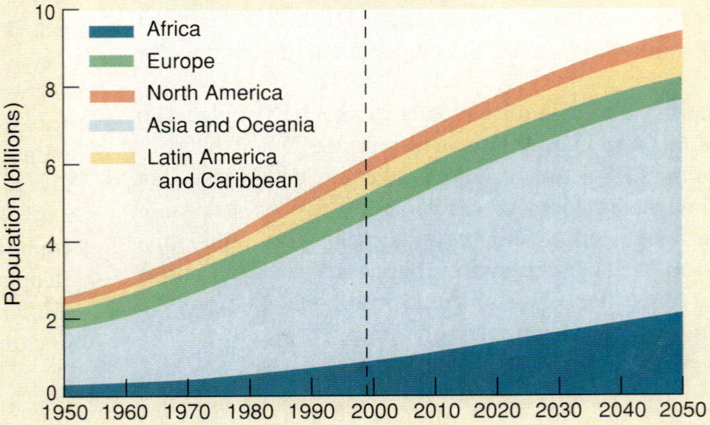

FIGURE 1 *The UN Population Division projects continued population growth, although at a gradually slowing rate, over the next 50 years.*
Source: World Resources Institute, *World Resources 1998–99*.

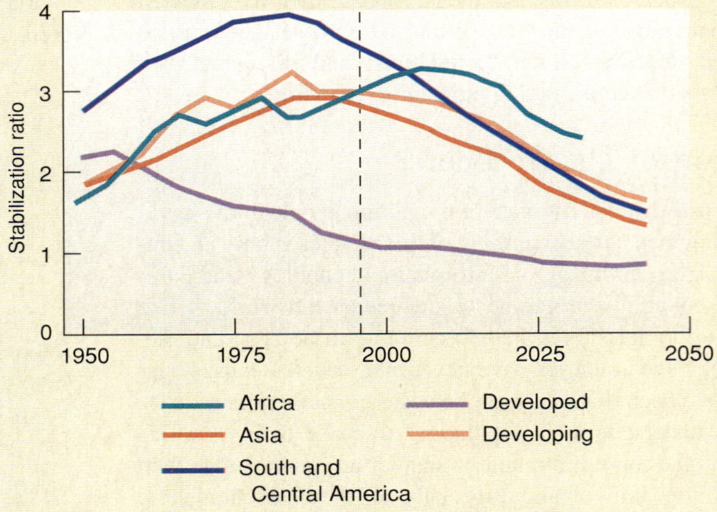

FIGURE 2 *The stabilization ratio is measured by dividing crude birth rate by crude death rate. A ratio of 1 indicates zero population growth.*
Source: United Nations (UN) Population Division, *World Population Prospects, 1950–2050 (The 1996 Revision)*. The United Nations, New York, 1996.

TABLE 4.2 The World's Largest Countries

IN 2002		IN 2050	
COUNTRY	POPULATION (IN MILLIONS)	COUNTRY	POPULATION (IN MILLIONS)
China	1,281	India	1,628
India	1,050	China	1,394
United States	287	United States	413
Indonesia	217	Pakistan	332
Brazil	174	Indonesia	316
Russia	144	Nigeria	304
Pakistan	144	Brazil	247
Bangladesh	134	Bangladesh	205
Nigeria	130	Congo, Dem. Rep. of	182
Japan	127	Ethiopia	173
Mexico	102	Mexico	151
Germany	82	Philippines	146
Philippines	80	Vietnam	117
Vietnam	80	Egypt	115
Egypt	71	Russia	102

Source: Data from Population Reference Bureau, 2003.

significantly over the next century. Japan, which has 126 million residents now, is expected to shrink to about 100 million by 2050. Europe, which now makes up about 12 percent of the world population, will constitute less than 7 percent in 50 years, if current trends continue. Even the United States and Canada would have nearly stable populations if immigration were stopped.

It isn't only wealthy countries that have declining populations. Russia, for instance, is now declining by nearly 1 million people per year as death rates have soared and birth rates have plummeted. A collapsing economy, hyperinflation, crime, corruption, and despair have demoralized the population. Horrific pollution levels left from the Soviet era, coupled with poor nutrition and health care, have resulted in high levels of genetic abnormalities, infertility, and infant mortality. Abortions are twice as common as live births, and the average number of children per woman is now 1.3, one of the lowest in the world. Death rates, especially among adult men, have risen dramatically. According to some medical experts, male life expectancy dropped from 68 years in 1990 to 58 years in 2000. After having been the fourth largest country in the world in 1950, Russia is expected to have a smaller population than Vietnam, the Philippines, or the Democratic Republic of Congo by 2050.

The situation is even worse in many African countries, where AIDS and other communicable diseases are killing people at a terrible rate. In Zimbabwe, Botswana, Zambia, and Namibia, for example, up to 30 percent of the adult population have AIDS or are HIV-positive. Health officials predict that more than two-thirds of the 15-year-olds now living in Botswana will die of AIDS before age 50. Many of these countries are soon expected to have declining populations. Overall, however, Africa is expected to grow by at least 1.5 billion over the next century.

The world population density map in Appendix 2 on p. 380 shows human population distribution around the world. Notice the high densities supported by fertile river valleys of the Nile, Ganges, Yellow, Yangtze, and Rhine Rivers and the well-watered coastal plains of India, China, and Europe. Historic factors, such as technology diffusion and geopolitical power, also play a role in geographic distribution.

Fertility and Birth Rates

Fecundity is the physical ability to reproduce, while fertility is the actual production of offspring. Those without children may be fecund but not fertile. The most accessible demographic statistic of fertility is usually the **crude birth rate,** the number of births in a year per thousand persons. It is statistically "crude" in the sense that it is not adjusted for population characteristics, such as the number of women of reproductive age.

The **total fertility rate** is the number of children born to an average woman in a population during her entire reproductive life. Upper-class women in seventeenth- and eighteenth-century Europe, whose babies were given to wet nurses immediately after birth and who were expected to produce as many children as possible, often had 25 or 30 pregnancies. The highest recorded total fertility rates for working-class people are among some Anabaptist agricultural groups in North America, who have averaged up to 12 children per woman. In most tribal or traditional societies, food shortages, health problems, and cultural practices limit total fertility to about six or seven children per woman, even without modern methods of birth control.

Fertility is usually calculated as births per woman because, in many cases, establishing paternity is difficult. Nevertheless, a few demographers argue that we should pay more attention to birth rates per male because, in some cultures men have far more children, on average, than do women. In Cameroon, for instance, due to multiple marriages, extramarital affairs, and a high rate of female mortality, men are estimated to have 8.1 children in their lifetime, while women average only 4.8.

Zero population growth (ZPG) occurs when births plus immigration in a population just equal deaths plus emigration. It takes several generations of replacement-level fertility (in which people just replace themselves) to reach ZPG. Where infant mortality rates are high, the replacement level may be 5 or more children per couple. In the more highly developed countries, however, this rate is usually about 2.1 children per couple because some people are infertile, have children who do not survive, or choose not to have children.

Fertility rates have declined dramatically in every region of the world except Africa over the past 50 years (fig. 4.5). In the 1960s, total fertility rates above 6 were common in many countries. The average family in Mexico in 1975, for instance, had 7 children. By 2000, however, the average Mexican woman had

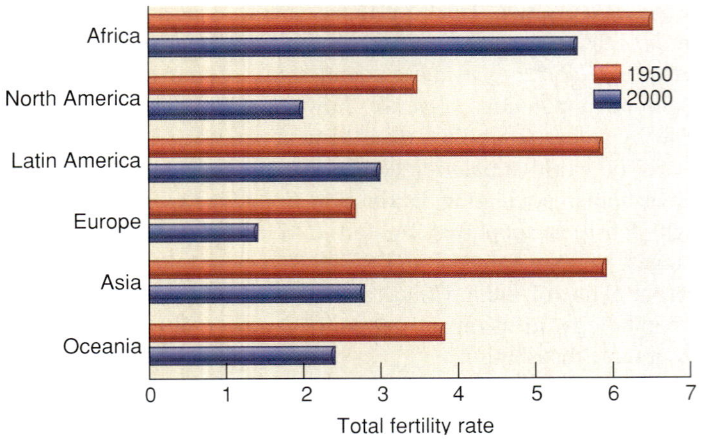

FIGURE 4.5 *Declines in fertility rates by region, 1950 and 2000.*
Source: Data from Population Reference Bureau, 2002.

only 2.5 children. According to the World Health Organization, 61 of the world's 190 countries are now at or below a replacement rate of 2.1 children per couple. The greatest fertility reduction has been in Southeast Asia, where rates have fallen by more than half, primarily in the past few decades. Contrary to what many demographers expected, some of the poorest countries in the world have been remarkably successful in lowering growth rates. Bangladesh, for instance, reduced its fertility rate from 6.9 in 1980 to only 3.1 children per woman in 1998.

China's one-child-per-family policy decreased the fertility rate from 6 in 1970 to 1.8 in 1990. This policy, however, has sometimes resulted in abortions, forced sterilizations, and even infanticide. Another adverse result is that the only children (especially boys) allowed to families may grow up to be spoiled "little emperors" who have an inflated impression of their own importance (fig. 4.6). Furthermore, there may not be enough workers to maintain the army, sustain the economy, or support retirees when their parents reach old age.

Although the number of boys and girls normally should be fairly balanced in a population, 20 years of female infanticides and sex-based abortions in China have created ratios as high as 140 boys to 100 girls in some regions. This shortage of women has created a flourishing trade in abducted brides. A crackdown in 2002 released 110,000 women who had been kidnapped and sold into marriage, but it's thought that the total number abducted is much higher.

While the world as a whole still has an average fertility rate of 2.7, growth rates are now lower than at any time since World War II. If fertility declines like those in Bangladesh and China were to occur everywhere in the world, our total population could begin to decline by the end of the twenty-first century. Interestingly, Spain and Italy, although predominately Roman Catholic, have the lowest reported fertility rates (1.2 children per woman) of any countries.

Mortality and Death Rates

A traveler to a foreign country once asked a local resident, "What's the death rate around here?" "Oh, the same as anywhere," was the reply, "about one per person." In demographics, however,

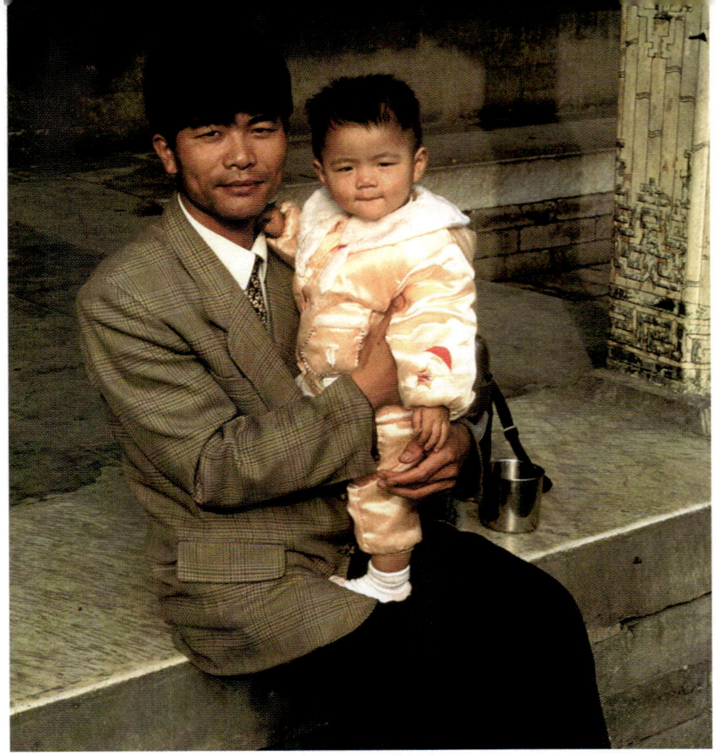

FIGURE 4.6 *China's one-child-per-family policy has been remarkably successful in reducing birth rates. It may, however, have created a generation of "little emperors," since parents and grandparents focus all their attention on an only child.*

crude death rates (or crude mortality rates) are expressed in terms of the number of deaths per thousand persons in any given year. Countries in Africa where health care and sanitation are limited may have mortality rates of 20 or more per 1,000 people. Wealthier countries generally have mortality rates around 10 per 1,000. The number of deaths in a population is sensitive to the population's age structure. Rapidly growing, developing countries, such as Belize or Costa Rica, have lower crude death rates (4 per 1,000) than do the more-developed, slowly growing countries, such as Denmark (12 per 1,000). This is because a rapidly growing country has proportionately more youths and fewer elderly than a more slowly growing country. Declining mortality, not rising fertility, was the primary cause of most population growth in the past 300 years. Crude death rates began falling in Western Europe during the late 1700s.

Life Span and Life Expectancy

Life span is the oldest age to which a species is known to survive. Although there are many claims in ancient literature of kings living for a thousand years or more, the oldest age that can be certified by written records was that of Jeanne Louise Calment of Arles, France, who was 122 years old at her death in 1997. While modern medicine has made it possible for many of us to survive much longer than our ancestors, it doesn't appear that the maximum life span has increased much at all. Apparently, cells in our bodies have a limited ability to repair damage and produce new components. Sooner or later they simply wear out, and we fall victim to disease, degeneration, accidents, or senility.

Life expectancy is the average age that a newborn infant can expect to attain in any given society. It is another way of expressing the average age at death. For most of human history, life expectancy in most societies probably has been 35 to 40 years. This doesn't mean that no one lived past age 40 but, rather, that many people died at earlier ages (mostly early childhood), which balanced out those who managed to live longer.

The twentieth century saw a global transformation in human health unmatched in history. This revolution can be seen in the dramatic increases in life expectancy in most places (table 4.3). Worldwide, the average life expectancy rose from about 40 to 65.5 years over the past century. The greatest progress was in developing countries. For example, in 1900, the average Indian man could expect to live less than 23 years, while the average woman would reach just over 23 years. By 2000, although India had an annual per capita income of less than $440 (U.S.), the average life expectancy for both men and women had nearly tripled and was very close to that of countries with ten times its income level. Longer lives were due primarily to better nutrition, improved sanitation, clean water, and education, rather than to miracle drugs or high-tech medicine. While the gains were not as great for the already industrialized countries, residents of the United States, Sweden, and Japan, for example, now live about half-again as long as they did at the beginning of the twentieth century, and they can expect to enjoy much of that life in relatively good health. The Disability Adjusted Life Years (DALYs, a measure of disease burden that combines premature death with loss of healthy life resulting from illness or disability) that someone living in Japan can expect is now 74.5 years, compared with only 64.5 DALYs two decades ago.

As figure 4.7 shows, annual income and life expectancy are strongly correlated up to about $4,000 (U.S.) per person. Beyond that level—which is generally enough for adequate food, shelter, and sanitation for most people—life expectancies level out at about 75 years for men and 85 for women.

Large discrepancies in how the benefits of modernization and social investment are distributed within countries are revealed in differential longevities of various groups. The greatest life

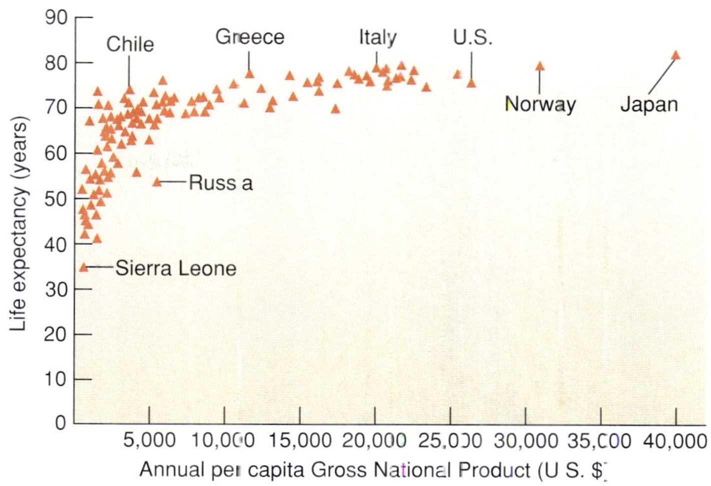

FIGURE 4.7 *As incomes rise, so does life expectancy up to about $4,000 (U.S.). In some countries, such as China and Cuba, however, people live as long as in richer countries, even though their income is less than one-tenth as much.*

Source: United Nations (UN) Population Division, *World Population Prospects, 1950–2050 (The 1996 Revision)*. The United Nations, New York, 1996

expectancy reported anywhere in the United States is for women in Stearns County, Minnesota, who live to an average age of 86. By contrast, Native American men on the Pine Ridge Indian Reservation in neighboring South Dakota live, on average, only to age 45. Only a few countries in Africa have a lower life expectancy. The Pine Ridge Reservation is the poorest area in America, with an unemployment rate near 75 percent and high rates of poverty, alcoholism, drug use, and alienation. Similarly, African-American men in Washington, D.C., live, on average, only 57.9 years, which is less than the life expectancy in Lesotho or Swaziland.

Living Longer: Demographic Implications

A population growing rapidly by natural increase has more young people than does a stationary population. One way to show these differences is to graph age classes in a histogram, as figure 4.8 shows. In Niger, which is growing at a rate of 3.5 percent per year, 47.8 percent of the population is in the prereproductive category (below age 15). Even if total fertility rates fell abruptly, the total number of births, and the population size, would continue to grow for some years as these young people entered reproductive age. This phenomenon is called population momentum.

By contrast, a country with a relatively stable population will have nearly the same number in most cohorts. Notice that females outnumber males in Sweden's oldest group because of differences in longevity between sexes. A rapidly declining population, such as Singapore's, can have a pronounced bulge in middle-age cohorts as fewer children are born than in their parents' generation.

Both rapidly growing countries and slowly growing countries can have a problem with their **dependency ratio,** or the number of nonworking compared with working individuals in a population. In Niger, for example, each working person supports

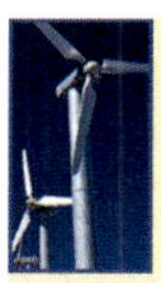

TABLE 4.3 Life Expectancy at Birth for Selected Countries in 1900 and 2000

	1900		2000	
COUNTRY	MALES	FEMALES	MALES	FEMALES
India	22.6	23.3	60.3	60.5
Japan	42.4	43.7	77.4	84.2
Russia	30.9	33.0	61.7	73.6
Sweden	56.6	59.5	77.0	82.1
United States	45.6	48.3	74.7	79.3

Source: Data from Population Reference Bureau, 2002.

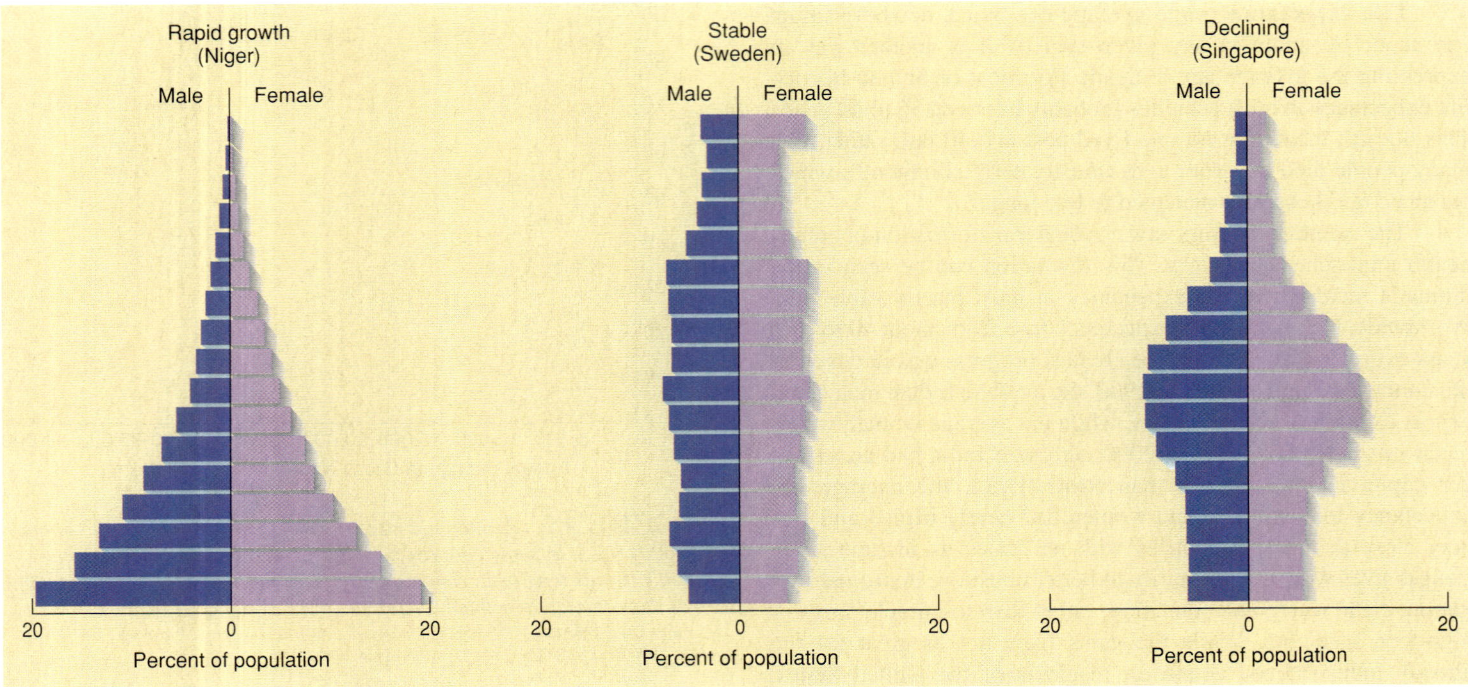

FIGURE 4.8 *Age structure graphs for rapidly growing, stable, and declining populations.*
Source: U.S. Census Bureau, 2003.

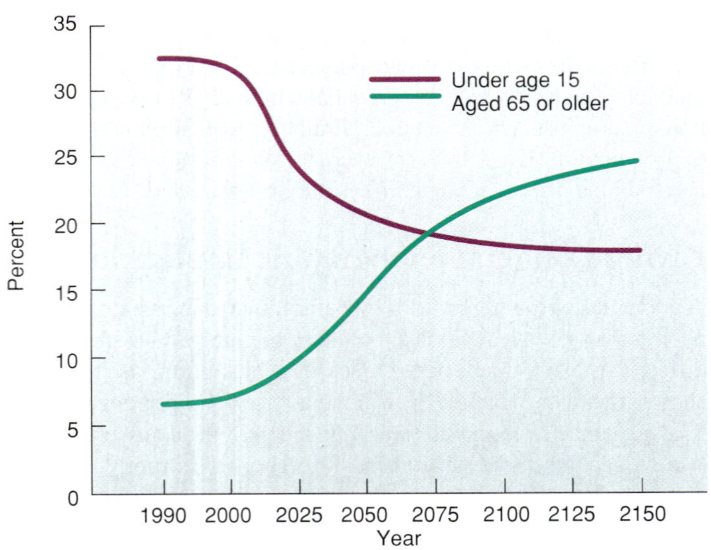

FIGURE 4.9 *Changing age structure of world population. In the twenty-first century, children under age 15 will make up a smaller percentage of world population, while people over age 65 will make up a rapidly rising share of the population.*

a high number of children. In the United States, by contrast, a declining working population is now supporting an ever larger number of retired persons. In 1970, the median age in the United States was 30, and there were four workers for every retired person. By 2050, if retirement age remains at 65, there could be more retired people than workers. Social Security wasn't designed to cope with a situation such as this. How will this affect your future?

This changing age structure and shifting dependency ratio are occurring worldwide (fig. 4.9). In 1950, there were only 130 million people in the world over 65 years old. In 2000, more than 420 million had reached this age. By 2150, those over 65 might make up 25 percent of the world population. Countries such as Japan, Singapore, and Taiwan already are concerned that they may not have enough young people to fill jobs and support their retirement system. They are encouraging couples to have more children and are recruiting immigrants who might bring down the average age of the population. A group of business leaders, including Federal Reserve Chairman Alan Greenspan, have called for increased immigration into the United States to fill jobs, prevent inflation, and boost economic productivity.

POPULATION GROWTH: OPPOSING FACTORS

A number of social and economic pressures affect decisions about family size, which in turn affects the population at large. In this section, we will examine both positive and negative pressures on reproduction.

Pronatalist Pressures

Factors that increase people's desires to have babies are called **pronatalist pressures.** Raising a family may be the most enjoyable and rewarding part of many people's lives. Children can be a source of pleasure, pride, and comfort. They may be the only source of support for elderly parents in countries without a social security system. Where infant mortality rates are high, couples may need to have many children to ensure that at least a few will survive to take care of them when they are old. Where there is little opportunity for upward mobility, children give status in society, express parental creativity, and provide a sense of continuity and accomplishment otherwise missing from life. Often children are valuable to the family not only for future income but even more as a source of current income and help with household chores. In much of the developing world, small children tend domestic animals and younger siblings, fetch water, gather firewood, help grow crops, or sell things in the marketplace (fig. 4.10). Parental desire for children rather than an unmet need for contraceptives may be the most important factor in population growth in many cases.

Society also has a need to replace members who die or become incapacitated. This need often is codified in cultural or religious values that encourage bearing and raising children. Some societies look upon families with few or no children with pity or contempt. The idea of deliberately controlling fertility may be shocking, even taboo. Women who are pregnant or have small children have special status and protection. Boys frequently are more valued than girls because they carry on the family name and are expected to support their parents in old age. Couples may have more children than they really want in an attempt to produce a son.

Male pride often is linked to having as many children as possible. In Niger and Cameroon, for example, men, on average, want 12.6 and 11.2 children, respectively. Women in these countries consider the ideal family size to be only about half of what their husbands desire. Even though a woman might desire fewer children, however, she may have few choices and little control over her own fertility. In many societies, a woman has no status outside of her role as wife and mother. Without children, she may have no source of support in her old age.

Birth Reduction Pressures

In more highly developed countries, many pressures tend to reduce fertility. Higher education and personal freedom for women often result in decisions to limit childbearing. A desire to spend time and money on other goods and activities offsets the desire to have children. When women have opportunities to earn a salary, they are less likely to stay home and have many children. Not only do many women find the challenge and variety of a career attractive, but the money that they earn outside the home becomes an important part of the family budget. Thus, education and socioeconomic status are usually inversely related to fertility in richer countries. In some developing countries, however, fertility initially increases as educational levels and socioeconomic status rise. With higher income, families are better able to afford the children they want. More money also means that women are healthier and therefore better able to conceive and carry a child to term. It may be a generation before this unmet desire for children abates.

In less-developed countries, where feeding and clothing children can be a minimal expense, adding one more child to a family usually doesn't cost much. By contrast, raising a child in a developed country can cost hundreds of thousands of dollars by the time the child finishes school and is independent. Under these circumstances, parents are more likely to choose to have one or two children on whom they can concentrate their time, energy, and financial resources.

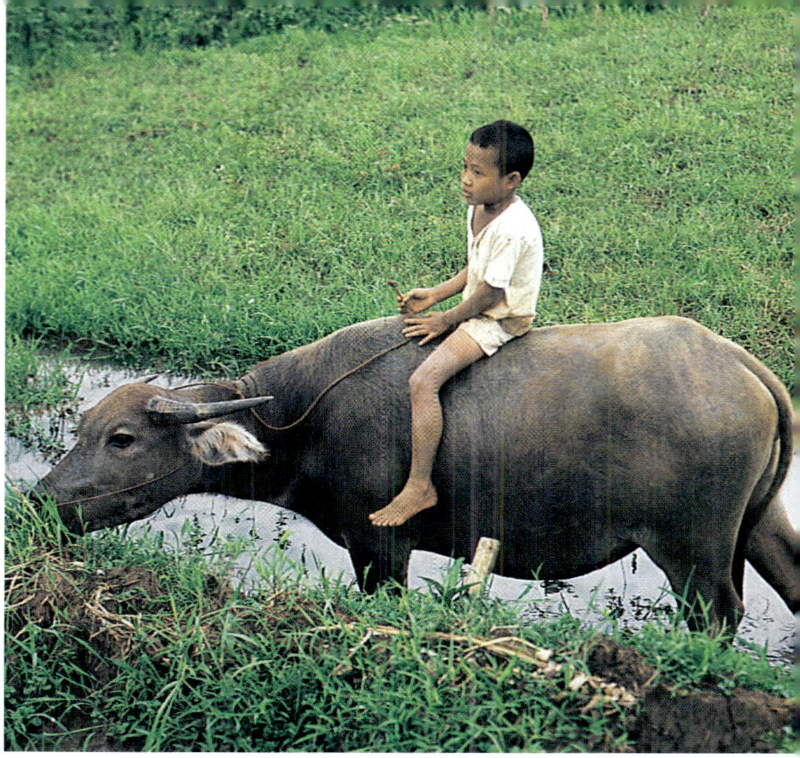

FIGURE 4.10 *Children in rural areas can help with many household chores, such as tending livestock or caring for younger children.*

Figure 4.11 shows U.S. birth rates between 1910 and 2000. As you can see, birth rates fell and rose in an irregular pattern. The period between 1910 and 1930 was a time of industrialization and urbanization. Women were getting more education than ever before and entering the workforce in large numbers. The Great Depression in the 1930s made it economically difficult for families to have children, and birth rates were low. The birth rate increased at the beginning of World War II (as it often does in wartime). For reasons that are unclear, a higher percentage of boys are usually born during war years.

A "baby boom" followed World War II, as couples were reunited and new families started. During this time, the government encouraged women to leave their wartime jobs and stay home. A high birth rate persisted through the times of prosperity and optimism of the 1950s but began to fall in the 1960s. Part of this decline was caused by the small number of babies born in the 1930s, which resulted in fewer young adults to give birth in the 1960s. Part was due to changed perceptions of the ideal family size. While in the 1950s women typically wanted four children or more, the norm dropped to one or two (or no) children in the 1970s. A small "echo boom" occurred in the 1980s, as baby boomers began to have babies, but changing economics and attitudes seem to have permanently altered our view of ideal family size in the United States.

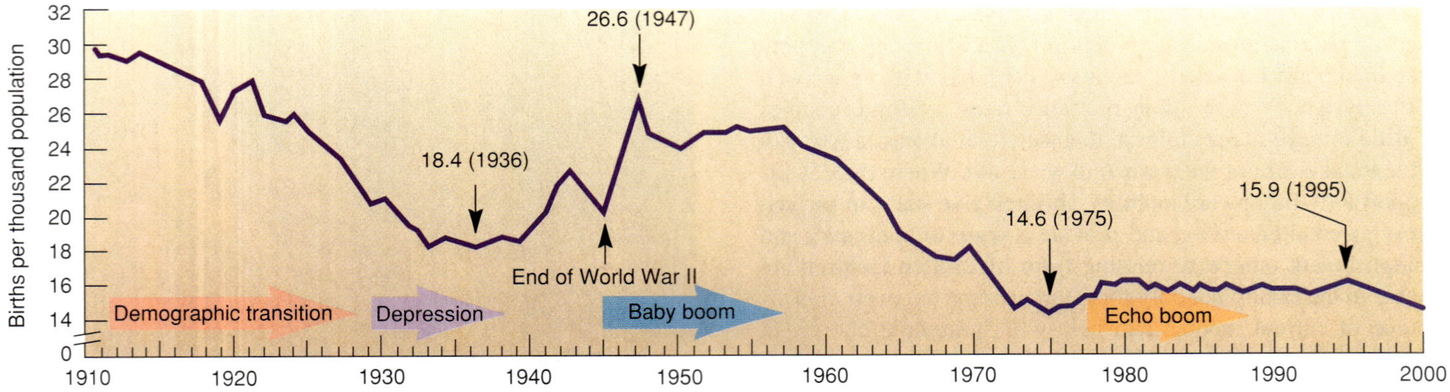

FIGURE 4.11 *Birth rates in the United States, 1910–2000. The falling birth rate from 1910 to 1929 represents a demographic transition from an agricultural to an industrial society. Note that this decline occurred before the start of the Great Depression. The baby boom following World War II lasted from 1945 to 1957. A much smaller "echo boom" occurred around 1980, when the baby boomers started to reproduce, but it produced far fewer births than anticipated.*

Source: Data from Population Reference Bureau and U.S. Census Bureau.

DEMOGRAPHIC TRANSITION

In 1945 demographer Frank Notestein pointed out that a typical pattern of falling death rates and birth rates due to improved living conditions usually accompanies economic development. He called this pattern the **demographic transition** from high birth and death rates to lower birth and death rates. Figure 4.12 shows an idealized model of a demographic transition. This model is often used to explain connections between population growth and economic development.

Development and Population

The left side of figure 4.12 represents the conditions in a premodern society. Food shortages, malnutrition, lack of sanitation and medicine, accidents, and other hazards generally keep death rates in such a society around 30 per 1,000 people. Birth rates are correspondingly high to keep population densities relatively constant. As economic development brings better jobs, medical care, sanitation, and a generally improved standard of living, death rates often fall very rapidly. Birth rates may actually rise at first as more money and better nutrition allow people to have the children they always wanted. Eventually, however, birth rates fall as people see that all their children are more likely to survive and that the whole family benefits from concentrating more resources on fewer children. Note that populations grow rapidly during the time that death rates have already fallen but birth rates remain high. Depending on how long it takes to complete the transition, the population may go through one or more rounds of doubling before coming into balance again.

The right-hand side of each curve in figure 4.12 represents conditions in many developed countries, where the transition is complete and both birth rates and death rates are low, often a third or less than those in the predevelopment era. The population comes into a new equilibrium in this phase, but at a much larger size than before. Most of the countries of northern and western Europe went through a demographic transition in the nineteenth or early twentieth century similar to the curves shown in figure 4.12. In countries such as Italy, where fertility levels have fallen below replacement rates, there are now fewer births than deaths, and the total population curve has started to decline.

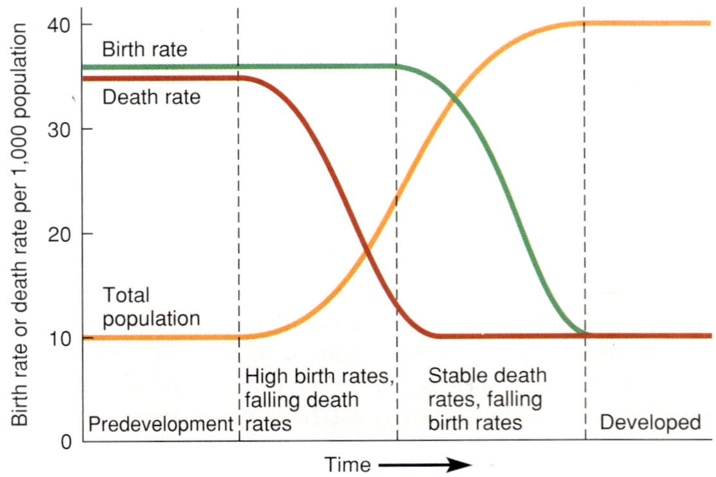

FIGURE 4.12 *Theoretical birth, death, and population growth rates in a demographic transition accompanying economic and social development.*

Many of the most rapidly growing countries in the world, such as Kenya, Yemen, Libya, and Jordan, now are in the middle phase of this demographic transition. Their death rates have fallen close to the rates of the fully developed countries, but birth rates have not fallen correspondingly. In fact, both their birth rates and total population are higher than those in most European countries when industrialization began 300 years ago. The large disparity between birth and death rates means that many developing countries now are growing at 3 to 4 percent per year. Such high growth rates in the Third World could boost total world population to 9 billion or more before the end of the twenty-first century. This raises what may be the two most important questions in this entire chapter: why are birth rates not yet falling in these countries, and what can be done about it?

An Optimistic View

Some demographers claim that a demographic transition already is in progress in most developing nations. They believe that problems in taking censuses and a normal lag between falling death and birth rates may hide this for a time but that the world population should stabilize sometime in the twenty-first century. Some evidence supports this view. As mentioned earlier in this chapter, fertility rates have fallen dramatically nearly everywhere in the world over the past half century.

Some countries have had remarkable success in population control. In Thailand, Indonesia, and Colombia, for instance, total fertility dropped by more than half in 20 years. Morocco, the Dominican Republic, Jamaica, Peru, and Mexico all have seen fertility rates fall between 30 and 40 percent in a single generation. Surprisingly, one of the most successful family planning programs in recent years has been in Iran (see Case Study, p. 89).

The following factors help stabilize populations:

- Growing prosperity and social reforms that accompany development reduce the need and desire for large families in most countries.
- Technology is available to bring advances to the developing world much more rapidly than was the case a century ago, and the rate of technology exchange is much faster than it was when Europe and North America were developing.
- Less-developed countries have historic patterns to follow. They can benefit from the mistakes of more-developed countries and chart a course to stability relatively quickly.
- Modern communications (especially television) have caused a revolution of rising expectations that act as stimuli to spur change and development.

A Pessimistic View

Economist Lester Brown of the Worldwatch Institute takes a more pessimistic view of world populations. He warns that many of the poorer countries of the world appear to be caught in a "demographic trap" that prevents them from escaping from the middle phase of the demographic transition. Their populations are now growing so rapidly that human demands exceed the sustainable yield of local forests, grasslands, croplands, and water resources. The resulting resource shortages, environmental deterioration, economic decline, and political instability may prevent these countries from ever completing modernization. Their populations may continue to grow until catastrophe intervenes.

Many people believe that the only way to break out of the demographic trap is to reduce population growth immediately and drastically by whatever means are necessary. They argue strongly for birth control education and bold national policies to encourage lower birth rates. Some agree with Malthus that helping the poor will simply increase their reproductive success and further threaten the resources on which we all depend. Author Garret Hardin described this view as lifeboat ethics:

> Each rich nation amounts to a lifeboat full of comparatively rich people. The poor of the world are in other much more crowded lifeboats. Continuously, so to speak, the poor fall out of their lifeboats and swim for a while, hoping to be admitted to a rich lifeboat, or in some other way to benefit from the goodies on board. . . . We cannot risk the safety of all the passengers by helping others in need. What happens if you share space in a lifeboat? The boat is swamped and everyone drowns. Complete justice, complete catastrophe.

A Social Justice View

A third view is that social justice (a fair share of social benefits for everyone) is the real key to successful demographic transitions. The world has enough resources for everyone, in this view, but inequitable social and economic systems cause maldistributions of those resources. Hunger, poverty, violence, environmental degradation, and overpopulation are symptoms of a lack of justice, rather than a lack of resources. Although overpopulation exacerbates other problems, a narrow focus on overpopulation alone encourages racism and hatred of the poor. Proponents of the social justice view argue that people in the richer nations should recognize our excess consumption levels and the impact that this consumption has on others. Figure 4.13 expresses the opinion of many people in less-developed countries about the relationship between resources and population.

Infant Mortality and Women's Rights

The 1994 International Conference on Population and Development in Cairo, Egypt, signaled a new approach to population issues. A broad consensus reached by the 180 participating countries agreed that responsible economic development, education and empowerment of women, and high-quality health care (including family planning services) must be accessible to everyone if population growth is to be slowed. Child survival is one of the most critical factors in stabilizing population. When infant and child mortality rates are high, as they are in much of the developing world, parents tend to have high numbers of children to ensure that some will survive to adulthood. There has never been a sustained drop in birth rates that was not first preceded by a sustained drop in infant and child mortality.

One of the most important distinctions in our demographically divided world is the high infant mortality rate in the less-developed countries. Better nutrition, improved health care, simple oral rehydration therapy, and immunization against infectious diseases (see chapter 8) have dramatically reduced child mortality rates, which have been accompanied in most regions by falling birth rates. Estimates indicate that saving 5 million children each year from easily preventable communicable diseases would avoid 20 or 30 million extra births.

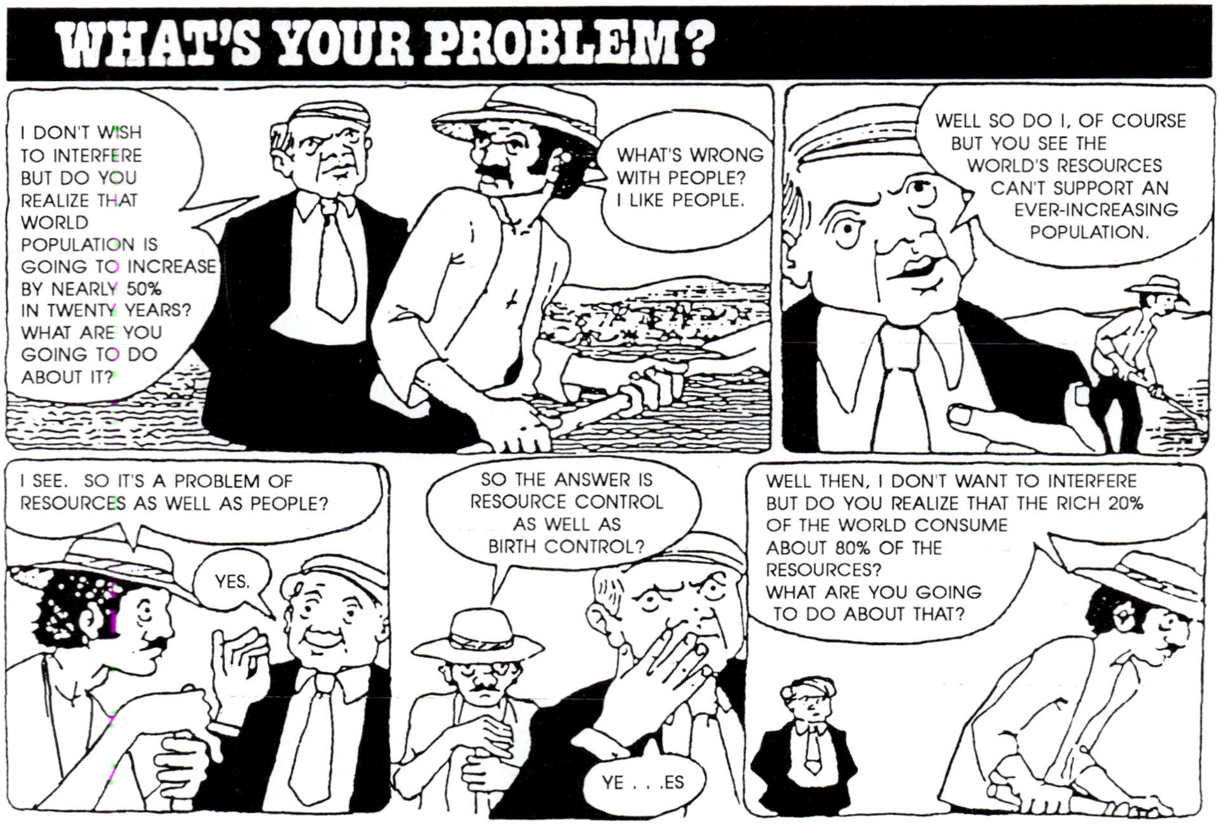
WHAT'S YOUR PROBLEM?
I DON'T WISH TO INTERFERE BUT DO YOU REALIZE THAT WORLD POPULATION IS GOING TO INCREASE BY NEARLY 50% IN TWENTY YEARS? WHAT ARE YOU GOING TO DO ABOUT IT?
WHAT'S WRONG WITH PEOPLE? I LIKE PEOPLE.
WELL SO DO I, OF COURSE BUT YOU SEE THE WORLD'S RESOURCES CAN'T SUPPORT AN EVER-INCREASING POPULATION.
I SEE. SO IT'S A PROBLEM OF RESOURCES AS WELL AS PEOPLE?
YES.
SO THE ANSWER IS RESOURCE CONTROL AS WELL AS BIRTH CONTROL?
YE . . .ES
WELL THEN, I DON'T WANT TO INTERFERE BUT DO YOU REALIZE THAT THE RICH 20% OF THE WORLD CONSUME ABOUT 80% OF THE RESOURCES? WHAT ARE YOU GOING TO DO ABOUT THAT?

FIGURE 4.13 *Controlling our population and resources—there may be more than one side to the issue.*
Used with permission of the Asian Cultural Forum on Development.

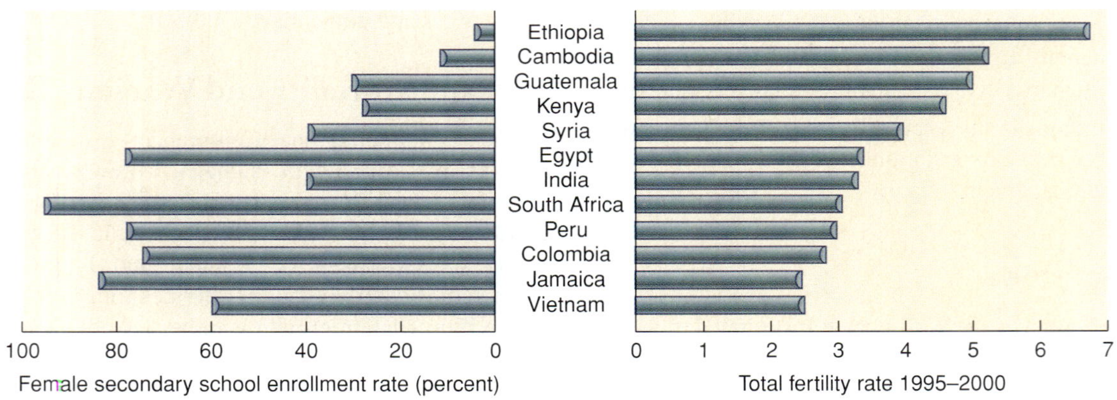

FIGURE 4.14 *Total fertility declines as women's education increases.*
Source: Data from Worldwatch Institute, 2002.

Increasing family income does not always translate into better welfare for children, since men in many cultures control most financial assets. As the UN Conference in Cairo noted, the best way to improve child survival often is to ensure the rights of mothers. Opportunities for women's education, for instance, as well as land reform, political rights, opportunities to earn an independent income, and improved health status of women often are better indicators of family welfare than is rising gross national product (fig. 4.14).

FAMILY PLANNING AND FERTILITY CONTROL

Family planning allows couples to determine the number and spacing of their children. It doesn't necessarily mean fewer children—people may use family planning to have the maximum number of children possible—but it does imply that the parents will control their reproductive lives and make rational, conscious decisions about how many children they will have and when those children

CASE STUDY

FAMILY PLANNING IN IRAN

After the Islamic Revolution in 1979, Iran had one of the world's highest population growth rates. In spite of civil war, large-scale emigration, and economic austerity, the country surged from 34 million to 63 million in just 20 years. A crude birth rate of 43.4 per 1,000 people and a total fertility rate of 5.1 per woman during this time resulted in an annual population growth of 3.9 percent and a doubling time of less than 18 years. Religious authorities exhorted couples to have as many children as Allah would give them. Any mention of birth control or family planning (other than to have as many children as possible) was forbidden, and the marriage age for girls was dropped to 9 years old. When a devastating war with Iraq in the 1980s killed at least 1 million young soldiers, producing more children to rebuild the army became a civic as well as religious duty.

In the late 1990s, however, the Iranian government became aware of the costs of such rapid population growth. With religious moderates gaining greater political power, public policy changed abruptly. Now the Iranian government is spending millions of dollars to lower birth rates. Couples must pass a national family planning course before they are allowed to marry. While it took a few years to convince people that this change will be long-lasting, most Iranian citizens are now eager for access to birth control information. Family planning classes are sought out both by engaged couples and those already married. A wide range of birth control methods are available. Implantable or injectable slow-release hormones, condoms, intrauterine devices (IUDs), pills, and male or female sterilization are free to all. Billboards, newspapers, television, and even water towers advertise this national program. Religious leaders have issued a *fatwah,* or command, that all faithful Muslims participate in family planning.

As a consequence, Iran has been remarkably successful in stemming its population growth. Between 1986 and 1996 the fertility rates for urban residents dropped almost by half, to less than three children per women, and the crude birth rate dropped from 43 to 18 per 1,000 people. By 2000 the average annual growth rate had fallen to 1.4 percent. While the population is still increasing, another decade of such progress would bring the country to a stable or even declining rate of growth.

Several societal changes have contributed to this rapid birth reduction. While the minimum marriage age has been returned to 15, couples are encouraged to wait until at least age 20 to begin their families. The educational benefits of concentrating the family resources on just one or two children are being promoted. Although women's roles are still highly restricted in the Islamic Republic, greater gender equity has given women more control over their reproductive lives. Access to modern, information-age jobs gives people an incentive to seek out education both for themselves and for their children.

The demographic transition hasn't spread to all levels of Iranian society, however. Rural families, ethnic minorities, and some urban poor still tend to have many children. Still, this example of how quickly both ideals of the perfect family size and information about modern birth control can spread through a society—even a highly religious, fundamentalist one—is encouraging for what might be accomplished worldwide in a surprisingly short time.

will be born, rather than leaving it to chance. As the desire for smaller families becomes more common, birth control often becomes an essential part of family planning. In this context, **birth control** usually means any method used to reduce births, including celibacy, delayed marriage, contraception, methods that prevent embryo implantation, and induced abortions.

Traditional Fertility Control

Evidence suggests that people in every culture and every historic period have used a variety of techniques to control population size. Studies of hunting and gathering people, such as the !Kung, or San, of the Kalahari Desert in southwest Africa, indicate that our early ancestors had stable population densities, not because they killed each other or starved to death regularly but because they controlled fertility.

For instance, San women breast-feed children for three or four years. When calories are limited, lactation depletes body fat stores and suppresses ovulation. Coupled with taboos against intercourse while breast-feeding, this is an effective way of spacing children. (However, breast-feeding among well-nourished women in modern societies doesn't necessarily suppress ovulation or prevent conception.) Other ancient techniques to control population size include celibacy, folk medicines, abortion, and infanticide. We may find some or all of these techniques unpleasant or morally unacceptable but we shouldn't assume that other people are too ignorant or too primitive to make decisions about fertility.

Current Birth Control Methods

Modern medicine gives us many more options for controlling fertility than were available to our ancestors. The major categories of birth control techniques include (1) avoidance of sex during fertile periods (for example, celibacy or the use of changes in body temperature or cervical mucus to judge when ovulation will occur), (2) mechanical barriers that prevent contact between sperm and egg (for example, condoms, spermicides, diaphragms, cervical caps, and vaginal sponges), (3) surgical methods that prevent release of sperm or egg (for example, tubal ligations in females and vasectomies in males), (4) chemicals that prevent maturation or release of sperm or eggs or that prevent embryo implantation in the uterus (for example, estrogen plus progesterone, or progesterone alone, for females; gossypol for males) (fig. 4.15), (5) physical barriers to implantation (for example, intrauterine devices), and (6) abortion.

Norplant, the trade name for flexible, matchstick-size silicon-rubber implants containing a slow-release analog of progesterone, is popular among women who want a reversible, semipermanent birth-control method. The implants are inserted under the skin, where they release hormones for up to five years. Depo-Provera, a progesterone analog, is given by injections four times a year. Both implants and injections have very low failure rates (0.3 percent, compared with about 1 percent for oral contraceptives) and eliminate the need to keep track of and take daily pills. They also can be used without knowledge of one's partner, who may oppose birth control. Some women experience increased vaginal bleeding or absence of menstrual periods from the injections or implants. Norplant may be linked to ovarian cysts, and the inserts have been difficult to remove in some cases.

Condom use more than doubled from 1980 to 2000, from about 3.5 million users in 1980 to 8 million in 2000. While condoms have about a 10 percent failure rate when used alone, their effectiveness is increased when used with spermicidal creams. Condoms also are important protection against sexually transmitted diseases. A condom for women consists of two flexible plastic rings connected by a strong, clear polyurethane sheath. One ring fits over the cervix much like a diaphragm, while the other remains outside the vagina. Each condom costs about $2 and is designed to be discarded after a single use. The six-month failure rate is about 12 percent, which means that 12 percent of women using only this device will get pregnant in six months. A female condom gives women control over their own reproduction, but some women find it difficult or unpleasant to use. None of these methods is perfect, and none suits every contraceptive need. Many require careful, conscientious use. Which choice is best for you depends on your life situation and your plans for the future.

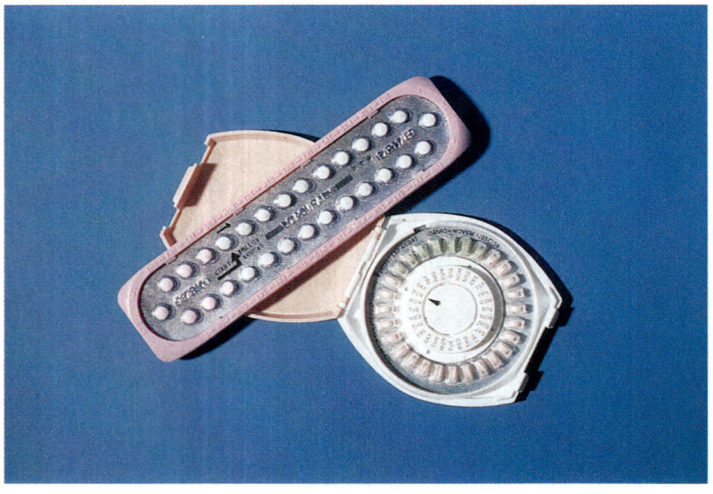

FIGURE 4.15 *Modern birth control methods can be highly effective when used properly.*

For nearly 20 years, the French drug RU486 (mifepristone or mifegyne) has been used as a "morning after" drug in Europe. RU486 blocks the effects of progesterone in maintaining the lining of the uterine wall. It is usually administered together with misoprostol (a prostaglandin analog), which causes uterine contraction and expulsion of the fetus. Interestingly, RU486 also appears to have promise in treating breast cancer, brain cancer, diabetes, and hypertension. RU486 has been approved for use in the United States, but restrictions on its use may make it unavailable for many women.

Recently a combination of two drugs previously on the market for other uses has been shown to be as safe and effective as RU486. Methotrexate and misoprostol are administered a week apart to induce abortion.

New Developments in Birth Control

More than 100 new contraceptive methods are now being studied, and some appear to have great promise. In the past two years, the U.S. Food and Drug Administration (FDA) approved five new birth control products:

- Ensure, a spring-like device that blocks the fallopian tubes in a noninvasive alternative to tubal ligation
- Mirena, a hormone-releasing intrauterine device that can stay in place for five years
- Lunelle, a hormone shot administered monthly
- NuvaRing, a hormonal vaginal ring changed every three weeks
- Ortho Evra, a hormone patch changed weekly

A group of drugs known as gonadotropin releasing-hormone agonists show promise in suppressing egg and sperm development. Some antipregnancy vaccines (immunization against chorionic gonadotropin—a hormone required to maintain the uterine lining) and antisperm vaccines are being tested that would use the immune system to prevent fertilization or embryonic implantation, but they are years away from the market. Clinical trials of hormone injections (progestin and testosterone) and calcium channel blockers (also used to treat high blood pressure) have shown some promise in suppressing sperm production, but it may be years before they are ready to market or before men will be willing to take them. A drug known as N-butyldeoxynorjirimycin, or NB-DJN, prevents sperm production in mice with no observed side effects. Whether it will prove effective in humans remains to be seen.

THE FUTURE OF HUMAN POPULATIONS

How many people will be in the world a century from now? Most demographers believe that world population will stabilize sometime during the twenty-first century. When we reach that equilibrium, the total number of humans is likely to be somewhere around 8 to 10 billion, depending on the success of family planning programs and the multitude of other factors affecting human populations. The United Nations Population Division projects three population scenarios (fig. 4.16). The optimistic (low) projection suggests that world population might stabilize by about 2030 and then drop back below current levels. The medium projection suggests that growth might continue to rise slowly until at least 2050 and then stabilize at about 9 billion. The most pessimistic (high) projection indicates that population growth will climb at present rates for 150 years or more.

Which of these scenarios will we follow? As you have seen in this chapter, population growth is a complex subject. Stabilizing or reducing human populations will require substantial changes from business as usual. One impediment is that the U.S. Congress refuses to make payments to the United Nations Family Planning Fund because some of the 135 countries that receive UN aid include abortion as part of population control programs. Population issues were conspicuously absent from the agenda of the UN Conference on Environment and Development in Rio de Janeiro (the Earth Summit) in 1992 because of opposition from religious groups and developing countries.

An encouraging sign is that worldwide contraceptive use has increased sharply in recent years. About half of the world's married couples used some family planning techniques in 2000, compared with only 10 percent 30 years earlier, but another 100 million couples say they want, but do not have access to, family planning. Contraceptive use varies widely by region, with high levels in Latin America and East Asia but relatively low use in much of Africa.

Figure 4.17 shows the unmet need for family planning among married women in some representative countries. When people in developing countries are asked what they want most, men say they want better jobs, but the first choice for a vast majority of women is family planning assistance. In general, a 15 percent increase in contraceptive use equates to about 1 fewer birth per woman per lifetime. In Chad, for example, where only 4 percent of all women use contraceptives, the average fertility is 6.6 children per woman. In Colombia, by contrast, where 77 percent of the women who would prefer not to be pregnant use contraceptives, the average fertility is 2.6 children.

Successful family planning programs often require significant societal changes. Among the most important of these are (1) improved social, educational, and economic status for women (birth control and women's rights are often interdependent); (2) improved status for children (fewer children are born if they are not needed as a cheap labor source) (3) acceptance of calculated choice as a valid element in life in general and in fertility in particular (the belief that we have no control over our lives discourages a sense of responsibility); (4) social security and political stability that give people the means and the confidence to plan for the future; and (5) the knowledge, availability, and use of effective and acceptable means of birth control. Concerted efforts to bring about these types of societal changes can be effective. Twenty years of economic development and work by voluntary family planning groups in Zimbabwe, for example, have lowered total fertility rates from 8.0 to 5.5 children per woman on average. Surveys show that desired family sizes have fallen nearly by half (9.0 to 4.6) and that nearly all women and 80 percent of men in Zimbabwe use contraceptives.

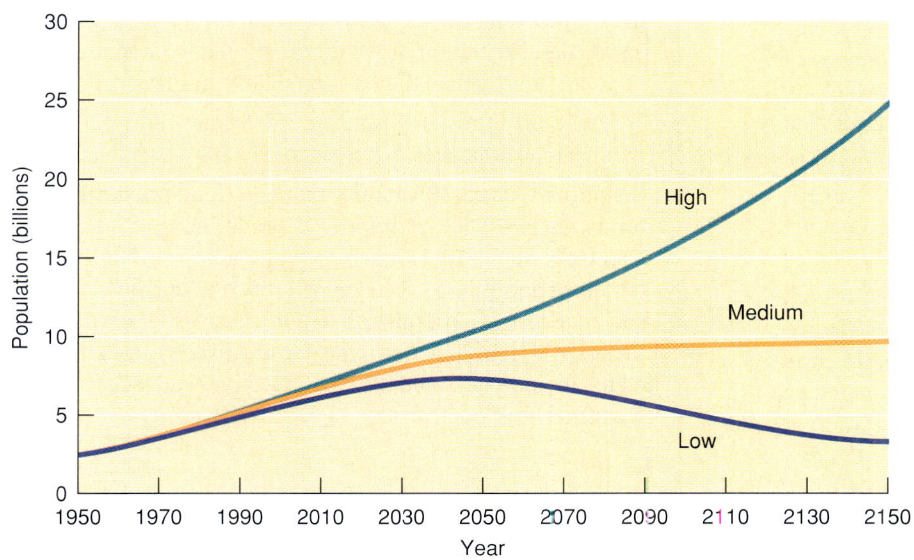

FIGURE 4.16 *Estimated and projected world population, 1950 to 2150, with different fertility levels.*
Source: Data from United Nations Population Division, 2003.

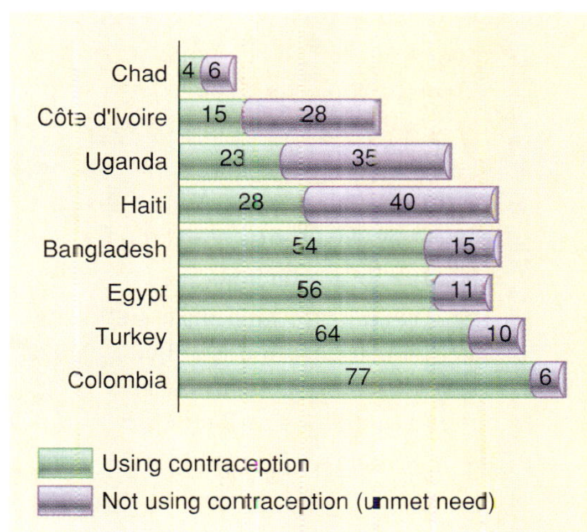

FIGURE 4.17 *Unmet need for family planning in selected countries. Globally, more than 100 million women in developing countries would prefer to avoid pregnancy but do not have access to family planning.*
Source: Data from Population Reference Bureau, 2003.

The current world average fertility rate of 2.8 births per woman is less than half what it was 50 years ago. If similar progress could be sustained for the next half century, fertility rates could fall to the replacement level of 2.1 children per woman (fig. 4.18). Whether this scenario comes true or not depends on choices that all of us make.

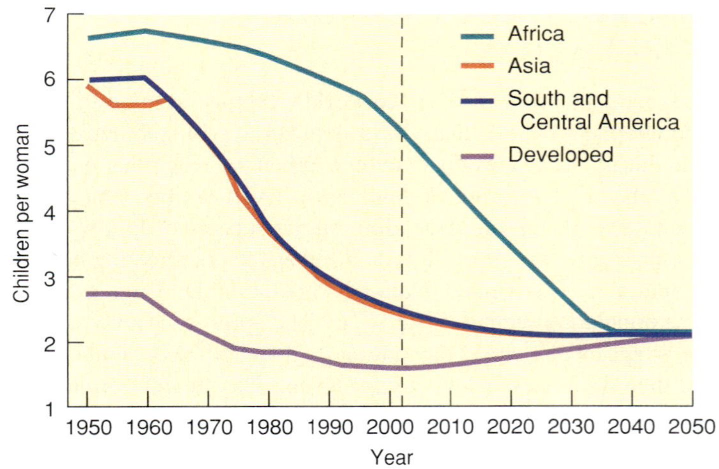

FIGURE 4.18 *Fertility declines, real and projected, 1950–2050.*
Source: Data from Population Reference Bureau, 2003.

SUMMARY

- Human populations have grown at an unprecedented rate over the past three centuries. In 2004 the world population stood at 6.4 billion people.
- If the current growth rate of 1.14 percent per year persists, the population will double in 61.4 years. Most of that growth will occur in the less-developed countries of Asia, Africa, and Latin America. There is a serious concern that the number of humans in the world and our impact on the environment will overload the life-support systems of the earth.
- The crude birth rate is the number of births in a year divided by the average population. A more accurate measure of growth is the general fertility rate, which takes into account the age structure and fecundity of the population.
- The crude birth rate minus the crude death rate gives the rate of natural increase. When this rate reaches a level at which people are just replacing themselves, zero population growth is achieved.
- The change from high birth and death rates that accompany industrialization is called a demographic transition. Many developing countries have already begun this transition. Death rates have fallen, but birth rates remain high.
- Some demographers believe that, as infant mortality drops and economic development progresses so that people in these countries can be sure of a secure future, they will complete the transition to a stable population. Others fear that excessive population growth and limited resources will catch many of the poorer countries in a demographic trap that could prevent them from ever achieving a stable population or a high standard of living.
- While larger populations bring many problems, they also may be a valuable resource of energy, intelligence, and enterprise that make it possible to overcome resource limitation problems. A social justice view argues that a more equitable distribution of wealth might reduce both excess population growth and environmental degradation.
- We have many more options now for controlling fertility than were available to our ancestors.
- Sometimes successful family planning requires deep cultural changes, such as improved social, educational, and economic status for women; higher values on individual children; acceptance of responsibility for our own lives; social security and political stability that give people the means and confidence to plan for the future; and knowledge, availability, and use of effective and acceptable means of birth control.

QUESTIONS FOR REVIEW

1. At what point in history did the world population pass its first billion? What factors restricted population before that time, and what factors contributed to growth after that point?
2. How might growing populations be beneficial in solving development problems?
3. Why do some economists consider human resources more important than natural resources in determining a country's future?
4. Where will most population growth occur during the twenty-first century? What conditions contribute to rapid population growth in some countries?
5. Define *crude birth rate, total fertility rate, crude death rate,* and *zero population growth.*
6. What is the difference between life expectancy and life span? Why are they different?
7. What is the dependency ratio, and how might it affect the United States in the future?
8. What factors increase or decrease people's desires to have babies?
9. Describe the conditions that lead to a demographic transition.
10. Describe the major choices in modern birth control.

THINKING SCIENTIFICALLY

1. Suppose that you were head of a family planning agency in India. How would you design a scientific study to determine the effectiveness of different approaches to population stabilization? How would you account for factors such as culture, religion, education, and economics?
2. Why do you suppose that the United Nations gives high, medium, and low projections for future population growth? Why not give a single estimate? What factors would you consider in making these projections?
3. Some demographers claim that the total world population has already begun to slow, while others dispute this claim. How would you recognize a true demographic transition, as opposed to mere random fluctuations in birth and death rates?
4. Why do we usually express crude birth and death rates per thousand people? Why not give the numbers per person or for the entire population?
5. In northern Europe, the demographic transition began in the early 1800s, a century or more before the invention of modern antibiotics and other miracle drugs. What factors do you think contributed to this transition? How would you use historical records to test your hypothesis?
6. In chapter 3, we discussed carrying capacities. What do you think the maximum and optimum carrying capacities for humans are? Why is this a more complex question for humans than it might be for other species? Why is designing experiments in human demography difficult?

KEY TERMS

birth control 89
crude birth rate 81
crude death rates 82
demographic transition 86
demography 79
dependency ratio 83
family planning 88
life expectancy 83
neo-Malthusians 78
pronatalist pressures 84
total fertility rate 81
zero population growth (ZPG) 81

SUGGESTED READINGS

Ashford, Lori. 2003. *Unmet Need for Family Planning: Recent Trends and Their Implications for Programs.* Population Reference Bureau. Published online at http://www.prb.org.

Dasgupta, Partha S. 1995. Population, poverty and the local environment. *Scientific American* (February 1995), pp. 40–45.

Ehrlich, Paul R. 2000. *Human Nature: Genes, Cultures, and the Human Prospect.* Island Press.

Hartmann, Betsy. 1999. Population, environment, and security: A new trinity. In *Dangerous Intersections: Feminist Perspectives on Population, Environment, and Development.* Jael Silliman and Ynestra King, eds. South End Press, pp. 1–23.

Pimentel, David, et al. 1999. Will limits of the earth's resources control human numbers? *Environment, Development and Sustainability* 1:19–39.

Sen, Amaryta. 1994. Population and reasoned agency: Food, fertility, and economic development. In *Population, Economic Development, and the Environment.* Kerstin Lindahl-Kiessling and Hans Landberg, eds. Oxford University Press, pp. 51–78.

Welcome to McGraw-Hill's Online Learning Center

http://www.mhhe.com/cunningham3e

WEB EXERCISES

Exponential and Logistic Growth

Find the Excel file Population_Growth.xls in the OLC, chapter 6, under Web Exercises. This file models and graphs growth since 1950, based on actual data, exponential growth, and logistic growth. Review these growth patterns in your text; then experiment with growth rates as follows:

1. Raise the growth rate *(r)*; then lower it, and watch how the curve changes. At 4 percent (comparable to the fastest growing countries), how many years does it take for the 1950 population to double? How many years at 3.5 percent? 0.5 percent? What rate brings the population closest to the projected curve for 2050?
2. Click on the Census Data tab (bottom of sheet). What is the range of actual rates? How have they changed over time?
3. Now look a the logistic curve. The key difference here is that growth rate decreases as the population approaches *K*. Set *r* to 1.4. Set *K* to 100. Do the logistic and exponential curves differ much? Reduce *K* to 80, then to 60, 40, and 20. When does the logistic curve fall below the projected curve? As implemented here, is the carrying capacity an abrupt population ceiling, or is it a density-dependent growth control?
4. Enter what you think would be a reasonable carrying capacity. What number have you entered? What population does this produce in 2050? How much does your restricted population vary from the U.S. Census' projection? What does *K* mean for humans, as compared with other populations?

Exploring Growth Factors in Population Data

How and why populations grow is a key question in environmental science. In this exercise, you examine and graph current world population data to explore which factors most strongly correlate with birth rates. Go to www.mhhe.com/cases.

There you will find an Excel data file named popdata.xls. Double-click on the file name to copy it to your hard disk. If you have Excel on your computer, you should be able to open the data file by double-clicking on it. (Other spreadsheet programs can also read this file, but you must open it from within your program, not by double-clicking.)

1. This file contains population data for the countries of the world, sorted by the United Nations Human Development Index (HDI) rank. First look at the top 20 countries. Where are they? What is the range of income levels (in GNP per capita) of the top 20? What is the range of income for the bottom 20 countries?
2. Now make an X,Y scatter graph of adult literacy and birth rate. (Detailed instructions for making graphs in Excel are included at the far right side of the spreadsheet page [column N].) How would you describe the relationship between these variables? How would you explain this relationship? Keep this graph in your spreadsheet while you make three more scatter graphs: (1) GNP per capita and birth rate, (2) life expectancy and birth rate, and (3) infant mortality and birth rate. Describe the trends you observe, and explain what they mean.
3. How would you compare the relative amount of scatter in each of your graphs? Why do some curves slope from right to left, while others slope in the opposite direction? If you draw a line through the middle of the dot cluster, some curve smoothly, while others seem to have a break or inflection point. How would you interpret these patterns?
4. Try changing the shape of your graphs. (See instructions on the right side of the spreadsheet to do this.) How does making the graphs taller or wider affect the way your trends look? How could you deliberately manipulate the graph shape to affect other people's interpretation of the data? Is this ethical? Have you ever seen it done?
5. Now make a dot graph of GNP per capita and adult literacy. Is there a linear relationship between the two variables? Why or why not?

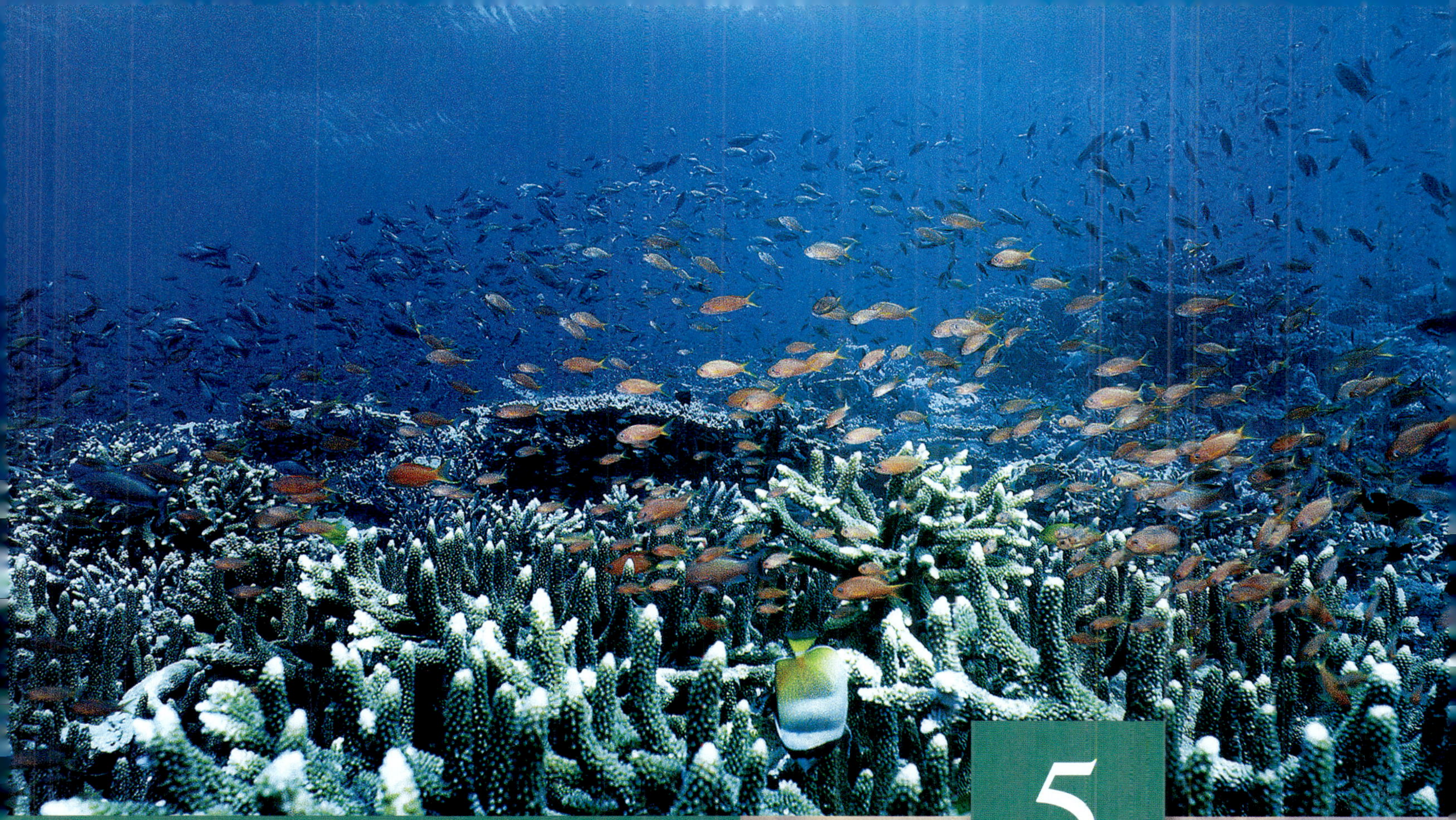

Biodiversity is essential for the ecological services on which we all depend.

5

Biomes and Biodiversity

In the end, we conserve only what we love.
We will love only what we understand.
We will understand only what we are taught.

–Baba Dioum

Welcome to McGraw-Hill's Online Learning Center
http://www.mhhe.com/cunningham3e

LEARNING ONLINE

Visit our webpage at www.mhhe.com/cunningham3e for data sources, further readings, additional case studies, current environmental news, and regional examples within the Online Learning Center to help you understand the material in this chapter. You'll also find active links to information pertaining to this chapter, including

Biomes
Global wetlands
Oceans and coastlines
Biological Resources Division, USGS
Biodiversity and endangered species
Biodiversity hot spots
Trade in endangered species

OBJECTIVES

After studying this chapter, you should be able to

- recognize the characteristics and general distribution of major biomes, and understand the most important factors that determine biome distributions.
- evaluate the degree of disturbance of major biomes, and identify the biomes that are most important for human activities and for biodiversity protection.
- define *biodiversity* and explain its importance.
- report on the total number and relative distribution of living species on the earth.
- describe how human activities cause biodiversity losses.
- identify regions and ecosystems of high biodiversity.
- evaluate the effectiveness of efforts to protect endangered species.

Coral Reefs Threatened

Often referred to as undersea gardens, coral reefs are among the most species-rich and productive ecosystems in the world. Ornate and visually stunning, the coral is vital to the health of the whole reef ecosystem. The reefs are colonies of minute, colonial animals, called polyps, that live symbiotically with photosynthetic algae. The calcium-rich framework created by the polyps provides structure to the reef, while the algae provide energy and nutrients. Fish, worms, crustaceans, sponges, sea fans, and myriad other creatures subsist on or hide within the reef. Scientists have identified some 4,000 species of fish and 800 species of reef-building coral, but the total number of species associated with reefs is probably more than 1 million.

Reefs grow slowly, as little as half an inch (1.25 cm) per year, and the coral needs just the right combination of light, warmth, and pure water to survive. Small changes in the reef environment can have disastrous effects on the health of the entire reef ecosystem. Although natural disturbances, such as hurricanes and typhoons, can cause severe changes in coral communities, humans have been linked to the vast majority of decreases in coral cover and general reef health. Among the most harmful human threats are coral mining for building materials, fishing with dynamite, deep-sea trawling, overfishing in general, and careless pleasure diving by tourists. Reefs also suffer from sediment from inland deforestation and removal of coastal mangroves, from industrial pollution, and from nutrient pollution created by sewage, fertilizers, and urban runoff.

A study of coral reef health conducted by the World Resources Institute recently concluded that nearly 60 percent of the world's reefs are at risk from human activities. The reefs of Southeast Asia, which are the most species-diverse in the world, are also the most threatened, with 86 percent at medium or high risk. The Pacific Ocean, on the other hand, which contains more reef area than any other region, is in much better shape, with just 10 percent of its reefs at high risk.

According to many marine biologists, global warming is the greatest long-term threat to coral reefs. When corals are stressed by elevated water temperatures, however, they often expel their symbiotic algae in a process called bleaching, which creates patches of bone-white reef. Some corals can acquire new algal partners, but many sicken and die. Once rare, bleaching has become common and widespread. In 1998 reefs from the Caribbean to Australia were hit by the worst coral bleaching episode in recorded history. On the 350,000-km^2 Great Barrier Reef, 60 percent of all corals—some of them 700 years old—died as a result. If the worst-case scenarios for global warming come true, some marine biologists predict all the remaining coral reefs in the world may be dead or dying in 50 years.

Coral reefs are only one of the many biological communities threatened by human actions. Habitat destruction, overharvesting of commercial species, pollution, introduction of exotic species, and global climate change threaten biologically rich communities from the Atlantic forest of Brazil to South Africa's Fynbos flora, to North America's tall grass prairie. A recent computer model study by researchers from the British Center for Biodiversity and Conservation warns that millions of species—perhaps up to 37 percent of all terrestrial plants and animals—could be forced into extinction by 2050 if the worst-case scenarios for global climate change come true. In this chapter, we'll survey some of the major terrestrial and aquatic biological communities as well as the biodiversity they harbor. We'll look at some of the benefits of biodiversity as well as the ways in which human activities endanger it.

TERRESTRIAL BIOMES

Although all local environments are unique, it is helpful to understand them in terms of a few general groups with similar climate conditions, growth patterns, and vegetation types. We call these broad types of biological communities **biomes.** Understanding the global distribution of biomes, and knowing the differences in what grows where and why, is essential to the study of global environmental science. Biological productivity—and ecosystem resilience—varies greatly from one biome to another. Human use of biomes and nature's ability to restore itself depend largely on those conditions. Clear-cut forests regrow relatively quickly in New England but very slowly in Siberia, where current logging is expanding. Some grasslands rejuvenate quickly after grazing, and some are slower to recover. Why these differences? The sections that follow seek to answer this question.

Temperature and precipitation are among the most important determinants in biome distribution on land (fig. 5.1). If we know the general temperature range and precipitation level, we can predict what kind of biological community is likely to occur there, in the absence of human disturbance. Landforms, especially mountains, and prevailing winds also exert important influences on biological communities.

It is helpful to understand biomes in terms of their global distribution (fig. 5.2). For example, a band of boreal (northern) forests crosses Canada and Siberia, tropical forests occur near the equator, and expansive grasslands lie near—or just beyond—the tropics. As you look at this map, which biomes do you think are most heavily populated by humans? Why? Look at the seasonal patterns of temperatures and moisture levels for some representative sites around the world (fig. 5.3). Does this help you understand patterns of both biome distribution and human habitation?

In this chapter, we'll examine the major terrestrial biomes; then we'll investigate ocean and freshwater communities and environments. Ocean environments are important because they cover two-thirds of the earth's surface, provide food for much of humanity, and help regulate our climate through photosynthesis. Wetlands are often small, but they have great influence on environmental health, biodiversity, and water quality. In chapter 6, we'll look at how we use these communities as well as how we preserve, manage, and restore them.

Deserts

You may think of deserts as barren and biologically impoverished. Their vegetation is sparse, but it can be surprisingly diverse, and most desert plants and animals are highly adapted to survive long droughts, extreme heat, and often extreme cold. **Deserts** occur where precipitation is rare and unpredictable, usually with less than 30 cm of rain per year. Adaptations to these conditions

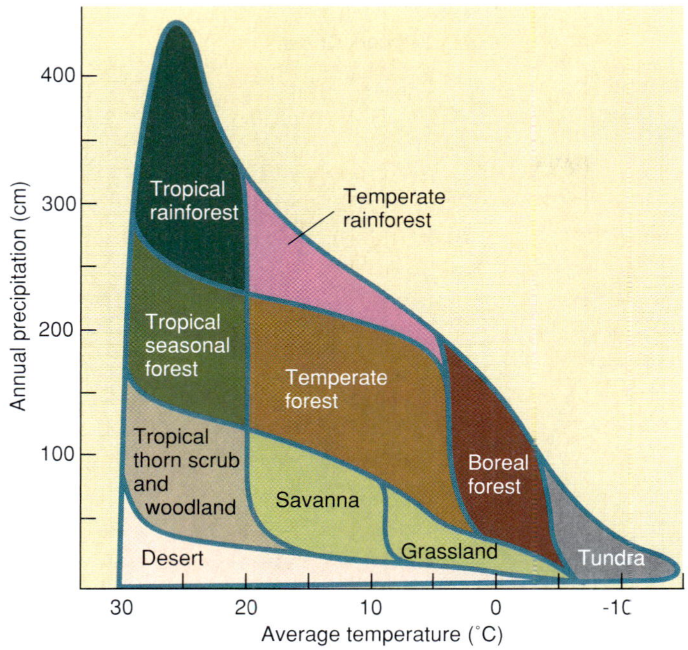

FIGURE 5.1 *Biomes most likely to occur in the absence of human disturbance or other disruptions, according to average annual temperature and precipitation.* Note: *This diagram does not consider soil type, topography, wind speed, or other important environmental factors. Still, it is a useful general guideline for biome location.*
Source: From *Communities and Ecosystems*, 2/e by R. H. Whitaker, © 1975. Reprinted by permission of Prentice Hall, Upper Saddle River, New Jersey.

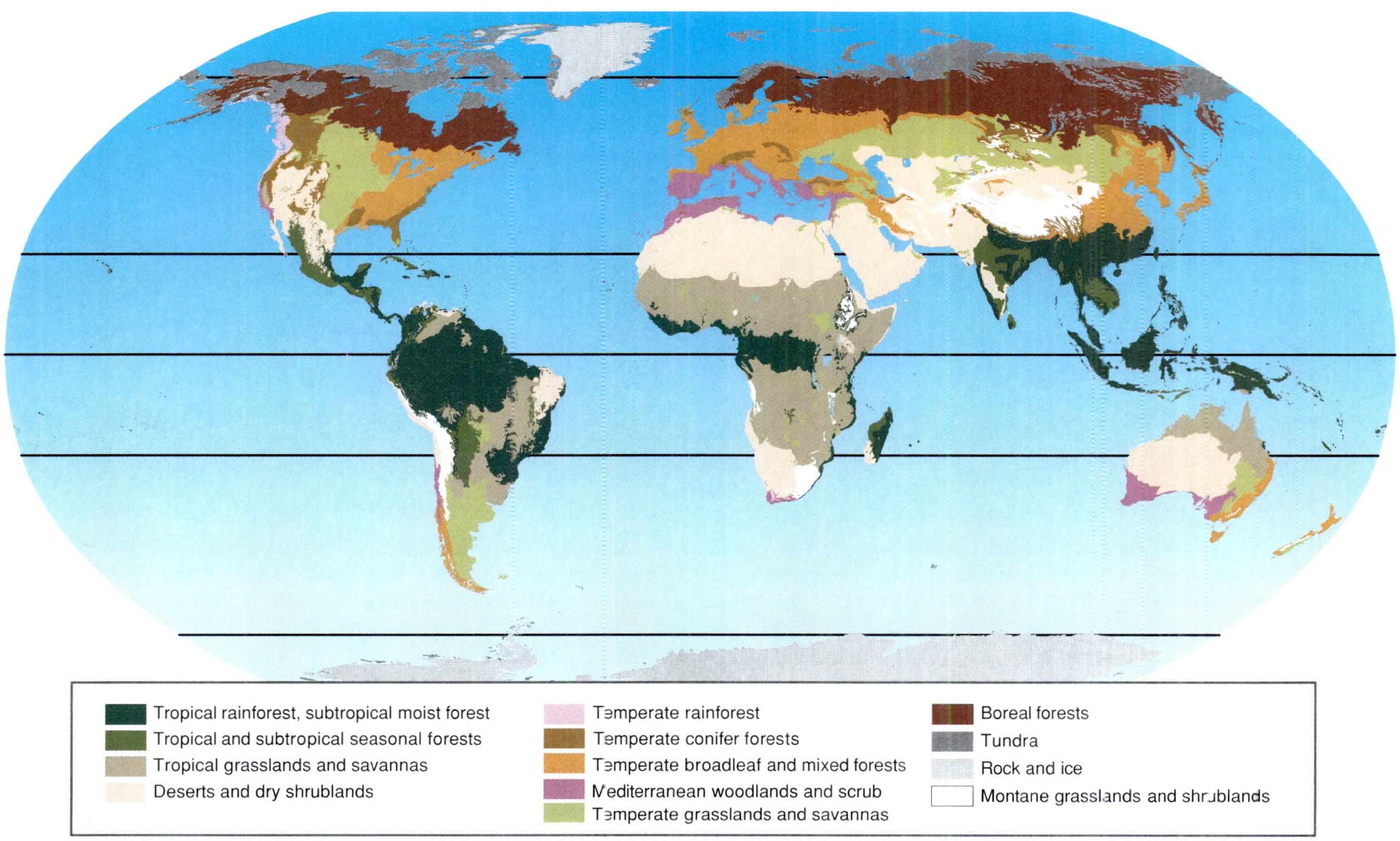

FIGURE 5.2 *Major world biomes. Compare this map with figure 5.1 for generalized temperature and moisture conditions that control biome distribution. Also compare it with the satellite image of biological productivity (fig. 5.12).*
Source: WWF Ecoregions.

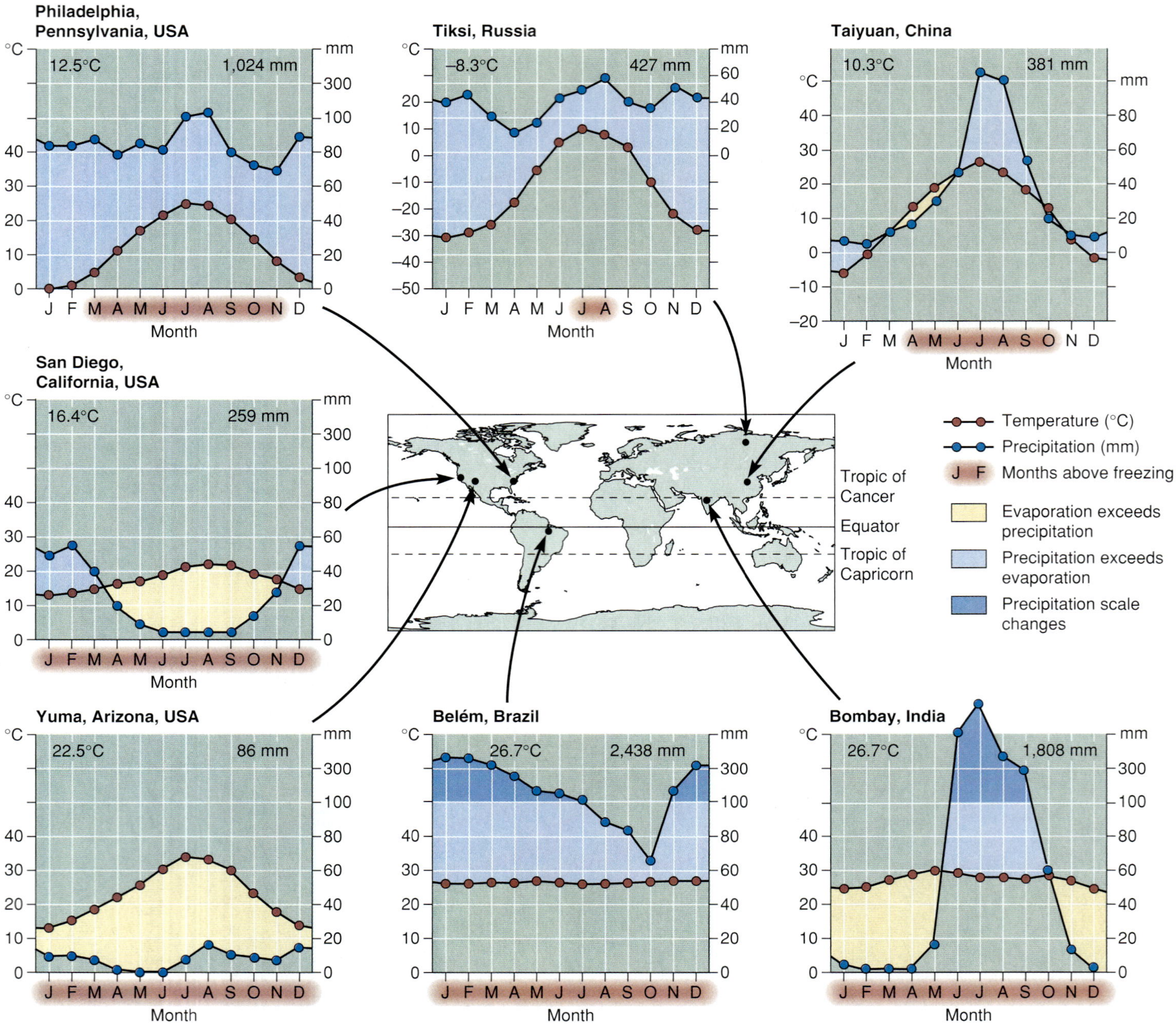

FIGURE 5.3 *Moisture availability depends on temperature as well as precipitation. The horizontal axis on these climate diagrams shows months of the year; vertical axes show temperature* (left side) *and precipitation* (right). *The number of dry months* (shaded yellow) *and wetter months* (blue) *varies with geographic location. Mean annual temperature (°C) and precipitation (mm) are shown at the top of each graph.*

include water-storing leaves and stems, thick epidermal layers to reduce water loss, and salt tolerance. Many desert plants are drought-deciduous; that is, they lose their leaves during the dry season (fig. 5.4). Most desert plants also bloom and set seed quickly when a spring rain does fall.

Like plants, animals in deserts are specially adapted. Many are nocturnal, spending their days in burrows to avoid the sun's heat and desiccation. Pocket mice, kangaroo rats, and gerbils can get most of their moisture from seeds and plants. Desert rodents also have highly concentrated urine and nearly dry feces, which allow them to eliminate body waste without losing precious moisture.

Deserts are more vulnerable than you might imagine. Sparse, slow-growing vegetation is quickly damaged by off-road vehicles. Desert soils recover slowly. Tracks left by army tanks practicing in California deserts during World War II can still be seen today.

Deserts are also vulnerable to overgrazing. In Africa's vast Sahel (the southern edge of the Sahara Desert), livestock are destroying much of the plant cover. Bare, dry soil becomes drift-

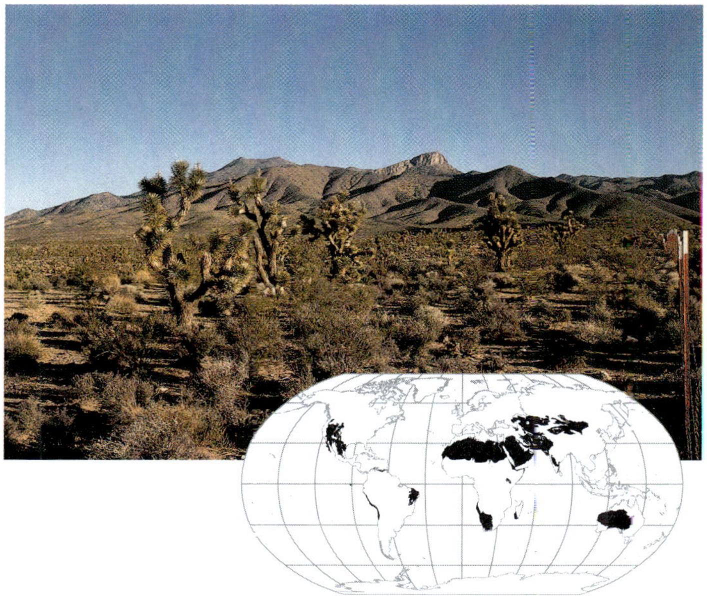

FIGURE 5.4 *World deserts* (top) *and a desert landscape in Joshua Tree National Park. Like most desert plants, these Joshua trees are adapted to conserve water and repel enemies.*

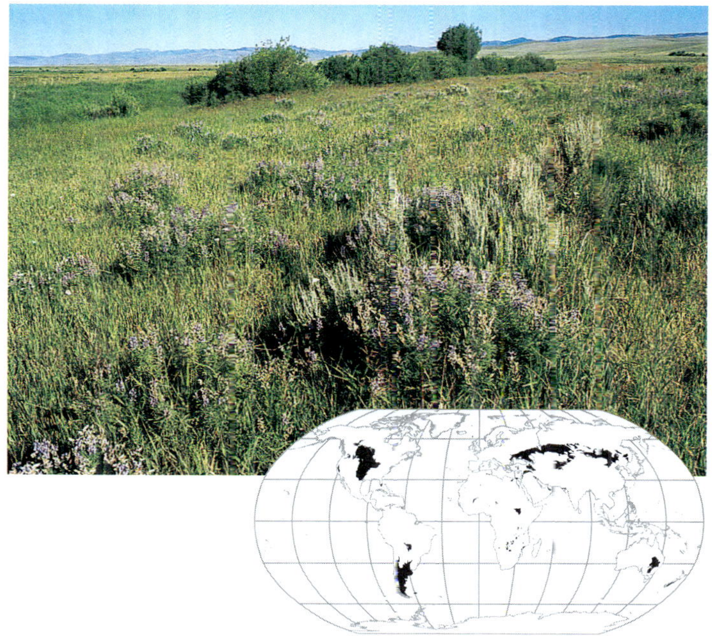

FIGURE 5.5 *Grasslands occur at midlatitudes on all continents. Kept open by extreme temperatures, dry conditions, and periodic fires, grasslands can have surprisingly high plant and animal diversity.*

ing sand, and restabilization is extremely difficult. Without plant roots and organic matter, the soil loses its ability to retain what rain does fall, and the land becomes progressively drier and more bare. Similar depletion of dryland vegetation is happening in many desert areas, including Central Asia, India, and the American Southwest and Plains states.

Grasslands: Prairies and Savannas

Grasslands occur where there is enough rain to support abundant grass but not enough for forests (fig. 5.5). Usually grasslands are a complex, diverse mix of grasses and flowering herbaceous plants, generally known as forbs. Black-eyed susan and purple coneflower are forbs that may be familiar to you. In drier grasslands, grasses and forbs may be less than half a meter tall. In wetter areas, grasses can exceed 2 m. Where scattered trees occur in a grassland, we call it a savanna.

Like desert plants, grassland and savanna vegetation is adapted to survive drought and extreme heat or cold. Most have deep, long-lived roots that seek groundwater and that persist when leaves and stems above ground die back. These deep roots, and annual accumulation of dead leaves on the surface, produce thick, organic-rich soils in many grasslands. Most grasslands are also adapted to survive fire. Fresh green shoots appear quickly after a fire, and migratory grazers, such as American bison, African wildebeest, and central Asian horses, thrive on this new growth.

Historically, the greatest threat to grasslands was conversion of the rich soils to farmland. The tallgrass prairies of the central Unites States and Canada are almost completely converted to corn, soy, and other crops. Remaining grasslands are mostly too dry for good farmland, so the greatest risk today is from overgrazing. As in a desert, excessive grazing eventually kills even deep-rooted plants. As groundcover disappears, soil erosion results, and unpalatable weeds, such as cheatgrass or leafy spurge, spread. An additional threat to remaining grasslands is fire suppression, which allows trees to encroach on former grasslands.

Tundra

Where temperatures are below freezing most of the year, only small, hardy vegetation can survive. **Tundra,** a treeless landscape that occurs at high latitudes or on mountaintops, has a growing season of only two to three months, and it may have frost any month of the year. Some people consider tundra a variant of grasslands because it has no trees; others consider it a very cold desert because water is unavailable (frozen) most of the year.

Arctic tundra is an expansive biome that has low productivity because it receives little light and has a short growing season (fig. 5.6). During midsummer, however, 24-hour sunshine supports a burst of plant growth and an explosion of insect life. Tens of millions of waterfowl, shorebirds, terns, and songbirds migrate to the Arctic every year to feast on the abundant invertebrate and plant life and to raise their young on the brief bounty. These birds then migrate to wintering grounds, where they may be eaten by local predators—effectively they carry energy and protein from high latitudes to low latitudes. Arctic tundra is essential for global biodiversity, especially for birds.

Alpine tundra, occurring on or near mountaintops, has environmental conditions and vegetation similar to arctic tundra. These areas have a short, intense growing season. Often one sees a

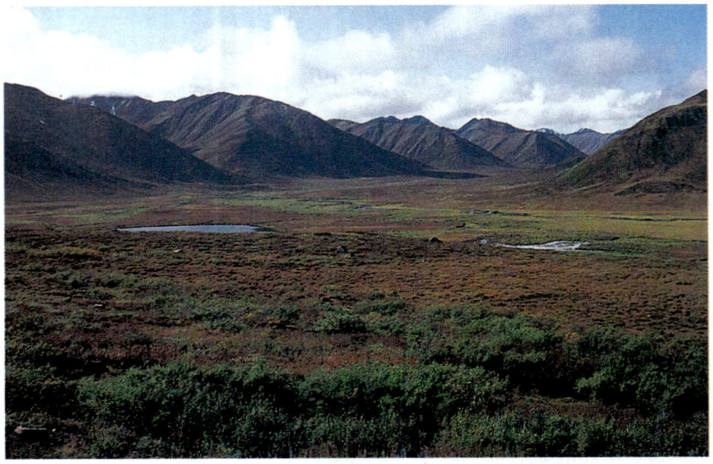

FIGURE 5.6 *Tundra ecosystems have short growing seasons and long, dark winters. Vegetation is mainly short and grows extremely slowly.*

splendid profusion of flowers in alpine tundra: this is because everything must flower at once in order to produce seeds in a few weeks before the snow comes again. Many alpine tundra plants also have deep pigmentation and leathery leaves to protect against the strong ultraviolet light in the thin mountain atmosphere.

Compared with other biomes, tundra has relatively low diversity. Dwarf shrubs, such as willows, sedges, grasses, mosses, and lichens, tend to dominate the vegetation. Migratory musk-ox, caribou, and alpine mountain sheep and mountain goats can live on the vegetation because they move frequently to new pastures.

Because these environments are too cold for most human activities, they are not as badly threatened as other biomes. There are important problems, however. Global climate change may be altering the balance of some tundra ecosystems, and air pollution from distant cities tends to accumulate at high latitudes (see chapter 9). In eastern Canada, coastal tundra is being badly depleted by overabundant populations of snow geese, whose numbers have exploded due to winter grazing on the rice fields of Arkansas and Louisiana. Oil and gas drilling—and associated truck traffic—threatens tundra in Alaska and Siberia. Clearly, this remote biome is not independent of human activities at lower latitudes.

APPLICATION: Comparing Biome Climates

Look back at the climate graphs for Yuma, Arizona, a desert region, and Tiksi, Russia, a tundra region (fig. 5.3). How much colder is Tiksi than Yuma in January? In July? Which location has the greater range of temperature through the year? How much do the two locations differ in precipitation during their wettest months?

Compare the temperature and precipitation in these two places with those in the other biomes shown. How wet are the wettest locations? Which biomes have distinct dry seasons? How do rainfall and length of warm seasons explain vegetation conditions in these biomes?

Answers: Tiksi is about 42°C colder in January, 25°C colder in June; Tiksi has the greater range of temperature; there is about 40 mm difference in precipitation in August.

Conifer Forests

Conifer (cone-bearing) forests occur in a wide range of temperate, or midlatitude, regions. Many grow where moisture is limited by sandy soil, and their thin, waxy leaves (needles) help them reduce moisture loss. In the United States, **southern pine forests** are one of the most important forest resources. These forests grow quickly, and they tolerate weathered, nutrient-poor soils. Bird and mammal diversity in these forests can be extremely high. Because these forests grow quickly in the warm, moist southern climate, though, many have been converted to plantations, with little plant or animal diversity.

Conifer needles can also survive the harsh winter of northern forests and mountains, so conifers tend to dominate high-latitude and high-altitude forests. The **boreal forest,** or northern conifer forest, stretches in a broad band around the world between about 45° and 60° north (fig. 5.7). Dominant trees are pine, hemlock, spruce, cedar, and fir. Some deciduous trees are also mixed in, such as maple, birch, aspen, and alder. In Siberia, Canada, and the western United States, conifer forests are also a key resource, on which large, regional economies depend.

The extreme, ragged edge of the boreal forest, where forest gradually gives way to tundra, is known by its Russian name, **taiga.** The extreme cold and short summer limit the growth rate of trees here. A 10-cm-diameter tree may be a century or two old in the far north.

The coniferous forests of the Pacific coast represent yet another special set of environmental circumstances. Mild year-

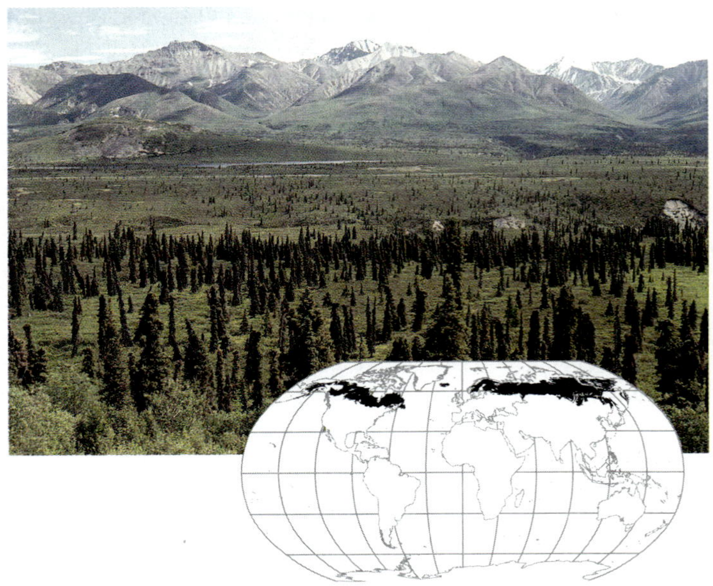

FIGURE 5.7 *Boreal forest. At the northern limit of the boreal forest in Alaska, we find small, widely spaced black spruce intermixed with willows and heather on a wet peatland.*

round temperatures and abundant rainfall, up to 250 cm (100 in.) per year, result in luxuriant plant growth and giant trees, such as the California redwoods, the largest trees in the world and the largest organism of any kind known to have ever existed. Redwoods once grew along the Pacific coast from California to Oregon, but logging has reduced them to a few small fragments.

The wettest coastal forests are known as the **temperate rainforest,** a cool, rainy forest often enshrouded in fog (fig. 5.8). Condensation in the canopy (leaf drip) is a major form of precipitation in the understory.

Because conifer forests are widespread and the trees are often large, they have been one of our most important natural resources. Remaining fragments of ancient forests are important areas of biodiversity, especially in North America and Europe. Recent battles over old-growth conservation (chapter 6) are focused mainly on these forests. Forest management policies are one of the more important, and perennial, political issues in the United States and Canada, and these issues are emerging in Russia.

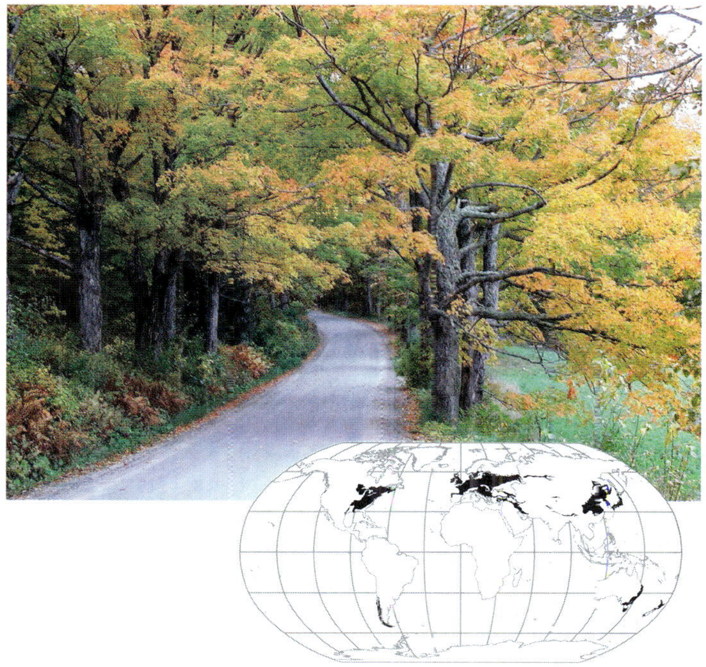

FIGURE 5.9 *Temperate deciduous forests lose their leaves, and often change to lovely colors, as freezing weather approaches*

Broad-Leaved Deciduous Forests

Broad-leaved forests occur throughout the world where rainfall is plentiful. In midlatitudes, these forests are **deciduous**; that is, they lose their leaves in winter (fig. 5.9). At warmer latitudes, broad-leaved trees may lose their leaves in a dry season, or they may retain most leaves most of the year. Southern live oaks and cypresses, for example, are broad-leaved evergreen trees.

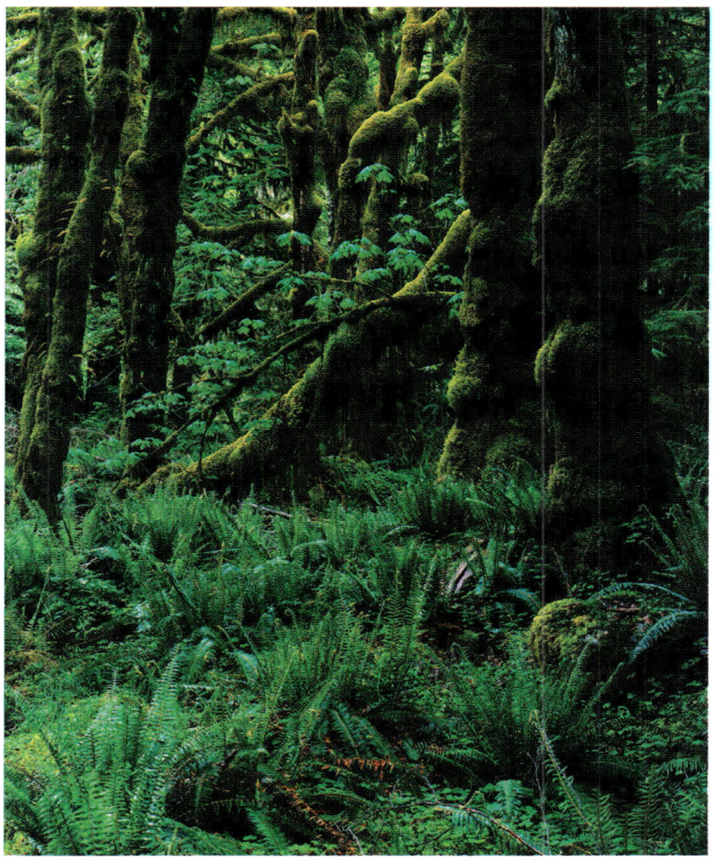

FIGURE 5.8 *Temperate rainforests, with towering conifers and a wet understory, are a very rainy variant of temperate coniferous biomes.*

Although these forests have a dense canopy in summer, they have a diverse understory that blooms in spring, before the trees leaf out. Spring ephemeral (short-lived) plants produce lovely flowers, and vernal pools support amphibians and insects. The middle layers and understory of these forests also harbor a great diversity of North American songbirds.

In North America, deciduous forests once covered most of what is now the eastern half of the United States and southern Canada. Most of western Europe was once deciduous forest. Most of this forest was cleared a thousand years ago. When European settlers first came to North America, they quickly settled and cut most of these forests for timber, firewood, industrial uses, or to make farmland.

Deciduous forests can regrow readily because they occupy a moist, moderate climate. But most of these forests have been occupied so long that human impacts are extensive, and most native species are at least somewhat threatened. Currently, the greatest threat to broad-leaved deciduous forests is in eastern Siberia, where deforestation is proceeding rapidly. Siberia may have the highest deforestation rate in the world. As forests disappear, so do Siberian tigers, bears, cranes, and a host of other endangered species.

Mediterranean/Chaparral/Thorn Scrub

Often, dry environments support drought-adapted shrubs and trees, as well as grass. These mixed environments can be highly variable. They can also be very rich biologically. Such conditions are often described as Mediterranean (with hot, dry summers and cool, moist winters). Evergreen shrubs with small, leathery, sclerophyllous (hard, waxy) leaves form dense thickets. Scrub oaks, drought-resistant pines, or other small trees often cluster in sheltered valleys. Periodic fires burn fiercely in this fuel-rich plant assemblage and are a major factor in plant succession. Annual spring flowers often bloom profusely, especially after fires. In California, this landscape is called **chaparral,** Spanish for thicket. Some typical animals include jackrabbits, kangaroo rats, mule deer, chipmunks, lizards, and many bird species. Very similar landscapes are found along the Mediterranean coast as well as southwestern Australia, central Chile, and South Africa. Although this biome doesn't cover a very large total area, it contains a high number of unique species and is often considered a hot spot for biodiversity. It also is highly desired for human habitation, often leading to conflicts with rare and endangered plant and animal species.

Areas that are drier year-round, such as the African Sahel (edge of the Sahara Desert), northern Mexico, or the American Intermountain West (or Great Basin), tend to have a more sparse, open scrubland, characterized by sagebrush (*Artemisia* sp.), chamiso (*Adenostoma* sp.), or saltbush (*Atriplex* sp.). In Africa, acacias and other spiny plants dominate this landscape, giving it the name **thorn scrub.** Some typical animals of this biome in America are a wide variety of snakes and lizards, rodents, birds, antelope, and mountain sheep. In Africa, this landscape is home to gazelle, rhinos, giraffes, and many other species (fig. 5.10).

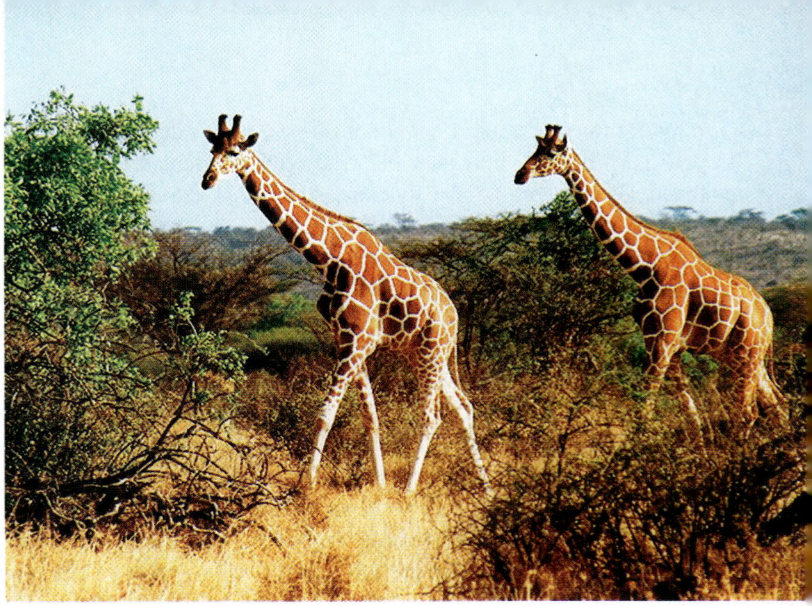

FIGURE 5.10 *The dry thorn scrub of East Africa is famous for its populations of large mammals.*

Tropical Moist Forests

The humid tropical regions of South and Central America, Africa, Southeast Asia, and some of the Pacific Islands support one of the most complex and biologically rich biome types in the world (fig. 5.11). Although there are several kinds of moist tropical forests, they share attributes of ample rainfall and uniform temperatures. Cool **cloud forests** are found high in the mountains where fog and mist keep vegetation wet all the time. **Tropical rainforests** occur where rainfall is abundant—more than 200 cm (80 in.) per year—and temperatures are warm to hot year-round.

The soil of both these tropical moist forest types tends to be old, thin, acidic, and nutrient-poor, yet the number of species present can be mind-boggling. For example, the number of insect species in the canopy of tropical rainforests has been estimated to be in the millions! It is estimated that one-half to two-thirds of all species of terrestrial plants and insects live in tropical forests.

The nutrient cycles of these forests also are distinctive. Almost all (90 percent) of the nutrients in the system are contained in the bodies of the living organisms. This is a striking contrast to temperate forests, where nutrients are held within the soil and made available for new plant growth. The luxuriant growth in tropical rainforests depends on rapid decomposition and recycling of dead organic material. Leaves and branches that fall to the forest floor decay and are incorporated almost immediately back into living biomass.

When the forest is removed for logging, agriculture, and mineral extraction, the thin soil cannot support continued cropping and cannot resist erosion from the abundant rains. And if the cleared area is too extensive, it cannot be repopulated by the rainforest community. Rapid deforestation is occurring in many tropical areas as people move into the forests to establish farms and ranches, but the land soon loses its fertility.

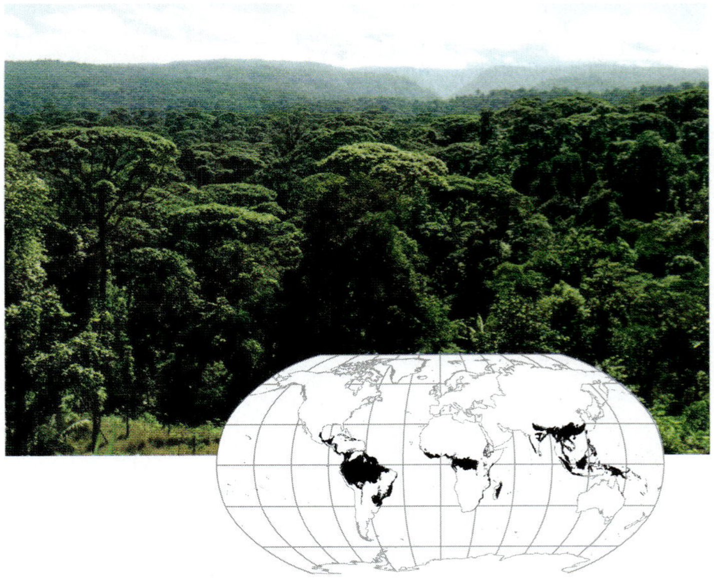

FIGURE 5.11 *Tropical rainforests, such as this one in Costa Rica, support a luxuriant profusion of life-forms. The canopies of tall trees harbor epiphytes and vines. Little light reaches the forest floor.*

Tropical Seasonal Forests

Many areas in India, Southeast Asia, Australia, West Africa, the West Indies, and South America have tropical regions characterized by distinct wet and dry seasons instead of uniform heavy rainfall throughout the year, although temperatures are hot year-round.

These areas have produced communities of **tropical seasonal forests:** semievergreen or partly deciduous forests tending toward open woodlands and grassy savannas dotted with scattered, drought-resistant tree species.

Tropical dry forests have typically been more attractive than wet forests for human habitation and have suffered greater degradation. Clearing a dry forest with fire is relatively easy during the dry season. Soils of dry forests often have higher nutrient levels and are more agriculturally productive than those of a rainforest. Finally, having fewer insects, parasites, and fungal diseases than a wet forest makes a dry or seasonal forest a healthier place for humans to live. Consequently, these forests are highly endangered in many places. Less than 1 percent of the dry tropical forests of the Pacific coast of Central America or the Atlantic coast of South America, for instance, remain in an undisturbed state.

MARINE ECOSYSTEMS

The biological communities in oceans and seas are poorly understood, but they are probably as diverse and as complex as terrestrial biomes. In this section, we will explore a few facets of these fascinating environments. Oceans cover nearly three-fourths of the earth's surface, and they contribute in important, although often unrecognized, ways to terrestrial ecosystems. Like land-based systems, most marine communities depend on photosynthetic organisms. Often it is algae, coral, or tiny, free-floating photosynthetic plants **(phytoplankton)** that support a marine food web, rather than the trees and grasses we see on land. In oceans, photosynthetic activity tends to be greatest near coastlines, where nitrogen, phosphorus, and other nutrients wash offshore and fertilize primary producers. Ocean currents also contribute to the distribution of biological productivity, as they transport nutrients and phytoplankton far from shore (fig. 5.12).

As plankton, algae, fish, and other organisms die, they sink toward the ocean floor. Deep-ocean ecosystems, consisting of crabs, filter-feeding organisms, strange phosphorescent fish, and many other life-forms, often rely on this "marine snow" as a primary nutrient source. Surface communities also depend on this material. Upwelling currents circulate nutrients from the ocean floor back to the surface. Along the coasts of South America, Africa, and Europe, these currents support rich fisheries.

Vertical stratification is a key feature of aquatic ecosystems. Light decreases rapidly with depth, and communities below the photic zone (light zone, often reaching about 20 m deep) must rely on energy sources other than photosynthesis to persist. Temperature also decreases with depth. Deep-ocean species often grow slowly in part because metabolism is reduced in cold conditions. In contrast, warm, bright, near-surface communities, such as coral reefs and estuaries, are among the world's most biologically productive environments. Temperature also affects the amount of oxygen and other elements that can be absorbed in water. Cold water holds abundant oxygen, so productivity is often high in cold oceans, as in the North Atlantic, North Pacific, and Antarctic.

Ocean systems can be described by depth and proximity to shore (fig. 5.13). In general, **benthic** communities occur on the bottom, and **pelagic** (from "sea" in Greek) zones are the water column. The epipelagic zone (*epi* = on top) has photosynthetic organisms. Below this are the mesopelagic (*meso* = medium) and bathypelagic (*bathos* = deep) zones. The deepest layers are the abyssal zone (to 4,000 m) and hadal zone (deeper than 6,000 m). Shorelines are known as littoral zones, and the area exposed by low tides is known as the intertidal zone. Often there is a broad, relatively shallow region along a continent's coast, which may reach a few kilometers or hundreds of kilometers from shore. This undersea area is the continental shelf.

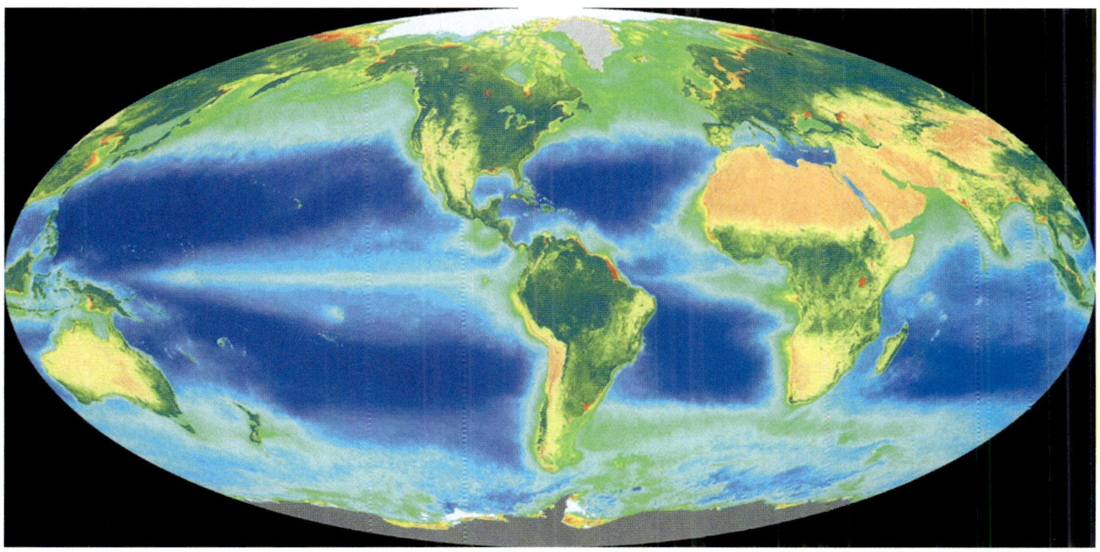

FIGURE 5.12 *Satellite measurements of chlorophyll levels in the oceans and on land. Dark green to blue land areas have high biological productivity. Dark blue oceans have little chlorophyll and are biologically impoverished. Light green to yellow ocean zones are biologically rich.* Courtesy SeaWiFS/NASA.

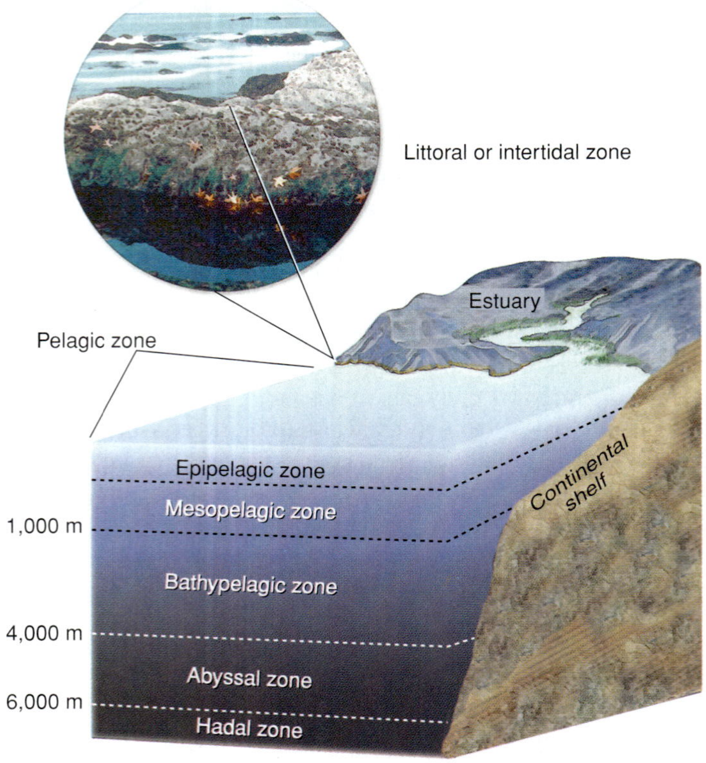

FIGURE 5.13 *Light penetrates only the top 10–20 m of the ocean. Below this level, temperatures drop and pressure increases. Nearshore environments include the intertidal zone and estuaries.*

The Open Ocean

The open ocean is often referred to as a biological desert because it has relatively low productivity. Fish and plankton abound in regions such as the equatorial Pacific and Antarctic oceans, where currents carry nutrients far from shore (fig. 5.12). Another notable exception, the Sargasso Sea in the western Atlantic, is known for its free-floating mats of brown algae. These algae mats support a phenomenal diversity of animals, including sea turtles, fish, and even eels that hatch amid the algae, then eventually migrate up rivers along the Atlantic coasts of North America and Europe.

Deep-sea thermal vent communities are another remarkable type of marine system that was completely unknown until 1977 explorations with the deep-sea submarine *Alvin*. These communities are based on microbes that capture chemical energy, mainly from sulfur compounds released from thermal vents—jets of hot water and minerals on the ocean floor. Magma below the ocean crust heats these vents. Tube worms, mussels, and microbes on these vents are adapted to survive both extreme temperatures, often above 350°C (700°F), and the intense water pressure at depths of 7,000 m (20,000 ft) or more. Oceanographers have discovered thousands of different types of organisms, most of them microscopic, in these communities.

Coastal Regions: Reefs, Estuaries, Shoals, and Mangroves

Runoff from adjacent land usually makes coastal areas much more nutrient-rich than the open ocean. In addition, if the water is sufficiently shallow and clear to allow sunlight to penetrate to the bottom, rooted plants, such as sea grass or kelp, or sedentary animals, such as corals, sponges, and sea fans, create a habitat structure that shelters myriad small organisms. Most pelagic fish (those living in the open ocean) use shallow shoals, reefs, or other coastal regions for spawning and juvenile development.

As the opening story of this chapter shows, coral reefs are highly endangered by damaging human action ranging from destructive fishing practices and global warming to smothering sediment and pollutants from land-based activities, such as farming, logging, construction, sewage disposal, and industrial wastes. Unfortunately, most other nearshore habitats are subjected to the same stresses. The biological losses from our abuses of oceans and coastlines are enormous.

Mangrove forests are a diverse group of salt-tolerant trees and other plants that grow in intertidal zones of tropical coastlines around the world (fig. 5.14). Mangrove forests are vital for healthy coastal ecosystems. Adapted to living in shallow, standing water or water-saturated mud, mangroves help stabilize shorelines, blunt the force of storms, and build land by trapping sediment and organic material. The forest detritus, consisting mainly of fallen leaves and branches from the mangroves, provides nutrients for

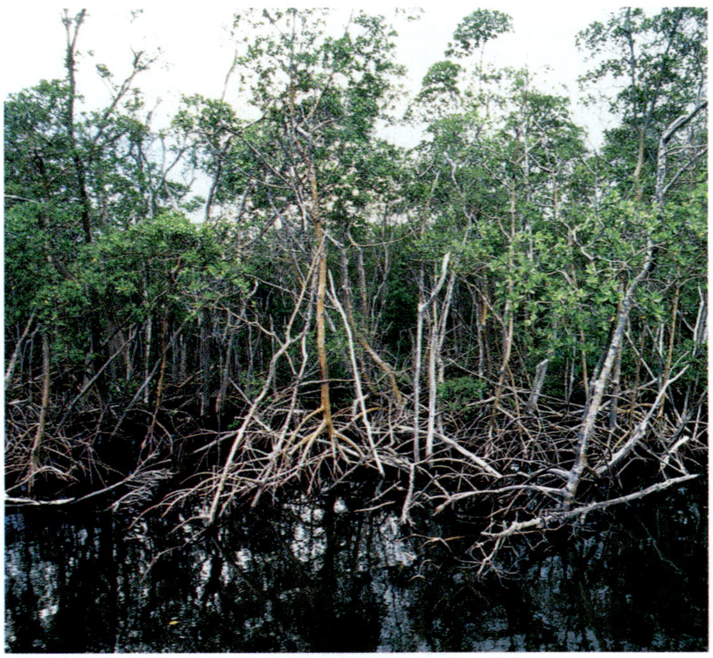

FIGURE 5.14 *Mangrove forests grow in intertidal zones of tropical or subtropical coasts around the world. They provide habitat and nutrients for many marine organisms. Unfortunately, many of these valuable forests have been damaged or destroyed by human actions.*

the marine environment and supports immense varieties of sea life in intricate food webs. Once estimated to cover 22 million hectares, more than half the world's original mangrove forests have been destroyed or degraded. They are clear-cut for timber and firewood or to provide room for aquaculture (fish or shrimp farming), poisoned by industrial toxins and sewage and dried out or flooded by altered water levels. It is estimated that parts of Southeast Asia and South America have lost 90 percent of their mangrove forests; most have been cleared to make room for shrimp and fish farms.

Tidal Environments and Barrier Islands

Among the many fascinating coastal communities are those occupying tidal zones. The rocky intertidal communities of the Pacific Northwest are excellent for "tide-pooling," or exploring the strange and beautiful animals and algae in the small pools left by a receding tide (fig. 5.15). These environments are distinctive largely because species are adapted to survive both the hammering of waves at high tide and the heat and desiccation of sunshine when the tide is out.

Estuaries are bays where rivers empty into the sea, mixing fresh water with salt water. Usually calm, warm, and nutrient-rich, estuaries are biologically diverse and productive. Rivers provide nutrients and sediments, and a muddy bottom supports emergent plants (whose leaves emerge from the water surface) as well as the young forms of crustaceans, such as crabs and shrimp, and molluscs, such as clams and oysters. Nearly two-thirds of all marine fish and shellfish rely on estuaries and saline wetlands for spawning and juvenile development. Estuaries and coastal wetlands also help stabilize shorelines and reduce storm damage inland.

The Chesapeake Bay, America's largest and most productive estuary, is a good example of the threats to coastal regions and the difficulty of restoring ecological health (see related story "Restoring the Chesapeake" at www.mhhe.com/cases).

Barrier islands are low, narrow, sandy islands that form parallel to a coastline. They occur where the continental shelf is shallow and rivers or coastal currents provide a steady source of sediments. They protect brackish (moderately salty), inshore lagoons and salt marshes from storms, waves, and tides. One of the world's most extensive sets of barrier islands lines the Atlantic coast from New England to Florida, as well as along the Gulf coast of Texas. Composed of sand that is constantly reshaped by wind and waves, these islands can be formed or removed by a single violent storm. Because they are mostly beach, barrier islands are also popular places for real estate development. About 20 percent of the barrier island surface in the United States has been developed. Barrier islands are also critical to preserving coastal shorelines, settlements, estuaries, and wetlands.

Unfortunately, human occupation often destroys the value that attracts us there in the first place. Barrier islands and beaches are dynamic environments, and sand is hard to keep in place. Wind and wave erosion is a constant threat to beach developments. Walking or driving vehicles over dune grass destroys the stabilizing vegetative cover and accelerates, or triggers, erosion. Cutting roads through the dunes further destabilizes these islands, making them increasingly vulnerable to storm damage. A single storm in 1962 caused $300 million in property damage along the East Coast and left hundreds of beach homes tottering into the sea (fig. 5.16). As barrier islands recede, inland waters and shorelines become increasingly exposed to ocean waves and wind.

Because of these problems, we spend billions of dollars each year building protective walls and barriers, pumping sand onto

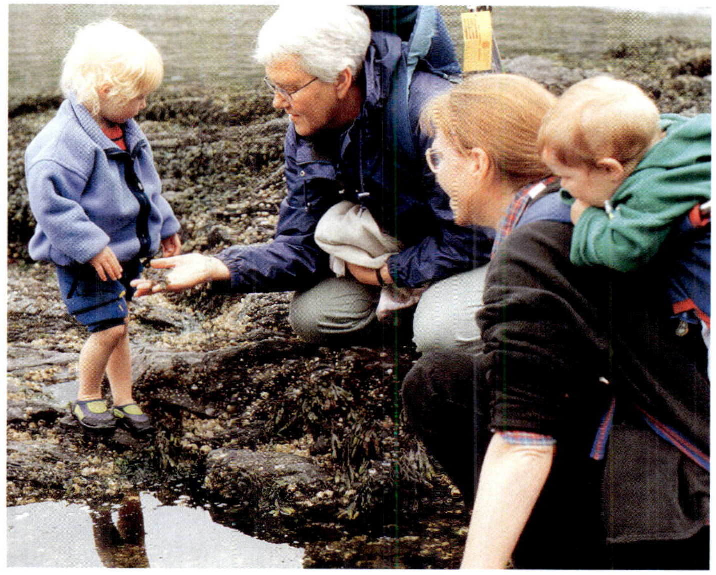

FIGURE 5.15 *Tide pools can povide a wonderful introduction to the beauty and amazing diversity of living organisms.*

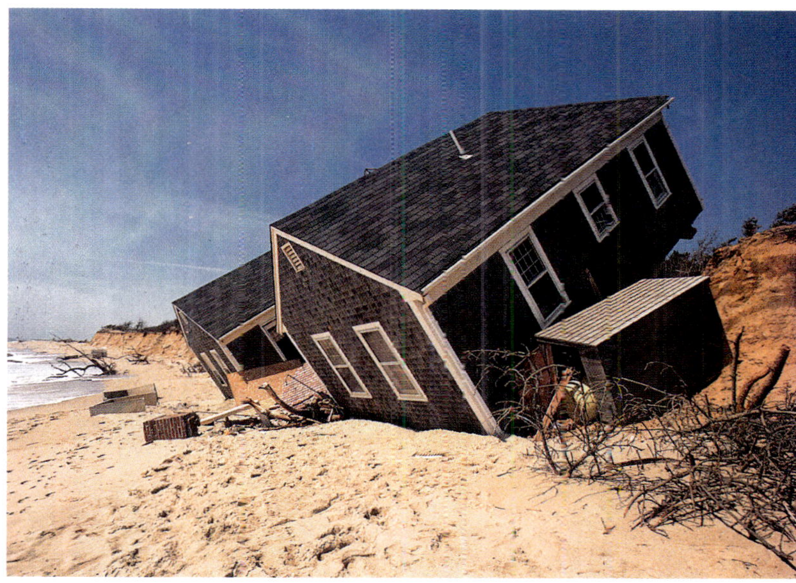

FIGURE 5.16 *Winter storms have eroded the beach and undermined the foundations of homes on this barrier island. Breaking through protective dunes to build such houses damages sensitive plant communities and exposes the whole island to storm sand erosion. Coastal zone management attempts to limit development on fragile sites.*

beaches from off-shore, and moving sand from one beach area to another. Insurance for beach structures is expensive, but many people can afford to pay high premiums for a coastal view and access to the water.

FRESHWATER ECOSYSTEMS

Freshwater environments are far less extensive than marine environments, but they are centers of biodiversity. Most terrestrial communities rely, to some extent, on freshwater environments. In deserts, isolated pools, streams, and even underground water systems support astonishing biodiversity as well as provide water to land animals. In Arizona, for example, many birds are found in trees and bushes surrounding the few available rivers and streams.

Lakes

Freshwater lakes, like marine environments, have distinct vertical zones (fig. 5.17). Near the surface a subcommunity of plankton, mainly microscopic plants, animals, and protists (single-celled organisms, such as amoebae), float freely in the water column. Insects such as water striders and mosquitoes also live at the air-water interface. Fish move through the water column, sometimes near the surface and sometimes at depth.

Finally, the bottom, or *benthos,* is occupied by a variety of snails, burrowing worms, fish, and other organisms. These make up the benthic community. Oxygen levels are lowest in the benthic environment, mainly because there is little mixing to introduce oxygen to this zone. Anaerobic (not using oxygen) bacteria may live in low-oxygen sediments. In the littoral zone, emergent plants, such as cattails and rushes, grow in the bottom sediment. These plants create important functional links between layers of an aquatic ecosystem, and they may provide the greatest primary productivity to the system.

Lakes, unless they are shallow, have a warmer upper layer that is mixed by wind and warmed by the sun. This layer is the *epilimnion.* Below the epilimnion is the hypolimnion (*hypo* = below), a colder, deeper layer that is not mixed. If you have gone swimming in a moderately deep lake, you may have discovered the sharp temperature boundary, known as the **thermocline,** between these layers. Below this boundary, the water is much colder. This boundary is also called the mesolimnion.

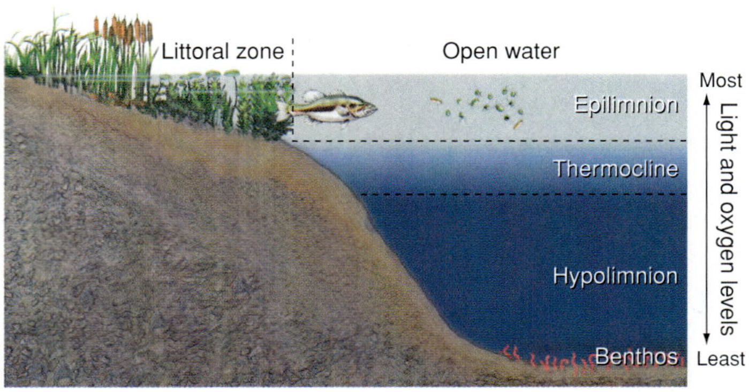

FIGURE 5.17 *The layers of a deep lake are determined mainly by gradients of light, oxygen, and temperature. The epilimnion is affected by surface mixing from wind and thermal convections, while mixing between the hypolimnion and epilimnion is inhibited by a sharp temperature and density difference at the thermocline.*

Local conditions that affect the characteristics of an aquatic community include (1) nutrient availability (or excess), such as nitrates and phosphates; (2) suspended matter, such as silt, that affects light penetration; (3) depth; (4) temperature; (5) currents; (6) bottom characteristics, such as muddy, sandy, or rocky floor; (7) internal currents; and (8) connections to, or isolation from, other aquatic and terrestrial systems.

Wetlands

Wetlands are shallow ecosystems in which the land surface is saturated or submerged at least part of the year. Wetlands have vegetation that is adapted to grow under saturated conditions. These legal definitions are important because, although wetlands make up only a small part of most countries, they are disproportionately important in conservation debates and are the focus of continual legal disputes in North America and elsewhere around the world. Beyond these basic descriptions, defining wetlands is a matter of hot debate. How often must a wetland be saturated, and for how long? How large must it be to deserve legal protection? Answers can vary, depending on political, as well as ecological, concerns.

These relatively small systems support rich biodiversity, and they are essential for both breeding and migrating birds. Although wetlands occupy less than 5 percent of the land in the United States, the Fish and Wildlife Service estimates that one-third of all endangered species spend at least part of their lives in wetlands. Wetlands retain storm water and reduce flooding by slowing the rate at which rainfall reaches river systems. Floodwater storage is worth \$3 billion to \$4 billion per year in the United States. As water stands in wetlands, it also seeps into the ground, replenishing groundwater supplies. Wetlands filter, and even purify, urban and farm runoff, as bacteria and plants take up nutrients and contaminants in water. They are also in great demand for filling and development. They are often near cities or farms, where land is valuable, and, once drained, wetlands are easily converted to more lucrative uses. At least half of all the existing wetlands in the United States when Europeans first arrived have been drained, filled, or degraded. In some major farming states, losses have been even greater. Iowa, for example, has lost 99 percent of its original wetlands.

Wetlands are described by their vegetation. **Swamps** are wetlands with trees. **Marshes** are wetlands without trees (fig. 5.18). **Bogs** are areas of water-saturated ground, and usually the ground is composed of deep layers of accumulated, undecayed vegetation known as peat. **Fens** are similar to bogs except that they are mainly fed by groundwater, so that they have mineral-rich water and specially adapted plant species. Bogs are fed mainly by precipitation. Swamps and marshes have high biological productivity. Bogs and fens, which are often nutrient-poor, have low biological productivity. They may have unusual and interesting species, though, such as sundews and pitcher plants, which are adapted to capture nutrients from insects rather than from soil.

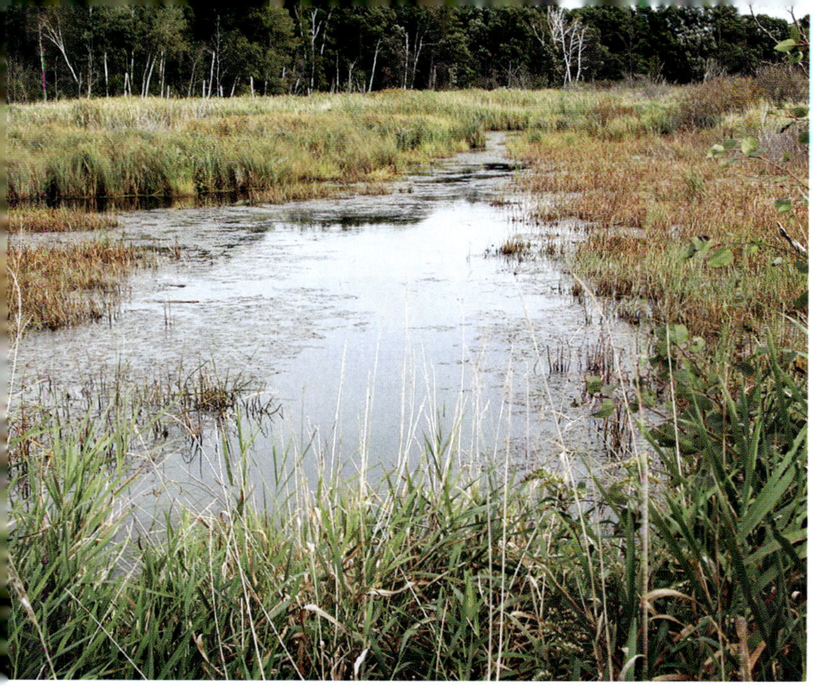

FIGURE 5.18 *Marshes are wetlands without trees. They provide a variety of valuable ecological services, including water storage and purification, wildlife habitat, and biomass production.*

The water in marshes and swamps usually is shallow enough to allow full penetration of sunlight and seasonal warming. These mild conditions favor great photosynthetic activity, resulting in high productivity at all trophic levels. In short, life is abundant and varied. Wetlands are major breeding, nesting, and migration staging areas for waterfowl and shorebirds.

Streams and Rivers

Streams form wherever precipitation exceeds evaporation and surplus water drains from the land. Within small streams, ecologists distinguish areas of riffles, where water runs rapidly over a rocky substrate, and pools, which are deeper stretches of slowly moving current. Water tends to be well mixed and oxygenated in riffles; pools tend to collect silt and organic matter. If deep enough, pools can have vertical zones similar to those of lakes. As streams collect water and merge, they form rivers, although there isn't a universal definition of when one turns into the other. Ecologists consider a river system to be a continuum of constantly changing environmental conditions and community inhabitants from the headwaters to the mouth of a drainage or watershed. The biggest distinction between stream and lake ecosystems is that, in a stream, materials, including plants, animals, and water, are continually moved downstream by flowing currents. This downstream drift is offset by active movement of animals upstream, productivity in the stream itself, and input of materials from adjacent wetlands or uplands.

BIODIVERSITY

The biomes you've just learned about shelter an astounding variety of living organisms. From the driest desert to the dripping rainforests, from the highest mountain peaks to the deepest ocean trenches, life occurs in a marvelous spectrum of sizes, colors, shapes, life cycles, and interrelationships. The varieties of organisms and complex ecological relationships give the biosphere its unique, productive characteristics. **Biodiversity,** the variety of living things, also makes the world a more beautiful and exciting place to live. Three kinds of biodiversity are essential to preserve ecological systems and functions: (1) *genetic diversity* is a measure of the variety of versions of the same genes within individual species; (2) *species diversity* describes the number of different kinds of organisms within individual communities or ecosystems; and (3) *ecological diversity* means the richness and complexity of a biological community, including the number of niches, trophic levels, and ecological processes that capture energy, sustain food webs, and recycle materials within this system.

How Many Species Are There?

The 1.7 million species presently known probably represent only a small fraction of the total number that exist (table 5.1). Based on the rate of new discoveries by research expeditions—especially in the tropics—taxonomists estimate that somewhere between 3 million and 50 million different species may be alive today. About 70 percent of all known species are invertebrates (animals without backbones, such as insects, sponges, clams, and worms) (fig. 5.19).

TABLE 5.1 Approximate Numbers of Known Living Species by Taxonomic Group

Group	Number
Bacteria and cyanobacteria	4,000
Protozoa (single-celled animals)	31,000
Algae (single-celled plants)	40,000
Fungi (molds, mushrooms)	72,000
Multicellular plants	270,000
Sponges	5,000
Jellyfish, corals, anemones	10,000
Flatworms (tapeworms, flukes)	12,000
Roundworms (nematodes, earthworms)	25,000
Clams, snails, slugs, squids, octopuses	70,000
Insects	1,025,000
Mites, ticks, spiders, crabs, shrimp, centipedes, other noninsect arthropods	110,000
Starfish, sea urchins	6,000
Fish and sharks	27,000
Amphibians	4,000
Reptiles	7,150
Birds	9,700
Mammals	4,650
Total	1,733,000

Source: Myers, Noman, et al. 2000. "Biodiversity hot spots for conservation priorities." *Nature* 403: 853–858.

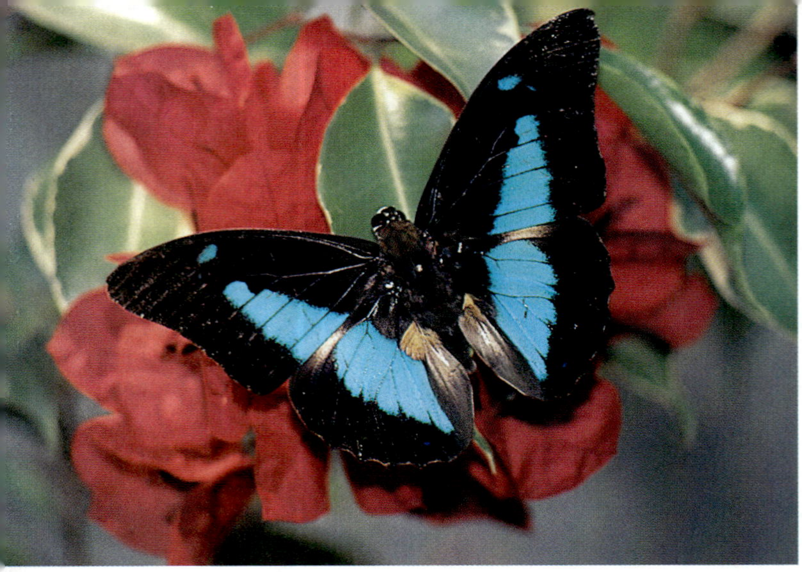

FIGURE 5.19 *Insects and other invertebrates make up more than half of all known species. Many, like this blue morpho butterfly, are beautiful as well as ecologically important.*

This group probably makes up the vast majority of organisms yet to be discovered and may constitute 90 percent of all species.

Biodiversity Hot Spots

Most of the world's biodiversity concentrations are near the equator, especially tropical rainforests and coral reefs (fig. 5.20). Of all the world's species, only 10 to 15 percent live in North America and Europe. Many of the organisms in megadiversity countries have never been studied by scientists. The Malaysian Peninsula, for instance, has at least 8,000 species of flowering plants, while Britain, with an area twice as large, has only 1,400 species. There may be more botanists in Britain than there are species of higher plants. South America, on the other hand, has fewer than 100 botanists to study perhaps 200,000 species of plants.

Areas isolated by water, deserts, or mountains can also have high concentrations of unique species and biodiversity. Madagascar, New Zealand, South Africa, and California are all midlatitude areas isolated by barriers that prevent mixing with biological communities from other regions and produce rich, unusual collections of species.

HOW DO WE BENEFIT FROM BIODIVERSITY?

We benefit from other organisms in many ways, some of which we don't appreciate until a particular species or community disappears. Even seemingly obscure and insignificant organisms can play irreplaceable roles in ecological systems or be the source of genes or drugs that someday may be indispensable.

Food

All of our food comes from other organisms. Many wild plant species could make important contributions to human food supplies either as they are or as a source of genetic material to improve domestic crops. Noted tropical ecologist Norman Myers estimates that as many as 80,000 edible wild plant species could be utilized by humans. Villagers in Indonesia, for instance, are

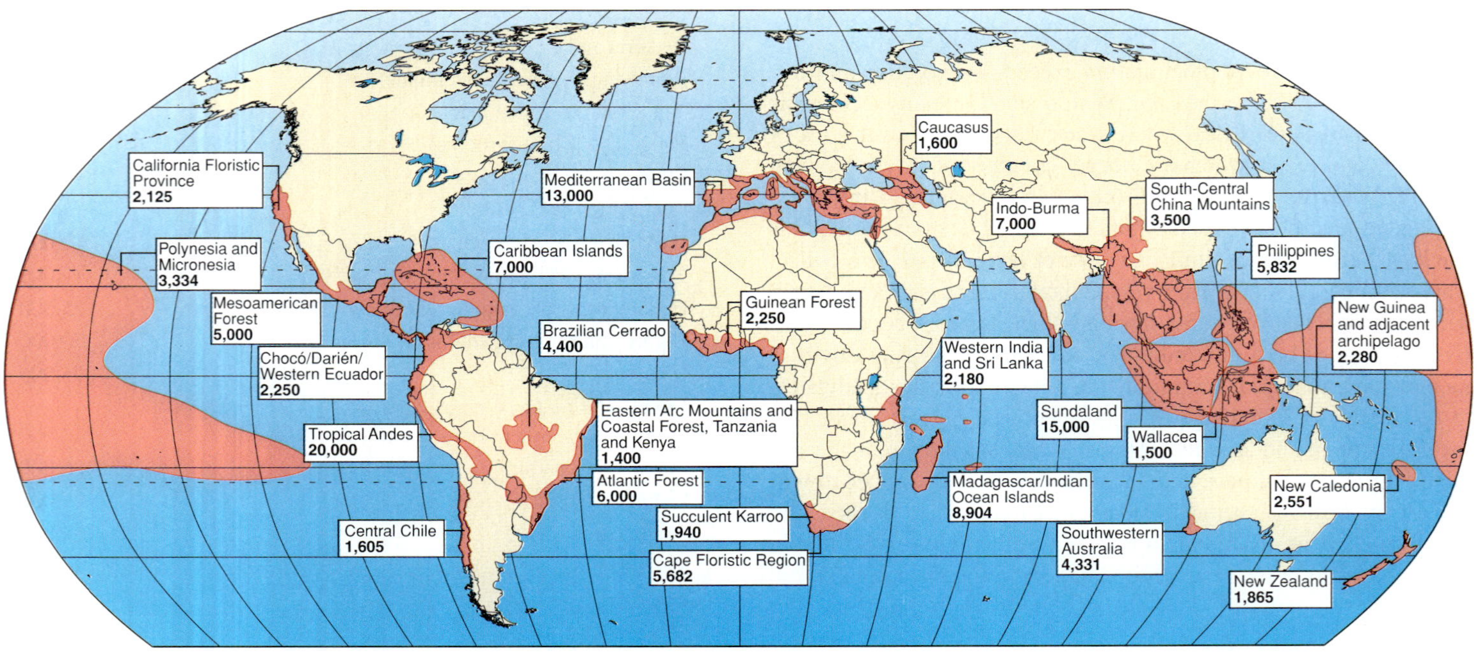

FIGURE 5.20 *Biodiversity hot spots identified by Conservation International tend to be in tropical or Mediterranean climates and on islands, coastlines, or mountains where many habitats exist and physical barriers encourage speciation. Numbers represent estimated endemic (locally unique) species in each area.*

Source: Data from Conservation International.

thought to use some 4,000 native plant and animal species for food, medicine, and other valuable products. Few of these species have been explored for possible domestication or more widespread cultivation. A 1975 study by the U.S. National Academy of Science found that Indonesia has 250 edible fruits, only 43 of which have been cultivated widely (fig. 5.21).

Drugs and Medicines

Living organisms provide us with many useful drugs and medicines (table 5.2). More than half of all prescriptions contain some natural products. The United Nations Development Programme estimates the value of pharmaceutical products derived from developing world plants, animals, and microbes to be more than $30 billion per year.

Consider the success story of vinblastine and vincristine. These anticancer alkaloids are derived from the Madagascar periwinkle *(Catharanthus roseus)*. They inhibit the growth of cancer cells and are very effective in treating certain kinds of cancer. Twenty years ago, before these drugs were introduced, childhood leukemias were invariably fatal. Now the remission rate for some childhood leukemias is 99 percent. Hodgkin's disease was 98 percent fatal a few years ago but is now only 40 percent fatal, thanks to these compounds. The total value of the periwinkle crop is roughly $15 million per year, although Madagascar gets little of those profits.

TABLE 5.2 Some Natural Medicinal Products

PRODUCT	SOURCE	USE
Penicillin	Fungus	Antibiotic
Bacitracin	Bacterium	Antibiotic
Tetracycline	Bacterium	Antibiotic
Erythromycin	Bacterium	Antibiotic
Digitalis	Foxglove	Heart stimulant
Quinine	Chincona bark	Malaria treatment
Diosgenin	Mexican yam	Birth control drug
Cortisone	Mexican yam	Anti-inflammation treatment
Cytarabine	Sponge	Leukemia cure
Vinblastine, vincristine	Periwinkle plant	Anticancer drugs
Reserpine	Rauwolfia	Hypertension drug
Bee venom	Bee	Arthritis relief
Allantoin	Blowfly larva	Wound healer
Morphine	Poppy	Analgesic

Ecological Benefits

Human life is inextricably linked to ecological services provided by other organisms. Soil formation, waste disposal, air and water purification, nutrient cycling, solar energy absorption, and food production all depend on biodiversity (see chapters 2 and 7). Total value of these ecological services is at least $33 trillion per year, or more than double total world GNP. In many environments, high diversity may help biological communities withstand environmental stress better and recover more quickly than those with fewer species.

Because we don't fully understand the complex interrelationships between organisms, we often are surprised and dismayed at the effects of removing seemingly insignificant members of biological communities. For instance, it is estimated that 95 percent of the potential pests and disease-carrying organisms in the world are controlled by natural predators and competitors. Maintaining biodiversity is essential to preserving these ecological services.

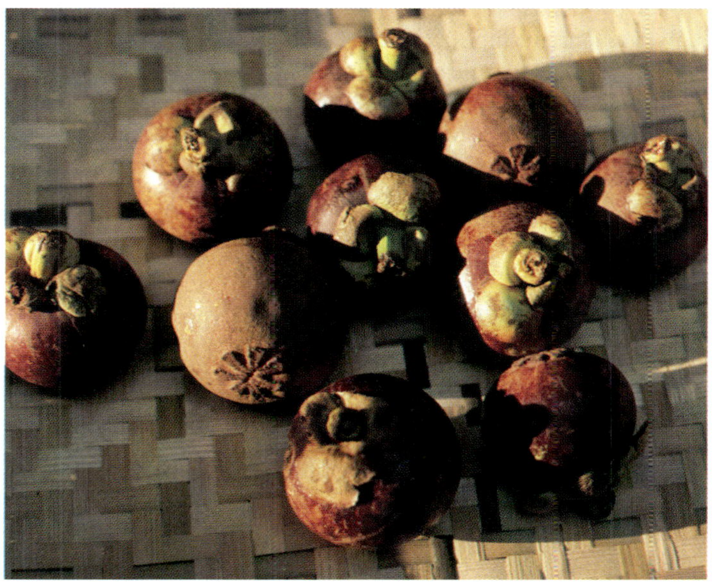

FIGURE 5.21 *Mangosteens from Indonesia have been called the world's best-tasting fruit, but they are practically unknown beyond the tropical countries where they grow naturally. There may be thousands of other traditional crops and world food resources that could be equally valuable but are threatened by extinction.*

Aesthetic and Cultural Benefits

Millions of people enjoy hunting, fishing, camping, hiking, wildlife watching, and other nature-based activities. These activities provide invigorating physical exercise, and contact with nature can be psychologically and emotionally restorative. In many cultures, nature carries spiritual connotations, and a particular species or landscape may be inextricably linked to a sense of identity and meaning. Observing and protecting nature has religious or moral significance for many people. Some religious organizations call for the protection of nature simply because it is God's creation.

Nature appreciation is economically important. The U.S. Fish and Wildlife Service estimates that Americans spend $104 billion every year on wildlife-related recreation (fig. 5.22). This compares to $81 billion spent each year on new automobiles.

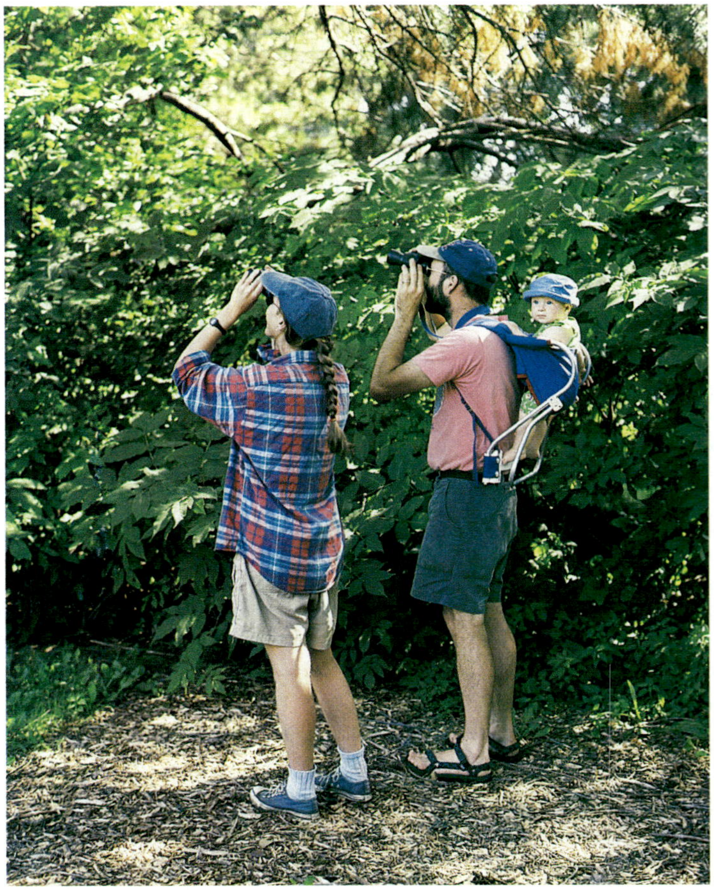

FIGURE 5.22 *Birdwatching and other wildlife observation contribute more than $29 million each year to the U.S. economy.*

Forty percent of all adults enjoy wildlife, including 39 million who hunt or fish and 76 million who watch, feed, or photograph wildlife. Many communities are finding that local biodiversity can bring cash to remote areas through ecotourism (see chapter 6).

For many people, the value of wildlife goes beyond the opportunity to photograph or shoot a particular species. They argue that existence value, the value of simply knowing that a species exists, is reason enough to protect and preserve it. Even if we never see a whooping crane or a redwood tree, many of us are happy to know that these species have not been destroyed.

WHAT THREATENS BIODIVERSITY?

Extinction, the elimination of a species, is a normal process of the natural world. Species die out and are replaced by others, often their own descendants, as part of evolutionary change. In undisturbed ecosystems, the rate of extinction appears to be about one species lost every decade. Over the past century, however, human impacts on populations and ecosystems have accelerated that rate, possibly causing thousands of species, subspecies, and varieties to become extinct every year. Ecologist E. O. Wilson estimates that we are losing 10,000 species or subspecies a year—that makes more than 27 per day! If present trends continue, we may destroy millions of kinds of plants, animals, and microbes in the next few decades. In this section, we will look at some ways we threaten biodiversity.

Natural Causes of Extinction

Studies of the fossil record suggest that more than 99 percent of all species that ever existed are now extinct. Most of those species were gone long before humans came on the scene. Periodically, mass extinctions have wiped out vast numbers of species and even whole families (table 5.3). The best studied of these events occurred at the end of the Cretaceous Period, when dinosaurs disappeared, along with at least 50 percent of existing species. An even greater disaster occurred at the end of the Permian Period, about 250 million years ago, when 90 percent of species and half of all families died out over a period of about 10,000 years—a mere moment in geologic time. Current theories suggest that these catastrophes were caused by climate changes, perhaps triggered when large asteroids struck the earth. Many ecologists worry that global climate change caused by our release of greenhouse gases in the atmosphere could have similarly catastrophic effects (see chapter 9).

HUMAN-CAUSED REDUCTIONS IN BIODIVERSITY

The rate at which species are disappearing has increased dramatically over the past 150 years. Between A.D. 1600 and 1850, human activities appear to have eliminated two or three species per decade, about double the natural extinction rate. In the past 150 years, the extinction rate has increased to thousands per decade. If present trends continue, biologist Paul Ehrlich warns, somewhere between one-third to two-thirds of all current species could be extinct by the middle of the twenty-first century. Conservation biologists call this the sixth mass extinction but note that this time it's not asteroids or volcanoes but human impacts that are responsible. E. O. Wilson summarizes human threats to biodiversity with the acronym **HIPPO,** which stands for Habitat destruction, Invasive species, Pollution, Population (human), and Overharvesting. Let's look in more detail at each of these issues.

TABLE 5.3 Mass Extinctions

HISTORIC PERIOD	TIME (BEFORE PRESENT)	PERCENT OF SPECIES EXTINCT
Ordovician	444 million	85
Devonian	370 million	83
Permian	250 million	95
Triassic	210 million	80
Cretaceous	65 million	76
Quaternary	Present	33–66

Source: Gibbs, W. W. 2001. "On the termination of species." *Scientific American* 285(5): 40–49.

Habitat Destruction

The most important extinction threat for most species—especially terrestrial ones—is habitat loss. Perhaps the most obvious example of habitat destruction is clear-cutting of forests and conversion of grasslands to crop fields (fig. 5.23). Over the past 10,000 years, humans have transformed billions of hectares of former forests and grasslands to croplands, cities, roads, and other uses. These human-dominated spaces aren't devoid of wild organisms, but they generally favor weedy species adapted to coexist with us.

Today, forests cover less than half the area they once did, and only around one-fifth of the original forest retains its old-growth characteristics. Species, such as the northern spotted owl *(Strix occidentalis caurina),* that depend on the varied structure and resources of old-growth forest vanish as their habitat disappears (chapter 6). Grasslands currently occupy about 4 billion ha (roughly equal to the area of closed-canopy forests). Much of the most highly productive and species-rich grasslands—for example, the tallgrass prairie that once covered the U.S. corn belt—has been converted to cropland. Much more may need to be used as farmland or pasture if human populations continue to expand.

Sometimes we destroy habitat as side effects of resource extraction, such as mining, dam-building, and indiscriminate fishing methods. Surface mining, for example, strips off the land covering along with everything growing on it. Waste from mining operations can bury valleys and poison streams with toxic material. Dam-building floods vital stream habitat under deep reservoirs and eliminates food sources and breeding habitat for some aquatic species. Our current fishing methods are highly unsustainable. One of the most destructive fishing techniques is bottom trawling, in which heavy nets are dragged across the ocean floor, scooping up every living thing and crushing the bottom structure to lifeless rubble. Marine biologist Jan Lubechenco says that trawling is "like collecting forest mushrooms with a bulldozer."

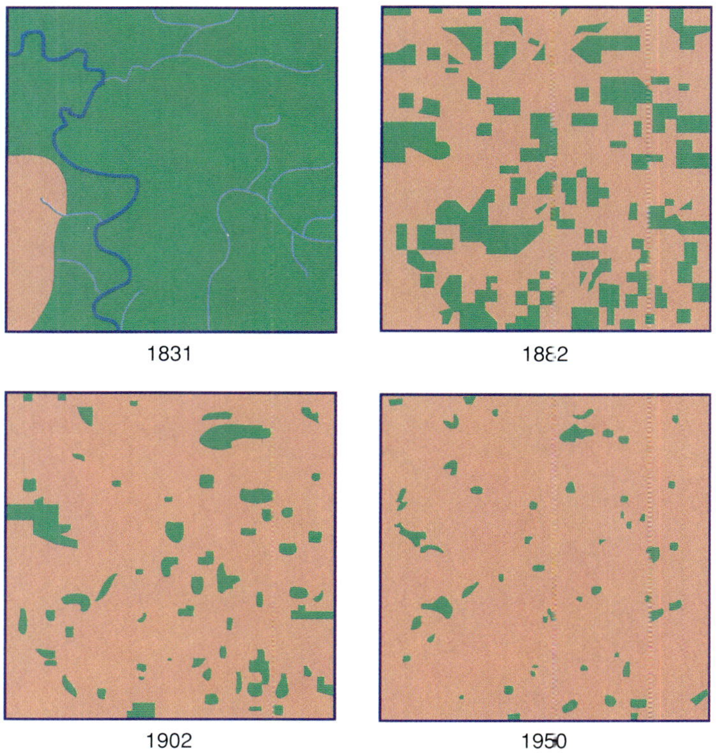

FIGURE 5.23 *Decrease in wooded area of Cadiz Township in southern Wisconsin during European settlement. Green areas represent the amount of land in forest each year.*

Fragmentation

In addition to the total area of loss habitat, another serious problem is habitat **fragmentation**—the reduction of habitat into small, isolated patches. Breaking up habitat reduces biodiversity because many species, such as bears and large cats, require large territories to subsist. Other species, such as forest interior birds, reproduce successfully only in deep forest far from edges and human settlement. Predators and invasive species often spread quickly into new regions following fragment edges.

Fragmentation also divides populations into isolated groups, making them much more vulnerable to catastrophic events, such as storms or diseases. A very small population may not have enough breeding adults to be viable even under normal circumstances. An important question in conservation biology is what is the **minimum viable population** size for various species.

Much of our understanding of fragmentation was elegantly outlined in the theory of **island biogeography,** developed by R. H. MacArthur and E. O. Wilson in the 1960s. Noticing that small islands far from a mainland have fewer terrestrial species than larger, nearer islands, MacArthur and Wilson proposed that species diversity is a balance between colonization and extinction rates. An island far from a population source naturally has a lower rate of colonization than a nearer island because it is harder for terrestrial organisms to reach. At the same time, fewer resources on small islands means that the population of any single species is likely to be small and more vulnerable to extinction. By contrast, a large island can support more individuals of a given species and is, therefore, less vulnerable to natural disasters, genetic problems, or demographic uncertainty (the chance that all the members of a single generation will be of the same sex).

Island biogeographic effects have been observed in many places. Cuba, for instance is 100 times as large and has about 10 times as many amphibian species as its Caribbean neighbor, Montserrat. Similarly, in a study of bird species on the California Channel Islands, Jared Diamond observed that, on islands with fewer than 10 breeding pairs, 39 percent of the populations went extinct over an 80-year period, while only 10 percent of populations between 10 and 100 pairs went extinct in the same time (fig. 5.24). Only one species numbering between 100 and 1,000 pairs went extinct and no species with over 1,000 pairs disappeared over this time.

Many of the parks and wildlife refuges we establish are effectively islands of good habitat surrounded by oceans of inhospitable territory. Like small, remote oceanic islands they are too isolated to be reached by new migrants, and they can't support large enough populations to survive catastrophic events or genetic problems. Large predators, such as tigers or wolves, need large expanses of contiguous range relatively free of human incursion to survive. Glacier National Park in Montana, for example, is excellent habitat for grizzly bears. It can support only about 100 bears, however, and if there isn't migration at least occasionally from other areas, this probably isn't a large enough population to survive in the long run (see Investigating Our Environment, p. 113).

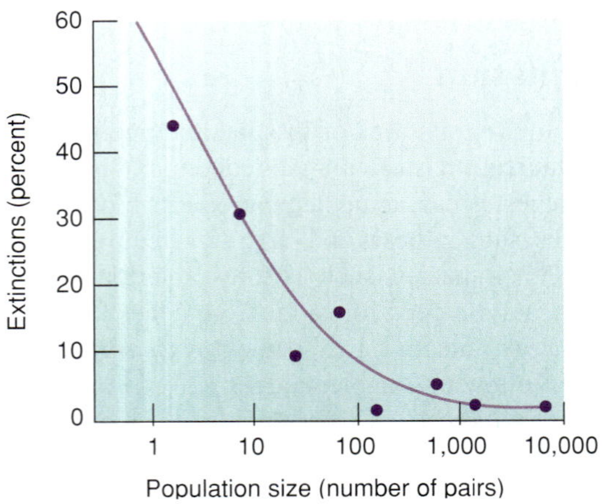

FIGURE 5.24 *Extinction rates of bird species on the California Channel Islands as a function of population size over 80 years.*
Source: Data from H. L. Jones and J. Diamond, "Short-term-base Studies of Turnover in Breeding Bird Populations on the California Coast Island," in *Condor,* vol. 78:526–549, 1976.

Invasive Species

A major threat to native biodiversity in many places is from accidentally or deliberately introduced species. Called a variety of names—alien, exotic, non-native, nonindigenous, unwanted, disruptive, or pests—**invasive species** are organisms that thrive in new territory where they are free of predators, diseases, or resource limitations that may have controlled their population in their native habitat. Although humans have probably transported organisms into new habitats for thousands of years, the rate of movement has increased sharply in recent years with the huge increase in speed and volume of travel by air, water, and land. We move species around the world in a variety of ways. Some are deliberately released because people believe they will be aesthetically pleasing or economically beneficial. Others hitch a ride in ship ballast water, in the wood of packing crates, inside suitcases or shipping containers, in the soil of potted plants, even on people's shoes.

Over the past 300 years, approximately 50,000 non-native species have become established in the United States. Many of these introductions, such as corn, wheat, rice, soybeans, cattle, poultry, and honeybees, have proved to be both socially and economically beneficial. At least 4,500 of these species have established free-living populations, of which 15 percent cause environmental or economic damage (fig. 5.25). Invasive species

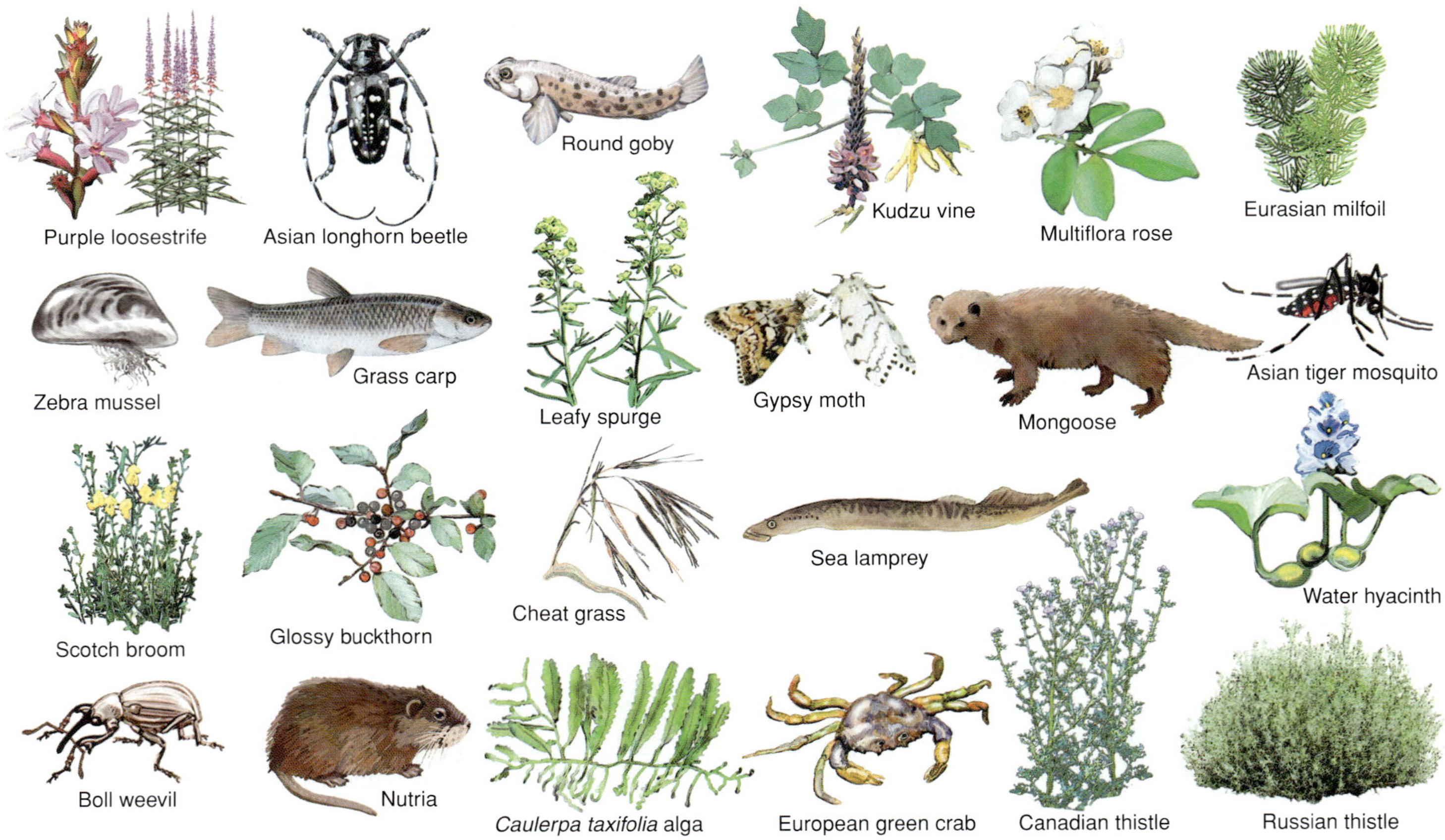

Purple loosestrife
Asian longhorn beetle
Round goby
Kudzu vine
Multiflora rose
Eurasian milfoil
Zebra mussel
Grass carp
Leafy spurge
Gypsy moth
Mongoose
Asian tiger mosquito
Scotch broom
Glossy buckthorn
Cheat grass
Sea lamprey
Water hyacinth
Boll weevil
Nutria
Caulerpa taxifolia alga
European green crab
Canadian thistle
Russian thistle

FIGURE 5.25 *A few of the approximately 50,000 invasive species in North America. Do you recognize any that occur where you live? What others can you think of?*

INVESTIGATING Our Environment

Using GIS to Protect Biodiversity

Investigating fragmentation, and many other biodiversity questions, requires information about the distribution of a species and its habitat. A researcher investigating grizzlies in Yellowstone, for example, needs to know where the bears are, where suitable habitat is, where sources of risk are (such as highways or towns), and where prey are abundant. Increasingly, all these maps are combined and analyzed using geographic information systems (GIS).

What is a GIS? It is software that makes maps from spatial data. Spatial data might show locations of animal observations, habitat boundaries, elevations and slopes, or other features. Land cover maps, showing the distribution of forests, lakes, farmlands, cities, and roads, help identify suitable habitat areas. By mapping all these features, scientists can investigate relationships among them.

You may have used a GIS: online mapping services, such as MapQuest, use digital data representing roads, cities, landmarks, and addresses to make maps on demand. While you might make a map showing the distance, direction, and driving routes to a destination, an ecologist might map animal locations, measure the size of habitat fragments, or monitor animal movements among habitat patches.

How does a GIS work? First it stores digital representations of features. Some representations are made up of fields of cells, as in a digital image. Imagine a digital picture of a daisy, for example: it is made up of a field of pixels (picture elements, or tiny squares). Some are coded white to represent petals; some are green to represent the stem and leaves. Now imagine a digital map of land cover. Some cells might be blue to represent water, some dark green to represent forest, some light green for grass, and some red for urban land uses. Another digital map might show different types of soils: brown for organic-rich fertile soils, yellow for sandy soils, gray for moist wetland soils. Alternatively, a GIS can have data encoded as points, lines, or polygons: a lake would be represented by a polygon, a stream by a line, and a water quality sampling station as a point.

Once data are encoded digitally, they can be overlaid or combined. An analyst can overlay land cover and soils layers, then calculate the amount of forests that occur on sandy soils, or the amount of urban land uses that have taken over arable organic-rich soils. Fragmentation problems can be investigated: how many forest fragments are there; how big are they, and how far apart? How close are urban areas to the best habitat areas—and how soon might we expect urban expansion to intrude into those habitat areas? To investigate biodiversity, one might ask, how many species observations have ocurred per habitat fragment? Once fragment size is calculated, how many species records are there per unit area? Do rare species occur only in the largest habitat fragments?

After analysis, a GIS makes maps to present data or results. Maps can be presented to the public for discussion, to policymakers for decisions, or to other researchers interested in similar problems.

GIS aids in studying many types of problems in many fields. Geographers, ecologists, urban planners, climatologists, sociologists, and many others are using maps and calculating measurements from digital data, to gain insight into their research questions.

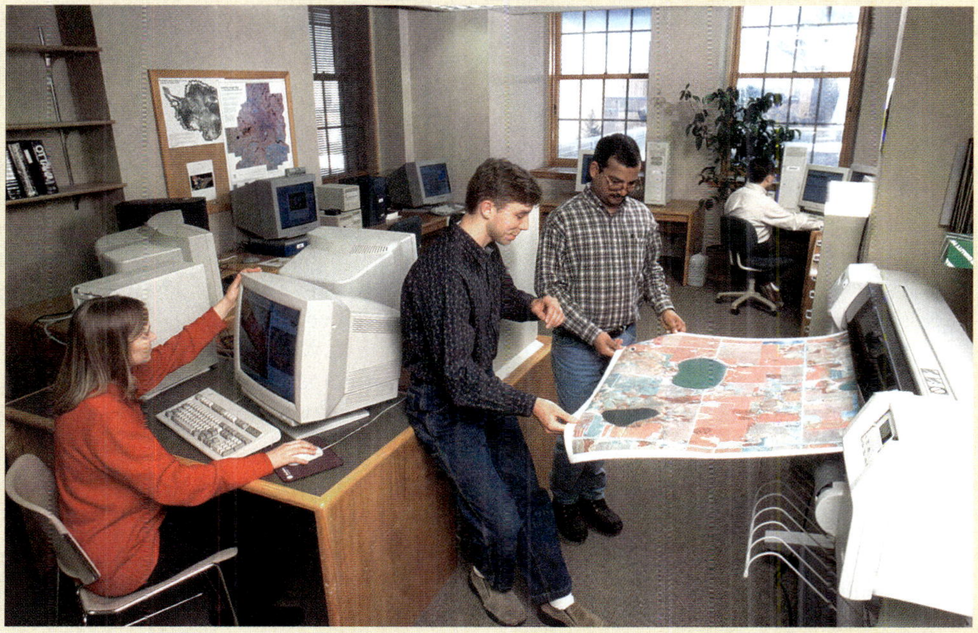

Gap analysis is an important example of using a geographic information system (GIS) for conserving biodiversity. Digital data help scientists quantify, analyze, and model environmental problems.

are estimated to cost the United States $138 billion annually and are forever changing a variety of ecosystems.

A few important examples of invasive species include the following:

- Eurasian milfoil (*Myriophyllum spicatum* L.) is an exotic aquatic plant native to Europe, Asia, and Africa. Scientists believe that milfoil arrived in North America during the late nineteenth century in shipping ballast. It grows rapidly and tends to form a dense canopy on the water surface, which displaces native vegetation, inhibits water flow, and obstructs boating, swimming, and fishing. Humans spread the plant between water body systems from boats and boat trailers carrying the plant fragments. Herbicides and mechanical harvesting are effective in milfoil control but can be expensive (up to $5,000 per hectare per year). There is also concern that the methods may harm nontarget organisms. A native milfoil weevil, *Euhrychiopsis lecontei,* is being studied as an agent for milfoil biocontrol.

- Water hyacinth *(Eichhornia crassipes)* is a free-floating aquatic plant that grows up to a meter in height. It has thick, waxy, dark green leaves with bulbous, spongy stalks. It grows a tall spike of lovely flowers with blue, lavender, or pink petals, some of which have yellow splotches. This South American native was introduced into the United States in the 1880s. Its growth rate is among the highest of any plant known: hyacinth populations can double in as little as 12 days. Many lakes and ponds are covered from shore to shore with up to 500 tons of hyacinths per hectare. Besides blocking boat traffic and preventing swimming and fishing, water hyacinth infestations also prevent sunlight and oxygen from getting into the water. Thus, water hyacinth infestations reduce fisheries, shade-out submersed plants, crowd-out immersed plants, and diminish biological diversity. Water hyacinth is controlled by using herbicides, machines, and biocontrol insects.
- Kudzu vine *(Pueraria lobata)* has blanketed large areas of the southeastern United States. Long cultivated in Japan for edible roots, medicines, and fibrous leaves and stems used for paper production, kudzu was introduced by the U.S. Soil Conservation Service in the 1930s to control erosion. Unfortunately, it succeeded too well. In the ideal conditions of its new home, kudzu can grow 18 to 30 m in a single season. Smothering everything in its path, it kills trees, pulls down utility lines, and causes millions of dollars in damage every year.
- Asian tiger mosquitoes *(Aedes albopictus)* are unusually aggressive species that now infest many coastal states in the United States. These species have apparently arrived on container ships carrying used tires, a notorious breeding habitat for mosquitoes. Asian tiger mosquitoes spread West Nile virus (another species introduced with the mosquitoes), which is deadly to many wild birds and occasionally to people and livestock.
- Purple loosestrife *(Lythrum salicaria)* grows in wet soil. Originally cultivated by gardeners for its bright purple flower spikes, this tall wetland plant escaped into New England marshes about a century ago. Spreading rapidly across the Great Lakes, it now fills wetlands across much of the northern United States and southern Canada. Because it crowds out indigenous vegetation and has few native predators or symbionts, it tends to reduce biodiversity wherever it takes hold.
- Zebra mussels *(Dreissena polymorpha)* probably made their way from their home in the Caspian Sea to the Great Lakes in ballast water of transatlantic cargo ships, arriving sometime around 1985. Attaching themselves to any solid surface, zebra mussels reach enormous densities—up to 70,000 animals per square meter—covering fish spawning beds, smothering native mollusks, and clogging utility intake pipes. Found in all the Great Lakes, zebra mussels have moved into the Mississippi River and its tributaries. Public and private costs for zebra mussel removal now amount to some $400 million per year. On the good side, mussels have improved water clarity in Lake Erie at least four-fold by filtering out algae and particulates.

Disease organisms, or pathogens, may also be considered predators. To be successful over the long term, a pathogen must establish a balance in which it is vigorous enough to reproduce, but not so lethal that it completely destroys its host. When a disease is introduced into a new environment, however, this balance may be lacking and an epidemic may sweep through the area.

The American chestnut was once the heart of many eastern hardwood forests. In the Appalachian Mountains, at least one of every four trees was a chestnut. Often over 45 m (150 ft) tall, 3 m (10 ft) in diameter, fast growing, and able to sprout quickly from a cut stump, it was a forester's dream. Its nutritious nuts were important for birds (such as the passenger pigeon), forest mammals, and humans. The wood was straight-grained, light, and rot-resistant, and it was used for everything from fence posts to fine furniture. In 1904 a shipment of nursery stock from China brought a fungal blight to the United States, and within 40 years, the American chestnut had all but disappeared from its native range. Efforts are now underway to transfer blight-resistant genes into the few remaining American chestnuts that weren't reached by the fungus or to find biological controls for the fungus that causes the disease.

The flow of organisms isn't just into America; we also send exotic species to other places. The Leidy's comb jelly, for example, which is native to the western Atlantic coast, has devastated the Black Sea, now making up more than 90 percent of all biomass at certain times of the year. Similarly, the bristle worm from North America has invaded the coast of Poland and now is almost the only thing living on the bottom of some bays and lagoons. A tropical seaweed named *Caulerpa taxifolia,* originally grown for the aquarium trade, has escaped into the northern Mediterranean, where it covers the shallow seafloor with a dense, meter-deep shag carpet from Spain to Croatia. Producing more than 5,000 leafy fronds per square meter, this aggressive weed crowds out everything in its path. Rarely growing in more than scattered clumps less than 25 cm (10 in.) high in its native habitat, this alga was transformed by aquarium breeding into a supercompetitor that grows over everything and can withstand a wide temperature range. Getting rid of these alien species once they dominate an ecosystem is difficult if not impossible.

Pollution

We have known for a long time that toxic pollutants can have disastrous effects on local populations of organisms. Pesticide-linked declines of fish-eating birds and falcons were well documented in the 1970s (fig. 5.26). Marine mammals, alligators, fish, and other declining populations suggest complex interrelations between pollution and health (chapter 8). Mysterious, widespread deaths of thousands of seals on both sides of the Atlantic in recent years are thought to be linked to an accumulation of persistent chlorinated hydrocarbons, such as DDT, PCBs, and dioxins, in fat, causing weakened immune systems that make animals vulnerable to infections. Similarly, mortality of Pacific sea lions, beluga whales in the St. Lawrence estuary, and striped dolphins in the Mediterranean is thought to be caused by accumulation of toxic pollutants.

Lead poisoning is another major cause of mortality for many species of wildlife. Bottom-feeding waterfowl, such as ducks,

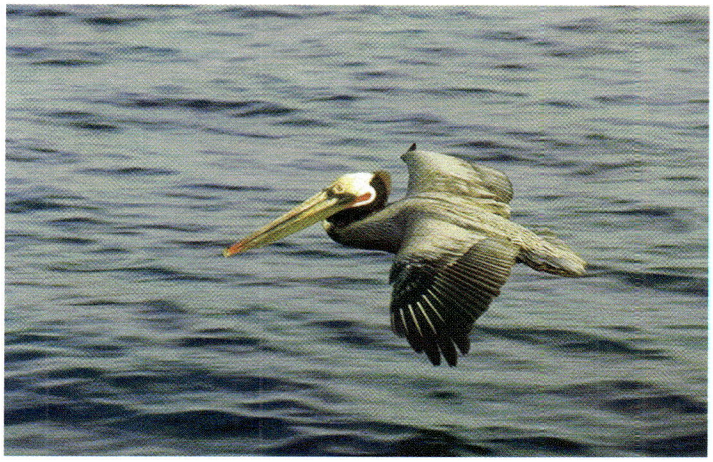

FIGURE 5.26 *Brown pelicans, and other bird species at the top of the food chain, were decimated by DDT in the 1960s. Pelicans and other species have largely recovered since DDT was banned in the United States.*

swans, and cranes, ingest spent shotgun pellets that fall into lakes and marshes. They store the pellets, instead of stones, in their gizzards and the lead slowly accumulates in their blood and other tissues. The U.S. Fish and Wildlife Service (USFWS) estimates that 3,000 metric tons of lead shot are deposited annually in wetlands and that between 2 and 3 million waterfowl die each year from lead poisoning.

Population

Human population growth represents a threat to biodiversity in several ways. If our consumption patterns remain constant, with more people we will need to harvest more timber, catch more fish, plow more land for agriculture, dig up more fossil fuels and minerals, build more houses, and use more water. All of these demands impact wild species. Unless we find ways to dramatically increase the crop yield per unit area, it will take much more land than is currently domesticated to feed everyone if our population grows to 8 to 10 billion, as current projections predict. This will be especially true if we abandon intensive (but highly productive) agriculture and introduce more sustainable practices. The human population growth curve is leveling off (chapter 4), but it remains unclear whether we can reduce global inequality and provide a tolerable life for all humans while also preserving healthy natural ecosystems and a high level of biodiversity.

Overharvesting

Overharvesting is responsible for depletion or extinction of many species. A classic example is the extermination of the American passenger pigeon *(Ectopistes migratorius)*. Even though it inhabited only eastern North America, 200 years ago this was the world's most abundant bird, with a population of between 3 and 5 billion animals (fig. 5.27). It once accounted for about one-quarter of all birds in North America. In 1830 John James Audubon saw a single flock of birds estimated to be ten miles wide, hundreds of

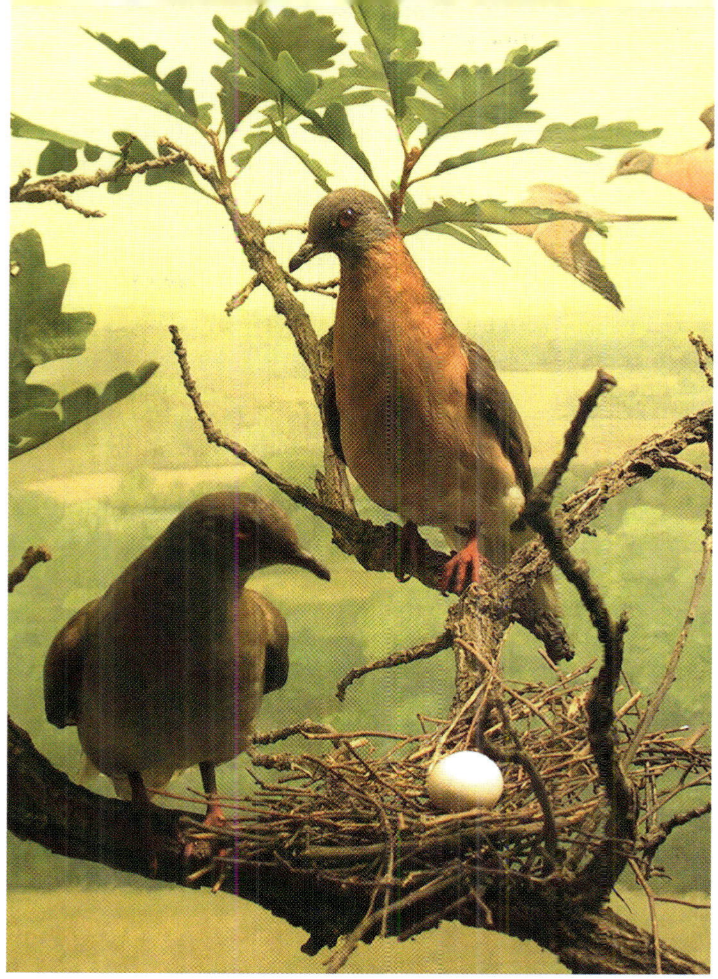

FIGURE 5.27 *A pair of stuffed passenger pigeons* (Ectopistes migratorius). *The last member of this species died in the Cincinnati Zoo in 1914.*

Courtesy of Bell Museum, University of Minnesota.

miles long, and thought to contain perhaps a billion birds. In spite of this vast abundance, market hunting and habitat destruction caused the entire population to crash in only about 20 years between 1870 and 1890. The last known wild bird was shot in 1900 and the last existing passenger pigeon, a female named Martha, died in 1914 in the Cincinnati Zoo.

At about the same time that passenger pigeons were being extirpated, the American bison, or buffalo *(Bison bison)*, was being hunted to near extinction on the Great Plains. In 1850 some 60 million bison roamed the western plains. Many were killed only for their hides or tongues, leaving millions of carcasses to rot. Much of the bison's destruction was carried out by the U.S. Army to deprive native peoples who depended on bison for food, clothing, and shelter of these resources, thereby forcing them onto reservations. After 40 years, there were only about 150 wild bison left and another 250 in captivity.

Fish stocks have been seriously depleted by overharvesting in many parts of the world. A huge increase in fishing fleet size and efficiency in recent years has led to a crash of many oceanic populations. Worldwide, 13 of 17 principal fishing zones are now reported to be commercially exhausted or in steep decline. At least three-quarters of all commercial oceanic species are overharvested.

Canadian fisheries biologists estimate that only 10 percent of the top predators, such as swordfish, marlin, tuna, and shark, remain in the Atlantic Ocean. Groundfish, such as cod, flounder, halibut, and hake, also are severely depleted. You can avoid adding to this overharvest by eating only abundant, sustainably harvested varieties.

Perhaps the most destructive example of harvesting terrestrial wild animal species today is the African bushmeat trade. Wildlife biologists estimate that 1 million tons of bushmeat, including antelope, elephants, primates, and other animals, are sold in African markets every year. For many poor Africans, this is the only source of animal protein in their diet. If we hope to protect the animals targeted by bushmeat hunters, we will need to help them find alternative livelihoods and replacement sources of high-quality protein. The emergence of SARS in 2003 (chapter 8) resulted from the wild food trade in China and Southeast Asia, where millions of civets, monkeys, snakes, turtles, and other animals are consumed each year as luxury foods.

Commercial Products and Live Specimens

In addition to harvesting wild species for food, we also obtain a variety of valuable commercial products from nature. Much of this represents sustainable harvest, but some forms of commercial exploitation are highly destructive, however, and represent a serious threat to certain rare species (fig. 5.28). Despite international bans on trade in products from endangered species, smuggling of furs, hides, horns, live specimens, and folk medicines amounts to millions of dollars each year.

Developing countries in Asia, Africa, and Latin America with the richest biodiversity in the world are the main sources of wild animals and animal products, while Europe, North America, and some of the wealthy Asian countries are the principal importers. Japan, Taiwan, and Hong Kong buy three-quarters of all cat and snake skins, for instance, while European countries buy a similar percentage of live birds. The United States imports 99 percent of all live cacti and 75 percent of all orchids sold each year.

The profits to be made in wildlife smuggling are enormous. Tiger or leopard fur coats can bring $100,000 in Japan or Europe. The population of African black rhinos dropped from approximately 100,000 in the 1960s to about 3,000 in the 1980s because of a demand for their horns. In Asia, where it is prized for its supposed medicinal properties, powdered rhino horn fetches $28,000 per kg. In Yemen, a rhino horn dagger handle can sell for up to $1,000.

Plants also are threatened by overharvesting. Wild ginseng has been nearly eliminated in many areas because of the Asian demand for the roots, which are used as an aphrodisiac and folk medicine. Cactus "rustlers" steal cacti by the ton from the American Southwest and Mexico. With prices as high as $1,000 for rare specimens, it's not surprising that many are now endangered.

The trade in wild species for pets is an enormous business. Worldwide, some 5 million live birds are sold each year for pets, mostly in Europe and North America. Currently, pet traders import (often illegally) into the United States some 2 million reptiles, 1 million amphibians and mammals, 500,000 birds, and 128 million tropical fish each year. About 75 percent of all saltwater tropical aquarium fish sold come from coral reefs of the Philippines and Indonesia.

Many of these fish are caught by divers using plastic squeeze bottles of cyanide to stun their prey (fig. 5.29). Far more fish die with this technique than are caught. Worst of all, it kills the coral animals that create the reef. A single diver can destroy all of the life on 200 m^2 of reef in a day. Altogether, thousands of divers currently destroy about 50 km^2 of reefs each year. Net fishing would prevent this destruction, and it could be enforced if pet owners would insist on net-caught fish. More than half the world's coral reefs are potentially threatened by human activities, with up to 80 percent at risk in the most populated areas.

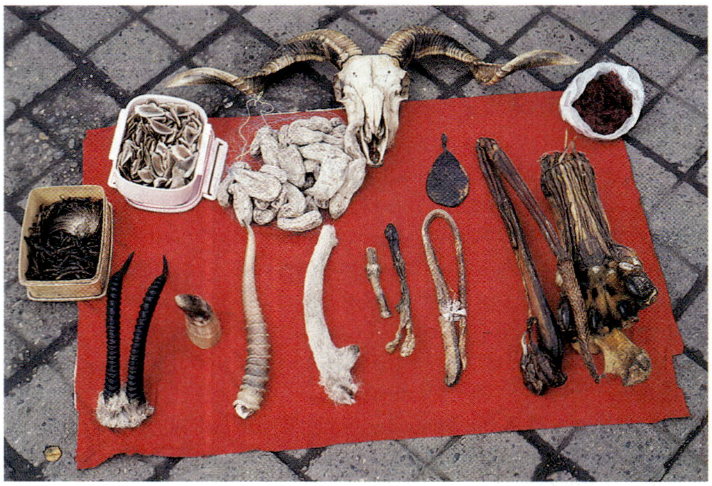

FIGURE 5.28 *Parts from rare and endangered species for sale on the street in China. Use of animal products in traditional medicine and prestige diets is a major threat to many species.*

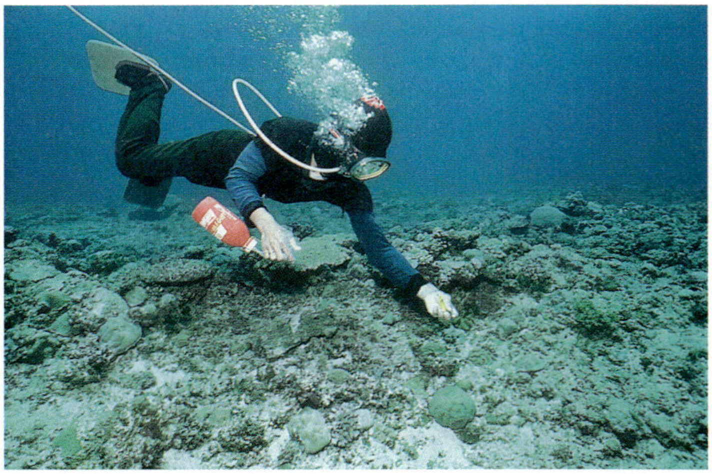

FIGURE 5.29 *A diver uses cyanide to stun tropical fish being caught for the aquarium trade. Many fish are killed by the method itself, while others die later during shipment. Even worse is the fact that cyanide kills the coral reef itself.*

Predator and Pest Control

Some animal populations have been greatly reduced, or even deliberately exterminated, because they are regarded as dangerous to humans or livestock or because they compete with our use of resources. Every year, U.S. government animal control agents trap, poison, or shoot thousands of coyotes, bobcats, prairie dogs, and other species considered threats to people, domestic livestock, or crops.

This animal control effort costs about $20 million in federal and state funds each year and kills some 700,000 birds and mammals, about 100,000 of which are coyotes. Defenders of wildlife regard this program as cruel, callous, and mostly ineffective in reducing livestock losses. Protecting flocks and herds with guard dogs or herders or keeping livestock out of areas that are home range of wild species would be a better solution, they believe. Ranchers and trappers, on the other hand, argue that, without predator control, western livestock operations would be uneconomical.

ENDANGERED SPECIES MANAGEMENT AND BIODIVERSITY PROTECTION

Over the years, we have gradually become aware of the harm we have done—and continue to do—to wildlife and biological resources. Slowly, we are adopting national legislation and international treaties to protect these irreplaceable assets. Parks, wildlife refuges, nature preserves, zoos, and restoration programs have been established to protect nature and rebuild depleted populations. There has been encouraging progress in this area, but much remains to be done. While most people favor pollution control or protection of favored species, such as whales or gorillas, surveys show that few understand what biological diversity is or why it is important.

Hunting and Fishing Laws

In 1874 a bill was introduced in the United States Congress to protect the American bison, whose numbers were already falling to dangerous levels. This initiative failed, however, because most legislators believed that all wildlife—and nature in general—was so abundant and prolific that it could never be depleted by human activity. As we discussed earlier in this chapter, however, by the end of the nineteenth century, bison had plunged from some 60 million to only a few hundred animals.

By the 1890s most states had enacted some hunting and fishing restrictions. The general idea behind these laws was to conserve the resource for future human use rather than to preserve wildlife for its own sake. The wildlife regulations and refuges established since that time have been remarkably successful for many species. A hundred years ago, there were an estimated half a million white-tailed deer in the United States; now there are some 14 million—more in some places than the environment can support. Wild turkeys and wood ducks were nearly gone 50 years ago. By restoring habitat, planting food crops, transplanting breeding stock, building shelters or houses, protecting these birds during breeding season, and using other conservation measures, we have restored populations of these beautiful and interesting birds to several million each. Snowy egrets, which were almost wiped out by plume hunters 80 years ago, are now common again.

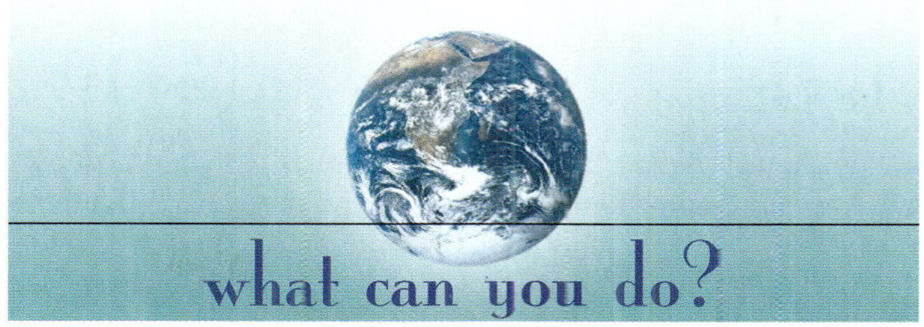

Don't Buy Endangered Species Products

You probably are not shopping for a fur coat from an endangered tiger, but there might be other ways you are supporting unsustainable harvest and trade in wildlife species. To be a sustainable consumer, you need to learn about the source of what you buy. Often plant and animal products are farm-raised, not taken from wild populations. But some commercial products are harvested in unsustainable ways. Here are a few products about which you should inquire before you buy:

Seafood includes many top predators that grow slowly and reproduce only when many years old. Despite efforts to manage many fisheries, the following have been severely, sometimes tragically, depleted:

- Top predators: swordfish, marlin, shark, bluefin tuna, albacore ("white") tuna
- Groundfish and deepwater fish: orange roughy, Atlantic cod, haddock, pollack (source of most fish sticks, artificial crab, generic fish products), yellowtail flounder, monkfish
- Other species, especially shrimp, yellowfin tuna, and wild sea scallops, are often harvested with methods that destroy other species or habitats

Pets and plants are often collected from wild populations, some sustainably and others not:

- Aquarium fish (often harvested by stunning with dynamite and squirts of cyanide, which destroy tropical reefs and many fish)
- Reptiles: snakes and turtles, especially, are often collected in the wild.
- Plants: orchids and cacti are the best-known, but not the only, groups collected in the wild.

Herbal products, such as wild ginseng and wild echinacea (purple coneflower), should be investigated before purchasing.

Do buy some of these sustainably harvested products:

- Shade-grown (or organic) coffee, nuts, and other sustainably harvested forest products
- Organic cotton, linen, and other fabrics
- Fish products that have relatively little environmental impact or fairly stable populations: farm-raised catfish, tilapia, trout, salmon, most mackerel, Pacific pollack, dolphinfish (mahimahi), squids, crabs, and crayfish
- Wild freshwater fish, such as bass, sunfish, pike, catfish, and carp, which are usually better managed than most ocean fish

See also What Can You Do? in chapter 6 (page 144).

The Endangered Species Act

Establishment of the U.S. Endangered Species Act (ESA) of 1973 and the Committee on the Status of Endangered Wildlife in Canada (COSEWIC) in 1976 represented powerful new approaches to wildlife protection. Where earlier regulations had been focused almost exclusively on "game" animals, these programs seek to identify all endangered species and populations and to save as much biodiversity as possible, regardless of its usefulness to humans. **Endangered species** are those considered in imminent danger of extinction, while **threatened species** are those that are likely to become endangered—at least locally—within the foreseeable future. Bald eagles, gray wolves, brown (or grizzly) bears, and sea otters, for instance, together with a number of native orchids and other rare plants, are considered to be locally threatened, even though they remain abundant in other parts of their former range. **Vulnerable species** are naturally rare or have been locally depleted by human activities to a level that puts them at risk. They often are candidates for future listing. For vertebrates, protected categories include species, subspecies, and local races or ecotypes.

The ESA regulates a wide range of activities involving endangered species, including "taking" (harassing, harming, pursuing, hunting, shooting, trapping, killing, capturing, or collecting) either accidentally or on purpose; importing into or exporting out of the United States; possessing, selling, transporting, or shipping; and selling or offering for sale any endangered species. Prohibitions apply to live organisms, body parts, and products made from endangered species. Violators of the ESA are subject to fines up to $100,000 and one-year imprisonment. Vehicles and equipment used in violations may be subject to forfeiture. In 1995 the Supreme Court ruled that critical habitat—habitat essential for a species' survival—must be protected, whether on public or private land.

Currently, the United States has 1,300 species on its endangered and threatened species lists and about 250 candidate species waiting to be considered. The number of listed species in different taxonomic groups reflects much more about the kinds of organisms that humans consider interesting and desirable than the actual number in each group. In the United States, invertebrates make up about three-quarters of all known species but only 9 percent of those deemed worthy of protection. Worldwide, the International Union for Conservation of Nature and Natural Resources (IUCN) lists a total of 16,496 endangered and threatened species, including nearly one-quarter of all known bird varieties (table 5.4).

Listing of new species in the United States has been very slow, generally taking several years from the first petition to final determination. Limited funding, political pressures, listing moratoria, and changing administrative policies have created long delays. In December 2000, flooded by lawsuits over species protection and badly underfunded, the USFWS stopped reviewing new cases altogether. Hundreds of species are classified as "warranted (deserving of protection) but precluded" for lack of funds or local support. At least 18 species have gone extinct since being nominated for protection. Advocates for listing insist that early action is far cheaper than last-ditch rescue efforts. Both environmentalists and property-rights advocates, however, tend to believe that the "single-species" approach is flawed and that efforts should be focused on multiple species and habitat protection.

TABLE 5.4 Endangered and Threatened Species Worldwide

Mammals	2,133
Birds	2,123
Reptiles	454
Amphibians	231
Fish	1,159
Insects and other invertebrates	3,374
Total fauna	9,474
Plants	7,022

Source: Data from *IUCN Red List*, 2003.

When Congress passed the original ESA, it probably intended to protect only a few charismatic species, such as birds and big game animals. Sheltering obscure species, such as the Delhi Sands flower-loving fly, the Coachella Valley fringe-toed lizard, Mrs. Furbisher's lousewort, or the orange-footed pimpleback mussel, most likely never occurred to those who voted for the bill. This raises some interesting ethical questions about the rights and values of seemingly minor species. Although uncelebrated, these species may be indicators of environmental health. Protecting them usually preserves habitat and a host of unlisted species.

Recovery Plans

Once a species is officially listed as endangered, the Fish and Wildlife Service is required to prepare a recovery plan detailing how populations will be rebuilt to sustainable levels. It usually takes years to reach agreement on specific recovery plans. Among the difficulties are costs, politics, interference on local economic interests, and the fact that, once a species is endangered, much of its habitat and ability to survive is likely compromised. The total cost of recovery plans for all currently listed species is estimated to be nearly $5 billion.

The United States currently spends about $150 million per year on endangered species protection and recovery. About half that amount is spent on a dozen charismatic species, such as the California condor and the Florida panther and grizzly bear, which receive around $13 million per year. By contrast, the 137 endangered invertebrates and 532 endangered plants get less than $5 million per year altogether. Our funding priorities often are based more on emotion and politics than biology. A variety of terms are used for rare or endangered species thought to merit special attention:

- *Keystone species* are those with major effects on ecological functions and whose elimination would affect many other members of the biological community; examples are prairie dogs *(Cynomys ludovicianus)* and bison *(Bison bison)*.

- *Indicator species* are those tied to specific biotic communities or successional stages or environmental conditions. They can be reliably found under certain conditions but not others; an example is brook trout *(Salvelinus fontinalis)*.
- *Umbrella species* require large blocks of relatively undisturbed habitat to maintain viable populations. Saving this habitat also benefits other species. Examples of umbrella species are the northern spotted owl *(Strix occidentalis caurina)* and tiger *(Panthera tigris)* (fig. 5.30).
- *Flagship species* are especially interesting or attractive organisms to which people react emotionally. These species can motivate the public to preserve biodiversity and contribute to conservation; an example is the giant panda *(Ailuropoda melanoleuca)*.

Some recovery plans have been gratifyingly successful. The American alligator was listed as endangered in 1967 because hunting (for meat, skins, and sport) and habitat destruction had reduced populations to precarious levels. Protection has been so effective that the species is now plentiful throughout its entire southern range. Florida alone estimates that it has at least 1 million alligators.

Twenty years ago, due mainly to DDT poisoning, only 800 bald eagles *(Haliaeetus leucocephalis)* remained in the contiguous United States. By 1994 the population had rebounded to more than 8,000 birds and the eagle's status was reduced from endangered to threatened. Bald eagles have been proposed for complete delisting, but disagreement over how they will be managed has delayed this step. Similarly, peregrine falcons, which had been down to only 39 breeding pairs in the 1970s, had rebounded to 1,650 pairs by 1999 and were taken off the endangered species list. Declaring the ESA a success, former Interior Secretary Bruce Babbit announced that 29 species, including mammals, fish, reptiles, birds, plants, and even one insect (the Tinian monarch) in addition to eagles and falcons have been removed or downgraded from the endangered species list.

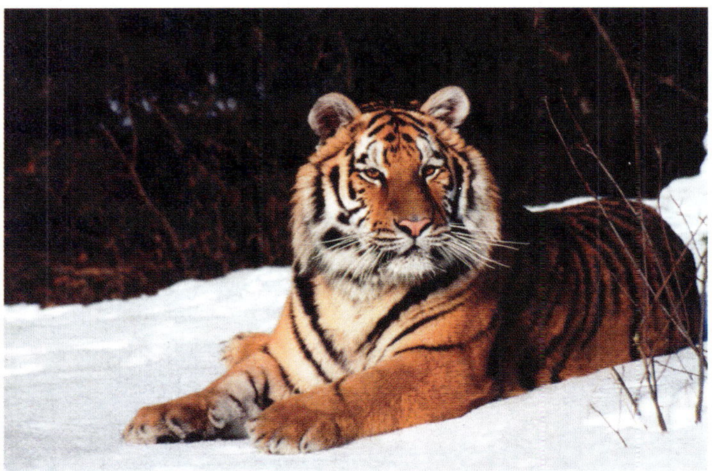

FIGURE 5.30 *Umbrella or flagship species generally are highly charismatic and can mobilize support to protect large blocks of habitat that benefit other creatures as well.*

Opponents of the ESA have repeatedly tried to require that economic costs and benefits be incorporated into endangered species planning. An important test of the ESA occurred in 1978 in Tennessee, where construction of the Tellico Dam threatened a tiny fish called the snail darter. As a result of this case, a federal committee (the so-called God Squad) was given power to override the ESA for economic reasons. Another important example is the case of the northern spotted owl (chapter 6), whose protection depends on preserving old-growth forest in the Pacific Northwest. Timber-industry economists estimate that saving a population of 1,600 to 2,400 owls would cost $33 billion, with most of the losses borne by local companies and residents of Washington and Oregon. Conservationists dispute these numbers and claim the owl is an umbrella species whose protection would aid many other organisms and resources (fig. 5.31).

An even more costly recovery program may be required for Columbia River salmon and steelhead endangered by hydropower dams and water storage reservoirs that block their migration to the sea. Opening floodgates to allow young fish to run downriver and

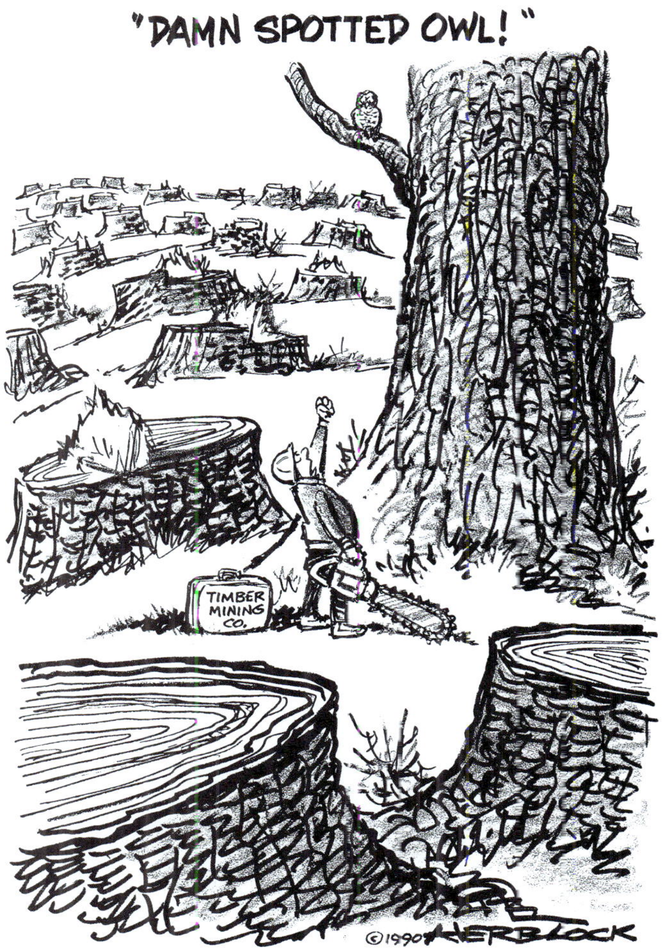

FIGURE 5.31 *Endangered species often serve as a barometer for the health of an entire ecosystem and as surrogate protector for a myriad of less well-known creatures.*

adults to return to spawning grounds would have high economic costs to barge traffic, farmers, and electric rate payers who have come to depend on abundant water and cheap electricity. On the other hand, commercial and sport fishing for salmon is worth $1 billion per year and employs about 60,000 people directly or indirectly.

Reauthorizing the Endangered Species Act

The ESA officially expired in 1992. Since then, Congress has debated many alternative proposals ranging from outright elimination to substantial strengthening of the act. Perhaps no other environmental issue divides Americans more strongly than the ESA. In the western United States, where traditions of individual liberty and freedom are strong and the federal government is viewed with considerable suspicion and hostility, the ESA seems to many to be a diabolical plot to take away private property and trample on individual rights. Many people believe that the law puts the welfare of plants and animals above that of humans. Farmers, loggers, miners, ranchers, developers, and other ESA opponents repeatedly have tried to scuttle the law or greatly reduce its power. Environmentalists, on the other hand, see the ESA as essential to protecting nature and maintaining the viability of the planet. They regard it as the single most effective law in their arsenal and want it enhanced and improved.

Proposals for a new ESA generally fall into one of two general categories. Environmentalists have repeatedly introduced versions that encourage an ecosystem and habitat protection approach rather than focusing on individual species. Reinforcing critical habitat protection and placing deadlines for listing and recovery plan completion, these bills would require that proposed recovery plans be independently peer-reviewed by qualified scientists. They also would expand citizen ability to enforce the law and increase civil and criminal penalties.

On the other side, ESA opponents want to protect private property rights and economic interests from what they see as unwarranted government actions. All recovery plan teams in their versions of the ESA would be required to include individuals with vested economic interests. Under these proposals, only the least costly, most cost-effective, or least burdensome measures would be taken to protect endangered organisms. Federal agencies would be allowed to do "self-consultation"—that is, to avoid consulting wildlife specialists from the Fish and Wildlife Service before undertaking projects. ESA opponents also would require notification and hearings in all states with resident candidate species and would give small-parcel landowners special exemptions from ESA regulations.

Habitat Protection

Over the past decade, growing numbers of scientists, land managers, policymakers, and developers have been making the case that it is time to focus on a rational, continentwide preservation of ecosystems that supports maximum biological diversity rather than a species-by-species battle for the rarest or most popular organisms. By focusing on populations already reduced to only a few individuals, we spend most of our conservation funds on species that may be genetically doomed no matter what we do. Furthermore, by concentrating on individual species, we spend millions of dollars to breed plants or animals in captivity that have no natural habitat where they can be released. While flagship species, such as mountain gorillas and Indian tigers, are reproducing well in zoos and wild animal parks, the ecosystems that they formerly inhabited have largely disappeared.

A leader of this new form of conservation is J. Michael Scott, who was project leader of the California condor recovery program in the mid-1980s and had previously spent ten years working on endangered species in Hawaii. In making maps of endangered species, Scott discovered that even Hawaii, where more than 50 percent of the land is federally owned, has many vegetation types completely outside of natural preserves (fig. 5.32). The gaps between protected areas may contain more endangered species than are preserved within them.

This observation has led to an approach called **gap analysis,** in which conservationists and wildlife managers look for unprotected landscapes, or gaps in the network of protected lands, that are rich in species. Gap analysis uses GIS (see Investigating Our Environment, p. 113) to overlay protected conservation areas with high-biodiversity areas. This overlay makes it easy to identify priority spots for conservation efforts. Maps also help biologists and land-use planners communicate about threats to biodiversity. This broad-scale, holistic approach seems likely to save more species than a piecemeal approach.

Conservation biologist R. E. Grumbine suggests four remanagement principles for protecting biodiversity in a large-scale, long-range approach:

1. Protect enough habitat for viable populations of all native species in a given region.
2. Manage at regional scales large enough to accommodate natural disturbances (fire, wind, climate change, etc.).

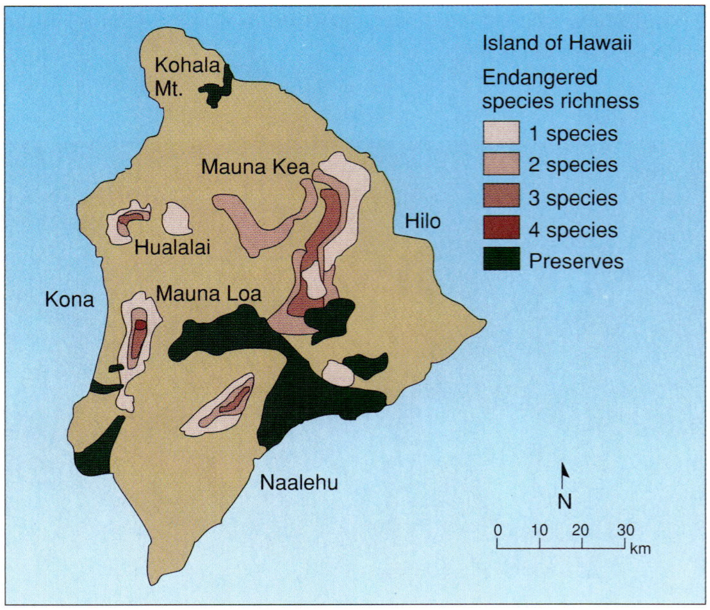

FIGURE 5.32 *Protected lands* (green) *are often different from biologically diverse areas* (red shades), *as shown here on the island of Hawaii.*

3. Plan over a period of centuries, so that species and ecosystems can continue to evolve.
4. Allow for human use and occupancy at levels that do not result in significant ecological degradation.

International Wildlife Treaties

The 1975 Convention on International Trade in Endangered Species (CITES) was a significant step toward worldwide protection of endangered flora and fauna. It regulated trade in living specimens and products derived from listed species, but it has not been foolproof. Species are smuggled out of countries where they are threatened or endangered, and documents are falsified to make it appear they have come from areas where the species are still common. Investigations and enforcement are especially difficult in developing countries where wildlife is disappearing most rapidly. Still, eliminating markets for endangered wildlife is an effective way of stopping poaching. Appendix I of CITES lists 700 species threatened with extinction by international trade.

SUMMARY

- Major ecosystem types, called biomes, are characterized by similar climates, soil conditions, and biological communities. Among the major terrestrial biomes are deserts, tundra, grasslands, temperate deciduous forests, temperate coniferous forests, tropical moist forests, and tropical seasonal forests.
- Aquatic ecosystems include oceans and seas, rivers, lakes, estuaries, marshes, swamps, bogs, fens, and reefs. Moisture and temperature are generally the most critical determinants for terrestrial biomes. Periodic natural disturbances, such as fires, play a major role in maintaining some biomes.
- Humans have disturbed, preempted, or damaged much—perhaps half or more—of all terrestrial biomes and now dominate about 40 percent of all net primary productivity on the land. Some of this disturbance and domination is permanent, but we have opportunities to apply ecological knowledge and practical experience to restoring and repairing ecosystems.
- Biomes shelter the world's biodiversity. Humans benefit from biodiversity in many ways, but we also threaten biodiversity through land conversion and other activities.
- Extinctions occur naturally, including ancient mass extinctions and evolutionary replacement. Among the human-caused threats to biodiversity are overharvesting of animals and plants for food and commercial products.
- Millions of live wild plants and animals are collected for pets, houseplants, and medical research. Among the greatest damage we do to biodiversity are habitat destruction, the introduction of exotic species and diseases, pollution of the environment, and genetic assimilation.
- The potential value of the species that may be lost if environmental destruction continues could be enormous. The changes we are causing could disrupt vital ecological services on which we all depend for life. The first hunting and fishing laws in the United States were introduced more than a century ago to restrict overexploitation and to preserve species for future uses. The Endangered Species Act and CITES represent a new attitude toward nature in which we protect organisms just because they are rare and endangered.
- Now we are expanding our concern from individual species to protecting habitat, threatened landscapes, and entire biogeographical regions. Social, cultural, and economic factors must also be considered if we want to protect biological resources on a long-term, sustainable basis.

QUESTIONS FOR REVIEW

1. Throughout the central portion of North America is a large biome once dominated by grasses. Describe how physical conditions and other factors control this biome.
2. What is taiga, and where is it found? Why might logging in taiga be more disruptive than in southern coniferous forests?
3. Describe four kinds of wetlands and four reasons they are valuable.
4. Define biodiversity, and give three types of biodiversity essential in preserving ecological systems and functions.
5. What is the range of estimates of the total number of species on the earth? Why is the range so great?
6. What group of organisms has the largest number of species?
7. Define *extinction*. What is the natural rate of extinction in an undisturbed ecosystem?
8. List at least five products derived from wild organisms.

9. What is the current rate of extinction, and how does this compare with past rates?
10. Compare the scope and effects of the Endangered Species Act and CITES.

THINKING SCIENTIFICALLY

1. Many poor tropical countries point out that a hectare of shrimp ponds can provide 1,000 times as much annual income as the same area in an intact mangrove forest. Debate this point with a friend or classmate. What are the arguments for and against saving mangroves?
2. Genetic diversity, or diversity of genetic types, is believed to enhance stability in a population. Most agricultural crops are genetically very uniform. Why might the usual importance of genetic diversity *not* apply to food crops? Why *might* it apply?
3. Scientists need to be cautious about their theories and assumptions. What arguments could you make for *and* against the statement that humans are causing extinctions unlike any in the history of the earth?
4. A conservation organization has hired you to lead efforts to reduce the loss of biodiversity in a tropical country. Which of the following problems would you focus on first and why: habitat destruction and fragmentation, hunting and fishing activity, harvesting of wild species for commercial sale, or introduction of exotic organisms?
5. Many ecologists and resource scientists work for government agencies to study resources and resource management. Do these scientists serve the public best if they try to do pure science, or if they try to support the political positions of democratically elected representatives, who, after all, represent the positions of their constituents?
6. You are a forest ecologist living and working in a logging community. An endangered salamander has recently been discovered in your area. What arguments would you make for and against adding the salamander to the official endangered species list?
7. A variety of environments are adapted to disturbance, including fire-adapted grasslands, fire-dependent forest types, and floodplains. How do you explain the difference between disturbance-adapted ecosystems and ecosystems that simply never mature and never reach climax conditions?

KEY TERMS

barrier islands 105
benthic 103
biodiversity 107
biomes 96
bogs 106
boreal forest 100
chaparral 102
cloud forests 102
conifer 100
deciduous 101
deserts 97
endangered species 118
estuaries 105
extinction 110
fens 106
fragmentation 111
gap analysis 120
grasslands 99
HIPPO 110
invasive species 112
island biogeography 111
mangrove forests 104
marshes 106
minimum viable population 111
overharvesting 115
pelagic 103
phytoplankton 103
southern pine forests 100
swamps 106
taiga 100
temperate rainforest 101
thermocline 106
thorn scrub 102
threatened species 118
tropical rainforests 102
tropical seasonal forests 103
tundra 99
vulnerable species 118
wetlands 106

SUGGESTED READINGS

du Toit, Johan T., et al. 2003. *The Kruger Experience: Ecology and Management of Savanna Heterogeneity.* Island Press.

Field, John G., et al., eds. 2002. *Oceans 2020: Science, Trends, and the Challenge of Sustainability.* Island Press.

Galindo-Leal, Carlos, and Ibsen de Gusmao Camara, eds. 2003. *The Atlantic Forest of South America: Biodiversity Status, Threats, and Outlook.* Island Press.

Jones, A. G., et al. 2003. "A review of conservation threats on Gough island: A case study for terrestrial conservation in the Southern Oceans." *Biological Conservation* 113(1):75–87.

Kalluri, S., et al. 2003. "The potential of remote sensing data for decision makers at the state, local and tribal level: Experiences from NASA's Synergy program." *Environmental Science and Policy* 6(6):487–500.

Quammen, David. 1997. *The Song of the Dodo: Island Biogeography in an Age of Extinctions.* Touchstone Books.

Tidwell, Mike. 2003. *Bayou Farewell: The Rich Life and Tragic Death of Louisiana's Cajun Coast.* Pantheon Books.

Woodward, Colin. 2003. "Saving Maine." *OnEarth* 25(2):14–22.

Welcome to McGraw-Hill's Online Learning Center

http://www.mhhe.com/cunningham3e

WEB EXERCISES

Mapping Biodiversity

Visit the following biodiversity website, maintained by a university in Bonn, Germany: www.botanik.uni-bonn.de/system/phytodiv.htm.

This site has excellent information on the nature of biodiversity worldwide. Look at the colored map of plant diversity as you answer the following questions. Note that you can also access a high-resolution image of the same map (click above the map or go to www.botanik.uni-bonn.de/system/globbiod.gif).

1. How many species/unit area are represented by the red color on the map? How many areas have this red color?
2. Look at the vegetation map in your text (p. 378). What kinds of vegetation regions occur in these zones of greatest diversity? Now look at a human population density map in your text (p. 380). In what ways do physiographic features or population density help explain regions of greatest biodiversity? Regions of least biodiversity?
3. What is the farthest north and south latitude range of the red regions? What is the range of species diversity north of 60° latitude?

Mapping Threatened Species: Marine Turtles

The World Conservation Monitoring Center (WCMC) monitors ecosystem health in key threatened environments. Go to the WCMC website http://ims.wcmc.org.uk, and click on IMAPS to find the link to marine turtle distribution in the Indian Ocean. This link produces an interactive map of sea turtles, of protected areas, and of critical coastal habitat—coral reefs and mangroves in the Indian and western Pacific oceans.

1. With the map at its full extent, click on the "draw" squares to draw flatback turtles; then add green turtles. What is the extent of the flatback's range (in yellow)? Which of the two species is more widespread? Now click on the protected areas (polygons). This shows all types of protected areas, inland as well as coastal. In which areas do turtle distributions and protected areas coincide best?
2. Check that the "Zoom in" button above the map is selected, then click on Indonesia on the map. Zoom in a second time in the eastern Indonesia/northern Australia region. At this closer scale, do conservation areas appear to cover turtle distributions better or worse than at the original scale? (You can move around the map and zoom in farther to see more detail.)
3. With the map zoomed in to eastern Indonesia and northern Australia, add mangroves by clicking on the square in the list of drawing features. Mangroves are flooded coastal forests that support many coastal marine ecosystems by sheltering young fish and crabs. Which countries in this area have the most mangroves? (Check the world political map in the back of your text to help identify countries.) How much mangrove area is protected? *Biodiversity is essential for the ecological services on which we all depend.*

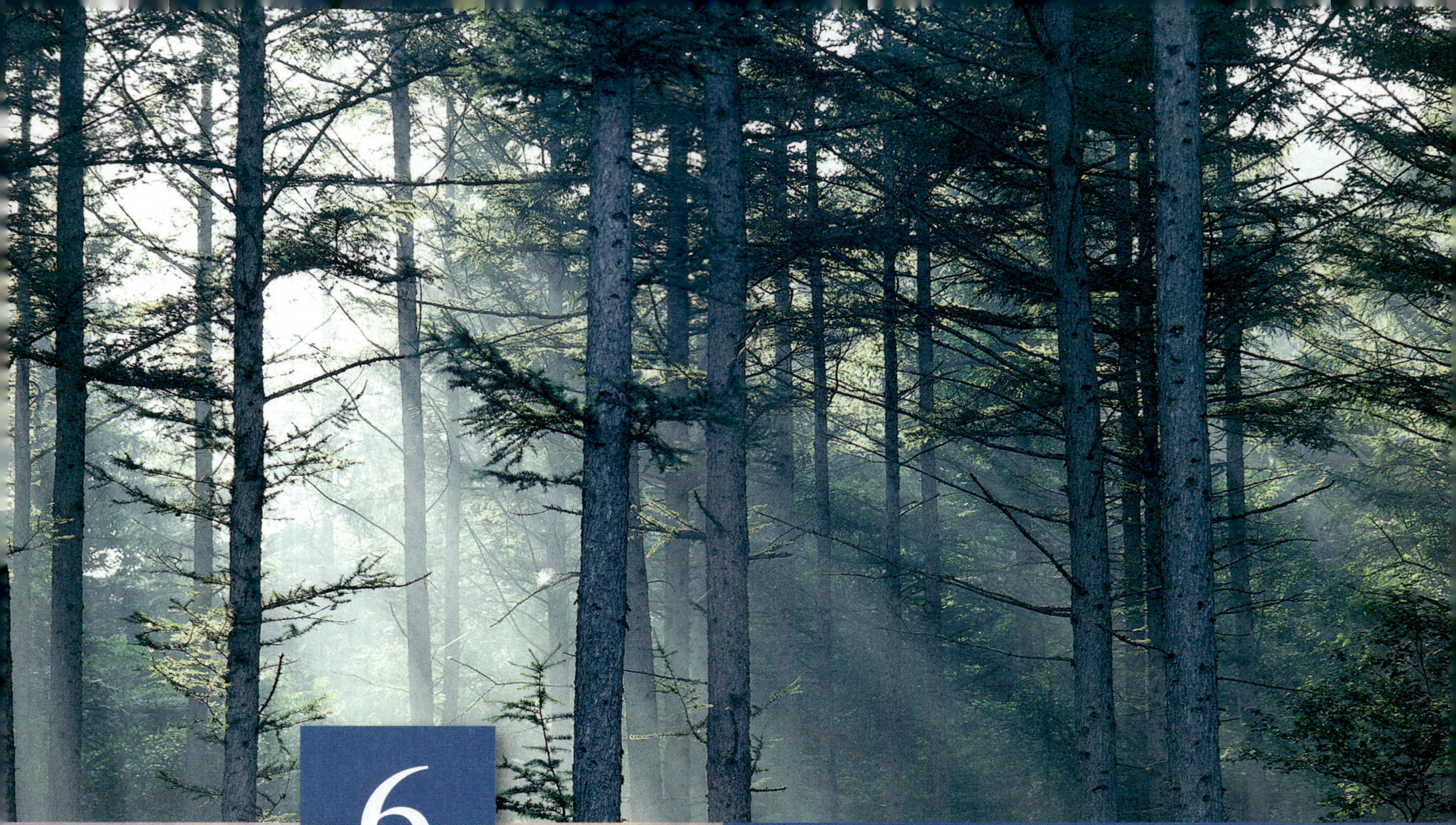

Forests and wildlands provide habitat for wildlife, ecological services that sustain us all, and a refuge for the human spirit.

6 Environmental Conservation: Forests, Grasslands, Parks, and Nature Preserves

What a country chooses to save
is what a country chooses to say about itself.
–Mollie Beatty, former director, U.S. Fish and Wildlife Service

Welcome to McGraw-Hill's Online Learning Center
http://www.mhhe.com/cunningham3e

LEARNING ONLINE

Visit our webpage at www.mhhe.com/cunningham3e for data sources, further readings, additional case studies, current environmental news, and regional examples within the Online Learning Center to help you understand the material in this chapter. You'll also find active links to information pertaining to this chapter, including

North American forests
Tropical forests
Sustainable forests
Grasslands and pastures
North American parks
World heritage areas and biosphere reserves
Wilderness areas
Ecotourism

OBJECTIVES

After studying this chapter, you should be able to

- discuss how and why old-growth temperate and tropical forests are being disturbed, as well as ways they might be preserved.
- explain why conservationists criticize large clear-cuts and forest road building.
- recount how overgrazing can lead to desertification in arid lands.
- understand the origins and current problems of national parks in America and other countries.
- evaluate the tension between conservation and economic development, and how the Man and Biosphere program and ecotourism projects address this tension.
- evaluate some of the controversy over wilderness area management, as well as how people in developing countries feel about the concept of wilderness.
- explain the need for, and problems with, wildlife refuges and nature preserves in the United States and elsewhere in the world.

Protecting Forests to Preserve Rain

How could cutting down trees in low-elevation forests affect tiny toads and beautiful birds on mountaintops many kilometers away? Recent climatological research in Costa Rica suggests a connection that may help solve a decade-old mystery. It may also suggest new conservation policies for the tropics as well as other parts of the world.

Monteverde, Costa Rica, is home to one of the world's best-known cloud forests. This lush mountaintop, continually bathed in fog and mist, is carpeted with a rich profusion of plants and is home to a host of rare birds, insects, and amphibians that inhabit the cool, moist forest. For decades, the Monteverde Cloud Forest Reserve has been an El Dorado for biologists and ecotourists eager to see the beautiful resplendent quetzal (*Pharomachrus mocinno*), Costa Rica's national symbol.

The reserve also is famous for the last known sighting of the glowing golden toad (*Bufo periglenes*), which disappeared abruptly in the late 1980s. Until 1987 the tiny toads congregated by the hundreds in rain pools on the cloud forest floor. In 1988, however, they were scarce, and the next year only a few, scattered individuals could be found. Since 1990 not a single golden toad has been seen anywhere in the world. What happened to them? No one knows for sure. Air pollution, waterborne contaminants, and diseases have been suggested as possible causes for their disappearance, but no conclusive evidence for any of these has been found. The forest itself still seems pristine and intact, having been protected from logging and grazing to preserve the watershed for lower-elevation villages.

Now scientists are realizing that mountaintops, like islands, may not be as isolated and independent as they seem. Satellite images show that the life-giving clouds that sustain Costa Rican mountain flora and fauna are disappearing, and the reason appears to be logging in far-distant lowlands. The clouds are formed as moisture-laden Caribbean winds sweep up the eastern slope of Costa Rica's central Cordillera de Tilarán range. When they reach high elevations, the winds cool and moisture condenses to form the fog and mist on which the biological community depends. Much of the moisture carried by the wind comes from the lowland rainforest over which it blows before reaching the mountains. When those forests are cut down, plant transpiration declines markedly. Furthermore, the pastures and croplands created by deforestation warm the air and dry it out even more.

After a century of logging and fires, only 18 percent of Costa Rica's lowland forest east of the mountains remains untouched. As a result, the air reaching the mountains is drier than normal, and clouds that once covered the mountaintops are sparse or even completely absent some times in the year. The bottoms of the clouds also are at much higher elevations, and areas once bathed continually in mist and fog are now dry for days at a time (fig. 6.1). If breeding pools disappear, the golden toads can't reproduce and the species quickly goes extinct. Similarly, if wild avocadoes, the quetzal's favorite food, fail to fruit because of dry conditions, the bird's survival may be threatened. If these trends continue, biologists worry that other rare and beautiful species that depend on the cloud forests may also disappear.

Although plants and animals within the Monteverde Reserve are protected from many types of abuse and misuse, we are discovering that park boundaries are not always enough to preserve a functioning ecosystem. Simply fencing a forest may not be sufficient to preserve it. Increasingly, we are recognizing that successful management of forests, parks, and reserves requires an understanding of the social, economic, and ecological context in which a reserve exists. In this chapter, we'll examine the strategies that have been used to conserve forests, rangelands, and areas of scenic beauty and biological importance.

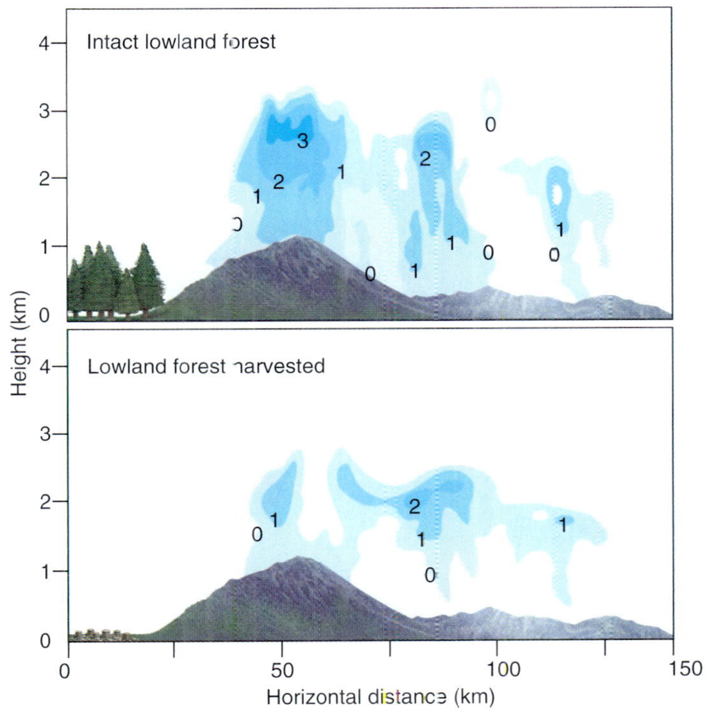

FIGURE 6.1 *Intact lowland forests supply moisture that maintains clouds and cool, wet cloud forests on Costa Rican mountain peaks. As lowland forests are harvested, mountain peaks warm and dry, adversely affecting many cloud forest species.*
Source: Data from R. O. Lawton et al., 2001.

WORLD FORESTS

As chapter 5 shows, forests and grasslands—especially in temperate regions—are among the most heavily disturbed by human activities of any terrestrial biomes. These ecosystems produce valuable materials, such as lumber, paper pulp, and domestic livestock, that are important in human culture. They also play vital roles in regulating climate, controlling water runoff, providing wildlife habitat, purifying the air, and providing a host of other ecological services. Furthermore, these terrestrial biomes have scenic, cultural, and historic values that deserve to be protected. In many cases, these competing land uses are incompatible. Much of the attention of environmental groups over the past century has been devoted to protecting forests, prairies, and other landscapes. This chapter will focus on how we now use and abuse these biological communities, as well as some of the ways they are being protected and conserved.

Forest Distribution

Figure 6.2 shows the main forest types around the world, while figure 6.3 presents the UN Food and Agriculture Program estimates of total forest area by continent as well as annual rates of forest change. The FAO Forest Resources Assessment defines *forest* as an area where trees cover 10 percent or more of the land. The 3.9 billion ha encompassed by this definition include open woodlands, thorn scrub, and savannas, as well as **closed-canopy forests,** where tree crowns create a more continuous groundcover. The largest forest area in this summary is in Europe, which includes Russia's vast boreal forest. The world's largest tropical forest area is in South America's Amazon basin. Note that the highest annual rates of forest losses are in Africa (especially tropical West Africa) and in South America. Southeast Asia also has high rates of deforestation—a great tragedy, considering the high level of biological diversity in the area.

The total above-ground forest biomass in the world is estimated to be about 422 billion metric tons, one-third of which is in South America. This biomass represents both an important economic resource and a huge carbon sink. Clearing and burning of forests releases much of this carbon into the atmosphere and contributes significantly to global climate change (see chapter 9).

Among the forests of greatest ecological importance are the remnants of primeval forests that are home to much of the world's biodiversity, endangered species, and indigenous human cultures.

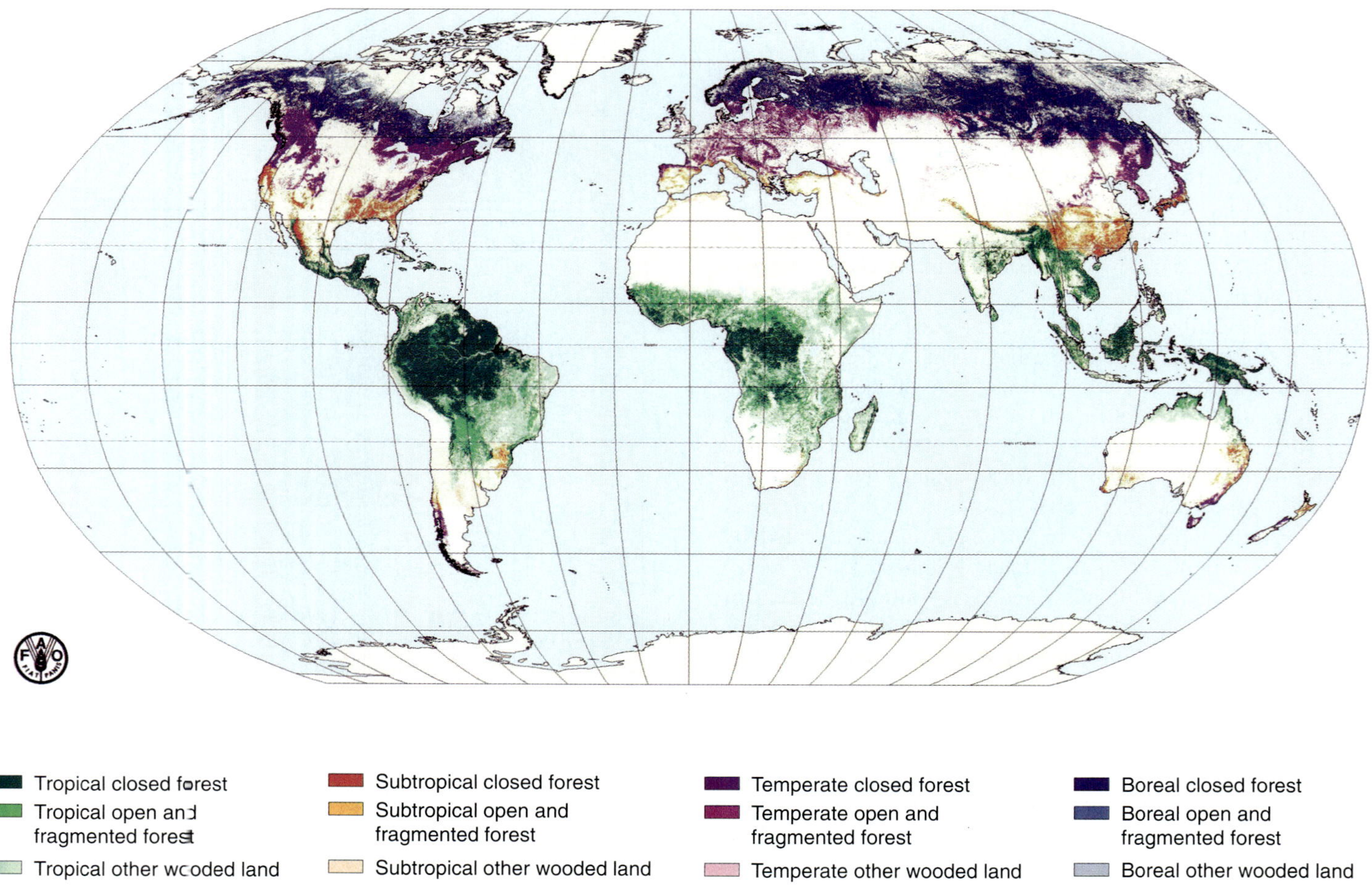

FIGURE 6.2 *Major forest types. Note that some of these forests are dense; others may have only 10 to 20 percent actual tree cover.*
Source: Data from United Nations Food and Agriculture Organization, 2002.

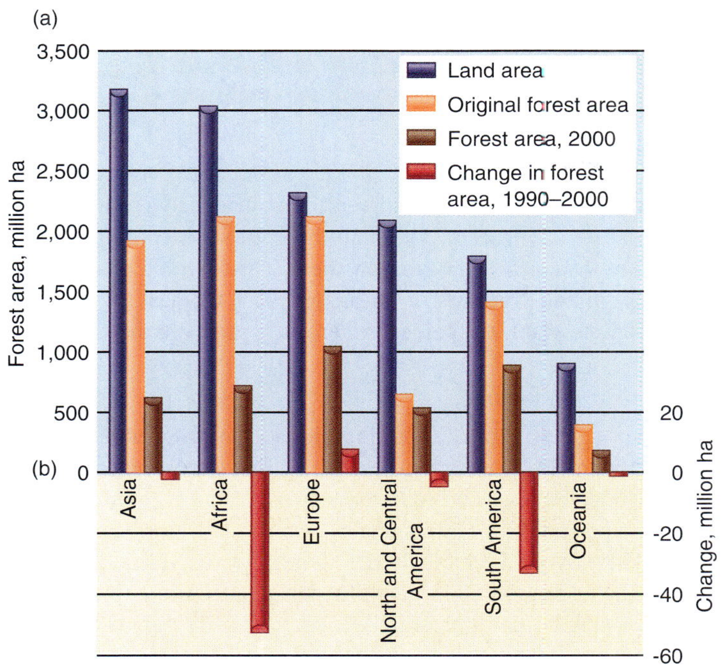

FIGURE 6.3 *Regional distribution of original and current forests* (a) *and regional forest losses, 1990 to 2000* (b). *Europe includes Russia's Siberian forests.*
Source: Data from United Nations Food and Agriculture Organization, 2002.

Sometimes called frontier forests, **old-growth forests** are those that cover a large enough area and have been undisturbed by human activities long enough that trees can live out a natural life cycle and ecological processes can occur in relatively normal fashion. That doesn't mean that all trees need be enormous or thousands of years old. In some old-growth forests, most trees live less than a century before being killed by disease or some natural disturbance, such as a fire. Nor does it mean that humans have never been present. Where human occupation entails relatively little impact, an old-growth forest may have been inhabited by people for a very long time. Even forests that have been logged or converted to cropland often can revert to old-growth characteristics if left alone long enough.

While forests still cover about half the area they once did worldwide, only one-quarter of those forests retain old-growth features. The largest remaining areas of old-growth forest are in Russia, Canada, Brazil, Indonesia, and Papua New Guinea. Together, these five countries account for more than three-quarters of all relatively undisturbed forests in the world. In general, remoteness rather than laws protect those forests. Although official data describe only about one-fifth of Russian old-growth forest as threatened, rapid deforestation—both legal and illegal—especially in the Russian Far East, probably put a much greater area at risk.

Forest Products

Wood plays a part in more activities of the modern economy than does any other commodity. There is hardly any industry that does not use wood or wood products somewhere in its manufacturing and marketing processes. Think about the amount of junk mail, newspapers, photocopies, and other paper products that each of us in developed countries handles, stores, and disposes of in a single day. Total annual world wood consumption is about 3.7 billion metric tons, or about 3.7 billion m^3. This is more than steel and plastic consumption combined. International trade in wood and wood products amounts to more than $100 billion each year (fig. 6.4). Developed countries produce less than half of all industrial wood but account for about 80 percent of its consumption. Less-developed countries, mainly in the tropics, produce more than half of all industrial wood but use only 20 percent.

The United States, Russia, and Canada are the largest producers of both industrial wood (lumber and panels) and paper pulp. Much of the industrial logging in North America and Europe occurs in managed forests, where cut trees are grown as a crop. In contrast, tropical hardwoods in Southeast Asia, Africa, and Latin America are being cut at an unsustainable rate, mostly from old-growth forests.

More than half of the people in the world depend on firewood or charcoal as their principal source of heating and cooking fuel (fig. 6.5). Consequently, fuelwood accounts for slightly more than half of all wood harvested worldwide. Unfortunately, burgeoning populations and dwindling forests are causing wood shortages in many less-developed countries. About 1.5 billion people who depend on fuelwood as their primary energy source have less than they need. At present rates of population growth and wood consumption, the annual deficit is expected to increase from 500 million m^3 in 2000 to 2,600 million m^3 in 2025. At that point, the demand would be twice the available fuelwood supply. The average amount of wood used for cooking and heating in 63 less-developed countries is about 1 m^3 per person per year,

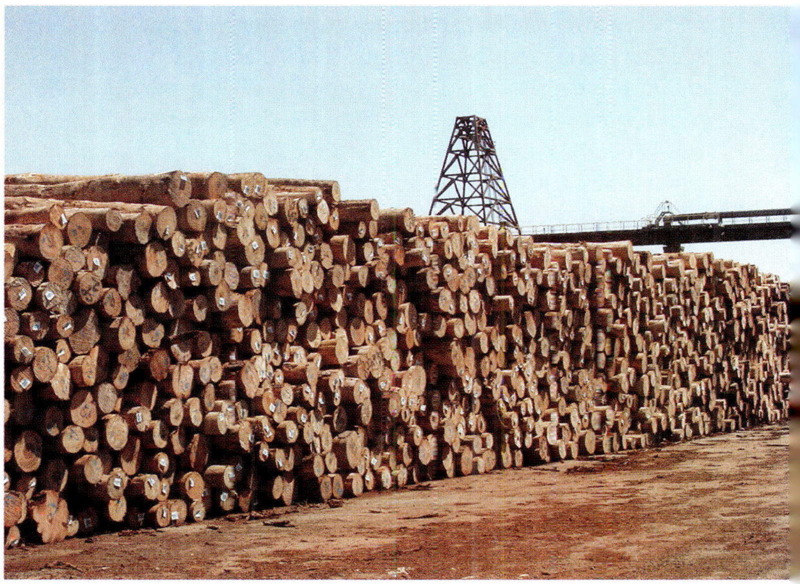

FIGURE 6.4 *Logs await shipment from a New Zealand port, part of the 1.5 billion m of industrial wood traded worldwide each year.*

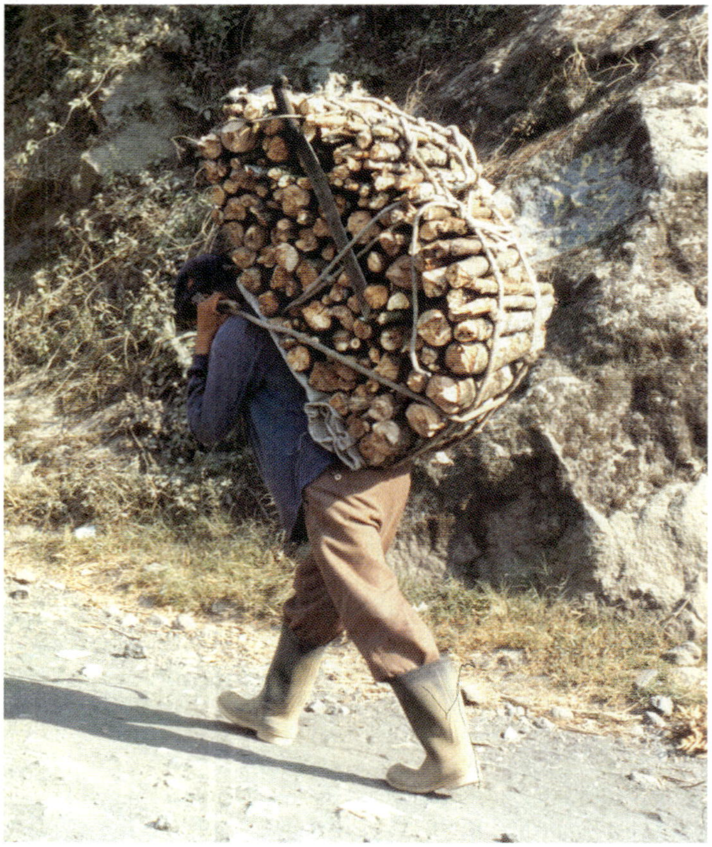

FIGURE 6.5 *Firewood accounts for almost half of all wood harvested worldwide and is the main energy source for nearly half of all humans.*

roughly equal to the amount of wood that each American consumes each year as paper products alone.

Approximately one-quarter of the world's forests are managed for wood production. Ideally, forest management involves scientific planning for sustainable harvests, with particular attention paid to forest regeneration. In temperate regions, according to the UN Food and Agriculture Organization (FAO), more land is being replanted or allowed to regenerate naturally than is being permanently deforested. Much of this reforestation, however, is in large plantations of single-species, single-use, intensive cropping called **monoculture forestry.** Although this produces rapid growth and easier harvesting than a more diverse forest, a dense, single-species stand often supports little biodiversity and does poorly in providing the ecological services, such as soil erosion control and clean water production, that may be the greatest value of native forests.

Some of the countries with the most successful reforestation programs are in Asia. China, for instance, cut down most of its forests 1,000 years ago and has suffered centuries of erosion and terrible floods as a consequence. Recently, however, timber cutting in the headwaters of major rivers has been outlawed, and a massive reforestation project has begun. In the 1990s, China planted 42 billion trees, mainly in Xinjiang Provence, to stop the spread of deserts. Korea and Japan also have had very successful forest restoration programs. After being almost totally denuded during World War II, both countries are now about 70 percent forested.

Tropical Forests

Some of the richest and most diverse terrestrial ecosystems on the earth are tropical forests. Although they now occupy less than 10 percent of the earth's land surface, these forests are thought to contain more than two-thirds of all higher plant biomass and at least half of all the plant, animal, and microbial species in the world.

Diminishing Forests

A century ago, an estimated 12.5 million km^2 of tropical lands were covered with closed-canopy forest. This was an area larger than the entire United States. The FAO estimates that about 9.2 million ha, or about 0.6 percent, of the remaining tropical forest is cleared each year.

There is considerable debate about current rates of deforestation in the tropics. In 2003, satellite data showed more than 30,000 fires in a single month in Brazil. Remote sensing experts calculate that 3 million ha per year are now being cut and burned in the Amazon basin alone. However, there are different definitions of *deforestation.* Some scientists insist that it means a complete change from forest to agriculture, urban areas, or desert. Others include any area that has been logged, even if the cut was selective and regrowth will be rapid. Furthermore, savannas, open woodlands, and succession following natural disturbance are hard to distinguish from logged areas. Consequently, estimates for total tropical forest losses range from about 5 million to more than 20 million ha per year. The FAO estimates of 12.3 million ha deforested per year are generally the most widely accepted. To put that figure in perspective, it means that about 1 acre—or the area of a football field—is cleared every second, on average, around the clock.

By most accounts, Brazil has the highest total deforestation rate in the world, but it also has by far the largest tropical forests. Indonesia and Malaysia together may be losing as much primary forest each year as Brazil, even though their original amount was far lower. In 1997 forest fires on Borneo and Sumatra, exacerbated by severe drought, burned 20,000 km^2 (8,000 mi^2). The fires reportedly were set both to clear land for agriculture and to hide illegal logging.

In Africa, the coastal forests of Senegal, Sierra Leone, Ghana, Madagascar, Cameroon, and Liberia already have been mostly destroyed. Haiti was once 80 percent forested; today, essentially all that forest has been destroyed, and the land lies barren and eroded. India, Burma, Kampuchea (Cambodia), Thailand, and Vietnam all have little old-growth lowland forest left. In Central America, nearly two-thirds of the original moist tropical forest has been destroyed, mostly within the past 30 years and primarily due to conversion of forest to cattle range. (See related story on "Disappearing Butterfly Forests" at www.mhhe.com/cases.)

Causes of Deforestation

A variety of factors contribute to deforestation, and, as figure 6.6 shows, different forces predominate in various parts of the world. Logging for valuable tropical hardwoods, such as teak and

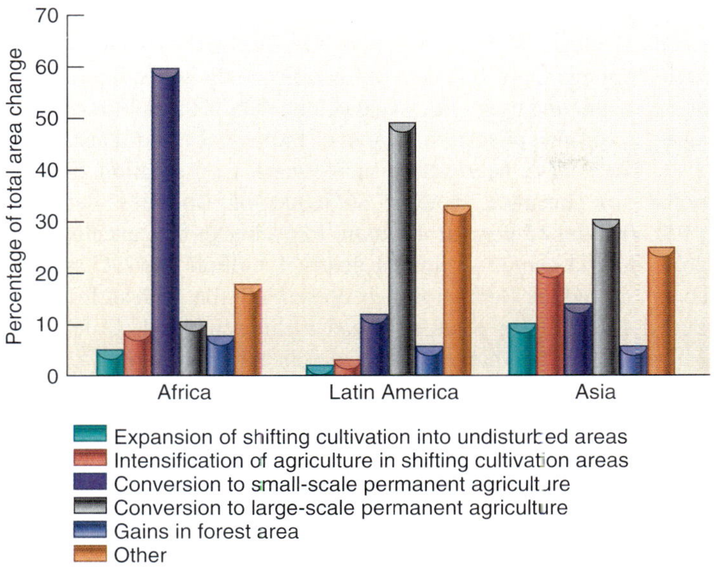

FIGURE 6.6 *Tropical forest losses by different processes.*
Source: Data from Food and Agriculture Organization of the United Nations, 2002.

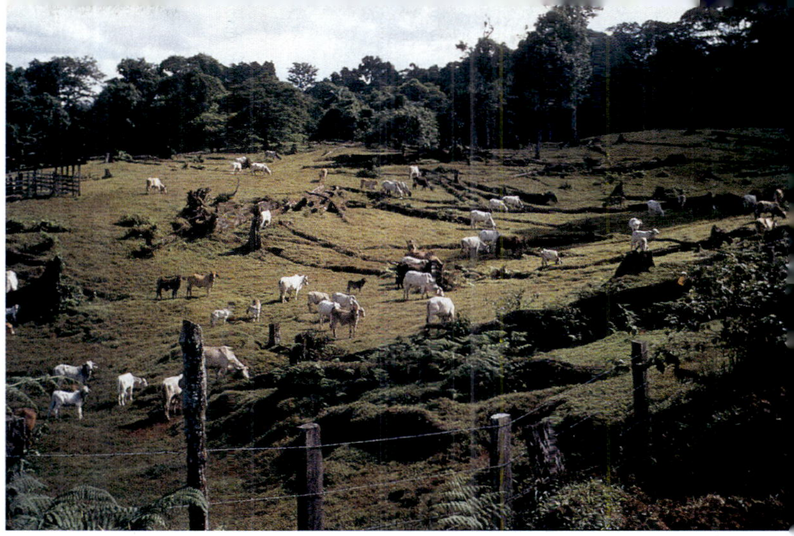

FIGURE 6.7 *Cattle graze on recently cleared tropical rainforest land. Millions of hectares have been cleared for pasture and cropland in recent decades. Unfortunately, the soil is poorly suited to grazing or farming, and new land must be cleared every few years.*

mahogany, is generally the first step. Although loggers may take only one or two of the largest trees per hectare, the canopy of tropical forests is usually so strongly linked by vines and interlocking branches that felling one tree can bring down a dozen others. Building roads to remove logs kills more trees, but even more important, it allows entry to the forest by farmers, miners, hunters, and others who cause further damage.

In Africa, conversion of forest into small-scale agriculture accounts for nearly two-thirds of all tropical forest destruction. In Latin America, poor, landless farmers often start the deforestation but are bought out—or driven out—after a few years by large-scale farmers or ranchers (fig. 6.7). The thin, nutrient-poor tropical forest soils frequently are worn out after a few years of cropping, and much of this land becomes unproductive pasture or impoverished scrubland. Shifting cultivation (sometimes called "slash and burn" or milpa farming) is often blamed for forest destruction. This practice can be sustainable where population densities are low and individual plots are allowed to regenerate for a decade or two between cultivation periods. In some Asian countries, however, growing populations and shrinking forests lead to short rotation cycles, and cropping intensification can lead to permanent deforestation.

As the opening story of this chapter shows, forest clearing can change regional rainfall patterns. A computer model created by Pennsylvania State University scientists suggests this phenomenon might create a kind of chain reaction. As forests are cut down, plant transpiration and rainfall decrease. Drought kills more vegetation, and fires become more numerous and extensive. In a worst-case scenario, an area as large as the entire Amazonian forest might be permanently damaged in just a few decades.

Forest Protection

What can be done to stop this destruction and encourage tropical forest protection? While much of the news is discouraging, there are some hopeful signs for forest conservation in the tropics. (See related story "Saving an African Eden" at www.mhhe.com/cases.) Many countries now recognize that forests are valuable resources. Intensive scientific investigations are underway to identify the best remaining natural areas.

About 12 percent of all world forests are in some form of protected status, but the effectiveness of that protection varies greatly. Costa Rica has one of the best plans for forest guardianship in the world. Attempts are being made there not only to rehabilitate the land (make an area useful to humans) but also to restore the ecosystems to naturally occurring associations. One of the best-known of these projects is Dan Janzen's work in Guanacaste National Park. Like many dry, tropical forests, the northwestern part of Costa Rica had been almost totally converted to ranchland. By controlling fires, however, Janzen and his coworkers are bringing back the forest. One of the keys to this success is involving local people in the project. Janzen also permits grazing in the park. The original forest evolved, he reasons, together with ancient grazing animals that are now extinct. Horses and cows can play a valuable role as seed dispersers.

People also are working on the grassroots level to protect and restore forests in other countries. India, for instance, has a long history of nonviolent, passive resistance movements—called *satyagrahas*—to protest unfair government policies. These protests go back to the beginning of Indian culture and often have been associated with forest preservation. Gandhi drew on this tradition in his protests of British colonial rule in the 1930s and 1940s. During the 1970s, commercial loggers began large-scale tree felling in the Garhwal region in the state of Uttar Pradesh in northern India. Landslides and floods resulted from stripping the forest cover from the hills. The firewood on which local people depended was destroyed, and the way of life of the traditional forest culture was threatened. In a remarkable display of courage and determination, the village women wrapped their arms around the trees to protect them, sparking the Chipko Andolan movement (literally, movement to hug trees). They prevented logging on 12,000 km^2 of

what can you do?

Lowering Your Forest Impacts

For most urban residents, forests—especially tropical forests—seem far away and disconnected from everyday life. There are things that each of us can do, however, to protect forests.

- Reuse and recycle paper. Make double-sided copies. Save office paper, and use the back for scratch paper.
- Use email. Store information in digital form, rather than making hard copies of everything.
- If you build, conserve wood. Use wafer board, particle board, laminated beams, or other composites, rather than plywood and timbers made from old-growth trees.
- Buy products made from "good wood" or other certified sustainably harvested wood.
- Don't buy products made from tropical hardwoods, such as ebony, mahogany, rosewood, or teak, unless the manufacturer can guarantee that the hardwoods were harvested from agroforestry plantations or sustainable-harvest programs.
- Don't patronize fast-food restaurants that purchase beef from cattle grazing on deforested rainforest land. Don't buy coffee, bananas, pineapples, or other cash crops if their production contributes to forest destruction.
- Do buy Brazil nuts, cashews, mushrooms, rattan furniture, and other nontimber forest products harvested sustainably by local people from intact forests. Remember that tropical rainforest is not the only biome under attack. Contact the Taiga Rescue Network (www. taigarescue.org) for information about boreal forests.
- If you hike or camp in forested areas, practice minimum-impact camping. Stay on existing trails, and don't build more or bigger fires than you absolutely need. Use only downed wood for fires. Don't carve on trees or drive nails into them.
- Write to your congressional representatives, and ask them to support forest protection and environmentally responsible government policies. Contact the U.S. Forest Service, and voice your support for recreation and nontimber forest values.

sensitive watersheds in the Alakanada basin. Today the Chipko Andolan movement has grown to more than 4,000 groups working to save India's forests.

Debt-for-Nature Swaps

Those of us in developed countries also can contribute toward saving tropical forests. Financing nature protection is often a problem in developing countries, where the need is greatest. One promising approach is called **debt-for-nature swaps.** Banks, governments, and lending institutions now hold nearly $1 trillion in loans to developing countries. There is little prospect of ever collecting much of this debt, and banks are often willing to sell bonds at a steep discount—perhaps as little as 10 cents on the dollar. Conservation organizations buy debt obligations on the secondary market at a discount and then offer to cancel the debt if the debtor country agrees to protect or restore an area of biological importance.

There have been many such swaps. Conservation International, for instance, bought $650,000 of Bolivia's debt for $100,000—an 85 percent discount. In exchange for canceling this debt, Bolivia agreed to protect nearly 1 million ha (2.47 million acres) around the Beni Biosphere Reserve in the Andean foothills. Ecuador and Costa Rica have had a different kind of debt-for-nature swap. They have exchanged debt for local currency bonds that fund activities of local private conservation organizations in the country. This has the dual advantage of building and supporting indigenous environmental groups while protecting the land. Critics, however, charge that these swaps compromise national sovereignty and do little to reduce Third World debt or to change the situations that led to environmental destruction in the first place.

Temperate Forests

Tropical countries aren't unique in harvesting forests at an unsustainable rate. Northern countries, such as the United States and Canada, also have allowed controversial forest management practices in many areas. For many years, the official policy of the U.S. Forest Service was "multiple use," which implied that the forests could be used for everything that we might want to do there simultaneously. Some uses are incompatible, however. Bird-watching, for example, isn't very enjoyable in a dirt bike racing course. And protecting species that need unbroken old-growth forest isn't feasible when you cut down the forest.

Old-Growth Forests

The most contentious forestry issues in the United States and Canada in recent years have centered on logging in old-growth forests in the Pacific Northwest. These forests have incredibly high levels of biodiversity, and they accumulate more total biomass in standing vegetation per unit area than any other ecosystem on earth (fig. 6.8). Many endemic species, such as the northern spotted owl (fig. 6.9), Vaux's swift, and the marbled murrelet, are so highly adapted to the unique conditions of these ancient forests that they live nowhere else.

Only a century ago, most of the coastal ranges of Washington, Oregon, northern California, British Columbia, and southeastern Alaska were clothed in a lush forest of huge trees, many a thousand years old or more. Today, less than 10 percent of the old-growth forest in the United States remains intact, and 80 percent of what is left is scheduled to be cut down in the near future. British Columbia has felled at least 60 percent of its richest and most productive ancient forests and is now cutting some 240 million ha (600 million acres) annually, about ten times the rate of old-growth harvest in the United States. At these rates, the only remaining ancient forests in North America in 50 years will be a fringe around the base of the mountains in a few national parks.

In 1989 environmentalists sued the U.S. Forest Service over logging rates in Washington and Oregon, arguing that northern

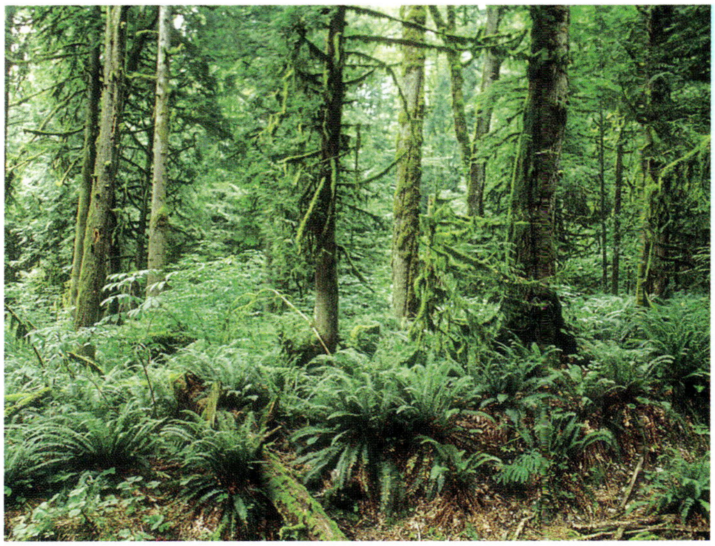

FIGURE 6.8 *The temperate rainforests of the Pacific Northwest have the highest biomass per hectare of any landscape in the world.*

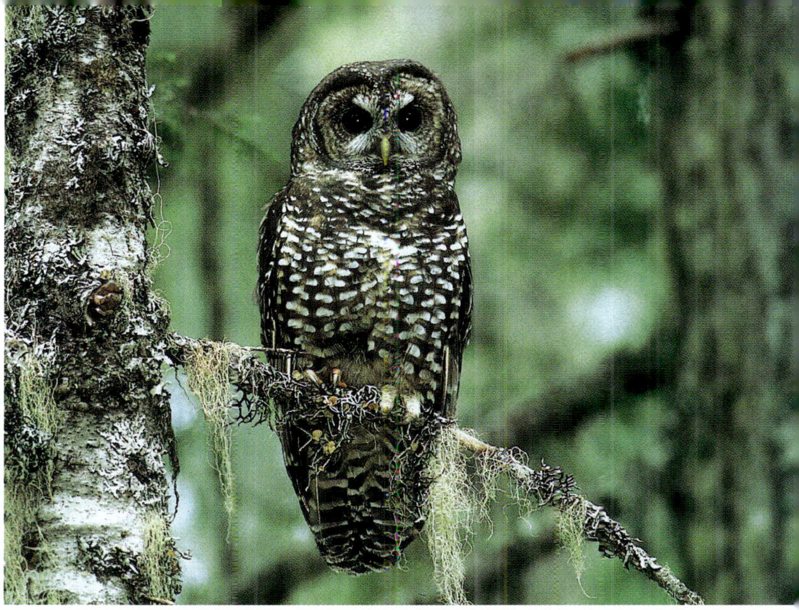

FIGURE 6.9 *Only about 2,000 pairs of northern spotted owls remain in the old-growth forests of the Pacific Northwest. Cutting old-growth forests threatens endangered species, but reduced logging threatens the jobs of many timber workers.*

spotted owls are endangered and must be protected under the Endangered Species Act. Federal courts agreed and ordered some 1 million ha (2.5 million acres) of ancient forest set aside to preserve the last 2,000 pairs of owls. This is about half the remaining virgin forest in Washington and Oregon. The timber industry claimed that 40,000 jobs would be lost, although economic studies show that most logging jobs were lost as a result of log exports and mechanization. Still, outrage in the logging communities was loud and clear. Convoys of logging trucks converged on protest sites, while angry crowds burned environmentalists in effigy. Bumper stickers urged, "Save a logger; eat an owl."

A compromise forest management plan was finally agreed upon that allows some continued logging but protects the most valuable forests, including selected old-growth preserves, riparian (streamside) buffer strips, and prime wildlife habitat. This plan may not be enough protection, however, to ensure the survival of endangered salmon and trout populations in northwestern rivers. An even bigger battle may be shaping up as specific fish populations are considered for listing as endangered species. Several salmon and steelhead trout populations were listed as endangered under the Clinton administration. These listings have been challenged by the timber industry, but the $1 billion-per-year fishing industry in the Pacific Northwest may be at least as powerful a constituency as were those concerned about spotted owls.

Harvest Methods

Most lumber and pulpwood in the United States and Canada currently are harvested by **clear-cutting,** in which every tree in a given area is cut, regardless of size (fig. 6.10). This method is effective for producing even-age stands of sun-loving species, such as aspen or pines, but often increases soil erosion and eliminates habitat for many forest species when carried out on large blocks. It was once thought that good forest management required immediate removal of all dead trees and logging residue. Research has shown, however, that standing snags and coarse woody debris play important ecological roles, including soil protection, habitat for a variety of organisms, and nutrient recycling.

Some alternatives to clear-cutting include **shelterwood harvesting,** in which mature trees are removed in a series of two or more cuts, and **strip-cutting,** in which all the trees in a narrow corridor are harvested. For many forest types, the least disruptive harvest method is **selective cutting,** in which only a small percentage of the mature trees are taken in each 10- or 20-year rotation. Ponderosa pine, for example, are usually selectively cut to thin stands and improve growth of the remaining trees. A forest managed by selective

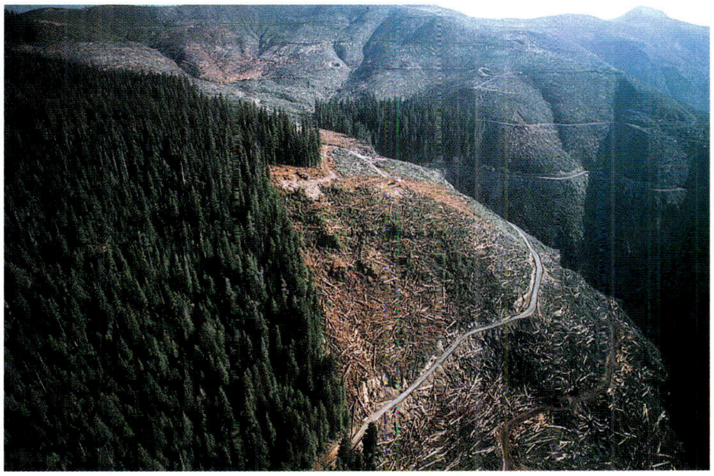

FIGURE 6.10 *This huge clear-cut in Washington's Gifford Pinchot National Forest threatens species dependent on old-growth forest and exposes steep slopes to soil erosion. Restoring something like the original forest will take hundreds of years.*

cutting can retain many of the characteristics of age distribution and groundcover of a mature old-growth forest. (See related story "Forestry for the Seventh Generation" at www.mhhe.com/cases.)

Should We Ban Logging and Roads in National Forests?

An increasing number of people in the United States are calling for an end to all logging on federal lands. In 2002 more than 220 scientists signed a letter to President Bush arguing that the value of timber produced from public lands is miniscule, compared with the environmental costs of harvests. American taxpayers, they argued, subsidize logging directly by charging less for timber sales than it costs to administer them, as well as indirectly because logging reduces the economic value of the forest for other uses. Just 4 percent of the nation's timber comes from national forests, they claimed, and this harvest adds about $4 billion to the American economy per year. In contrast, recreation, fish and wildlife, clean water, and other ecological services provided by the forest, by their calculations, are worth at least $224 billion each year. Timber industry officials, on the other hand, dispute these claims, arguing that logging not only provides jobs and supports rural communities but also keeps forests healthy. What do you think? Could we make up for decreased timber production from public lands by more intensive management of private holdings and by substitution or recycling of wood products? Are there alternative ways you could suggest to support communities now dependent on timber harvesting?

Roads on public lands are another controversy. Over the past 40 years, the Forest Service has expanded its system of logging roads more than ten-fold, to a current total of nearly 550,000 km (343,000 mi), or more than ten times the length of the interstate highway system. Government economists regard road building as a benefit because it opens up the country to motorized recreation and industrial uses. Wilderness enthusiasts and wildlife supporters, however, see this as an expensive and disruptive program. In 2001 the Clinton administration announced a plan to protect 23.7 million ha (58.5 million acres) of de facto wilderness from roads. Timber, mining, and oil companies protested this rule. In 2002 a federal judge in Idaho ruled that blocking road construction would do "irreparable harm" to the forest. He also ruled that the 600 public meetings held over a 12-month period to discuss this plan, and the record 1.6 million written comments gathered (90 percent of which supported increased protection), did not represent adequate public input. The Bush administration overturned the "roadless rule" and ordered resource managers to expedite logging, mining, and motorized recreation. What do you think? How much of the remaining old growth should be protected as ecological reserves?

Fire Management

Following a series of disastrous fire years in the 1930s, in which hundreds of millions of hectares of forest were destroyed, whole towns burned to the ground, and several hundred people died, the U.S. Forest Service adopted a policy of aggressive fire control in which every blaze on public land was to be out before 10 A.M. Smokey Bear was adopted as the forest mascot and warned us that "only you can prevent forest fires." Recent studies, however, of fire's ecological role suggest that our attempts to suppress all fires may have been misguided. Many biological communities are fire-adapted and require periodic burning for regeneration. Furthermore, eliminating fire from these forests has allowed woody debris to accumulate, greatly increasing the chances of a very big fire (fig. 6.11).

Forests that once were characterized by 50 to 100 mature, fire-resistant trees per hectare and an open understory now have a thick tangle of up to 2,000 small, spindly, mostly dead saplings in the same area. The U.S. Forest Service estimates that 33 million ha (73 million acres), or about 40 percent of all federal forestlands, are at risk of severe fires. To make matters worse, Americans increasingly live in remote areas where wildfires are highly likely. Because there haven't been fires in many of these places in living memory, many people assume there is no danger, but by some estimates, 40 million U.S. residents now live in areas with high wildfire risk.

A recent prolonged drought in the western United States has heightened fire danger. In 2002 more than 88,000 wildfires burned 2.8 million ha (6.9 million acres) of forests and grasslands in the United States. Federal agencies spent about $1.6 billion to fight these fires, nearly four times the previous ten-year average.

The dilemma is how to undo years of fire suppression and fuel buildup. Fire ecologists favor small, prescribed burns to clean out debris. Loggers decry this approach as a waste of valuable timber, and local residents of fire-prone areas fear that prescribed fires will escape and threaten them. Recently the Forest Service proposed a massive new program of forest thinning and emergency salvage operations (removing trees and flammable material from mature or recently burned forests) on 16 million ha (40 million acres) of national forest. Carried out over a 20-year period, this program could cost as much as $12 billion and would open up much roadless, de facto wilderness to large-scale logging. Critics

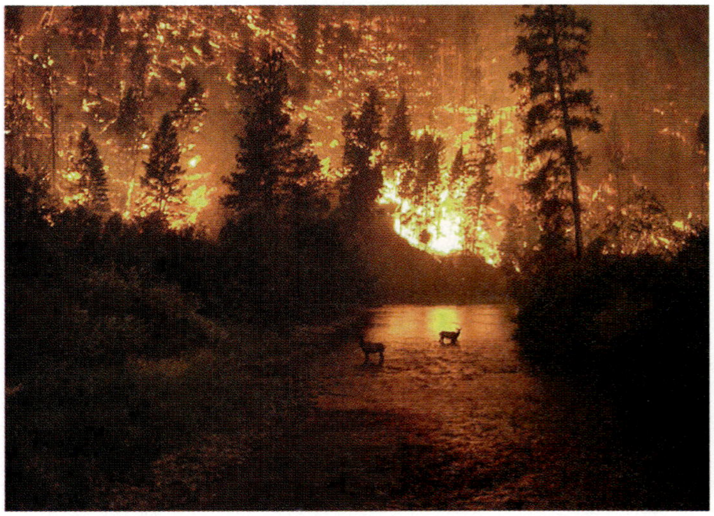

FIGURE 6.11 *By suppressing fires and allowing fuel to accumulate, we make major fires such as this more likely. The safest and most ecologically sound management policy for some forests may be to allow natural or prescribed fires, which don't threaten property or human life, to burn periodically.*

INVESTIGATING Our Environment

Forest Thinning and Salvage Logging

For more than 70 years, firefighting has been a high priority for forest managers. Unfortunately, our efforts have been so successful that dead wood and brush have now built up to dangerous levels in many forests. Lands that would once have been cleaned out by frequent low-temperature ground fires now have so much accumulated fuel that a catastrophic wildfire is all but inevitable. To make matters worse, increasing numbers of people are building cabins and homes in remote, fire-prone areas, where they expect to be protected from unavoidable risks.

People living in or near national forests demand protection from wildfires. In response, federal agencies are starting thinning programs to remove excess fuel. To make it profitable for loggers to remove fire-prone dead wood, small trees, and brush, the government is allowing them to harvest large, valuable, and fire-resistant trees located in the backcountry, often miles away from the nearest communities. And to avoid what many loggers claim is "red tape and litigation" that have tied up forest managers in "analysis paralysis," most thinning projects are exempt from public comment and administrative appeals, as well as from environmental reviews under the National Environmental Policy Act (NEPA).

Environmental groups denounce these projects as merely logging without laws. Thinning, they argue, looks very much like clear-cutting. Forest ecologists argue that thinning, unless it is repeated every few years, actually makes the forests more, rather than less, fire-prone. Removing big, old trees opens up the forest canopy and encourages growth of brush and new tree seedlings. Furthermore, logging compacts soil and introduces invasive species. Many forest ecologists maintain that small, prescribed burns can reduce fuel and produce healthier forests than commercial logging.

Other research calls into question a main justification for thinning: protecting housing that has proliferated around the edges of federal forests. The only thinning needed to protect houses, according to fire experts, is within about 60 m around the building. Regardless of how intense the fire is, building damage can be minimized by installing a metal roof, clearing pine needles and brush around the house, and removing trees immediately around the building.

After a fire has burned a forest, local residents often call for emergency salvage logging to utilize dead trees before they fall and become fuel for future fires. Foes say that salvage sales allow timber companies to cut many trees that survive the flames and, like thinning, leave roads and scars from heavy equipment that last far longer than any effects of the fires themselves. And, critics contend, the salvage contracts rarely require timber companies to remove the very fuel that stokes wildfires—the underbrush and downed timber for which there is little or no market. The result, some conservationists say, is the ecological equivalent of mugging a fire victim.

What do you think? How can we get out of the crisis we've created by preventing fires and letting dead wood accumulate? If you were a forest manager, would you authorize thinning and salvage logging, or can you think of other ways to remove forest fuels in an ecologically and economically sustainable manner? What research projects would you direct your staff to undertake in order to inform your decision in this dilemma?

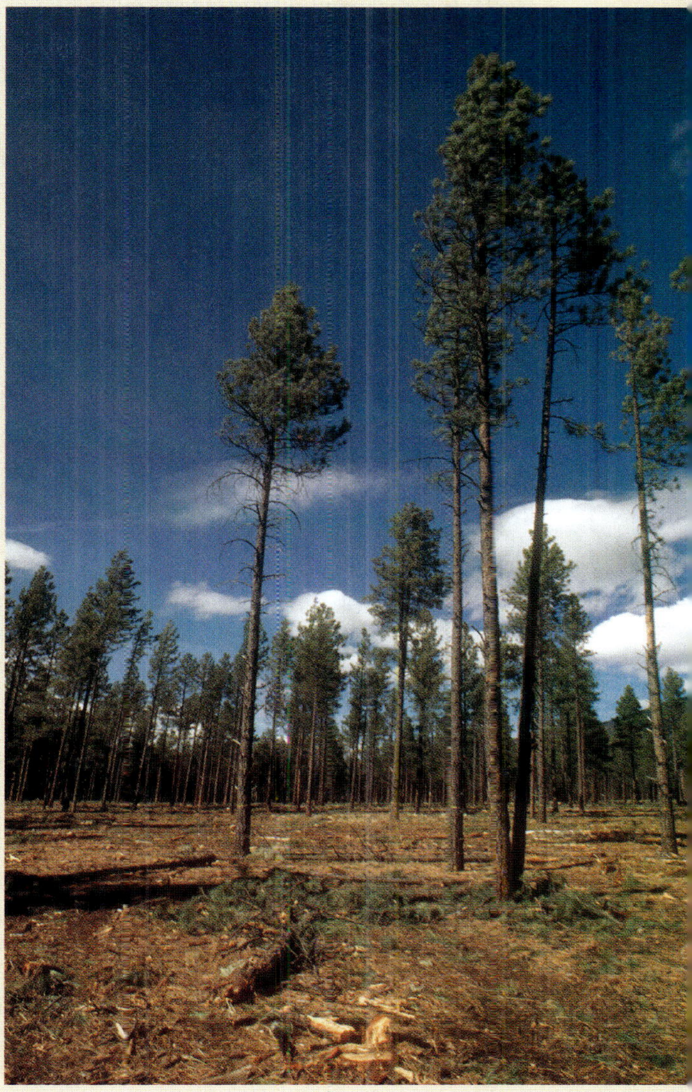

Demonstration forest thinning (or fuel reduction) project in the Coconino National Forest, Arizona. "Exactly this kind of treatment has to happen across the western U.S.," said Forest Service chief Dale Bosworth. "We have only 20 years to treat 30 million acres."

complain that this program is ill advised and environmentally destructive. Proponents argue that the only way to save the forest is to log it (see Investigating Our Environment, above, and related story "The Quincy Library Group" at www.mhhe.com/cases).

Ecosystem Management

In the 1990s the U.S. Forest Service began to shift its policies from a timber production focus to **ecosystem management,** which attempts to integrate sustainable ecological, economic, and social goals in a unified, systems approach. Some of the principles of this new philosophy include

- Managing across whole landscapes, watersheds, or regions over ecological time scales
- Considering human needs and promoting sustainable economic development and communities

- Maintaining biological diversity and essential ecosystem processes
- Utilizing cooperative institutional arrangements
- Generating meaningful stakeholder and public involvement and facilitating collective decision making
- Adapting management over time, based on conscious experimentation and routine monitoring

Some critics argue that we don't understand ecosystems well enough to make practical decisions in forest management on this basis. They argue we should simply set aside large blocks of untrammeled nature to allow for chaotic, catastrophic, and unpredictable events. Others see this new approach as a threat to industry and customary ways of doing things. Still, elements of ecosystem management appear in the *National Report on Sustainable Forests* prepared by the U.S. Forest Service. Based on the Montreal Working Group criteria and indicators for forest health, this report suggests goals for sustainable forest management (table 6.1).

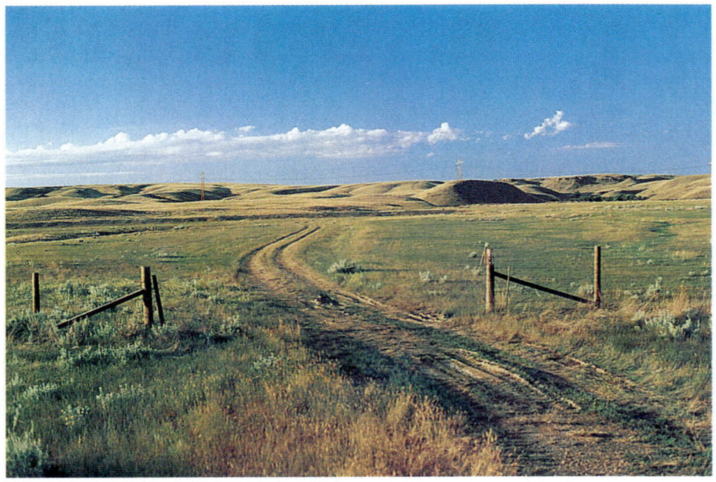

FIGURE 6.12 *This short-grass prairie in northern Montana is too dry for trees but, nevertheless, supports a diverse biological community.*

RANGELANDS

After forests, grasslands are among the biomes most heavily used by humans. Prairies, savannas, steppes, open woodlands, and other grasslands occupy about one-quarter of the world's land surface. Much of the U.S. Great Plains and the Prairie Provinces of Canada fall in this category (fig. 6.12). The 3.8 billion ha (12 million mi^2) of pastures and grazing lands in this biome make up about twice the area of all agricultural crops. When you add to this about 4 billion ha of other lands (forest, desert, tundra, marsh, and thorn scrub) used for raising livestock, more than half of all land is used at least occasionally for grazing. More than 3 billion cattle, sheep, goats, camels, buffalo, and other domestic animals on these lands make a valuable contribution to human nutrition. Sustainable pastoralism can increase productivity while maintaining biodiversity in a grassland ecosystem.

Because grasslands, chaparral, and open woodlands are attractive for human occupation, they frequently are converted to cropland, urban areas, or other human-dominated landscapes. Worldwide the rate of grassland disturbance each year is three times that of tropical forest. Although they may appear to be uniform and monotonous to the untrained eye, native prairies can be highly productive and species-rich. According to the U.S. Department of Agriculture, more threatened plant species occur in rangelands than in any other major American biome.

Range Management

By carefully monitoring the numbers of animals and the condition of the range, ranchers and **pastoralists** (people who live by herding animals) can adjust to variations in rainfall, seasonal plant conditions, and the nutritional quality of forage to keep livestock healthy and avoid overusing any particular area. Conscientious management can actually improve the quality of the range.

When grazing lands are abused by overgrazing—especially in arid areas—rain runs off quickly before it can soak into the soil to nourish plants or replenish groundwater. Springs and wells dry up. Seeds can't germinate in the dry, overheated soil. The barren ground reflects more of the sun's heat, changing wind patterns, driving away moisture-laden clouds, and leading to further desiccation. This process of conversion of once fertile land to desert is called **desertification.**

This process is ancient, but in recent years it has been accelerated by expanding populations and the political conditions that force people to overuse fragile lands. According to the International Soil Reference and Information Centre in the Netherlands, nearly three-quarters of all rangelands in the world show signs of either degraded vegetation or soil erosion. Overgrazing is responsible for about one-third of that degradation (fig. 6.13). The highest percentage of moderate, severe, and extreme land degradation is in Mexico and Central America, while the largest total area is in Asia, where the world's most extensive grasslands occur. Can we reverse this process? In some places, people are reclaiming deserts and repairing the effects of neglect and misuse.

TABLE 6.1 Draft Criteria for Sustainable Forestry

1. Conservation of biological diversity
2. Maintenance of productive capacity of forest ecosystems
3. Maintenance of forest ecosystem health and vitality
4. Maintenance of soil and water resources
5. Maintenance of forest contribution to global carbon cycles
6. Maintenance and enhancement of long-term socioeconomic benefits to meet the needs of legal, institutional, and economic framework for forest conservation and sustainable management

Source: Data from USFS, 2002.

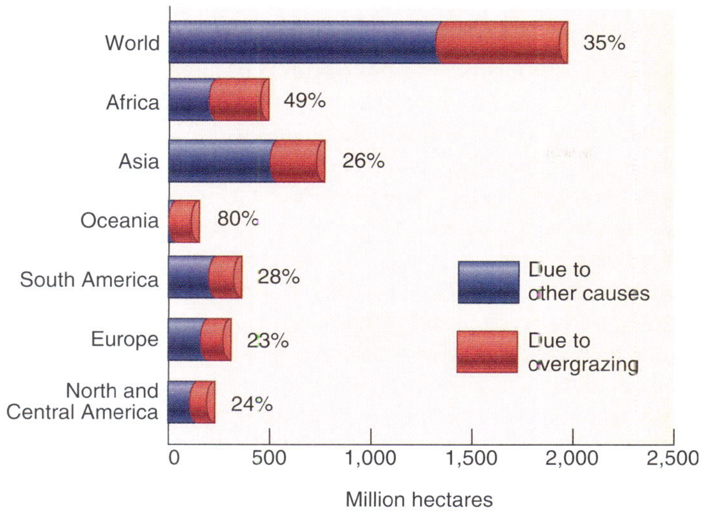

FIGURE 6.13 *Rangeland soil degradation due to overgrazing and other causes. Notice that, in Europe, Asia, and the Americas, farming, logging, mining, urbanization, and so on are responsible for about three-quarters of all soil degradation. In Africa and Oceania, where more grazing occurs and desert or semiarid scrub make up much of the range, grazing damage is higher.*
Source: Data from World Resource Institute.

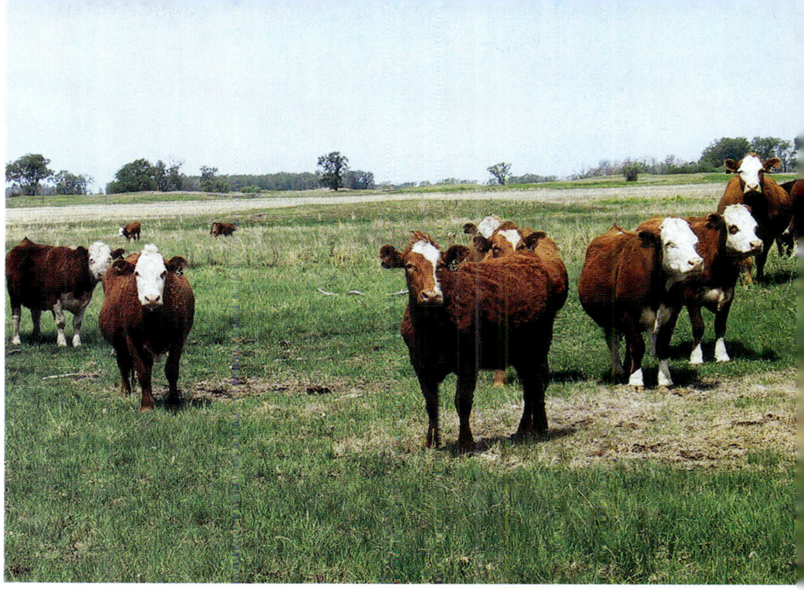

FIGURE 6.14 *More than half of all publicly owned grazing land in the United States is in poor or very poor condition. Overgrazing and invasive weeds are the biggest problems.*

Rangelands in the United States

The health of most public grazing lands in the United States is not good. Political and economic pressures encourage managers to increase grazing allotments beyond the carrying capacity of the range. Lack of enforcement of existing regulations and limited funds for range improvement have resulted in overgrazing, loss of native forage species, and erosion. The Natural Resources Defense Council claims that only 30 percent of public rangelands are in fair condition, and 55 percent are poor or very poor (fig. 6.14).

Overgrazing has allowed populations of unpalatable or inedible species, such as sage, mesquite, cheatgrass, and cactus, to build up on both public and private rangelands. Wildlife conservation groups regard cattle grazing as the most ubiquitous form of ecosystem degradation and the greatest threat to endangered species in the southwestern United States. They call for a ban on cattle and sheep grazing on all public lands, noting that it provides only 2 percent of the total forage consumed by beef cattle and supports only 2 percent of all livestock producers.

Like federal timber management policy, grazing fees charged for use of public lands often are far below market value and represent an enormous hidden subsidy to western ranchers. Holders of grazing permits generally pay the government less than 25 percent the amount of leasing comparable private land. The 31,000 permits on federal range bring in only $11 million in grazing fees but cost $47 million per year for administration and maintenance. The $36 million difference amounts to a massive "cow welfare" system of which few people are aware.

On the other hand, ranchers defend their way of life as an important part of western culture and history. Although few cattle go directly to market from their ranches, they produce almost all the beef calves subsequently shipped to feedlots. And without a viable ranch economy, they claim, even more of the western landscape would be subdivided into small ranchettes to the detriment of both wildlife and environmental quality. What do you think? How much should we subsidize extractive industries to preserve rural communities and traditional occupations?

New Approaches to Ranching

Where a small number of livestock are free to roam a large area, they generally eat the tender, best-tasting grasses and forbs first, leaving the tough, unpalatable species to flourish and gradually dominate the vegetation. In some places, farmers and ranchers find that short-term, intensive grazing helps maintain forage quality. As South African range specialist Allan Savory observed, wild ungulates (hoofed animals), such as gnus or zebras in Africa or bison (buffalo) in America, often tend to form dense herds that graze briefly but intensively in a particular location before moving on to the next area. Rest alone doesn't necessarily improve pastures and rangelands. Short-duration, **rotational grazing**—confining animals to a small area for a short time (often only a day or two) before shifting them to a new location—simulates the effects of wild herds (fig. 6.15). Forcing livestock to eat everything equally, to trample the ground thoroughly, and to fertilize heavily with manure before moving on helps keep weeds in check and encourages the growth of more desirable forage species. This approach doesn't work everywhere, however. Many plant communities in the U.S. desert Southwest, for example, apparently evolved in the absence of large, hoofed animals and can't withstand intensive grazing.

Another approach to ranching in some areas is to raise wild species, such as red deer, impala, wildebeest, or oryx (fig. 6.16). These animals forage more efficiently, resist harsh climates, often are more pest- and disease-resistant, and fend off predators better than usual domestic livestock. Native species also may have different feeding preferences and needs for water and shelter than

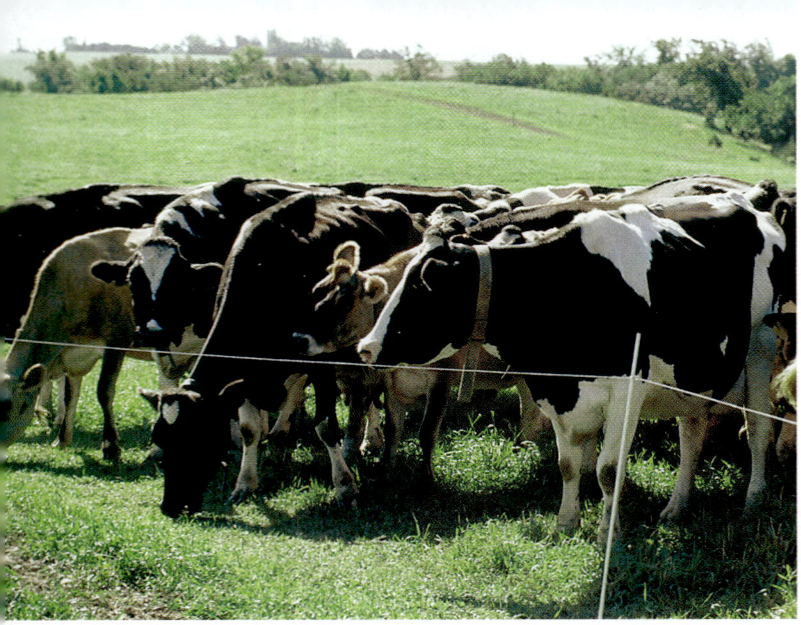

FIGURE 6.15 *Intensive, rotational grazing encloses livestock in a small area for a short time (often only one day) within a movable electric fence to force them to eat vegetation evenly and fertilize the area heavily.*

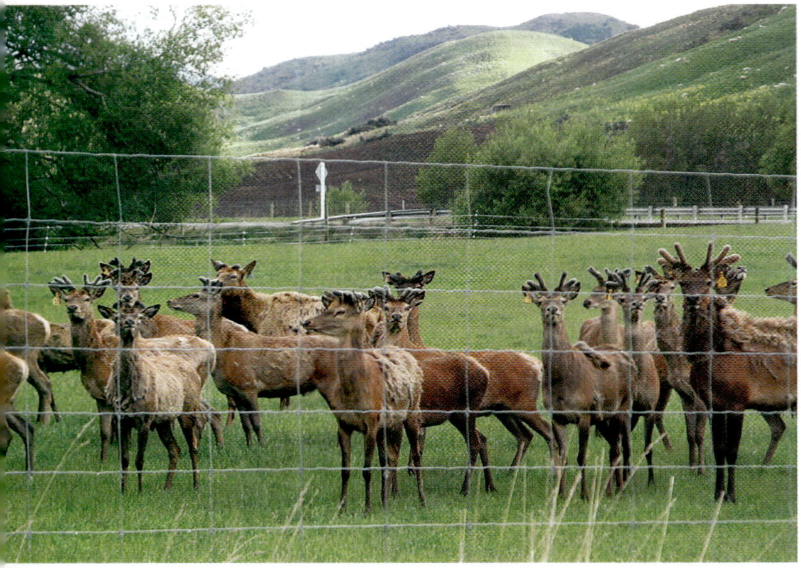

FIGURE 6.16 *Red deer* (Cervus elaphus) *are raised in New Zealand for antlers and venison.*

cows, goats, or sheep. The African Sahel, for instance, can provide only enough grass to raise about 20 to 30 kg (44 to 66 lbs) of beef per hectare. Ranchers can produce three times as much meat with wild native species in the same area because these animals browse on a wider variety of plant materials.

In the United States, ranchers find that elk, American bison, and a variety of African species take less care and supplemental feeding than cattle or sheep and result in a better financial return because their lean meat can bring a better market price than beef or mutton. Media mogul Ted Turner has become both the biggest private landholder in the United States and the owner of more American bison than anyone other than the government.

PARKS AND NATURE PRESERVES

Since ancient times, sacred groves have been set aside for religious purposes and hunting preserves or pleasuring grounds for royalty. These lands tended to be open only to elite members of society, but they helped preserve biodiversity and natural landscapes. Perhaps the first public parks open to ordinary citizens were the grand esplanades and the tree-sheltered agora that served as a gathering place in planned Greek cities. The modern design movement that incorporated Greek and Roman city planning principles in the redevelopment of European cities in the sixteenth and seventeenth centuries brought nature and beauty into the city in the form of parks, boulevards, and public gardens. It has been only in the past 130 years or so that we have begun to think about preserving wild places for the sake of wildlife and scenic beauty.

Parks serve a variety of purposes. They can teach us about our past and provide sanctuaries where nature is allowed to evolve in its own way. They are havens not only for wild plants and animals but also for the human spirit. Canada and the United States have greater total amounts of land dedicated to protected areas than any country except Denmark (which protects vast areas of Greenland's ice and snow) and Australia (which has designated great expanses of outback as aboriginal lands and parks). Although Mexico's parks are newer and less extensive than its wealthy neighbors, they contain far more biological and cultural diversity than do parks in either the United States or Canada.

North American Parks

In 1872 President Ulysses S. Grant signed an act designating about 800,000 ha (almost 2 million acres) of land in the Wyoming, Montana, and Idaho territories as Yellowstone National Park, the first national park in the world. Although the initial interest of both the founders and early visitors to Yellowstone were the curiosity of geysers, hot springs, and other odd features (fig. 6.17), the park

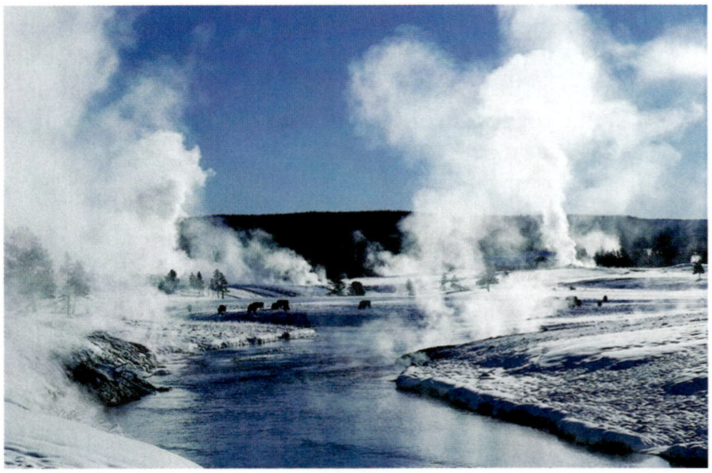

FIGURE 6.17 *Yellowstone National Park, established in 1872, is regarded as the first national park in the world. Although initial interest focused on the park's natural curiosities and wonders, Yellowstone has come to be appreciated for its beauty and wilderness values.*

was large enough to encompass and preserve wilderness. As it became apparent that places of wild nature, scenic beauty, and cultural importance were rapidly disappearing with the closing of the North American frontier, the drive to set aside more national parks accelerated. Canada's Banff National Park was established in 1885. In the United States, Crater Lake, Mesa Verde, Grand Canyon, Glacier, and Rocky Mountain National Parks all were created between 1900 and 1915.

The U.S. national park system has grown to more than 280,000 km^2 (108,000 mi^2) in 376 parks, monuments, historic sites, and recreation areas. Each year about 300 million visitors enjoy this system. The most heavily visited units are the urban recreation areas, parkways, and historic sites (fig. 6.18). What most people imagine when they think of a national park, however, are the great wilderness parks of the West. While these parks preserve areas of great natural beauty, they often have far more rocks, ice, and snow than biodiversity or ecological complexity. When the U.S. public domain was being carved up over a century ago, the most productive land generally ended up in private hands.

Most of our national parks are intended to preserve an area as we believe it looked before any human habitation. Often this is an illusion because people have inhabited and affected the land for thousands of years. Furthermore, the idea of maintaining a static equilibrium in nature is based on ideas of climax communities discarded by most ecologists today. What would it mean for park management if we conceived of biological communities as constantly changing mosaics of chance associations of plants and animals (including humans)?

Canada has a total of 1,471 parks and protected areas occupying about 150,000 km^2. Among this group are national parks, provincial parks, outdoor recreation parks, and historic parks. They range in size from vast wilderness expanses, such as Wood Buffalo National Park in northern Manitoba or Ellesmere National Park Reserve in Nunavut Territory, to tiny pockets of cultural or natural history occupying only a few hectares. Kluane National Park in the Yukon, together with the Tatshenshini-Alsek Wilderness in British Columbia, the adjoining Wrangell-St. Elias National Park, and Glacier Bay National Park in Alaska, encompass an area of about 10 million ha (24.7 million acres), roughly the size of Belgium or ten times as big as Yellowstone National Park. While many ecological reserves in Canada enforce strictly controlled access, other reserves encourage intensive recreation; allow hunting, logging, or mining; and permit environmental manipulation for management purposes.

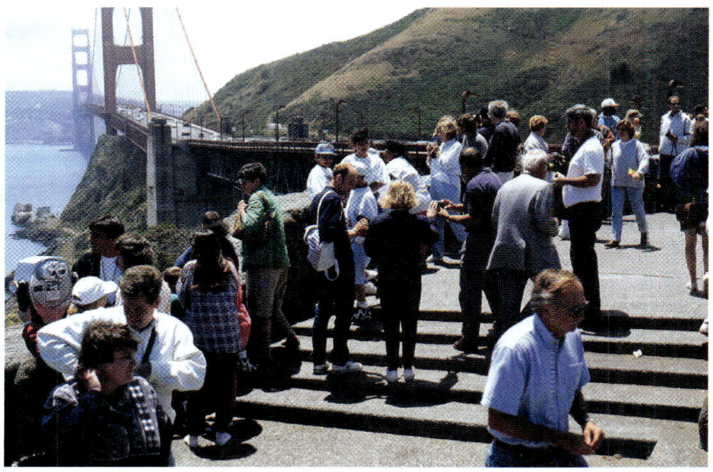

FIGURE 6.18 *Golden Gate National Recreation Area, the largest urban park in the world, gets more than 13 million recreational visits per year.*

Park Problems

Originally the great wilderness parks of Canada and the United States were fortresses protected from development or exploitation by legal boundaries and diligent park rangers. Most were buffered from human impacts by their remote location and the wild lands surrounding them. Today the situation has changed. Many parks have become islands of nature surrounded and threatened by destructive land uses and burgeoning human populations that crowd park boundaries. Forests are clear-cut right up to the edges of some parks, while mine drainage contaminates streams and groundwater. Garish tourist traps clustered at park entrances detract from the beauty and serenity that most visitors seek.

Some popular parks, such as Yosemite and Grand Canyon, have become so crowded that managers have had to restrict automobile access and institute mass-transit systems to reduce traffic jams and pollution. Sometimes trails are so packed with tourists that they seem more like city streets than wilderness refuges. Visitors demand services, such as golf courses, laundries, video arcades, bars, grocery stores, and other facilities, that intrude on the solitude and natural beauty that parks were established to protect. Park rangers often spend more time on crime prevention and crowd control than natural history.

In many parks, dune buggies, dirt bikes, and off-road vehicles (ORV) run over fragile landscapes, disturbing vegetation and wildlife and destroying the aesthetic experience of those who come to enjoy nature (fig. 6.19). The U.S. Park Service has proposed plans to exclude snowmobiles and personal watercraft (jet skis and waverunners) from many parks, but these plans have been challenged by manufacturers and owners' groups. Yellowstone National Park is a case in point. On a typical winter weekend in 2000, more than 1,000 snowmobiles entered the park. Air pollution from their engines was so bad that rangers at the west Yellowstone entry point were forced to wear respirators. Although the snowmobile phase-out plan was based on 22 public hearings and 65,000 written comments (a majority of which favored a ban), Secretary of the Interior Gale Norton ordered the Park Service to continue to allow snowmobile use. A federal court judge then ruled, however, the secretary's ruling lacked merit and ordered the park to ban snowmobiles. At the time of this writing, the issue was still being contested. Ask your instructor what has happened recently.

Air pollution has become a serious threat to other parks as well. Sulfate concentrations in Shenandoah and Great Smoky Mountains National Parks are five times human health standards, and ozone levels in Acadia National Park in Maine exceed primary air quality standards by as much as 50 percent on some summer

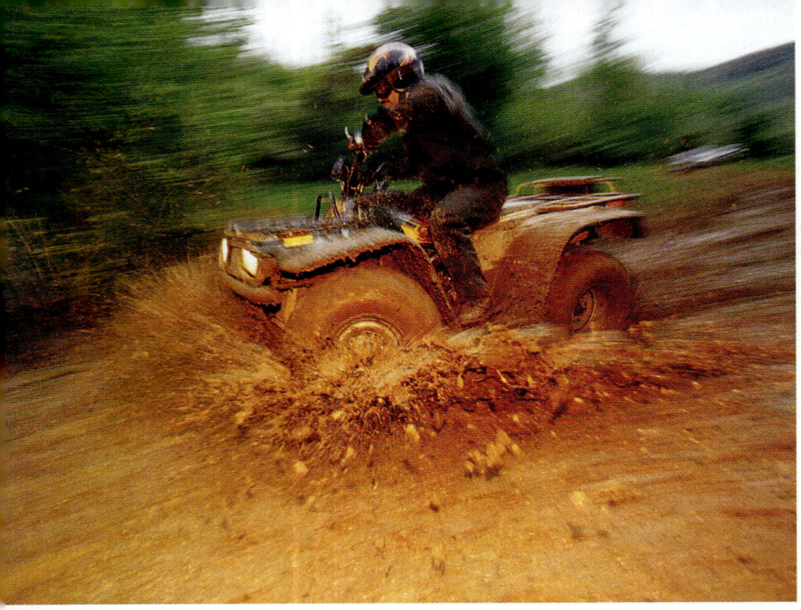

FIGURE 6.19 *Off-road vehicles cause severe, long-lasting environmental damage when driven through wetlands.*

days. Visitors to the Grand Canyon once could see mountains 160 km (100 mi) away; now the air is so smoggy you can't see from one rim to the other during one-third of the year because of soot and sulfate aerosols from nearby power plants in Utah and Arizona.

Mining and oil interests continue to push for permission to dig and drill in the parks, especially on the 3 million acres of private **inholdings** (private lands) in the parks. Oil and gas wells recently have been drilled in Padre Island National Seashore, Big Cypress National Preserve, and the Upper Missouri River Breaks National Monument.

Wildlife Issues

Wildlife is at the center of many arguments regarding whether the purpose of the parks is to preserve nature or to provide entertainment for visitors (fig. 6.20). In the early days of the parks, "bad" animals (such as wolves and mountain lions) were killed, so that populations of "good" animals (such as deer and elk) would be high. Rangers cut trees to improve views, put out salt blocks to lure animals to good viewing points close to roads, and otherwise manipulated nature to provide a more enjoyable experience for the guests.

Critics of this policy claim that favoring some species over others has unbalanced ecosystems and created a sad illusion of a natural system. They claim that excessively large deer and elk populations in Yellowstone and Grand Teton National Parks, for instance, have degraded the range so badly that massive die-offs have occurred in severe winters. Park rangers tried hiring professional hunters to reduce the herds, but a storm of protest was raised. Sportsmen want to be able to hunt the animals themselves, animal lovers don't want the animals to be killed at all, and wilderness advocates don't like the precedent of hunting in national parks. Proposals to reduce elk and bison populations by reintroducing predators, such as wolves and mountain lions, have been highly controversial (see Case Study, p. 139).

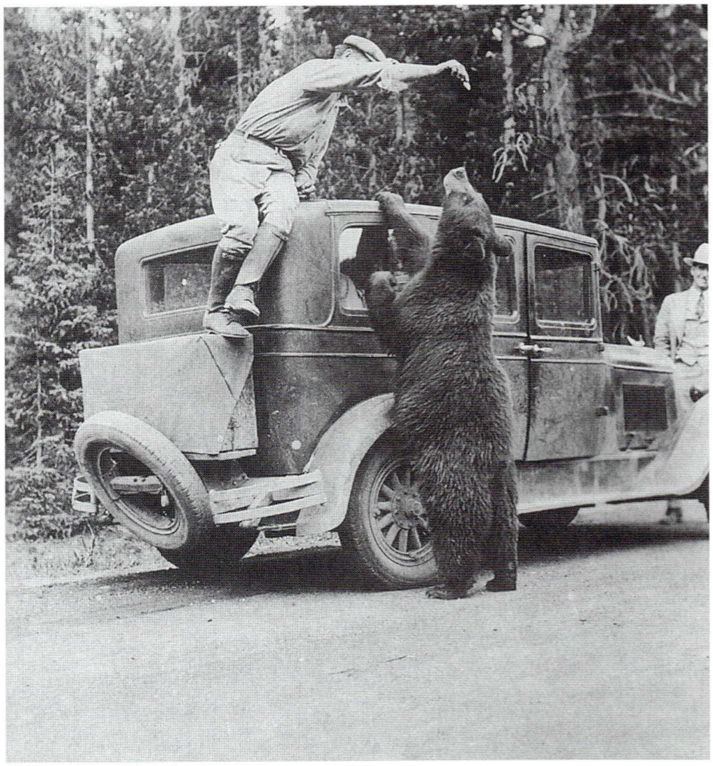

FIGURE 6.20 *Wild animals have always been one of the main attractions in national parks. Many people lose all common sense when interacting with big, dangerous animals. This is not a petting zoo.*

Parks as Ecosystems

One of the biggest problems with managing parks and nature preserves is that boundaries usually are based on political rather than ecological considerations. Airsheds, watersheds, and animal territories or migration routes often extend far beyond official boundaries and yet profoundly affect communities that we are attempting to preserve. Yellowstone and Grand Teton National Parks in northwestern Wyoming are examples of this dilemma. Although about 1 million ha (2.47 million acres) in total size, these parks probably cannot preserve viable populations of large predators, such as grizzly bears and mountain lions, completely within their borders. Management policies in the surrounding national forests and private lands seriously affect conditions in the park (fig. 6.21). The natural **biogeographical area** (an entire ecosystem and its associated land, water, air, and wildlife resources) must be managed as a unit if we are to preserve all its values.

The International Union for the Conservation of Nature and Natural Resources (IUCN) (also known as the World Conservation Union) divides protected areas into five categories, with increasing levels of protection and decreasing human impacts (table 6.2). Many of our parks have tried to meet all these goals simultaneously but may have to select those of highest value. Most parks limit the number of overnight visitors. The time may

CASE STUDY

REINTRODUCING WOLVES TO YELLOWSTONE

A little more than a century ago, an estimated 100,000 gray, or timber, wolves (*Canis lupis*) roamed the western United States. As farmers and ranchers moved west, however, wolves were poisoned, shot, and trapped wherever they could be found. The last wolves were eliminated from the northern Rocky Mountains in the early 1900s. Without a predator to restrain their numbers, elk and deer populations expanded rapidly. In Yellowstone National Park, for instance, the elk herd grew to some 25,000 animals, probably four or five times the vegetation's carrying capacity. Vegetation was overgrazed, and populations of smaller animals, such as ground squirrels, declined. For several decades, ecologists urged that wolves be reintroduced to control prey populations. These proposals brought howls of angry protest from local ranchers, who see wolves as sinister killers that threaten children, pets, livestock, and the ranching way of life. It took more than 20 years to get approval for wolf reintroduction.

In 1995 wolves were trapped in western Canada and relocated to Yellowstone. Once in the park, wolves became established surprisingly quickly. Taking advantage of the abundant food supply, they tripled their population in just three years. The effects on the ecosystem were immediate and striking. Biodiversity increased noticeably. Fewer elk, deer, and moose meant more food for squirrels, gophers, voles, and mice. Abundant small prey, in turn, led to increased numbers of eagles, hawks, fox, pine martens, and weasels. Large animal carcasses left by the wolves provided a feast for scavengers, such as bears, ravens, and magpies. Nearly half the coyotes, which had become common in the wolf's absence, were killed by their larger cousins. This helped small mammals that once were coyote prey. Plants such as grasses, forbs, willows, and aspen flourished in the absence of grazing and browsing pressure. Rangers and naturalists were delighted that the ecosystem was back in balance once again, while tourists were thrilled to catch a glimpse of a wolf or to hear them howl.

By 2004 researchers counted about 160 wolves in 22 packs in Yellowstone, well beyond the recovery goal of 10 packs for three consecutive years. Not everyone was happy, however, with the reintroduction program. Ranchers continue to regard wolves as a threat to their way of life. And some animal rights groups object to a policy that allows any wolf to be shot if it strays from the park and attacks livestock.

Wolf reintroduction raises some important questions about the purposes of parks. Are they recreational areas or refuges for nature? What responsibilities do parks have to their neighbors (and vice versa)? What role should science play in this dispute? Suppose you were a wildlife biologist charged with designing an acceptable wolf management program in Yellowstone. What strategies would you use, and where would you start?

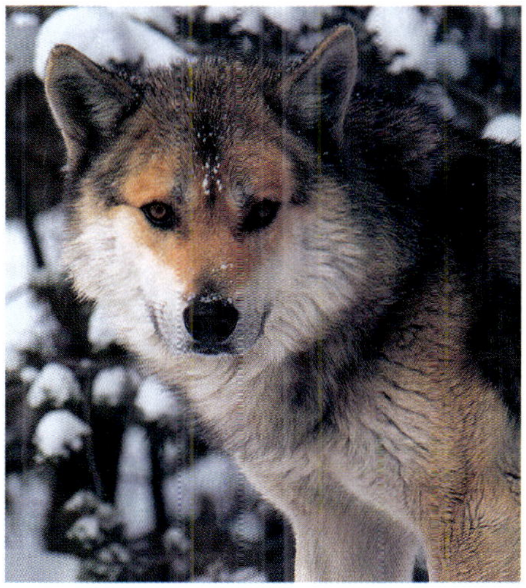

Are wolves beautiful, thrilling symbols of wild nature or ruthless killers? Reintroduction of these top predators into Yellowstone National Park has enthusiastic support from environmental groups but passionate opposition from local ranchers and hunters.

come when park permits will need to be reserved years in advance, and visits to certain parks will be limited to once in a lifetime! How would you feel about such a policy? Would you rather visit a pristine, uncrowded park only once or a less perfect place whenever you wanted?

One solution to congestion and overuse of our parks is to create new ones to distribute the load. This would also allow us to protect and enjoy other magnificent areas that deserve preservation in their own right. At the end of his term in office, President Bill Clinton created ten new parks and national monuments, protecting nearly 2 million ha (about 5 million acres) in western states. Environmentalists celebrated protection of these areas; local residents, however, generally opposed what they feared would be increased restrictions on their use of the land and its resources. The Bush administration promised to give local residents and officials unprecedented input in devising management plans for these new parklands and monuments.

Canada's Green Plan, released in 1990, called for a doubling of protected areas to a total of 12 percent of total land surface. Representative samples of every ecoregion should be included in this network, including cultural landscapes and marine ecosystems.

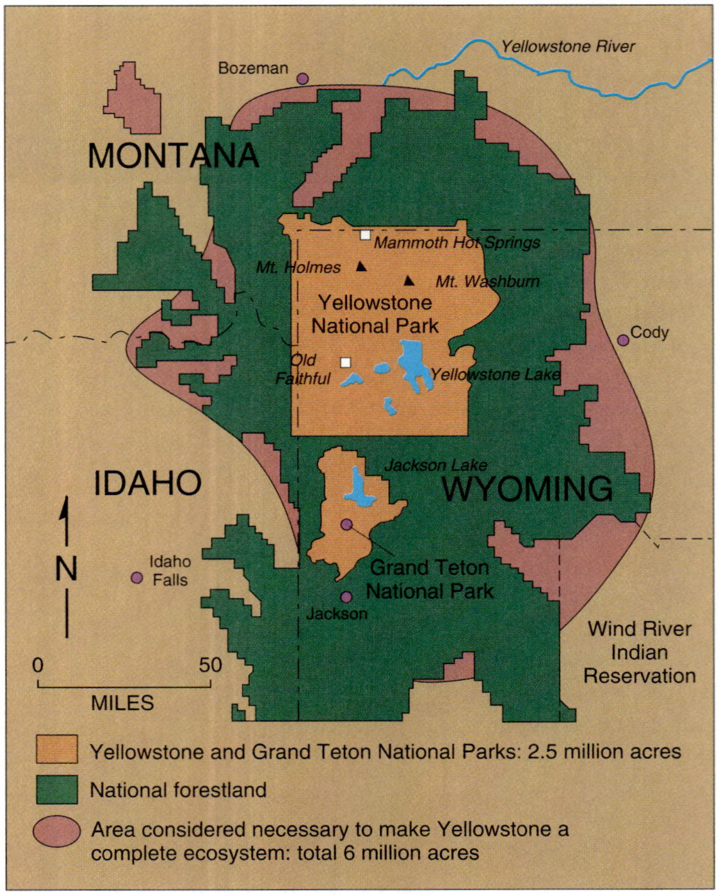

FIGURE 6.21 *This map shows the Yellowstone ecosystem complex, or biogeographical region, which extends far beyond the park's boundaries. Park managers and ecologists believe that it is necessary to manage the entire region if the park itself is to remain biologically viable.*

WORLD PARKS AND PRESERVES

Global parks and preserves face innumerable challenges, but the statistics have been improving in recent years. The idea of setting aside nature preserves has spread rapidly over the past 50 years, as people around the world have become aware of the growing scarcity of wildlife and wild places. There are several reasons for a global increase in protected areas. International nongovernment organizations have developed a range of tactics, including debt-for-nature swaps to establish preserves. Consumer pressure has forced logging and mining companies to collaborate in preserving forests. And governments are increasingly interested in slowing resource depletion and in gaining status by protecting lands. Currently some 1.3 billion ha (about 10 percent of the earth's land area) is in some form of protected status.

Within the past several years, Brazil, for example, has pledged to protect 12 percent of its Amazon rainforest, some 500,000 km^2, and both Brazil and Bolivia are working to protect the Pantanal region, the world's largest freshwater wetland complex. Mexico has increased protection for its biosphere reserve at Laguna San Ignacio, the breeding ground for gray whales. Mozambique, despite extreme poverty, has created two new national parks to protect dugongs, sea turtles, elephants, and other wildlife.

Regions with the most dramatic increases in protected areas have been Asia, North America, and Latin America (fig. 6.22). Among the individual countries with the most admirable plans to protect natural resources are Costa Rica, Tanzania, Rwanda, Botswana, Benin, Senegal, Central African Republic, Zimbabwe, Bhutan, and Switzerland, each of which has designated 10 percent or more of its land as ecological protectorates.

So far, however, many of these areas are parks in name only. Lacking guards, visitor centers, administrative personnel, or even boundary fences, many are vulnerable to poaching by hunters and loggers, as well as to encroachment by settlers. In many countries it is easier to declare a new park than to protect and manage it.

TABLE 6.2 IUCN Categories of Protected Areas

CATEGORY	ALLOWED HUMAN IMPACT OR INTERVENTION
1. Ecological reserves and wilderness areas	Little or none
2. National parks	Low
3. Natural monuments and archaeological sites	Low to medium
4. Habitat and wildlife management areas	Medium
5. Cultural or scenic landscapes, recreation areas	Medium to high

Source: Data from World Conservation Union, 1990.

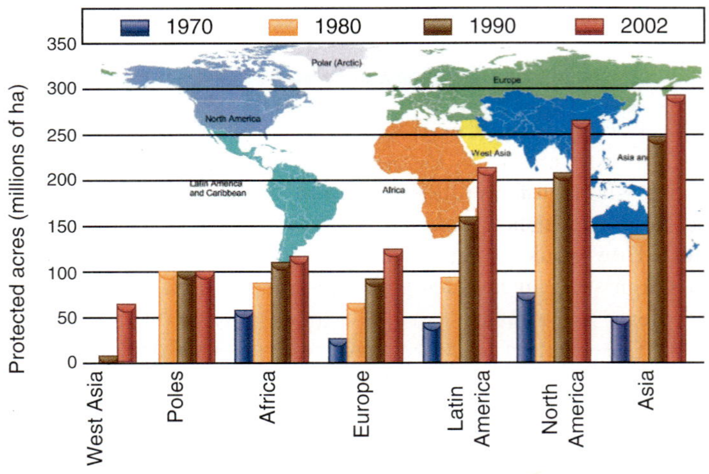

FIGURE 6.22 *Change in amount of protected areas by region.*
Source: Data from UN Environmental Program, 2003.

Often parks are created where people already live, farm, and hunt. The needs of these people must be accounted for if a protected area is to work on the ground, rather than just on paper.

Marine Preserves

As ocean fish stocks become increasingly depleted globally (see chapter 9), biologists are calling for protected areas where marine organisms are sheltered from destructive harvest methods. Research has shown that "no-take" refuges not only protect the species living within them but also serve as nurseries for nearby areas. In a study of 100 of these refuges around the world, researchers found that, on average, the number of organisms inside refuges was twice as high as surrounding areas where harvest was allowed. In addition, the biomass of organisms was three times as great and individual animals were, on average, 30 percent larger inside the refuge, compared with outside. The size necessary for a safe haven to protect flora and fauna and replenish the area around it depends on the species involved, but some marine biologists have called on nations to protect at least 20 percent of their nearshore territory as marine refuges.

Coral reefs are among the most threatened marine ecosystems in the world (see chapter 5). Recent remote sensing surveys show that living coral covers only about 285,000 km^2 (110,000 mi^2), or an area about the size of Nevada. This is less than half of previous estimates, and 90 percent of all reefs face threats from sea temperature change, destructive fishing methods, coral mining, sediment runoff, and other human disturbance. In many ways, coral reefs are the old-growth rainforests of the ocean. Biologically rich, these sensitive habitats can take a century or more to recover from damage. If current trends continue, some researchers predict that in 50 years there will be no viable coral reefs anywhere in the world.

What can be done to reverse this trend? Among the national monuments created by President Bill Clinton are three that preserve coral reefs: the U.S. Virgin Islands Coral Reef National Monument, The Pacific Ocean Preserve northwest of Hawaii, and the Tortugas Refuge within the Florida Keys National Marine Sanctuary. Together, these refuges protect 90 percent of all coral in U.S. territory. All are closed to commercial fishing, and the Tortugas reefs are completely protected as a "no-take" zone. Unfortunately, most reefs lack such protection. A survey of marine biological resources identified the ten richest and most threatened hot spots, which are the Philippines, the Gulf of Guinea and Cape Verde Islands (off the west coast of Africa), Indonesia's Sunda Islands, the Mascarene Islands in the Indian Ocean, South Africa's coast, southern Japan and China, the western Caribbean, and the Red Sea and Gulf of Aden. We urgently need a system of underwater national parks and preserves like those established to protect terrestrial biomes.

Protecting Natural Heritage

Even parks and preserves with protective systems in place are not always safe from exploitation or changes in political priorities. Many problems threaten natural resources and environmental quality in these areas. In Greece, the Pindus National Park is threatened by plans to build a hydroelectric dam in the center of the park. Furthermore, excessive stock grazing and forestry exploitation in the peripheral zone are causing erosion and loss of wildlife habitat. In Colombia, the Paramillo National Park also is threatened by dam building. Oil exploration along the border of the Yasuni National Park in Ecuador pollutes water supplies, while miners and loggers in Peru have invaded portions of Huascarán National Park. In Palau, coral reefs identified as a potential biosphere reserve are damaged by dynamiting, while on some beaches in Indonesia, every egg laid by endangered sea turtles is taken by egg hunters. These are just a few of the many problems around the world. Often countries with the most important biomes lack funds, trained personnel, and experience to manage some of the areas under their control.

The IUCN has developed a **world conservation strategy** for natural resources that includes the following three objectives: (1) to maintain essential ecological processes and life-support systems (such as soil regeneration and protection, nutrient recycling, and water purification) on which human survival and development depend; (2) to preserve genetic diversity essential for breeding programs to improve cultivated plants and domesticated animals; and (3) to ensure that any utilization of wild species and ecosystems is sustainable. These goals are further elaborated in the ecological plan of action adopted by the IUCN and shown in table 6.3.

Size and Design of Nature Preserves

What is the optimum size and shape of a nature preserve? For many years, conservation biologists have disputed whether it is better to have a *single large or several small* reserves (the SLOSS debate). Ideally, a reserve should be large enough to support viable populations of endangered species, keep ecosystems intact, and

TABLE 6.3 IUCN Ecological Plan of Action

1. Launch a consciousness-raising exercise to bring the issue of biological resources to the attention of policymakers and the public at large.
2. Design national conservation strategies that take explicit account of the values at stake.
3. Expand our network of parks and preserves to establish a comprehensive system of protected areas.
4. Undertake a program of training in the fields relevant to biological diversity to improve the scientific skills and technological grasp of those charged with its management.
5. Work through conventions and treaties to express the interest of the community of nations in the collective heritage of biological diversity.
6. Establish a set of economic incentives to make species conservation a competitive form of land use.

Source: Data from International Union for Conservation and National Resources.

isolate critical core areas from damaging external forces. But as gaps are opened in habitat by human disturbance and areas are fragmented into isolated islands (see chapter 5), edge effects may eliminate core characteristics everywhere.

To satisfy the conflicting needs and desires of humans and nature, we may need a spectrum of preserves with decreasing levels of interference and management, including (1) recreation areas, designed primarily for human entertainment, aesthetics, and enjoyment; (2) historic areas, intended to preserve a landscape as we imagine it looked in a previous time, such as presettlement or pioneer days; (3) conservation reserves, set aside to maintain essential ecological functions, preserve biodiversity, or protect a particular species or group of organisms; (4) pristine research areas, to serve as a baseline of undisturbed nature; and (5) inviolable preserves, for sensitive species and from which all human entrance is strictly prohibited.

For some species with small territories, several small, isolated refuges can support viable populations and provide insurance against a disease or another calamity that might wipe out a single population. But small preserves can't support species, such as elephants or tigers, that need large amounts of space. Given human needs and pressures, however, big preserves aren't always possible. Establishing **corridors** of natural habitat to allow movement of species from one area to another (fig. 6.23) can help maintain genetic exchange and prevent the high extinction rates often characteristic of isolated and fragmented areas. Some animals, however, don't use corridors and so large, contiguous areas may be the only way to save them.

An interesting experiment funded by the World Wildlife Fund and the Smithsonian Institution is being carried out in the Brazilian rainforest to determine the effects of shape and size on biological reserves. Twenty-three test sites, ranging in size from 1 ha (2.47 acres) to 10,000 ha have been established. Some areas are surrounded by clear-cuts and newly created pastures (fig. 6.24), while others remain connected to the surrounding forest. Selected species are regularly inventoried to monitor their dynamics after disturbance. As expected, some species disappear very quickly, especially from small areas. Sun-loving species flourish in the newly created forest edges, but deep-forest, shade-loving species move out, particularly when size or shape reduces the distance from the edge to the center below a certain minimum. This demonstrates the importance of surrounding some reserves with buffer zones that maintain the balance of edge and shade species.

Conservation and Economic Development

Many of the most seriously threatened species and ecosystems of the world are in the developing countries, especially in the tropics. This situation concerns us all because these countries are the guardians of biological resources that may be vital to all of us. Unfortunately, where political and economic systems fail to provide people with land, jobs, and food, disenfranchised citizens turn to legally protected lands, plants, and animals for their needs. Immediate human survival always takes precedence over long-term environmental goals. Clearly, the struggle to save species and unique ecosystems cannot be divorced from the broader struggle to achieve a new world order in which the basic needs of all are met.

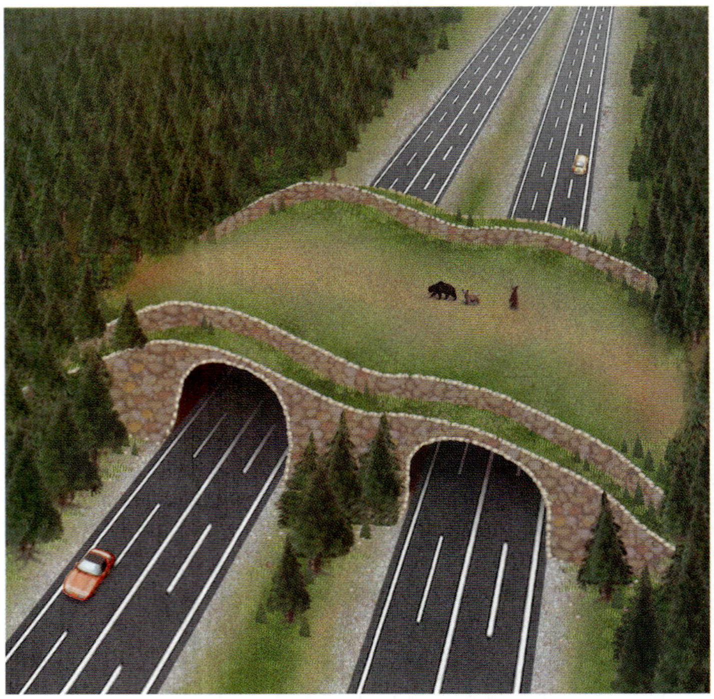

FIGURE 6.23 *Corridors link together fragmented habitats and allow wildlife to move from one place to another. In Baniff National Park, specially constructed bridges allow animals to cross a busy freeway.*

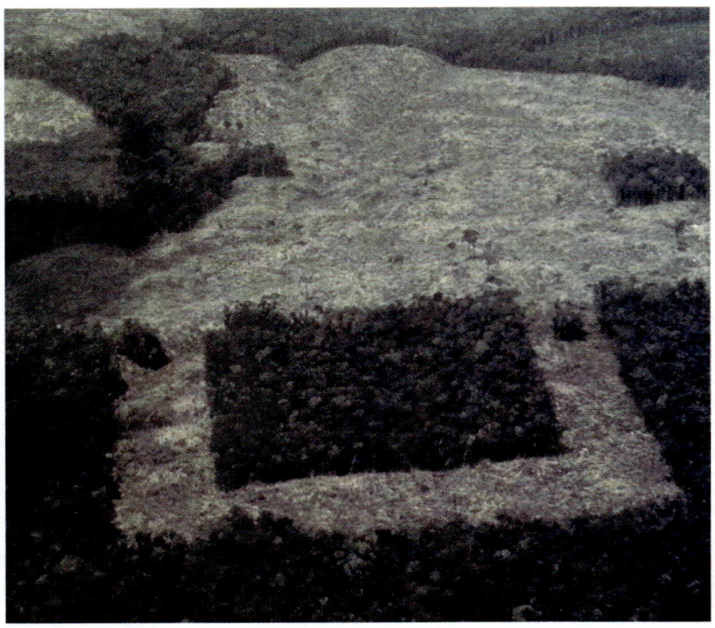

FIGURE 6.24 *How small can a nature preserve be? In an ambitious research project, scientists in the Brazilian rainforest are carefully tracking wildlife in plots of various sizes, either connected to existing forests or surrounded by clear-cuts. As you might expect, the largest and most highly specialized species are the first to disappear.*

People in some developing countries are beginning to realize that the biological richness of their environment may be their most valuable resource and that its preservation is vital for sustainable development. **Ecotourism** (tourism that is ecologically and socially sustainable) can be more beneficial to many of these countries over the long term than extractive industries, such as logging and mining (fig. 6.25). The what can you do? box (p. 318) suggests some ways to ensure that your vacations are responsible ecotourism.

At the 1982 World Congress on National Parks in Bali, 500 scientists, managers, and politicians discussed the design and location of biological reserves and the ecological, economic, and social factors that impinge on wildlife preservation. They concluded that conservation and rural development are not necessarily incompatible. In many cases, sustainable production of food, fiber, medicines, and water in rural areas depends on ecosystem services derived from adjacent conservation reserves. Tourism associated with wildlife watching and outdoor recreation can be a welcome source of income for underdeveloped countries. If local people share in the benefits of saving wildlife, they probably will cooperate, and the programs will be successful. To reformulate Thoreau's famous dictum, "In broadly shared economic progress is preservation of the wild."

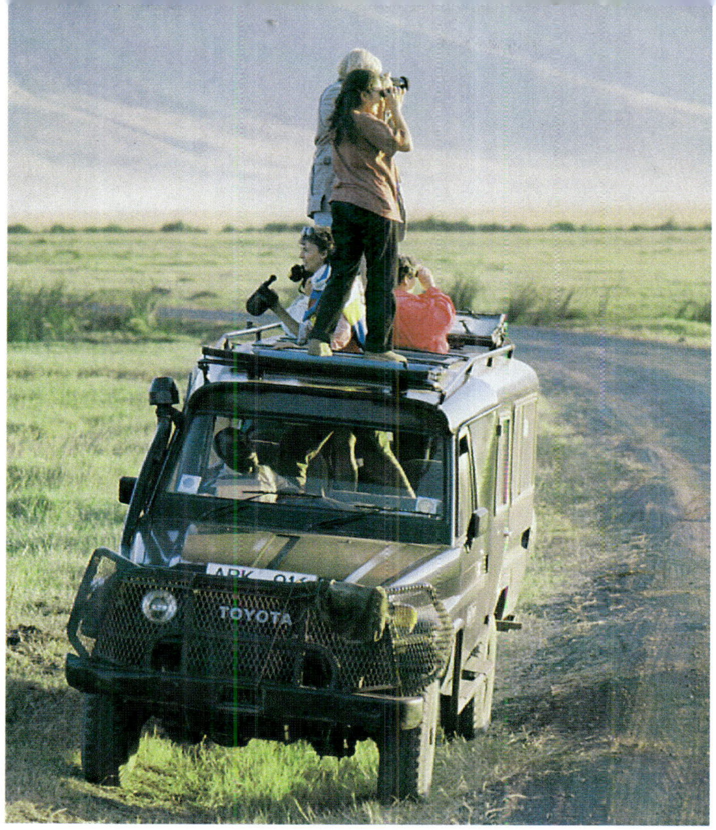

FIGURE 6.25 *Ecotourism can be a sustainable resource use. If local communities share in the revenue, ecotourism gives them an incentive to value and protect biodiversity and natural beauty.*

Indigenous Communities and Biosphere Reserves

Areas chosen for nature preservation are often traditional lands of indigenous people who cannot simply be ordered out. Finding ways to integrate human needs with those of wildlife is essential for local acceptance of conservation goals in many countries. In 1986 UNESCO (United Nations Educational, Scientific, and Cultural Organization) initiated its **Man and Biosphere (MAB) program,** which encourages the division of protected areas into zones with different purposes. Critical ecosystem functions and endangered wildlife are protected in a central core region, where limited scientific study is the only human access allowed. Ecotourism and research facilities are located in a relatively pristine buffer zone around the core, while sustainable resource harvesting and permanent habitation are allowed in multiple-use peripheral regions (fig. 6.26).

Mexico's 545,000-ha (2,100-mi^2) Sian Ka'an Reserve on the Caribbean coast is a good example of an MAB reserve. The core area includes 528,000 ha (1.3 million acres) of coral reef and adjacent bays, marshes, and lowland tropical forest. More than 335 bird species have been observed within the reserve, along with endangered manatees, five types of jungle cats, spider and howler monkeys, and four species of increasingly rare sea turtles. Approximately 25,000 people live in communities in peripheral regions around the reserve, and the resort developments of Cancún are located just to the north. In addition to tourism, the economic base of the area includes lobster fishing, small-scale farming, and coconut cultivation.

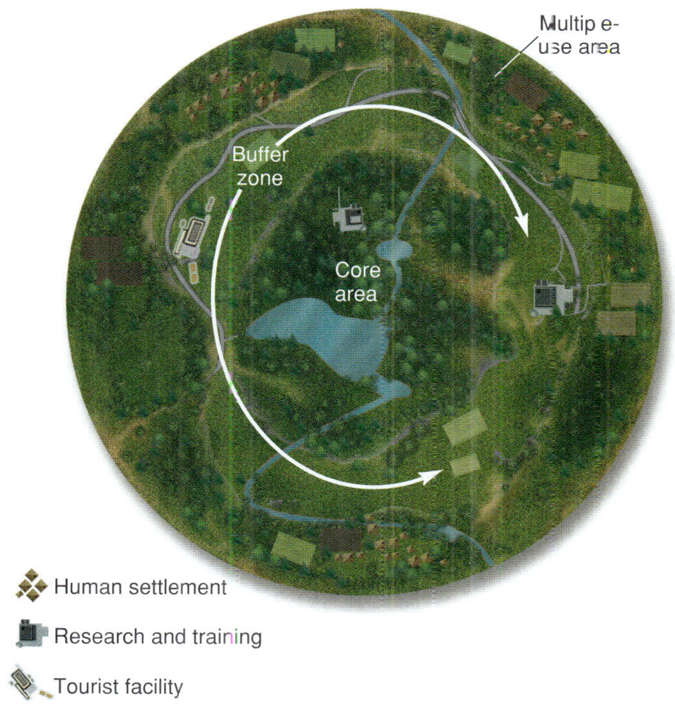

FIGURE 6.26 *A model biosphere reserve. Critical ecosystem is preserved in the core. Research and tourism are allowed in the buffer zone, while sustainable resource harvesting and permanent habitations are located in the multiple-use area around the perimeter.*

The Amigos de Sian Ka'an, a local community organization, played a central role in establishing the reserve and is working to protect the resource base while it improves living standards for

what can you do?

Being a Responsible Ecotourist

1. *Pretrip preparation.* Learn about the history, geography, ecology, and culture of the area you will visit. Understand the do's and don'ts that will keep you from violating local customs and sensibilities.
2. *Environmental impact.* Stay on designated trails and camp in established sites, if available. Take only photographs and memories and leave only goodwill wherever you go.
3. *Resource impact.* Minimize your use of scarce fuels, food, and water resources. Do you know where your wastes and garbage go?
4. *Cultural impact.* Respect the privacy and dignity of those you meet and try to understand how you would feel in their place. Don't take photos without asking first. Be considerate of religious and cultural sites and practices. Be as aware of cultural pollution as you are of environmental pollution.
5. *Wildlife impact.* Don't harass wildlife or disturb plant life. Modern cameras make it possible to get good photos from a respectful, safe distance. Don't buy ivory, tortoise shell, animal skins, feathers, or other products taken from endangered species.
6. *Environmental benefit.* Is your trip strictly for pleasure, or will it contribute to protecting the local environment? Can you combine ecotourism with work on cleanup campaigns or delivery of educational materials or equipment to local schools or nature clubs?
7. *Advocacy and education.* Get involved in letter writing, lobbying, or educational campaigns to help protect the lands and cultures you have visited. Give talks at schools or to local clubs after you get home to inform your friends and neighbors about what you have learned.

local people. New intensive farming techniques and sustainable harvesting of forest products enable people to make a living without destroying the resource base. Better lobster harvesting techniques developed at the reserve have improved the catch without depleting native stocks. Local people now see the preserve as a benefit rather than an imposition from outside. Unfortunately, the government has very limited funds to develop or patrol the reserve. (See related story "Ecotourism on the Roof of the World" at www. mhhe.com/cases.)

WILDERNESS AREAS

Although indigenous people had lived in the Americas for thousands of years before the first Europeans arrived, introduced diseases killed up to 90 percent of the existing population, so that the continent appeared a vast, empty wilderness to early explorers. As historian Frederick Jackson Turner pointed out in a series of articles and speeches at the beginning of the twentieth century, a belief that wilderness is not only a source of wealth but also the origin of strength, self-reliance, wisdom, and character is deeply embedded in our culture. The frontier was seen as a place for the continuous generation of democracy, social progress, economic growth, and national energy. A number of authors, including Henry Thoreau, Aldo Leopold, Sigurd Olson, Edward Abbey, and Wallace Stegner, have written about the physical, mental, and social benefits for modern people of rediscovering solitude and challenge in wilderness (fig. 6.27).

Beginning with designated primitive and roadless areas in a few national forests in the 1920s, the United States has established a system of 264 wilderness areas, encompassing nearly 40 million ha (100 million acres). These wilderness areas are found in national parks, national forests, wildlife refuges, and lands administered by the Bureau of Land Management (BLM).

The 1964 Wilderness Act, which is the basis for much of this system, defined **wilderness** as "an area of undeveloped land affected primarily by the forces of nature, where man is a visitor who does not remain; it contains ecological, geological, or other features of scientific or historic value; it possesses outstanding opportunities for solitude or a primitive and unconfined type of recreation; and it is an area large enough so that continued use will not change its unspoiled, natural conditions." Most of the areas meeting these standards are in the western states and Alaska.

Additional wilderness areas continue to be evaluated for protected status. Conservation groups argue that another 80 million ha (200 million acres), half of it in Alaska, should be added to the wilderness system. A prolonged battle has been waged over these de facto wilderness areas, pitting environmental groups who want more wilderness against loggers, miners, ranchers, and others who want less wilderness. The arguments for saving wilderness are that it provides (1) a refuge for endangered wildlife, (2) an opportunity for solitude and primitive recreation, (3) a baseline for ecological research, and (4) an area where we have chosen simply to leave things in their natural state.

Among the most common arguments against more wilderness are that timber, energy resources, and critical minerals contained on these lands are essential for economic development in local communities, while people want access for motorized recreation, such as off-road vehicles, snowmobiles, and motorboats. For many people living in remote areas, jobs, personal freedom, and local control of resources seem more important than abstract values of wilderness. They often see themselves as an embattled minority trying to protect an endangered, traditional way of life against a wealthy elite who want to lock up huge areas for recreation or aesthetic purposes. Wilderness proponents point out that 96 percent of the country already is open for resource exploitation; the remaining 4 percent is mostly land that developers didn't want, anyway.

For many people, especially those in developing countries, the idea of pristine wilderness untouched by humans is neither very important nor very interesting. In most places, all land is occupied fully—if sparsely—by indigenous people. To them, the area is home, no matter how empty it may look to outsiders. From

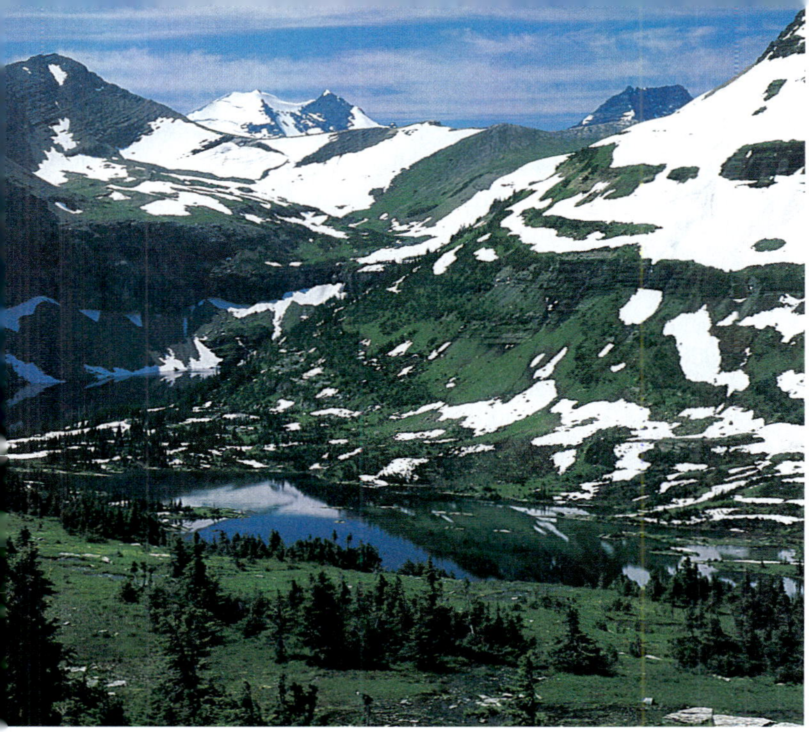

FIGURE 6.27 *Wilderness provides opportunities for solitude, self-propelled recreation, and undisturbed nature.*

this perspective, preserving biological diversity, scenic beauty, and other natural resources may be a good idea, but excluding humans and human features from the land does not necessarily make it more valuable. In fact, saving cultural heritage, working landscapes, and historical evidence of early human occupation can often be among the most important reasons to protect an area.

WILDLIFE REFUGES

In 1901 President Teddy Roosevelt established 51 national **wildlife refuges,** the first in an important but troubled system for wildlife preservation in the United States. There are now 511 wildlife refuges in this system, encompassing nearly 40 million ha of land and water and representing every major biome in North America. They range in size from less than 1 ha (2.47 acres) for the tiny Mille Lacs Refuge in Minnesota to 7.3 million ha (18 million acres) in the Arctic National Wildlife Refuge of Alaska. Altogether, about 1 percent of U.S. surface area is designated as wildlife refuge. Every state has at least one refuge. Ostensibly, wildlife refuges are our most direct efforts to protect wildlife. Many of these sanctuaries are managed, however, primarily to produce game species for hunters.

Over the years, a number of problematic uses have become accepted in wildlife refuges, including oil drilling, cattle grazing, snowmobiling, motorboating, off-road vehicle use, timber harvesting, hay cutting, trapping, and military exercises. A U.S. General Accounting Office report found that 60 percent of all refuges allow activities that are harmful to wildlife. The biggest current battle over U.S. wildlife refuges concerns proposals for oil and gas drilling in the Arctic National Wildlife Refuge on the north slope of Alaska's Brooks Range.

Refuges also face threats from external activities. More than three-quarters of all U.S. refuges have water pollution problems, two-thirds of which are serious enough to affect wildlife. A notorious example is the former Kesterson Wildlife Refuge in California, where selenium-contaminated irrigation water drained from farm fields turned the marsh into a death trap for wildlife, rather than a sanctuary. Eventually, the marsh had to be drained and capped with clean soil to protect wildlife. Subsequent research has shown that at least 20 wildlife refuges in western states have toxic metal pollution caused by agricultural and industrial activities outside the refuge.

International Wildlife Preserves

As we saw earlier in this chapter, most developing countries rarely have separate systems of parks and wildlife refuges. Many nature preserves are set up primarily to protect wildlife, however. An outstanding example of both the promise and the problems in managing parks in the less-developed countries is seen in the Serengeti ecosystem in Kenya and Tanzania. This area of savanna, thorn woodland, and volcanic highland lying between Lake Victoria and the Great Rift Valley in East Africa is home to the highest density of ungulates (hoofed grazing animals) in the world. Over 1.5 million wildebeests (or gnus) graze on the savanna in the wet season, when grass is available, and then migrate through the woodlands into the northern highlands during the dry season. The ecosystem also supports hundreds of thousands of zebras, gazelles, impalas, giraffes, and other beautiful and intriguing animals. The herbivores, in turn, support lions and a variety of predators and scavengers, such as leopards, hyenas, cheetahs, wild dogs, and vultures. This astounding diversity and abundance is surely one of the greatest wonders of the world.

Tanzania's Serengeti National Park was established in 1940 to protect 15,000 km^2 (5,700 mi^2), an area about the size of Connecticut, or twice as big as Yellowstone National Park. It is bordered on the east by the much smaller Ngorongoro Conservation Area and Lake Manyara National Park. Kenya's Masa Mara National Reserve borders the Serengeti on the north. Rapidly growing human populations push against the boundaries of the park on all sides. Herds of domestic cattle compete with wild animals for grass and water. Agriculturalists clamor for farmland, especially in the temperate highlands along the Kenya-Tanzania border. So many tourists flock to these parks that the vegetation is ground to dust by hundreds of sight-seeing vans, and wildlife find it impossible to carry out normal lives.

Perhaps the worst problem in Africa is **poaching** by illegal hunters who massacre wildlife for valuable meat, horns, and tusks. Where there once were about 1 million rhinos in Africa, the population had dropped by the mid-1980s to fewer than 10,000 animals. Antipoaching efforts have allowed the population to recover to about 15,000 currently.

Elephants are under a similar assault. Thirty years ago, there were no elephants in the Serengeti, but perhaps 3 million in all of Africa (fig. 6.28). Since then, about 80 percent of the African elephants have been killed—mainly for their ivory—at a rate of 100,000 each year. The 2,000 elephants now in Serengeti National Park were driven there by hunting pressures elsewhere. Fortunately,

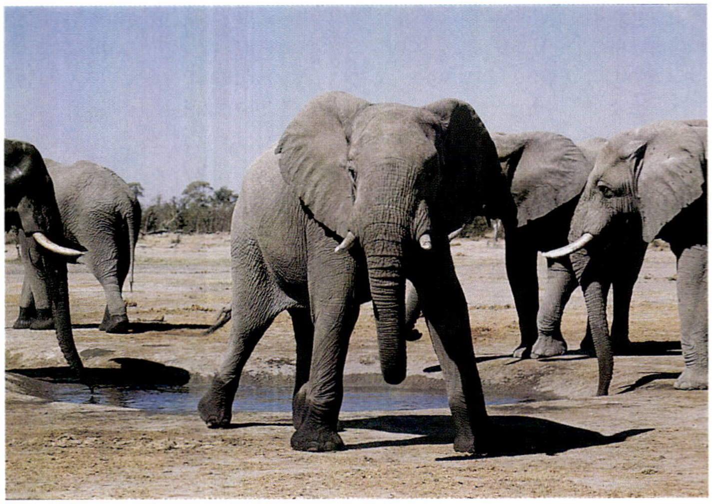

FIGURE 6.28 *Elephant populations have been decimated throughout the world. The biggest threat is from poachers, who kill for the elephants' valuable ivory.*

the elephants find refuge in the park and add to the pleasure of tourists who go to see the wildlife; however, they are changing the ecosystem. Crowded into inadequate space, the elephants smash down the acacia trees, turning the woodland and mixed savanna into continuous grassland. This is beneficial for some animals, but not for others.

Poachers continue to pursue the elephants and rhinos, even in the park. Armed with high-powered rifles and even machine guns and bazookas from the many African wars in the past decade, the poachers take a terrible toll on the wildlife. Park rangers try to stop the carnage, but they often are outgunned by the poachers. The parks are beginning to resemble war zones, with fierce, lethal firefights rather than peace and tranquility.

Still, as ecotourism grows in importance in national budgets, both local residents and governments are coming to recognize that protecting wildlife and natural resources makes economic sense. Although wildlife has been decimated in many areas, vast numbers remain an inspiring spectacle elsewhere. With careful stewardship, we may be able to protect much of what's left of nature's diversity and abundance.

SUMMARY

- Temperate broad-leaved forests and grasslands (biomes that make up most of North America and Europe) are among the most heavily human-dominated habitat type on the earth. The most biologically rich forests are the old-growth forests filled with ancient trees and relatively undisturbed ecological processes. While forests still cover about half the area worldwide that they did before humans became the dominant species on the planet, only about 22 percent of those forests retain old-growth characteristics.
- Wood plays a larger part in the modern economy than does any other commodity. Total annual wood consumption is around 3.7 billion m^3. More than half of all humans depend on firewood or charcoal for cooking and heating.
- An innovative program for habitat and biodiversity protection involves debt-for-nature swaps, in which long-term debt is forgiven if a country or a company agrees to protect natural areas. Many such arrangements have been worked out for developing countries. Conservationists are especially concerned about huge clear-cuts, in which all vegetation is removed over a large area. This method drives out wildlife and exposes soil to erosion.
- Seventy years of fire suppression in U.S. forests have allowed fuel to build up, so that we now worry about huge conflagrations. Prescribed fires to reduce fuel loads would help solve the problem, but the public fears that even small fires could escape and threaten them.
- Grasslands are among the most human-dominated of any biome. More than 3 billion domestic animals raised on pastures and grazing lands make a valuable contribution to human nutrition. Sustainable pastoralism can maintain ecosystem health on many grasslands, but too often overgrazing leads to habitat degradation and desertification. In some areas, rotational grazing and ranching of wild species can be useful approaches.
- Parks, wildlife refuges, wilderness areas, and nature preserves occupy a small percentage of the earth's total land area but protect valuable cultural resources and representative samples of the earth's species and ecosystems. Parks are havens for wildlife and places for healthful outdoor recreation. Many are overcrowded, misused, and neglected, however. Pollution and incompatible uses outside parks threaten the values that we seek to protect. Wildlife is at the center of many park controversies. Is the purpose of parks to preserve wild nature or provide entertainment for visitors?
- Marine refuges can protect the sensitive old-growth habitats along coastlines and islands that serve as nurs-

eries for a large percentage of oceanic biodiversity. No-take zones in these refuges not only serve as a sanctuary for threatened species but also replenish nearby areas open to harvesting. Coral reefs are among the most biologically rich but threatened habitats in the world.

- The optimum size for nature preserves depends on the terrain and the values they are intended to protect, but in general, the larger the reserve, the more species it can protect. Establishing corridors to link separate areas can be a good way to increase effective space and to allow migration from one area to another. Economic development and nature protection can go hand in hand. Ecotourism may be the most lucrative and long-lasting way to use resources in many developing countries.
- Areas chosen for preservation often are lands of indigenous people. Careful planning and zoning can protect nature and allow sustainable use of resources. Man and Biosphere (MAB) reserves provide for multiple use in some areas, but strict conservation in others.
- Wilderness areas are defined as those where humans are visitors who do not remain. Wilderness areas possess outstanding opportunities for solitude and primitive recreation. Wildlife refuges were intended to be sanctuaries for wildlife, but over the years, many improbable and damaging uses have become established in them.

QUESTIONS FOR REVIEW

1. How could protecting lowland forests help preserve mountaintop fauna?
2. Which continents have the largest forest area, and which have the highest net rate of forest change?
3. Why is there disagreement over the amount of deforestation in the tropics?
4. What is a debt-for-nature swap? How does it work?
5. What are clear-cuts, and why are they criticized?
6. Summarize the state of rangelands in the United States.
7. List some problems and threats from inside and outside national parks and preserves.
8. Why is the reintroduction of wolves into Yellowstone National Park a controversial issue?
9. List the three main points in the IUCN world conservation strategy and the six steps in the action plan to meet these goals.
10. What is a Man and Biosphere reserve, and what problems is it designed to solve?

THINKING SCIENTIFICALLY

1. Suppose you were assigned to study the relation among lowland forest harvesting, cloud forest climate, and populations of rare cloud forest species, such as golden toads. How would you proceed? What evidence would you examine, and how might you test the validity of your hypotheses?
2. Conservationists argue that we could reduce or redirect the demand for wood products; timber companies claim that continued production is essential for jobs and the economy. What evidence would you need to make a decision in this case, and where might you get it?
3. Brazil needs cash to pay increasing foreign debts and to fund needed economic growth. Why shouldn't it harvest its forests and mineral resources to gain the foreign currency it wants and needs? If we want Brazil to save its forests, what can or should we do to encourage conservation?
4. The U.S. government has kept timber prices and grazing leases low to maintain low lumber and meat prices for consumers and to help support rural communities and traditional ways of life. If you were a forest supervisor, how would you weigh those human interests against the ecological values of forests and rangelands?
5. There is considerable uncertainty about the extent of desertification of grazing lands or destruction of tropical rainforests. If you were evaluating these data, what evidence would you want to see, or how would you appraise conflicting evidence?
6. Is "contrived" naturalness a desirable feature in parks and nature preserves? How much human intervention do you think is acceptable in trying to make nature more beautiful, safe, comfortable, or attractive to human visitors? Think of some specific examples that you would or would not accept.
7. If you were superintendent of Yellowstone National Park, how would you determine the park's carrying capacity for elk? If there were too many elk, how would you thin the herd?
8. Why do you suppose that dry tropical forests and tundra are well represented in protected areas, while grasslands and wetlands are rarely protected? Consider social, cultural, and economic as well as biogeographical reasons in your answer.
9. Oil and gas companies want to drill in several parks, monuments, and wildlife refuges. Do you think this should be allowed? If so, under what conditions or restrictions?

KEY TERMS

biogeographical area 138
clear-cutting 131
closed-canopy forests 126
corridors 142
debt-for-nature swaps 130
desertification 134
ecosystem management 133
ecotourism 143
inholdings 138
Man and Biosphere (MAB) program 143
monoculture forestry 128
old-growth forests 127
pastoralists 134
poaching 145
rotational grazing 135
selective cutting 131
shelterwood harvesting 131
strip-cutting 131
wilderness 144
wildlife refuges 145
world conservation strategy 141

SUGGESTED READINGS

Arno, Stephen F., and Steven Allison-Bunnell. 2002. *Flames in Our Forest: Disaster or Renewal?* Island Press.

Dombeck, Michael P., Christopher A. Wood, and Jack E. Williams. 2003. *From Conquest to Conservation: Our Public Lands Legacy.* Island Press.

Fischman, Robert L. 2004. *The National Wildlife Refuges: Coordinating a Conservation System Through Law.* Island Press.

Havlick, David G. 2002. *No Place Distant: Roads and Motorized Recreation on America's Public Lands.* Island Press.

Honey, Martha. 2002. *Ecotourism and Certification: Setting Standards in Practice.* Island Press.

Knight, Richard L., Wendell C. Gilgert, and Ed Marston. 2002. *Ranching West of the 100th Meridian: Culture Ecology and Economic.* Island Press.

Lawton, R. O., et al. 2001. "Climate Impact of Tropical Lowland Deforestation on Nearby Montane Cloud Forests." *Science* 294:584–87.

Lindenmayer, David B., and Jerry F. Franklin, eds. 2003. *Towards Forest Sustainability: Regional, National, and Global Perspectives.* Island Press.

Mittermeir, R. A., et al. 2003. "Wilderness and biodiversity conservation." *Proceedings of the National Academy of Sciences of the United States of America* 100(18):10309–13.

Terbogh, J. 2000. "The fate of tropical forests: A matter of stewardship." *Conservation Biology* 14(5):1358–61.

Welcome to McGraw-Hill's Online Learning Center

http://www.mhhe.com/cunningham3e

WEB EXERCISES

Graph and Map World Land Uses

How can you map international changes in forest or grassland cover yourself? Believe it or not, it's easy. The United Nations Environment Program (UNEP) and UN Food and Agriculture Organization (FAO) are among the most important sources for global environmental data. Even more important, these organizations provide their data at http://geodata.grid.unep.ch. Go to this website. (Note: the .ch in the address indicates that the site comes from Switzerland, where these programs are based.)

There are five steps to make a graph. First, enter a search term: enter *forest* in the space provided; then click on the *continue* button near the bottom of the window. Second, select one of the variables available to show distribution of forests or grasslands and press *continue* again. Third, select all the years available and press *continue* again. Fourth, select the *draw graph* option. Finally, you'll have to select a country and a graph type. Since you're interested first in change over time, choose a country that you suspect has lost forest, and select the *line graph* option. Use all years, so that you can see the change in forest area over time. Now click on the *make new graph* button. Were you right in your expectations for this country? How much was there in the first year shown, compared with the last year? Calculate the percentage change: divide last year's value (on the vertical axis) by the first year's value to find the relative amount lost or gained.

Now find another country that you suspect has lost forest area. Select that country and make a new graph. Were you right? Try to find a country that has *gained* forests. Which region would you most likely look in for this?

Now try selecting two countries that you think might have different rates of forest change. Select just two dates (early and recent); then select the *bar graph* option and make a new graph. Were you right in your expectations?

Note that this webpage lets you make maps or graphs of many variables. Explore and experiment a bit to see what you can learn.

World Protected Areas

The United Nations Environment Program (UNEP) is one of the main sources of information on the global environment. You can map (or graph) protected areas on the UNEP website. Go to http://geodata.grid.unep.ch/. You'll see an option to "search the GEO database." In the search space, enter *protected areas.* The search should return a list of variables, such as extent of protected mangroves (by number of sites or by total area), number or area of marine protected areas, and so on. Some of these variables are grouped by country, some by region (e.g., Africa), and some by subregion (e.g., southern Africa).

Select *Mangroves, Forest Extent* (at the national level). Then click *continue.* The next window asks you to select a year to map, but you have only one option, so click *continue* again. Next select the *Draw Map* option. Look at the legend below the map, showing ranges in extent of protected mangroves. Which countries have the most protected mangroves?

Zoom in on Indonesia (using the *Basic Tools, Zoom In* option). As you zoom in, you should see the shape of the ocean floor. Can you see the flat shelves around Indonesia where mangroves might flourish?

Now check which countries have the maximum amount of protected mangroves: click on the *show extremes* box; then click on the map to redraw. Which five countries have the most?

Go back to the Geo Data Portal website, and you can return to the list of data sets by clicking on *2. Dataset,* just above the *Draw Map* option. Select another variable to map. Protected Areas (IUCN Categories I–VI) is a good option. After you've made your map, you can use the *show extremes* option again. Which countries have the most protected areas? Which have the least? Can you think of some explanations for these extremes?

Note that you can make bar graphs to compare selected countries; you can look at (and download) data tables; and if you select a variable with multiple dates, you can draw a line graph showing change over time.

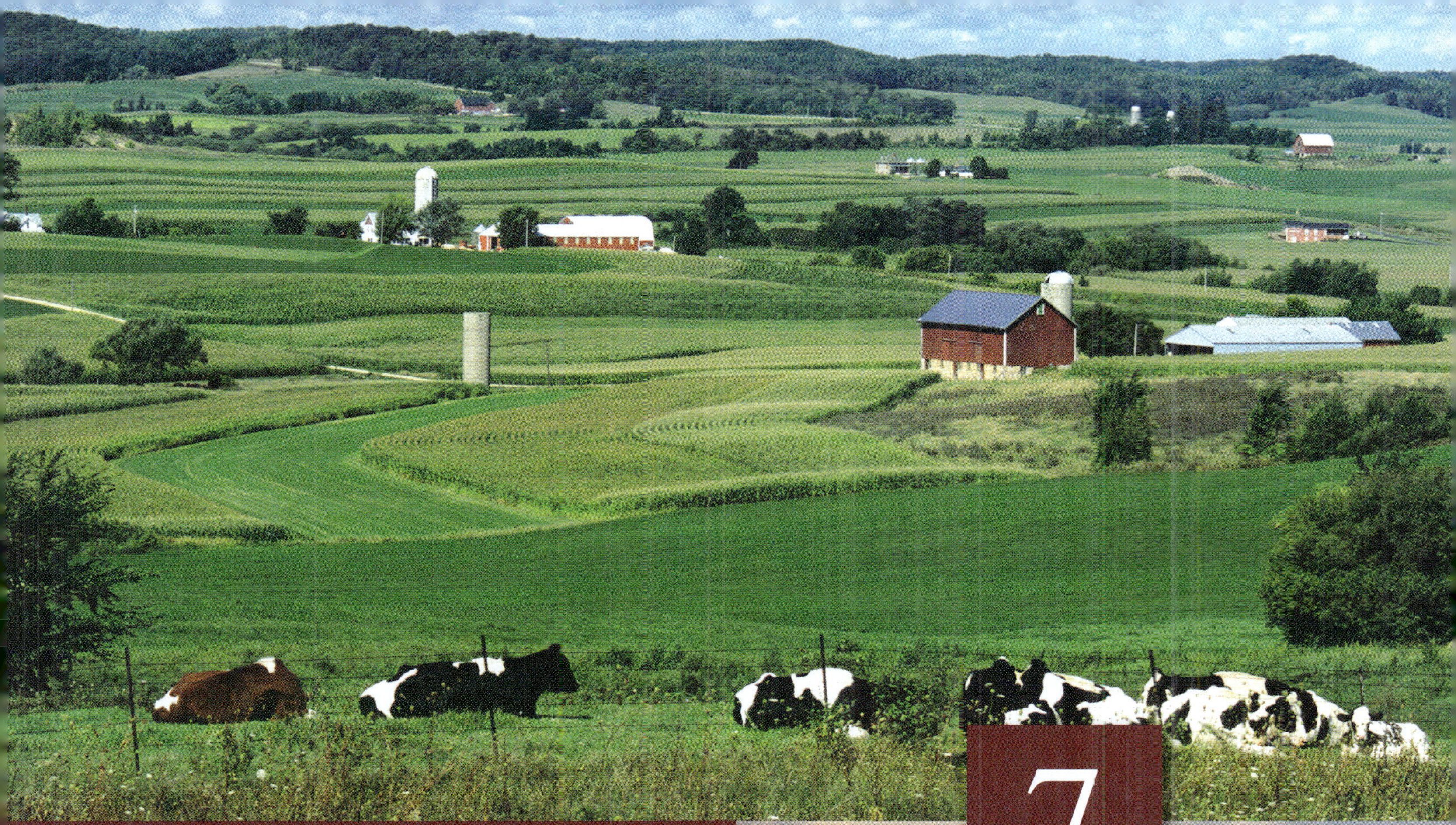

Soil conservation practices can protect air and water quality and preserve wildlife habitat.

7 Food and Agriculture

> We abuse the land because we regard it as a commodity belonging to us. When we see land as a community to which we belong, we may begin to use it with love and respect.
>
> *–Aldo Leopold*

Welcome to McGraw-Hill's Online Learning Center

http://www.mhhe.com/cunningham3e

LEARNING ONLINE

Visit our webpage at www.mhhe.com/cunningham3e for data sources, further readings, additional case studies, current environmental news, and regional examples within the Online Learning Center to help you understand the material in this chapter. You'll also find active links to information pertaining to this chapter, including

World hunger and nutrition
Soil science and soil types
Soil conservation
Agriculture and trade policy
Agricultural research
Sustainable agriculture
Genetic engineering
Pesticides and pest control
Integrated pest management
Persistent organic pollutants (POPs)

OBJECTIVES

After studying this chapter, you should be able to

- describe world food supplies and some causes of chronic hunger in the midst of growing food surpluses.
- explain some major human nutritional requirements, as well as the consequences of deficiencies in those nutrients.
- differentiate between famine and chronic undernutrition, and understand the relation between natural disasters and social or economic forces in triggering food shortages.
- sketch the roles of living organisms, physical forces, and other factors in creating and maintaining fertile soil.
- differentiate between the sources and effects of land degradation, including erosion, nutrient depletion, waterlogging, and salinization.
- analyze some of the promises and perils of genetic engineering.
- explain the need for water, energy, and nutrients for sustained crop production, as well as some limits on our use of these resources.
- recognize the potential for low-input, sustainable, regenerative agriculture.

Golden Rice

Every year more than a million children die and another 350,000 go blind from the effects of vitamin A deficiency. Can modern science help find a solution to this tragedy? Swiss researcher Ingo Potrykus thinks so. For the past decade, Potrykus, of the Swiss Federal Institute of Technology in Zurich, and his colleague, Peter Beyer of the University of Freiburg in Germany, have been working on a crop that could improve the lives of millions of the poorest people in the world. Using genetic engineering techniques, they moved the genes that make daffodils yellow into *Oryza sativa,* the rice species eaten as a staple food by about half the people in the world (fig. 7.1).

The problem is that the poorest people often live on only a bowl or two of rice per day. Rice is low in beta carotene, the precursor for vitamin A. While rice, like all green plants, makes light-absorbing carotenes in its leaves, no known member of the *Oryza* genus stores these compounds in its seeds. Thus, ordinary techniques of plant breeding don't offer a way to enrich the crop. Extracting carotene genes from daffodils, and promoters (DNA segments that regulate gene expression) from bacteria, Potrykus and Beyer constructed a plasmid (a naked DNA loop) that was innoculated into the soil bacterium *Agrobacterium tumefaciens.* The transgenic agrobacteria were then incubated with rice embryos in a plant tissue culture medium. As the bacteria infect rice cells, they also transfer the genes that encode instructions for making beta carotene. When the embryos grow into mature plants, they make beta carotene in all their tissues—including the endosperm that fills the golden rice grains. These plants can be crossbred with rice varieties adapted to a variety of local conditions and made available to poor farmers around the world.

In 2000, after nearly ten years of work and $2.6 million in support from the Swiss government, the European Union, and the Rockefeller Foundation, Potrykus and his colleagues had grain ready to distribute for free to developing countries. To their surprise, however, the researchers found themselves embroiled in heated controversy. While they felt they had made a scientific breakthrough to save millions of lives and incalculable suffering, bioengineering opponents regarded their creation as unholy tinkering with nature and a sinister threat to our diet, traditional farming, and the health of the world environment. Opponents of genetically modified organisms (GMOs) objected that this rice would be a first step toward making farmers dependent on multinational seed producers. They also questioned whether there might be unforeseen ecological consequences of releasing newly created plants around the world. Activists threatened to destroy experimental crops and to mount protests against companies or governments attempting to introduce what they considered to be "Frankenfoods," the unnatural creations of agricultural biotechnology.

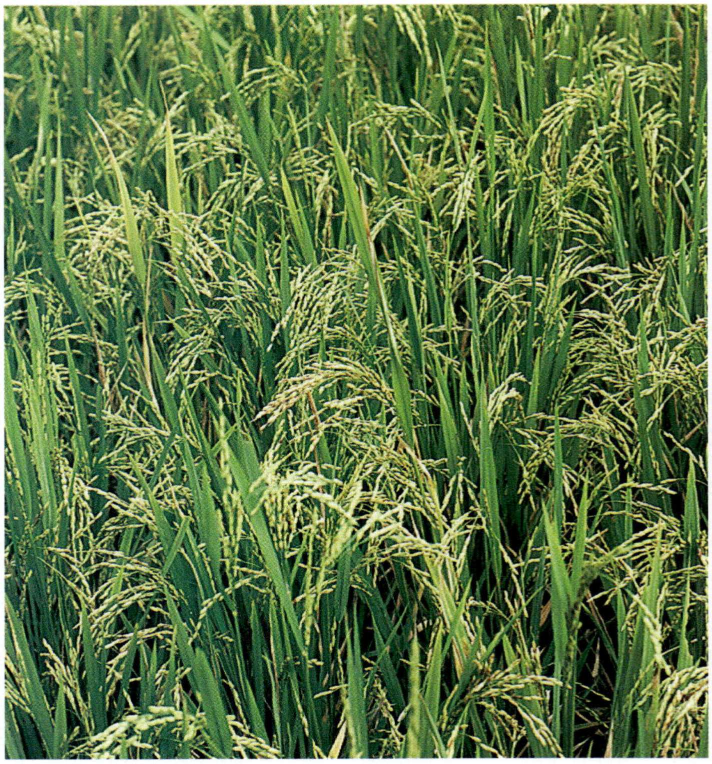

FIGURE 7.1 *Rice makes up a major part of the diet for half the people in the world. Unless supplemented with other sources of vitamins, minerals, and protein, however, rice alone doesn't constitute a healthy diet.*

Even some who don't oppose genetic engineering per se argue that technological solutions aren't the answer to poverty and malnutrition. There are better ways, they claim, to provide a nutritious diet to poor children. Furthermore, the families whose children are the most likely to suffer vitamin deficiencies often are landless peasants who can't grow the golden grain for themselves. Will they be able to buy the new varieties, or will they continue to subsist on the cheapest, least nutritious foods that barely keep them alive?

This dilemma illustrates the complexity of food security issues, and it raises several important questions for environmental science. (1) Will there be enough nutritious food for everyone in the world? (2) Will that food be safe to eat? (3) What will be the environmental consequences of raising the food we need? Science plays an important role in answering these questions, but it can't be separated from controversies about human society and access to resources. In this chapter, we'll look at world food supplies, hunger, nutrition, and agricultural systems that contribute to or help solve these difficult questions.

FOOD AND NUTRITION

Despite dire predictions that runaway population growth would soon lead to terrible famines (see chapter 4), world food supplies have more than kept up with increasing human numbers over the past two centuries. The past 40 years have seen especially encouraging strides in reducing world hunger. While population growth averaged 1.7 percent per year during that time, world food production increased an average of 2.2 percent. Increased use of irrigation, improved crop varieties, more readily available fertilizers, and distribution systems to transport food from regions with surpluses to those in need have brought improved nutrition to billions of people. In this section, we'll look at the causes and effects of remaining chronic and acute food shortages, as well as recommendations for a balanced, healthful diet.

Chronic Hunger and Food Security

In 1960 nearly 60 percent of the residents of developing countries were considered **chronically undernourished,** meaning their diet didn't provide the 2,200 kcal per day, on average, considered necessary for a healthy, productive life. Today, despite the fact that their population has doubled over the past 40 years, the proportion in these countries suffering from chronic caloric deficiency has fallen to less than 15 percent.

The UN Food and Agriculture Organization (FAO) expects agricultural production to continue to grow over the next few decades. Where the current world food supply would be sufficient, if equitably distributed, to provide an average of 2,800 kcal per person per day, the FAO predicts that, by 2030, there will be enough food available to supply 3,050 kcal per day to everyone, or about 30 percent more than most of us need. In countries such as the United States, the problem already has become what to do with surplus food. Farmers in these countries are paid billions of dollars per year not to grow crops.

Still, in a world of surplus food, some 840 million people don't have enough to eat. Figure 7.2 shows countries with the highest risk of food shortages. As you can see, most of sub-Saharan Africa, South and Southeast Asia, and parts of Latin America fall in this category. Ninety-five percent of the chronically undernourished are in developing countries, but an increasing number are in transition countries (primarily states of the former Soviet Union and its allies undergoing a change from socialism to market economies) where bad weather, poor management, and social crises have resulted in sharply falling agricultural production (fig. 7.3). Even in the richest countries, where excess calories are the greatest problem for the majority, some 11 million people don't have enough to eat.

Poverty is the greatest threat to **food security,** or the ability to obtain sufficient food on a day-to-day basis. The 1.4 billion people in the world who live on less than $1 per day all too often can't buy the food they need and don't have access to resources to grow it for themselves. Food security occurs at multiple scales. In the poorest countries, hunger may affect nearly everyone. In other countries, although the average food availability may be satisfactory, some individual communities or families may not have enough to eat. And within families, males often get both the largest share and the most nutritious food, while women and children—who need food most—all too often get the poorest diet. At least 6 million children under 5 years old die every year of diseases exacerbated by hunger and malnutrition. Providing a healthy diet might eliminate as much as 60 percent of all premature deaths worldwide.

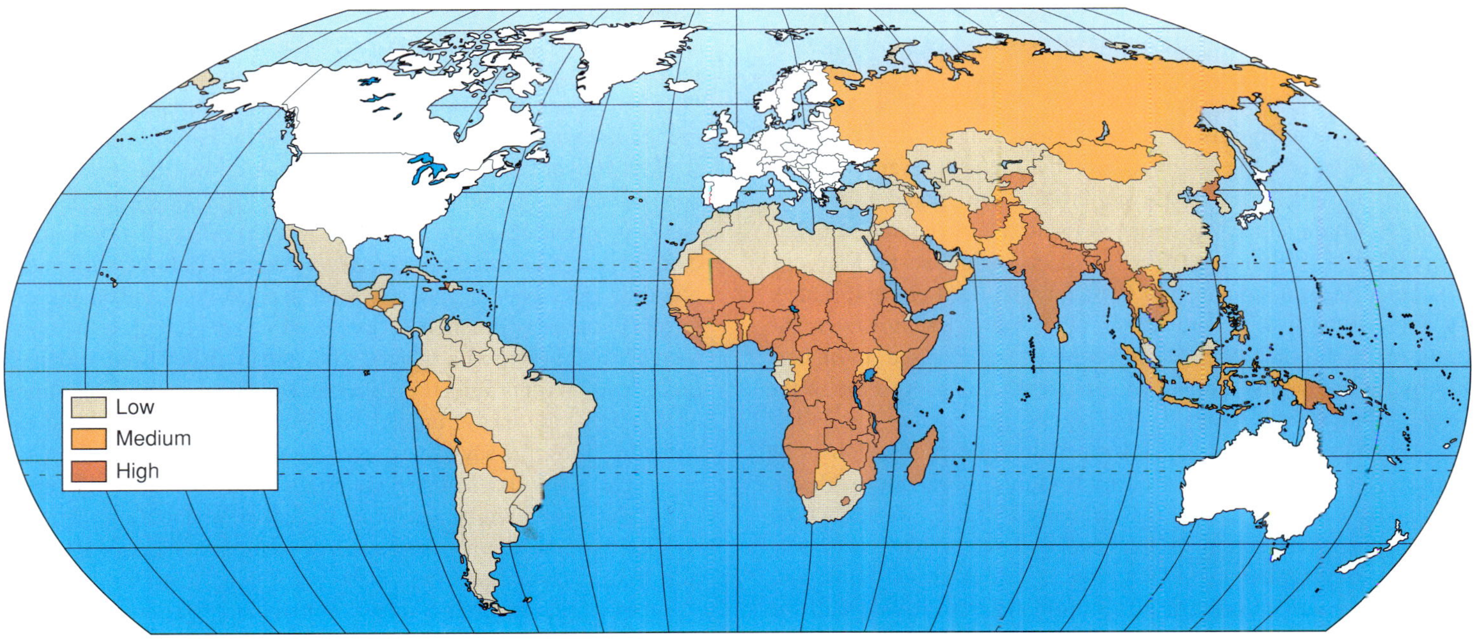

FIGURE 7.2 *Countries with populations at risk for inadequate nutrition. The United States, Canada, Europe, Japan, and Australia have little risk.*
Source: World Resources 1998–99, World Resource Institute. Reprinted by permission.

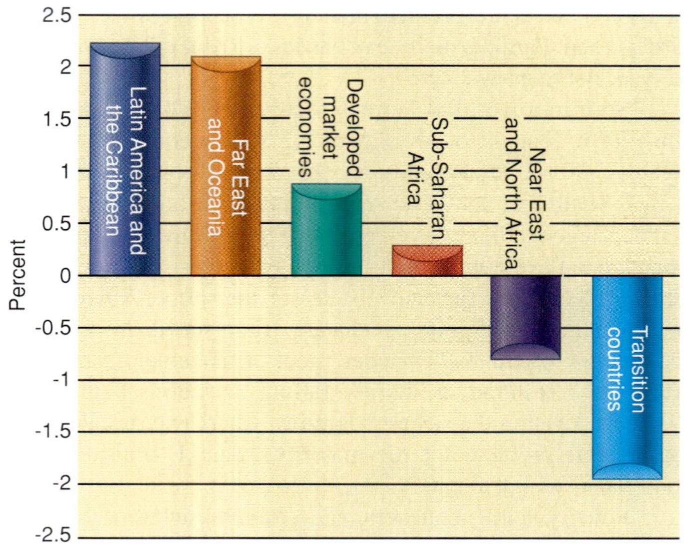

FIGURE 7.3 *Changes in agricultural production in 2000. Transition countries are states from the former Soviet Union undergoing a change from socialism to capitalism.*
Source: Data from Food and Agriculture Organization (FAO), 2002.

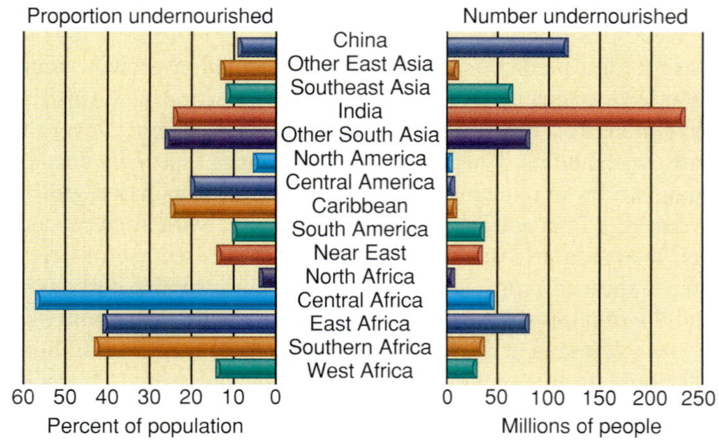

FIGURE 7.4 *Number and percent of population chronically undernourished by region in the developing world.*
Source: Data from Food and Agriculture Organization (FAO), 2002.

Hungry people can't work their way out of poverty, the Nobel Prize–winning economist Robert Fogel points out. He estimates that in 1790 about 20 percent of the population of England and France was effectively excluded from the labor force because they were too weak and hungry to work. Improved nutrition, he calculates, accounted for about half of all European economic growth during the nineteenth century. Since many developing countries are as poor now (in relative terms) as Britain and France were in 1790, his analysis suggests that reducing hunger could yield more than \$120 billion (U.S.) in economic growth produced by longer, healthier, more productive lives for several hundred million people.

The 2003 UN World Food Summit reaffirmed the goal set by previous conventions of reducing the number of chronically undernourished people to 400 million by 2015. We aren't on track to meet that goal, but some countries have made impressive progress. China, alone, has reduced its number of undernourished people by 74 million over the past decade. Indonesia, Vietnam, Thailand, Nigeria, Ghana, and Peru each reduced chronic hunger by about 3 million people. In 47 other countries, however, the numbers of chronically underfed people have increased. India now has by far the largest number of persistently hungry people in the world, while central Africa has the highest percentage (fig. 7.4).

Recognizing the role of women in food production is an important step toward food security for all. Throughout the developing world, women do 50 to 70 percent of all farm work but control only a tiny fraction of the land and rarely have access to capital or developmental aid. In Nigeria, for example, home gardens occupy only 2 percent of all cropland but provide half the food families eat. Making land, credit, education, and access to markets available to women could contribute greatly to family nutrition.

Famines and Acute Food Shortages

Famines are characterized by large-scale food shortages, massive starvation, social disruption, and economic chaos. Starving people eat their seed grain and slaughter their breeding stock in a desperate attempt to keep themselves and their families alive. Even if better conditions return, they have often sacrificed their productive capacity and will take a long time to recover. Famines often trigger mass migrations, as starving people travel to refugee camps in search of food and medical care (fig. 7.5). Many die on the way or fall prey to robbers.

In 2004 the United Nations reported that approximately 60 million people in 30 countries needed emergency food aid. What causes these emergencies? Environmental conditions are usually the immediate trigger, but politics and economics are often equally important in preventing people from getting the food they need. Drought, floods, insect outbreaks, and other natural disasters cause crop failures and create food shortages. But the Nobel Prize–winning work of Harvard economist Amartya K. Sen shows that these factors have often been around for a long time, and local people usually have ways to get through hard times if they aren't thwarted by inept or corrupt governments and greedy elites. National politics, commodity hoarding, price gouging, poverty, wars, landlessness, and other social factors often conspire, so that poor people can neither grow their own food nor find jobs to earn money to buy the food they need. Professor Sen points out that armed conflict and political oppression almost always are at the root of famine. No democratic country with a relatively free press, he says, has ever had a major famine.

The aid policies of rich countries often serve more to get rid of surplus commodities and make us feel good about our generosity than to eliminate the root causes of starvation. Crowding people into feeding camps generally is the worst thing to do for them. The stress of getting there kills many of them, and the density and lack of sanitation in the camps expose them to epidemic diseases. There are no jobs in refugee camps, so people can't support themselves if they try. Social chaos and family breakdown expose the weakest to

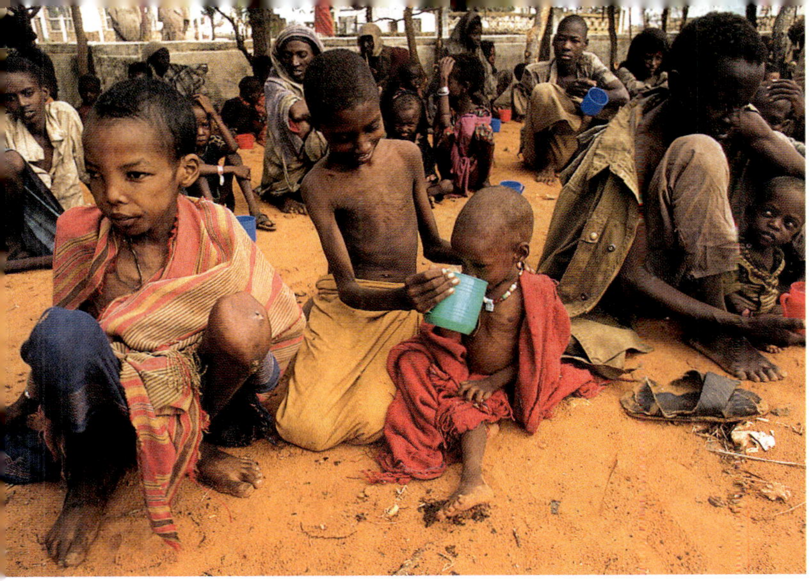

FIGURE 7.5 *Children wait for their daily ration of porridge at a feeding station in Somalia. When people are driven from their homes by hunger or war, social systems collapse, diseases spread rapidly, and the situation quickly becomes desperate.*

robbery and violence. Having left their land and tools behind, people can't replant crops when the weather returns to normal.

Malnutrition and Obesity

In addition to energy (calories), we also need specific nutrients in our diet, such as proteins, vitamins, and certain trace minerals. You might have more than enough calories and still suffer from **malnourishment,** a nutritional imbalance caused by a lack of specific dietary components or an inability to absorb or utilize essential nutrients. Those of us in richer countries often eat too much meat, salt, and fat and too little fiber, vitamins, trace minerals, and other components lost from highly processed foods. On average, we consume about one-third more calories than we need and get too little exercise. Food provides solace in stressful lives, and we're constantly bombarded with advertising tempting us to consume more. According to the U.S. surgeon general, 64 percent of all adult Americans are overweight, up from 40 percent only a decade ago, and about one-third of us are seriously overweight or **obese**—generally considered to be a body mass greater than 30 kg/m^2, or roughly 30 pounds above normal for an average person.

Being overweight substantially raises your risk for hypertension, diabetes, heart attacks, stroke, gallbladder disease, osteoarthritis, respiratory problems, and certain cancers. Every year, about 400,000 in the United States die from illnesses related to obesity. This number is approaching the 435,000 annual deaths from diseases related to smoking. Paradoxically, food insecurity and poverty can contribute to obesity. In one study, more than half of the women who reported not having enough to eat were overweight, compared with one-third of the food-secure women. Lack of time for cooking and access to healthy food choices, along with ready availability of fast-food snacks and calorie-laden drinks, lead to dangerous dietary imbalances for many people.

This trend isn't limited to richer countries. Obesity is spreading around the world (fig. 7.6). For the first time in history, there are probably more overweight people (more than 1 billion) than underweight. As chapter 8 points out, Western diets and lifestyles are being adopted by many in the developing world, and diseases such as heart attack, stroke, diabetes, and depression, which once were thought to afflict only wealthy nations, are now becoming the most prevalent causes of death and disability everywhere.

Many poor people can't afford meat, fruits, and vegetables that would provide a balanced diet. The FAO estimates that nearly 3 billion people (half the world population) suffer from vitamin, mineral, or protein deficiencies. This results in devastating illnesses and deaths, as well as reduced mental capacity, developmental abnormalities, and stunted growth. Altogether, these problems bring an incalculable loss of human potential and social capital.

Anemia (low hemoglobin levels in the blood, usually caused by dietary iron deficiency) is the most common nutritional problem in the world. According to the FAO, more than 2 billion people (52 percent are pregnant women and 39 percent are children under 5) suffer from iron deficiencies. The problem is most severe in India, where more than 80 percent of all pregnant women are anemic. Anemia increases the risk of maternal deaths from hemorrhage in childbirth and affects childhood development. Red meat, eggs, legumes, and green vegetables all are good sources of dietary iron.

Iodine is essential for synthesis of thyroxin, an endocrine hormone that regulates metabolism and brain development, among other things. Chronic iodine deficiency causes goiter (a swollen thyroid gland, fig. 7.7), stunted growth, and reduced mental ability. The FAO estimates that 740 million people—mainly in South and Southeast Asia—suffer from iodine deficiency and that 177 million children have stunted growth and development. Adding a few pennies worth of iodine to our salt has largely eliminated this problem in developed countries.

Starchy foods, such as maize (corn), polished rice, and manioc (tapioca), which form the bulk of the diet for many poor people, tend to be low in several essential vitamins as well as minerals. According to the FAO, vitamin A deficiencies affect between 100 and 140 million children at any given time. As mentioned in the

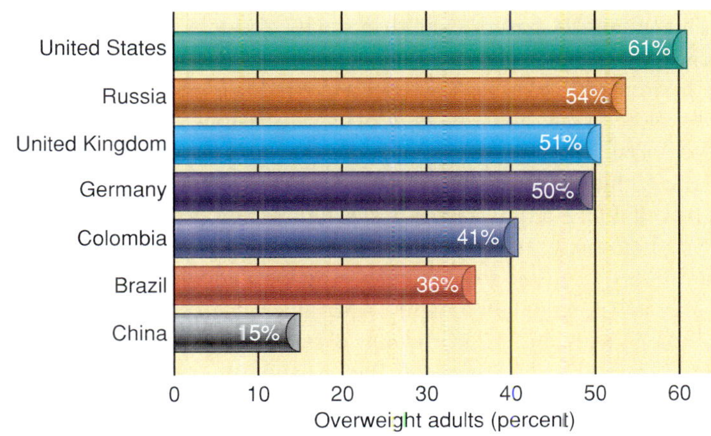

FIGURE 7.6 *While nearly a billion people are chronically undernourished, people in wealthier countries are at risk from eating too much.*
Source: Data from Worldwatch Institute, 2001.

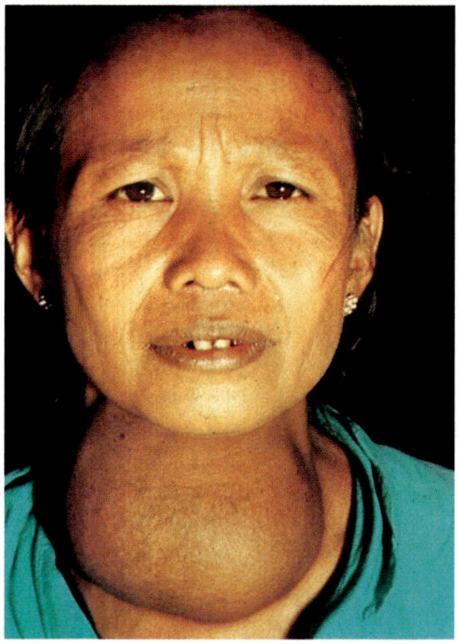

FIGURE 7.7 *Goiter, a swelling of the thyroid gland at the base of the neck, is often caused by an iodine deficiency. It is a common problem in many parts of the world, particularly where soil iodine is low and seafood is unavailable.*

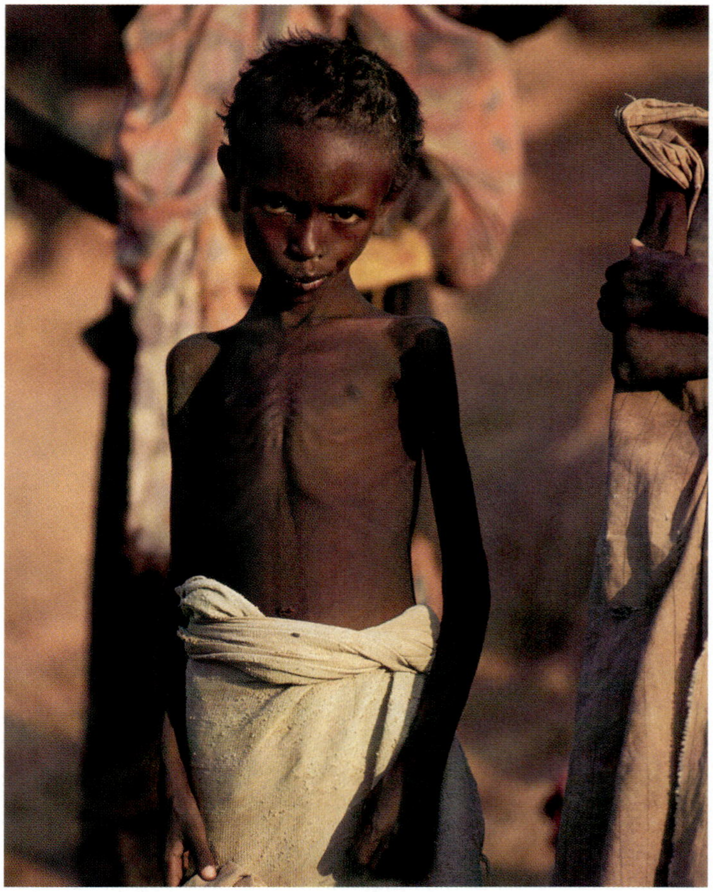

FIGURE 7.8 *Marasmus is caused by combined energy (calorie) and protein deficiencies. Children with marasmus have the wizened look and dry, flaky skin of an old person.*

story "Golden Rice" at the beginning of this chapter, more than a million of those children die and another 350,000 go blind every year from the effects of this vitamin shortage. Folic acid (found in dark green, leafy vegetables) is essential for early fetal development. Folic acid deficiencies have been linked to neurological problems in babies, including microencephaly (an abnormally small head) or even anencephaly (lacking a brain).

Protein also is essential for normal growth and development. The two most widespread human protein deficiency diseases are kwashiorkor and marasmus. **Kwashiorkor** is a West African word meaning "displaced child." (A young child is displaced—and deprived of nutritious breast milk—when a new baby is born.) This condition occurs mainly in young children who eat mostly cheap, starchy food and don't get enough good-quality protein. Children with kwashiorkor often have reddish-orange hair; puffy, discolored skin; and a bloated belly. **Marasmus** (from the Greek "to waste away") is caused by a diet low in both calories and protein. A child suffering from severe marasmus is generally thin and shriveled, like a tiny, very old, starving person (fig. 7.8). Children with both these deficiencies have low resistance to infections and are likely to suffer from stunted growth, mental retardation, and other developmental problems. Altogether, the FAO estimates, the annual losses due to deaths and diseases caused by calorie and nutrient deficiencies are equivalent to 46 million years of productive life (see more in chapter 8 on disability-adjusted life years).

Eating a Balanced Diet

What's the best way to be sure you're getting a healthy diet? Generally, it isn't necessary to take synthetic dietary supplements. Eating a good variety of foods should give you all the nutrients you need. For years, Americans were advised to eat daily servings of four major food groups: meat, dairy products, grains, and fruits and vegetables. These recommendations were revised in 1992 to emphasize only sparing servings of meat, dairy, fats, and sweets.

Some nutritionists believe that the 1992 recommendations for 6 to 11 servings a day of bread, cereal, rice, and pasta still provide too many simple sugars (or starches that are quickly converted to sugar). Based on observations of the health effects of Mediterranean diets, as well as a long-term study of 140,000 U.S. health professionals, Drs. Walter Willett and Meir Stampfer of Harvard University recommended a new dietary pyramid (fig. 7.9). Both red meat and starchy food, such as white rice, white bread, potatoes, and pasta, should be eaten sparingly. Nuts, legumes (beans, peas, and lentils), fruit, vegetables, and whole-grain foods form the basis of this diet. Unsaturated plant oils should make up 30 to 40 percent of dietary calories, according to this view. Trans fat (the kind found in hydrogenated margarine), on the other hand, is not recommended at all. Combined with regular, moderate exercise, this food selection should provide most people with all the nutrition they need.

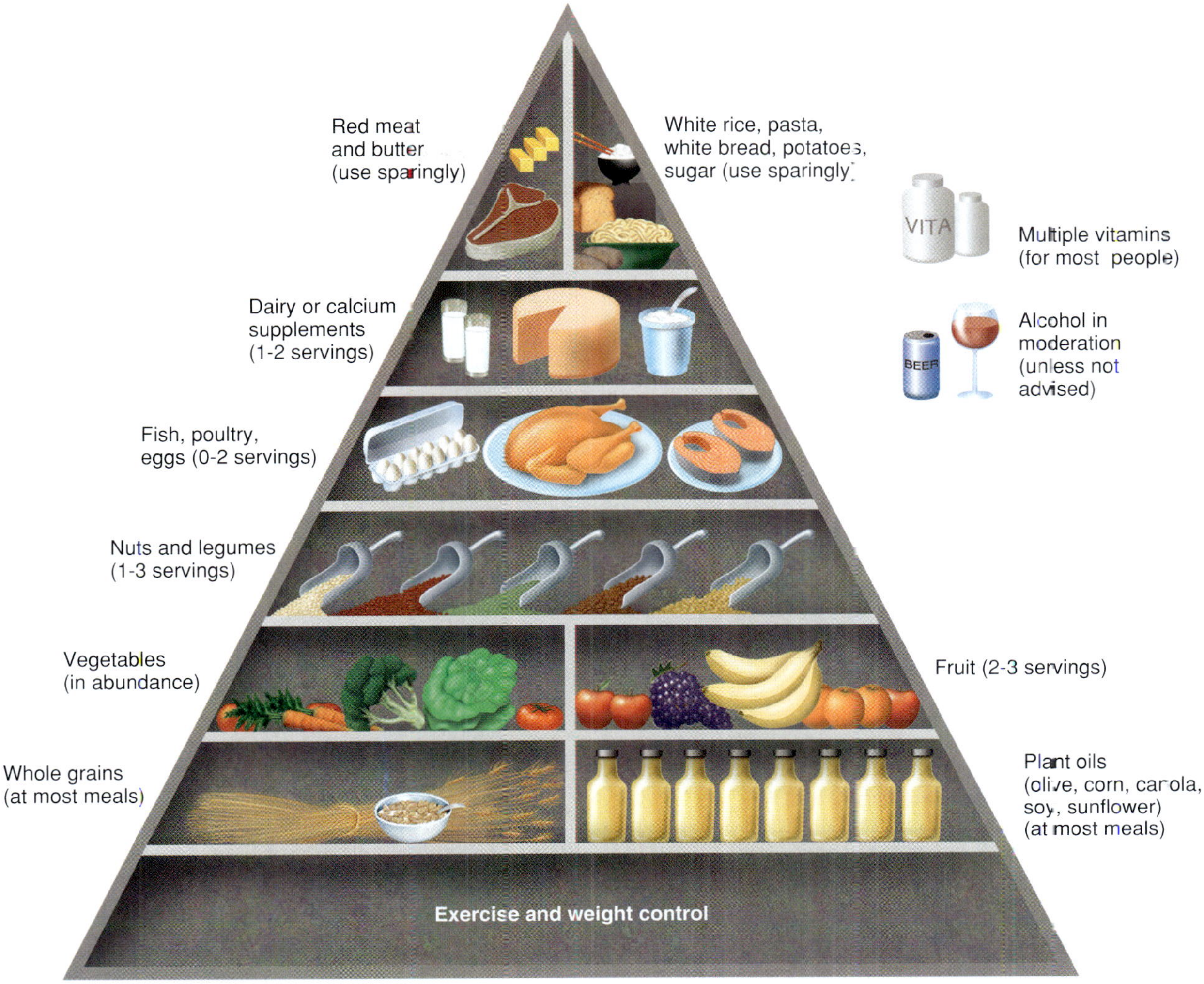

FIGURE 7.9 *The food pyramid proposed by Drs. Walter Willett and Meir Stampfer deemphasizes consumption of red meat, butter, white rice, potatoes, and pasta and suggests a diet rich in whole grains, unsaturated plant oils, fruits, and vegetables.*
Source: Data from Willett and Stampfer, 2002.

MAJOR FOOD SOURCES

Of the thousands of edible plants and animals in the world, only about a dozen types of seeds and grains, three root crops, twenty or so common fruits and vegetables, six mammals, two domestic fowl, and a few fish and other forms of marine life make up almost all of the food humans eat. Table 7.1 shows annual production of some important foods in human diets. In this section, we will highlight sources and characteristics of those foods.

Major Crops

The three crops on which humanity depends for the majority of its nutrients and calories are wheat, rice, and maize. Together, about 2,100 million metric tons of these three grains are grown each year. Wheat and rice are especially important, since they are the staple foods for most of the 5 billion people in the developing countries. These two grass species supply around 60 percent of the calories that humans consume directly.

Potatoes, barley, oats, and rye are staples in mountainous regions and high latitudes (northern Europe, North Asia) because they grow well in cool, moist climates. Cassava, sweet potatoes, and other roots and tubers grow well in warm, wet areas and are staples in Amazonia, Africa, Melanesia, and the South Pacific. Sorghum and millet are drought-resistant and are staples in the dry regions of Africa.

Fruits and vegetables—including vegetable oils—make a surprisingly large contribution to human diets. They are especially welcome because they typically contain high levels of vitamins, minerals, dietary fiber, and complex carbohydrates.

Meat and Dairy

Protein-rich foods are prized by people nearly everywhere. In the past, the rich countries consumed a vast majority of the meat and dairy traded internationally. The four-fifths of the world's people in less-developed countries generally raised 60 percent of the 3 billion domestic ruminants and 6 billion poultry in the world but consumed only one-fifth of all commercial animal products. The

TABLE 7.1 Some Important Food Sources

CROP	2002 YIELD (MILLION METRIC TONS)
Wheat	603
Rice (paddy)	593
Maize (corn)	933
Potatoes	308
Barley and oats	168
Soybeans	177
Cassava and sweet potatoes	315
Sugar (cane and beet)	141
Pulses (beans, peas)	54
Oil seeds	324
Vegetables and fruits	905
Meat and milk	735
Fish and seafood	140

Source: Data from Food and Agriculture Organization (FAO), 2003.

APPLICATION: Mapping Your Food Supply

Make a list of all the food you ate on a recent day. Insofar as you are able, map where each of those food items came from. For raw materials, you may have to make an educated guess. If you live in North America, for instance, the wheat in baked goods probably came from the upper Great Plains or Prairie Provinces; corn syrup in prepared foods probably came from the corn belt; cane sugar is mostly from Florida; beet sugar is mostly from the Red River Valley of the north. What was the average distance traveled by each food item from its source to your table that day? What do you know about the growing conditions or social circumstances at the source of your food? Are there pesticide controls, for instance, where your food originated? How many calories did you eat that day?

FAO reports, however, that, as incomes rise in developing countries, food choices throughout the world are shifting toward higher-quality and more expensive foods. Meat consumption in developing countries, for example, has risen from only 10 kg per person annually in the 1960s to 26 kg currently (fig. 7.10). By 2030, average annual meat consumption in those countries is expected to be nearly 40 kg per person. Far more cereal grain will be needed to raise livestock if this trend continues.

Most of the livestock grown in North America is confined in concentrated animal feeding operations for part or all of the animals' lifetime. A diet rich in grain, oil, and protein fattens animals quickly and produces meat preferred by many consumers. Globally, some 660 million metric tons of cereals are used as livestock feed each year, representing just over a third of the world total cereal use. It's often pointed out that we could feed about ten times as many people if we ate grain directly rather than feeding it to livestock. Surprisingly, the FAO claims that using cereals as animal feed does not contribute to hunger and undernutrition. Given current agricultural economics, if these cereals were not used as animal feed, they would probably not be produced at all and thus would not be available as food. According to this view, if everyone became a vegetarian, the lack of demand for cereals for livestock production would simply lead to lower crop production, not more food for the hungry.

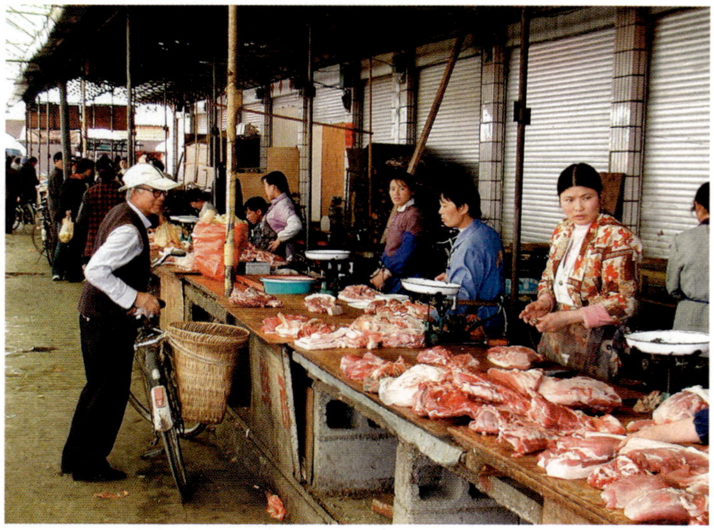

FIGURE 7.10 *Meat and dairy consumption has quadrupled in the past 40 years, and China represents about 40 percent of that increased demand.*

The rapid proliferation of large-scale animal confinement operations raises a number of social and environmental questions. Up to 10,000 hogs enclosed in a giant barn, or 100,000 cattle in a single feedlot complex, can cause serious local air and water pollution (fig. 7.11). Animal waste often is stored in enormous open lagoons, which can leak or rupture, contaminating both surface waters and groundwater supplies. When Hurricane Floyd dumped torrential rains on North Carolina in 1999, an estimated 10 million m^3 (2.5 billion gal) of hog and poultry waste overflowed from storage lagoons into local rivers (see related story "Flood of Pigs" at www.mhhe.com/cases). The high density of animals in these facilities and the rich diet they're fed to speed weight gain require a constant use of antibiotics and growth hormones. More than half of all antibiotics used in the United States are administered to livestock, mostly in confinement facilities. A big part of the rapid rise in antibiotic-resistant pathogens is due to this massive and constant dosing with drugs. Emergent diseases (see chapter 8) are having significant impacts on our diet. In 2004 mad cow disease, avian flu, rabies, and other infectious diseases blocked an estimated one-third of all global meat exports. The FAO estimated losses of $10 billion (U.S.). The impacts on many farmers were catastrophic. It's estimated that one-quarter of all U.S. cattle have

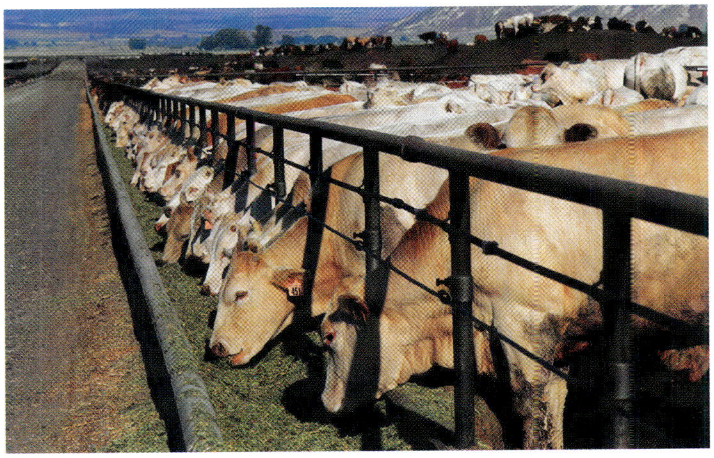

FIGURE 7.11 *Up to 100,000 cattle may be confined in a single feedlot operation. Note the animals in the background standing on a manure mound.*

the deadly bacterium *E. coli* 0157-H7 in their gut. As few as two or three of these cells can kill you.

Seafood

The 140 million metric tons of seafood we eat every year is an important part of our diet. Seafood provides about 15 percent of all animal protein eaten by humans, and it is the main animal protein source for about 1 billion people in developing countries. Unfortunately, overharvesting and habitat destruction threaten most of the world's wild fisheries (see related story "Shark Finning" at www.mhhe.com/cases). Annual catches of ocean fish rose by about 4 percent annually between 1950 and 1988. Since 1989, however, 13 of 17 major marine fisheries have declined dramatically or become commercially unsustainable. According to the United Nations, three-quarters of the world's edible ocean fish, crustaceans, and mollusks are declining and in urgent need of managed conservation.

The problem is too many boats using efficient but destructive technology to exploit a dwindling resource base. Boats as big as ocean liners travel thousands of kilometers and drag nets large enough to scoop up a dozen jumbo jets, sweeping a large patch of ocean clean of fish in a few hours. Long-line fishing boats set cables up to 10 km long with hooks every 2 meters that catch birds, turtles, and other unwanted "by-catch" along with targeted species. Trawlers drag heavy nets across the bottom, scooping up everything indiscriminately and reducing broad swaths of habitat to rubble. One marine biologist compared the technique to harvesting apples with a chainsaw. In some operations, up to 15 kg of dead and dying by-catch are dumped back into the ocean for every kilogram of marketable food. The FAO estimates that operating costs for the 4 million boats now harvesting wild fish exceed sales by $50 billion (U.S.) per year. Countries subsidize fishing fleets to preserve jobs and to ensure access to this valuable resource.

Aquaculture is providing an increasing share of the world's seafood. Fish can be grown in farm ponds that take relatively little space but are highly productive. Cultivation of high-value carnivorous species, however, such as salmon, sea bass, and tuna, threaten wild stocks exploited to stock captive operations or to provide fish food. Building coastal fish-rearing ponds causes destruction of hundreds of thousands of hectares of mangrove forests and wetlands, which serve as irreplaceable nurseries for marine species. Net pens anchored in nearshore areas allow spread of diseases, escape of exotic species, and release of feces, uneaten food, antibiotics, and other pollutants into surrounding ecosystems.

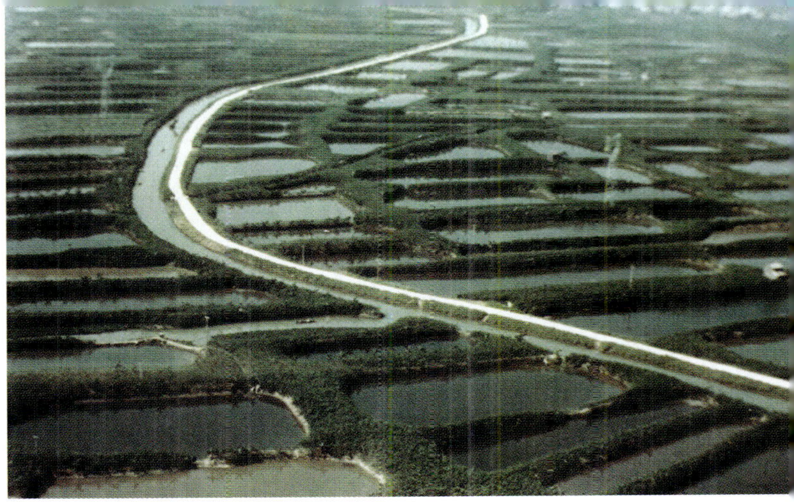

FIGURE 7.12 *Fish ponds are interspersed with mulberry plantations in China. Dead tree leaves fertilize the ponds and silkworms provide fish food, while enriched pond water irrigates the trees.*

Polyculture systems of mixed species of herbivores or filter feeders can alleviate many aquaculture problems. Raising species in enclosed, land-based ponds or warehouses can eliminate the pollution problems associated with net pens in lakes or oceans. In China, for example, most fish are raised in ponds or rice paddies (fig. 7.12). One ecologically balanced system uses four carp species that feed at different levels of the food chain. The grass carp, as its name implies, feeds largely on vegetation, while the common carp is a bottom feeder, living on detritus that settles to the bottom. Silver carp and bighead carp are filter feeders that feed on phytoplankton and zooplankton, respectively. Agricultural wastes, such as manure, dead silkworms, and rice straw, fertilize ponds and encourage phytoplankton growth. All these carp species are considered dangerous invasive species in North America. Still, these integrated polyculture systems typically boost fish yields per hectare by 50 percent or more, compared with monoculture farming. Of the top ten seafood species recommended by the Monterey Aquarium as ecologically acceptable, six are farmed (see related story "Are Shrimp Safe to Eat?" at www.mhhe.com/cases).

SOIL: A RENEWABLE RESOURCE

Growing the food and fiber needed to support human life is a complex enterprise that requires knowledge from many different fields and cooperation from many different groups of people. In this section, we will survey some of the principles of soil science and look at some of the inputs necessary for continued agricultural production.

Of all the earth's crustal resources, the one we take most for granted is soil. We are terrestrial animals and depend on soil for life, yet most of us think of it only in negative terms. English is unique in using *soil* as an interchangeable word for earth and excrement. *Dirty* has a moral connotation of corruption and impurity. Perhaps these uses of the word enhance our tendency to abuse soil without scruples; after all, it's only dirt.

The truth is that **soil** is a marvelous substance, a living resource of astonishing beauty, complexity, and frailty. It is a complex mixture of weathered mineral materials from rocks, partially decomposed organic molecules, and a host of living organisms. It can be considered an ecosystem by itself. Soil is an essential component of the biosphere, and it can be used sustainably, or even enhanced, under careful management.

There are at least 20,000 different soil types in the United States and many thousands more worldwide. They vary because of the influences of parent material, time, topography, climate, and organisms on soil formation. There are young soils that, because they have not weathered much, are rich in soluble nutrients. There are old soils, such as the red soils of the tropics, from which rainwater has washed away most of the soluble minerals and organic matter, leaving behind clay and rust-colored oxides.

To understand the potential for feeding the world on a sustainable basis, we need to know how soil forms, how it is lost, and what we can do to protect and rebuild good agricultural soil. With careful husbandry, soil can be replenished and renewed indefinitely. Many farming techniques deplete soil nutrients, however, and expose the soil to the erosive forces of wind and moving water. As a result, in many places we are essentially "mining" this resource and using it much faster than it is being replaced.

Building good soil is a slow process. Under the best circumstances, good **topsoil** accumulates at a rate of about 10 tons per ha (2.5 acres) per year—enough soil to make a layer about 1 mm deep when spread over a hectare. Under poor conditions, it can take thousands of years to build that much soil. Perhaps one-third to one-half of the world's current croplands are losing topsoil faster than it is being replaced. In some of the worst spots, erosion carries away about 2.5 cm (1 in.) of topsoil per year. With losses like that, agricultural production has already begun to fall in many areas.

Soil Organisms

Without soil organisms, the earth would be covered with sterile mineral particles far different from the rich, living soil ecosystems on which we depend for most of our food. The activity of the myriad organisms living in the soil helps create structure, fertility, and tilth (condition suitable for tilling or cultivation).

Soil organisms usually stay close to the surface, but that thin living layer can contain thousands of species and billions of individual organisms per hectare. Algae live on the surface, while bacteria and fungi flourish in the top few centimeters of soil (fig. 7.13).

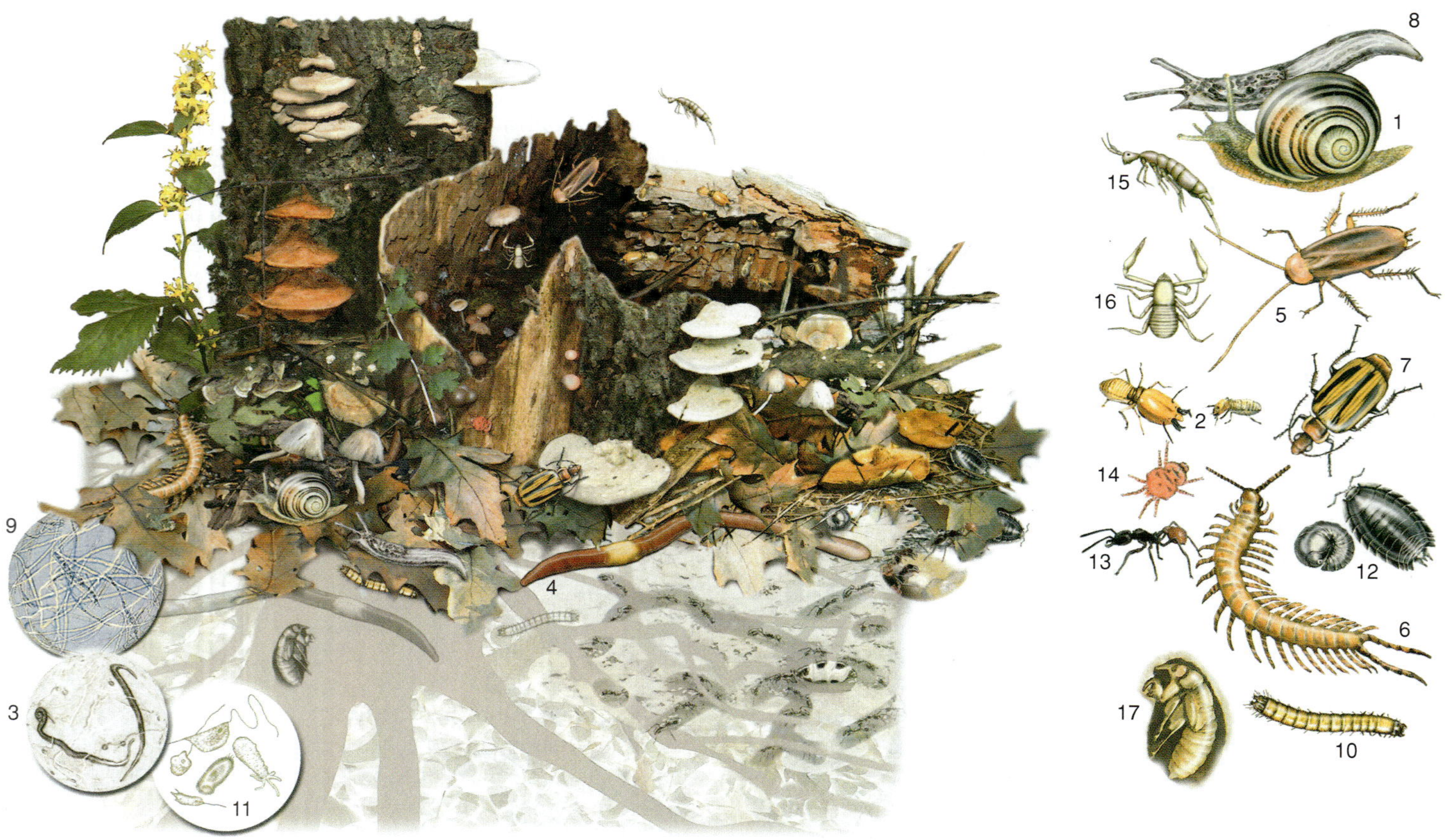

FIGURE 7.13 *Soil ecosystems include numerous consumer organisms, as depicted here: (1) snail, (2) termite, (3) nematode and nematode-killing constricting fungus, (4) earthworm, (5) wood roach, (6) centipede, (7) carabid (ground) beetle, (8) slug, (9) soil fungus, (10) wireworm (click beetle larva), (11) soil protozoan, (12) sow bug, (13) ant, (14) mite, (15) springtail, (16) pseudoscorpion, and (17) cicada nymph.*

A single gram of soil (about one-half teaspoon) can contain hundreds of millions of these microscopic cells. Worms and nematodes process plant roots and litter. Bacteria and fungi decompose organic detritus and recycle nutrients that plants can use for additional growth. The sweet aroma of freshly turned soil is caused by actinomycetes, bacteria that grow in fungus-like strands and give us the antibiotics streptomycin and tetracycline.

Soil Profiles

Most soils are stratified into horizontal layers called **soil horizons,** which reveal much about the soil's history and usefulness. The thickness, color, texture, and composition of each horizon are used to classify the soil. A cross-sectional view of the horizons in a soil is called a soil profile. Figure 7.14 shows the series of horizons generally seen in a soil profile. Soil scientists give each horizon a letter or descriptive name. Soils usually have one to seven or more horizons with different properties, depending on the soil type and history of a specific area.

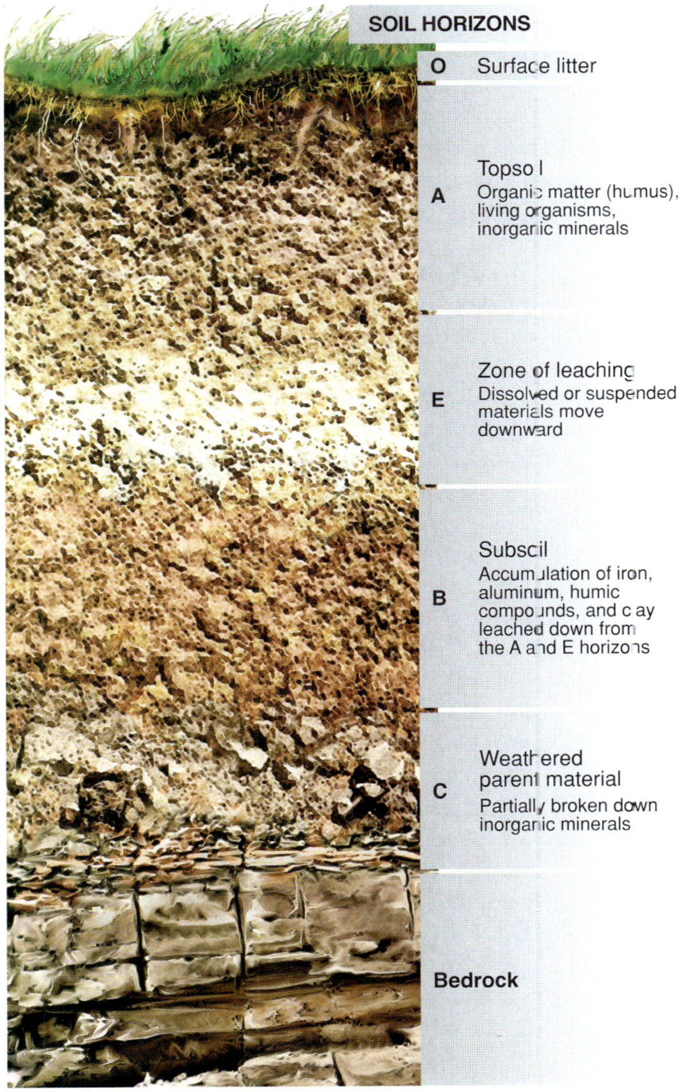

FIGURE 7.14 *Soil profile showing possible soil horizons. The actual number, composition, and thickness of these layers vary in different soil types.*

The soil surface is often covered with a layer of leaf litter, crop residues, or other fresh or partially decomposed organic material (O horizon). Under this organic layer is the surface horizon, usually an A horizon or topsoil, composed of mineral particles mixed with organic material. The A horizon ranges from a thickness of several meters under virgin prairie to zero in some deserts. The surface horizon contains most of the living organisms and organic material in the soil, and it is in this layer that most plants spread their roots to absorb water and nutrients. The surface horizon often blends into another horizon (the E horizon), which is subject to leaching (removal of soluble nutrients) by water percolating through it. This zone of leaching may have a very different appearance and composition from horizons above or below it.

Beneath the surface horizons, the subsurface horizons, or **subsoil**, usually have a lower organic content and higher concentrations of mineral particles. Under the subsoil is the parent material, or C horizon, made of weathered rock fragments with very little organic material. Weathering of this layer produces new soil particles and allows downward expansion of the horizons above. About 70 percent of all the parent horizon material in the United States was transported to its present site by geologic forces (glaciers, wind, and water) and is not directly related to the bedrock below it.

Soil Types

Soils are classified according to their structure and composition into orders, suborders, great groups, subgroups, families, and series. The richest farming soils are the mollisols (formed under grasslands) and alfisols (formed under moist, deciduous forests). North America is fortunate to have extensive areas of these fertile soils.

WAYS WE USE AND ABUSE SOIL

Only about 11 percent of the earth's land area (14.66 million km^2 out of a total of 132.4 million km^2) is currently in agricultural production. Perhaps four times as much land could be converted to cropland, but much of this land serves as a refuge for cultural or biological diversity or suffers from constraints, such as steep slopes, shallow soils, poor drainage, tillage problems, low nutrient levels, metal toxicity, or excess soluble salts or acidity, that limit the types of crops that can be grown there (fig. 7.15).

Land Resources

In parts of Canada and the United States, temperate climates, abundant water, and high soil fertility produce high crop yields that contribute to high standards of living. Other countries, although rich in land area, lack suitable soil, topography, water, or climate to sustain our levels of productivity.

Arable land shrank from 0.38 ha (0.94 acre) per person in 1970 to 0.23 ha (0.56 acre) in 2000. If current population projections are correct, the amount of cropland per person will decline to

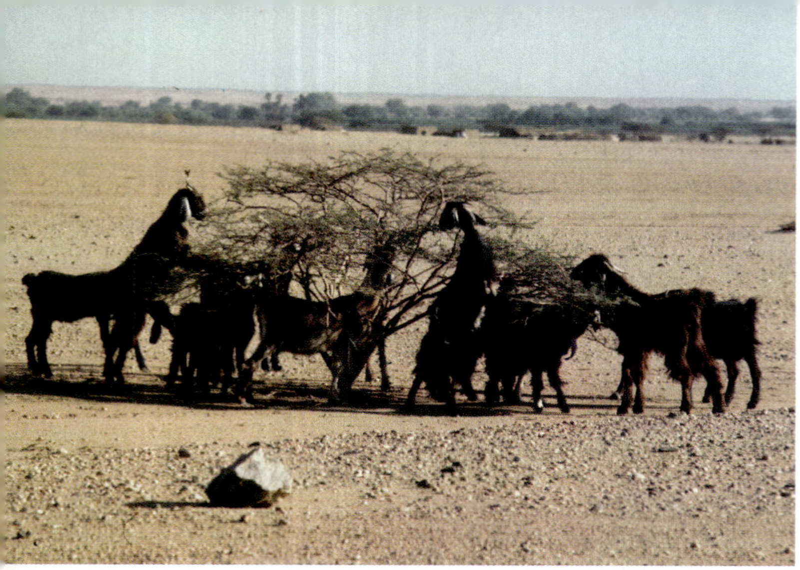

FIGURE 7.15 *In many areas, soil or climate constraints limit agricultural production. These hungry goats in Sudan feed on a solitary Acacia shrub.*

0.15 ha (0.37 acre) by 2050. In Asia, cropland will be even more scarce—0.09 ha (0.22 acre) per person—in 50 years. If you live on a typical quarter-acre suburban lot, look at your yard and imagine feeding yourself for a year on what you could produce there.

In the developed countries, 95 percent of agricultural growth in the twentieth century came from improved crop varieties or increased fertilization, irrigation, and pesticide use, rather than from bringing new land into production. In fact, less land is being cultivated now than 100 years ago in North America, or 600 years ago in Europe. As more effective use of labor, fertilizer, and water and improved seed varieties have increased in the more-developed countries, productivity per unit of land has increased, and marginal land has been retired, mostly to forests and grazing lands. In many developing countries, land continues to be cheaper than other resources, and new land is still being brought under cultivation, mostly at the expense of forests and grazing lands. Still, at least two-thirds of recent production gains have come from new crop varieties and more intense cropping, rather than expansion into new lands.

The largest increases in cropland over the past 30 years have occurred in South America and Oceania, where forests and grazing lands are rapidly being converted to farms. Many developing countries are reaching the limit of lands that can be exploited for agriculture without unacceptable social and environmental costs, but others still have considerable potential for opening new agricultural lands. East Asia, for instance, already uses about three-quarters of its potentially arable land. Most of its remaining land has severe restrictions for agricultural use. Further increases in crop production will probably have to come from higher yields per hectare. Latin America, by contrast, uses only about one-fifth of its potential land, and Africa uses only about one-fourth of the land that theoretically could grow crops. However, there would be serious ecological trade-offs in putting much of this land into agricultural production.

While land surveys tell us that much more land in the world could be cultivated, not all of that land necessarily should be farmed. Much of it is more valuable in its natural state. The soils over much of tropical Asia, Africa, and South America are old, weathered, and generally infertile. Most of the nutrients are in the standing plants, not in the soil. In many cases, clearing land for agriculture in the tropics has resulted in tragic losses of biodiversity and the valuable ecological services that it provides. Ultimately, much of this land is turned into useless scrub or semidesert.

On the other hand, there are large areas of rich, subtropical grassland and forest that are well watered, have good soil, and could become productive farmland without unduly reducing the world's biological diversity. Argentina, for instance, has pampas grasslands about twice the size of Texas that closely resemble the American Midwest a century ago in climate and potential for agricultural growth. Some of this land could probably be farmed with relatively little ecological damage if it were done carefully.

Land Degradation

Agriculture both causes and suffers from environmental degradation. The International Soil Reference and Information Centre in the Netherlands estimates that, every year, 3 million ha (7.4 million acres) of cropland are ruined by erosion, 4 million ha are turned into deserts, and 8 million ha are converted to nonagricultural uses, such as homes, highways, shopping centers, factories, and reservoirs. Over the past 50 years, some 1.9 billion ha of agricultural land (an area greater than that now in production) have been degraded to some extent. About 300 million ha of this land are strongly degraded (meaning that the soil has deep gullies, severe nutrient depletion, or poor crop growth or that restoration is difficult and expensive). Some 910 million ha—about the size of China—are moderately degraded. Nearly 9 million ha of former croplands are so degraded that they no longer support any crops at all. The causes of this extreme degradation vary: in Ethiopia, it is water erosion; in Somalia, it is wind; and in Uzbekistan, salt and toxic chemicals are responsible.

Definitions of degradation are based on both biological productivity and our expectations about what the land should be like. Often this is a subjective judgment, and it is difficult to distinguish between human-caused deterioration and natural conditions, such as drought. We generally consider the land degraded when the soil is impoverished or eroded, water runs off or is contaminated more than normal, vegetation is diminished, biomass production is decreased, or wildlife diversity diminishes. On farmlands, this results in lower crop yields. On ranchlands, it means that fewer livestock can be supported per unit area. On nature reserves, it means lower biological diversity.

The amount and degree of land degradation vary by region and country. About 20 percent of land in Africa and Asia is degraded, but most is in either the light or the moderate category. In Central America and Mexico, by contrast, 25 percent of all vegetated land suffers moderate to extreme degradation. Figure 7.16 shows some areas of greatest concern for soil degradation, as well as the major mechanisms for this problem. Water and wind erosion provide the motive force for the vast majority of all soil degradation worldwide. Chemical degradation includes nutrient depletion, salt accumulation, acidification, and pollution. Physical degrada-

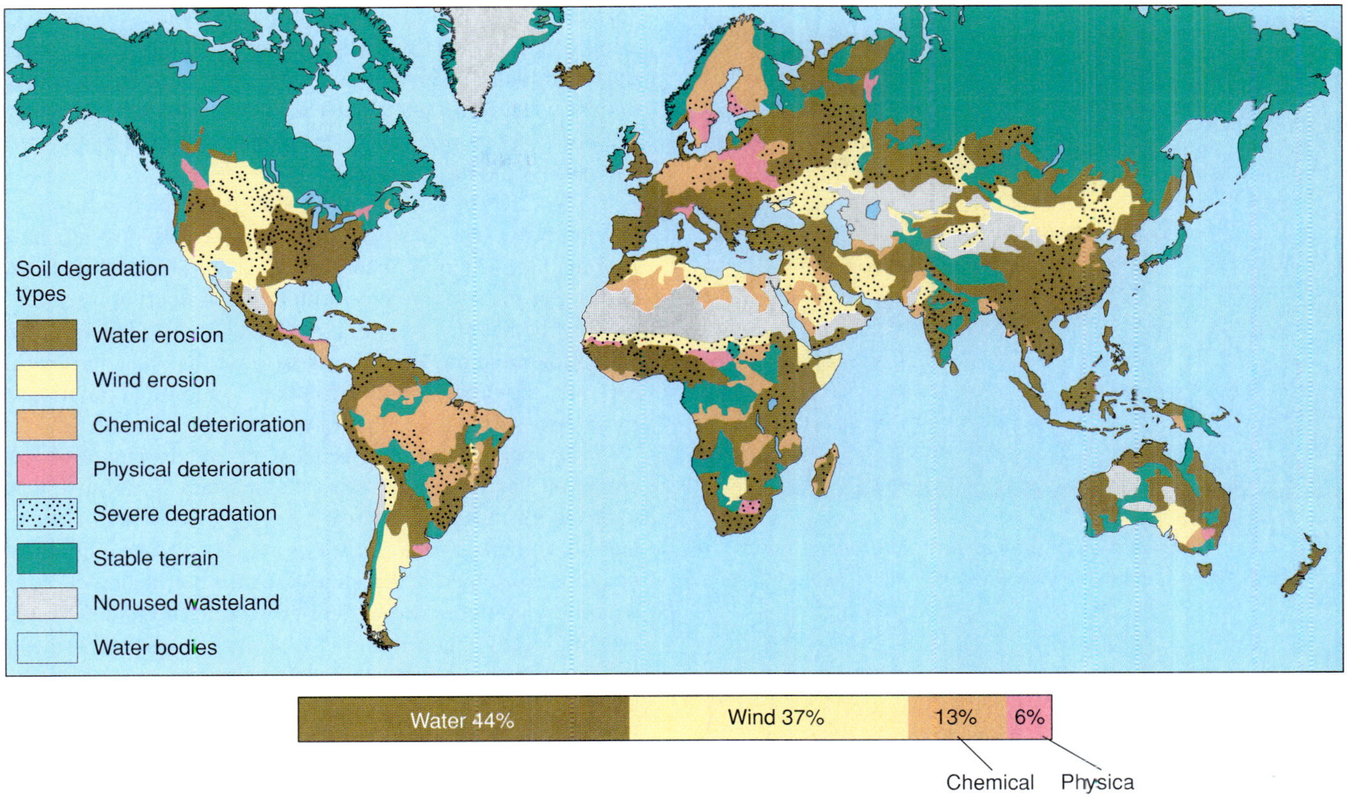

FIGURE 7.16 *Causes and locations of global soil degradation.*
Source: Data from Food and Agriculture Organization (FAO), 2003.

tion includes compaction by heavy machinery or trampling by cattle, water accumulation from excess irrigation and poor drainage, and laterization (solidification of iron and aluminum-rich tropical soil when exposed to sun and rain).

Erosion: The Nature of the Problem

Erosion is an important natural process, resulting in the redistribution of the products of geologic weathering, and it is part of both soil formation and soil loss. The world's landscapes have been sculpted by erosion. When the results are spectacular enough, we enshrine them in national parks, as we did with the Grand Canyon.

Where erosion has worn down mountains and spread soil over the plains or deposited rich alluvial silt in river bottoms, we farm it. Erosion is a disaster only when it occurs in the wrong place at the wrong time.

In some places, erosion occurs so rapidly that anyone can see it happen. Deep gullies are created where water scours away the soil, leaving fenceposts and trees sitting on tall pedestals as the land erodes away around them. In most places, however, erosion is more subtle. It is a creeping disaster that occurs in small increments. A thin layer of topsoil washes off of fields year after year until, eventually, nothing is left but poor-quality subsoil that requires more and more fertilizer and water to produce any crop at all.

It's estimated that 25 billion metric tons of soil are lost from croplands every year due to wind and water erosion. The net effect, worldwide, of this widespread topsoil erosion is a reduction in crop production equivalent to removing about 1 percent of the world's cropland each year. Many farmers are able to compensate for this loss by applying more fertilizer and by bringing new land into cultivation. Continuation of current erosion rates, however, could reduce agricultural production by 25 percent in Central America and Africa and by 20 percent in South America by 2020. The total annual soil loss from croplands is thought to be 25 billion metric tons. About twice that much soil is lost from rangelands, forests, and urban construction sites each year.

In addition to reduced land fertility, erosion results in sediment loading of rivers and lakes, siltation of reservoirs and harbors, smothering of wetlands and coral reefs, creation of "dead zones" in coastal regions, and clogging of water intakes and waterpower turbines.

Mechanisms of Erosion

Wind and water are the main agents that move soil around (see fig. 7.16). Water flowing across a gently sloping, bare field removes a thin, uniform layer of soil in what is known as **sheet erosion.** When little rivulets of running water gather together and cut small channels in the soil, the process is called **rill erosion** (fig. 7.17). If rills enlarge to form bigger channels or ravines that are too large to be removed by normal tillage operations, we call the process **gully erosion** (fig. 7.18). Streambank erosion is the washing away of soil

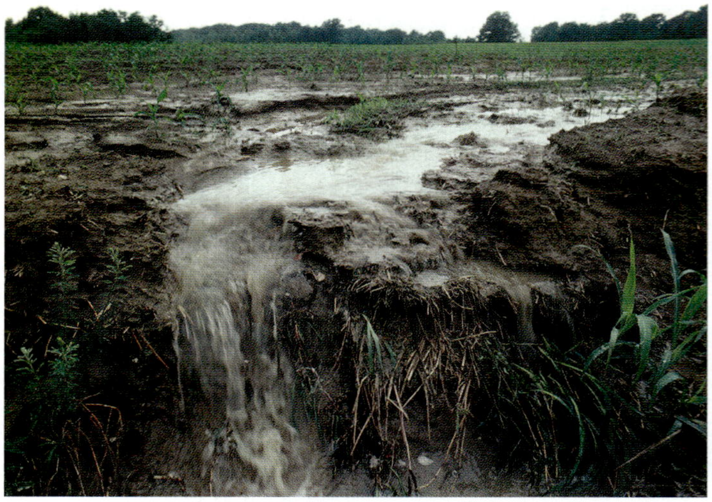

FIGURE 7.17 *Sheet and rill erosion remove soil from the entire surface of a field, cutting small channels in the soil, which generally are erased by plowing.*

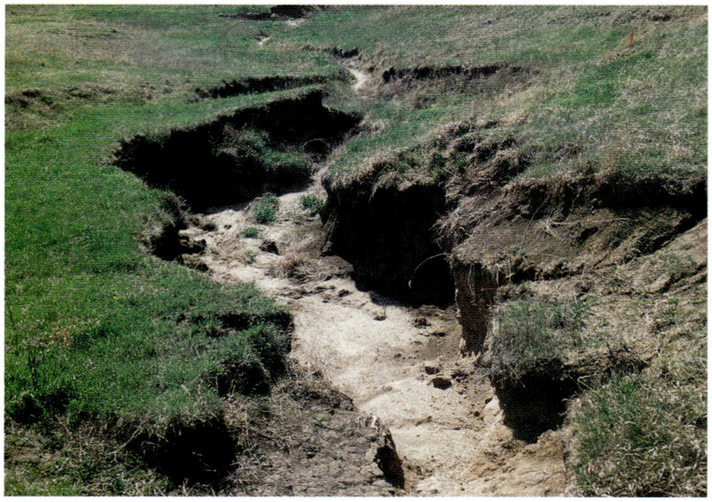

FIGURE 7.18 *Uncontrolled erosion has cut a deep gully through this Kansas pasture.*

from the banks of established streams, creeks, or rivers, often as a result of removing trees and brush along streambanks and of cattle damaging the banks.

Most soil erosion on agricultural land is rill erosion. Large amounts of soil can be transported a little bit at a time without being very noticeable. A farm field can lose 20 metric tons of soil per hectare during winter and spring runoff in rills so small that they are erased by the first spring cultivation. That represents a loss of only a few millimeters of soil over the whole surface of the field, hardly apparent to any but the most discerning eye. But it doesn't take much mathematical skill to see that, if you lose soil twice as fast as it is being replaced, it eventually will run out.

Wind can equal or exceed water in erosive force, especially in a dry climate and on relatively flat land. When plant cover and surface litter are removed from the land by agriculture or grazing, wind lifts loose soil particles and sweeps them away. Windborne dust is sometimes transported from one continent to another. Scientists in Hawaii can tell when spring plowing begins in China because dust from Chinese farmland is carried by winds all the way across the Pacific Ocean.

Some areas of the United States and Canada have very high erosion rates. The U.S. Department of Agriculture reports that 69 million ha (170 million acres) of U.S. farmland and range are eroding at rates that reduce long-term productivity. Eleven metric tons per hectare (5 tons per acre) is generally considered the maximum tolerable rate of soil loss because that is generally the highest rate at which soil forms under optimum conditions. Some farms lose soil at twice that rate or more.

Intensive farming practices are largely responsible for this situation. Row crops, such as corn and soybeans, leave soil exposed for much of the growing season (fig. 7.19). Deep plowing and heavy herbicide applications create weed-free fields that look neat but are subject to erosion. Because big machines cannot easily follow contours, they often go straight up and down the hills, creating ready-made gullies for water to follow. Farmers sometimes plow through grass-lined watercourses (low areas where water runs off after a rain) and pull out windbreaks and fencerows to accommodate the large machines and to get every last square meter into production. Consequently, wind and water carry away the topsoil.

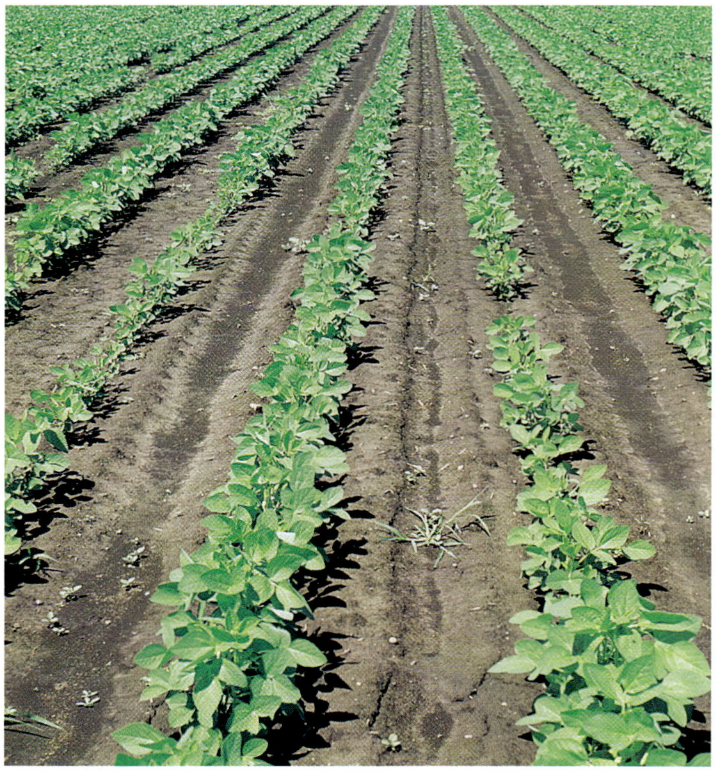

FIGURE 7.19 *Annual row crops leave soil bare and exposed to erosion for most of the year, especially when fields are plowed immediately after harvest, as this one always is.*

Erosion Hot Spots

Data on soil conditions and soil erosion often are incomplete, but it is evident that many places have problems as severe as, or perhaps worse than, those found in the United States and Canada. China, for example, has a large area of loess (windblown silt) deposits on the North China Plain that once was covered by forest and grassland. The forests were cut down, and the grasslands were converted to cropland. This plateau is now scarred by gullies 30 to 40 m (100 to 130 ft) deep, and the soil loss is thought to be at least 480 metric tons per ha per year, equivalent to 3 cm (1.2 in.) of topsoil lost per year.

One way to estimate soil loss is to measure the sediment load carried by rivers draining an area. China's Huang (Yellow) River, which flows through the loess plateau, transports 1.6 billion tons of sediment every year. Although its drainage basin is only one-fifth as big as that of the Mississippi River, the Huang carries more than four times as much soil each year. This suggests that the average soil loss per ha in northern China may be 20 times that in the United States.

OTHER AGRICULTURAL RESOURCES

Soil is only part of the agricultural resource picture. Agriculture is also dependent upon water, nutrients, favorable climates to grow crops, productive crop varieties, and the mechanical energy to tend and harvest the crops.

Water

All plants need water to grow (fig. 7.20). Agriculture accounts for the largest single share of global water use. At least two-thirds of all fresh water withdrawn from rivers, lakes, and groundwater supplies is used for irrigation (see chapter 10). Irrigation increases yields of most crops by 100 to 400 percent. Although estimates vary widely (as do definitions of irrigated land), about 15 percent of all cropland, worldwide, is irrigated.

Some countries are water rich and can readily afford to irrigate farmland, while other countries are water poor and must use water very carefully. The efficiency of irrigation water use varies greatly. High evaporative and seepage losses from unlined and uncovered canals in some places can mean that as much as 80 percent of water withdrawn for irrigation never reaches its intended destination. Poor farmers may overirrigate because they lack the technology to meter water and distribute just the amount needed.

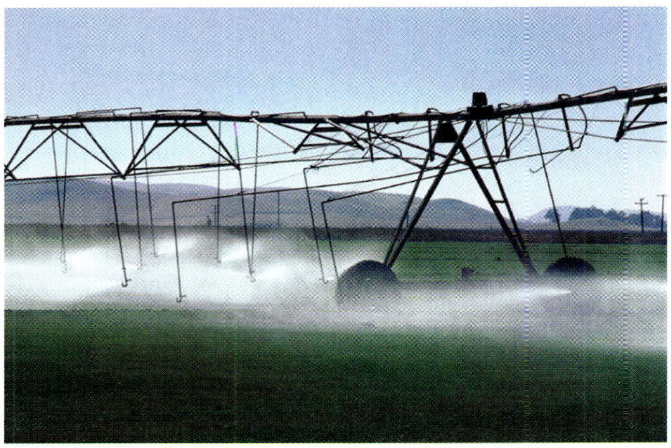

FIGURE 7.20 *Downward-facing sprinklers on this center-pivot irrigation system deliver water more efficiently than upward-facing sprinklers.*

Excessive use not only wastes water but also often results in **waterlogging.** Waterlogged soil is saturated with water, and plant roots die from lack of oxygen. **Salinization,** in which mineral salts accumulate in the soil, is often a problem when irrigation water dissolves and mobilizes salts in the soil. As the water evaporates, it leaves behind a salty crust on the soil surface that is lethal to most plants. Flushing with excess water can wash away this salt accumulation, but the result is even more saline water for downstream users.

The FAO estimates that 20 percent of all irrigated land is damaged to some extent by waterlogging or salinity. Water conservation techniques can greatly reduce problems arising from excess water use. Conservation also makes more water available for other uses or for expanded crop production where water is in short supply (see chapter 10).

Fertilizer

In addition to water, sunshine, and carbon dioxide, plants need small amounts of inorganic nutrients for growth. The major elements required by most plants are nitrogen, potassium, phosphorus, calcium, magnesium, and sulfur. Calcium and magnesium often are limited in areas of high rainfall and must be supplied in the form of lime. Lack of nitrogen, potassium, and phosphorus often limits plant growth even more. Adding these elements in fertilizer usually stimulates growth and greatly increases crop yields. A good deal of the doubling in worldwide crop production since 1950 has come from increased inorganic fertilizer use. In 1950 the average amount of fertilizer used was 20 kg per ha. In 2000 this had increased to an average of 90 kg per ha worldwide.

Farmers may overfertilize because they are unaware of the specific nutrient content of their soils or the needs of their crops. While European farmers use more than twice as much fertilizer per hectare as do North American farmers, their yields are not proportionally higher. Phosphates and nitrates from farm fields and cattle feedlots are a major cause of aquatic ecosystem pollution. Nitrate levels in groundwater have risen to dangerous levels in many areas where intensive farming is practiced. Young children are especially sensitive to the presence of nitrates. Using nitrate-contaminated water to mix infant formula can be fatal for newborns.

What are some alternative ways to fertilize crops? Manure and green manure (crops grown specifically to add nutrients to the soil) are important natural sources of soil nutrients. Nitrogen-fixing bacteria living symbiotically in root nodules of legumes are valuable for making nitrogen available as a plant nutrient (see chapter 2). Interplanting and rotating beans or some other leguminous crop with such crops as corn and wheat are traditional ways of increasing nitrogen availability.

There is considerable potential for increasing the world's food supply by increasing fertilizer use in low-production countries if ways can be found to apply fertilizer more effectively and to reduce pollution. Africa, for instance, uses an average of only

19 kg of fertilizer per ha (17 lbs per acre), or about one-fourth of the world average. It has been estimated that the developing world could at least triple its crop production by raising fertilizer use to the world average.

Energy

Farming as it is generally practiced in the industrialized countries is highly energy-intensive. Fossil fuels supply almost all of this energy. Between 1920 and 1980, direct energy use on farms rose as gasoline and diesel fuels were consumed by increasing mechanization of agriculture. Indirect energy use, in the form of synthetic fertilizers, pesticides, and other agricultural chemicals, increased even more, especially after World War II. On intensively fertilized farms, indirect energy use may be five times that of direct energy. The energy price shocks of the 1970s encouraged energy conservation that has reduced farm energy use, even though total food production has continued to rise.

After crops leave the farm, additional energy is used in food processing, distribution, storage, and cooking. It has been estimated that the average food item in the American diet travels 2,000 km (1,250 mi) between the farm that grew it and the person who consumes it. The energy required for this complex processing and distribution system may be five times as much as is used directly in farming. As a whole, the food system in the United States consumes about 16 percent of the total energy we use. Most of our foods require more energy to produce, process, and get to market than they yield when we eat them.

Clearly, unless we find some new energy sources, our present system is unsustainable. As fossil fuels become more scarce, we may need to adopt farming methods that are self-supporting. Is it possible that we may need to go back to using draft animals that can eat crops grown on the farm? Could we reintroduce natural methods of pest control, fertilization, crop drying, and irrigation? Or can we develop alternative energy sources to run our farming enterprise?

Pest Control

Biological pests reduce crop yields and spoil as much as half of the crops harvested every year in some areas. Modern agriculture largely depends on toxic chemicals to kill or drive away these pests, but there are many serious concerns about the types and amounts of pesticides now in use.

There are many traditional methods for protecting crops from pests, but our war against unwanted organisms entered a new phase in the twentieth century with the invention of synthetic organic chemicals, such as DDT (dichlorodiphenyltrichloroethane). These chemicals have been an important part of our increased crop production and have helped control many disease-causing organisms. It's estimated that up to half our current crop yields might be lost if we had no pesticides to protect them. Indiscriminate and profligate pesticide use, however, also has caused many problems, such as killing nontarget species, creating new pests of organisms that previously were not a problem, and causing widespread pesticide resistance among pest species (fig. 7.21). Often highly persistent and mobile in the environment, many pesticides have moved through air, water, and soil and bioaccumulated or bioconcentrated in food chains, nearly exterminating several top predators, such as peregrine falcons.

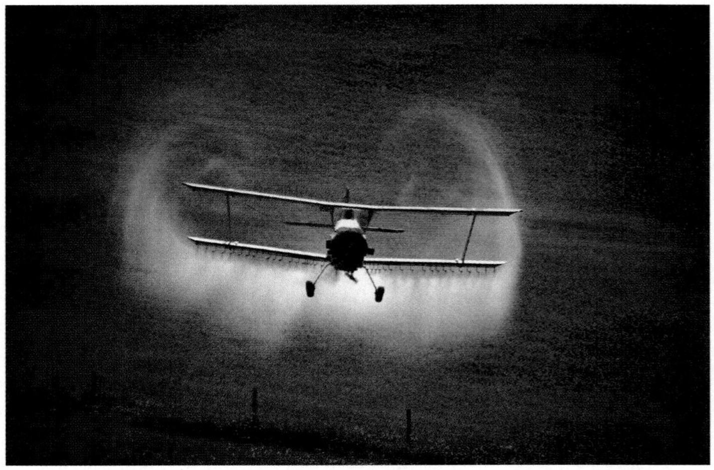

FIGURE 7.21 *Spraying pesticides by air is quick and cheap, but toxins often drift to nearby fields.*

Your exposure to pesticides is probably higher than you suspect. A study by the U.S. Department of Agriculture found that 73 percent of conventionally grown foods (out of 94,000 samples assayed) had residues from at least one pesticide. By contrast, only 23 percent of the organic samples of the same food groups had any residues. It is now clear that humans suffer adverse health effects from persistent organic pollutants (POPs), such as pesticides. In fact, most of the "dirty dozen" POPs recently banned globally are pesticides. See chapter 8 for more on health effects of POPs.

In 2002 Swiss researchers published results of a two-decades-long comparison of organic and conventional farming. Crops grown without synthetic fertilizers or pesticides produced, on average, about a 20 percent lower yield than similar crops grown by conventional methods, but they more than made up the difference with lower operating costs, premium crop prices, less ecological damage, and healthier farm families.

Some alternatives for reducing our dependence on dangerous chemical pesticides include management changes, such as using cover crops and mechanical cultivation, and planting mixed polycultures rather than vast monoculture fields. Consumers may have to learn to accept less than perfect fruits and vegetables if we want to avoid toxic chemicals in our diet. Biological controls, such as insect predators, pathogens, or natural poisons specific for a particular pest, can help reduce chemical use. Genetic breeding and biotechnology can produce pest-resistant crop and livestock strains as well. Integrated pest management (IPM) is a relatively new science that combines all of these alternative methods, together with judicious use of synthetic pesticides under precisely controlled conditions. There are ways that you can minimize pesticides in your diet (see What Can You Do? page 165).

what can you do?

Reducing the Pesticides in Your Food

If you want to reduce the amount of pesticide residues and other toxic chemicals in your diet, follow these simple rules.

- Wash and scrub all fresh fruits and vegetables thoroughly under running water.
- Peel fruits and vegetables when possible. Throw away the outer leaves of leafy vegetables, such as lettuce and cabbage.
- Store food carefully so it doesn't get moldy or pick up contaminants from other foods. Use food as soon as possible to ensure freshness.
- Cook or bake foods that you suspect have been treated with pesticides to break down chemical residues.
- Trim the fat from meat, chicken, and fish. Eat lower on the food chain when possible to reduce bioaccumulated chemicals.
- Don't pick and eat berries or other wild foods that grow on the edges of roadsides where pesticides may have been sprayed.
- Grow your own fruits and vegetables without using pesticides or with minimal use of dangerous chemicals.
- Ask for organically grown food at your local grocery store, or shop at a farmer's market or co-op where you can get such food

NEW CROPS AND GENETIC ENGINEERING

Although at least 3,000 species of plants have been used for food at one time or another, most of the world's food now comes from only 16 widely grown crops. Many new or unconventional varieties might be valuable human food supplies, however, especially in areas where conventional crops are limited by climate, soil, pests, or other problems. Among the plants now being investigated as potential additions to our crop roster is the winged bean, a perennial plant that grows well in hot climates where other legumes will not grow. It is totally edible (pods, mature seeds, shoots, flowers, leaves, and tuberous roots), resistant to diseases, and enriches the soil. Another promising crop is triticale, a hybrid between wheat (*Triticum*) and rye (*Secale*) that grows in light, sandy, infertile soil. It is drought-resistant, has nutritious seeds, and is being tested for salt tolerance for growth in saline soils or irrigation with seawater. Some traditional crop varieties grown by Native Americans, such as tepary beans, amaranth, and Sonoran panic grass, are being collected by seed conservator Gary Nabhan, both as a form of cultural revival for native people and as possible food crops for harsh environments.

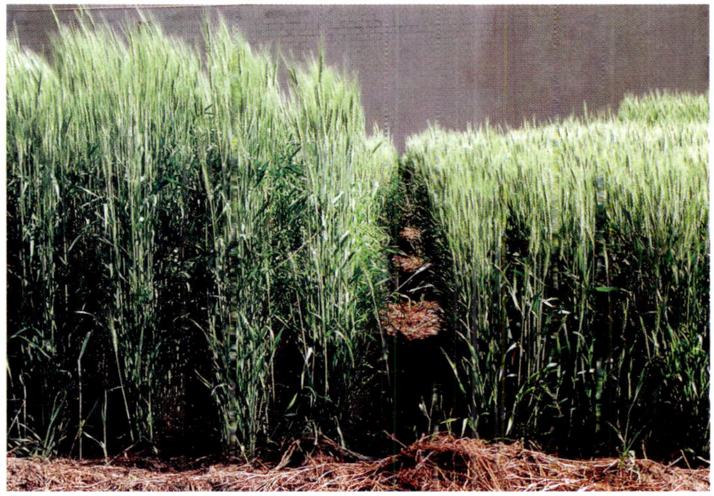

FIGURE 7.22 *Semidwarf wheat* (right), *bred by Norman Borlaug, has shorter, stiffer stems and is less likely to lodge (fall over) when wet than its conventional cousin* (left). *This "miracle" wheat responds better to water and fertilizer and has played a vital role in feeding a growing human population.*

The Green Revolution

So far, the major improvements in farm production have come from technological advances and modification of a few well-known species. Yield increases often have been spectacular. A century ago, when all maize (corn) in the United States was open pollinated, average yields were about 25 bushels per acre (bu/acre). In 2000 the average yield from rainfed fields in Iowa was 138 bu/acre, and irrigated maize in Arizona averaged 208 bu/acre. The highest yield ever recorded in field production was 370 bu/acre on an Illinois farm, but theoretical calculations suggest that 500 bu/acre (32 metric tons per hectare) could be possible. Most of this gain was accomplished by use of synthetic fertilizers along with conventional plant breeding: geneticists laboriously hand-pollinating plants and looking for desired characteristics in the progeny.

Starting about 50 years ago, agricultural research stations began to breed tropical wheat and rice varieties that would provide food for growing populations in developing countries. The first of the "miracle" varieties was a dwarf, high-yielding wheat developed by Norman Borlaug (who received a Nobel Peace Prize for his work) at a research center in Mexico (fig. 7.22). At about the same time, the International Rice Institute in the Philippines developed dwarf rice strains with three or four times the production of varieties in use at the time. The spread of these new high-yield varieties around the world has been called the **green revolution.** It is one of the main reasons that world food supplies have more than kept pace with the growing human population over the past few decades.

Most green revolution breeds really are "high responders," meaning that they yield more than other varieties if given optimum levels of fertilizer, water, and protection from pests and diseases (fig. 7.23). Under suboptimum conditions, on the other hand, high responders may not produce as well as traditional varieties. Poor farmers who can't afford the expensive seed, fertilizer, and water required to become part of this movement usually are left out of the green revolution. In fact, they may be driven out of farming altogether as rising land values and falling commodity prices squeeze them from both sides.

Genetic Engineering

Genetic engineering, splicing a gene from one organism into the chromosome of another, has the potential to greatly increase both the quantity and the quality of our food supply. It is now possible to build entirely new genes, and even new organisms, often called "transgenic" organisms or **genetically modified organisms (GMOs),** by taking a bit of DNA from here, a bit from there, and even synthesizing artificial sequences to create desired characteristics in engineered organisms (fig. 7.24).

Proponents predict dramatic benefits from this new technology. Research is now underway to improve yields and create crops that resist drought, frost, or diseases. Other strains are being developed to tolerate salty, waterlogged, or low-nutrient soils, allowing degraded or marginal farmland to become productive. All of these could be important for reducing hunger in developing countries. Plants that produce their own pesticides might reduce the need for toxic chemicals, while engineering for improved protein or vitamin content could make our food more nutritious (see opening story in this chapter). Attempts to remove specific toxins or allergens from crops also could make our food safer. Crops such as bananas and tomatoes have been altered to contain oral vaccines that can be grown in developing countries where refrigeration and sterile needles are unavailable. Plants have been engineered to make industrial oils and plastics. Animals, too, are being genetically modified to grow faster, gain weight on less food, and produce pharmaceuticals, such as insulin, in their milk. It may even be possible to create animals with human cell-recognition factors that could serve as organ donors.

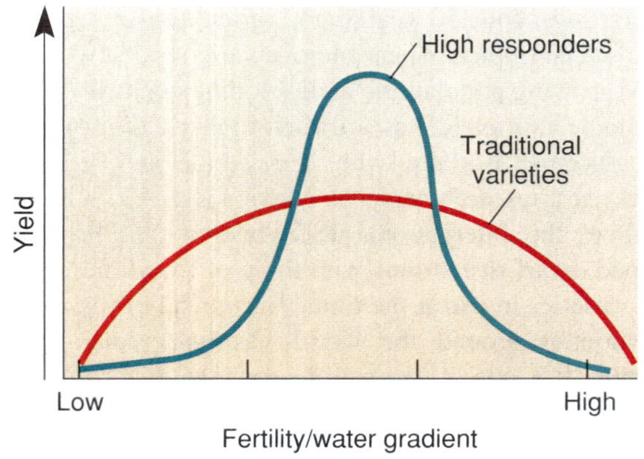

FIGURE 7.23 *Green revolution miracle crops are really high responders, meaning that they have excellent yields under optimum conditions. For poor farmers who can't afford the fertilizer and water needed by high responders, traditional varieties may produce better yields.*

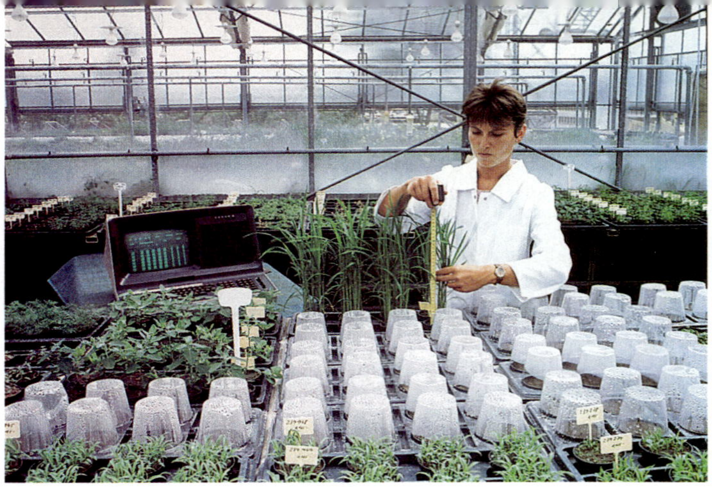

FIGURE 7.24 *A researcher measures growth of genetically engineered rice plants. Superior growth and yield, pest resistance, and other useful traits can be moved from one species to another by molecular biotechnology.*

Opponents worry that moving genes willy-nilly could create a host of problems, some of which we can't even imagine. GMOs themselves might escape and become pests or they might interbreed wild relatives. In either case, we may create superweeds or reduce native biodiversity. Constant presence of pesticides in plants could accelerate pesticide resistance in insects or leave toxic residues in soil or our food. Genes for toxicity or allergies could be transferred along with desirable genes, or novel toxins could be created as genes are mixed together. This technology may be available only to the richest countries or the wealthiest corporations, making family farms uncompetitive and driving developing countries even further into poverty.

Both the number of GMO crops and the acreage devoted to growing them is increasing rapidly. Between 1987 and 2003, more than 8,800 field tests for some 750 different crop varieties were carried out in the United States (fig. 7.25). Hawaii is the most popular site for GMO testing, with about 1,500 field releases over the past 16 years. Illinois, Iowa, California, and Puerto Rico each had more than 1,000 tests during that time. Worldwide, 53 million ha (131 million acres) were planted with GMO crops in 2003. The United States accounted for 68 percent of that acreage, followed by Argentina with 23 percent. Canada, Australia, Mexico, China, and South Africa together make up 9 percent of all transgenic cropland.

Some transgenic crops have reached mainstream status. About 82 percent of all soybeans, one-quarter of all maize (corn), and 71 percent of all cotton grown in the United States are now GMOs. You've already probably eaten some genetically modified food. Estimates are that at least 60 percent of all processed food in America contains GMO ingredients. Since the United States, Argentina, and Brazil account for 90 percent of international trade in maize and soybeans (in which GMOs often are mixed with other grains), a large fraction of the world most likely has been exposed to some GMO products.

Pest Resistance and Weed Control

Biotechnologists have created plants with genes for endogenous insecticides. *Bacillus thuringiensis* (Bt), a bacterium, makes tox-

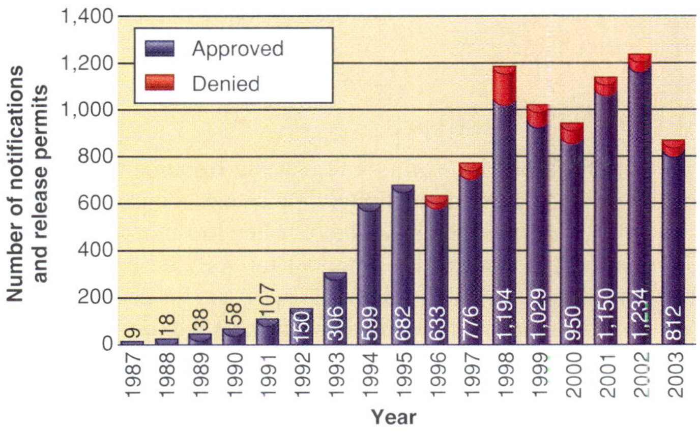

FIGURE 7.25 *Transgenic crop field releases in the United States 1987–2003.*

Source: Data from Information Systems for Biotechnology, Virginia Tech University.

ins lethal to Lepidoptera (butterfly family) and Coleoptera (beetle family). The genes for some of these toxins have been transferred into crops such as maize (to protect against European cutworms), potatoes (to fight potato beetles), and cotton (to protect against boll weevils). This allows farmers to reduce insecticide spraying. Arizona cotton farmers, for example, report reducing their use of chemical insecticides by 75 percent.

Most European nations have not approved Bt-containing varieties. Fear of transgenic products has been a sticking point in agricultural trade between the United States and the European Union.

In 2001 Starlink, a Bt-containing maize variety that had not yet been approved for human consumption, was found mixed into a wide variety of consumer products. By the time food was made from Starlink, no Bt could be detected, only the genes that code for it. There is no evidence that Bt is harmful to humans, but the form in Starlink may be allergenic. In fact, Bt is one of the few insecticides approved for organic farmers. Nevertheless, a public outcry ensued and seed companies, farmers, shippers, and food processors spent more than $1 billion trying to remove it from the food chain. What do you think: was the fear of Starlink justified?

Entomologists worry that Bt plants churn out toxin throughout the growing season, regardless of the level of infestation, creating perfect conditions for selection of Bt resistance in pests. Already 500 species of insect, mite, or tick are resistant to one or more pesticides. Having Bt constantly available can only aggravate this dilemma. One solution is to plant at least a part of every field in non-Bt crops that will act as a refuge for nonresistant pests. The hope is that interbreeding between these "wild-type" bugs and those exposed to Bt will dilute out recessive resistance genes. Deliberately harboring pests and letting them munch freely on crops is something that many farmers find hard to do. In addition, devoting a significant part of their land to nonproductive crops lowers the total yield and counteracts the profitability of engineered seed.

The other major group of transgenic crops is engineered to tolerate high doses of herbicides. The two dominant products in this category are Monsanto's "Roundup Ready" crops—so-called because they can withstand treatment with Monsanto's best-selling herbicide, Roundup (glyphosate)—and AgrEvo's "Liberty Link" crops, which resist that company's Liberty (glufosinate) herbicide. Because crops with these genes can grow in spite of high herbicide doses, farmers can spray fields heavily to exterminate weeds. This allows for conservation tillage and leaving more crop residue on fields to protect topsoil from erosion—both good ideas—but it also can mean using more herbicide in higher doses than might otherwise be done.

Is Genetic Engineering Safe?

Ever since scientists discovered how to move genes from one organism to another, critics have worried about irresponsible use of this technology or unforeseen consequences arising from novel combinations of genetic material. Greenpeace and several other environmental groups have campaigned against transgenic organisms, labeling them "Frankenfoods." Industry groups, on the other hand, describe their critics as Neo-Luddites, who blindly oppose any new technology. How can we decide what to believe in this welter of claims and counterclaims?

At the base of some people's unease with genetic modification is a feeling that it simply isn't right to mess with nature. It doesn't seem proper to recombine genes any way we want. Doing so raises specters of gruesome monsters stitched together from spare parts, like Mary Shelley's Frankenstein. Is this merely a fear of science, or is it a valid ethical issue?

The U.S. Food and Drug Administration declined to require labeling of foods containing GMOs, saying that these new varieties are "substantially equivalent" to related varieties bred via traditional practices. After all, proponents say, we have been moving genes around for centuries through plant and animal breeding. All domesticated organisms should be classified as genetically modified, some people argue. Biotechnology may be a more precise way of creating novel organisms than normal breeding procedures, its supporters suggest. We're moving only a few genes—or even part of one gene—at a time with biotechnology, rather than hundreds of unknown genes through classical techniques.

But what if GMOs escape and crossbreed with native species? In a ten-year study of genetically modified crops, a group from Imperial College, London, concluded that GMOs tested so far do not survive well in the wild and are no more likely to invade other habitats than their unmodified counterparts.

On the other hand, there is already evidence that some GMO crops can spread their genes to nearby fields. Normal rape seed (canola oil) varieties in Canada were found to contain genes from genetically modified varieties in nearby fields. It isn't clear, however, if the genes involved will have any adverse affect or whether they will persist for many generations. In 2001 researchers reported finding traces of genetically modified corn in wild relatives in Mexico, which supposedly has banned planting of GMOs, especially in regions where species were thought to have originated. This report was later withdrawn due to criticism of the techniques used to detect genetic markers, but it gave an interesting insight into the politics and sociology of science.

The first genetically modified animal designed to be eaten by humans is an Atlantic salmon (*Salmo salar*) containing extra growth hormone genes from an oceanic pout (*Macrozoarces americanus*). The greatest worry from this fish is not that it will introduce extra hormones into our diet—that's already being done by chickens and beef that get extra growth hormone via injections or their diet—but, rather, the ecological effects if the fish escape from captivity. The transgenic fish grow seven times faster and are more attractive to the opposite sex than a normal salmon. If they escape from captivity, they may outcompete already endangered wild relatives for food, mates, and habitat. Fish farmers say they will grow only sterile females and will keep them in secure net pens. Opponents point out that salmon frequently escape from aquaculture operations and that, if just a few fertile transgenic fish break out, it could be catastrophic for wild stocks.

Many scientists argue that we should take a better-safe-than-sorry "precautionary approach" that errs—if at all—on the side of safety. The 5,000-member Society of Toxicology recently concluded that, "based on available tests, there's no reason to suspect that transgenic plants differ in any substantive way from traditional varieties." On the other hand, a panel of biologists and agricultural scientists convened by the U.S. National Academy of Sciences urged the government to more carefully, and more publicly, review the potential environmental impacts of genetically modified plants and animals before approving them for commercial use.

Finally, there are social and economic implications of GMOs. Will they help feed the world, or will they lead to a greater consolidation of corporate power and economic disparity? Might higher yields and fewer losses to pests and diseases allow poor farmers in developing countries to stop using marginal land and avoid cutting down forests to create farmland? Is this simply a technological fix, or could it help promote agricultural sustainability? Critics suggest that there are simpler and cheaper ways other than high-tech crop varieties to provide vitamin A to children in developing countries or to increase the income of poor rural families. Adding a cow or a fishpond or training people in water harvesting or regenerative farming techniques (as we'll discuss in the next section) may have a longer-lasting impact than selling them expensive new seeds.

On the other hand, if we hope to reduce malnutrition and feed eight billion people in 50 years, maybe we need all the tools we can get. Where do you stand in this debate? What additional information would you need to reach a reasoned judgment about the risks and benefits of this new technology?

SUSTAINABLE AGRICULTURE

How, then, shall we feed the world? Can we make agriculture compatible with sustainable ecological and social systems? Having discussed some of the problems that beset modern agriculture, we now consider some suggested ways to overcome problems and make farming and food production just and lasting enterprises. This goal is usually termed **sustainable agriculture,** or **regenerative farming,** both of which aim to produce food and fiber on a sustainable basis and repair the damage caused by destructive practices. Some alternative methods are developed through scientific research; others are discovered in traditional cultures and practices nearly forgotten in our mechanization and industrialization of agriculture.

Soil Conservation

With careful husbandry, soil is a renewable resource that can be replenished and renewed indefinitely. Since agriculture is the area in which soil is most essential and most often lost through erosion, agriculture offers the greatest potential for soil conservation and rebuilding. Some rice paddies in Southeast Asia, for instance, have been farmed continuously for a thousand years without any apparent loss of fertility. The rice-growing cultures that depend on these fields have developed management practices that return organic material to the paddies and carefully nurture the soil's ability to sustain life.

While American agriculture hasn't reached that level of sustainability, there is evidence that soil conservation programs are having a positive effect. In one Wisconsin study, erosion rates in one small watershed were 90 percent less in 1975–1993 than they were in the 1930s. Among the most important elements in soil conservation are topography management, ground cover, and reduced tillage.

Managing Topography

Water runs downhill. The faster it runs, the more soil it carries off the fields. Comparisons of erosion rates in Africa have shown that a 5 percent slope in a plowed field has three times the water runoff volume and eight times the soil erosion rate of a comparable field with a 1 percent slope. Water runoff can be reduced by grass strips in waterways and by **contour plowing**—that is, plowing across the hill rather than up and down. Contour plowing is often combined with **strip-farming,** the planting of different kinds of crops in alternating strips along the land contours (fig. 7.26). When one crop is harvested, the other is still present to protect the soil and keep water from running straight downhill. The ridges created by cultivation make little dams that trap water and allow it to seep into the soil, rather than running off. In areas where rainfall is very heavy, tied ridges are often useful. This method involves a series of ridges running at right angles to each other, so that water runoff is blocked in all directions and is encouraged to soak into the soil.

Terracing involves shaping the land to create level shelves of earth to hold water and soil (fig. 7.27). The edges of the terrace are planted with soil-anchoring plant species. This is an expensive procedure, requiring either much hand labor or expensive machinery, but it makes farming of very steep hillsides possible. The rice terraces in the Chico River Valley in the Philippines rise as much as 300 m (1,000 ft) above the valley floor. They are considered one of the wonders of the world.

Planting **perennial species** (plants that grow for more than two years) is the only suitable use for some lands and some soil types. Establishing forest, grassland, or crops such as tea, coffee, or other crops that do not have to be cultivated every year may be necessary to protect certain unstable soils on sloping sites or watercourses. The $180 billion U.S. Farm Bill passed in 2002 includes $17 billion (over ten years) to encourage soil, water, and wildlife conservation.

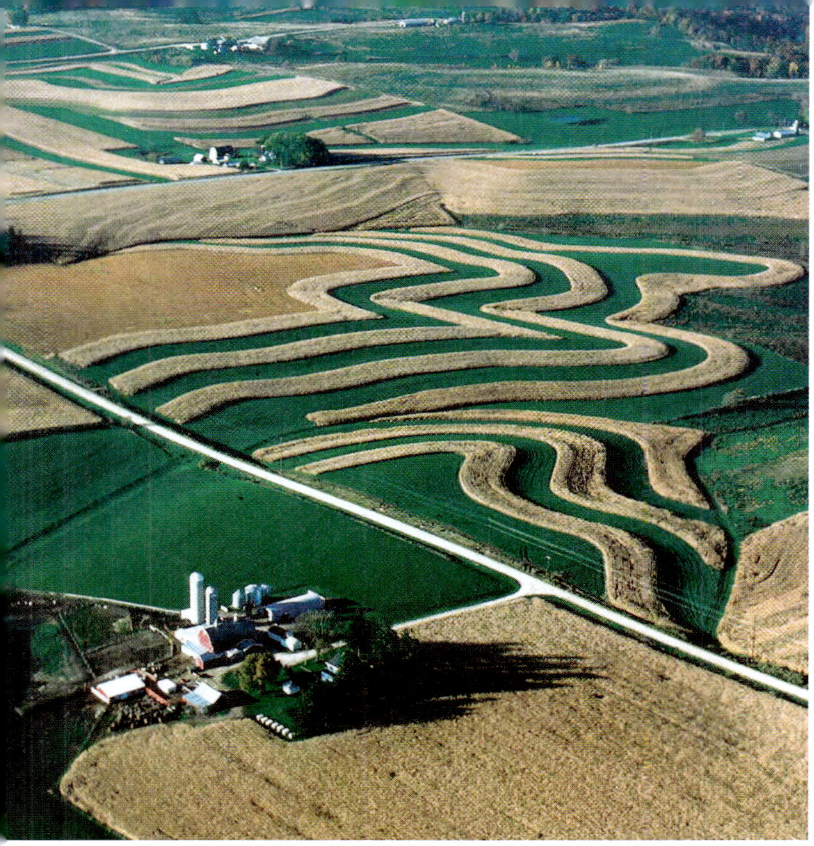

FIGURE 7.26 *Contour plowing and strip cropping help prevent soil erosion on hilly terrain, as well as create a beautiful landscape.*

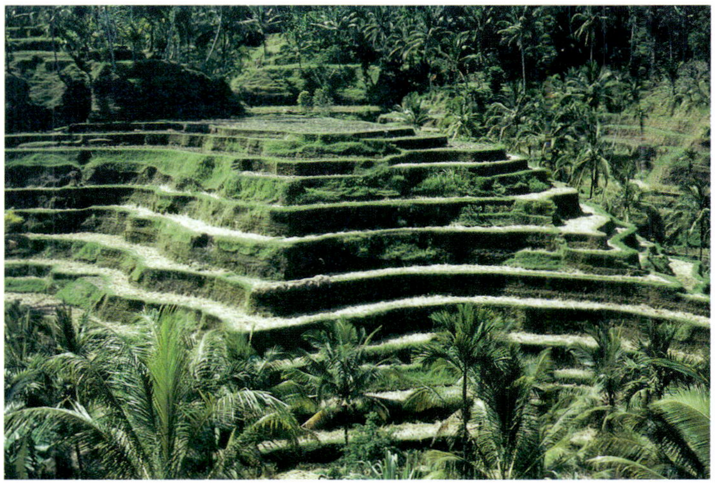

FIGURE 7.27 *Rice terraces in Indonesia. Some rice paddies have been cultivated for hundreds or even thousands of years without any apparent loss of productivity.*

Providing Groundcover

Annual row crops, such as corn or beans, generally cause the highest erosion rates because they leave soil bare for much of the year (table 7.2). Often the easiest way to provide cover that protects soil from erosion is to leave crop residues on the land after harvest. They not only cover the surface to break the erosive effects of wind and water but also reduce evaporation and soil temperature in hot climates and protect ground organisms that help aerate and rebuild soil. In some experiments, 1 ton of crop residue per acre (0.4 ha) increased water infiltration 99 percent, reduced runoff 99 percent, and reduced erosion 98 percent. Leaving crop residues on the field also can increase disease and pest problems, however, and may require increased use of pesticides and herbicides.

TABLE 7.2 Soil Cover and Soil Erosion

CROPPING SYSTEM	AVERAGE ANNUAL SOIL LOSS (TONS/HECTARE)	PERCENT RAINFALL RUNOFF
Bare soil (no crop)	41.0	30
Continuous corn	19.7	29
Continuous wheat	10.1	23
Rotation: corn, wheat, clover	2.7	14
Continuous bluegrass	0.3	12

Source: Based on 14 years of data from Missouri Experiment Station, Columbia, Missouri.

Where crop residues are not adequate to protect the soil or are inappropriate for subsequent crops or farming methods, such **cover crops** as rye, alfalfa, and clover can be planted immediately after harvest to hold and protect the soil. These cover crops can be plowed under at planting time to provide green manure. Another method is to flatten cover crops with a roller and drill seeds through the residue to provide a continuous protective cover during early stages of crop growth.

In some cases, interplanting of two different crops in the same field not only protects the soil but also is a more efficient use of the land, providing double harvests. Native Americans and pioneer farmers, for instance, planted beans or pumpkins between the corn rows. The beans provided nitrogen needed by the corn, the pumpkins crowded out weeds, and both crops provided foods that nutritionally balance corn. Traditional swidden (slash-and-burn) cultivators in Africa and South America often plant as many as 20 different crops together in small plots. The crops mature at different times, so that there is always something to eat, and the soil is never exposed to erosion for very long. Shade-grown coffee and cocoa can play important roles in conserving biodiversity (see Case Study, p. 170).

Mulch is a general term for a protective groundcover that includes manure, wood chips, straw, seaweed, leaves, and other natural products. For some high-value crops, such as tomatoes, pineapples, and cucumbers, it is cost-effective to cover the ground with heavy paper or plastic sheets to protect the soil, save water, and prevent weed growth. Israel uses millions of square meters of plastic mulch to grow crops in the Negev Desert.

Reduced Tillage

Farmers have traditionally used a moldboard plow to till the soil, digging a deep trench and turning the topsoil upside down. In the

CASE STUDY

SHADE-GROWN COFFEE AND COCOA

Has it ever occurred to you that your purchases of coffee and chocolate may be contributing to the protection or destruction of tropical forests? Both coffee and cocoa are examples of food products grown exclusively in the Third World but consumed almost entirely in the First World (vanilla and bananas are some other examples). Coffee grows in cool, mountain areas of the tropics, while cocoa is native to the warm, moist lowlands. Both are small trees of the forest understory, adapted to low light levels.

Until a few decades ago, most of the world's coffee and cocoa were **shade-grown** under a canopy of large forest trees. Recently, however, new varieties of both crops have been developed that can be grown in full sun. Because more coffee or cocoa trees can be crowded into these fields, and they get more solar energy than in a shaded plantation, yields for sun-grown crops are higher.

There are costs, however, in this new technology. Sun-grown trees die earlier from the stress and diseases common in these fields. Furthermore, ornithologists have found that the number of bird species can be cut in half in full-sun plantations, and the number of individual birds may be reduced by 90 percent. Shade-grown coffee and cocoa generally require fewer pesticides (or sometimes none) because the birds and insects residing in the forest canopy eat many of the pests. Shade-grown plantations also need less chemical fertilizer because many of the plants in these complex forests add nutrients to the soil. In addition, shade-grown crops rarely need to be irrigated because heavy leaf fall protects the soil, while forest cover reduces evaporation.

Currently, about 40 percent of the world's coffee and cocoa plantations have been converted to full-sun varieties and another 25 percent are in process. Traditional techniques for coffee and cocoa production are worth preserving. Thirteen of the world's 25 biodiversity hot spots occur in coffee or cocoa regions. If all the 20 million ha (49 million acres) of coffee and cocoa plantations in these areas are converted to monocultures, an incalculable number of species will be lost.

The Brazilian state of Bahia is a good example of both the ecological importance of these crops and how they might help preserve forest species. At one time, Brazil produced much of the world's cocoa, but in the early 1900s, the crop was introduced into West Africa. Now Côte d'Ivoire alone grows more than 40 percent of the world total, and the value of Brazil's harvest has dropped by 90 percent. Côte d'Ivoire is aided in this competition by a labor system that reportedly includes widespread child slavery. Even adult workers in Côte d'Ivoire get only about \$165 (U.S.) per year (if they get paid at all), compared with a minimum wage of \$850 (U.S.) per year in Brazil. As African cocoa production ratchets up, Brazilian landowners are converting their plantations to pastures or other crops.

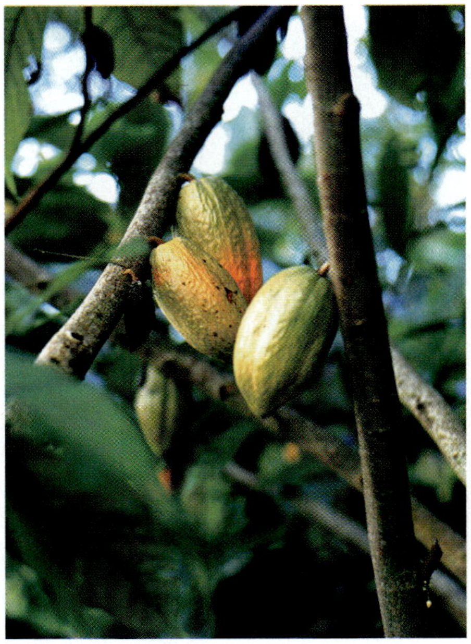

Cocoa pods grow directly on the trunk and large branches of cocoa trees.

The area of Bahia where cocoa was once king is part of Brazil's Atlantic Forest, one of the most threatened forest biomes in the world. Only 8 percent of this forest remains undisturbed. Although cocoa plantations don't represent the full diversity of intact forests, they protect a surprisingly large sample of what once was there. And shade-grown cocoa can provide an economic rationale for preserving that biodiversity. Brazilian cocoa will probably never compete with that from other areas for lowest cost. There is room in the market, however, for specialty products. If consumers were willing to pay a small premium for organic, fair-trade, shade-grown chocolate and coffee, it might provide the incentive needed to preserve biodiversity. Wouldn't you like to know that your chocolate or coffee wasn't grown with child slavery and is helping protect plants and animal species that might otherwise go extinct?

1800s it was shown that tilling a field fully—until it was "clean"—increased crop production. It helped control weeds and pests, reducing competition; it brought fresh nutrients to the surface, providing a good seedbed; and it improved surface drainage and aerated the soil. This is still true for many crops and many soil types, but it is not always the best way to grow crops. Less plowing and cultivation often improves water management, preserves soil, saves energy, and increases crop yields.

There are three major **reduced tillage systems.** *Minimum till* involves reducing the number of times a farmer disturbs the soil by plowing, cultivating, and so on. This often involves a disc or chisel plow rather than a traditional moldboard plow. A chisel plow is a curved, chisel-like blade that doesn't turn the soil over but creates ridges on which seeds can be planted. It leaves up to 75 percent of plant debris on the surface between the rows, preventing erosion (fig. 7.28). *Conserv-till* farming uses a coulter (a sharp, disc like a pizza cutter), which slices through the soil, opening up a furrow, or slot, just wide enough to insert seeds. This disturbs the soil very little and leaves almost all plant debris on the surface. *No-till* planting is accomplished by drilling seeds into the ground directly through mulch and groundcover. This allows a cover crop to be interseeded with a subsequent crop.

Farmers who use these conservation tillage techniques often must depend on pesticides (insecticides, fungicides, and herbicides) to control insects and weeds. Increased use of toxic agricultural chemicals is a matter of great concern. Massive use of pesticides is not, however, a necessary corollary of soil conservation. It is possible to combat pests and diseases with integrated pest management that combines crop rotation, trap crops, natural repellents, and biological controls.

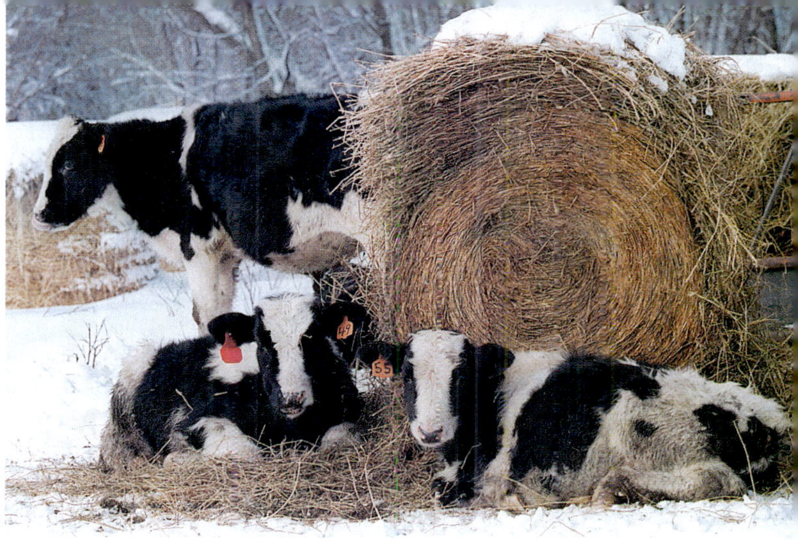

FIGURE 7.29 *On the Minar family's 230-acre dairy farm near New Prague, Minnesota, cows and calves spend the winter outdoors in the snow, bedding down on hay. Dave Minar is part of a growing counterculture that is seeking to keep farmers on the land and bring prosperity to rural areas.*

Low-Input Sustainable Agriculture

In contrast to the trend toward industrialization and dependence on chemical fertilizers, pesticides, antibiotics, and artificial growth factors common in conventional agriculture, some farmers are going back to a more natural, agroecological farming style. Finding that they can't—or don't want to—compete with factory farms, these folks are making money and staying in farming by returning to small-scale, low-input agriculture. The Minar family, for instance, operates a highly successful 150-cow dairy operation on 97 ha (240 acres) near New Prague, Minnesota. No synthetic chemicals are used on their farm. Cows are rotated every day between 45 pastures or paddocks to reduce erosion and maintain healthy grass. Even in the winter, livestock remain outdoors to avoid the spread of diseases common in confinement (fig. 7.29). Antibiotics are used only to fight diseases. Milk and meat from this operation are marketed through co-ops and a community-supported agriculture (CSA) program. Sand Creek, which flows across the Minar land, has been shown to be cleaner when leaving the farm than when it enters.

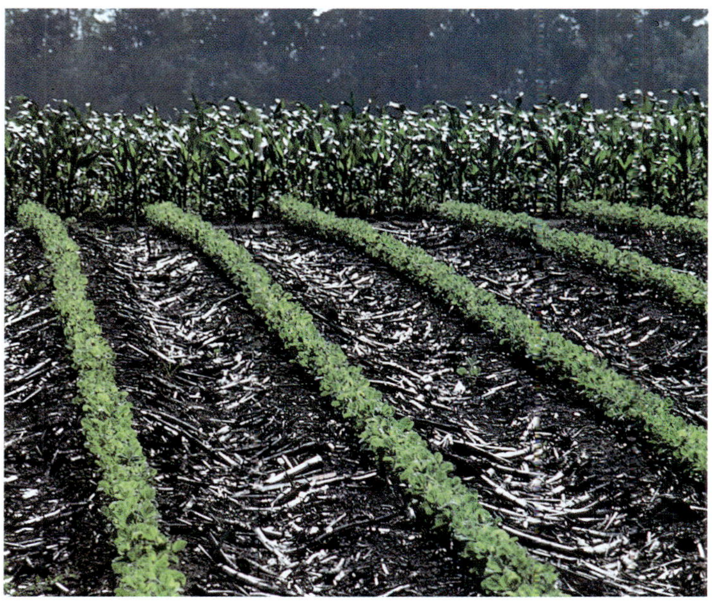

FIGURE 7.28 *In ridge-tilling, a chisel plow is used to create ridges on which crops are planted and shallow troughs filled with crop residue. Less energy is used on plowing and cultivation, and weeds are suppressed and moisture is retained by the groundcover, or crop residue, left on the field.*

Similarly, the Franzen family, who raise livestock on their organic farm near Alta Vista, Iowa, allow their pigs to roam in lush pastures, where they can supplement their diet of corn and soybeans with grasses and legumes. Housing for these happy hogs is in spacious, open-ended hoop structures. As fresh layers of straw are added to the bedding, layers of manure beneath are composted, breaking down into odorless organic fertilizer.

Low-input farms such as these typically don't turn out the quantity of meat or milk that their intensive agriculture neighbors do, but their production costs are lower, and they get higher prices for their crops, so that the all-important net gain is often higher. The Franzens, for example, calculate that they pay 30 percent less for animal feed, 70 percent less for veterinary bills, and half as much for buildings and equipment as their neighboring confinement operations. And on the Minar's farm, erosion after an especially heavy rain was measured to be 400 times lower than on a conventional farm nearby.

Preserving small-scale family farms also helps preserve rural culture. As Marty Strange of the Center for Rural Affairs in Nebraska asks, "Which is better for the enrollment in rural schools, the membership of rural churches, and the fellowship of rural communities—two farms milking 1,000 cows each or twenty farms milking 100 cows each?" Family farms help keep rural towns alive by purchasing machinery at the local implement dealer, gasoline at the neighborhood filling station, and groceries at the mom-and-pop grocery store.

One way to support local agriculture is to shop at a farmers' market (fig. 7.30). The produce is fresh, and profits go directly to the farmer who grows the crop. A local food co-op or owner-operated grocery store also is likely to buy from local farmers and to feature pesticide-free foods. Many co-ops and buyers' associations sign contracts directly with producers to grow the types of food they want to eat. This benefits both parties. Producers are guaranteed a local market for organic food or specialty items. Consumers can be assured of quality and can even be involved in production.

Many large supermarkets also now carry organic produce and other foods. If yours doesn't, why not ask the manager to look into it? Organic foods are becoming increasingly accepted—and profitable—as their benefits become more widely understood.

Agroecology, or sustainable farming using ecological knowledge, also can be applied effectively in poorer countries. Brian Haliweil, of the Worldwatch Institute, reports that farmers in the Guatemalan Highlands raised their crop yields ten-fold without the use of chemical fertilizers or pesticides. Encouraged by World Neighbors, a nongovernmental development organization, to find innovative, local solutions to their problems, the farmers came up with low-cost techniques, such as planting cover crops and grass strips to reduce erosion and rotating corn with beans, peas, and other legumes to add nitrogen to the soil. Corn harvests increased from 0.4 tons to 4.5 tons per hectare, yields comparable with those of many richer countries.

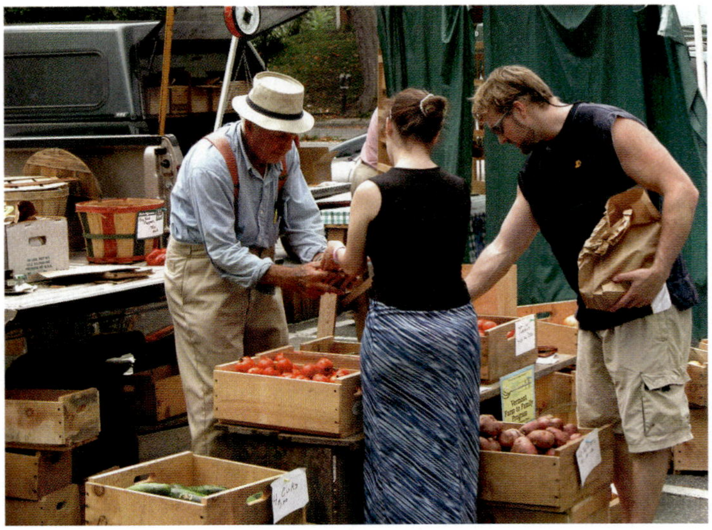

FIGURE 7.30 *Your local farmers' market is a good source of locally grown organic produce.*

One of the largest experiments in low-input farming is currently taking place in Cuba, where loss of aid from the former Soviet Union coupled with a trade embargo imposed by the United States have forced farmers to turn to organic, nonmechanized agriculture (see related story "Organic Farming in Cuba" at www.mhhe.com/cases).

SUMMARY

- Forty years ago, 60 percent of the developing world was considered undernourished, meaning their diet didn't provide the average 2,200 kcal per day considered necessary for a healthy, productive life. Today, despite the fact that world population has doubled since 1960, less than 15 percent of the population suffers from chronic caloric deficiency. However, that means that 840 million people still don't have enough to eat.
- Poverty is the greatest threat to food security, or the ability to obtain sufficient food on a day-to-day basis. The 1.4 billion people in the world who live on less than $1 (U.S.) per day all too often can't buy the food they need and don't have access to resources to grow it for themselves. Even in communities or families where, on average, there would be enough for everyone, those with lowest status (women and children) may not get the food they need for a healthy life.
- An epidemic of obesity is spreading around the world as more of us eat too much meat, salt, and saturated fat and get too little exercise. Being overweight raises the risk for hypertension, diabetes, heart attacks, stroke, and many other diseases, which are becoming the leading causes of death and disability everywhere.
- A few crop species provide almost all the food humans eat. Wheat, rice, and maize supply the majority of the nutrients and calories for the vast majority of the world. Meat, dairy, and seafood consumption are rising rapidly as more people can afford these foods. Growing animals in dense concentrations in confinement operations can cause serious environmental and social problems.
- Soil is a marvelous, complex substance. Thousands of specific soil types exist in the world, having arisen from different parent material under diverse ecological conditions. Some are fertile, tillable, and wonderfully suited for agriculture. Others may need a great deal of husbandry to become useful.
- Large areas of the world suffer soil degradation caused by erosion, nutrient depletion, salinization, waterlogging, or

other symptoms of abuse. It's estimated that 25 billion metric tons of soil are lost from cropland every year due to wind and water erosion. This erosion causes pollution and siltation of rivers, lakes, reservoirs, wetlands, and coastal ocean areas.

- The FAO predicts that most future production growth will come from higher yields and new crop varieties rather than expansion of arable lands. Genetic engineering involves removing genetic material from one organism and splicing it into the chromosomes of another. This new technology has the potential to greatly increase both the quantity and the quality of our food supply, but there are worries about both the ecological safety and the possible health effects of genetic modification of organisms.
- Sustainable agriculture, agroecology, or regenerative farming all aim to produce food and fiber on a sustainable basis and to repair damage caused by destructive practices. Soil conservation provides techniques to preserve, protect, and rebuild this precious resource. Small-scale, low-input farming offers an alternative to industrial, chemically intensive agriculture. Even in very poor countries, using ecological knowledge and local initiatives can increase yields and improve profits.

QUESTIONS FOR REVIEW

1. How many people in the world are chronically undernourished, and where do they live?
2. What is food security, and what threatens it?
3. Define *malnutrition* and *obesity*. How many Americans are considered overweight?
4. How have recommendations for a balanced diet changed over the years?
5. What is the composition of soil? Why are soil organisms so important?
6. How much soil erodes from cropland each year? What are some effects of this loss?
7. What is meant by "green revolution"?
8. What is genetic engineering, or biotechnology, and how might it help or hurt agriculture?
9. What is sustainable agriculture?
10. What can farmers do to increase agricultural production without increasing land use?

THINKING SCIENTIFICALLY

1. Suppose that you were engaged in biotechnology, or genetic engineering; what environmental safeguards would you impose on your own research? Are there experiments that would be ethically off-limits for you?
2. Debate the claim that famines are caused more by human actions (or inactions) than by environmental forces. What scientific evidence would you need to have to settle this question? What hypotheses could you test to help resolve the debate?
3. Should farmers be forced to use ecologically sound techniques that serve farmers' best interests in the long run, regardless of short-term consequences? How could we mitigate hardships brought about by such policies?
4. How would you provide assurance to consumers, government officials, and other interested parties that new genetically engineered products were environmentally and socially safe? What experiments would you set up to test for unknown unknowns?
5. Former U.S. President Jimmy Carter said, "Responsible biotechnology is not the enemy; starvation is." Do you agree?
6. Some rice paddies in Southeast Asia have been cultivated continuously for a thousand years or more without losing fertility. How could we in other countries adapt these techniques to our own agricultural systems?
7. Shade-grown coffee and chocolate might help protect endangered tropical forest species. If you were buying these products for your local co-op, what characteristics would you look for, and how much of a premium would you pay?

KEY TERMS

SUGGESTED READINGS

Bailey, Britt, and Marc Lappé. 2002. *Engineering the Farm: The Social and Ethical Aspects of Agricultural Biotechnology.* Island Press.

Brown, Kathryn. 2001. Seeds of concern. *Scientific American* 284(4):50–57.

Ellis, Richard. 2003. *The Empty Ocean.* Island Press.

Food and Agriculture Organization (UN). 2002. *The State of Food Insecurity in the World.* Food and Agriculture Organization of the United Nations.

Halweil, Brian. 2002. Farming in the public interest. *State of the World 2002.* W.W. Norton & Co. for the Worldwatch Institute.

Helvarg, David. 2003. The last fish. *Earth Island Journal* 18(1): 26–30.

Jackson, Dana L., and Laura L. Jackson. 2002. *Farm as Natural Habitat: Reconnecting Food Systems with Ecosystems.* Island Press.

Tillman, David, et al. 2002. Agricultural sustainability and intensive production practices. *Nature* 418:671–77.

Willett, Walter C., and Meir J. Stampfer. 2003. Rebuilding the food pyramid. *Scientific American* 288(1):64–71.

Welcome to McGraw-Hill's Online Learning Center

http://www.mhhe.com/cunningham3e

WEB EXERCISE

Learning about Agricultural Biotechnology

Genetic engineering is one of the hottest topics of current public debate in environmental science. Proponents portray this science as a technological leap that will bestow incalculable benefits on us, while opponents claim this is a slippery slope toward ecological and economic ruin. You will find a plethora of information pro and con about this topic on the Internet. Visit some of the sites listed in "Learning Online" at the beginning of this chapter, or find other sites by conducting a web search for the terms *genetic engineering, gene transfer,* and *genetically modified organisms.* Find at least one source on each side of this controversy, and analyze their arguments. Don't take any single source or study as the last word on a subject. Remember that for every expert or fact there is always an equal and opposite expert or fact.

1. What sources are quoted or what links to other pages are referenced in the information you have found?
2. Are scientific studies quoted as evidence for the authors' positions? Where were they published? Were the studies peer reviewed? What is the reputation of the journal being quoted?
3. Are the presentations moderate and balanced or shrill, strident calls to action? Are they attempting to sway your emotions with loaded terms such as *Frankenfoods* or *Terminator genes?* Is useful information obscured by technical jargon?
4. Who is responsible for the pages you've found? What do you know about the political agendas of these groups? Remember that environmental or social activism groups aren't necessarily unbiased. They may want to scare you to persuade you to support their cause or to donate money to support their organization.
5. Look for deceptive names of groups that aren't what they seem. Innocuous-sounding names such as Committee for the Environment or the Environmental Health Organization could be industry fronts attempting to push a self-interested agenda.
6. After reviewing the information you found, what is your assessment of biotechnology? What limits—if any—to research and application in this area would you want to see imposed? Should some areas of science be out of bounds? Would you eat genetically modified foods?

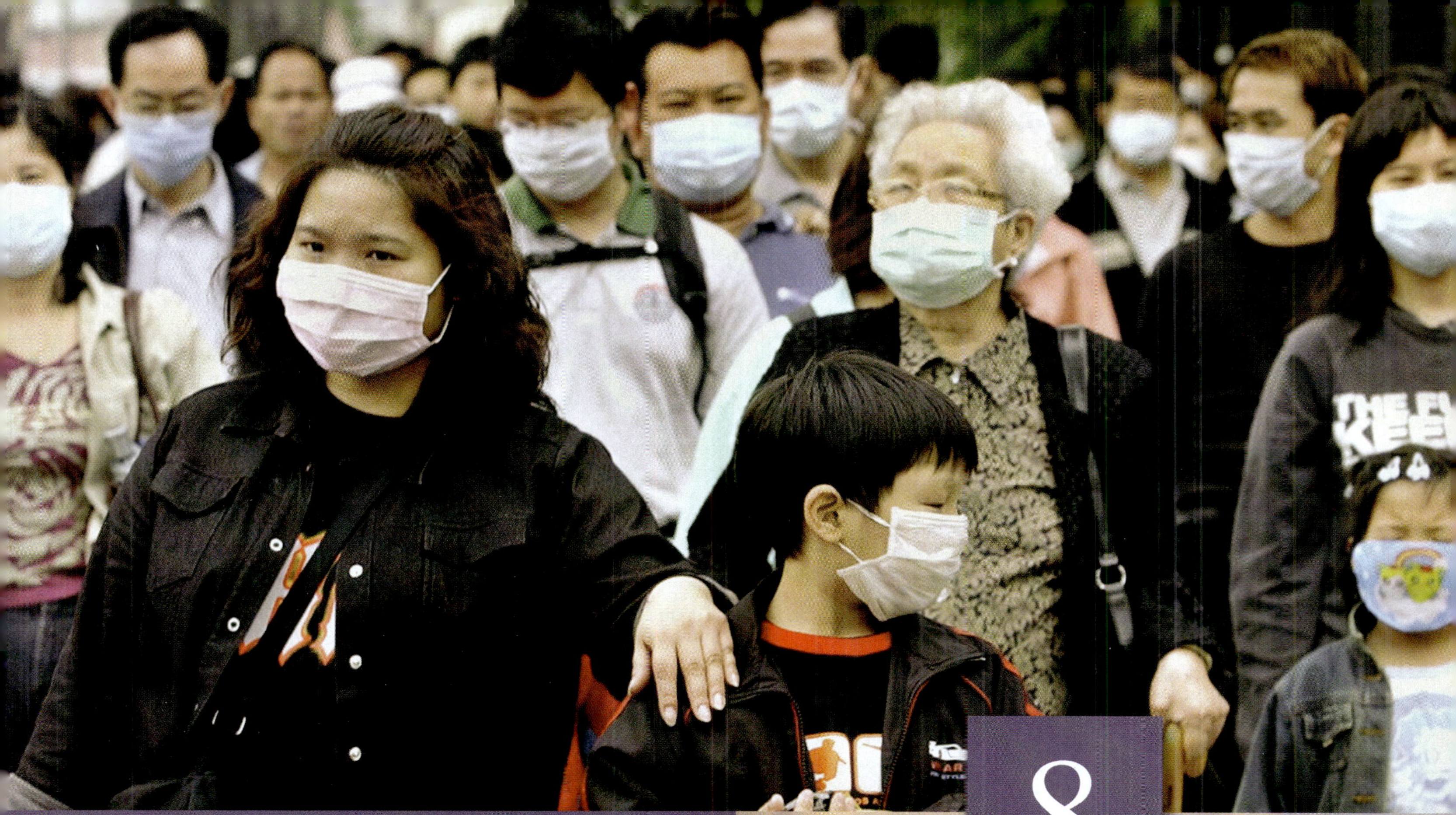

Hong Kong residents protect themselves from severe acute respiratory syndrome (SARS), a highly infectious, pneumonia-like emergent disease.

8

Environmental Health and Toxicology

To wish to become well is a part of becoming well.

–Seneca

Welcome to McGraw-Hill's Online Learning Center

http://www.mhhe.com/cunningham3e

LEARNING ONLINE

Visit our webpage at www.mhhe.com/cunningham3e for aids to help you study this chapter. You'll find practice quizzes, key term flashcards, career information, case studies, current environmental news, and regional examples of important environmental issues. You'll also discover active links to valuable web pages, including

International health
Emergent and ecological diseases
Centers for Disease Control and Prevention
National Institutes of Health
U.S. National Library of Medicine

OBJECTIVES

After studying this chapter, you should be able to

- define *health* and *disease* and describe how global disease burden is now changing.
- identify some major infectious organisms and hazardous agents that cause environmental diseases.
- identify examples of emergent human and ecological diseases.
- distinguish between toxic and hazardous chemicals and between chronic and acute exposures and responses.
- compare factors that affect toxin movement and persistence in the environment as well as routes of entry and effects in our bodies.
- evaluate the major environmental risks we face and how risk assessment and risk acceptability are determined.

The Cough Heard Round the World

Early in 2003 news began to trickle out of China that a very infectious "atypical pneumonia" was spreading rapidly in hospitals around Guangzhou (formerly known as Canton) in Guangdong Province. Symptoms included fever, chills, headaches, muscle pains, and a dry cough, but in many patients, especially the elderly, the disease would quickly turn into a deadly pneumonia. In February of 2003 a doctor from Guangzhou, who had contracted this disease from his patients, traveled to Hong Kong. There he passed the infection to other travelers, who carried what is now know as severe acute respiratory syndrome (SARS) to Beijing, Canada, Taiwan, Singapore, and Vietnam.

Within six months, SARS spread to 31 countries around the world, where more than 8,500 probable cases and 812 deaths were reported. Fear of SARS traveled even faster and farther than the disease itself. Rumors multiplied across the Internet as conferences and sporting events were canceled, factories closed, and tourism to China fell by as much as 85 percent after the epidemic was revealed. The economic impact of SARS is estimated to be at least $30 billion (U.S.) in 2003 alone. By July 2003 the World Health Organization (WHO) declared the outbreak contained but suggested that the world remain alert for further infections. In 2004 a few more SARS cases were found in China and Taiwan, but better vigilance prevented another widespread outbreak.

The rapid transmission of this disease shows how interconnected we all are. A virus can travel in just a few days anywhere a plane flies. One flight attendant is thought to have been the source of infection for 160 people in seven countries. SARS also points to the need for better communication and identification of new diseases. Because the Chinese government hid the extent and severity of the disease for several months, patients with this highly infectious disease mingled with the general hospital population, spreading the illness. Medical professionals, not knowing how serious the infection was, treated patients without wearing protective clothing. Major hospitals in Beijing, Taipei, Hong Kong, and Singapore were closed because so many staff members were sick, making treatment of the contagion even more difficult.

While globalization helped spread SARS, it also helped in rapid recognition and treatment of the disease. It took centuries to discover the cause of cholera. Identifying the virus that causes AIDS took two years. But within weeks after the WHO issued its first warning about SARS, electron microscopists at the Centers for Disease Control in Atlanta had photographs of the SARS virus. Less than a month later, labs from Vancouver to Singapore were sequencing its RNA. And, within a few weeks, scientists at Hong Kong University identified a coronavirus nearly identical to those from SARS patients in civets, badgers, and raccoon dogs being sold in Guangdong meat markets.

Wild species had been suspected as a source of the SARS virus, since some of the first infections occurred among chefs and animal merchants. Exotic animals are regarded as delicacies in southern China, where they are featured at banquets and dinners at expensive restaurants. After discovery of the SARS source, Chinese police raided animal markets and hotels and restaurants, seizing 838,500 animals, including many rare and endangered species. The emergence of SARS may reduce animal smuggling, but the existence of a reservoir of this virus in the wild may also mean that it will be impossible to completely eradicate the disease.

SARS deaths, so far, are relatively insignificant, compared with the 3 million people who die from AIDS or the 1 million who die from malaria every year, but we tend to fear new risks with unknown causes, while ignoring more routine but perhaps more dangerous risks that we believe we can control. Still, the emergence of SARS reminds us how susceptible we remain to infectious diseases in an interconnected world. Dr. Jong-wook Lee, the head of the WHO said, "SARS is the first new disease of the twenty-first century, but it will not be the last." The U.S. Institute of Medicine warns that gaps in our defenses against biological assault from both terrorists and natural sources makes us vulnerable to other deadly epidemics. In this chapter, we'll look at some principles of environmental health to help you understand some of the risks we face and what we might do about them.

ENVIRONMENTAL HEALTH

What is health? The World Health Organizaion (WHO) defines **health** as a state of complete physical, mental, and social well-being, not merely the absence of disease or infirmity. By that definition, we all are ill to some extent. Likewise, we all can improve our health to live happier, longer, more productive, and more satisfying lives if we think about what we do.

What is disease? A **disease** is an abnormal change in the body's condition that impairs important physical or psychological functions. Diet and nutrition, infectious agents, toxic substances, genetics, trauma, and stress all play roles in **morbidity** (illness) and **mortality** (death). **Environmental health** focuses on external factors that cause disease, including elements of the natural, social, cultural, and technological worlds in which we live. Figure 8.1 shows some major environmental disease agents, as well as the media through which we encounter them. Ever since the publication of Rachel Carson's *Silent Spring* in 1962, the discharge, movement, fate, and effects of synthetic chemical toxins have been a special focus of environmental health. Later in this chapter, we'll study these topics in detail. First, however, let's look at some of the major causes of illness worldwide.

Global Disease Burden

In the past, health organizations have focused on the leading causes of death as the best summary of world health. Mortality data, however, fail to capture the impacts of nonfatal outcomes of disease and injury, such as dementia or blindness, on human well-being. When people are ill, work isn't done, crops aren't planted or harvested, meals aren't cooked, and children can't study and learn. Health agencies now calculate **disability-adjusted life years (DALYs)** as a measure of disease burden. DALYs combine premature deaths and loss of a healthy life resulting from illness or disability. This is an attempt to evaluate the total cost of disease, not simply how many people die. Clearly, many more years of expected life are lost when a child dies of neonatal tetanus than when an 80-year-old dies of pneumonia. Similarly, a teenager permanently paralyzed by a traffic accident will have many more years of suffering and lost potential than will a senior citizen who has a stroke. According to the WHO, chronic diseases now account for nearly 60 percent of the 56.5 million total deaths worldwide each year and about half of the global disease burden.

The world is now undergoing a dramatic epidemiological transition. Chronic conditions, such as cardiovascular disease

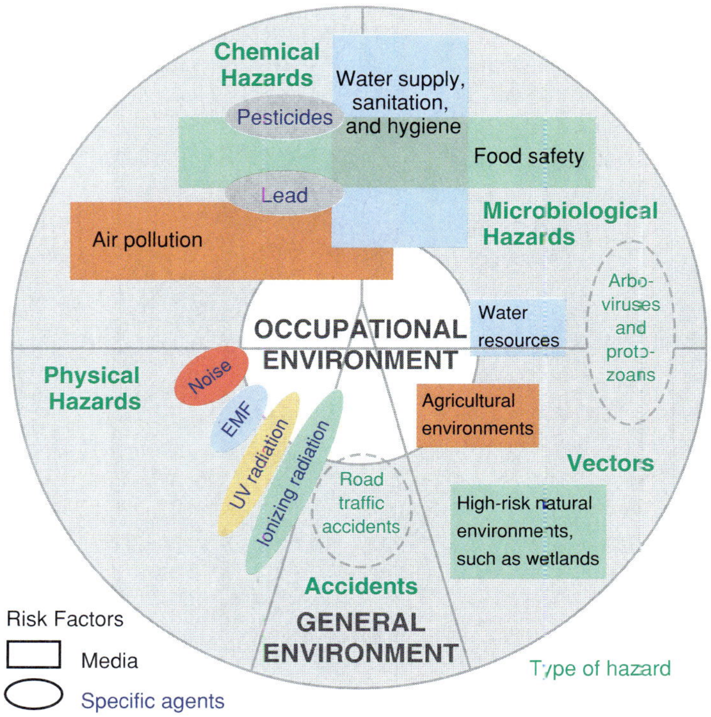

FIGURE 8.1 *Major sources of environmental health risks.*
Source: Data from World Health Organization, 2002.

TABLE 8.1 Leading Causes of Global Disease Burden

RANK	1990	RANK	2020
1	Pneumonia	1	Heart disease
2	Diarrhea	2	Depression
3	Perinatal conditions	3	Traffic accidents
4	Depression	4	Stroke
5	Heart disease	5	Chronic lung disease
6	Stroke	6	Pneumonia
7	Tuberculosis	7	Tuberculosis
8	Measles	8	War
9	Traffic accidents	9	Diarrhea
10	Birth defects	10	HIV/AIDS
11	Chronic lung disease	11	Perinatal conditions
12	Malaria	12	Violence
13	Falls	13	Birth defects
14	Iron anemia	14	Self-inflicted injuries
15	Malnutrition	15	Respiratory cancer

Source: Data from World Health Organization, 2002.

and cancer, no longer afflict only wealthy people. Marvelous progress in eliminating communicable diseases, such as smallpox, polio, and malaria, is allowing people nearly everywhere to live longer. As chapter 7 points out, over the past century the average life expectancy worldwide has risen by about two-thirds. In some poorer countries, such as India, life expectancies nearly tripled in the twentieth century. Although the traditional killers in developing countries—infections, maternal and perinatal (birth) complications, and nutritional deficiencies—still take a terrible toll, diseases such as depression and heart attacks that once were thought to occur only in rich countries are rapidly becoming the leading causes of disability and premature death everywhere.

In 2020, the WHO predicts, heart disease, which was fifth in the list of causes of global disease burden a decade ago, will be the leading source of disability and deaths worldwide (table 8.1). Most of that increase will be in the poorer parts of the world where people are rapidly adopting the lifestyles and diet of the richer countries. Similarly, global cancer rates will increase by 50 percent. By 2020 it's expected that 15 million people will have cancer and 9 million will die from it.

Ask American women what disease they're most afraid of and a majority will probably answer breast cancer. What many don't realize is that cardiovascular disease is the leading cause of death among U.S. women. While focusing on the 40,000 women who die each year from breast cancer, we aren't aware of the 500,000 who die in the same time from heart attacks and strokes. For reasons we don't fully understand, women are far more likely than men to be disabled or die as a result of heart attack or stroke. Forty-six percent of women are seriously disabled by their first heart attack, for instance, compared with only 22 percent of men. Smoking, diabetes, high blood pressure, high cholesterol, excess weight, and lack of physical activity increase cardiovascular disease risks in both women and men, but women are less likely than men to be aware of the importance of these health factors.

Taking disability as well as death into account in our assessment of disease burden reveals the increasing role of mental health as a worldwide problem. WHO projections suggest that psychiatric and neurological conditions could increase their share of the global burden from 10 percent currently to 15 percent of the total load by 2020. Again, this isn't just a problem of the developed world. Depression is expected to be the second largest cause of all years lived with disability worldwide, as well as the cause of 1.4 percent of all deaths. For women in both developing and developed regions, depression is the leading cause of disease burden, while suicide, which often is the result of untreated depression, is the fourth largest cause of female deaths.

Notice in table 8.1 that diarrhea, which was the second leading cause of disease burden in 1990, is expected to be ninth on the list in 2020, while measles and malaria are expected to drop out of the top 15 causes of disability. Tuberculosis, which is becoming resistant to antibiotics and is spreading rapidly in many areas (especially in Russia), is the only infectious disease whose ranking is not expected to change over the next 20 years. Traffic accidents are now soaring as more people drive. War, violence, and self-inflicted injuries similarly are becoming much more important health risks than ever before.

Chronic obstructive lung diseases (e.g., emphysema, asthma, and lung cancer) are expected to increase from eleventh to fifth in disease burden by 2020. A large part of the increase is due to rising use of tobacco in developing countries, sometimes called "the tobacco epidemic." Every day about 100,000 young people—most of them in poorer countries—become addicted to tobacco. At least 1.1 billion people now smoke, and this number is expected to increase at least 50 percent by 2020. If current patterns persist, about 500 million people alive today will eventually be killed by tobacco. This is expected to be the biggest single cause of death worldwide (because illnesses such as heart attack and depression are triggered by multiple factors). In 2003 the World Health Assembly adopted a historic tobacco-control convention that requires countries to impose restrictions on tobacco advertising, establish clean indoor air controls, and clamp down on tobacco smuggling. Dr. Gro Harlem Brundtland, former director-general of the WHO, predicted that the convention, if ratified by enough nations, could save billions of lives.

As chapter 7 points out, the world is now experiencing an epidemic of obesity. Poor diet and lack of exercise are now the second leading underlying cause of death in America, causing at least 400,000 deaths per year. Obesity is expected to overtake tobacco soon as the largest single health risk in many countries.

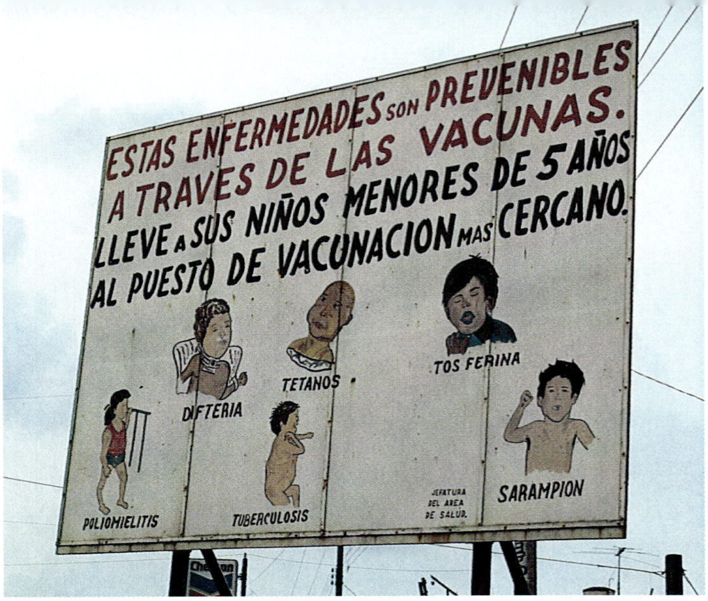

ESTAS ENFERMEDADES SON PREVENIBLES
A TRAVES DE LAS VACUNAS.
LLEVE A SUS NIÑOS MENORES DE 5 AÑOS
AL PUESTO DE VACUNACION MAS CERCANO.
DIFTERIA
TETANOS
TOS FERINA
POLIOMIELITIS
TUBERCULOSIS
JEFATURA DEL AREA DE SALUD
SARAMPION

FIGURE 8.2 *Millions of children die each year from easily prevented childhood diseases. This Guatemalan billboard urges that children be vaccinated against polio, diphtheria, TB, tetanus, pertussis (whooping cough), and scarlet fever* (left to right).

Emergent and Infectious Diseases

Although the ills of modern life have become the leading killers almost everywhere in the world, communicable diseases still are responsible for about one-third of all disease-related mortality. Diarrhea, acute respiratory illnesses, malaria, measles, tetanus, and a few other infectious diseases kill about 11 million children under age five every year in the developing world. Better nutrition, clean water, improved sanitation, and inexpensive inoculations could eliminate most of those deaths (fig. 8.2).

A wide variety of **pathogens** (disease-causing organisms) afflict humans, including viruses, bacteria, protozoans (single-celled animals), parasitic worms, and flukes (fig. 8.3). Probably the greatest loss of life from an individual disease in a single year was the great influenza epidemic of 1918. Nearly every year a new version of the flu virus appears, but most are merely unpleasant rather than fatal for healthy adults. In 1918, however, a particularly virulent flu spread rapidly across the globe, killing around 30 million people in less than 12 months. This was more than the total number killed in all the battles of World War I, which was raging at the time.

Every year there are 76 million cases of foodborne illnesses in the United States, resulting in 300,000 hospitalizations and 5,000 deaths. *Giardia,* a parasitic intestinal protozoan, is thought to be the largest single cause of diarrhea in the United States. It is spread from human feces through food and water. You may think of this as a wilderness disease, but researchers report that the best place to find the pathogens is day care centers and nursery schools. At any given time, around 2 billion people—one-third of the world population—suffer from worms, flukes, and other internal parasites. Guinea worms (*Dracunculus medinesis*) are round worms transmitted via contaminated water. After a year of migrating through the body, the adult, which can be 1 meter long, emerges to lay eggs (fig. 8.3c). A campaign to eradicate this scourge has eliminated it from most countries. (See related story "Fighting the Fiery Serpent" at www.mhhe.com/cases.)

Malaria is one of the most prevalent remaining infectious diseases. Every year about 300 million new cases of this disease occur, and about 1 million people die from it. The territory infected by this disease is expanding as global climate change allows mosquito vectors to move into new territory. Simply providing insecticide-treated bed nets and a few dollars worth of chloroquine pills could prevent tens of millions of cases of this debilitating disease every year. Tragically, some of the countries where malaria is most widespread tax both bed nets and medicine as luxuries, placing them out of reach for ordinary people.

Emergent diseases are those not previously known or that have been absent for at least 20 years. The story of SARS that introduced this chapter is a good example of an emergent disease. Although coronaviruses have long been known to cause a variety of diseases—some lethal—in animals, and two members of this virus family cause about 30 percent of all human colds, the particularly virulent form that appears to have jumped from wild animals to humans in southern China had been previously unknown to science. Similarly, in 2004 an avian flu spread from domestic poultry to humans and then spread rapidly through Southeast Asia. Although only about 24 people died, millions of ducks and chickens were slaughtered to stop the spread of the disease. Altogether, one-third of all global meat exports were banned in 2004 due to bird flu and other emergent diseases. Figure 8.4 shows some recent outbreaks of emergent diseases around the world.

Health experts point out that West Nile virus is the most virulent and rapidly moving disease to hit the United States in recent years. West Nile belongs to a family of mosquito-transmitted viruses that cause encephalitis (brain inflammation). Although rec-

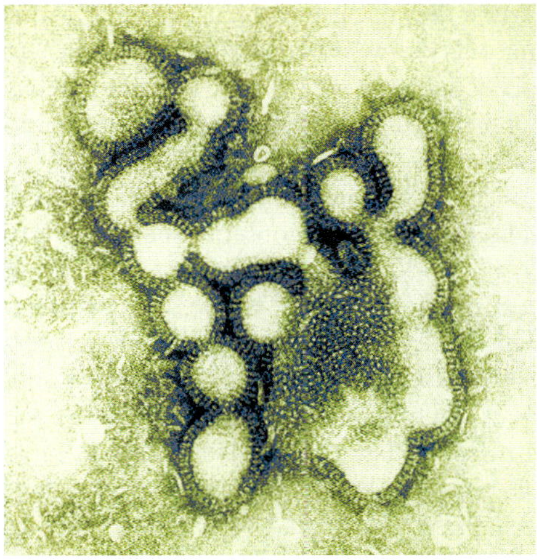

(a)

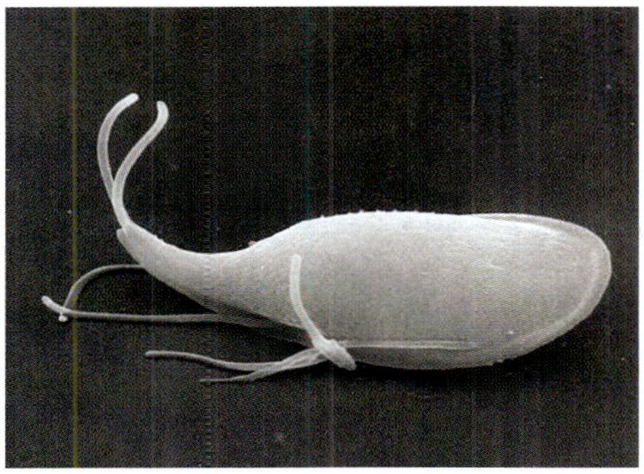

(b)

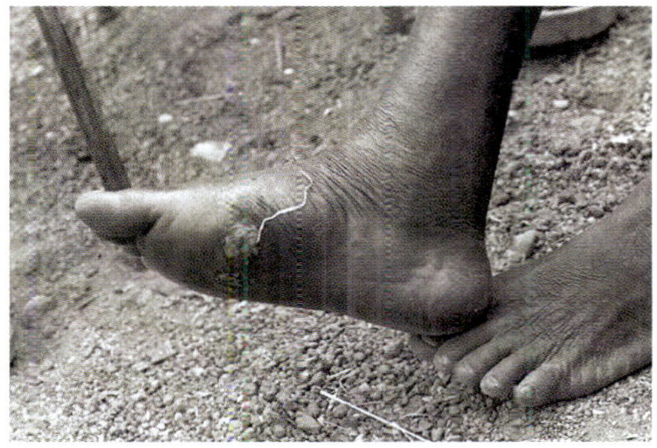

(c)

FIGURE 8.3 (a) *A group of influenza viruses magnified about 300,000 times.* (b) Giardia, *a parasitic intestinal protozoan, magnified about 10,000 times.* (c) *A guinea worm emerges from the foot of an infected person.*

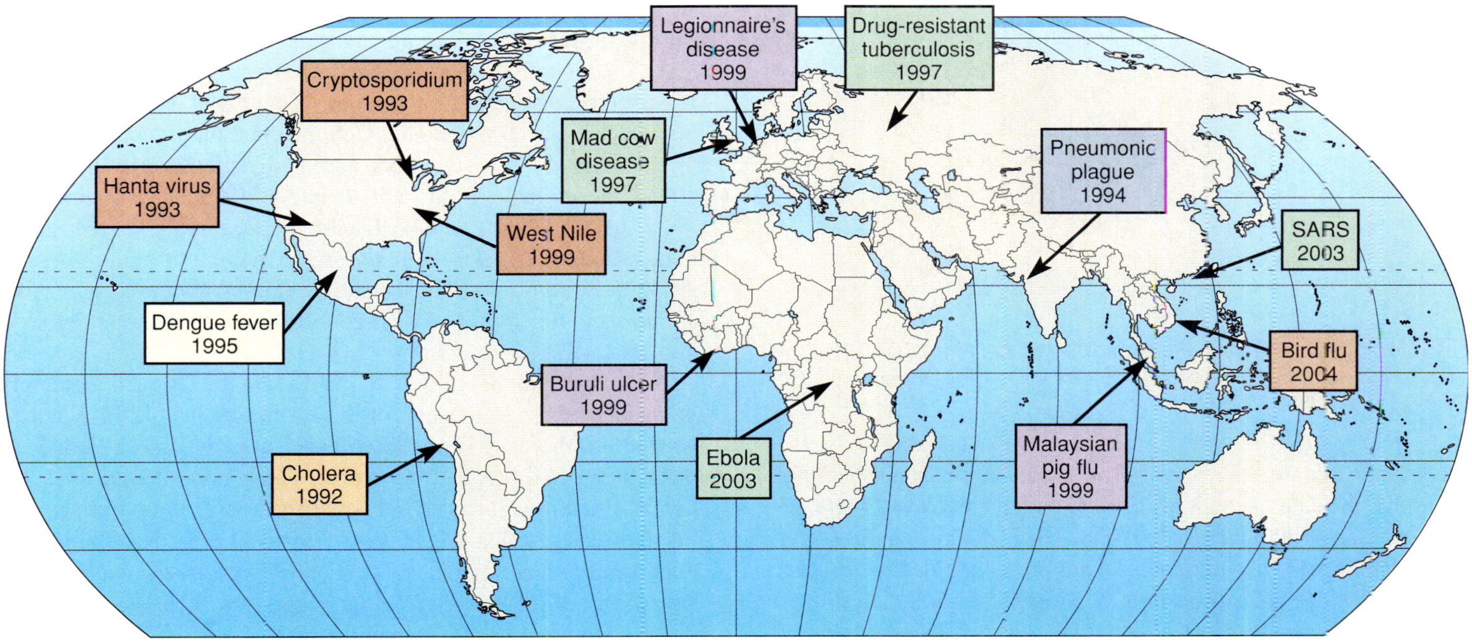

FIGURE 8.4 *Some recent outbreaks of highly lethal infectious diseases. Why are supercontagious organisms emerging in so many different places?*
Source: Data from U.S. Centers for Disease Control and Prevention.

ognized in Africa in 1937, the West Nile virus was absent from North America until 1999, when it apparently was introduced by a bird or mosquito from the Middle East. The disease spread from New York, where it was first reported, throughout the eastern United States in only two years (fig. 8.5). The virus infects 230 species of animals, including 130 bird species. In 2002 more than 4,000 people contracted the disease and 284 died in the United States. There's a worry that, if the disease reaches Hawaii, it could completely eradicate rare species, such as the Hawaiian crow and several types of honeycreeper.

The largest recent human death toll from an emergent disease is due to HIV/AIDS. Although it was first recognized in the early 1980s, acquired immune deficiency syndrome has now become the fifth greatest cause of contagious deaths. The WHO estimates that 60 million people are now infected with the human immune-deficiency virus and that 3 million die every year from AIDS complications. Although two-thirds of all current HIV infections are now in sub-Saharan Africa, the disease is spreading rapidly in South and East Asia. Over the next 20 years, there could be an additional 65 million AIDS deaths. In Botswana, health officials estimate about 40 percent of all adults are HIV-positive and that two-thirds of all current 15-year-olds will die of AIDS before age 50. Without AIDS, the life expectancy in Botswana would be expected to be 69.7 years. With AIDS, Botswana's average life

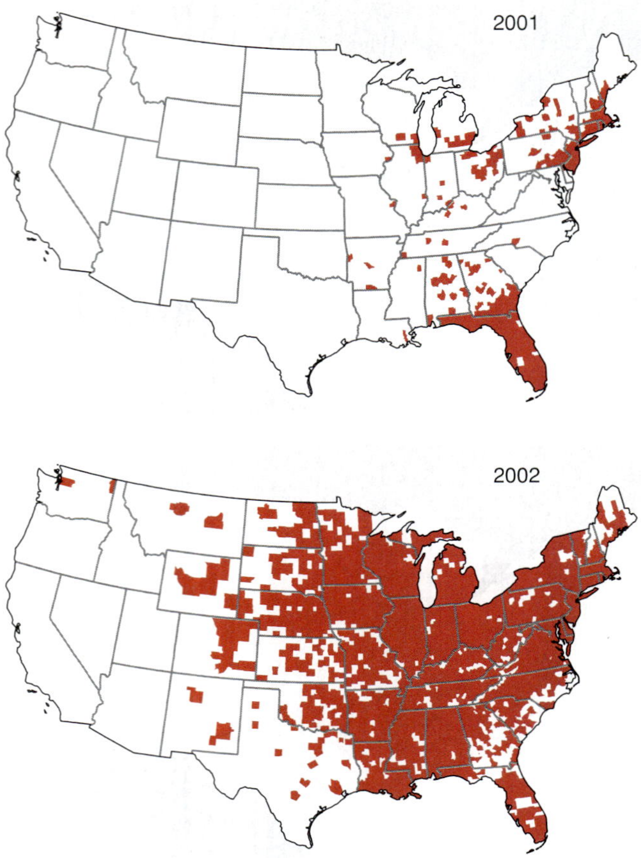

FIGURE 8.5 *The spread of West Nile virus in birds, 2001–2002.*
Source: Data from U.S. Centers for Disease Control and U.S. Geological Survey.

expectancy is now 36.1 years. Worldwide, more than 14 million children—the equivalent of every child under age five in America—have lost one or both parents to AIDS. The economic costs of treating patients and lost productivity from premature deaths resulting from this disease are estimated to be at least $35 billion (U.S.) per year, or about one-tenth of the total GDP of sub-Saharan Africa.

Funding Health Care

The heaviest burden of illness is borne by the poorest people, who can afford neither a healthy environment nor adequate health care. Women in sub-Saharan Africa, for example, suffer six times the disease burden per 1,000 population of women in most European countries. The WHO estimates that 90 percent of all disease burden occurs in developing countries, where less than one-tenth of all health care dollars is spent. The group Medecins Sans Frontieres (MSF, or Doctors without Borders) calls this the 10/90 gap. While wealthy nations pursue drugs to treat baldness and obesity, depression in dogs, and erectile dysfunction, billions of people are sick or dying from treatable infections and parasitic diseases to which little attention is paid. Worldwide, only 2 percent of the people with AIDS have access to modern medicines. Every year, some 600,000 infants acquire HIV—almost all of them through mother-to-child transmission during birth or breast-feeding. Antiretroviral therapy costing only a few dollars can prevent most of this transmission. The Bill and Melinda Gates Foundation has pledged $200 million for medical aid to developing countries to help fight AIDS, TB, and malaria.

Dr. Jeffrey Sachs of the Columbia University Earth Institute says that disease is as much a cause as a consequence of poverty and political unrest, yet the world's richest countries now spend just $1 per person per year on global health. He predicts that raising our commitment to about $25 billion annually (about 0.1 percent of the annual GDP of the 20 richest countries) would not only save about 8 million lives each year but also would boost the world economy by billions of dollars. There also would be huge social benefits for the rich countries in not living in a world endangered by mass social instability; the spread of pathogens across borders; the spread of other ills, such as terrorism; and drug trafficking caused by social problems. Sachs also argues that reducing disease burden would help reduce population growth. When parents believe their offspring will survive, they have fewer children and invest more in food, health, and education for smaller families.

The United States is among the least generous of the world's rich countries, donating only about 12 cents per $100 of GDP on international development aid. Could this country do better? During this time of fear of terrorism and rising anti-American feelings around the globe, it's difficult to interest legislators in international aid, yet helping reduce disease might win the United States more friends and make the nation safer than buying more bombs and bullets. Improved health care in poorer countries may also help prevent the spread of emergent diseases, such as SARS, in a globally interconnected world.

At the 2003 meeting of the Global Health Council, epidemiologists noted that almost all of the 2.2 billion people expected to be added to the world population in the next 30 years will live in megacities of the developing world. The economic and environmental conditions in those cities will have a profound impact on global disease burden. Madagascar President Marc Ravalomanana urged conference attendees—and the world—to address the "lethal disease of poverty." More discussion of urban areas and their problems is presented in chapter 14.

Ecological Diseases

Humans aren't the only ones to suffer from new and devastating diseases. Domestic animals and wildlife also experience sudden and widespread epidemics. In 1998, for example, a distemper virus killed half the seals in Western Europe. It's thought that toxic pollutants and hormone-disrupting environmental chemicals might have made seals and other marine mammals susceptible to infections.

Chronic wasting disease (CWD) is spreading through deer and elk populations in North America (fig. 8.6). Caused by a strange protein called a prion, CWD is one of a family of irreversible, degenerative neurological diseases known as transmissible spongiform encephalopathies (TSE), which include mad cow disease in cattle, scrapie in sheep, and Creutzfelt-Jacob disease in humans. CWD probably started when elk ranchers fed contaminated animal by-products to their herds. Infected animals were

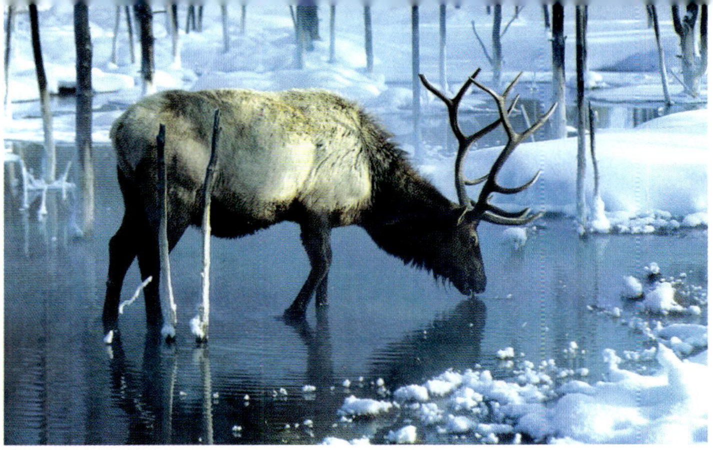

FIGURE 8.6 *Wild elk and deer are widely affected by chronic wasting disease, which probably originated with domestic herds.*

sold to other ranches, and now the disease has spread to wild populations. First recognized in 1967 in Saskatchewan, CWD has been identified in wild deer populations and ranch operations in at least eight American states and two Canadian provinces.

The Canadian government is estimated to have spent $65 million in an attempt to stop the spread of CWD. In 2002, Wisconsin encouraged hunters to kill some 20,000 deer in an area near Madison in an effort to contain the disease. No humans are known to have contracted TSE from deer or elk, but there is a concern that we might see something like the mad cow disaster that afflicted Europe in the 1990s. At least 100 people died, and nearly 5 million European cattle and sheep were slaughtered in an effort to contain that disease.

Currently, California oak trees are dying from a fast-spreading new disease known as sudden oak death syndrome (SODS). The disease is caused by a fungus-like organism known as *Phytophthora ramorum,* part of a group known as water molds. Possibly imported with Asian rhododendrons shipped from European plant nurseries, this organism is a close relative of the pathogen that caused Ireland's potato blight and another species that has wiped out vast swaths of forest in western Australia. Recently, foresters reported that Douglas fir, one of the nation's most economically important timber species, and California coast redwood also can be infected with SODS. In addition to being beautiful trees and dominant members of forest communities, these species provide commercial products worth more than a billion dollars per year in the United States.

Starting in the early 1970s, an illness called black-band disease has been attacking corals throughout the Caribbean. A cyanophyte alga (*Phormidium corallyticum*) actually kills the coral polyps. As the black ring of dead polyps spreads through the colony, it leaves behind a bleached coral skeleton. Researchers have found pathogenic bacteria from human feces associated with dying corals and think that they may play a role in triggering the algal attack. Coliform bacteria are present on reefs far from any human occupation. These pathogens may be carried by dust storms from as far away as Africa. Coral subjected to environmental stressors, such as nutrient imbalance or elevated seawater temperatures, may be especially susceptible to infection.

In 2003 a naturally occurring but deadly toxin produced by sea algae killed record numbers of dolphins and sea lions along sections of California's southern coast. More than 1,000 marine mammals were found stranded or dead on state beaches. Hundreds of seabirds, including endangered brown pelicans, grebes, and loons, also were affected. The animals are being poisoned by domoic acid, a nerve toxin produced by certain algae. First detected on the west coast of the United States in 1991, domoic acid is a naturally occurring product of the diatom species *Pseudo-nitzschia.* Marine animals and seabirds are poisoned by eating small fish that have consumed diatoms. Filter-feeding animals, such as mussels, also feed on the toxin-laced algae. Humans who eat toxin-contaminated fish or shellfish contract an illness called amnesic shellfish poisoning (ASP). Symptoms include vomiting, nausea, diarrhea, and abdominal cramps. In more severe cases, confusion, seizures, cardiac arrhythmia, and coma can occur. People poisoned with very high doses of the toxin can die. The exact cause of the toxin increase is a mystery, but scientists speculate that the algae may be thriving on nutrients from agricultural runoff or sewage. Weather patterns could also play a role.

One thing all of these diseases have in common is human-made environmental changes that stress biological communities and upset normal ecological relationships. How many other ways might we be altering the world around us, and what might the consequences be for both ourselves and other species?

Antibiotic and Pesticide Resistance

Malaria, the most deadly of all insectborne diseases, is an example of the return of a disease that once was thought to be nearly vanquished. Malaria now claims about a million lives every year—90 percent in Africa, and most of them children. With the advent of modern medicines and pesticides, malaria had nearly been wiped out in many places but recently has come roaring back. The protozoan parasite that causes the disease is now resistant to most antibiotics, while the mosquitoes that transmit it have developed resistance to many insecticides. Spraying of DDT in India and Sri Lanka, for instance, reduced malaria from millions of infections per year to only a few thousand in the 1950s and 1960s. Now South Asia is back to its pre-DDT level of about half a million new cases of malaria every year. Other places that never had malaria cases now have them as a result of climate change and habitat alteration.

Why have vectors, such as mosquitoes, and pathogens, such as the malaria parasite, become resistant to pesticides and antibiotics? Part of the answer is natural selection and the ability of many organisms to evolve rapidly. Another factor is the human tendency to use control measures carelessly. When we discovered that DDT and other insecticides could control mosquito populations, we spread them everywhere. This not only harmed wildlife and beneficial insects but also created perfect conditions for natural selection. Many pests and pathogens were exposed only minimally to control measures, allowing those with natural resistance to survive and spread their genes through the population (fig. 8.7). After repeated cycles of exposure and selection, many microorganisms and their vectors have become insensitive to almost all our weapons against them.

Raising huge numbers of cattle, hogs, and poultry in densely packed barns and feedlots is another reason for widespread antibiotic resistance in pathogens. Confined animals are dosed constantly

FIGURE 8.7 *How microbes acquire antibiotic resistance.* (a) *Random mutations make a few cells resistant. When challenged by antibiotics, only those cells survive to give rise to a resistant colony.* (b) *Sexual reproduction (conjugation) or plasmid transfer moves genes from one strain or species to another.*

Source: © 1994 Time Inc. Reprinted by permission.

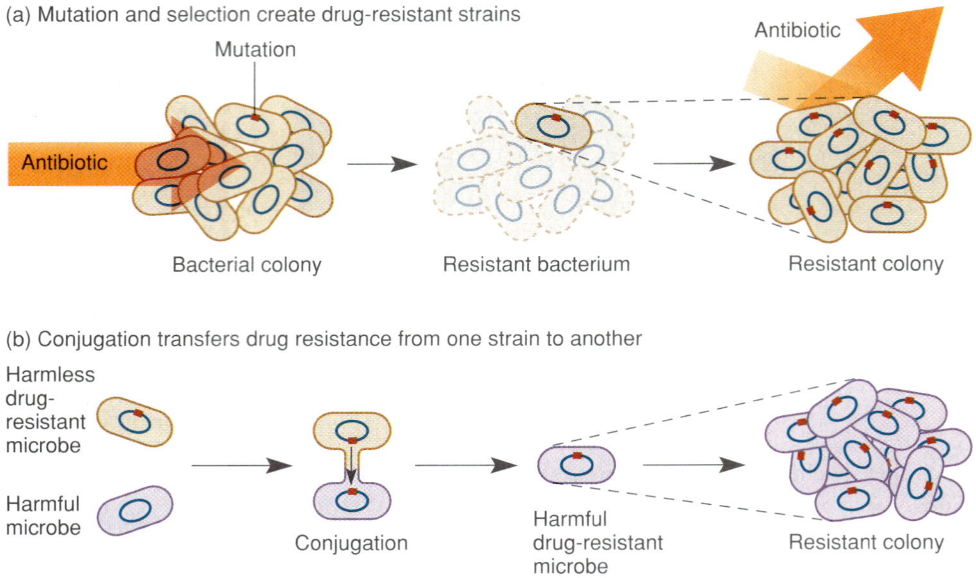

with antibiotics and steroid hormones to keep them disease-free and to make them gain weight faster. More than half of all antibiotics used in the United States each year are fed to livestock. A significant amount of these antibiotics and hormones are excreted in urine and feces, which are spread, untreated, on the land or discharged into surface water, where they contribute further to the evolution of supervirulent pathogens.

At least half of the 100 million antibiotic doses prescribed for humans every year in the United States are unnecessary or are the wrong ones. Furthermore, many people who start a course of antibiotic treatment fail to carry it out for the time prescribed. For your own health and that of the people around you, if you are taking an antibiotic, follow your doctor's orders. Finish your prescribed doses and don't stop taking the medicine as soon as you start feeling better.

Diet

Diet also has an important effect on health. For instance, there is a strong correlation between cardiovascular disease and the amount of salt and saturated fat in one's diet. Lack of physical activity and poor diet are now the second leading causes of preventable death (after smoking) in the United States. Highly processed foods, fat, and smoke-cured, high-nitrate meats also seem to be associated with cancer.

Fruits, vegetables, whole grains, complex carbohydrates, and dietary fiber (plant cell walls), on the other hand, often have beneficial health effects. Certain dietary components—such as pectins; vitamins A, C, and E; substances produced in cruciferous vegetables (cabbage, broccoli, cauliflower, brussels sprouts); and selenium, which we get from plants—seem to have anticancer effects.

Eating too much food is a significant dietary health factor in developed countries and among the well-to-do everywhere. Nearly two-thirds of all Americans are considered overweight, and the worldwide total of obese or overweight people is estimated to be over 1 billion. Every year in the United States, 300,000 deaths are linked to obesity.

The U.S. Centers for Disease Control in Atlanta warn that one in three U.S. children will become diabetic unless many more people start eating less and exercising more. The odds are worse for Black and Hispanic children: nearly half of them are likely to develop the disease. And among the Pima tribe of Arizona, nearly 80 percent of all adults are diabetic. Some goals for reducing obesity and other diet-related problems are shown in table 8.2. More information about food and its health effects is available in chapter 7.

TOXICOLOGY

Toxicology is the study of **toxins** (poisons) and their effects, particularly on living systems. Because many substances are known to be poisonous to life (whether plant, animal, or microbial), toxicology is a broad field, drawing from biochemistry, histology, pharmacology, pathology, and many other disciplines. Toxins damage or kill living organisms because they react with cellular

TABLE 8.2 National Health Recommendations and Diet Goals

1. Balance the food you eat with physical activity to maintain or improve your weight.
2. Choose a diet with plenty of grain products, vegetables, and fruits.
3. Choose a diet low in fat, saturated fat, and cholesterol.
4. Eat a variety of foods.
5. Choose a diet moderate in salt and sodium.
6. Choose a diet moderate in sugars.
7. If you drink alcoholic beverages, do so in moderation.

Source: Data from U.S. Department of Health and Human Services, 1995.

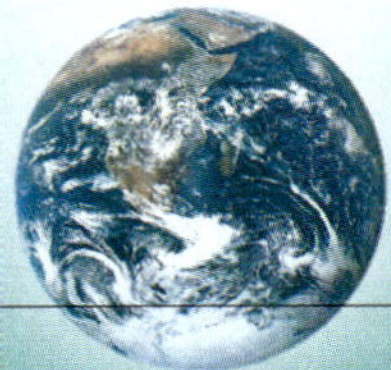

what can you do?

Tips for Staying Healthy

- Eat a balanced diet with plenty of fresh fruits, vegetables, legumes, and whole grains. Wash fruits and vegetables carefully; they may have come from a country where pesticide and sanitation laws are lax.
- Use unsaturated oils, such as olive or canola, rather than hydrogenated or semisolid fats, such as margarine.
- Cook meats and other foods at temperatures high enough to kill pathogens; clean utensils and cutting surfaces; store food properly.
- Wash your hands frequently. You transfer more germs from hand to mouth than any other means of transmission.
- When you have a cold or flu, don't demand antibiotics from your doctor—they aren't effective against viruses.
- If you're taking antibiotics, continue for the entire time prescribed—quitting as soon as you feel well is an ideal way to select for antibiotic-resistant germs.
- Practice safe sex.
- Don't smoke; avoid smoky places.
- If you drink, do so in moderation. Never drive when your reflexes or judgment are impaired.
- Exercise regularly: walk, swim, jog, dance, garden. Do something you enjoy that burns calories and maintains flexibility.
- Get enough sleep. Practice meditation, prayer, or some other form of stress reduction. Get a pet.
- Make a list of friends and family who make you feel more alive and happy. Spend time with one of them at least once a week.

components to disrupt metabolic functions. Because of this reactivity, toxins often are harmful even in extremely dilute concentrations. In some cases, billionths, or even trillionths, of a gram can cause irreversible damage.

All toxins are hazardous, but not all hazardous materials are toxic. Some substances, for example, are dangerous because they're flammable, explosive, acidic, caustic, irritants, or sensitizers. Many of these materials must be handled carefully in large doses or high concentrations, but they can be rendered relatively innocuous by dilution, neutralization, or other physical treatment. They don't react with cellular components in ways that make them poisonous at low concentrations.

Environmental toxicology, or ecotoxicology, specifically deals with the interactions, transformation, fate, and effects of natural and synthetic chemicals in the biosphere, including individual organisms, populations, and whole ecosystems. In aquatic systems the fate of the pollutants is primarily studied in relation to mechanisms and processes at interfaces of the ecosystem components. Special attention is devoted to the sediment/water, water/organisms, and water/air interfaces. In terrestrial environments, the emphasis tends to be on effects of metals on soil fauna community and population characteristics.

Table 8.3 is a list of the top 20 toxins compiled by the U.S. Environmental Protection Agency from the 275 substances regulated by the Comprehensive Environmental Response, Compensation, and Liability Act (CERCLA), commonly known as the Superfund Act. These materials are listed in order of assessed importance in terms of human and environmental health.

Allergens are substances that activate the immune system. Some allergens act directly as **antigens;** that is, they are recognized as foreign by white blood cells and stimulate the production of specific antibodies (proteins that recognize and bind to foreign cells or chemicals). Other allergens act indirectly by binding to and changing the chemistry of foreign materials so they become antigenic and cause an immune response.

Formaldehyde is a good example of a widely used chemical that is a powerful sensitizer of the immune system. It is directly allergenic and can trigger reactions to other substances. Widely used in plastics, wood products, insulation, glue, and fabrics, formaldehyde concentrations in indoor air can be thousands of times higher than in normal outdoor air. Some people suffer from what is called **sick building syndrome**: headaches, allergies, and chronic fatigue caused by poorly vented indoor air contaminated by molds, carbon monoxide, nitrogen oxides, formaldehyde, and other toxic chemicals released by carpets, insulation, plastics, building materials, and other sources (fig. 8.8). The Environmental Protection Agency

TABLE 8.3 Top 20 Toxic and Hazardous Substances

1. Arsenic
2. Lead
3. Mercury
4. Vinyl chloride
5. Polychlorinated biphenyls (PCBs)
6. Benzene
7. Cadmium
8. Benzo(a)pyrene
9. Polycyclic aromatic hydrocarbons
10. Benzo(b)fluoranthene
11. Chloroform
12. DDT
13. Aroclor 1254
14. Aroclor 1260
15. Trichloroethylene
16. Dibenz(a,h)anthracene
17. Dieldrin
18. Chromium, hexavalent
19. Chlordane
20. Hexachlorobutadiene

Source: Data from U.S. Environmental Protection Agency, 2003.

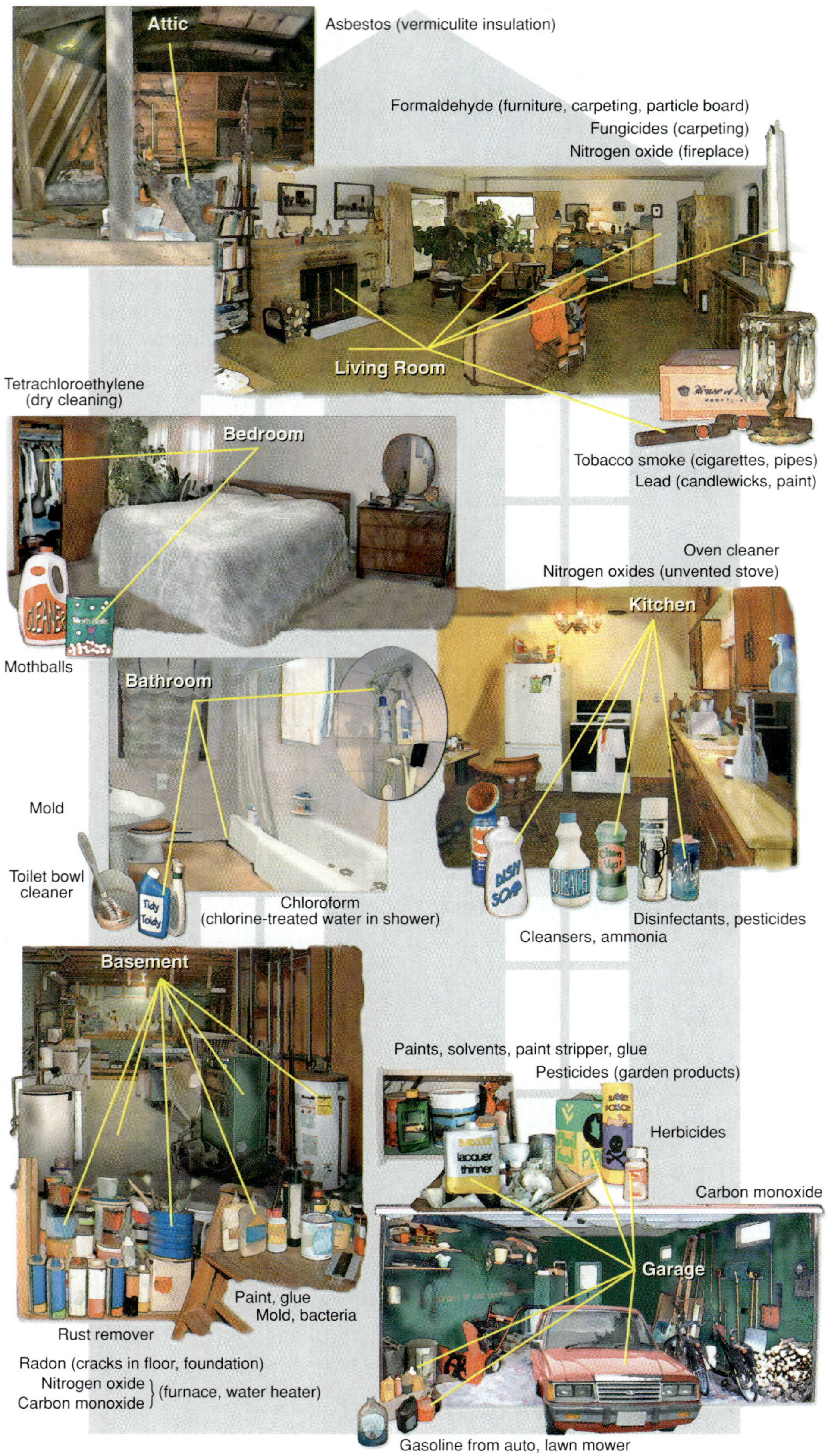

FIGURE 8.8 *Some sources of toxic and hazardous substances in a typical home.*

estimates that poor indoor air quality may cost the nation $60 billion a year in absenteeism and reduced productivity.

Neurotoxins are a special class of metabolic poisons that specifically attack nerve cells (neurons). The nervous system is so important in regulating body activities that disruption of its activities is especially fast-acting and devastating. Different types of neurotoxins act in different ways. Heavy metals, such as lead and mercury, kill nerve cells and cause permanent neurological damage. Anesthetics (ether, chloroform, halothane, etc.) and chlorinated hydrocarbons (DDT, Dieldrin, Aldrin) disrupt nerve cell membranes necessary for nerve action. Organophosphates (Malathion, Parathion) and carbamates (carbaryl, zeneb, maneb) inhibit acetylcholinesterase, an enzyme that regulates signal transmission between nerve cells and the tissues or organs they innervate (for example, muscle). Most neurotoxins are both acute and extremely toxic. More than 850 compounds are now recognized as neurotoxins.

Mutagens are agents, such as chemicals and radiation, that damage or alter genetic material (DNA) in cells. This can lead to birth defects if the damage occurs during embryonic or fetal growth. Later in life, genetic damage may trigger neoplastic (tumor) growth. When damage occurs in reproductive cells, the results can be passed on to future generations. Cells have repair mechanisms to detect and restore damaged genetic material, but some changes may be hidden, and the repair process itself can be flawed. It is generally accepted that there is no "safe" threshold for exposure to mutagens. Any exposure has some possibility of causing damage.

Teratogens are chemicals or other factors that specifically cause abnormalities during embryonic growth and development. Some compounds that are not otherwise harmful can cause tragic problems in these sensitive stages of life. Perhaps the most prevalent teratogen in the world is alcohol. Drinking during pregnancy can lead to **fetal alcohol syndrome**—a cluster of symptoms including craniofacial abnormalities, developmental delays, behavioral problems, and mental defects, that last throughout a child's life. Even one alcoholic drink a day during pregnancy has been associated with decreased birth weight.

Carcinogens are substances that cause **cancer**—invasive, out-of-control cell growth that results in malignant tumors. Cancer rates rose in most industrialized countries during the twentieth century, and cancer is now the second leading cause of death in the United States, killing more than half a million people in 2000. Twenty-three of the 28 compounds listed by the U.S. EPA as greatest risk to human health are probable or possible human carcinogens. More than 200 million people live in areas where the combined upper limit lifetime cancer risk from these carcinogens exceeds 10 in 1 million, or 10 times the risk normally considered acceptable.

The American Cancer Society calculates that one in two males and one in three females in the United States will have some form of cancer in their lifetime. Some authors blame this cancer increase on toxic synthetic chemicals in our environment and diet. Others argue that it is attributable mainly to lifestyle (smoking, sunbathing, drinking alcohol) or simply living longer.

Endocrine Hormone Disrupters

One of the most recently recognized environmental health threats are **endocrine hormone disrupters,** chemicals that disrupt normal endocrine hormone functions. Hormones are chemicals released into the bloodstream by glands in one part of the body to regulate the development and function of tissues and organs elsewhere in the body (fig. 8.9). You undoubtedly have heard about sex hormones and their powerful effects on how we look and behave, but these are only one example of the many regulatory hormones that rule our lives.

We now know that some of the most insidious effects of persistent chemicals, such as DDT and PCBs, are that they interfere with normal growth, development, and physiology of a variety of animals—presumably including humans—at very low doses. In some cases, picogram concentrations (trillionths of a gram per liter) may be enough to cause developmental abnormalities in sensitive organisms. These chemicals are sometimes called environmental estrogens or androgens, because they often cause sexual dysfunction (reproductive health problems in females or feminization of males, for example). They are just as likely, however, to disrupt thyroxin functions or those of other important regulatory molecules as they are to obstruct sex hormones.

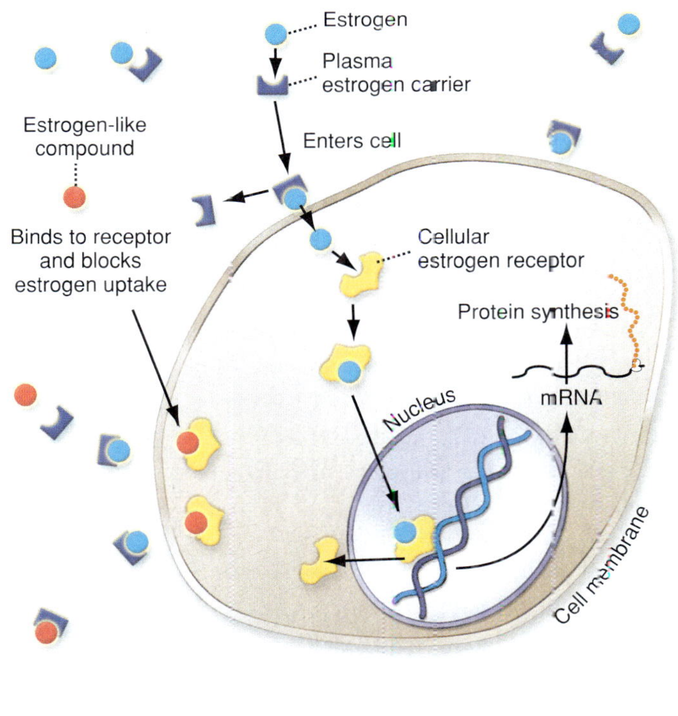

FIGURE 8.9 *Steroid hormone action. Plasma hormone carriers deliver regulatory molecules to the cell surface, where they cross the cell membrane. Intracellular carriers deliver hormones to the nucleus, where they bind to and regulate expression of DNA.*

MOVEMENT, DISTRIBUTION, AND FATE OF TOXINS

There are many sources of toxic and hazardous chemicals in the environment and many factors related to each chemical itself, its route or method of exposure, and its persistence in the environment, as well as characteristics of the target organism (table 8.4), that determine the danger of the chemical. We can think of both individuals and an ecosystem as sets of interacting compartments between which chemicals move, based on molecular size, solubility, stability, and reactivity (fig. 8.10). The dose (amount), route of entry, timing of exposure, and sensitivity of the organism all play important roles in determining toxicity. In this section, we will consider some of these characteristics and how they affect environmental health.

Solubility and Mobility

Solubility is one of the most important characteristics in determining how, where, and when a toxic material will move through the environment or through the body to its site of action. Chemicals can be divided into two major groups: those that dissolve more readily in water and those that dissolve more readily in oil. Water-soluble compounds move rapidly and widely through the environment because water is ubiquitous. They also tend to have ready access to most cells in the body because aqueous solutions bathe all our cells.

TABLE 8.4 Factors in Environmental Toxicity

FACTORS RELATED TO THE TOXIC AGENT

1. Chemical composition and reactivity
2. Physical characteristics (such as solubility, state)
3. Presence of impurities or contaminants
4. Stability and storage characteristics of toxic agent
5. Availability of vehicle (such as solvent) to carry agent
6. Movement of agent through environment and into cells

FACTORS RELATED TO EXPOSURE

1. Dose (concentration and volume of exposure)
2. Route, rate, and site of exposure
3. Duration and frequency of exposure
4. Time of exposure (time of day, season, year)

FACTORS RELATED TO THE ORGANISM

1. Resistance to uptake, storage, or cell permeability of agent
2. Ability to metabolize, inactivate, sequester, or eliminate agent
3. Tendency to activate or alter nontoxic substances so they become toxic
4. Concurrent infections or physical or chemical stress
5. Species and genetic characteristics of organism
6. Nutritional status of subject
7. Age, sex, body weight, immunological status, and maturity

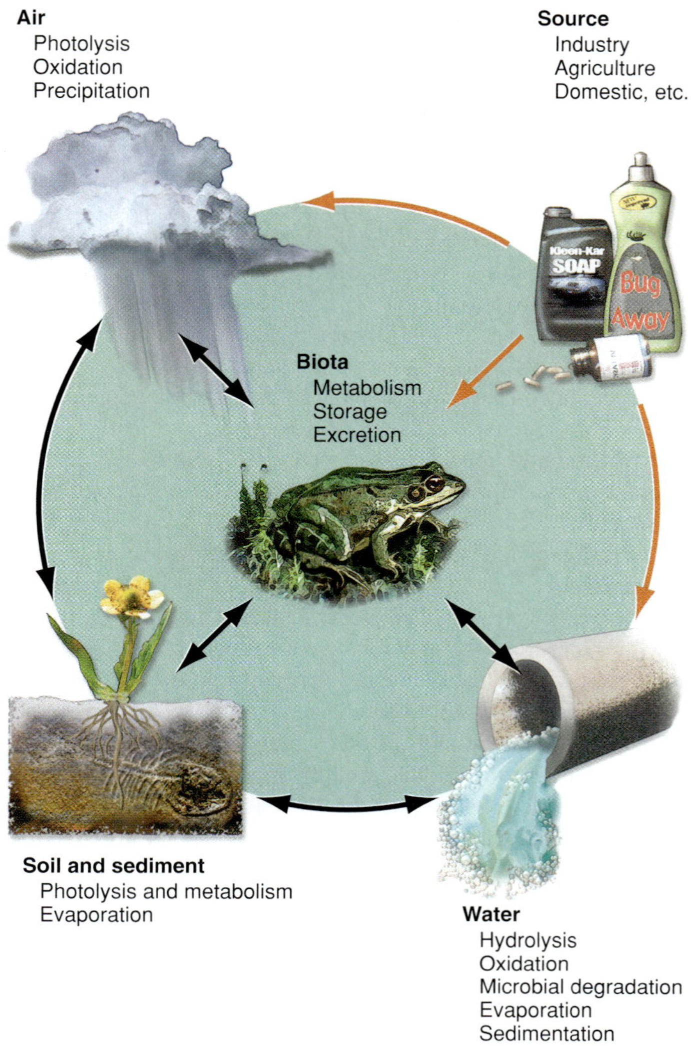

FIGURE 8.10 *Movement and fate of chemicals in the environment. Processes that modify, remove, or sequester compounds are shown below each compartment. Toxins also move directly from a source to soil and sediment.*

Molecules that are oil- or fat-soluble (usually organic molecules) generally need a carrier to move through the environment and into or within the body. Once inside the body, however, oil-soluble toxins penetrate readily into tissues and cells because the membranes that enclose cells are themselves made of similar oil-soluble chemicals. Once inside cells, oil-soluble materials are likely to accumulate and to be stored in lipid deposits, where they may be protected from metabolic breakdown and persist for many years.

Exposure and Susceptibility

Just as there are many sources of toxins in our environment, there are many routes for entry of dangerous substances into our bodies (fig. 8.11). Airborne toxins generally cause more ill health than any other exposure source. We breathe far more air every day than the volume of food we eat or water we drink. Furthermore, the lining of our lungs, which is designed to exchange gases very effi-

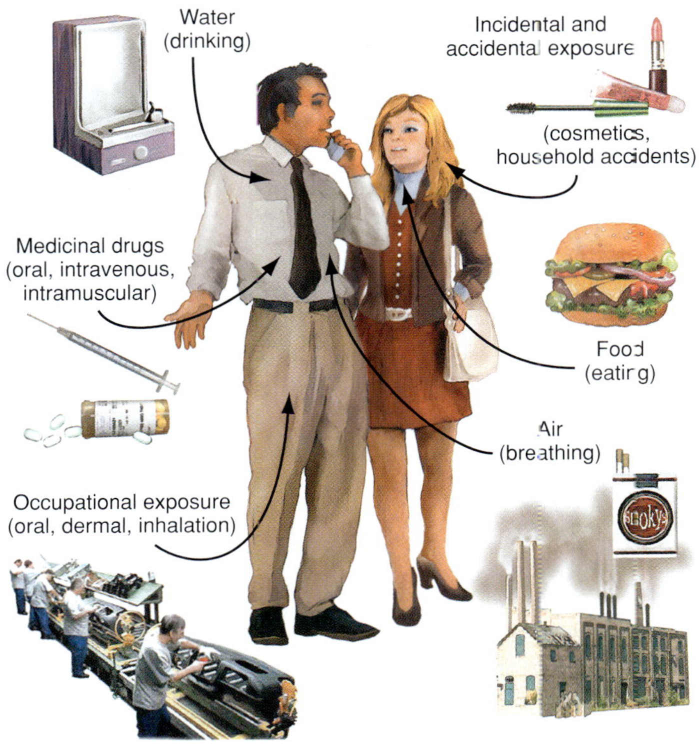

FIGURE 8.11 *Routes of exposure to toxic and hazardous environmental factors.*

ciently, also absorbs toxins very well. Still, food, water, and skin contact also can expose us to a wide variety of toxins. The largest exposures for many toxins are found in industrial settings, where workers may encounter doses thousands of times higher than would be found anywhere else. The European Agency for Safety and Health at Work warns that 32 million people (20 percent of all employees) in the European Union are exposed to unacceptable levels of carcinogens and other toxins in their workplace.

Condition of the organism and timing of exposure also have strong influences on toxicity. Healthy adults, for example, may be relatively insensitive to doses that would be very dangerous for young children or for someone already weakened by disease (What Do You Think? p. 188). Similarly, exposure to a toxin may be very dangerous at certain stages of developmental or metabolic cycles but may be innocuous at other times. A single dose of the notorious teratogen thalidomide, for example, taken in the third week of pregnancy (a time when many women aren't aware they're pregnant) can cause severe abnormalities in fetal limb development. A complication in measuring toxicity is that great differences in sensitivity exist among species. Thalidomide was tested on a number of laboratory animals without any deleterious effects. Unfortunately, however, it is a powerful teratogen in humans.

Bioaccumulation and Biomagnification

Cells have mechanisms for **bioaccumulation,** the selective absorption and storage of a great variety of molecules. This allows them to accumulate nutrients and essential minerals, but at the same time, they also may absorb and store harmful substances through the same mechanisms. Toxins that are rather dilute in the environment can reach dangerous levels inside cells and tissues through this process of bioaccumulation.

The effects of toxins also are magnified in the environment through food webs. **Biomagnification** occurs when the toxic burden of a large number of organisms at a lower trophic level is accumulated and concentrated by a predator in a higher trophic level. Phytoplankton and bacteria in aquatic ecosystems, for instance, take up heavy metals or toxic organic molecules from water or sediments (fig. 8.12). Their predators—zooplankton and small fish—collect and retain the toxins from many prey organisms, building up higher concentrations of toxins. The top carnivores in the food chain—game fish, fish-eating birds, and humans—can accumulate such high toxin levels that they suffer adverse health effects.

One of the first known examples of bioaccumulation and biomagnification was DDT, which accumulated through food chains, so that by the 1960s it was shown to be interfering with reproduction of peregrine falcons, brown pelicans, and other predatory birds at the top of their food chains.

Persistence

Some chemical compounds are very unstable and degrade rapidly under most environmental conditions, so that their concentrations decline quickly after release. Most modern herbicides and pesticides, for instance, quickly lose their toxicity. Other substances are more persistent and last for years or even centuries in the environment. PVC plastics chlorinated hydrocarbon pesticides, and asbestos are valuable because they are resistant to degradation, among other properties. This stability, however, also causes problems because these materials persist in the environment and have unexpected effects far from the sites of their original use.

Some **persistent organic pollutants (POPs)** have become extremely widespread, being found now from the tropics to the Arctic. They often accumulate in food webs and reach toxic concentrations in long-living top predators, such as humans, sharks, raptors, swordfish, and bears. Some of greatest current concerns are

- Polybrominated diphenyl ethers (PBDE) are widely used as flame-retardants in textiles, foam in upholstery, and plastic in appliances and computers. This compound was first reported accumulating in women's breast milk in Sweden in the 1990s. It was subsequently found in humans and other species everywhere from Canada to Israel. Nearly 150 million metric tons (330 million lbs) of PBDEs are used every year worldwide. The toxicity and environmental persistence of PBDE are much like those of PCBs, to which it is closely related chemically. The dust at ground zero in New York City after September 11 was heavily laden with PBDE. The European Union has already banned this compound.
- Perfluorooctane sulfonate (PFOS) and perfluorooctanoic acid (PFOA, also known as C8) are members of a chemical family used to make nonstick, waterproof, and stain-resistant products such as Teflon, Gortex, Scotchguard, and Stainmaster.

what do you think?

Children's Health

Increasing evidence shows that children are much more vulnerable than adults to environmental toxins. Pound for pound, children drink more water, eat more food, and breathe more air than do adults. Constantly putting fingers, toys, and other objects into their mouths increases children's exposure to toxins in dust or soil. Compared with adults, children generally have less developed protective mechanisms, such as immune systems or metabolic processes to degrade or excrete toxins. Rapid growth and development in childhood makes their metabolism and maturation highly susceptible to disruption. And because children have more years of life remaining than do most adults, they have more time to develop chronic diseases, such as cancer, that may require decades to be expressed.

Childhood cancer incidence has risen 1 percent per year since the early 1970s. Asthma also is up sharply. Some 6.3 million children now suffer from this disease, a four-fold increase over the past 30 years. Asthmatic attacks, which cause blockage of the airways and result in coughing, wheezing, and difficulty breathing, are now the fourth-ranking cause of childhood hospitalization. Inner-city children seem to be particularly at risk for this disease. One study found that 25 percent of all children in New York City's central Harlem suffer from asthma. Scientists believe genetic predisposition plays an important role in this disease but that environmental exposure to factors such as dust, cockroaches and mites, cigarette smoke, mold and mildew, and diesel engine fumes also act as a trigger.

Currently, about 430,000 American children between the ages of 1 and 5 have elevated blood lead levels that can cause irreversible disabilities, such as lower IQ and neurological damage. Autism and attention-deficit hyperactivity disorder (ADHD) are reported to have increased sharply in the past 20 years, although increasing awareness and diagnosis of these conditions may be partly responsible for this increase. A growing percentage of boys with reproductive tract defects also has been reported.

A recently recognized environmental hazard for children is the chromated copper arsenate (CCA)-treated lumber often used to build rot-resistant decks, sidewalks, and playground equipment. All three metals are toxic. Arsenic, the worst of the three, can leach out of weathered wood and has been shown to cause muscle damage as well as lung, bladder, and skin cancer. CCA-treated wood is being phased out in the United States, but not fast enough, according to some groups.

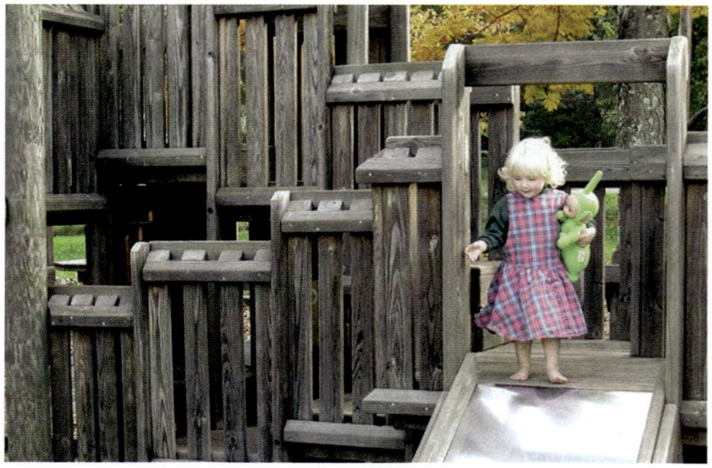

Should all arsenic-treated lumber be removed from places where children play?

In 2003 the U.S. EPA issued its first guidelines to define the greater risks that children face from environmental toxins. According to these proposed rules, regulators should assume that children have ten times the exposure risk of adults to cancer-causing chemicals. Some health groups criticized these guidelines as not being strong enough, pointing out that certain chemicals, such as vinyl chloride (used in PVC plastics), diethylnitrosamine (from tobacco smoke), and polychlorinated biphenyls (PCBs, in electrical transformers), can be up to 65 times more potent in infants and toddlers than in adults.

To study connections between environmental exposures and potential health effects issues, the U.S. government has started a landmark National Children's Study, which will follow 100,000 children from birth to age 18. In establishing this study, former EPA Administrator Christie Whitman said, "Children represent 25 percent of our population, but 100 percent of the future."

What do you think? What would be the best way to safeguard children from environmental hazards? Would you ban CCA-treated lumber completely, or just remove it from playgrounds and other places in which children might be exposed? How would you distinguish between the effects of poverty and environmental hazards for inner-city children? Might it be more effective to focus on providing them with better housing, nutrition, and education than on protecting them from environmental chemicals? What research would you request if you were an environmental regulator?

Industry makes use of their slippery, heat-stable properties to manufacture everything from airplanes and computers to cosmetics and household cleaners. Now these chemicals—which are reported to be infinitely persistent in the environment—are found throughout the world, even the most remote and seemingly pristine sites. Almost all Americans have one or more perfluorinated compounds in their blood. Heating some non-stick cooking pans above 260°C (500°F) can release enough PFOA to kill pet birds. This chemical family has been shown to cause liver damage as well as various cancers and reproductive and developmental problems in rats. Exposure may be especially dangerous to women and girls, who may be 100 times more sensitive than men to these chemicals.

- Phthalates (pronounced *thalates*) are found in cosmetics, deodorants, and many plastics (such as soft polyvinyl chloride, or PVC) used for food packaging, children's toys, and medical devices. Some members of this chemical family are known to be toxic to laboratory animals, causing kidney and liver damage and possibly some cancers. In addition, many phthalates act as endocrine hormone disrupters and have been linked to reproductive abnormalities and decreased fertility. A correlation has been found between phthalate levels in urine and low sperm numbers and decreased sperm motility in men. Nearly everyone in the United States has phthalates in his or her body at levels reported to cause these problems. While not yet conclusive,

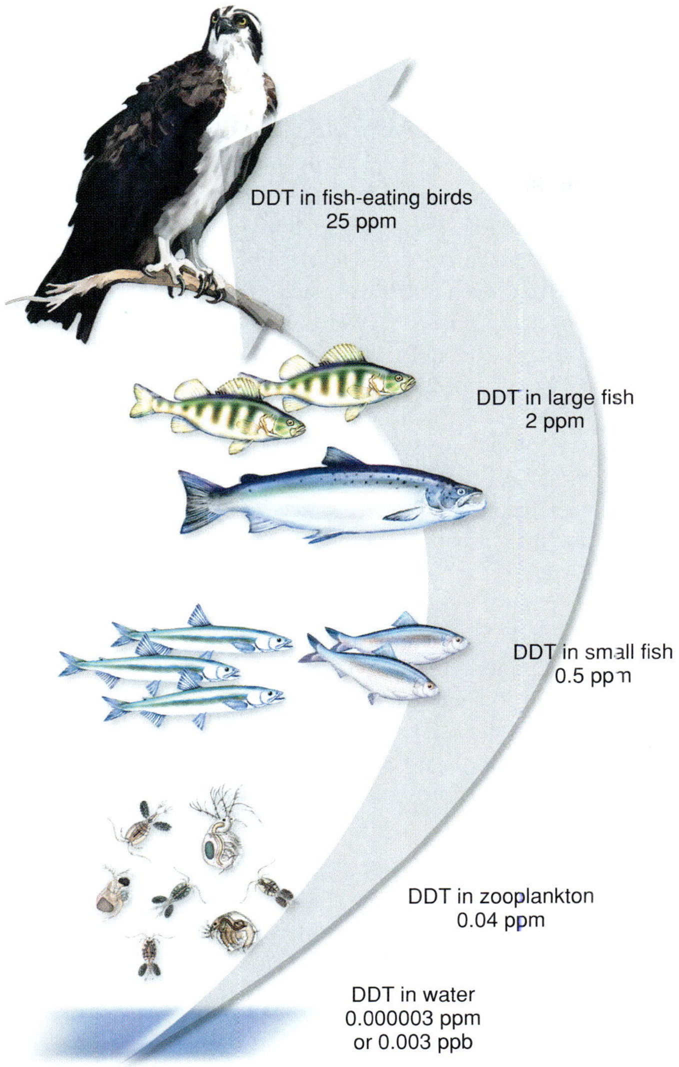

FIGURE 8.12 *Bioaccumulation and biomagnification. Organisms lower on the food chain take up and store toxins from the environment. They are eaten by larger predators, who are eaten, in turn, by even larger predators. The highest members of the food chain can accumulate very high levels of the toxin.*

these results could help explain a 50-year decline in semen quality in most industrialized countries.

- Bisphenol A (BPA), a prime ingredient in polycarbonate plastic (commonly used for products ranging from water bottles to tooth-protecting sealants), has been widely found in humans, even those who have no known exposure to these chemicals. So far, there is little direct evidence linking BPA exposure to human health risks, but studies in animals have found that the chemical can cause abnormal chromosome numbers, a condition called aneuploidy, which is the leading cause of miscarriages and several forms of mental retardation. It also is an environmental estrogen and may alter sexual development in both males and females.
- Atrazine, one of the most widely used herbicides in the midwestern corn belt, has been shown to cause abnormal development and sexual dysfunction in frogs. Farmers who use Atrazine heavily have high rates of certain lymphomas, but these farmers are generally exposed to other toxic compounds as well. A study of farm families in northwestern Minnesota found considerably higher rates of birth defects than in urban families. "The data is associative," said Dr. Vince Gary, who directed the research. No definitive cause and effect can be shown with any particular pesticide, but the sensitivity of other species raises concerns.

Chemical Interactions

Some materials produce *antagonistic* reactions. That is, they interfere with the effects or stimulate the breakdown of other chemicals. For instance, vitamins E and A can reduce the response to some carcinogens. Other materials are *additive* when they occur together in exposures. Rats exposed to both lead and arsenic show twice the toxicity of only one of these elements. Perhaps the greatest concern is synergistic effects. **Synergism** is an interaction in which one substance exacerbates the effects of another. For example, occupational asbestos exposure increases lung cancer rates 20-fold. Smoking increases lung cancer rates by the same amount. Asbestos workers who also smoke, however, have a 400-fold increase in cancer rates. How many other toxic chemicals are we exposed to that are below threshold limits individually but combine to give toxic results?

MECHANISMS FOR MINIMIZING TOXIC EFFECTS

A fundamental concept in toxicology is that every material can be poisonous under some conditions, but most chemicals have a safe level or threshold below which their effects are undetectable or insignificant. Each of us consumes lethal doses of many chemicals over the course of a lifetime. One hundred cups of strong coffee, for instance, contain a lethal dose of caffeine. Similarly, 100 aspirin tablets, 10 kg (22 lbs) of spinach or rhubarb, or a liter of alcohol would be deadly if consumed all at once. Taken in small doses, however, most toxins can be broken down or excreted before they do much harm. Furthermore, the damage they cause can be repaired. Sometimes, however, mechanisms that protect us from one type of toxin or at one stage in the life cycle become deleterious with another substance or in another stage of development. Let's look at how these processes help protect us from harmful substances, as well as how they can go awry.

Metabolic Degradation and Excretion

Most organisms have enzymes that process waste products and environmental poisons to reduce their toxicity. In mammals, most of these enzymes are located in the liver, the primary site of detoxification of both natural wastes and introduced poisons. Sometimes, however, these reactions work to our disadvantage. Compounds such as benzepyrene, for example, that are not toxic in their original form are processed by the same liver enzymes into cancer-causing carcinogens. Why would we have a system that makes a chemical more dangerous? Evolution and natural selection are expressed through reproductive success or failure. Defense mechanisms that protect us from toxins and hazards early in life are "selected for" by evolution. Factors or conditions that affect postreproductive ages (such as cancer or premature senility) usually don't affect reproductive success or exert "selective pressure."

We also reduce the effects of waste products and environmental toxins by eliminating them from the body through excretion. Volatile molecules, such as carbon dioxide, hydrogen cyanide, and ketones, are excreted via breathing. Some excess salts and other substances are excreted in sweat. Primarily, however, excretion is a function of the kidneys, which can eliminate significant amounts of soluble materials through urine formation. Toxin accumulation in the urine can damage this vital system, however, and the kidneys and bladder often are subjected to harmful levels of toxic compounds. In the same way, the stomach, intestine, and colon often suffer damage from materials concentrated in the digestive system and may be afflicted by diseases and tumors.

Repair Mechanisms

In the same way that individual cells have enzymes to repair damage to DNA and protein at the molecular level, tissues and organs that are exposed regularly to physical wear-and-tear or to toxic or hazardous materials often have mechanisms for damage repair. Our skin and the epithelial linings of the gastrointestinal tract, blood vessels, lungs, and urogenital system have high cellular reproduction rates to replace injured cells. With each reproduction cycle, however, there is a chance that some cells will lose normal growth controls and run amok, creating a tumor. Thus, any agent, such as smoking or drinking, that irritates tissues is likely to be carcinogenic. And tissues with high cell-replacement rates are among the most likely to develop cancers.

APPLICATION: Assessing Toxins

The earliest studies of human toxicology came from experiments in which volunteers (usually students or prisoners) were given measured doses of suspected toxins. Today it is considered neither ethical nor humane to deliberately expose individuals to danger, even if they volunteer. Toxicology is now done in either retrospective or prospective studies. In a **retrospective study,** you identify a group of people who have been exposed to a suspected risk factor and then compare their health with that of a control group who are as nearly identical as possible to the experimental group, except for exposure to that particular factor. Unfortunately, people often can't remember where they were or what they were doing many years ago. In a **prospective study,** you identify a study group and a control group and then keep track of everything they do and how it affects their health. Then you watch and wait for years to see if a response appears in the study group but not in the control group. This kind of study is expensive because you may need a very large group to study a rare effect, and it is still difficult to distinguish among many simultaneous variables.

Suppose that you and your classmates have been chosen to be part of a prospective study of the health risks of a particular soft drink.

1. The researchers can't afford to keep records of everything that you do or are exposed to over the next 20 or 30 years. What do you think would be the most important factors and/or effects to monitor?
2. In a study group of a hundred students, how many would have to get sick to convince you that the soft drink was a risk factor? (Remember that there are many potential variables in the health of your study group.)

MEASURING TOXICITY

In 1540 the Swiss scientist Paracelsus said, "The dose makes the poison," by which he meant that almost everything is toxic at some level. This remains the most basic principle of toxicology. Sodium chloride (table salt), for instance, is essential for human life in small doses. If you were forced to eat a kilogram of salt all at once, however, it would make you very sick. A similar amount injected into your bloodstream would be lethal. How a material is delivered—at what rate, through which route of entry, and in what medium—plays a vital role in determining toxicity.

This does not mean that all toxins are identical, however. Some are so poisonous that a single drop on your skin can kill you. Others require massive amounts injected directly into the blood to be lethal. Measuring and comparing the toxicity of various materials are difficult because species differ in sensitivity, and individuals within a species respond differently to a given exposure. In this section, we will look at methods of toxicity testing and at how results are analyzed and reported.

Animal Testing

The most commonly used and widely accepted toxicity test is to expose a population of laboratory animals to measured doses of a specific substance under controlled conditions. This procedure is expensive, time-consuming, and often painful and debilitating to the animals being tested. It commonly takes hundreds—or even thousands—of animals, several years of hard work, and hundreds of thousands of dollars to thoroughly test the effects of a toxin at very low doses. More humane toxicity tests using computer simulations of model reactions, cell cultures, and other substitutes for whole living animals are being developed. However, conventional large-scale animal testing is the method in which scientists have the most confidence and on which most public policies about pollution and environmental or occupational health hazards are based.

In addition to humanitarian concerns, several other problems in laboratory animal testing trouble both toxicologists and policymakers.

One problem is differences in toxin sensitivity among the members of a specific population. Figure 8.13 shows a typical dose/response curve for exposure to a hypothetical toxin. Some individuals are very sensitive to the toxin, while others are insensitive. Most, however, fall in a middle category, forming a bell-shaped curve. The question for regulators and politicians is whether we should set pollution levels that will protect everyone, including the most sensitive people, or only aim to protect the average person. It might cost billions of extra dollars to protect a very small number of individuals at the extreme end of the curve. Is that a good use of resources?

Dose/response curves are not always symmetrical, making it difficult to compare toxicity of unlike chemicals or different species of organisms. A convenient way to describe toxicity of a chemical is to determine the dose to which 50 percent of the test population is sensitive. In the case of a lethal dose (LD), this is called the **LD50** (fig. 8.14).

Unrelated species can react very differently to the same toxin, not only because body sizes vary but also because physiology and metabolism differ. Even closely related species can have very dissimilar reactions to a particular toxin. Hamsters, for instance, are nearly 5,000 times less sensitive to some dioxins than are guinea pigs. Of 226 chemicals found to be carcinogenic in either rats or mice, 95 cause cancer in one species but not the other. These variations make it difficult to estimate the risks for humans, since we don't consider it ethical to perform controlled experiments in which we deliberately expose people to toxins.

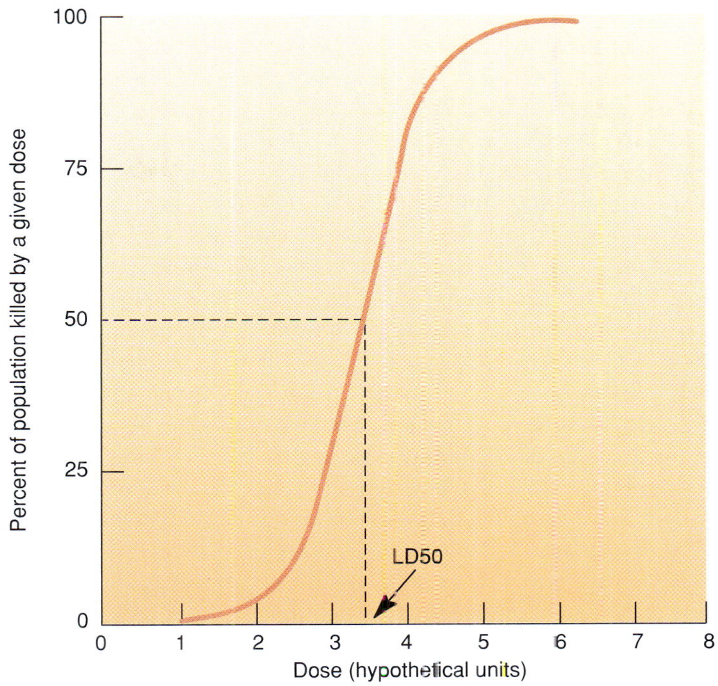

FIGURE 8.14 *Cumulative population response to increasing doses of a toxin. The LD50 is the dose that is lethal to half the population.*

Toxicity Ratings

It is useful to group materials according to their relative toxicity. A moderate toxin takes about 1 g per kg of body weight (about 2 oz for an average human) to make a lethal dose. Very toxic materials take about one-tenth that amount, while extremely toxic substances take one-hundredth as much (only a few drops) to kill most people. Supertoxic chemicals are extremely potent; for some, a few micrograms (millionths of a gram—an amount invisible to the naked eye) make a lethal dose. These materials are not all synthetic. One of the most toxic chemicals known, for instance, is ricin, a protein found in castor bean seeds. It is so toxic that 0.3 billionths of a gram given intravenously will kill a mouse. If aspirin were this toxic for humans, a single tablet, divided evenly, could kill 1 million people.

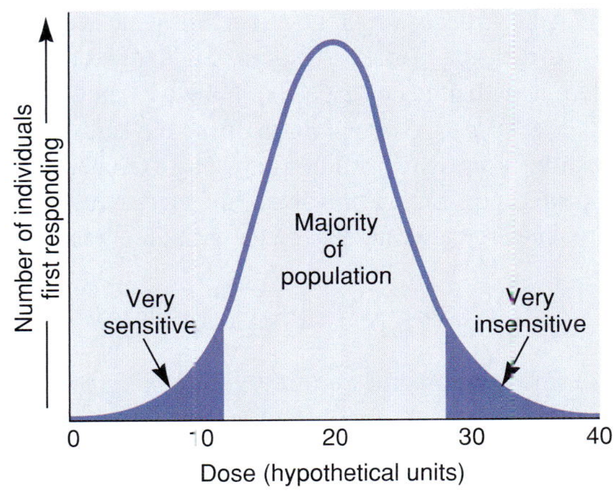

FIGURE 8.13 *Probable variations in sensitivity to a toxin within a population. Some members of a population may be very sensitive to a given toxin, while others are much less sensitive. The majority of the population falls somewhere between the two extremes.*

Many carcinogens, mutagens, and teratogens are dangerous at levels far below their direct toxic effect because abnormal cell growth exerts a kind of biological amplification. A single cell, perhaps altered by a single molecular event, can multiply into millions of tumor cells or an entire organism. Just as there are different levels of direct toxicity, however, there are different degrees of carcinogenicity, mutagenicity, and teratogenicity. Methanesulfonic acid, for instance, is highly carcinogenic, while the sweetener saccharin is a possible carcinogen whose effects may be vanishingly small.

Acute versus Chronic Doses and Effects

Most of the toxic effects that we have discussed so far have been **acute effects.** That is, they are caused by a single exposure to the toxin and result in an immediate health crisis. Often, if the individual experiencing an acute reaction survives this immediate crisis, the effects are reversible. **Chronic effects,** on the other hand, are long-lasting, perhaps even permanent. A chronic effect can result from a single dose of a very toxic substance, or it can be the result of a continuous or repeated sublethal exposure.

We also describe long-lasting exposures as chronic, although their effects may or may not persist after the toxin is removed. It usually is difficult to assess the specific health risks of chronic exposures because other factors, such as aging or normal diseases, act simultaneously with the factor under study. It often requires very large populations of experimental animals to obtain statistically significant results for low-level chronic exposures. Toxicologists talk about "megarat" experiments in which it might take a million rats to determine the health risks of some supertoxic chemicals at very low doses. Such an experiment would be terribly expensive for even a single chemical, let alone for the thousands of chemicals and factors suspected of being dangerous.

An alternative to enormous studies involving millions of animals is to give massive amounts—usually the maximum tolerable dose—of a toxin being studied to a smaller number of individuals and then to extrapolate what the effects of lower doses might have been. This is a controversial approach because it is not clear that responses to toxins are linear or uniform across a wide range of doses.

Figure 8.15 shows three possible results from low doses of a toxin. Curve (a) shows a baseline level of response in the population, even at zero dose of the toxin. This suggests that some other factor in the environment also causes this response. Curve (b) shows a straight-line relationship from the highest doses to zero exposure. Many carcinogens and mutagens show this kind of response. Any exposure to such agents, no matter how small, carries some risks. Curve (c) shows a threshold for the response where some minimal dose is necessary before any effect can be observed. This generally suggests the presence of a defense mechanism that prevents the toxin from reaching its target in an active form or repairs the damage that the toxin causes. Low levels of exposure to the toxin in question may have no deleterious effects, and it might not be necessary to try to keep exposures to zero.

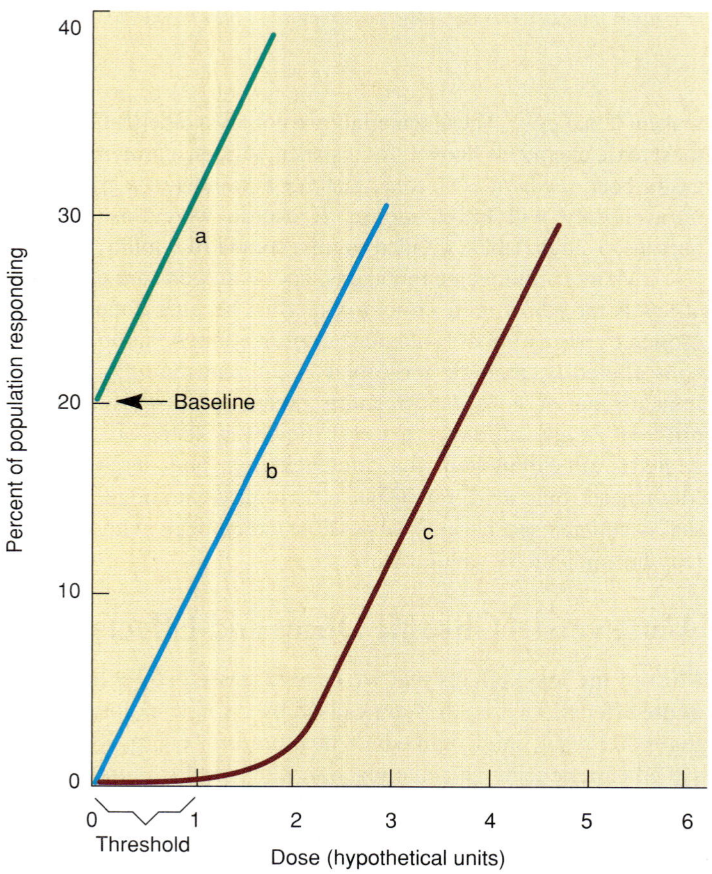

FIGURE 8.15 *Three possible dose-response curves at low doses.* (a) *Some individuals respond, even at zero dose, indicating that some other factor must be involved.* (b) *Response is linear down to the lowest possible dose.* (c) *Threshold must be passed before any response is seen.*

Which, if any, environmental health hazards have thresholds is an important but difficult question. The 1958 Delaney Clause to the U.S. Food and Drug Act forbids the addition of any amount of known carcinogens to food and drugs, based on the assumption that any exposure to these substances represents unacceptable risks. This standard was replaced in 1996 by a "no reasonable harm" requirement, defined as less than one cancer for every million people exposed over a lifetime. This change was supported by a report from the National Academy of Sciences concluding that synthetic chemicals in our diet are unlikely to represent an appreciable cancer risk. We will discuss risk analysis in the section "Risk Assessment and Acceptance."

Detection Limits

You may have seen or heard dire warnings about toxic materials detected in samples of air, water, or food. A typical headline announced recently that 23 pesticides were found in 16 food samples. What does that mean? The implication seems to be that any amount of dangerous materials is unacceptable and that counting the numbers of compounds detected is a reliable way to establish danger. We have seen, however, that the dose makes the poison. It matters not only what is there but also how much, where it is located, how accessible it is, and who is exposed. At some level, the mere presence of a substance is insignificant.

Toxins and pollutants may seem to be more widespread now than in the past, and this is surely a valid perception for many substances. The daily reports we hear of new materials found in new places, however, are also due, in part, to our more sensitive measuring techniques. Twenty years ago, parts per million were generally the limits of detection for most chemicals. Anything below that amount was often reported as "zero" or "absent," rather than more accurately as "undetected." A decade ago, new machines and techniques were developed to measure parts per billion. Suddenly, chemicals were found where none had been suspected. Now we can detect parts per trillion or even parts per quadrillion in some cases. Increasingly sophisticated measuring capabilities may lead us to believe that toxic materials have become more prevalent. In fact, our environment may be no more dangerous; we are just better at finding trace amounts.

RISK ASSESSMENT AND ACCEPTANCE

Even if we know with some certainty how toxic a specific chemical is in laboratory tests, it still is difficult to determine **risk** (the probability of harm times the probability of exposure) if that chemical is released into the environment. As we have seen, many factors complicate the movement and fate of chemicals both around us and within our bodies. Furthermore, public perception of relative dangers from environmental hazards can be skewed so that some risks seem much more important than others.

Understanding Risks

A number of factors influence how we perceive relative risks associated with different situations.

- People with social, political, or economic interests—including environmentalists—tend to downplay certain risks and emphasize others that suit their own agendas. We do this individually as well, building up the dangers of things that don't benefit us, while diminishing or ignoring the negative aspects of activities we enjoy or profit from.
- Most people have difficulty understanding and believing probabilities. We feel that there must be patterns and connections in events, even though statistical theory says otherwise. If the coin turned up heads last time, we feel certain that it will turn up tails next time. In the same way, it is difficult to understand the meaning of a 1-in-10,000 risk of being poisoned by a chemical.
- Our personal experiences often are misleading. When we have not personally experienced a bad outcome, we feel it is more rare and unlikely to occur than it actually may be. Furthermore, the anxieties generated by life's gambles make us want to deny uncertainty and to misjudge many risks.
- We have an exaggerated view of our own abilities to control our fate. We generally consider ourselves above-average drivers, safer than most when using appliances or power tools, and less likely than others to suffer medical problems, such as heart attacks. People often feel they can avoid hazards because they are wiser or luckier than others.
- News media give us a biased perspective on the frequency of certain kinds of health hazards, overreporting some accidents or diseases, while downplaying or underreporting others. Sensational, gory, or especially frightful causes of death, such as murders, plane crashes, fires, or terrible accidents, receive a disproportionate amount of attention in the public media. Heart disease, cancer, and stroke kill nearly 15 times as many people in the United States as do accidents and 75 times as many people as do homicides, but the emphasis placed by the media on accidents and homicides is nearly inversely proportional to their relative frequency, compared with either cardiovascular disease or cancer. This gives us an inaccurate picture of the real risks to which we are exposed.
- We tend to have an irrational fear or distrust of certain technologies or activities that leads us to overestimate their dangers. Nuclear power, for instance, is viewed as very risky, while coal-burning power plants seem to be familiar and relatively benign; in fact, coal mining, shipping, and combustion cause an estimated 10,000 deaths each year in the United States, compared with none known so far for nuclear power generation. An old, familiar technology seems safer and more acceptable than does a new, unknown one.
- Alarmist myths and fallacies spread through society, often fueled by xenophobia, politics, or religion. For example, the World Health Organization campaign to eradicate polio worldwide has been thwarted by religious leaders in northern Nigeria—the last country where the disease remains widespread—who claim that oral vaccination is a U.S. plot to spread AIDS or infertility among Muslims.

Accepting Risks

How much risk is acceptable? How much is it worth to minimize and avoid exposure to certain risks? Most people will tolerate a higher probability of occurrence of an event if the harm caused by that event is low. Conversely, harm of greater severity is acceptable only at low levels of frequency. A 1-in-10,000 chance of being killed might be of more concern to you than a 1-in-100 chance of being injured. For most people, a 1-in-100,000 chance of dying from some event or some factor is a threshold for changing what they do. That is, if the chance of death is less than 1 in 100,000, we are not likely to be worried enough to change our ways. If the risk is greater, we will probably do something about it. The Environmental Protection Agency generally assumes that a risk of 1 in 1 million is acceptable for most environmental hazards. Critics of this policy ask, acceptable to whom?

For activities that we enjoy or find profitable, we are often willing to accept far greater risks than this general threshold. Conversely, for risks that benefit someone else, we demand far higher protection. For instance, your chance of dying in a motor vehicle accident in any given year are about 1 in 5,000, but that doesn't deter many people from riding in automobiles. Your chances of dying from lung cancer if you smoke one pack of cigarettes per day are about 1 in 1,000. By comparison, the risk from drinking water with the EPA limit of trichloroethylene is about 2 in 1 billion. Strangely, many people demand water with zero levels of trichloroethylene while continuing to smoke cigarettes.

More than 1 million Americans are diagnosed with skin cancer each year. Some of these cancers are lethal, and most are disfiguring,

APPLICATION: Calculating Probabilities

You can calculate the statistical danger of a risky activity by multiplying the probability of danger by the frequency of the activity. For example, in the United States, 1 person in 3 will be injured in a car accident in their lifetime (so the probability of injury is 1 per 3 persons, or $^1/_3$). In a population of 30 car-riding people, the cumulative risk of injury is 30 people × (1 injury/3 people) = 10 injuries over 30 lifetimes.

1. If the average person takes 50,000 trips in a lifetime, and the accident risk is $^1/_3$ per lifetime, what is the probability of an accident per trip?
2. If you have been riding safely for 20 years, what is the probability of an accident during your next trip?

Answers: *1.* Probability of injury per trip = (1 injury/3 lifetimes) × (1 lifetime/50,000 trips) = 1 injury/150,000 trips. *2.* 1 in 150,000. Statistically, you have the same chance each time.

yet only one-third of teenagers routinely use sunscreen. Tanning beds more than double your chances of cancer, especially if you're young, but about 10 percent of all teenagers admit regularly using these devices.

Table 8.5 lists lifetime odds of dying from some leading causes. These are statistical averages, of course, and there clearly are differences in where one lives and how one behaves that affect the danger level of these activities. Although the average lifetime chance of dying in an automobile accident is 1 in 100, there are clearly things you can do—such as wearing a seat belt, driving defensively, and avoiding risky situations—to improve your odds. Still, it is interesting how we readily accept some risks while shunning others.

Our perception of relative risks is strongly affected by whether risks are known or unknown, whether we feel in control of the outcome, and how dreadful the results are. Risks that are unknown or unpredictable and results that are particularly gruesome or disgusting seem far worse than those that are familiar and socially acceptable.

Studies of public risk perception show that most people react more to emotion than to statistics. We go to great lengths to avoid some dangers while gladly accepting others. Factors that are involuntary, unfamiliar, undetectable to those exposed or catastrophic; those that have delayed effects; and those that are a threat to future generations are especially feared. Factors that are voluntary, familiar, detectable, or immediate cause less anxiety. Even though the actual number of deaths from automobile accidents, smoking, or alcohol, for instance, is thousands of times greater than those from pesticides, nuclear energy, or genetic engineering, the latter group preoccupies us far more than the former.

TABLE 8.5 Lifetime Chances of Dying in the United States

SOURCE	ODDS (1 IN *x*)
Heart disease	2
Cancer	3
Smoking	4
Lung disease	15
Pneumonia	30
Automobile accident	100
Suicide	100
Falls	200
Firearms	200
Fires	1,000
Airplane accident	5,000
Jumping from high places	6,000
Drowning	10,000
Lightning	56,000
Hornets, wasps, bees	76,000
Dog bite	230,000
Poisonous snakes, spiders	700,000
Botulism	1 million
Falling space debris	5 million
Drinking water with EPA limit of trichloroethylene	10 million

Source: Data from U.S. National Safety Council, 2003.

ESTABLISHING PUBLIC POLICY

Risk management combines principles of environmental health and toxicology with regulatory decisions based on socioeconomic, technical, and political considerations (fig. 8.16). The biggest problem in making regulatory decisions is that we are usually exposed to many sources of harm, often unknowingly. It is difficult to separate the effects of all these different hazards and to evaluate their risks accurately, especially when the exposures are near the threshold of measurement and response. In spite of often vague and contradictory data, public policymakers must make decisions.

The case of the sweetener saccharin is a good example of the complexities and uncertainties of risk assessment in public health. Studies in the 1970s at the University of Wisconsin and the Canadian Health Protection Branch suggested a link between saccharin and bladder cancer in male rats. Critics of these studies pointed out that humans would have to drink 800 cans of diet soda *per day* to get a saccharin dose equivalent to that given to the rats. Furthermore, they argued this response may be unique to male rats. In 2000 the U.S. Department of Health concluded a study that found no association between saccharin and cancer in humans. Congress ordered that all warnings be removed from saccharin-containing products. Still, some groups, such as the Center for Science in the Public Interest, consider this sweetener dangerous and urge us to avoid it if possible.

In setting standards for environmental toxins, we need to consider (1) combined effects of exposure to many different sources of damage, (2) different sensitivities of members of the

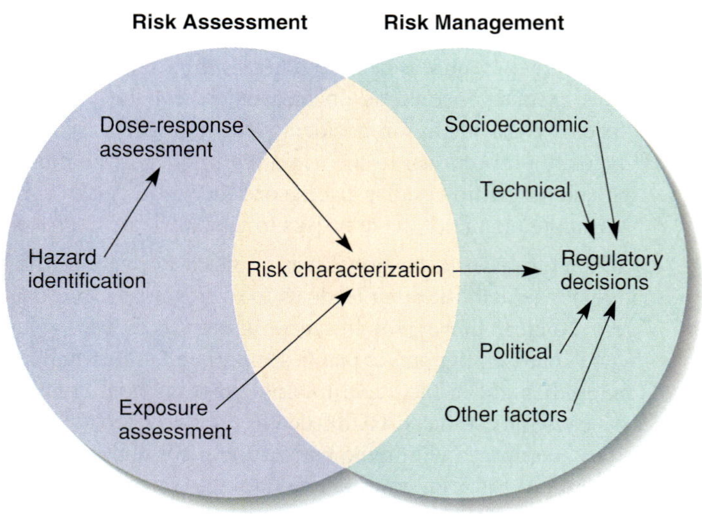

FIGURE 8.16 *Risk assessment organizes and analyzes data to determine relative risk. Risk management sets priorities and evaluates relevant factors to make regulatory decisions.*
Source: Data from D. E. Patton, "USEPA's Framework for Ecological Risk Assessment" in *Human Ecological Risk Assessment,* Vol. 1, No. 4.

population, and (3) effects of chronic as well as acute exposures. Some people argue that pollution levels should be set at the highest amount that does *not* cause measurable effects. Others demand that pollution be reduced to zero if possible, or as low as is technologically feasible. It may not be reasonable to demand that we be protected from every potentially harmful contaminant in our environment, no matter how small the risk. As we have seen, our bodies have mechanisms that enable us to avoid or repair many kinds of damage, so that most of us can withstand a minimal level of exposure without harm (fig. 8.17).

On the other hand, each challenge to our cells by toxic substances represents stress on our bodies. Although each individual stress may not be life-threatening, the cumulative effects of all the environmental stresses, both natural and human-caused, to which we are exposed may seriously shorten or restrict our lives. Furthermore, some individuals in any population are more susceptible to those stresses than others. Should we set pollution standards so that no one is adversely affected, even the most sensitive individuals, or should the acceptable level of risk be based on the average member of the population?

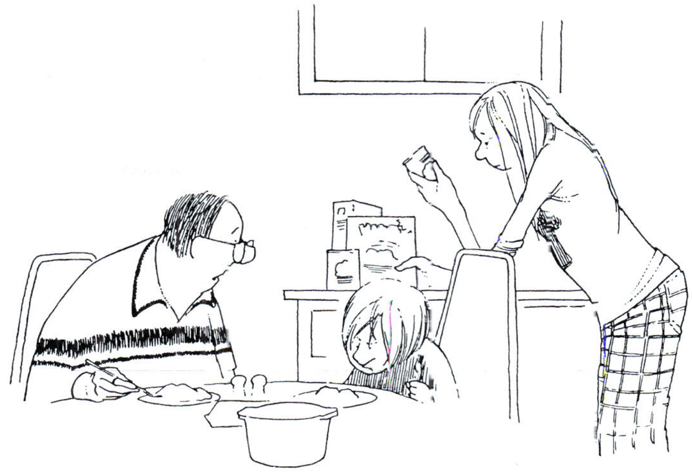

FIGURE 8.17 *"Do you want to stop reading those ingredients while we're trying to eat?"*
Source: Reprinted with permission of the *Star-Tribune*, Minneapolis-St. Paul.

Finally, policy decisions about hazardous and toxic materials also need to be based on information about how such materials affect the plants, animals, and other organisms that define and maintain our environment. In some cases, pollution can harm or destroy whole ecosystems with devastating effects on the life-supporting cycles on which we depend. In other cases, only the most sensitive species are threatened. Table 8.6 shows the Environmental Protection Agency's assessment of relative risks to human welfare. This ranking reflects a concern that our exclusive focus on reducing pollution to protect human health has neglected risks to natural ecological systems. While there have been many benefits from a case-by-case approach in which we evaluate the health risks of individual chemicals, we have often missed broader ecological problems that may be of greater ultimate importance.

TABLE 8.6 Relative Risks to Human Welfare

RELATIVELY HIGH-RISK PROBLEMS	RELATIVELY MEDIUM-RISK PROBLEMS	RELATIVELY LOW-RISK PROBLEMS
Habitat alteration and destruction	Herbicides/pesticides	Oil spills
Species extinction and loss of biological diversity	Toxins and pollutants in surface waters	Groundwater pollution
Stratospheric ozone depletion	Acid deposition	Radionuclides
Global climate change	Airborne toxins	Thermal pollution

Source: Data from U.S. Environmental Protection Agency.

SUMMARY

- Health is a state of physical, mental, and social well-being, not merely the absence of disease or infirmity. Environmental health focuses on health risks in the natural, social, cultural, and technological worlds in which we live.
- The world is now undergoing a dramatic epidemiological transition. The traditional killers—infectious diseases, maternal and perinatal complications, and nutritional deficiencies—still take a terrible toll in the developing world, but health problems such as heart attack, depression, and traffic accidents, once thought to occur only in rich countries, are now becoming the leading killers everywhere as people live longer and adopt Western lifestyles and diets.

- Disability-adjusted life years (DALYs) measure the disease burden arising from both premature deaths and the loss of healthy life resulting from illness and disability.
- Emergent diseases are those not previously known or that have been absent for at least 20 years. Some examples are SARS (severe acute respiratory syndrome), West Nile virus, and AIDS (acquired immune deficiency syndrome). AIDS is currently the most deadly of these diseases, infecting about 65 million people and killing some 3 million every year.
- Only 10 percent of all medical expenditures go to the major diseases that affect 90 percent of the world population. Currently, the United States donates only 0.01 percent of its GDP for health care in the developing world. Investing more would not only save millions of lives but could also boost the world economy significantly.
- CWD (chronic wasting disease), a rapidly spreading brain disease in deer, is an emergent ecological disease. Some other examples are sudden oak death syndrome in California, black-band disease in the Caribbean, and domoic acid poisoning, which is killing marine mammals in the Pacific.
- Toxins are poisons. They can be very specific because they interact with and disrupt the metabolic machinery that keeps cells alive. Some materials are so supertoxic that a single molecule can cause cell death.
- Allergens, carcinogens, mutagens, neurotoxins, teratogens, and endocrine disrupters all are examples of toxins that cause specific health problems. Diet, also, is an important health factor.
- Solubility, persistence, chemical reactivity, and bioaccumulation all are important factors in toxicity, as are timing, dose, and route of exposure. Characteristics and condition of the target organism also are very influential in determining effects of toxins.
- Children are much more sensitive to most toxins than are adults. Pound for pound, children drink more water, eat more food, and breathe more air than adults. How best to protect children from environmental hazards is a difficult, but important, question.
- Some persistent organic pollutants (POPs), such as PBDE, PFOS, PFOA, and BPA, are now found throughout the world. Every human has them in his or her blood. The health effects of these compounds are not yet known, but there are concerns about chronic exposures.
- We depend on animal testing for much of our assessment of toxins, but great differences in sensitivity between species makes risk evaluation difficult. Just because something can be detected doesn't mean that it's present in a dangerous form or concentration.
- Our perception of risk is strongly influenced by emotion and factors such as whether the hazard is voluntary or familiar, whether it has a lag before its effects are known, and whether those at risk benefit from the source of exposure.
- Health experts generally regard a 1 in 1 million risk of death to be acceptable, but some people ask, "Acceptable to whom?" We often disregard familiar but serious risks while demanding protection from other, highly improbable risks.

QUESTIONS FOR REVIEW

1. What is SARS? How is it thought to have started?
2. Define the terms *disease* and *health*.
3. What were some of the most serious diseases in the world in 1990? How is this list expected to change in the next 20 years?
4. What are emergent diseases? Give a few examples, and describe their causes and effects.
5. How do bacteria acquire antibiotic resistance? What might we do about this?
6. What is the difference between toxic and hazardous? Give some examples of materials in each category.
7. How do the physical and chemical characteristics of materials affect their movement, persistence, distribution, and fate in the environment?
8. What is the difference between acute and chronic toxicity?
9. Define *carcinogenic, mutagenic, teratogenic,* and *neurotoxic.*
10. What are the relative risks of smoking, driving a car, and drinking water with the maximum permissible levels of trichloroethylene? Are these relatively equal risks?

THINKING SCIENTIFICALLY

1. What consequences (positive or negative) do you think might result from defining *health* as a state of complete physical, mental, and social well-being? Who might favor or oppose such a definition?
2. Do rich countries bear any responsibilities if the developing world adopts unhealthy lifestyles or diets? What could (or should) we do about it?
3. Why do we spend more money on heart or cancer research than on childhood illnesses?
4. How much do you think the United States should donate for health care in developing countries? What evidence would you offer to support your position?
5. Some people seem to have a poison paranoia about synthetic chemicals. Why do we tend to assume that natural chemicals are benign while industrial chemicals are evil?
6. Analyze the claim that we are exposed to thousands of times more natural carcinogens in our diet than industrial ones. Is this a good reason to ignore pollution?

7. Are good health and a clean environment basic human rights or merely things for which we should strive?
8. What are the premises in the discussion of assessing risk? Could conflicting conclusions be drawn from the facts presented in this section? What is your perception of risk from your environment?
9. Should pollution levels be set to protect the average person in the population or the most sensitive? Why not have zero exposure to all hazards?
10. What level of risk is acceptable to you? Are there some things for which you would accept more risk than others?

KEY TERMS

acute effects 191
allergens 183
antigens 183
bioaccumulation 187
biomagnification 187
cancer 185
carcinogens 185
chronic effects 191
disability-adjusted life years (DALYs) 176
disease 176
emergent diseases 178
endocrine hormone disrupters 185
environmental health 176
fetal alcohol syndrome 185
health 176
LD50 191
morbidity 176
mortality 176
mutagens 185
neurotoxins 185
pathogens 178
persistent organic pollutants (POPs) 187
prospective study 190
retrospective study 190
risk 192
sick building syndrome 183
synergism 189
teratogens 185
toxins 182

SUGGESTED READINGS

Calabrese, E. J., and L. A. Baldwin. 2003. Toxicology rethinks its central belief. *Nature* 421:691–92.

Daszak, P., et al. 2000. Emerging infectious diseases of wildlife—Threats to biodiversity and human health. *Science* 287:443–49.

Donnelly, C. A., et al. 2003. Epidemiological determinants of spread of causal agent of severe acute respiratory syndrome in Hong Kong. *Lancet* 361:111–34.

Hughes, J. M. 2001 Emerging infectious diseases: A CDC perspective. *Emerging Infectious Diseases* 7(3) Supplement: 494–96.

Klaassen, Curtis D., ed. 2001. *Casarett & Doull's Toxicology: The Basic Science of Poisons,* 6th ed. McGraw-Hill.

Koop, C. Everett, et al. 2002. *Critical Issues in Global Health.* Jossey-Bass.

Landrigan, Phillip, et al. 2002. *Raising Healthy Children in a Toxic World: 101 Smart Solutions for Every Family.* Rodale Press.

Miller, Judith, Stephen Engelberg, and William J. Broad. 2001. *Germs: Biological Weapons and America's Secret War.* Simon & Schuster.

Slovic, Paul. 2000. *The Perception of Risk.* Earthscan.

Woloshin, S., et al. 2002. Risk charts: Putting cancer in context. *Journal of the National Cancer Institute* 94(11):799–840.

World Health Organization. 2003. *World Health Report.* Oxford University Press.

Yam, Philip. 2003. Shoot this deer. *Scientific American* 288(6):38–43.

Welcome to McGraw-Hill's Online Learning Center

http://www.mhhe.com/cunningham3e

WEB EXERCISE

Learning about Diseases

The World Health Organization has a wealth of information about mortality, disability burdens, life expectancies, demographics, and other topics related to environmental health. For information about specific diseases, go to www.who.int/health-topics/en/. Look up the current status of ebola and SARS, and compare them with a disease that occurs closer to where you live (consult fig. 8.4 in this chapter). For more information about SARS, consult www3.who.int/whosis/menu.cfm and click on *statistics by topic*. From this page, you can also link to information about other diseases by clicking on *statistics by disease or condition* and then *tropical diseases.* What organisms cause these diseases? What is their current distribution and prevalance? What environmental and social factors contribute to their spread? What treatment (if any) exists for these diseases, and how might they be prevented? See links on this webpage for the newsletter *Action against Infection* for up-to-date information about efforts to stop the spread of contagious diseases

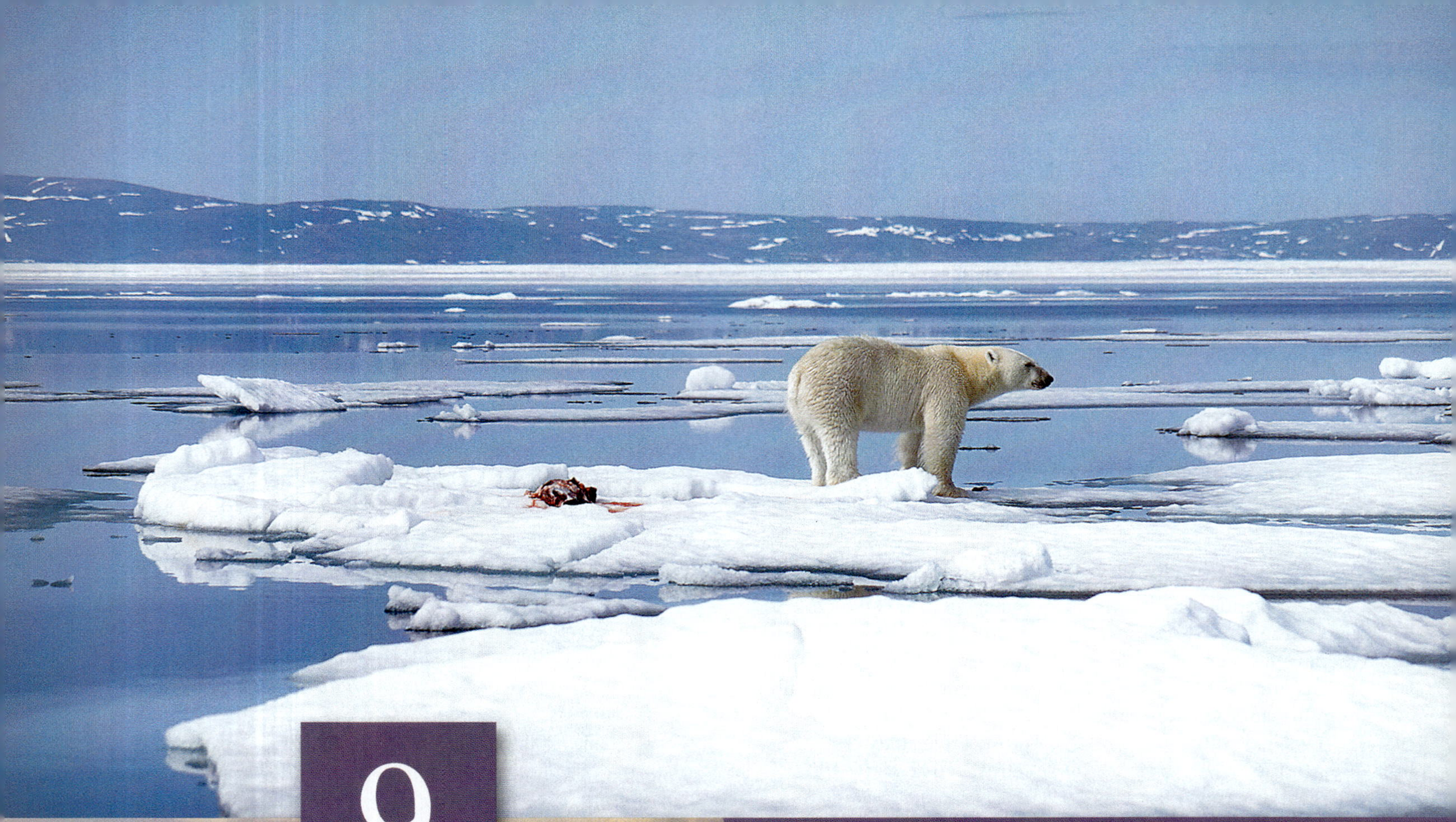

Dramatic reductions in sea ice are preventing polar bears from hunting seals.

9

Air: Climate and Pollution

Climate is an angry beast, and we are poking it with sticks.
–Wallace Broekcer

LEARNING ONLINE

Visit our webpage at www.mhhe.com/cunningham3e for data sources, further readings, additional case studies, current environmental news, and regional examples within the Online Learning Center to help you understand the material in this chapter. You'll also find active links to information pertaining to this chapter, including

National Oceanic and Atmospheric Administration (NOAA)
Tropical Prediction Center/National Hurricane Center
National Weather Service Page
Weather sites
Air pollution
United States Environmental Protection Agency
National Vehicle and Fuel Emissions Laboratory
Ozone depletion

OBJECTIVES

After studying this chapter, you should be able to

- summarize the structure and composition of the atmosphere.
- explain how jet streams, seasonal winds, and global climate patterns determine local weather.
- understand El Niño cycles and the causes of natural climate change.
- debate the hypothesis that human actions are altering the global climate.
- describe the major categories and sources of air pollution.
- evaluate the dangers of stratospheric ozone depletion.
- understand how air pollution damages human health, vegetation, and building materials.
- judge how air quality around the world has improved or degraded, and suggest what we might do about problem areas.

What's Happening to Our Weather?

What do skinny polar bears and drowned seal pups, Peruvian cholera epidemics, the melting of Mt. Kilimanjaro's famous snows, Chinese drinking-water shortages, unusually severe Bangladeshi floods, coastal erosion in Louisiana, and the disappearance of Edith's Checkerspot butterfly in southern California have in common? All these phenomena are thought to be signs of human-caused global climate change, which may well be the most critical issue in environmental science today.

The problem is that we are adding greenhouse gases—pollutants that trap in the earth's heat—to the atmosphere at a faster rate than at any time over the past several thousand years. Essentially, we are conducting a giant experiment to see what will happen if we alter atmospheric chemistry. So far, the results don't look very good. All around us, evidence suggests we are modifying our climate on both a local and a global scale. The twentieth century was the warmest in the past 1,000 years. The 10 hottest years in the 143 years for which we have instrument readings have all been since 1990, with the three highest being 1998, 2002, and 2001.

Polar regions are changing even faster than the rest of the globe. According to Environment Canada, parts of the Arctic coast have warmed as much as 7.5°C (13.5°F) since 1970. Sea ice forms later in the fall and melts earlier in the spring, giving polar bears a shorter seal-hunting season. Hudson's Bay polar bears now weigh as much as 100 kg (220 lbs) less than in the 1960s. In 2002 early melting of ice floes in Canada's Gulf of St. Lawrence appeared to have drowned nearly all of the 200,000 to 300,000 harp seal pups normally born there.

Glaciers are disappearing on every continent. Mt. Kilimanjaro has lost 85 percent of its ice cap since 1915. By 2015 all permanent ice on the mountaintop is expected to be gone. Alpine glaciers feed rivers, such as the Indus, Ganges, Yangtze, Yellow, and Mekong, that supply drinking water and irrigation to more than a billion people in South and East Asia, where water is already becoming a source of conflict. Ocean warming is causing severe storms and heavy monsoon rains that result in flooding in Bangladesh as well as erosion in Louisiana, where rising sea levels have inundated low-lying costal marshes. And Edith's Checkerspot is only one of many species of mammals, birds, amphibians, fish, insects, and plants that are reported to have moved their territory or migration patterns or to have disappeared altogether as a result of changing climate.

Higher temperatures apparently are allowing disease-causing bacteria, viruses, and fungi to move into new areas where they may harm species as diverse as lions, snails, butterflies, and humans. Climate changes are thought to have contributed to an epidemic of avian malaria that wiped out thousands of birds in Hawaii, the spread of distemper in African lions, and the bleaching of coral reefs around the globe. Unusually warm water off the coast of South America is thought to be responsible for the reappearance of cholera in humans during the 1990s after nearly a century of absence.

What do all these changes mean? Taken individually, it's hard to say; they may just be random events in a notoriously variable system. Viewed altogether, however, it seems increasingly evident that we are changing our climate with results we don't yet fully comprehend. Learning something about our atmosphere and how it produces our weather and climate is essential if we are to understand how changing climate might affect us, and what we might do to counter those effects. In this chapter, we'll look at how greenhouse gases and other air pollutants affect human and natural systems, and we'll examine some of the international politics of this crucial topic.

THE ATMOSPHERE AND CLIMATE

We live at the bottom of a virtual ocean of air that extends upward about 500 km (300 mi). In the lowest 18 to 8 km, a layer known as the troposphere, the air moves ceaselessly, flowing, swirling, and continually redistributing heat and moisture from one part of the globe to another. The composition and behavior of the troposphere and other layers control our **weather** (daily temperature and moisture conditions in a place) and our **climate** (long-term weather patterns).

The earth's earliest atmosphere probably consisted mainly of hydrogen and helium. Over billions of years, most of that hydrogen and helium diffused into space. Volcanic emissions added carbon, nitrogen, oxygen, sulfur, and other elements to the atmosphere. Virtually all of the molecular oxygen (O_2) we breathe was probably produced by photosynthesis in blue-green bacteria, algae, and green plants.

Clean, dry air is mostly nitrogen and oxygen (table 9.1). Water vapor concentrations vary from near 0 to 4 percent, depending on air temperature and available moisture. Minute particles and liquid droplets—collectively called **aerosols**—also are suspended in the air. Atmospheric aerosols play important roles in the earth's energy budget and in rain production.

The atmosphere has four distinct zones of contrasting temperature, due to differences in absorption of solar energy (fig. 9.1). The layer of air immediately adjacent to the earth's surface is called the **troposphere** (*tropein* means to turn or change, in Greek). Within the troposphere, air circulates in great vertical and horizontal **convection currents,** constantly redistributing heat and moisture around the globe. The troposphere ranges in depth from about 18 km (11 mi) over the equator to about 8 km (5 mi) over the poles, where air is cold and dense. Because gravity holds most air molecules close to the earth's surface, the troposphere is much denser than the other layers: it contains about 75 percent of the total mass of the atmosphere. Air temperature drops rapidly with increasing altitude in this layer, reaching about –60°C (–76°F) at the top of the troposphere. A sudden reversal of this temperature

TABLE 9.1 Present Composition of the Lower Atmosphere*		
GAS	SYMBOL OR FORMULA	PERCENT BY VOLUME
Nitrogen	N_2	78.08
Oxygen	O_2	20.94
Argon	Ar	0.934
Carbon dioxide	CO_2	0.035
Neon	Ne	0.00182
Helium	He	0.00052
Methane	CH_4	0.00015
Krypton	Kr	0.00011
Hydrogen	H_2	0.00005
Nitrous oxide	N_2O	0.00005
Xenon	Xe	0.000009

*Average composition of dry, clean air.

gradient creates a sharp boundary called the tropopause, which limits mixing between the troposphere and upper zones.

The **stratosphere** extends from the tropopause up to about 50 km (31 mi). It is vastly more dilute than the troposphere, but it has a similar composition—except that it has almost no water vapor and nearly 1,000 times more **ozone** (O_3). This ozone absorbs some wavelengths of ultraviolet solar radiation, known as UV-B (290–330 nm, see fig. 2.10). This absorbed energy makes the atmosphere warmer toward the top of the stratosphere. Since UV radiation damages living tissues, this UV absorption in the stratosphere also protects life on the surface. Recently discovered depletion of stratospheric ozone, especially over Antarctica, is allowing increased amounts of UV radiation to reach the earth's surface. If observed trends continue, this radiation could cause higher rates of skin cancer, genetic mutations, crop failures, and disruption of important biological communities, as you will see later in this chapter.

Unlike the troposphere, the stratosphere is relatively calm. There is so little mixing in the stratosphere that volcanic ash and human-caused contaminants can remain in suspension there for many years.

Above the stratosphere, the temperature diminishes again, creating the mesosphere, or middle layer. The thermosphere (heated layer) begins at about 50 km. This is a region of highly ionized (electrically charged) gases, heated by a steady flow of high-energy solar and cosmic radiation. In the lower part of the thermosphere, intense pulses of high-energy radiation cause electrically charged particles (ions) to glow. This phenomenon is what we know as the *aurora borealis* and *aurora australis,* or northern and southern lights.

No sharp boundary marks the end of the atmosphere. Pressure and density decrease with distance from the earth until they become indistinguishable from the near vacuum of interstellar space.

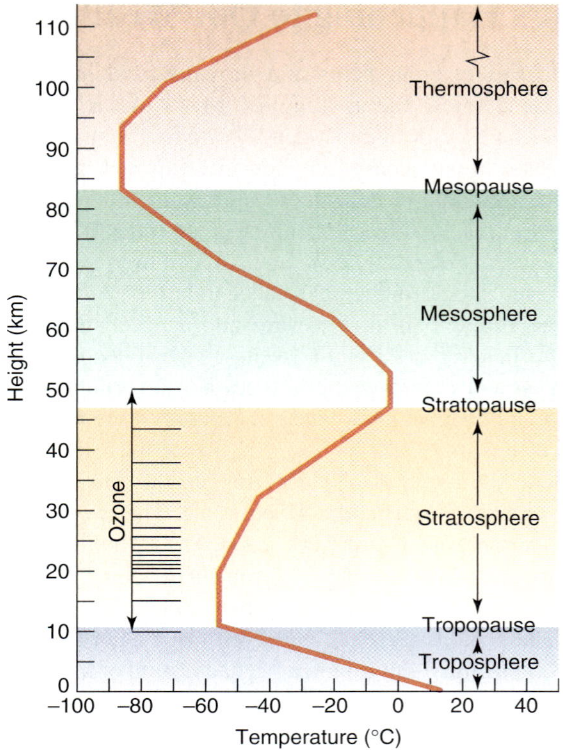

FIGURE 9.1 *Temperatures change drastically in the four layers of the atmosphere. Bars in the ozone graph represent relative concentrations of stratospheric ozone with altitude.*
Source: Courtesy of Dr. William Culver, St. Petersburg Junior College.

Energy and the "Greenhouse Effect"

The sun supplies the earth with an enormous amount of energy, but that energy is not evenly distributed over the globe. Incoming solar radiation (insolation) is much stronger near the equator than at high latitudes. Of the solar energy that reaches the outer atmosphere, about one-quarter is reflected by clouds and atmospheric gases, and another quarter is absorbed by carbon dioxide, water vapor, ozone, methane, and a few other gases (fig. 9.2). This energy absorption warms the atmosphere slightly. About half of incoming solar radiation (insolation) reaches the earth's surface. Most of this energy is in the form of light or infrared (heat) energy (see fig. 2.10). Some of this energy is reflected by bright surfaces, such as snow, ice, and sand. The rest is absorbed by the earth's surface and by water. Surfaces that *reflect* energy have a high **albedo** (reflectivity). Most of these surfaces appear bright to us because they reflect light as well as other forms of radiative energy. Surfaces that *absorb* energy have a low albedo and generally appear dark. Black soil, asphalt pavement, and dark green vegetation, for example, have low albedos (table 9.2).

Absorbed energy heats the absorbing surface (such as an asphalt parking lot in summer), evaporates water, and provides the energy for photosynthesis in plants. Following the second law of thermodynamics, absorbed energy is gradually reemitted as lower-quality heat energy. A brick building, for example, absorbs energy in the form of light and reemits that energy in the form of heat.

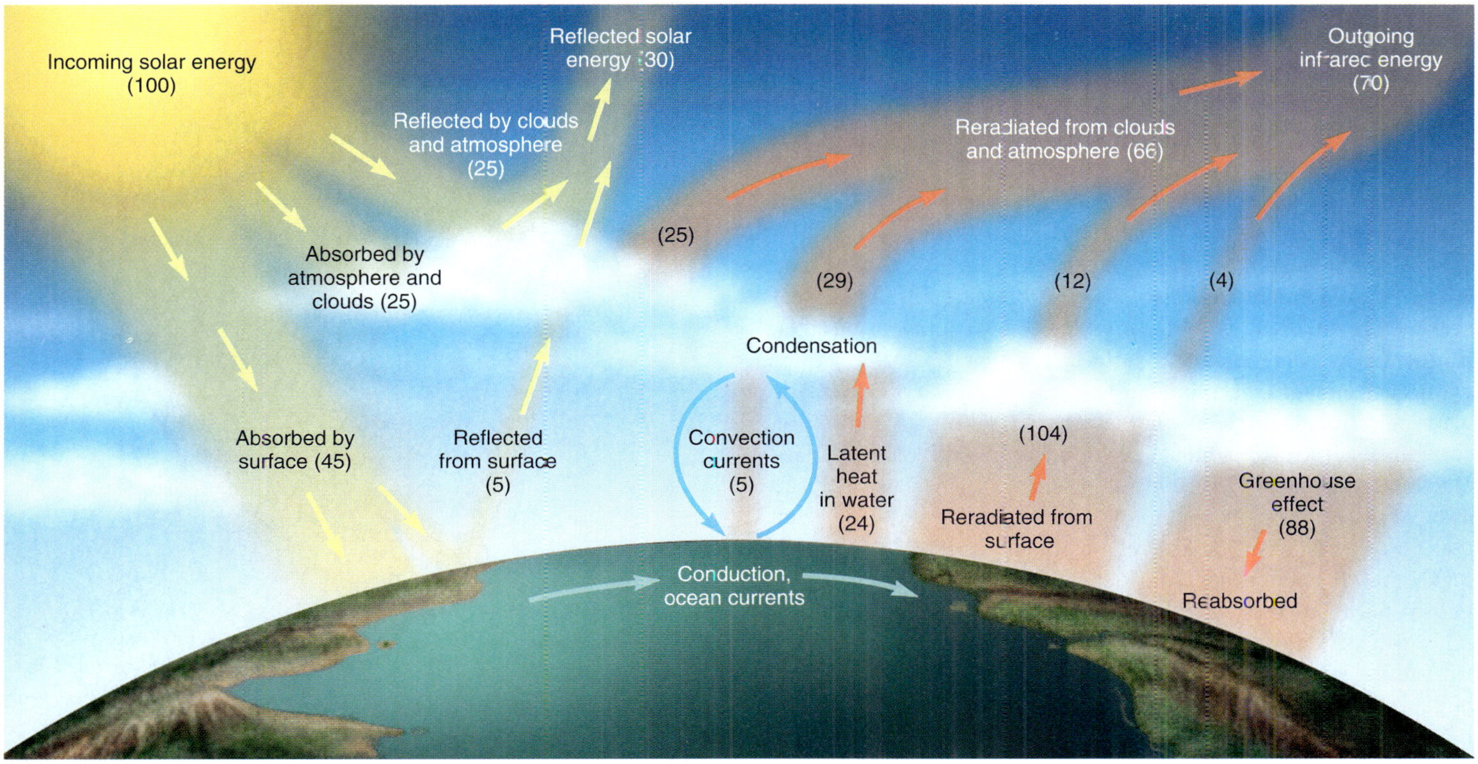

FIGURE 9.2 *Energy balance between incoming and outgoing radiation. The atmosphere absorbs or reflects about half of the solar energy reaching the earth. Most of the energy reemitted from the earth's surface is long-wave, infrared energy. Most of this infrared energy is absorbed by aerosols and gases in the atmosphere and is re-radiated toward the planet, keeping the surface much warmer than it would otherwise be. This is known as the greenhouse effect.*

TABLE 9.2 Albedo (Reflectivity) of Surfaces

SURFACE	ALBEDO (%)
Fresh snow	80–85
Dense clouds	70–90
Water (low sun)	50–80
Sand	20–30
Water (sun overhead)	5
Forest	5–10
Black soil	3
Earth/atmosphere average	30

The change in energy quality is very important because the atmosphere selectively absorbs longer wavelengths. Most solar energy comes in the form of intense, high-energy light or near-infrared wavelengths. This short-wavelength energy passes relatively easily through the atmosphere to reach the earth's surface. Energy re-released from the earth's warmed surface is lower-intensity, longer-wavelength energy in the far-infrared part of the spectrum. Atmospheric gases, especially carbon dioxide and water vapor, absorb much of this long-wavelength energy, re-releasing it in the lower atmosphere and letting it leak out to space only slowly. This re-irradiated energy provides most of the heat in the lower atmosphere. If the atmosphere were as transparent to infrared radiation as it is to visible light, the earth's average surface temperature would be about –18°C (0°F)—33°C (59°F) colder than it is now.

This phenomenon is called the **greenhouse effect** because the atmosphere, loosely comparable to the glass of a greenhouse, transmits sunlight while trapping heat inside. The greenhouse effect is a natural atmospheric process that is necessary for life as we know it. However, too much greenhouse effect, caused by burning of fossil fuels and deforestation, may cause harmful environmental change.

Convection and Atmospheric Pressure

Much of the incoming solar energy is used to evaporate water. Every gram of evaporating water absorbs 580 calories of energy as it transforms from liquid to gas. Globally, water vapor contains a huge amount of stored energy, known as **latent heat.** When water vapor condenses, returning from a gas to a liquid form, the 580 calories of heat energy are released. Imagine the sun shining on the Gulf of Mexico in the winter. Warm sunshine and plenty of water allow continuous evaporation that converts an immense amount of solar (light) energy into latent heat stored in evaporated water. Now imagine a wind blowing the humid air north from the Gulf toward Canada. The air cools as it moves north (especially if it encounters cold air moving south). Cooling causes the water vapor to condense. Rain (or snow) falls as a consequence. Note that it is not only water that has moved from the Gulf to the Midwest: 580 calories of heat have also moved with every gram of moisture. The heat and water have moved from a place with strong incoming solar energy to a place with much less solar energy and much less water. The redistribution of heat and water around the globe is essential to life on earth.

Uneven heating, with warm air close to the equator and colder air at high latitudes, also produces pressure differences that cause wind, rain, storms, and everything else we know as weather. As the sun warms the earth's surface, the air nearest the surface warms and expands, becoming less dense than the air above it. The warm air must then rise above the denser air. Vertical convection currents result, which circulate air from warm latitudes to cool latitudes and vice versa. These convection currents can be as small and as localized as a narrow column of hot air rising over a sun-heated rock, or they can cover huge regions of the earth. At the largest scale, the convection cells are described by a simplified model known as Hadley cells, which redistribute heat globally (fig. 9.3).

Where air rises in convection currents, air pressure at the surface is low. Where air is sinking, or subsiding, air pressure is high. On a weather map these high and low pressure centers, or rising and sinking currents of air, move across continents. In most of North America, they generally move from west to east. Rising air tends to cool with altitude, releasing latent heat, which causes further rising. Very warm and humid air can rise very vigorously, especially if it is rising over a mass of very cold air. Storms associated with low pressure and rising air are known as cyclonic storms. These include some of the most violent storms we know: hurricanes, tornadoes, and intense rain and hail (fig. 9.4).

Pressure differences are an important cause of wind. There is always someplace with sinking (high-pressure) air and someplace with rising (low-pressure) air. Air moves from high-pressure centers toward low-pressure areas, and we call this movement wind.

Why Does It Rain?

To understand why it rains, remember two things: water condenses as air cools, and air cools as it rises. Anytime air is rising, clouds, rain, or snow might form. Cooling occurs because of

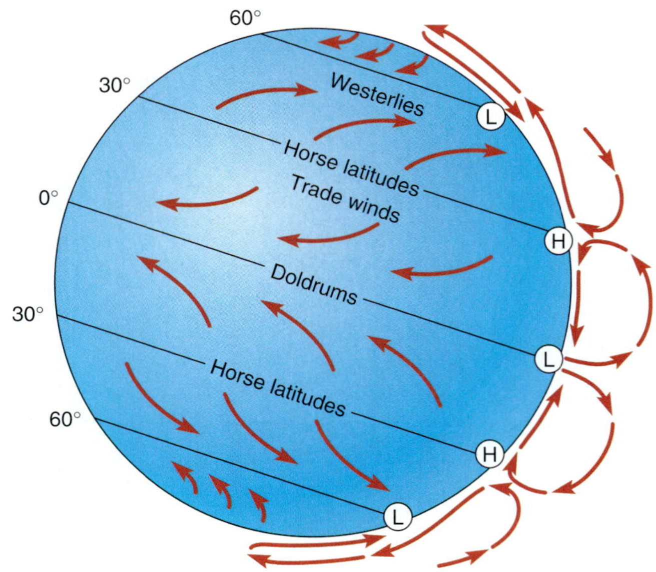

FIGURE 9.3 *General circulation patterns redistribute heat and moisture around the globe. The approximate locations of vertical convection currents, generally referred to as Hadley cells, are noted on the right side. Low-pressure belts* (L) *occur at latitudes where air rises. High-pressure belts* (H) *occur where air sinks. Dominant winds, such as trade winds and westerlies, also occur in latitudinal bands.*

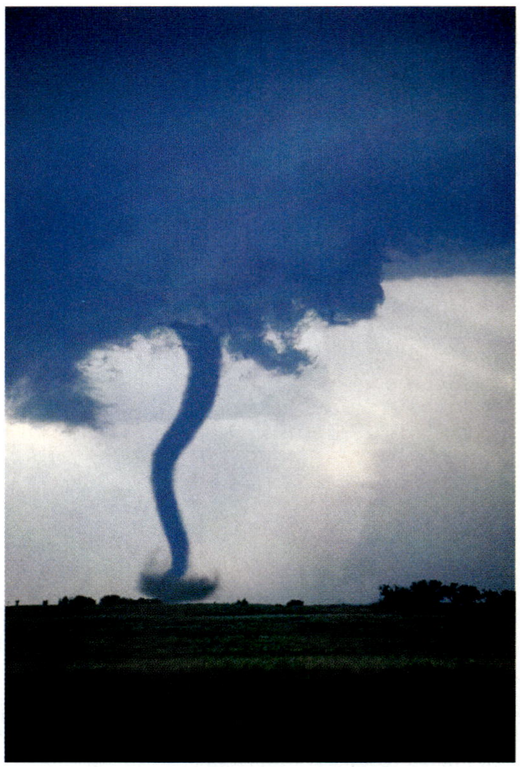

FIGURE 9.4 *Tornadoes are local cyclonic storms caused by rapid mixing of cold, dry air and warm, wet air. Wind speeds in the swirling funnel can reach 320 km/hr (200 mph).*

APPLICATION: How Much Heat Is Released in a 1-in. Rainstorm in Your Neighborhood?

Most Americans measure rainfall in inches, but centimeters are easier to calculate. A 1-in. rainfall is about 2.54 cm of rain. Suppose your neighborhood is a 1 km × 1 km square. If rain releases 580 cal/cm^3, how much heat is released by this rainstorm?

Answer: $\frac{25.4 \text{ cm of rain}}{1} \times \frac{100{,}000 \text{ cm}}{\text{km}} \times \frac{100{,}000 \text{ cm}}{\text{km}} \times \frac{580 \text{ cal}}{\text{cm}^3 \text{ of rain}} = 17.2 \times 10^{12}$ cal.

changes in pressure with altitude: air cools as it rises (as pressure decreases); air warms as it sinks (as pressure increases). Air rises in convection currents where solar heating is intense, such as over the equator. Moving masses of air also rise over each other and cool. Air also rises when it encounters mountains. If the air is moist (if it has recently come from over an ocean or an evaporating forest region, for example), condensation and rainfall are likely as the air is lifted (fig. 9.5). Regions with intense solar heating, frequently colliding air masses, or mountains tend to receive a great deal of precipitation.

Where air is sinking, on the other hand, it tends to warm because of increasing pressure. As it warms, available moisture evaporates. Rainfall occurs relatively rarely in areas of high pressure. High pressure and clear, dry conditions occur where convection currents are sinking. High pressure also occurs where air sinks after flowing over mountains. Figure 9.3 shows sinking, dry air at about 30º north and south latitudes. If you look at a world map, you will see a band of deserts at approximately these latitudes.

Another ingredient is usually necessary to initiate condensation of water vapor: condensation nuclei. Tiny particles of smoke, dust, sea salts, spores, and volcanic ash all act as condensation nuclei. These particles form a surface on which water molecules can begin to coalesce. Without them even supercooled vapor can remain in gaseous form. Even apparently clear air can contain large numbers of these particles, which are generally too small to be seen by the naked eye.

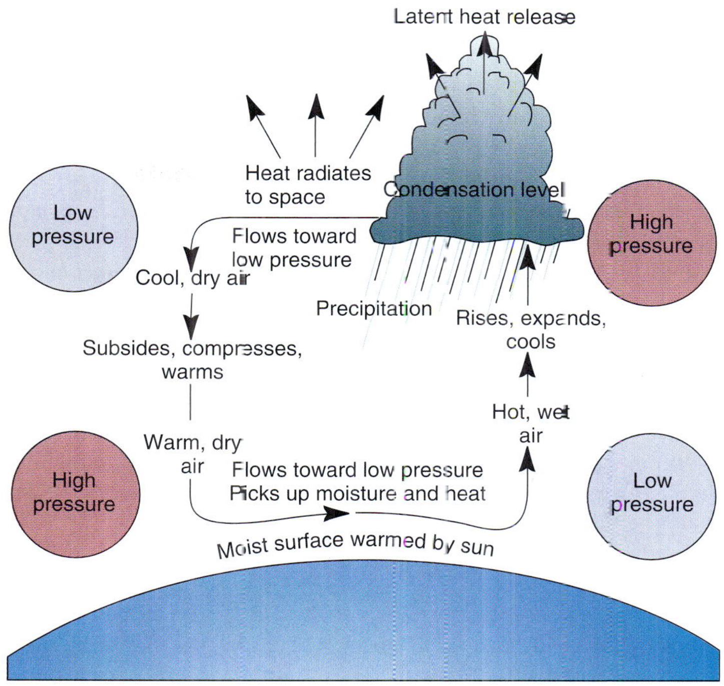

FIGURE 9.5 *Convection currents and latent energy cause atmospheric circulation and redistribution of heat and water around the globe.*

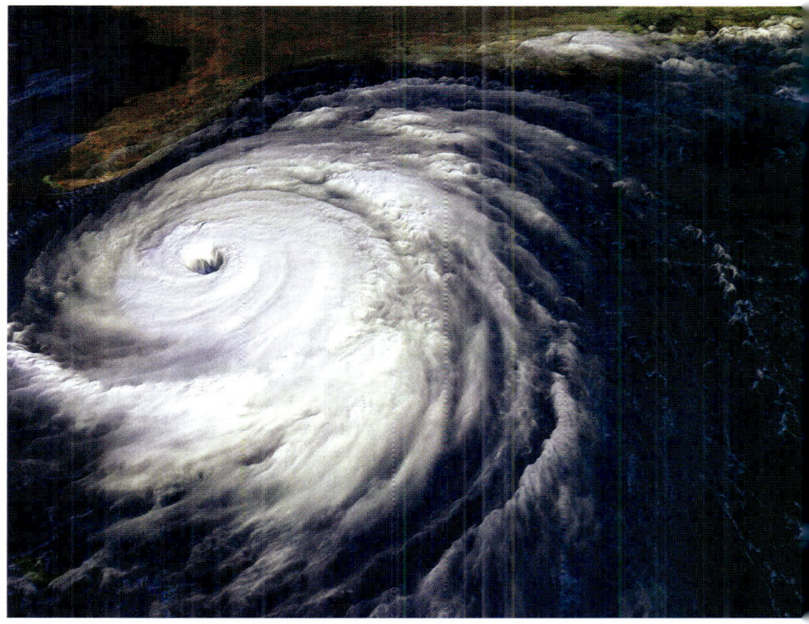

FIGURE 9.6 *You can clearly see the Coriolis effect as winds swirl counterclockwise around the low-pressure center of Hurricane Floyd as it approached Florida in 1999.*

The Coriolis Effect and Jet Streams

Large-scale winds tend not to move in a straight line across the earth's surface. In the Northern Hemisphere, they generally bend clockwise (right), and in the Southern Hemisphere, they bend counterclockwise (left). This curving pattern results from the fact that the earth rotates in an eastward direction as the winds move above the surface. The apparent curvature of the winds is known as the **Coriolis effect.** On a global scale, this effect produces steady, reliable wind patterns, such as the trade winds and the midlatitude westerlies (see fig. 9.3). Ocean currents similarly curve clockwise in the Northern Hemisphere and counterclockwise in the south (see appendix 3, p. 382). On a regional scale, the Coriolis effect produces cyclonic winds, or wind movements controlled by the earth's spin. Cyclonic winds spiral clockwise out of an area of high pressure in the Northern Hemisphere and counterclockwise into a low-pressure zone (fig. 9.6). If you look at a weather map in the newspaper, can you find this counterclockwise spiral pattern?

Why does this curving or spiraling motion occur? Imagine you were looking down on the North Pole of the rotating earth. Now imagine that the earth is a merry-go-round in a playground, with the North Pole at its center and the equator around the edge. As it spins counterclockwise (eastward), the spinning edge moves very fast (a full rotation, 39,800 km, every 24 hours for the real earth, or more than 1,600 km/hour). Near the center, though, there is very little eastward velocity. If you threw a ball from the edge toward the center, it would be traveling faster (edge speed) than the middle. It would appear, to someone standing on the merry-go-round, to curve toward the right. If you threw the ball from the center toward the edge, it would start out with no eastward velocity, but the surface below it would spin eastward, making the ball end up, to a person on the merry-go-round, west of its starting point. Winds move above the earth's surface much as the ball does. If you were looking down at the South Pole, you would see the earth spinning clockwise, and winds—or thrown balls—would appear to bend left. Incidentally, this effect does not apply to drains in your house. Their movement is far too small to be affected by the spinning of the earth. And, contrary to popular myth, there is no significant difference in sink draining between the Northern and Southern Hemispheres.

At the top of the troposphere are **jet streams,** hurricane-force winds that circle the earth. These powerful winds follow an undulating path approximately where the vertical convection currents known as the Hadley and Ferrell cells meet. Although we can't perceive jet streams on the ground, they are important to us because they greatly affect weather patterns. Sometimes jet streams dip down near the top of the world's highest mountains, exposing mountain climbers to violent, brutally cold winds.

Ocean Currents

Warm and cold ocean currents strongly influence climate conditions on land. Surface ocean currents result from wind pushing on the ocean surface. As surface water moves, deep water wells up to replace it, creating deeper ocean currents. Differences in water density—depending on the temperature and saltiness of the water—also drive ocean circulation. Huge cycling currents called gyres carry water north and south, redistributing heat from low latitudes to high latitudes (see appendix 3, p. 382, global climate map). The Alaska current, flowing from Alaska southward to California, keeps San Francisco cool and foggy during the summer. The Gulf Stream, one of the best known currents, carries warm Caribbean water north past Canada's maritime provinces to northern Europe. This current is immense, some 800 times the volume of the Amazon, the world's largest river. The heat transported from the Gulf keeps Europe much warmer than it should be for its latitude. As the warm Gulf Stream passes Scandinavia and swirls around Iceland, the water cools and evaporates, becomes dense and salty, and plunges downward, creating a strong, deep, southward current.

Ocean circulation patterns were long thought to be unchanging, but now oceanographers believe that currents can shift abruptly. For example, melting ice at the North Pole could create a flood of cold, fresh water, disrupting the Gulf Stream and causing rapid, drastic cooling in Europe. This shift may have happened in geologic history, and many climatologists fear it could occur again if global warming melts arctic ice again.

Seasonal Winds and Monsoons

While figure 9.3 shows regular global wind patterns, large parts of the world, especially the tropics, receive seasonal winds and rainy seasons that are essential for sustaining both ecosystems and human life. Sometimes these seasonal rains are extreme, causing disastrous flooding. (See related story "Floods in Mozambique" at www.mhhe.com/cases.)

Sometimes the rains fail, causing crop failures and famine. The most regular seasonal winds and rains are known as **monsoons.** In India and Bangladesh, monsoon rains come when seasonal winds blow hot, humid air from the Indian Ocean (fig. 9.7). Strong convection currents lift this air, causing heavy rain across the subcontinent. When the rising air reaches the Himalayas, it rises even farther, creating some of the heaviest rainfall in the world. During the five-month rainy season of 1970, a weather station in the foothills of the Himalayas recorded 25 m (82 ft) of rain!

Tropical and subtropical regions around the world have seasonal rainy and dry seasons (see the discussion of tropical biomes, chapter 5). The main reason for this variable climate is that the region of most intense solar heating and evaporation shifts through the year. Remember that the earth's axis of rotation is at an angle. Sometimes the sun hits the surface just south of the equator, and sometimes it hits just north of the equator. Wherever the sun shines most directly, evaporation and convection currents—and rainfall and thunderstorms—are very strong. As the earth orbits the sun, different regions fall below the sun, and different regions receive seasonal rain and winds. These seasonal rains support seasonal tropical forests, and they fill some of the world's greatest rivers, including the Ganges and the Amazon. As the year shifts from summer to winter, solar heating weakens, the rainy season ends, and little rain may fall for months.

During the 1970s and 1980s, rains failed repeatedly in parts of the Sahel in northern Africa. Although rains have often been irregular in this region, increasing populations and civil disorder made these droughts result in widespread starvation and death (fig. 9.8).

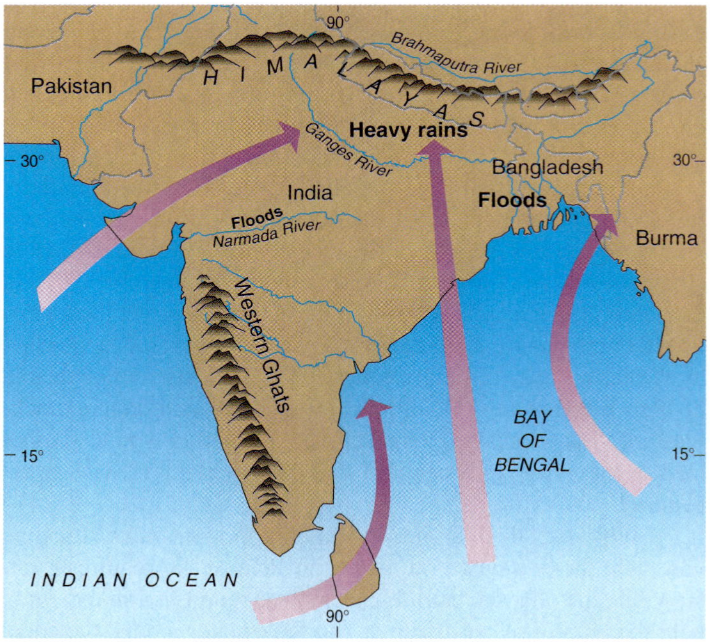

FIGURE 9.7 *Summer monsoon air flows over the Indian subcontinent. Warming air rises over the plains of central India in the summer, creating a low-pressure cell that draws in warm, wet, oceanic air. As this moist air rises over the Western Ghats or the Himalayas, it cools, and heavy rains result. These monsoon rains flood the great rivers, bringing water for agriculture but also causing much suffering.*

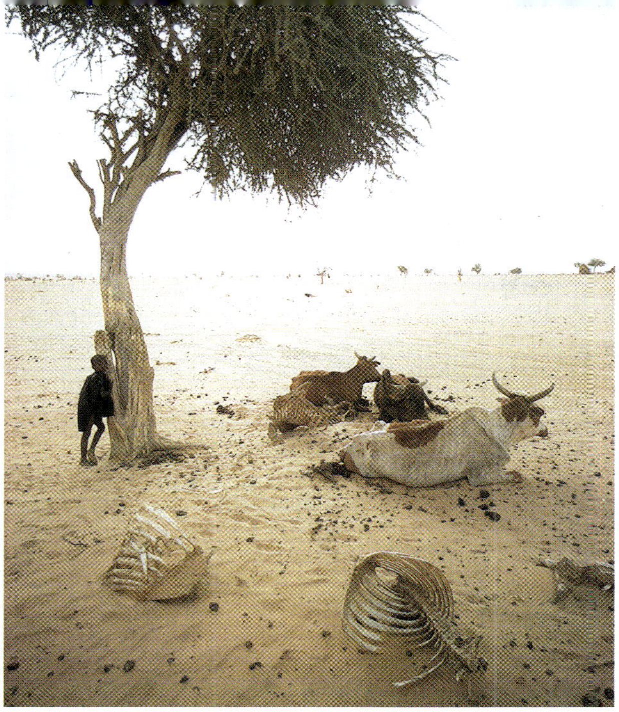

FIGURE 9.8 *Failure of monsoon rains brings drought, starvation, and death to both livestock and people in the Sahel desert margin of Africa. Although drought is a fact of life in Africa, many governments fail to plan for it, and human suffering is much worse than it needs to be.*

CLIMATE CHANGE

Both global and local climate can be highly variable, often over relatively short time scales (fig. 9.9). Note the close correlation between climate and atmospheric chemistry. It isn't yet clear, however, which is cause and which is effect. These abrupt climate changes can be disastrous for biological organisms. A sudden cooling 65 million years ago, for example, is thought to have ended the age of dinosaurs, along with 75 percent of the species existing at the time. There may have been a dozen such mass extinctions (see table 5.3). On a shorter time scale, several ice ages, each lasting hundreds of thousands of years, have come and gone in the past 2 million years. Even shorter climate shifts occur, such as the "little ice age," which began in the 1300s and caused crop failures throughout Europe for the next two centuries. On a scale of decades there seem to be approximately 20-year drought cycles in North America.

What causes these climate shifts at these different time scales? One explanation is periodic changes in sunlight intensity resulting from **Milankovitch cycles.** These cycles, named for the Serbian scientist who first described them in the 1920s, include (1) the shape of the earth's orbit around the sun elongates and shortens in a 100,000-year cycle, (2) the axis of rotation changes its angle of tilt in a 40,000-year cycle, and (3) over a 26,000-year period, the axis wobbles like an out-of-balance spinning top (fig. 9.10). Worldwide expansion of glaciers every 100,000 years or so could result from the orbital shifts. Decadal droughts, meanwhile, may be explained by 11-year sunspot cycles, shifts in stormy activity on the sun's surface.

Climate does not necessarily change gradually. Atmospheric gas bubbles from ice cores drilled in polar ice caps suggest that, during the last major interglacial period 135,000 to 115,000 years ago, temperatures flipped suddenly over a period of years or decades, rather than centuries. Meteor impacts and sudden shifts in ocean currents, which redistribute heat around the globe, could have also

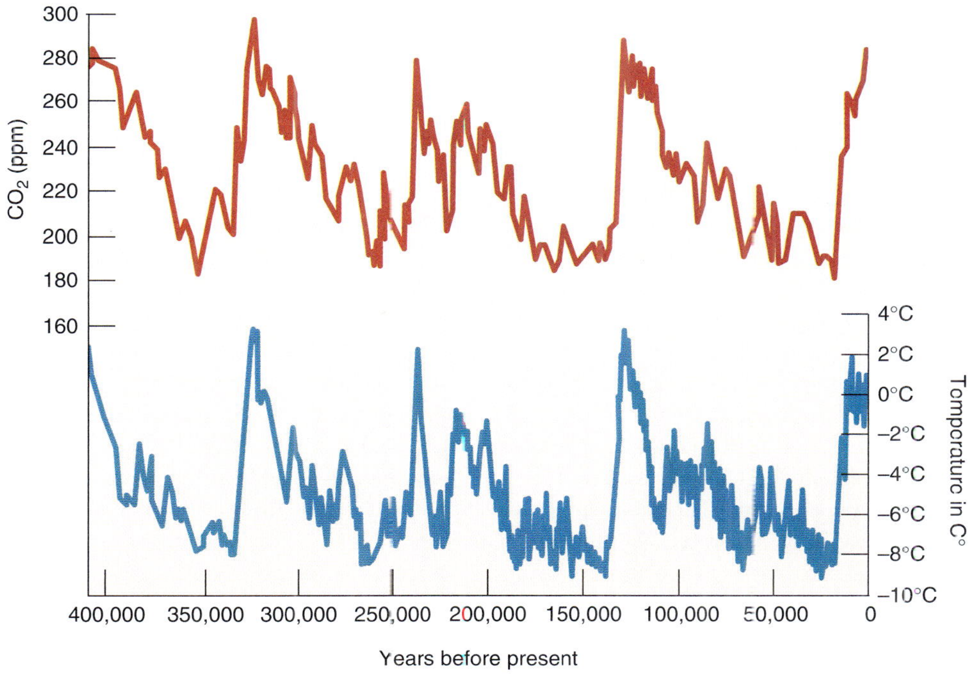

FIGURE 9.9 *Atmospheric CO_2 concentrations and global mean temperatures estimated from the Antarctic Vostok ice core. Note the relatively rapid changes and close correlation in both climate and atmospheric chemistry.*
Source: Data from United Nations Environment Programme.

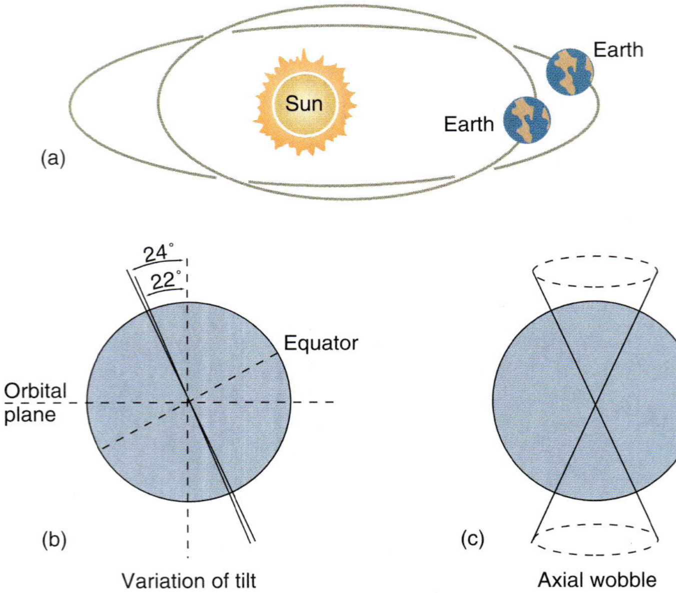

FIGURE 9.10 *Milankovitch cycles that may affect long-term climate conditions:* (a) *changes in the occupancy of the earth's orbit,* (b) *shifting tilt of the axis, and* (c) *wobble of the earth.*

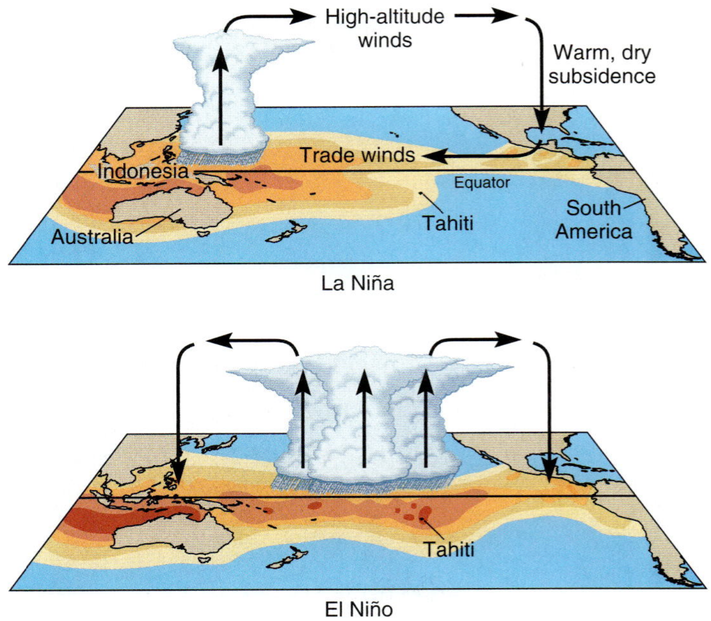

FIGURE 9.11 *The El Niño/La Niña/Southern Oscillation cycle. Every three to five years, surface trade winds that normally push warm water westward toward Indonesia weaken and allow this pool of water to flow eastward toward South America.*

caused rapid climate changes. Some climatologists suspect that rapid releases of methane trapped beneath the ocean floor, a "big burp," may have produced a sudden warming that caused the mass extinction 183 million years ago. This theory raises questions about the stability of methane deposits currently stored beneath the seafloor.

Two important shorter-term climate changes, El Niño and anthropogenic global warming, are discussed in the next sections.

El Niño/Southern Oscillation

El Niño, *La Niña,* and the *Southern Oscillation* are all terms referring to a major ocean-current/climate connection that affects weather throughout the Pacific—and possibly throughout the world. The core of this system is a huge pool of warm surface water in the Pacific Ocean that sloshes slowly back and forth between Indonesia and South America like water in a giant bathtub. Most years, this pool is held in the western Pacific by steady equatorial trade winds that push ocean surface currents westward (fig. 9.11). From Southeast Asia to Australia, this concentration of warm equatorial water provides latent heat (water vapor) that drives strong upward convection (low pressure) in the atmosphere. Heavy rain results, supporting dense tropical forests. On the other side of the Pacific, the westward-moving surface waters are replaced by cold water welling up along the South American coast. Cold, nutrient-rich waters support dense schools of anchovies and other fish. While the trade winds blow westward on the ocean's surface, returning winds high in the troposphere flow back from Indonesia to Chile and to Mexico and southern California. There the returning air sinks, creating dry, desert conditions.

Every three to five years, for reasons that we don't fully understand, the Indonesian low-pressure system collapses, and the mass of warm surface water surges back east across the Pacific. One theory is that the high cirrus clouds block enough sunshine to cool the ocean surface in Asia. Convection would then weaken, and trade winds—and ocean currents—would reverse, flowing eastward instead of westward. Another theory is that eastward-flowing deep currents called baroclinic waves periodically interfere with coastal upwelling, warming the sea surface off South America and eliminating the temperature gradient across the Pacific.

Fishermen in Peru were the first to notice irregular cycles of rising ocean temperatures because the fish disappeared when the water warmed. They named this event El Niño (Spanish for the Christ child) because they often occur around Christmastime. The counterpart to El Niño, when the eastern tropical Pacific cools, has come to be called La Niña (little girl). Together, these cycles are called the El Niño Southern Oscillation (ENSO).

ENSO cycles have far-reaching effects. During an El Niño year, the northern jet stream—which is normally over Canada—splits and is drawn south over the United States. This pulls moist air from the Pacific and Gulf of Mexico inland, bringing intense storms and heavy rains from California across the midwestern states. The intervening La Niña years bring hot, dry weather to the same areas. Oregon, Washington, and British Columbia, on the other hand, tend to have warm, sunny weather in El Niño years rather than their usual rain. Droughts in Australia and Indonesia during El Niño episodes cause disastrous crop failures and forest fires, including one in Borneo in 1983 that burned 3.3 million ha (8 million acres).

Some climatologists believe that ENSO events are becoming stronger or more frequent because of global climate change.

There are signs that warm ocean-surface temperatures are spreading, which could contribute to El Niño strength or frequency. On the other hand, increased cloud cover over warmer oceans could raise global albedo, and strong convection currents generated by these storms could pump heat into the stratosphere. This might have an overall cooling effect and act as a safety valve for global warming.

Human-Caused Global Climate Change

As the opening vignette in this chapter shows, most scientists now regard anthropogenic (human-caused) global climate change to be the most important environmental issue of our times. The possibility that humans might alter world climate is not a new idea. In 1895 Svante Arrhenius, who subsequently received a Nobel Prize for his work in chemistry, predicted that CO_2 released by coal burning could cause global warming. Most of Arrhenius' contemporaries dismissed his calculations as impossible, but his work seems remarkably prescient now.

The first evidence that human activities are increasing atmospheric CO_2 came from an observatory on top of the Mauna Loa volcano in Hawaii. The observatory was established in 1957 as part of an International Geophysical Year and was intended to provide data on air chemistry in a remote, pristine environment. Surprisingly, measurements showed CO_2 levels increasing about 0.5 percent per year, rising from 315 ppm in 1958 to 378 ppm in 2004 (fig. 9.12). This increase isn't a straight line, however. Because a majority of the world's land and vegetation are in the Northern Hemisphere, northern seasons dominate the signal. Every May, CO_2 levels drop slightly as plant growth on northern continents uses CO_2 in photosynthesis. During the northern winter, levels rise again as respiration releases CO_2.

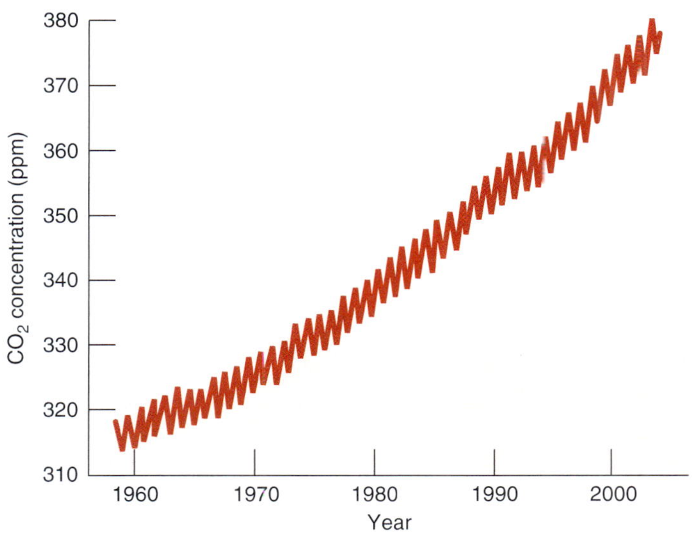

FIGURE 9.12 *Carbon dioxide concentrations at Mauna Loa Observatory in Hawaii have increased dramatically since 1958. Annual fluctuations reflect differences in photosynthesis and respiration between winter and summer.*
Source: Data from Dave Keeling and Tim Whorf, Scripps Institute of Oceanography.

In 1988 the United Nations Environment Programme and World Meteorological Organization formed the **Intergovernmental Panel on Climate Change (IPCC).** This panel brings together scientists from many nations and a wide variety of fields to assess the current state of knowledge about climate change. The IPCC's First Assessment Report played an important role in adoption of the UN Framework Convention on Climate Change at the Rio Earth Summit in 1992. In 2001 the IPCC released its third climate report, which said "with a high degree of confidence" that "recent changes in the world's climate have had discernible impacts on physical and biological systems." For this report, more than 700 scientists representing 100 countries reviewed results from some 3,000 scientific studies, which showed changes in 420 different physical and biological systems.

Noting that the earth's surface temperature has risen by about 0.6°C (1.1°F) over the past century, with most of that warming occurring in the previous two decades, the IPCC concluded that human activities must be at least partially responsible. Separating the impact of human activity from natural climate variation is extremely difficult. Nonetheless, the IPCC claims, the observed global warming is unlikely to be the result of natural variability alone. "We have altered the chemical composition of the atmosphere through the buildup of greenhouse gases—primarily carbon dioxide, methane, and nitrous oxide," the report declared. "The heat-trapping property of these gases is undisputed although uncertainties exist about exactly how earth's climate responds to them."

Climate Skeptics

Not everyone agrees with the IPCC conclusions or its method of reaching them. Dr. Frederick Seitz, president emeritus of Rockefeller University and former president of the U.S. National Academy of Sciences, for example, charged that bureaucrats and politicians altered the report in ways that didn't represent the consensus agreed upon by scientists. Others claim we don't know enough yet to make predictions about what may be happening to our global climate. While much of the dissenting views come from industry lobbying groups, some prominent scientists also hold that dire predictions about climate change may be overblown (see What Do You Think? p. 208). John Cristy of the University of Alabama, for example, says that the upper trophosphere isn't warming as fast as the earth's surface, perhaps showing that our current ideas about global climate are incorrect.

Richard Lindzen of MIT contends that current computer models don't adequately account for cloud effects. Higher evaporation rates, he believes, could produce more clouds that reflect sunlight and balance the greenhouse effect. And Vincent Gray, a climate consultant from New Zealand, contends that CO_2 concentrations measured at Mauna Loa have increased at a remarkably constant rate over the past 42 years, despite the fact that worldwide fossil fuel consumption has increased almost 50 percent during that time. Something is missing from our models, he claims.

Sources of Greenhouse Gases

Since preindustrial times, atmospheric concentrations of CO_2, CH_4, and N_2O have climbed by over 31 percent, 151 percent, and 17 percent, respectively. Carbon dioxide is by far the most important

what do you think?

Science and Uncertainty in Climate Change

Why is there so much disagreement about whether human activities are causing global climate change? A big part of the problem is that weather and climate are complex and highly variable. Making predictions about what we might expect over the long term is difficult even in normal conditions. Many scientists agree, for example, that mean global temperatures will probably warm 1.5° to 6°C (2.7° to 11°F) over the next century. They can't say, however, whether particular regions will be warmer or cooler, and for many regions they are even unable to state whether a wetter or a drier climate is more likely. Virtually all published estimates of how the climate could change are the results of computer models of the atmosphere known as "general circulation models." These complicated mathematical models are able to simulate many features of the climate, but they are still not accurate enough to provide reliable forecasts of specific climatic conditions. In fact, different models often yield contradictory results. Given the unreliability of these models, researchers trying to understand the future impacts of climate change generally analyze different scenarios from several different climate models. The hope is that, by using a wide variety of climate models, one's analysis can include the entire range of scientific uncertainty. Climatologists warn us that projections of climate change in specific areas are not forecasts but are reasonable examples of what might happen.

The U.S. EPA lists several reasons for caution in interpreting climate models:

1. The cooling effects of sulfate aerosols (from volcanoes and burning fossil fuels) could make a big difference in local conditions. Introducing aerosol effects into some models, for instance, changes precipitation predictions from a decline of 15 percent to an increase of 18 percent.
2. Most models focus on a doubling of CO_2, but we may very well be forced to cope with three or four times the current CO_2 concentrations over the longer term.
3. Nature may produce major surprises. If ocean currents are disrupted, for example, some parts of the world may actually need to deal with a substantially cooler rather than warmer climate.
4. Climate may not change in a "linear" fashion. This assumed gradualness underlies the assumption that society will have time to adjust. Some evidence suggests that climate has changed in a rather abrupt and chaotic fashion in the past.
5. Climate model simulations of today's regional climates are often inaccurate. This could be due simply to a lack of computational power to allow for local variations, or it could indicate a serious flaw in the models.

In the face of scientific uncertainty, interpretations of the costs and benefits of actions will vary. If you think major climate change is highly probable, then inaction is perilous. If you think that changes, if any, are likely to be small and gradual, then changing current policies may be unacceptable. For example, some economists (using models themselves) project that strict emission controls would cost the U.S. economy 10,000 jobs and $30 billion per year. It would be cheaper, they argue, to adapt to climate change than to try to prevent it. Ecological economists, meanwhile, argue that the costs of action need not be so high. They point out that we could cut emissions by 30 percent simply by improving efficiency and using newer technology. Further, leading the development of efficient technology will create jobs. These calculations also involve uncertainty, of course; economic models differ just as widely in their predictions as climate models do.

It's important to think about who bears the costs and who enjoys the benefits of any particular policy. Mandating energy conservation would be good for those selling renewable energy but would be painful for those whose livelihoods depend on fossil fuels. And assuming that it will be cheaper to adapt to climate changes in the future rather than change our habits now means shifting the costs to future generations. Is that fair?

If you were in Congress and had to vote on whether or not to mandate greenhouse gas reductions, how would you use scenarios from climate models? What additional information would you need to make a decision in this issue? How would you weigh the risks of inaction compared with the immediate pain of making changes in our society and technology?

---

cause of anthropogenic climate change (table 9.3). Burning fossil fuels, making cement, burning forests and grasslands, and other human activities release nearly 30 billion tons of CO_2 every year, on average, containing some 8 billion tons of carbon (fig. 9.13). About 3 billion tons of this excess carbon is taken up by terrestrial ecosystems, and around 2 billion tons are absorbed by the oceans, leaving an annual atmospheric increase of some 3 billion tons per year. If current trends continue, CO_2 concentrations could reach about 500 ppm (approaching twice the preindustrial level of 280 ppm) by the end of the twenty-first century.

Although rarer than CO_2, methane absorbs 20 to 30 times as much infrared and is accumulating in the atmosphere about twice as fast as CO_2. Methane is released by ruminant animals, wet-rice paddies, coal mines, landfills, and pipeline leaks. Chloroflurocarbons (CFCs) also are powerful infrared absorbers. CFC releases have declined since many of their uses were banned, but the CFCs already in the atmosphere will persist for many years. Nitrous oxide is produced by burning organic material and by soil denitrification. As table 9.3 shows, CFCs and N_2O together are thought to account for only about 17 percent of human-caused global warming.

TABLE 9.3 Proportion of Global Warming Caused by Four Greenhouse Gases

GAS	PERCENTAGE
Carbon dioxide (CO_2)	64
Methane (CH_4)	19
Chlorofluorocarbons (CFCs)	11
Nitrous oxide (N_2O)	6
Sulfur hexafluoride	0.4

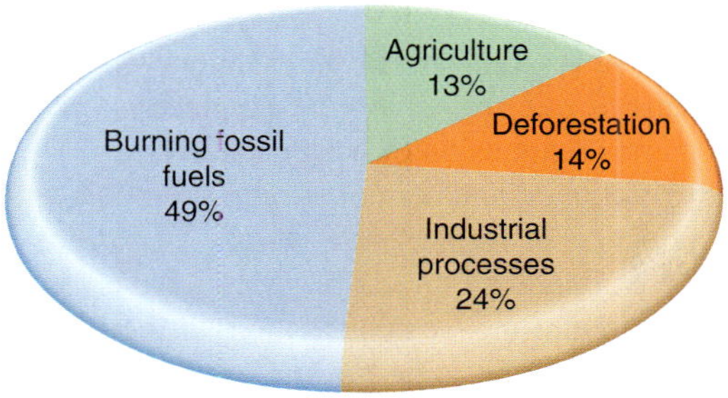

FIGURE 9.13 *Contributions to global warming by different types of human activities.*
Source: Data from World Resources Institute, 2001.

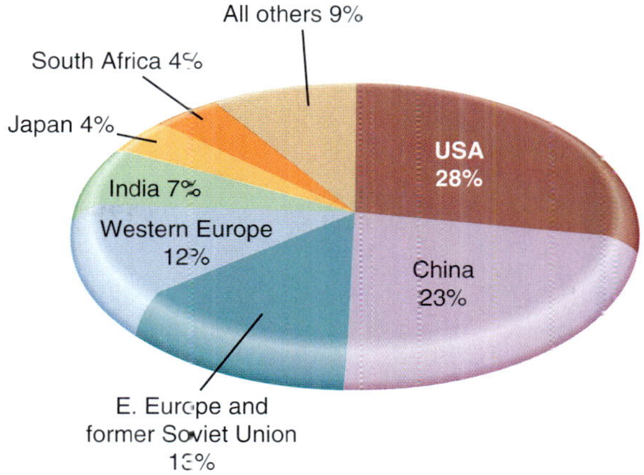

FIGURE 9.14 *Sources of anthropogenic CO_2 by country or region in 2000.*
Source: Data from World Resources Institute, 2001.

Aerosols have a tendency to counteract the effects of greenhouse gases, on local and sometimes global scales. Sulfate aerosols and soot produced by some of the same activities that release CO_2 can shade urban air, for example, and reduce air temperatures by as much or more than greenhouse gases increase them. The 1991 eruption of Mt. Pinatubo in the Philippines ejected enough ash and sulfate particles to cool the global climate about 1°C, but this cooling lasted for only about a year.

The United States, with less than 5 percent of the world's population, produces 28 percent of all anthropogenic CO_2 (fig. 9.14). China, with 1.3 billion people, is second in total CO_2 emissions, but fourteenth in per capita production. Japan and Western Europe, which by most measures have standards of living at least equal to the United States, produce only half as much CO_2 per person. Eastern Europe and the former Soviet Union have many old, inefficient factories and coal-buring power plants that emit high CO_2 levels with relatively little economic return.

Current Evidence of Climate Change

Increasingly, evidence from around the world suggests that global climate is already changing as a result of human actions. Precipitation has increased by about 1 percent over the world's continents in the past century. High latitudes are tending to see more rainfall, while precipitation has actually declined in some tropical areas (fig. 9.15). Warmer temperatures apparently are causing more water evaporation. We expect this to produce more severe storms. Hurricanes, typhoons, tornadoes, severe rainstorms, and flooding seem to be more frequent and more damaging, although part of the increased damage results from more people living in dangerous

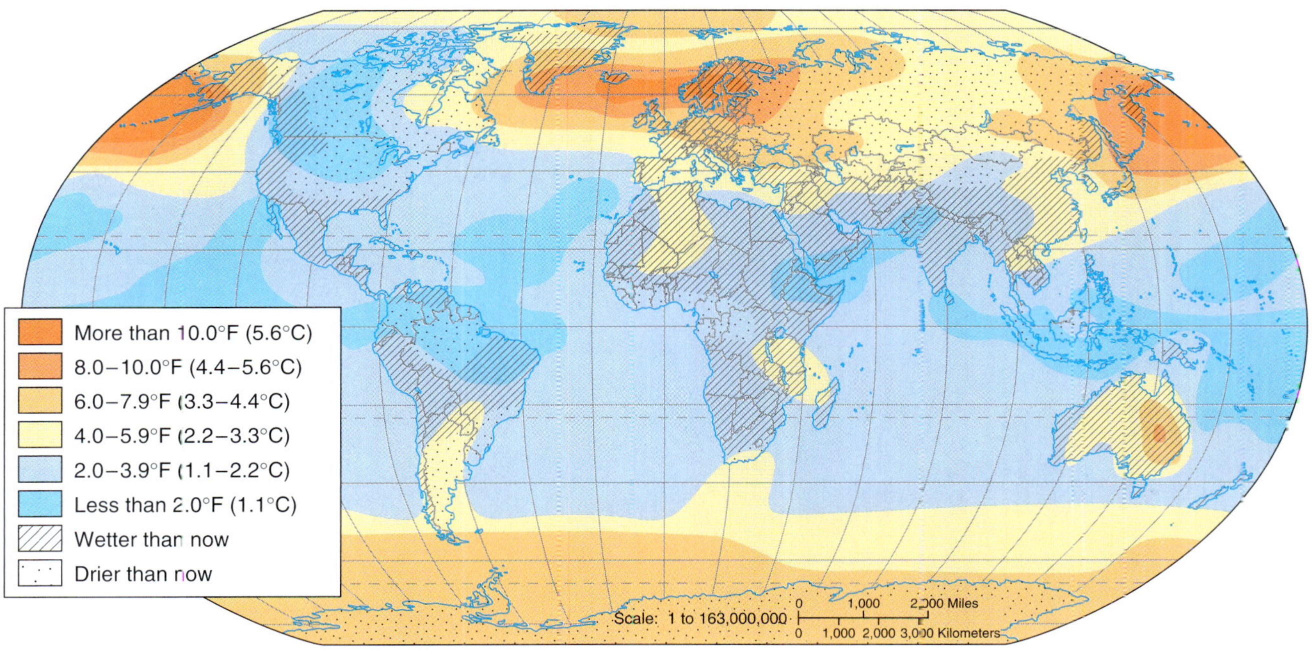

FIGURE 9.15 *Potential global temperature and precipitation change by 2050. Note that most of the United States and Canada are expected to be drier* (stippled areas) *while most tropical countries will probably be wetter* (diagonal lines).
Source: Data from National Oceanic and Atmospheric Administration, 2001.

locations along coasts and in floodplains. In 2003 at least 30,000 people died in Europe's hottest summer since 1540. Climate models predict that temperature extremes such as this will become increasingly common by the end of this century, if greenhouse gas emissions aren't reduced.

Satellite images and surface temperature data show that growing seasons are now as much as three weeks longer in a band across northern Eurasia than they were 30 years ago (see fig 1.15). Arctic sea ice is 40 percent thinner now, and the edge of the Arctic sea ice pack averages about 500 km (312 mi) farther north than it was a century ago. Arctic wildlife, including polar bears, walruses, beluga whales, caribou, and musk oxen, is declining or changing migration and feeding patterns as a result of changing climate conditions. In the south, the West Antarctic Ice Sheet has shrunk 25 percent over the past 25 years, including several giant icebergs—the largest about the size of Delaware—that have calved off in recent years (see Investigating Our Environment, p. 211). In 2002 a huge section of the Larsen B ice shelf along the coast of the Antarctic Peninsula suddenly collapsed and broke into innumerable small bergs. Although the ice shelves were known to be breaking up, the disintegration of an area nealry the size of Connecticut in just a few weeks was unprecedented (see related story "Collapse of the Larsen B" at www.mhhe.com/cases). Here, too, wildlife is suffering from loss of habitat and diminishing food supplies. Adele penguins, for instance, are declining precipitously across the Antarctic as the ice on which they rest and lay their eggs is disappearing.

Alpine glaciers everywhere are retreating rapidly (fig. 9.16). In 1972 Venezuela had six glaciers; now it has only two. All the glaciers in Montana's Glacier National Park will be gone by 2070, if current trends continue. Over the next 50 years, at least half of all alpine glaciers in the world could disappear. Without this resource, agriculture, industry, power generation, and drinking-water supplies will suffer. About 1.7 billion people now live in areas where water supplies are tight. This number could increase to 5.4 billion by 2025. Sea level has risen worldwide approximately 15–20 cm (6–8 in.) in the past century. About one-quarter of this increase is due to melting alpine glaciers; roughly half is caused by thermal expansion of ocean water.

Many wild plant and animal species are being forced out of their current ranges as the climate warms. In Europe and North America, for example, 57 butterfly species have died out at the southern end of their range, extended their northern limits, or both. Given enough time and a route for migration, these species might adapt to new conditions, but we now are forcing them to move at least ten times the rate many achieved at the end of the last ice age (fig. 9.17). The disappearance of amphibians, such as the beautiful golden toads, from the cloud forests of Costa Rica or western toads from Oregon's Cascade Range are thought to have been caused at least in part by changing weather patterns.

Around the world, coral reefs are bleaching because of higher water temperatures. Rivaling tropical rainforests in their biological diversity and net productivity, coral reefs already are threatened by human activities, such as dynamite fishing and limestone excavation. If sea temperatures continue to rise, most coral reefs will be wiped out in the next 50 years. Similarly, the Cape Floral Kingdom of South Africa, one of the most unique terrestrial ecosystems in the world, could disappear due to changing weather patterns.

In a broad study of tropical plants and animals, British scientists warned that even the lowest estimates of potential climate change suggest that 1 million species could be driven into extinction by 2050. If migration to more suitable habitat is blocked by fragmentation, more than half of all tropical species might be eliminated.

Winners and Losers

Local climate changes could well have severe effects on human societies, agriculture, and natural ecosystems. In many cases, both organisms and human infrastructure will not be able to move or

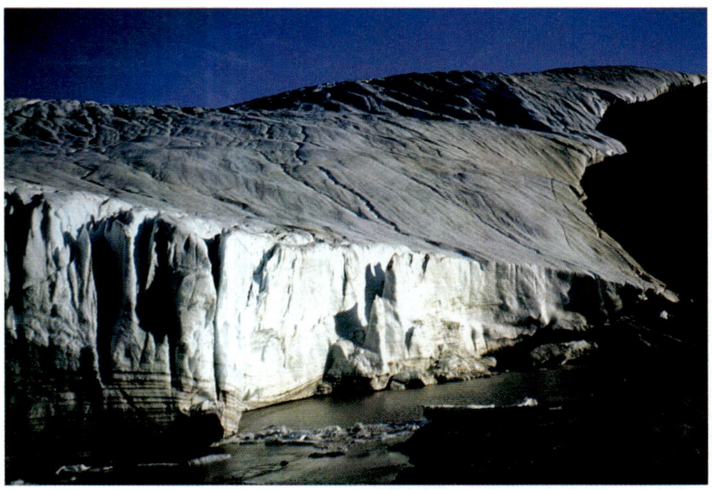

FIGURE 9.16 *Alpine glaciers are retreating rapidly nearly everywhere in the world. For the billions of people whose drinking water comes from glacial-fed rivers, this could be a serious threat.*

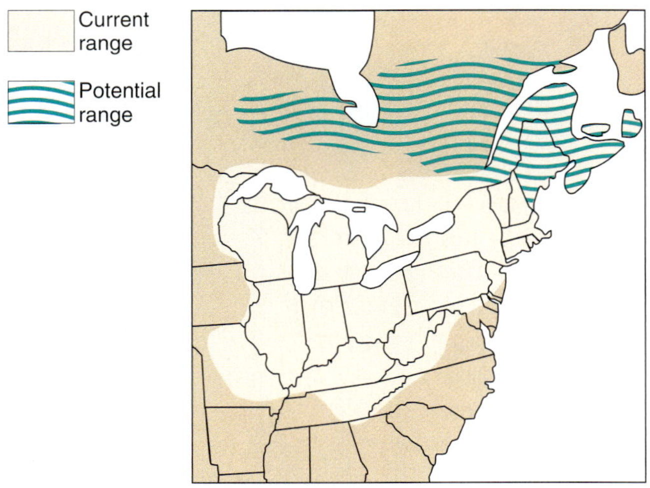

FIGURE 9.17 *Change in suitable range for sugar maple trees, according to the climate change model.*

Source: Data from Margaret Davis and Catherine Zabriskie in *Global Warming and Biological Diversity,* ed. by Peters and Lovejoy, 1991, Yale University Press.

INVESTIGATING Our Environment

Satellite Images

How do we measure widespread phenomena such as El Niños, climate change, and weather? Some information can be gathered from ground-based observatories, but these facilities only tell us about a scattering of isolated points. To detect patterns on a global scale, a more distant view is useful, and that is why so much environmental science now involves remote sensing.

Remote sensing is a general term for data gathered from satellites, or sometimes by sensors on airplanes. Just as a camera is a sensor that captures light energy reflected from objects, sensors on satellites capture energy wavelengths reflected from the earth's surface, from clouds, or from the atmosphere. Some satellites detect infrared wavelengths, which indicate warm areas in the oceans, on ice caps, or on land. Others might detect selected wavelengths of visible light, such as green or blue, or microwaves, which provide images of cloud cover and precipitation (see fig. 2.10). Our current understanding of the Antarctic ozone hole comes from satellites that detect near-ultraviolet wavelengths, which are absorbed by ozone in the atmosphere.

There are now many different satellites orbiting the earth in order to monitor environmental conditions. Most satellites carry several sensors, each designed to collect specific wavelengths for specific monitoring purposes. Perhaps the best-known satellites are the *Landsat* series (currently *Landsat 7* is in operation) sent up to capture land cover and vegetation information. Each pixel represents about 30 x 30 m on the ground, so the images are highly detailed. Another important group of satellites, the Earth Observing System (EOS), collects coarser pictures more frequently—250 to 1,000 m pixel resolution images taken every day, instead of every two weeks for *Landsat*. The EOS satellites collect 36 energy bands, from ultraviolet to infrared. Bands are selected to detect land/sea boundaries, differences in temperature, phytoplankton concentrations, atmospheric water vapor, atmospheric chemistry, and other characteristics of the earth's surface and atmosphere. These satellites orbit the earth, approximately pole to pole. In contrast, there are "geostationary" satellites that are "parked" over the earth, orbiting with the planet to maintain a constant position over the Pacific or Atlantic Ocean. These collect data on atmospheric conditions more than once an hour, so they are good for monitoring the movement of clouds and storm systems.

There are more than 7,000 satellites orbiting the earth. Most are used for communication—to reflect radio, telephone, or TV signals. Others are spy satellites collecting highly detailed images of strategic areas. The closest satellites, including the EOS satellites, are less than 1,000 km above the earth's surface. TV satellites and geostationary weather satellites are more than 35 km up. When you look up at the sky at night, you might see some of the closest satellites, gathering data to give us the "big picture" of environmental change as they travel across the sky.

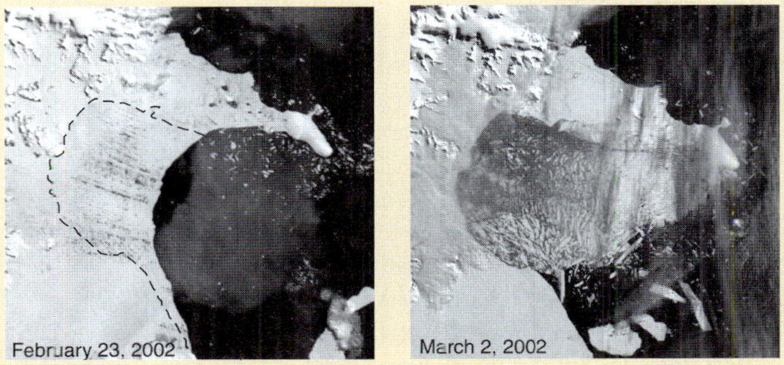

In early 2002, satellite images showed a Rhode Island–sized section of the Larsen B ice shelf on the Antarctic Peninsula disintegrated into shards. Satellite images show 3,250 km² that collapsed into the ocean.
Source: National Snow and Ice Data Center/University of Colorado/NOAA.

adapt quickly enough to accommodate the rates at which climate seems to be changing.

Does anyone win in these scenarios? Residents of northern Canada, Siberia, and Alaska probably would enjoy warmer temperatures, longer growing seasons, and longer ice-free shipping seasons from their ports. Stronger monsoons bringing more moisture to parts of Central Africa and South Asia could increase crop yields. But soils in some areas may not be suitable for crops no matter how agreeable the climate. Carbon dioxide is a fertilizer for plants, and higher CO_2 levels bring faster growth with less water for many plant species. Sherwood Idso of the U.S. Department of Agriculture says that increased CO_2 concentrations could trigger lush plant growth that would make crops abundant.

Enough water is stored in glacial ice caps in Greenland and Antarctica to raise sea levels around 100 meters (330 feet) if they all melt. About one-third of the world's population now live in areas that would be flooded if that happened. Even the 75 cm (30 in.) sea-level rise expected by 2050 will flood much of south Florida, Bangladesh, Pakistan, and many other low-lying coastal areas. Most of the world's largest urban areas are on coastlines. Wealthy cities, such as New York or London, can probably afford to build dikes to keep out rising seas, but poorer cities, such as Jakarta, Calcutta, or Manila, might simply be abandoned as residents flee to higher ground. Several small island countries, such as the Maldives, the Bahamas, Kiribati, and the Marshall Islands, could become uninhabitable if sea levels rose a meter or more. In 2002 the South Pacific nation of Tuvalu announced that it was abandoning its island homeland. All 11,000 residents will move to New Zealand, perhaps the first of many climate change refugees.

Insurance companies worry that the $2 trillion in insured property along U.S. coastlines could be at risk from a combination of high seas and catastrophic storms. Some 87,000 homes in the United States within 150 m (500 ft) of a shoreline are in danger of coastal erosion or flooding in the next 50 years. Accountants state that loss of land and structures to flooding and coastal erosion together with damage to fishing stocks, agriculture, and water supplies could raise worldwide insurance claims from about $50 billion per year in the 1970s to a projected $150 billion per year in 2010. Some of this increase in insurance claims is because more people are living in dangerous places, but extra-severe storms and rising sea levels only exacerbate this problem.

Infectious diseases are likely to increase as the insects, rodents, and ticks that carry them spread to new areas. Already we have seen diseases such as malaria, dengue fever, and West Nile virus appear in parts of North America where they had never before been reported. Coupled with the movement of hundreds of millions of environmental refugees and greater crowding as people are forced out of areas made uninhabitable by rising seas and changing climates, the spread of epidemic diseases will also increase.

Permafrost is already beginning to melt in the Arctic, causing roads to buckle and houses to sink into the mud. An ominous possibility from this melting is the release of vast stores of methane hydrate now locked in frozen ground and in sediments in the ocean floor. Together with the increased oxidation of high-latitude peat lands potentially caused by warmer and dryer conditions, release of these carbon stores could add as much CO_2 to the atmosphere as all the fossil fuels ever burned. We could trigger a disastrous positive feedback loop in which the effects of warming cause even more warming.

Another potentially catastrophic outcome of global climate change is that greater terrestrial runoff from increased rainfall might suddenly change ocean circulation patterns that now moderate northern climates (see appendix 3, p. 382). On the other hand, increased ocean evaporation might intensify snowfall at high latitudes so that Arctic glaciers and snow pack would increase rather than decrease. Ironically, the increased albedo (reflectivity) of colder, snow-covered surfaces might then trigger a new ice age.

International Climate Negotiations

One of the centerpieces of the 1992 United Nations Earth Summit meeting in Rio de Janeiro was the Framework Convention on Climate Change, which set an objective of stabilizing greenhouse gas emissions to reduce the threats of global warming. At a follow-up conference in Kyoto, Japan, in 1997, 160 nations agreed to roll back CO_2, methane, and nitrous oxide emissions about 5 percent below 1990 levels by 2012. Three other greenhouse gases, hydrofluorocarbons, perfluorocarbons, and sulfur hexafluoride, would also be reduced, although from what level was not decided. Known as the **Kyoto Protocol,** this treaty sets different limits for individual nations, depending on their output before 1990. Poorer nations, such as China and India, were exempted from emission limits to allow development to increase their standard of living. Wealthy countries created the problem, the poorer nations argue, and the wealthy should deal with it.

Although the United States took a lead role in negotiating a compromise at Kyoto that other countries could accept, President George W. Bush refused to honor U.S. commitments. Claiming that reducing carbon emissions would be too costly for the U.S. economy, he said, "We're going to put the interests of our own country first and foremost."

Meanwhile, 126 countries have ratified the Kyoto Protocol. With the addition of Russia to this list in 2004, the provisions became legally binding on all signatories whether they ratify the protocol or not. If the U.S. continues to refuse to comply, it could have severe ramifications on U.S. corporations engaged in international business. Thousands of American businesses—including most of the largest ones—fall into this category. Having to modify their products and practices for overseas markets while not doing so for domestic sales would be expensive and would put them at a disadvantage with competitors not subject to these costs. Moreover, because Kyoto is based on a global cap-and-trade program, companies that get in on it early will have an advantage—they can buy cheap emissions credits before the price gets bid up.

Even if the United States joins the rest of the world in accepting the Kyoto provisions, however, many climatologists argue that much more will have to be done to combat global warming. According to some calculations, we will have to reduce CO2 emissions by 60 percent or more to stabilize atmospheric concentrations. In the next section, we'll look at some of the ways we might accomplish this.

Controlling Greenhouse Emissions

In spite of U.S. intransigence, progress already is being made in many places toward reducing greenhouse emissions. The United Kingdom, for example, had already rolled CO_2 emissions back to 1990 levels by 2000 and vowed to reduce them 60 percent by 2050. Britain already has started to substitute natural gas for coal, promote energy efficiency in homes and industry, and raise its already high gasoline tax. Plans are to "decarbonize" British society and to decouple GNP growth from CO_2 emissions. A revenue-neutral carbon levy is expected to lower CO_2 releases and trigger a transition to renewable energy over the next five decades. Greenhouse gas emissions trading, which has already started in the U.K., is expected to reach $10 billion (U.S.) in 2005.

Germany, also, has reduced its CO_2 emissions at least 10 percent by switching from coal to gas and by encouraging energy efficiency throughout society. Atmospheric scientist Steve Schneider calls this a "no regrets" policy; even if we don't need to stabilize our climate, many of these steps save money, conserve resources, and have other environmental benefits. Nuclear power also is being promoted as an alternative to fossil fuels. It's true that nuclear reactions don't produce greenhouse gases, but security worries and unresolved problems of how to store wastes safely make this option unacceptable to many people.

Renewable energy sources offer a better solution to climate problems, many people believe (fig. 9.18). Chapter 12 discusses options for conserving energy and switching to renewable sources, such as solar, wind, geothermal, biomass, and fuel cells. Denmark, the world's leader in wind power, now gets 20 percent of its electricity from windmills. Plans are to generate half of the nation's electricity from offshore wind farms by 2030. Even China reduced its CO_2 emissions 17 percent between 1997 and 1999 through greater efficiency in coal burning and industrial energy use. The U.S. energy plan, meanwhile, is to burn more coal, drill for gas

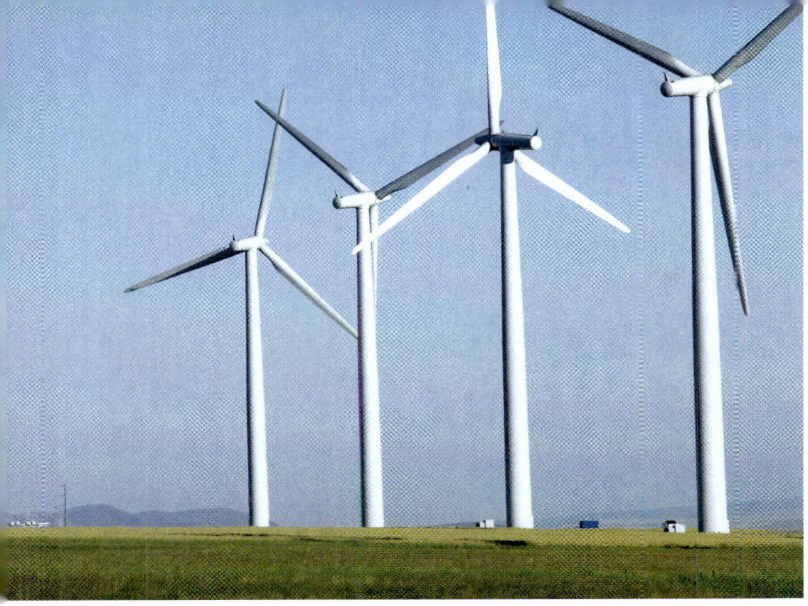

FIGURE 9.18 *Renewable energy sources, such as wind, solar energy, geothermal power, and biomass crops, could eliminate our dependence on fossil fuels and prevent extreme global climate change, if we act quickly.*

and oil in wildlife refuges and wilderness areas, and build more nuclear plants.

In addition to reducing its output, there are options for capturing and storing CO_2. Planting trees can be effective if they're allowed to mature to old-growth status or are made into products, such as window frames and doors, that will last for many years before they're burned or recycled. Farmland also can serve as a carbon sink if farmers change their crop mixture and practice minimum till cultivation that keeps carbon in the soil. In 1988 John H. Martin suggested that phytoplankton growth in the ocean may be limited by iron deficiency. This theory was tested in 2000, when researchers spread about 3.5 tons of dissolved iron over 75 km^2 of the South Pacific. Monitored by satellite, a ten-fold rise in chlorophyll concentration eventually spread over about 1,700 km^2 and was calculated to have pulled several thousand tons of CO_2 out of the air. Still, some ecologists warn about such large-scale tinkering. We don't know whether the carbon fixed by phytoplankton growth will be stored in sediments or simply eaten by predators and returned immediately to the atmosphere. It's possible that dying algae might create an anoxic zone that would devastate oceanic food webs.

Another way to store CO_2 is to inject it into underground strata or deep ocean waters. Since 1996, Norway's Statoil has been pumping more than 1 million metric tons of CO_2 per year into an aquifer 1,000 m below the seafloor at a North Sea gas well. It is economical to do so because otherwise the company would have to pay a $50 per ton carbon tax on its emissions. Around the world, deep, briny aquifers could store a century worth of CO_2 output at current fossil fuel consumption rates. It might also be possible to pump liquid CO_2 into deep ocean trenches, where it would form lakes contained by enormous water pressures. There are worries, however, about what this might do to deep ocean fauna and what might happen if earthquakes or landslides caused a sudden release of this CO_2. In Canada, an Alberta power plant is injecting CO_2 into a coal seam too deep to be mined. The CO_2 releases natural gas, which is burned to produce electricity and more CO_2. Proponents of **carbon management,** as these various projects are called, argue that it may be cheaper to clean up fossil fuel effluents than to switch to renewable energy sources.

Most attention is focused on CO_2 because it lasts in the atmosphere, on average, for about 120 years. Methane and other greenhouse gases are much more powerful infrared absorbers but remain in the air for a much shorter time. NASA's Dr. James Hansen made a controversial suggestion, however, that the best short-term attack on warming might come by focusing not on carbon dioxide but on methane. Reducing gas pipeline leaks would conserve this valuable resource as well as help the environment.

Methane from landfills, oil wells, and coal mines that once would have been simply vented into the air is now being collected and used to generate electricity. Rice paddies are a major methane source. Changing flooding schedules and fertilization techniques can reduce anoxia (oxygen depletion) that produces marsh gas. Finally, ruminant animals (such as cows, camels, and buffalo) create large amounts of digestive system gas. Modified diets can reduce flatulence significantly. In 2003 New Zealand passed a tax on ruminants as a way to meet its Kyoto Obligations. Farmers were outraged by what they derided as a "fart tax" and got it repealed.

Soot, while not mentioned in the Kyoto Protocol, might also be important in global warming. Dark, airborne particles absorb both ultraviolet and visible light, converting them to heat energy. According to some calculations, reducing soot from diesel engines, coal-fired generators, forest fires, and wood stoves might reduce net global warming by 40 percent within three to five years. Curbing soot emissions would also have beneficial health effects.

Some individual cities and states have announced their own plans to combat global warming. Among the first of these were Toronto, Copenhagen, and Helsinki, which pledged to reduce CO_2 emissions 20 percent from 1990 levels by 2010. Portland, Oregon, was the first U.S. city to implement a CO_2-reduction strategy. States with plans to limit greenhouse gas emissions include California, New York, and New Hampshire. Some corporations are following suit. British Petroleum has set a goal of cutting CO_2 releases from all its facilities by 10 percent before 2010. In 2000 BP, Alcan, DuPont, and other companies joined with the Environmental Defense Fund to launch a partnership for climate action, pledging to meet or exceed Kyoto requirements. Each of us can make a contribution in this effort. Chapter 12 discusses ways we can cut our individual energy consumption, the principal cause of greenhouse gas emissions (see p. 289).

CLIMATE AND AIR POLLUTION

As the global warming debate shows, human activities can influence climate processes. In this section, we will discuss ways that human activities affect air quality and environmental processes on a more local scale.

According to the Environmental Protection Agency (EPA), Americans release some 147 million metric tons of air pollution (not counting carbon dioxide or wind-blown soil) each year.

Worldwide emissions of these pollutants are around 2 billion metric tons per year. Even remote, pristine wilderness areas are now affected. Over the past 20 years, however, air quality has improved in most cities in Western Europe, North America, and Japan. Many young people might be surprised to learn that, a generation ago, most American cities were much dirtier than they are today. The EPA estimates that, since 1990, when regulation of the most hazardous materials began, air toxics emissions have been reduced more than 1 million tons per year. This is almost ten times the reductions achieved in the previous 20 years. Since the 1970s, the levels of major pollutants monitored by the EPA have decreased in the United States, despite population growth of more than 30 percent (table 9.4). Pollution reductions have resulted mainly from greater efficiency and pollution-control technologies in factories, power plants, and automobiles. Our success in controlling some of the most serious air pollutants gives us hope for similar progress in other environmental problems.

While developed countries have been making progress, however, air quality in the developing world has been getting much worse. Especially in the burgeoning megacities of rapidly industrializing countries (see chapter 14), air pollution often exceeds World Health Organization standards by large margins. In Lahore, Pakistan, and Xi'an, China, for instance, airborne dust, smoke, and dirt often are ten times higher than levels considered safe for human health (fig. 9.19).

Studies of air pollutants over southern Asia reveal that a 3 km (2 mi) thick toxic cloud of ash, acids, aerosols, dust, and photochemical reactants covers the entire Indian subcontinent for much of the year. Nobel laureate Paul Crutzen estimates that up to 2 million people in India alone die each year from atmospheric pollution. Produced by forest fires, the burning of agricultural wastes, and dramatic increases in the use of fossil fuels, the Asian smog layer cuts the amount of solar energy reaching the earth's surface beneath it by up to 15 percent. Meteorologists suggest that the cloud—80 percent of which is human-made—could disrupt monsoon weather patterns and cut rainfall over northern Pakistan,

TABLE 9.4 Reductions in U.S. Pollution Emissions, 1970–1997

POLLUTANT	PERCENT CHANGE IN ANNUAL EMISSIONS
Carbon monoxide	–32
Lead[1]	–98
Nitrogen oxides[2]	+11
Ozone	–37
Particulate matter	–75
Sulfur dioxide	–35

Source: Data from U.S. Environmental Protection Agency.

[1] Reduction due mainly to elimination of leaded gasoline.

[2] Increase mainly from more vehicle emissions.

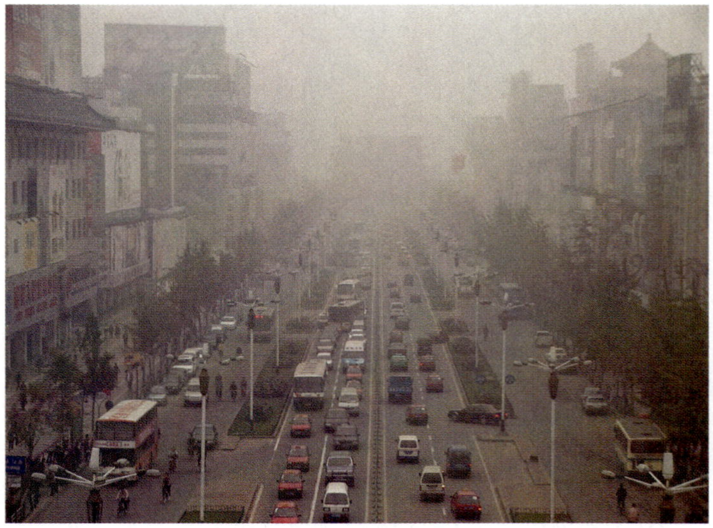

FIGURE 9.19 *While air quality is improving in many industrialized countries, newly developing countries have growing pollution problems. Xi'an, China, often has particulate levels above 300 μg/m^3.*

Afghanistan, western China, and central Asia by up to 40 percent. Shifting monsoon flows may also have contributed to the catastrophic floods in Nepal, Bangladesh, and eastern India in 2002 that killed at least 1,000 people and left more than 25 million homeless.

When this "Asian Brown Cloud" drifts out over the Indian Ocean at the end of the monsoon season, it cools sea temperatures and may be changing El Niño/Southern Oscillation patterns in the Pacific Ocean as well. As UN Environment Programme Executive Director Klaus Töpfer said, "There are global implications because a pollution parcel like this, which stretches 3 km high, can travel half way round the globe in a week."

Major Kinds of Pollutants

In the United States, principal pollutants are identified and regulated by the Clean Air Act of 1970. Primary pollutants are released in a harmful form (fig. 9.20). Secondary pollutants, by contrast, become hazardous after reactions in the air. **Photochemical oxidants** (compounds formed with solar energy) and atmospheric acids are probably the most important secondary pollutants. **Fugitive emissions** are those that do not go through a smokestack. By far the most massive example of this category is dust from soil erosion, strip mining, rock crushing, and building construction (and destruction). Leaking valves and pipe joints contribute as much as 90 percent of the hydrocarbons and volatile organic chemicals emitted from oil refineries and chemical plants.

Conventional, or **criteria, pollutants** are a group of seven major pollutants (sulfur dioxide, carbon monoxide, particulates, volatile organic compounds, nitrogen oxides, ozone, and lead) that contribute the largest volume of air-quality degradation and are considered the most serious threat of all air pollutants to human health and welfare. Figure 9.21 shows the main sources of six of these criteria pollutants. Since 1970 the Clean Air Act has man-

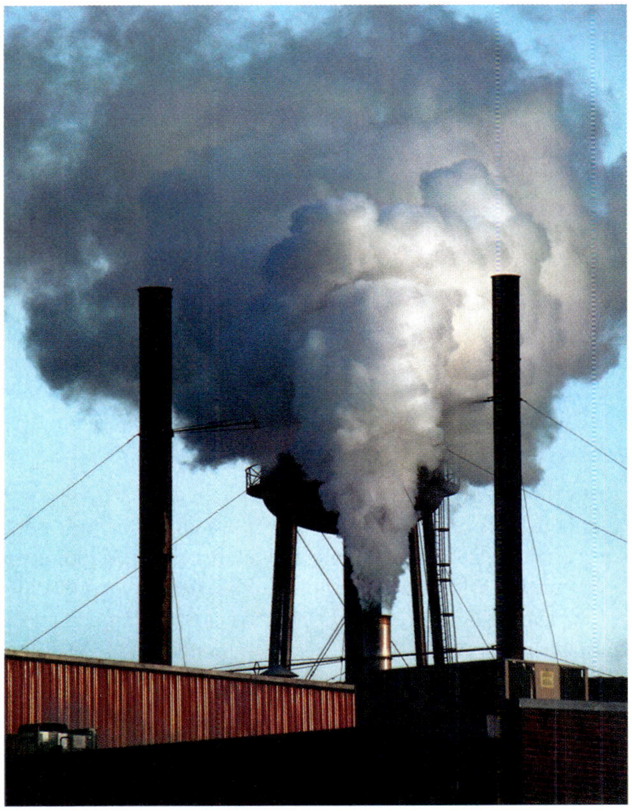

FIGURE 9.20 *Primary pollutants are released directly from a source into the air. A point source is a specific location of highly concentrated discharge, such as this smokestack.*

dated that the EPA set allowable limits for concentrations of these pollutants in **ambient air** (the air around us), especially in cities.

The EPA also monitors **unconventional pollutants,** compounds that are produced in less volume than conventional pollutants but that are especially toxic or hazardous. Among these are asbestos, benzene, beryllium, mercury, polychlorinated biphenyls (PCBs), and vinyl chloride. Most of these materials have no natural source in the environment (to any great extent) and are, therefore, only anthropogenic in origin.

Aesthetic degradation is another important form of pollution. Noise, odors, and light pollution may not be life threatening, but they reduce the quality of our lives. In most urban areas, it is difficult or impossible to see stars in the sky at night because of dust in the air and stray light from buildings, outdoor advertising, and streetlights.

Sources and Problems of Major Pollutants

Most conventional pollutants are produced primarily from burning fossil fuels, especially in coal-powered electric plants and in cars and trucks, as well as in processing natural gas and oil. Others, especially sulfur and metals, are by-products of mining and manufacturing processes. Of the 188 air toxics listed in the Clean Air Act, about two-thirds are volatile organic compounds (VOCs), and most of the rest are metal compounds. In this section we will discuss the characteristics and origin of the major pollutants.

Sulfur dioxide (SO_2) is a colorless, corrosive gas that damages both plants and animals. Once in the atmosphere, it can be further oxidized to sulfur trioxide (SO_3), which reacts with water vapor or dissolves in water droplets to form sulfuric acid (H_2SO_4),

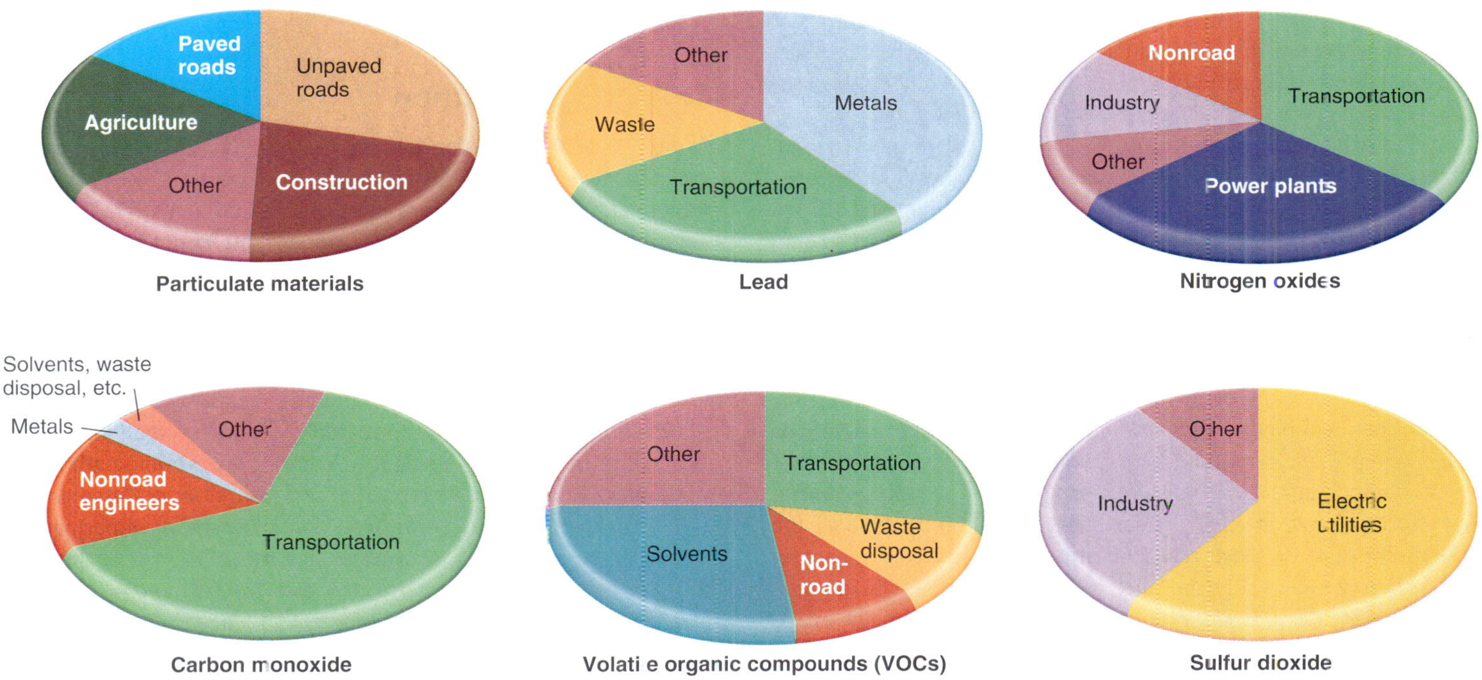

FIGURE 9.21 *Anthropogenic sources of six of the primary criteria air pollutants in the United States.*

Source: Data from Joyce E. Penner, "Atmospheric Chemistry and Air Quality" in W. B. Meyer and B. L. Turner (eds.), *Changes in Land Use and Land Cover: A Global Perspective,* 1994. Cambridge University Press and UNEP, 1999.

a major component of acid rain. Sulfur dioxide and sulfate ions are probably second only to smoking as causes of air-pollution–related health damage. Sulfate particles and droplets also reduce visibility in the United States by as much as 80 percent.

Nitrogen oxides (NO_x) are highly reactive gases formed when combustion initiates reactions between atmospheric nitrogen and oxygen. The initial product, nitric oxide (NO), oxidizes further in the atmosphere to nitrogen dioxide (NO_2), a reddish-brown gas that gives photochemical smog its distinctive color. Because these gases convert readily from one form to the other, the general term NO_x is used to describe these gases. Nitrogen oxides combine with water to form nitric acid (HNO_3), which is also a major component of acid precipitation. Excess nitrogen in water is causing eutrophication of inland waters and coastal seas. It may also encourage the growth of weedy species that crowd out native plants.

Carbon monoxide (CO) is less common than the principal form of atmospheric carbon, carbon dioxide (CO_2), but more dangerous. CO is a colorless, odorless, but highly toxic gas produced mainly by incomplete combustion of fuel (coal, oil, charcoal, wood, or gas). CO inhibits respiration in animals by binding irreversibly to hemoglobin. In the United States, two-thirds of the CO emissions are created by internal combustion engines in transportation. Land-clearing fires and cooking fires also are major sources. About 90 percent of the CO in the air is consumed in photochemical reactions that produce ozone.

Particulate material includes dust, ash, soot, lint, smoke, pollen, spores, algal cells, and many other suspended materials. Aerosols, or extremely minute particles or liquid droplets suspended in the air, are included in this class. Particulates often are the most apparent form of air pollution, since they reduce visibility and leave dirty deposits on windows, painted surfaces, and textiles. Breathable particles smaller than 2.5 μm are among the most dangerous of this group because they can damage lung tissues. Asbestos fibers and cigarette smoke are among the most dangerous respirable particles in urban and indoor air because they are carcinogenic.

Volatile organic compounds (VOCs) are organic gases. Plants, bogs, and termites are the largest sources of VOCs, especially isoprenes (C_5H_8), terpenes ($C_{10}H_{15}$), and methane (CH_4). These volatile hydrocarbons are generally oxidized to CO and CO_2 in the atmosphere.

More dangerous synthetic organic chemicals, such as benzene, toluene, formaldehyde, vinyl chloride, phenols, chloroform, and trichloroethylene, are released by human activities. Principal sources are incompletely burned fuels from vehicles, power plants, chemical plants, and petroleum refineries. These chemicals play an important role in the formation of photochemical oxidants.

Photochemical oxidants are products of secondary atmospheric reactions driven by solar energy (table 9.5). One of the most important of these reactions involves formation of singlet (atomic) oxygen by splitting nitrogen dioxide (NO_2). This atomic oxygen then reacts with another molecule of O_2 to make ozone (O_3). Although ozone is important in the stratosphere, in ambient air it is highly reactive and damages vegetation, animal tissues, and building materials. Ozone's acrid, biting odor is a distinctive characteristic of photochemical smog.

TABLE 9.5 Photochemical Oxidant Production

STEPS	PHOTOCHEMICAL PRODUCTS
1. $NO + VOC \rightarrow$	NO_2 (nitrogen dioxide)
2. NO_2 + UV sunlight $\rightarrow$	$NO + O$ (nitric oxide + atomic oxygen)
3. $O + O_2 \rightarrow$	O_3 (ozone)
4. $NO_2 + VOC \rightarrow$	PAN (peroxyacetyl nitrate)

Lead and Other Toxic Elements

Toxic metals and halogens are chemical elements that are toxic when concentrated and released in the environment. Principal metals of concern are lead, mercury, arsenic, nickel, beryllium, cadmium, thallium, uranium, cesium, and plutonium. Halogens (fluorine, chlorine, bromine, and iodine) are highly reactive toxic elements. Most of these materials are mined and used in manufacturing. Metals commonly occur as trace elements in fuels, especially coal.

Lead and mercury are widespread neurotoxins that damage the nervous system. By some estimates, 20 percent of all inner-city children suffer some degree of developmental retardation from high environmental lead levels. Long-range transport of lead and mercury through the air is causing bioaccumulation in remote aquatic ecosystems, such as arctic lakes and seas. Chlorine is a toxic halogen widely used in bleach, plastics, and other products. Methyl bromide (a powerful fungicide used in agriculture) and **chlorofluorocarbons** (propellants and refrigerants) are also implicated in ozone depletion.

Indoor Air Pollution

We have spent a considerable amount of effort and money to control the major outdoor air pollutants, but we have only recently become aware of the dangers of indoor air pollutants. The EPA has found that indoor concentrations of toxic air pollutants are often higher than outdoors. Furthermore, people generally spend more time inside than out and therefore are exposed to higher doses of these pollutants. In some cases, indoor air in homes has chemical concentrations that would be illegal outside or in the workplace. Under some circumstances, compounds such as chloroform, benzene, carbon tetrachloride, formaldehyde, and styrene can be 70 times higher in indoor air than in outdoor air. Molds, pathogens, and other biohazards also represent serious indoor pollutants.

Cigarette smoke is without doubt the most important air contaminant in developed countries in terms of human health. The U.S. surgeon general has estimated that 430,000 people die each year in the United States from emphysema, heart attacks, strokes, lung cancer, or other diseases caused by smoking. These diseases are responsible for 20 percent of all mortality in the United States, or four times as much as infectious agents. Total costs for early deaths and smoking-related illnesses are estimated to be $100 billion per year. Eliminating smoking probably would save more lives than any other pollution-control measure.

In the less-developed countries of Africa, Asia, and Latin America, where such organic fuels as firewood, charcoal, dried dung, and agricultural wastes make up the majority of household energy, smoky, poorly ventilated heating and cooking fires represent the greatest source of indoor air pollution (fig. 9.22). The World Health Organization (WHO) estimates that 2.5 billion people—nearly half the world's population—are adversely affected by pollution from this source. In particular, women and small children spend long hours each day around open fires or unventilated stoves in enclosed spaces.

INTERACTIONS BETWEEN CLIMATE PROCESSES AND AIR POLLUTION

Physical processes in the atmosphere transport, concentrate, and disperse air pollutants. To comprehend the global effects of air pollution, it is necessary to understand how climate processes interact with pollutants. Global warming in which pollutants are altering the earth's energy budget, is the best-known case of interaction between anthropogenic pollutants and the atmosphere. In this section we will survey other important climate-pollution interactions.

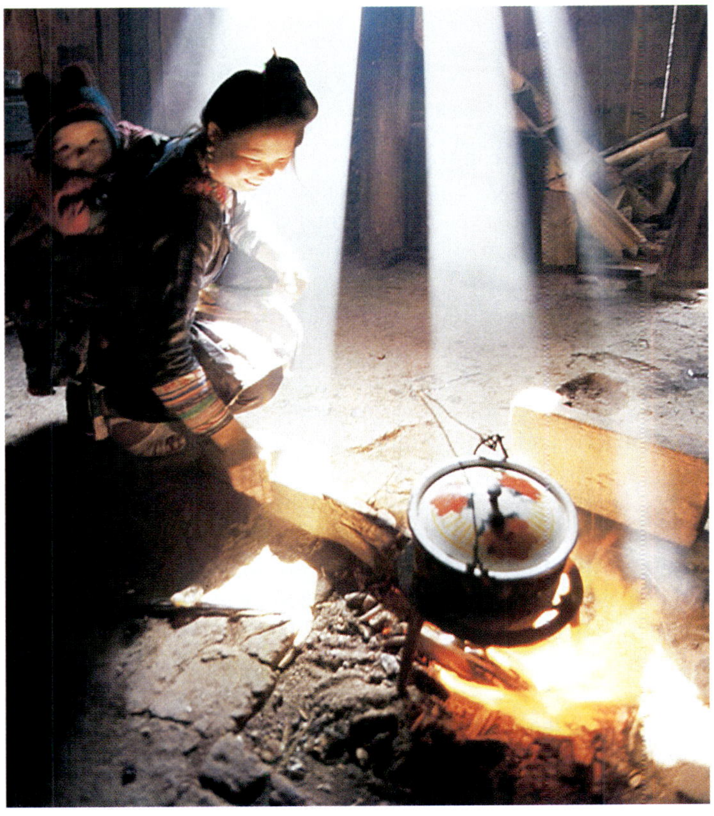

FIGURE 9.22 *Some 2.5 billion people, mainly women and children, spend hours each day in poorly ventilated kitchens and living spaces where carbon monoxide, particulates, and cancer-causing hydrocarbons often reach dangerous levels.*

Long-Range Transport

Dust and fine aerosols can be carried great distances by the wind. Pollution from the industrial belt between the Great Lakes and the Ohio River Valley regularly contaminates the Canadian Maritime Provinces and sometimes can be traced as far as Ireland (fig. 9.23). Similarly, dust storms from China's Gobi and Takla Makan Deserts routinely close schools, factories, and airports in Japan and Korea, and often reach western North America. In one particularly severe dust storm in 1998, chemical analysis showed that 75 percent of the particulate pollution in Seattle, Washington, air came from China.

Increasingly sensitive monitoring equipment has begun to reveal industrial contaminants in places usually considered among the cleanest in the world. Samoa, Greenland, and even Antarctica and the North Pole all have heavy metals, pesticides, and radioactive elements in their air. Since the 1950s, pilots flying in the high Arctic have reported dense layers of reddish-brown haze clouding the arctic atmosphere. Aerosols of sulfates, soot, dust, and toxic heavy metals, such as vanadium, manganese, and lead, travel to the pole from the industrialized parts of Europe and Russia.

In a process called "grasshopper" transport, or atmosphere distillation, volatile compounds evaporate from warm areas, travel through the atmosphere, then condense and precipitate in cooler regions. Over several years, contaminants accumulate in the coldest places, generally at high latitudes, where they bioaccumulate in food chains. Whales, polar bears, sharks, and other top carnivores in polar regions have been shown to have dangerously high levels of pesticides, metals, and other hazardous air pollutants in their bodies. The Inuit people of Broughton Island, well above the Arctic Circle, have higher levels of polychlorinated biphenyls (PCBs) in their blood than any other known population, except victims of industrial accidents. Far from any source of this industrial by-product, these people accumulate PCBs from the flesh of fish, caribou, and other animals they eat.

Stratospheric Ozone Depletion

Long-range pollution transport and the chemical reactions of atmospheric gases and pollution produce the phenomenon known as the ozone hole (fig. 9.24). The ozone "hole," really a thinning of ozone concentrations in the stratosphere was discovered in 1985 but has probably been developing since at least the 1960s. Chlorine-based aerosols, especially chlorofluorocarbons (CFCs) and other halon gases, are the principal agents of ozone depletion. Nontoxic, nonflammable, chemically inert, and cheaply produced, CFCs were extremely useful as industrial gases and in refrigerators, air conditioners, styrofoam inflation, and aerosol spray cans for many years. From the 1930s until the 1980s, CFCs were used all over the world and widely dispersed through the atmosphere.

Although ozone is a pollutant in the ambient air, ozone in the stratosphere is important because it absorbs much of the ultraviolet (UV) radiation entering the atmosphere. UV radiation harms plant and animal tissues, including the eyes and the skin. A 1 percent loss of ozone could result in about a million extra human

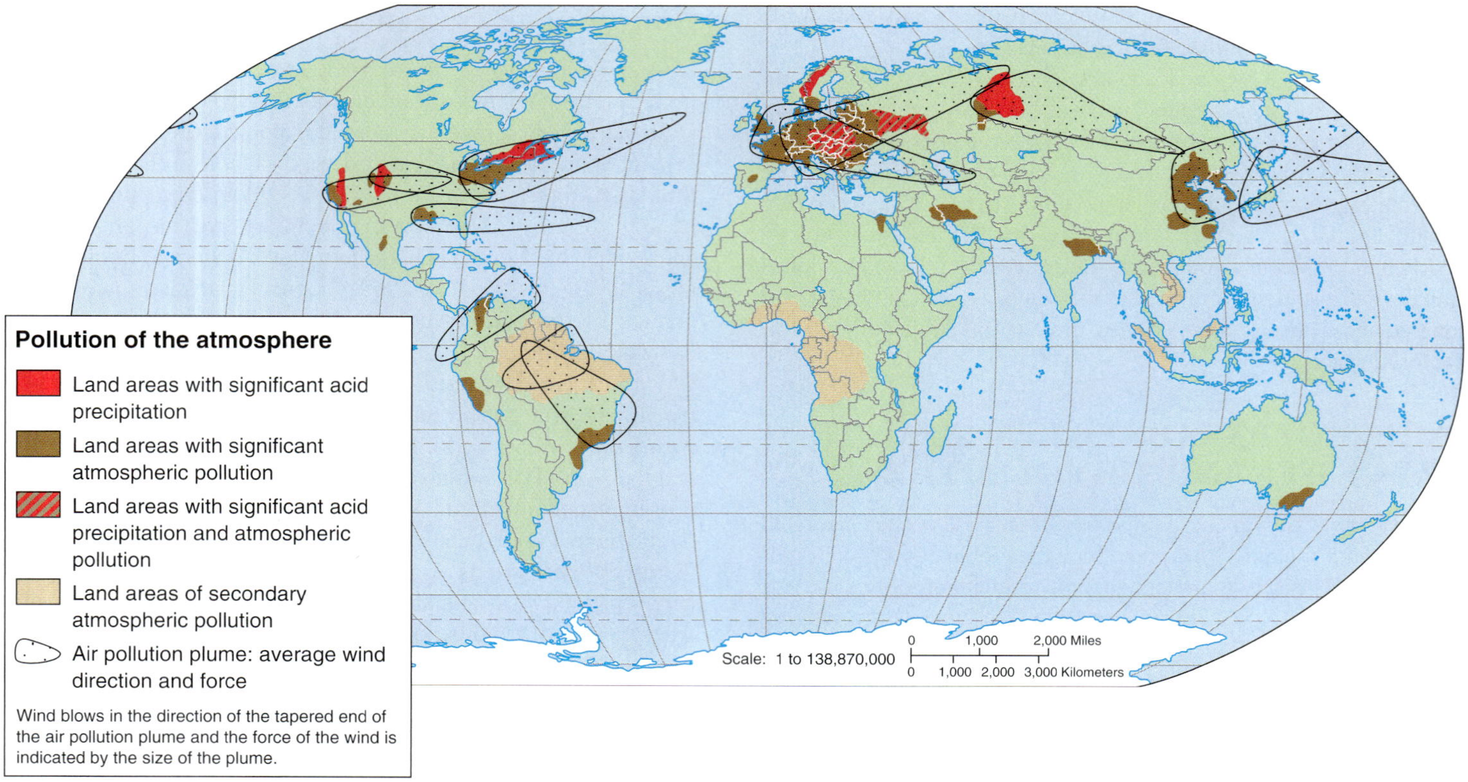

FIGURE 9.23 *Long-range transport carries air pollution from source regions thousands of kilometers away into formerly pristine areas. Secondary air pollutants can be formed by photochemical reactions far from primary emissions sources.*
Source: J. Allen, *World Geography,* 2003.

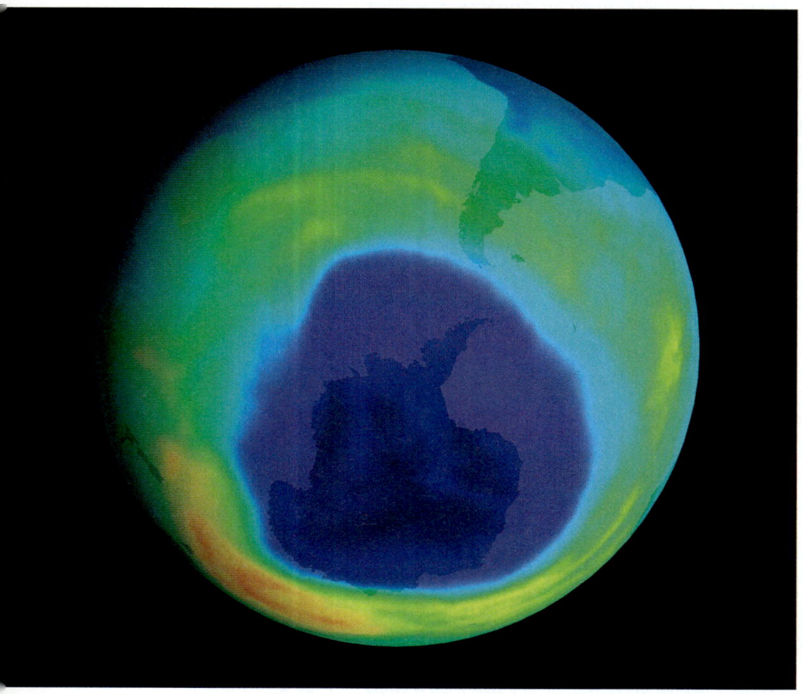

FIGURE 9.24 *In 2003 stratospheric ozone was depleted over an area* (dark, irregular circle) *that covered 28.5 million square kilometers, or more than the entire Antarctic continent. Although CFC production is declining, this was the second highest area ever recorded.*

skin cancers per year worldwide if no protective measures are taken. Excessive UV exposure could reduce agricultural production and disrupt ecosystems. Scientists worry, for example, that high UV levels in Antarctica could reduce populations of plankton, the tiny floating organisms that form the base of a food chain that includes fish, seals, penguins, and whales in Antarctic seas.

Antarctica's exceptionally cold winter temperatures (–85° to –90°C) help break down ozone. During the long, dark, winter months, strong winds known as the circumpolar vortex isolate Antarctic air and allow stratospheric temperatures to drop low enough to create ice crystals at high altitudes—something that rarely happens elsewhere in the world. Ozone and chlorine-containing molecules are absorbed on the surfaces of these ice particles. When the sun returns in the spring, it provides energy to liberate chlorine ions, which readily bond with ozone, breaking it down to molecular oxygen (table 9.6). It is only during the Antarctic spring (September through December) that conditions are ideal for rapid ozone destruction. During that season, temperatures are still cold enough for high-altitude ice crystals, but the sun gradually becomes strong enough to drive photochemical reactions.

As the Antarctic summer arrives, temperatures moderate somewhat, the circumpolar vortex breaks down, and air from warmer latitudes mixes with Antarctic air, replenishing ozone concentrations in the ozone hole. Slight decreases worldwide result from this mixing, however. Ozone re-forms naturally, but not nearly as fast as it is destroyed. Since the chlorine atoms are not

TABLE 9.6 Stratospheric Ozone Destruction by Chlorine Atoms and UV Radiation

STEP	PRODUCTS
1. $CFCl_3$ (chlorofluorocarbon) + UV energy	$CFCl_2 + Cl$
2. $Cl + O_3$	$ClO + O_2$
3. O_2 + UV energy	2O
4. ClO + 2O	$O_2 + Cl$
5. Return to step 2	

themselves consumed in reactions with ozone, they continue to destroy ozone for years, until they finally precipitate or are washed out of the air. Almost every year since it was discovered, the Antarctic ozone hole has grown. In 2000 the region of ozone depletion covered 29.8 million km^2 (about the size of North America). In 2003 the hole was nearly as large.

Ominously, this phenomenon is now spreading to other parts of the world as well. About 10 percent of all stratospheric ozone worldwide has been destroyed in recent years, and levels over the Arctic have averaged 40 percent below normal. Ozone depletion has been observed over the North Pole as well, although it is not as concentrated as that in the south.

Signs of Progress

The discovery of stratospheric ozone losses brought about a remarkably quick international response. In 1987 an international meeting in Montreal, Canada, produced the Montreal Protocol, the first of several major international agreements on phasing out most use of CFCs by 2000. As evidence accumulated, showing that losses were larger and more widespread than previously thought, the deadline for the elimination of all CFCs (halons, carbon tetrachloride, and methyl chloroform) was moved up to 1996, and a $500 million fund was established to assist poorer countries in switching to non-CFC technologies. Fortunately, alternatives to CFCs for most uses already exist. The first substitutes are hydrochlorofluorocarbons (HCFCs), which release much less chlorine per molecule. Eventually, scientists hope to develop halogen-free molecules that work just as well and are no more expensive than CFCs.

There is some evidence that the CFC ban is already having an effect. CFC production in most industrialized countries has fallen sharply since 1989 (fig. 9.25), and CFCs are now being removed from the atmosphere more rapidly than they are being added. In 50 years or so, stratospheric ozone levels are expected to be back to normal. Unfortunately, there may be a downside to stopping ozone destruction. Ozone is a potent greenhouse gas. Some models suggest that lower ozone levels have been offsetting the effects of increased CO_2. When ozone is restored, global warming may be accelerated. As so often is the case, when we disturb one environmental factor, we affect others as well.

Urban Climates

Temperature inversions can concentrate dangerous levels of pollutants within cities. Normally, air temperatures decrease with elevation above the earth's surface. An inversion reverses these conditions, with cool, dense air lying below a warmer, lighter layer. In these very stable conditions, convection currents cannot develop, and there is no mechanism for dispersing pollutants. The most stable inversion conditions are usually created by rapid nighttime cooling in a valley or basin where air movement is restricted. Los Angeles is a classic example of an area with conditions that

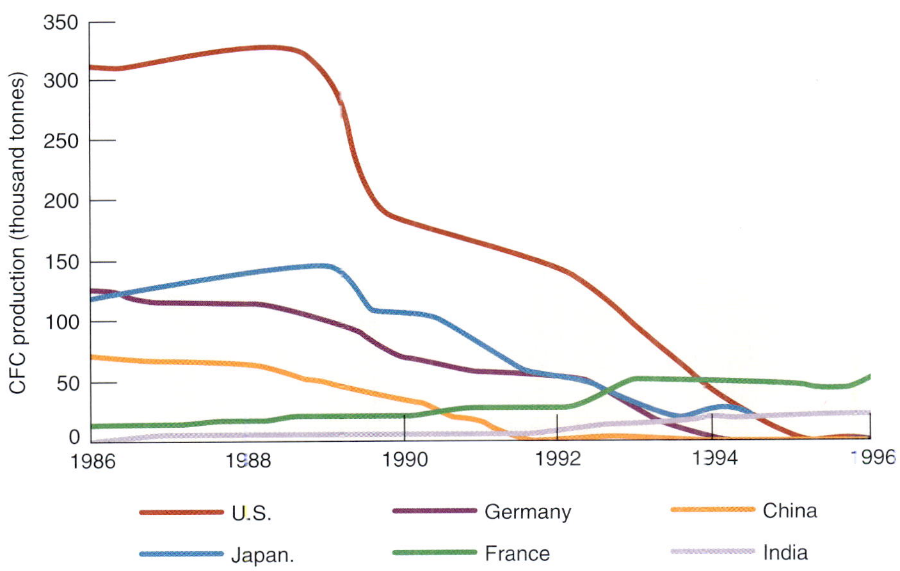

FIGURE 9.25 *Production of chlorofluorocarbons has fallen sharply in many countries since the Montreal Protocol was passed in 1987.*
Source: Data from United Nations Environment Programme.

create temperature inversions and photochemical smog. Mountains surround the city on three sides, reducing wind movement; the climate is sunny; and heavy traffic creates high pollution levels. Skies are generally clear at night, allowing rapid radiant heat loss, and the ground cools quickly. Surface air layers are cooled by conduction, while upper layers remain relatively warm. Density differences retard vertical mixing. During the night, cool, humid, onshore breezes slide in under the contaminated air, squeezing it up against the cap of warmer air above and concentrating the pollutants accumulated during the day.

Morning sunlight initiates photochemical oxidation in the concentrated aerosols and gaseous chemicals in the inversion layer. A toxic brew of hazardous chemicals, especially ozone and nitrogen dioxide, quickly develops. On summer days, ozone concentrations in the Los Angeles basin can reach 0.34 ppm or more by late afternoon, and the pollution index can be 300, the stage considered a health hazard.

Heat islands and *dust domes* occur in cities even without inversion conditions. With their low albedo, concrete and brick surfaces in cities absorb large amounts of solar energy. A lack of vegetation or water results in very slight evaporation (latent heat production); instead, available solar energy is turned into heat. As a result, temperatures in cities are frequently 3° to 5°C (5° to 9°F) warmer than in the surrounding countryside, a condition known as an urban heat island. Tall buildings create convective updrafts that sweep pollutants into the air. Stable air masses created by this heat island over the city concentrate pollutants in a dust dome.

EFFECTS OF AIR POLLUTION

Air pollution is equally serious for ecosystem health and for human health. In this section we will review the most important effects of air pollution.

Human Health

Consequences of breathing dirty air include increased probability of heart attacks, respiratory diseases, and lung cancer. This can mean as much as a five- to ten-year decrease in life expectancy if you live in the worst parts of Los Angeles or Baltimore, for example. Of course, the intensity and duration of your exposure, as well as your age and general health, are extremely important: you are much more likely to be at risk if you are very young, very old, or already suffering from some respiratory or cardiovascular disease. Bronchitis and emphysema are common chronic conditions resulting from air pollution. The U.S. Office of Technology Assessment estimates that 250,000 people suffer from pollution-related bronchitis and emphysema in the United States, and some 50,000 excess deaths each year are attributable to complications of these diseases, which are probably second only to heart attack as a cause of death.

Conditions are often much worse in developing countries. The United Nations estimates that at least 1.3 billion people around the world live in areas where the air is dangerously polluted. In the "black triangle" region of Poland, Hungary, the Czech Republic, and Slovakia, for example, respiratory ailments, cardiovascular diseases, lung cancer, infant mortality, and miscarriages are as much as 50 percent higher than in cleaner parts of those countries. And in China, city dwellers are four to six times more likely than country folk to die of lung cancer. The World Health Organization estimates that 4 million people die each year from diseases exacerbated by air pollution.

How does air pollution cause these health effects? Because they are strong oxidizing agents, sulfates, SO_2, NO_x, and O_3 irritate and damage delicate tissues in the eyes and lungs. Fine, suspended particulate materials penetrate deep into the lungs, causing irritation, scarring, and even tumor growth. Heart stress results from impaired lung functions. Carbon monoxide binds to hemoglobin, reducing oxygen flow to the brain. Headaches, dizziness, and heart stress result. Lead also binds to hemoglobin, damaging critical neurons in the brain and resulting in mental and physical impairment and developmental retardation.

Plant Pathology

In the early days of industrialization, fumes from furnaces, smelters, refineries, and chemical plants often destroyed vegetation and created desolate, barren landscapes around mining and manufacturing centers. The copper-nickel smelter at Sudbury, Ontario, is a spectacular example. Starting in 1886, open-bed roasting was used to purify sulfide ores of nickel and copper. The resulting sulfur dioxide and sulfuric acid destroyed almost all

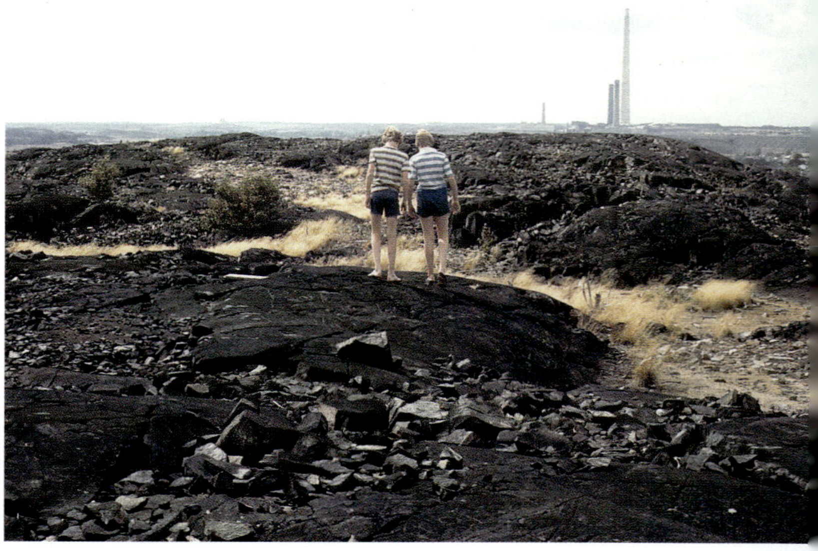

FIGURE 9.26 *Sulfur dioxide emissions and acid precipitation from the International Nickel Company copper-nickel smelter* (background) *killed all vegetation over a large area near Sudbury, Ontario. Even the pink granite bedrock was burned black. The installation of scrubbers has dramatically reduced sulfur emissions. The ecosystem farther away from the smelter is slowly beginning to recover.*

plant life within about 30 km (18.6 mi) of the smelter. Rains washed away the exposed soil, leaving a barren moonscape of blackened bedrock (fig. 9.26). Recently, emission controls have been introduced, and the environment is beginning to recover.

There are two probable ways that air pollutants damage plants. They can damage sensitive cell membranes, much as irritants do in human lungs. Toxic levels of oxidants produce discoloration (destruction of chlorophyll) and then necrotic (dead) spots. Often, however, the symptoms are vague and difficult to separate from diseases or insect damage. Pollutants can also act as hormones, disrupting plant metabolism, growth, and development. Ethylene, a volatile organic compound released in automobile exhaust and from petroleum refineries and chemical plants, often injures plants around roads and factories.

Certain combinations of environmental factors have synergistic effects in which the injury caused by exposure to two factors together is more than the sum of exposure to each factor individually. For instance, white pine seedlings exposed to subthreshold concentrations of ozone and sulfur dioxide individually do not suffer any visible injury. If the same concentrations of pollutants are given together, however, visible damage occurs.

Pollutant levels too low to produce visible symptoms of damage may still have important effects. Field studies show that yields in some crops, such as soybeans, may be reduced as much as 50 percent by currently existing levels of oxidants in ambient air. Some plant pathologists suggest that ozone and photochemical oxidants are responsible for as much as 90 percent of agricultural, ornamental, and forest losses from air pollution. The total costs of this damage may be as much as $10 billion per year in North America alone.

Visibility Reduction

We have only recently realized that pollution affects rural areas as well as cities. Even supposedly pristine places such as our national parks are suffering from air pollution. Grand Canyon National Park, where maximum visibility used to be 300 km (185 mi), is now so smoggy on some winter days that visitors can't see the opposite rim only 20 km (12.5 mi) across the canyon. Mining operations, smelters, and power plants (some of which were moved to the desert to improve air quality in cities such as Los Angeles) are the main culprits. Huge regions are affected by pollution. A gigantic "haze blob" as much as 3,000 km (about 2,000 mi) across covers much of the eastern United States in the summer, cutting visibility as much as 80 percent. People become accustomed to these conditions and don't realize that the air once was clear. Studies indicate, however, that, if all human-made sources of air pollution were shut down, the air would clear up in a few days, and there would be about 150-km (90-mi) visibility nearly everywhere, rather than the 15 km to which we have become accustomed.

Acid Deposition

Acid precipitation, the deposition of wet, acidic solutions or dry, acidic particles from the air, became widely recognized as a pollution problem only in the last 20 years. But the concept has been recognized since the 1850s. We describe acidity in terms of pH, with substances below pH 7 being acidic (see chapter 2). Normal, unpolluted rain generally has a pH of about 5.6 due to carbonic acid created when rainwater reacts with CO_2 in the air. Downwind of industrial areas, rainfall acidity can reach levels below pH 4.3, more than ten times as acidic as normal rain. Acid fog, snow, mist, and dew can deposit damaging acids on plants, in water systems, and on buildings. Furthermore, fallout of dry sulfate and nitrate particles can account for as much as half of the acidic deposition in some areas.

A vigorous program of pollution control has been undertaken by Canada, the United States, and several European countries since the widespread recognition of acid rain. SO_2 and NO_x emissions from power plants have decreased dramatically over the past three decades over much of Europe and eastern North America as a result of pollution-control measures. However, rain falling in these areas remains acidic (fig. 9.27). Apparently, alkaline dust that would once have neutralized acids in air has been depleted by years of acid rain and is now no longer effective.

Aquatic Effects of Acid Deposition

Aquatic ecosystems in Scandinavia were among the first discovered to be damaged by acid precipitation. Prevailing winds from Germany, Poland, and other parts of Europe deliver acids generated by industrial and automobile emissions—principally H_2SO_4 and HNO_3. The thin, acidic soils and nutrient-poor lakes and streams in the mountains of southern Norway and Sweden have been severely affected by this acid deposition. Most noticeable is the reduction of trout, salmon, and other game fish, whose eggs and fry die below pH 5. Aquatic plants, insects, and invertebrates also suffer. Some 18,000 lakes in Sweden are now so acidic that they will no longer support game fish or other sensitive aquatic organisms. Large parts of Europe and eastern North America are similarly affected by acid precipitation.

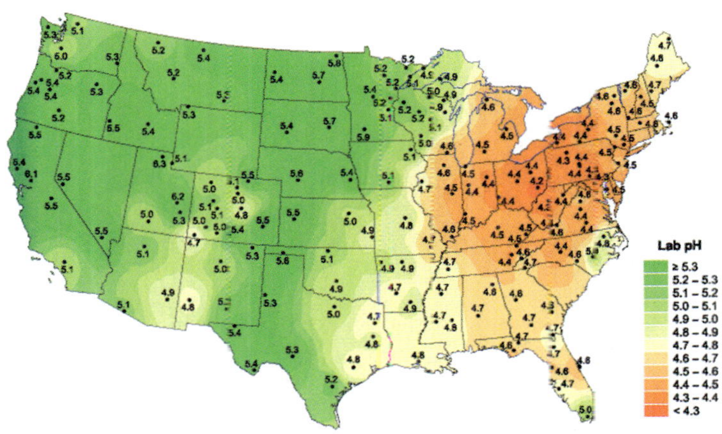

FIGURE 9.27 *Acid precipitation over the United States, 2000.*
Source: Data from National Acid Deposition Program, 2001.

Forest Damage

Since the early 1980s observers have documented forest declines apparently related to acid damage in both Europe and North America. A detailed 1980 ecosystem inventory on Camel's Hump Mountain in Vermont found that seedling production, tree density, and viability of spruce-fir forests at high elevations had declined about 50 percent in 15 years. On Mount Mitchell in North Carolina, nearly all the trees above 2,000 m (6,000 ft) are losing needles, and about half of them are dead (fig. 9.28). Damage has been reported throughout Europe, from the Netherlands to Switzerland, as well as in China and the states of the former Soviet Union. In 1985 West German foresters estimated that about half the total forest area in West Germany (more than 4 million ha) was declining. The loss to the forest industry is estimated to be about 1 billion DM (deutsche marks) per year.

High-elevation forests are most severely affected. Mountain tops often have thin, acidic soils under normal conditions, with little ability to buffer, or neutralize, acid precipitation. Acidic fog and mist frequently rest on mountaintops, lengthening plants' exposure to acidity. Mountaintops also catch more rain and snow than lowlands, so they are more exposed to acidic precipitation.

The most visible mechanism of forest decline is direct damage to plant tissues and seedlings. Nutrient availability in forest soils is also depleted, however. Acids can also dissolve and mobilize toxic metals, such as aluminum, and weakened trees become susceptible to diseases and insect pests.

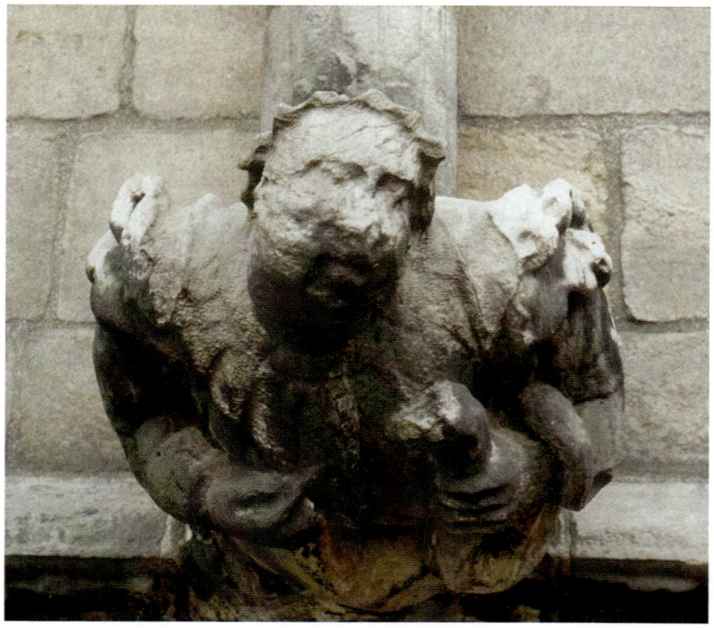

FIGURE 9.29 *Atmospheric acids, especially sulfuric and nitric acids, have almost completely eaten away the face of this medieval statue. Each year, the total losses from air pollution damage to buildings and materials amount to billions of dollars.*

Buildings and Monuments

In cities throughout the world, air pollution is destroying some of the oldest and most glorious buildings and works of art. Smoke and soot coat buildings, paintings, and textiles. Acids dissolve limestone and marble, destroying features and structures of historic buildings (fig. 9.29). The Parthenon in Athens, the Taj Mahal in Agra, the Coliseum in Rome, medieval cathedrals in Europe, and the Washington Monument in Washington, D.C., are slowly dissolving and flaking away because of acidic fumes in the air. On a more mundane level, air pollution and acid precipitation corrode steel in reinforced concrete, weakening buildings, roads, and bridges. Limestone, marble, and some kinds of sandstone flake and crumble. The Council on Environmental Quality estimates that U.S. economic losses from architectural damage caused by air pollution amount to about $4.8 billion in direct costs and $5.2 billion in property-value losses each year.

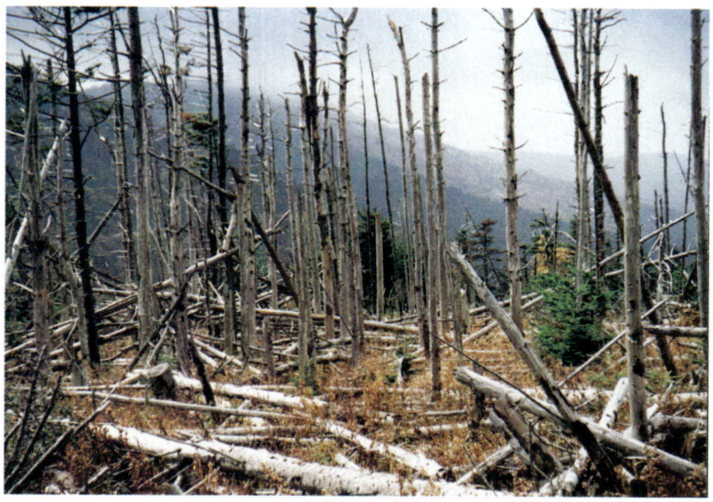

FIGURE 9.28 *A Fraser fir forest on Mount Mitchell, North Carolina, killed by acid rain, insect pests, and other stressors.*

AIR POLLUTION CONTROL

"Dilution is the solution to pollution" was one of the early approaches to air pollution control. Tall smokestacks were built to send emissions far from the source, where they became unidentifiable and largely untraceable. But dispersed and diluted pollutants are now the source of some of our most serious pollution problems. We are finding that there is no "away" to which we can throw our waste products.

Reducing Production

The most effective strategy for controlling pollution is to minimize polluting activities. Since most air pollution in the developed world is associated with transportation and energy production, the most effective strategy would be conservation: reducing electricity consumption, insulating homes and offices, and developing better public transportation could all greatly reduce air pollution in the United States, Canada, and Europe. Alternative energy sources, such as wind and solar power, produce energy with little or no pollution, and these and other technologies are becoming economically competitive (see chapter 12). In addition to conservation, pollution can be controlled by technological innovation.

Particulate removal involves filtering air emissions. Filters trap particulates in a mesh of cotton cloth, spun glass fibers, or asbestos-cellulose. Industrial air filters are generally giant bags 10 to 15 m long and 2 to 3 m wide. Effluent gas is blown through the bag, much like the bag on a vacuum cleaner. Every few days or weeks, the bags are opened to remove the dust cake. Electrostatic precipitators are the most common particulate controls in power plants. Ash particles pick up an electrostatic surface charge as they pass between large electrodes in the effluent stream (fig. 9.30). Charged particles then collect on an oppositely charged collecting plate. These precipitators consume a large amount of electricity, but maintenance is relatively simple, and collection efficiency can be as high as 99 percent. The ash collected by both of these techniques is a solid waste (often hazardous due to the heavy metals and other trace components of coal or other ash source) and must be buried in landfills or other solid waste disposal sites.

Sulfur removal is important because sulfur oxides are among the most damaging of all air pollutants in terms of human health and ecosystem viability. Switching from soft coal with a high sulfur content to low-sulfur coal is the surest way to reduce sulfur emissions. High-sulfur coal is frequently politically or economically expedient, however. In the United States, Appalachia, a region of chronic economic depression, produces mostly high-sulfur coal. In China, much domestic coal is rich in sulfur. Switching to cleaner oil or gas would eliminate metal effluents as well as sulfur. Cleaning fuels is an alternative to switching. Coal can be crushed, washed, and gasified to remove sulfur and metals before combustion. This improves heat content and firing properties but may replace air pollution with solid waste and water pollution problems; furthermore, these steps are expensive.

Sulfur can also be removed to yield a usable product instead of simply a waste disposal problem. Elemental sulfur, sulfuric acid, and ammonium sulfate can all be produced using catalytic converters to oxidize or reduce sulfur. Markets have to be reasonably close and fly ash contamination must be reduced as much as possible for this procedure to be economically feasible.

Nitrogen oxides (NO_x) can be reduced in both internal combustion engines and industrial boilers by as much as 50 percent by carefully controlling the flow of air and fuel. Staged burners, for example, control burning temperatures and oxygen flow to prevent formation of NO_x. The catalytic converter on your car uses platinum-palladium and rhodium catalysts to remove up to 90 percent of NO_x, hydrocarbons, and carbon monoxide at the same time.

Hydrocarbon controls mainly involve complete combustion or the control of evaporation. Hydrocarbons and volatile organic compounds are produced by incomplete combustion of fuels or by solvent evaporation from chemical factories, paints, dry cleaning, plastic manufacturing, printing, and other industrial processes. Closed systems that prevent escape of fugitive gases can reduce many of these emissions. In automobiles, for instance, positive crankcase ventilation (PCV) systems collect oil that escapes from around the pistons and unburned fuel and channels them back to the engine for combustion. Controls on fugitive losses from industrial valves, pipes, and storage tanks can have a significant impact on air quality. Afterburners are often the best method for destroying volatile organic chemicals in industrial exhaust stacks.

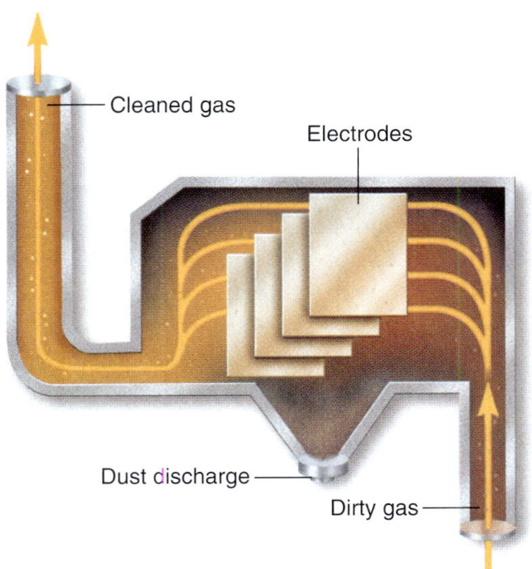

FIGURE 9.30 *An electrostatic precipitator traps particulate material on electrically charged plates as effluent makes its way to the smokestack.*

CLEAN AIR LEGISLATION

Throughout history, countless ordinances have prohibited the emission of objectionable smoke, odors, and noise. Air pollution traditionally has been treated as a local problem, however. The Clean Air Act of 1963 was the first national legislation in the United States aimed at air pollution control. The act provided federal grants to states to combat pollution but was careful to preserve states' rights to set and enforce air quality regulations. It soon became obvious that some pollution problems cannot be solved on a local basis.

In 1970 an extensive set of amendments essentially rewrote the Clean Air Act. These amendments identified the criteria pollutants discussed earlier in this chapter and established primary and secondary standards for ambient air quality. Primary standards (table 9.7) are intended to protect human health, while secondary standards are set to protect materials, crops, climate, visibility, and personal comfort.

Since 1970 the Clean Air Act has been modified, updated, and amended. The most significant amendments were in the 1990 update. Amendments have involved acrimonious debate, with bills sometimes languishing in Congress from one session to the next because of disputes over burdens of responsibility and cost and definitions of risk. Some of the principal problems that have been addressed in amendments include the following:

- Acid rain: reductions in sulfur dioxide and nitrogen oxides
- Urban smog: lower vehicle emissions, alternative fuels in the smoggiest cities
- Toxic air pollutants: controls on 188 airborne toxins from about 250 types of sources

TABLE 9.7 National Ambient Air Quality Standards (NAAQS)

POLLUTANT	PRIMARY (HEALTH-BASED) AVERAGING TIME	STANDARD CONCENTRATION
TSP[1]	Annual geometric mean[2]	50 $\mu g/m^3$
	24 hours	150 $\mu g/m^3$
SO_2	Annual arithmetic mean[3]	80 $\mu g/m^3$ (0.03 ppm)
	24 hours	120 $\mu g/m^3$ (0.14 ppm)
CO	8 hours	10 mg/m^3 (9 ppm)
	1 hour	40 mg/m^3 (35 ppm)
NO_2	Annual arithmetic mean	80 $\mu g/m^3$ (0.05 ppm)
O_3	Daily max 8 hours avg.	157 $\mu g/m^3$ (0.08 ppm)
Lead	Maximum quarterly avg.	1.5 $\mu g/m^3$

[1]Total suspended particulate material.

[2]The geometric mean is obtained by taking the *n*th root of the product of *n* numbers. This tends to reduce the impact of a few very large numbers in a set.

[3]An arithmetic mean is the average determined by dividing the sum of a group of data points by the number of points.

- Ozone protection: phasing out CFCs, carbon tetrachloride, and other compounds (smuggling from developing countries such as Mexico, where CFCs are still cheap and legal, has become a serious problem)
- Marketing pollution rights: allowing corporations to avoid pollution reduction by buying, selling, and "banking" pollution rights from other factories
- Fugitive emissions of volatile organic compounds (VOCs): detailed standards for manufacture, use, and storage methods
- Ambient ozone, soot, and dust: reduced-sulfur gasoline, cleaner smokestacks and cars
- NO_x emissions: improved standards for sport-utility vehicles, personal watercraft, and other polluting vehicles

A 2002 report concluded that, simply by enforcing existing clean air legislation, the United States could save at least another 6,000 lives per year and prevent 140,000 asthma attacks.

Clear Skies

In 2002 President Bush announced his "Clear Skies" plan, calling it the "most aggressive initiative in American history to cut power plant emissions." Supporters applauded his declared intent to eliminate "outdated and obstructive features" of the Clean Air Act and to establish a market-based approach for controlling three key air pollutants (sulfur dioxide, nitrogen oxide, and mercury). Opponents, however, criticized the plan as "the biggest rollback of the Clean Air Act in history."

The most controversial aspect of Bush's plan is elimination of the "new source review," which was established in 1977. This provision was originally adopted because industry argued that it would be intolerably expensive to install new pollution-control equipment on old power plants and factories that were about to close down, anyway. Congress agreed to "grandfather" or exempt existing equipment from new pollution limits with the stipulation that, when they were upgraded or replaced, more stringent rules would apply. The result was that owners kept old facilities operating precisely because they were exempted from pollution control. In fact, corporations poured millions into aging power plants and factories, expanding their capacity rather than building new ones. A quarter of a century later, most of those grandfathered plants are still going strong and continue to be among the biggest contributors to smog and acid rain.

In 1999 the Clinton administration sued 51 power plants and dozens of other industrial facilities for illegally making major upgrades without installing the necessary pollution controls. In response, utilities in Ohio, Virginia, and Florida agreed to make billion-dollar investments to reduce pollution. Two years later, President Bush said that determining which facilities are new, and which are not, represents a cumbersome and unreasonable imposition on industries (many of which contributed generously to his election campaign). The EPA subsequently announced it would abandon new source reviews, depending instead on voluntary emissions controls and a trading program for air pollution allowances. Several of the utilities that had already agreed to install new pollution controls immediately put their plans on hold.

Environmental groups generally agree that cap-and-trade (which sets maximum amounts for pollutants and then lets facilities facing costly cleanup bills pay others with lower costs to reduce emissions on their behalf) has worked fairly well for sulfur dioxide. When trading began in 1990, economists estimated that eliminating 10 million tons of sulfur dioxide would cost \$15 billion per year. Left to find the most economical ways to reduce emissions, however, utilities have been able to reach clean air goals for one-tenth that price. A serious shortcoming of this approach is that, while trading has resulted in overall pollution reduction, some local "hot spots" remain where owners have found it cheaper to pay someone else to reduce pollution than to do it themselves. Knowing that the average person is enjoying cleaner air isn't much comfort if you're living in one of the persistently dirty areas.

Critics also complained that, while the Bush administration moved quickly to abandon the new source review, legislation for replacing it with market-based controls was slow in coming. Nine northeastern states, which find themselves on the receiving end of acid rain and air pollution from grandfathered power plants and factories in the Midwest, sued the EPA for abandoning one of the few effective programs for combating dirty air. In 2003 the EPA agreed to reconsider its revisions of the new source review. Many environmentalists would also like any market-based plan to take a "four pollutant" approach, adding carbon dioxide to sulfur dioxide, nitrogen oxide, and mercury regulations. President Bush, who continues to maintain that global warming remains an uncertain theory, resists calls for expensive greenhouse gas restrictions.

CURRENT CONDITIONS AND FUTURE PROSPECTS

Although the United states has not yet achieved the Clean Air Act goals in many parts of the country, air quality has improved dramatically in the past decade in terms of the major large-volume pollutants. For 23 of the largest U.S. cities, the number of days each year in which air quality reached the hazardous level is down 93 percent from a decade ago. Of 97 metropolitan areas that failed to meet clean air standards in the 1980s, 41 were in compliance in 1991–1992. For many cities, this was the first time they met air quality goals in 20 years. Still, the EPA estimates that some 86 million Americans breathe unhealthy air at least part of the time.

The EPA estimates that, between 1970 and 1994, lead fell 98 percent, SO_2 declined 35 percent, and CO shrank 32 percent (fig. 9.31). Filters, scrubbers, and precipitators on power plants and other large stationary sources are responsible for most of the particulate and SO_2 reductions. Catalytic converters on automobiles are responsible for most of the CO and O_3 reductions.

The only conventional criteria pollutants that have not dropped significantly are particulates and NO_x. Because automobiles are the main source of NO_x, cities such as Nashville, Tennessee, and Atlanta, Georgia, where pollution comes largely from traffic, still have serious air-quality problems. Particulate matter (mostly dust and soot) is produced by agriculture, fuel combustion, metal smelting, concrete manufacturing, and other activities. Industrial cities, such as Baltimore, Maryland, and Baton Rouge, Louisiana, also have continuing problems. In 1999, for the first time in many years, Houston passed Los Angeles as having the worst air quality in the country. Eighty-five other urban areas are still considered nonattainment regions. In spite of these local failures, however, 80 percent of the United States now meets the National Ambient Air Quality Standards. This improvement in air quality is perhaps the greatest environmental success story in our history.

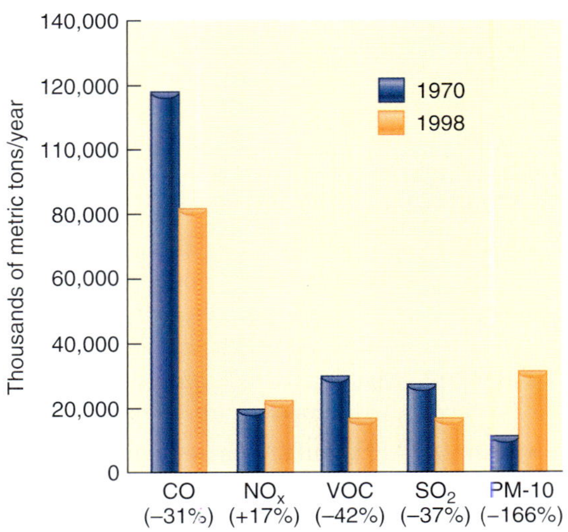

FIGURE 9.31 *Air pollution trends in the United States, 1970 to 1998. Although population and economic activity increased during this period, emissions of all criteria air pollutants, except for nitrogen oxides and particulate matter, decreased significantly.*
Source: Data from U.S. Environmental Protection Agency, 2002.

Air Pollution in Developing Countries

The outlook is not as encouraging in other parts of the world. The major metropolitan areas of many developing countries are growing at explosive rates to incredible sizes (see chapter 14), and environmental quality is abysmal in many of them. Mexico City remains notorious for bad air. Pollution levels exceed WHO health standards 350 days per year, and more than half of all city children have lead levels in their blood high enough to lower intelligence and retard development. Mexico City's 131,000 industries and 2.5 million vehicles spew out more than 5,500 tons of air pollutants daily. Santiago, Chile, averages 299 days per year on which suspended particulates exceed WHO standards of 90 mg/m^3.

While there are few statistics on China's pollution situation, it is known that many of China's 400,000 factories have no air pollution controls. Experts estimate that home coal burners and factories emit 10 million tons of soot and 15 million tons of sulfur dioxide annually and that emissions have increased rapidly over the past 20 years. Sheyang, an industrial city in northern China, is thought to have the world's worst continuing particulate problem, with peak winter concentrations over 700 mg/m^3 (nine times U.S. maximum standards). Airborne particulates in Sheyang exceed WHO standards on 347 days per year. Beijing, Xi'an, and Guangzhou are nearly as bad (see fig. 9.19). The high incidence of cancer in Shanghai is thought to be linked to air pollution.

As political walls came down across Eastern Europe and the Soviet Union at the end of the 1980s, horrifying environmental conditions in these centrally planned economies were revealed. Inept industrial managers, a rigid bureaucracy, and lack of democracy have created ecological disasters. Where governments own, operate, and regulate industry, there are few checks and balances or incentives to clean up pollution. Much of the Eastern bloc depends heavily on soft, brown coal for its energy, and pollution controls are absent or highly inadequate.

Southern Poland, the northern Czech Republic, and Slovakia are covered most of the time by a cloud of smog from factories and power plants. Acid rain is eating away historic buildings and damaging already inadequate infrastructures. Home gardening has been banned in Katowice, Poland, because vegetables raised there have unsafe levels of lead and cadmium. For miles around the infamous Romanian "black town" of Copsa Mica, the countryside is so stained by soot that it looks as if someone poured black ink over everything. Birth defects afflict ten percent of infants in northern Bohemia. Workers in factories there get extra hazard pay—burial money, they call it. Life expectancy in these industrial towns is as much as ten years less than the national average.

Signs of Hope

Not all is pessimistic, however. There have been some spectacular successes in air pollution control. Sweden and West Germany (countries affected by forest losses due to acid precipitation) cut their sulfur emissions by two-thirds between 1970 and 1985. Austria and Switzerland have gone even further, regulating even motorcycle emissions. The Global Environmental Monitoring System (GEMS) reports declines in particulate levels in 26 of 37 cities worldwide. Sulfur dioxide and sulfate particles, which cause acid rain and respiratory disease, have declined in 20 of these cities.

Twenty years ago, Cubatao, Brazil, was described as the "Valley of Death," one of the most dangerously polluted places in the world. Steel mills, oil refineries, and fertilizer and chemical factories churned out thousands of tons of air pollutants every year (fig. 9.32). Trees died on the surrounding hills. Birth defects and respiratory diseases were alarmingly high. Since then, however, the citizens of Cubatao have made remarkable progress in cleaning up their environment. The end of military rule and the restoration of democracy allowed residents to publicize their complaints. The environment became an important political issue. The state of São Paulo invested about $100 million and the private sector spent twice as much to clean up most pollution sources in the valley. Particulate pollution was reduced 75 percent, ammonia emissions were reduced 97 percent, hydrocarbons that cause ozone and smog were cut 86 percent, and sulfur dioxide production fell 84 percent. Fish are returning to the rivers, and forests are regrowing on the mountains. Progress is possible! We hope that similar success stories will be obtainable elsewhere.

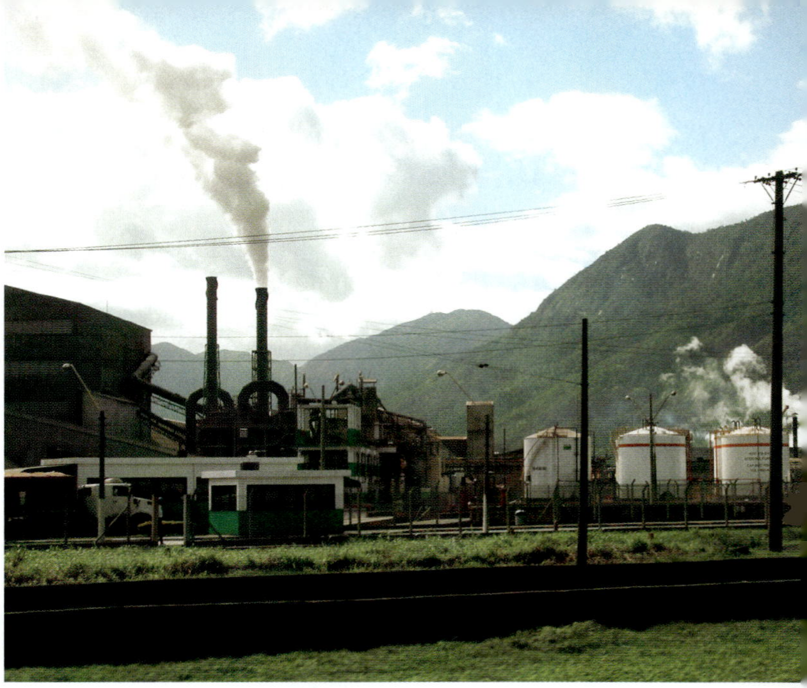

FIGURE 9.32 *Cubatao, Brazil was once considered one of the most polluted cities in the world. Better environmental regulations and enforcement along with massive investments in pollution control equipment have improved air quality significantly.*

SUMMARY

- The atmospheric gases in our air are relatively transparent to the visible light that warms the earth's surface and supports photosynthesis. The same gases trap outgoing energy, keeping the earth warm enough for life as we know it. Excessive greenhouse gases, though, appear to be causing global warming, which will have complex effects.
- When air is warmed by the earth's surface, it expands and rises, creating convection currents. These vertical updrafts carry water vapor aloft and initiate circulation patterns that redistribute energy and water from areas of surplus to areas of deficit. Pressure gradients created by this circulation drive great air masses around the globe and generate winds that determine both immediate weather and long-term climate.
- The earth's climate changes over time. The El Niño/Southern Oscillation (ENSO) is an important example. ENSO cycles involve a complex interaction between oceans and atmosphere that has far-reaching climatic, ecological, and social effects.
- Anthropogenic global warming is another important climate change. International agreements, including the Kyoto Protocol, have sought to limit CO_2 production, but so far, economic concerns have prevented adoption in America, the world's largest CO_2 producer. Numerous changes, especially at high latitudes, suggest that global warming already has begun, but doubters claim these may all be merely natural climate anomalies.
- Air pollution interacts with climate in important ways: climate patterns concentrate or distribute pollution around the globe, and air pollution can alter climate conditions. Among the most important of these processes are long-range transport of pollutants and photochemical reactions in trapped inversion layers over urban areas.
- The Clean Air Act regulates major types and sources of air pollution in the United States, and this law has dramatically improved ambient air quality in the past 30 years.

- Encouraging improvements have been made in ambient outdoor air quality over most of the United States in the past few decades. We have made considerable progress in designing and installing pollution-control equipment to reduce the major conventional pollutants.
- Much remains to be done, especially in developing countries and in Eastern Europe, but air pollution control is, perhaps, our greatest success in environmental protection and an encouraging example of what can be accomplished in this field.

QUESTIONS FOR REVIEW

1. What is the greenhouse effect?
2. What is the ENSO cycle?
3. What are some theories explaining major climate changes?
4. Define *primary* and *secondary air pollutants*.
5. What are the seven criteria pollutants in the original Clean Air Act? Why were they chosen?
6. What is an atmospheric inversion, and how does it trap air pollutants?
7. What is acid deposition? What causes it?
8. Which of the conventional, or criteria, pollutants has decreased most in the recent past, and which has decreased least?

THINKING SCIENTIFICALLY

1. El Niño is a natural climate process, but some scientists suspect it is changing because of global warming. What sort of evidence would you look for to decide if El Niño has gotten stronger recently?
2. If you look at the map of long-range transport (fig. 9.23), which regions produce pollutants that will affect your area?
3. Global warming appears to be warming night temperatures more than day temperatures, and it is warming winter weather more than summer. Given what you know about global warming, how can you explain this?
4. Explain the process of photochemical oxidation. How does it work? What are important examples?
5. One of the problems with the Kyoto Protocol and with the Clean Air Act is that economists and scientists define problems differently and have contrasting priorities. How would an economist and an ecologist explain disputes over the Kyoto Protocol differently?
6. Economists and scientists often have difficulty reaching common terms for defining and solving issues such as the Clean Air Act renewal. How might their conflicting definitions be reshaped to make the discussion more successful?

KEY TERMS

acid precipitation 221
aerosols 199
albedo 200
ambient air 215
carbon management 213
carbon monoxide 216
chlorofluorocarbons 216
climate 199
convection currents 199
conventional (criteria) pollutants 214
Coriolis effect 203
El Niño 206
fugitive emissions 214
greenhouse effect 201
Intergovernmental Panel on Climate Change (IPCC) 207
jet streams 204
Kyoto Protocol 212
latent heat 201
Milankovitch cycles 205
monsoons 204
nitrogen oxides 215
ozone 200
particulate material 216
photochemical oxidants 214
stratosphere 200
sulfur dioxide 215
troposphere 199
unconventional pollutants 215
volatile organic compounds 216
weather 199

SUGGESTED READINGS

Adams, J. B. "Proxy evidence for an El Niño-like response to volcanic forcing." *Nature* 426:274–78.

Baldasano, J. M., et al. 2003. "Air quality data from large cities." *The Science of the Total Environment* 307(1–3):141–65.

Bindschadler, Robert A., and Charles R. Bently. 2002. "On Thin Ice?" *Scientific American* 287(6):98–105.

Davis, Devra. 2002. *When Smoke Ran Like Water: Tales of Environmental Deception and the Battle against Pollution*. Basic Books.

Gupta, J., et al. 2003. "The role of scientific uncertainty in compliance with the Kyoto Protocol to the Climate Change Convention." *Environmental Science and Policy* 6(6):475–86.

Intergovernmental Panel on Climate Change (IPCC). 2001. *Climate Change IPCC Third Assessment.*

Karl, T. R., and K. E. Trenberth. 2003. "Modern global climate change." *Science* 302:1175–77.

Lindzen, R. S., M-D. Chou, and A. Y. Hou. 2001. "Does the Earth have an adaptive infrared iris?" *Bulletin of the American Meteorological Society* 82:417–32.

Mims, S. A., and F. M. Mims. 2004. "Fungal spores are transported long distances in smoke from biomass fires." *Atmospheric Environment* 38(5):651–55.

Parmesan, Camille, and Gary Yohe. 2003. "A globally coherent fingerprint of climate change impacts across natural systems." *Nature* 421:37–42.

Stott L., et al. 2002. "Super ENSO and global climate oscillations at millennial time scales." *Science* 297:222–26.

Welcome to McGraw-Hill's Online Learning Center

http://www.mhhe.com/cunningham3e

WEB EXERCISES

El Niño and Ocean/Climate Conditions

Before doing this exercise, review the El Niño discussion, p. 206. Then visit the website www.ssmi.com/ssmiMonthly.html.

Satellite images are one of the principal ways scientists map and monitor environmental conditions worldwide. This exercise uses satellite data gathered by the U.S. government for a variety of environmental monitoring purposes. This website is one of many excellent sources providing up-to-date environmental data. The monthly "static data" website provides graphic images of satellite data. If you are using a slow server, you may want to save a few of the images on your computer for answering the questions that follow.

For the following questions you will mostly be looking at *atmospheric water vapor,* or humidity. Keep this in mind: humidity is higher where evaporation is high, so *high humidity* indicates *warm water;* low humidity indicates cooler water.

The Special Sensor Microwave Imager (SSMI) monthly data page lets you select a month and year to view and provides four types of atmospheric information.

1. What are the four types of information shown? What units are used to measure these data types? (How fast is 1 wind-speed unit, compared with how fast you walk?)
2. Look at the Atmospheric Water Vapor map for the current month. Bright red and yellow colors indicate high humidity in the air—and high temperatures. Where is the greatest concentration of red and yellow?
3. Look at November 1998. Then change to November 1997. (Each time you change years or months, you must click on the "Update Display" button to redraw.) Sketch on a piece of paper the general location of the red concentration in the Indian and Pacific Oceans in 1998 and in 1997. How do the two years differ?
4. Now look at the surface wind-speed maps for 1998 and 1997. Which year has the lowest wind speeds in the Pacific Ocean? In the Indian Ocean? Can you think of how wind speeds and ocean temperatures might be related?
5. Go backward, year by year, to see how the concentration of red changes over the years. For each year, mark an *X* on the following graph to show the approximate location of the biggest red concentration in the Pacific Ocean. During which years does the region of strong red/yellow expand farthest eastward?

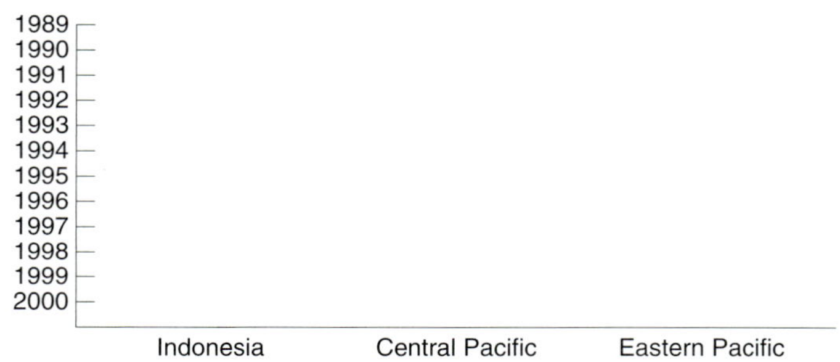

6. If you have a fast network connection, start with January 1997 (or an earlier year) and hit the "next month" button to watch conditions change through the years. During which months do the 1998 El Niño conditions really start to develop?

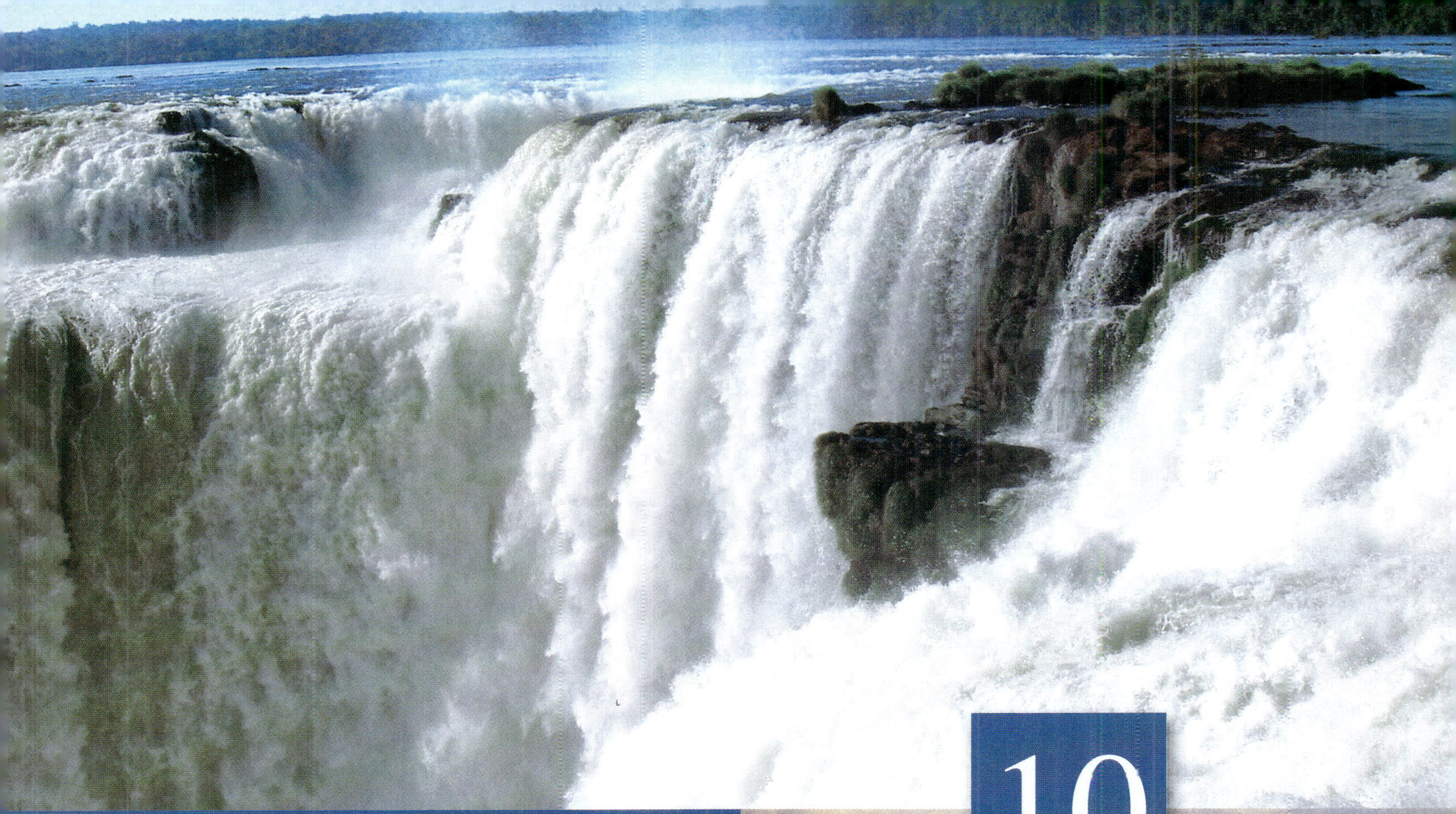

Iguazu Falls on the Brazil/Argentina border has 275 individual falls spread along a 4-km-long cliff.

10

Water:
Resources and Pollution

If there is magic on this planet, it is in water.
–Loren Eisley

Welcome to McGraw-Hill's Online Learning Center

http://www.mhhe.com/cunningham3e

LEARNING ONLINE

Visit our webpage at www.mhhe.com/cunningham3e for data sources further readings, additional case studies, current environmental news, and regional examples within the Online Learning Center to help you understand the material in this chapter. You'll also find active links to information pertaining to this chapter, including

USGS—water resources of the United States
Bureau of Reclamation
National Wetlands Inventory homepage
World water supplies
Water pollution
Water quality/pollution control
River basins and watersheds
International Rivers Network

OBJECTIVES

After studying this chapter, you should be able to

- describe the important sources of water and the major ways we use it.
- appreciate the causes and consequences of water shortages around the world and what they mean in people's lives in water-poor countries.
- debate the merits of proposals to increase water supplies and manage demand.
- apply some water conservation methods in your own life.
- define *water pollution* and describe the sources and effects of some major types.
- appreciate why access to sewage treatment and clean water are important to people in developing countries.
- explain ways to control water pollution, including technological and legal solutions.

Sharing the Chattahoochee

Beginning from a small spring in northern Georgia's Blue Ridge Mountains, the Chattahoochee River provides drinking water, irrigation, hydropower, wildlife habitat, and recreation for millions of people. As it tumbles down from the mountains, the Chattahoochee is a clean, cool, swift-flowing stream, a popular destination for fishing, swimming, and boating. Far downstream, the Chattahoochee joins the Flint to form the Apalachicola River, which flows across the Florida Panhandle into Apalachicola Bay, in the Gulf of Mexico (fig. 10.1). Together, the Apalachicola, Chattahoochee, and Flint (ACF) watershed supports rich and diverse ecosystems, including valuable marine fisheries for oysters, shrimp, and finfish.

But between the mountains and the sea, the Chattahoochee River passes through Atlanta, where it undergoes dramatic changes. Atlanta is one of America's fastest-growing cities. Expanding suburbs and industries crowd the Chattahoochee's banks, producing runoff of silt, salts, and yard fertilizers that wash into the river. Growing households and industries withdraw water from the river, which becomes lower, slower, and warmer. Additional contaminants mix with remaining water—oils, metals, and dust from city streets and storm sewers, as well as chlorine and other contaminants from sewage treatment plants. The warm, shallow, turbid water holds less oxygen and supports fewer of the river's native plants and animals. The Environmental Protection Agency has named the 100 km of the Chattahoochee south of Atlanta one of the five most polluted river segments in the United States.

In an effort to force action, the EPA has levied millions of dollars in fines on Atlanta for polluting the river. Atlanta dilutes the contaminated waters by releasing more clean water from reservoirs upstream, but the city government says little can be done to prevent widespread runoff from the large and growing city. Meanwhile, Alabama and Florida complain that Georgia is taking too much water. They say the 2.3 billion liters (600 million gal) of water withdrawn each year in Georgia is needed downstream for homes, industries, and farms. Low river flows and contaminated water also threaten wildlife, shipping, and recreation. The Apalachicola Bay is particularly endangered. Pollution, reduced river flow, and increasing salinity in the estuary jeopardize the bay's multimillion-dollar-per-year fishing and tourism industries.

Atlanta recognized the looming problem of water supplies in the 1970s, and the city has been working with the Army Corps of Engineers to develop additional water supplies. In 2004 Georgia

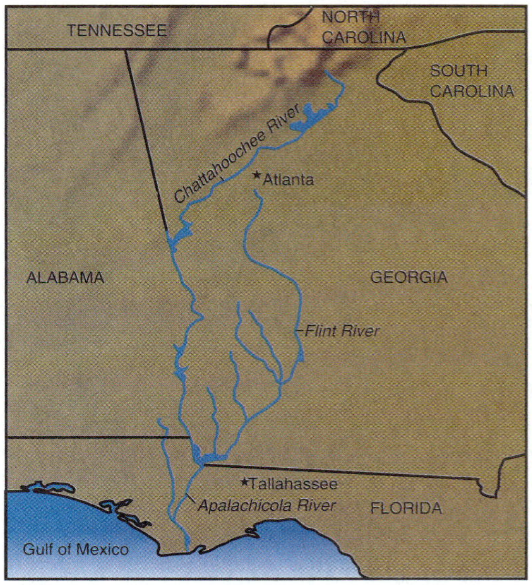

FIGURE 10.1 *Rising in the mountains of northern Georgia, the Chattahoochee flows south through Atlanta before joining the Flint to form the Apalachicola River.*

began working on a comprehensive state water plan, which is scheduled to be completed in 4 years. Ecologists worry that wildlife and biodiversity won't be adequately represented in this planning. Meanwhile, hydrologists point out that climate change could result in more erratic, less dependable rainfall in the future (see chapter 9). If river flows become more unpredictable as a result, water management could become an even more urgent and difficult concern.

In the United States, water shortages have long been a western problem, with growing cities in California and other western states struggling to acquire enough water without destroying river ecosystems. But like Atlanta, many growing metropolitan areas in other regions are increasingly competing with other users for water. Around the world, cities are experiencing water shortages, while pollution makes the water we do have less useful. The United Nations warns that water supplies are likely to become one of the most pressing environmental issues of the twenty-first century. By 2025 two-thirds of all humans could be living in countries where water resources are inadequate. In this chapter, we'll look at where our fresh water comes from, what we do with it, and how we can protect its quality and extend its usefulness.

WATER RESOURCES

Water is a marvelous substance—flowing, swirling, seeping, constantly moving from sea to land and back again. It shapes the earth's surface and moderates our climate. Water is essential for life. It is the medium in which all living processes occur (see chapter 2). Water dissolves nutrients and distributes them to cells, regulates body temperature, supports structures, and removes waste products. About 60 percent of your body is water. You could survive for weeks without food, but only a few days without water. Water also is needed for agriculture, industry, transportation, and a host of other human uses. In short, clean freshwater is one of our most vital natural resources.

Where Does Our Water Come From?

The water we use cycles endlessly through the environment. The total amount of water on our planet is immense—more than 1,404 million km^3 (370 billion billion gal) (table 10.1). This water evaporates from moist surfaces, falls as rain or snow, passes through living organisms, and returns to the ocean in a process known as the **hydrologic cycle** (see fig. 2.18). Every year, about 500,000 km^3, or a layer 1.4 m thick, evaporates from the oceans. More than 90 percent of that moisture falls back on the ocean. The 47,000 km^3 carried onshore joins some 72,000 km^3 that evaporate from lakes, rivers, soil, and plants to become our annual, renewable freshwater supply. Plants play a major role in the hydrologic cycle, absorbing groundwater and pumping it into the atmosphere by transpiration (transport plus evaporation). In tropical forests, as much as 75 percent of annual precipitation is returned to the atmosphere by plants.

Solar energy drives the hydrologic cycle by evaporating surface water, which becomes rain and snow. Because water and sunlight are unevenly distributed around the globe, water resources are very uneven. At Iquique in the Chilean desert, for instance, no rain has fallen in recorded history. At the other end of the scale, 22 m (72 ft) of rain was recorded in a single year at Cherrapunji in India. Figure 10.2 shows broad patterns of precipitation around the world. Most of the world's rainiest regions are tropical, where heavy rainy seasons occur, or in coastal mountain regions. Most of the driest areas are in the high-pressure bands of deserts (see chapter 9). Deserts occur on every continent just outside the tropics (the Sahara, the Namib, the Gobi, the Sonoran, and many others). Rainfall is also slight at very high latitudes, another high-pressure region.

TABLE 10.1 Units of Water Measurement

One cubic kilometer (km^3) equals 1 billion cubic meters (m^3), 1 trillion liters, or 264 billion gal.

One acre-foot is the amount of water required to cover an acre of ground 1 ft deep. This is equivalent to 325,851 gal, or 1.2 million liters, or 1,234 m^3, approximately the amount consumed annually by a family of four in the United States.

One cubic foot per second of river flow equals 28.3 liters per second, or 449 gal per minute.

Mountains also influence moisture distribution. The windward sides of mountain ranges, including the Pacific Northwest and the flanks of the Himalayas, are typically wet and have large rivers; on the leeward sides of mountains, in areas known as the rain shadow, dry conditions dominate, and water can be very scarce. The windward side of Mount Waialeale on the island of Kauai, for example, is one of the wettest places on earth, with an annual rainfall around 1,200 cm (460 in.). The leeward side, only a few kilometers away, has an average yearly rainfall of only 46 cm (18 in.).

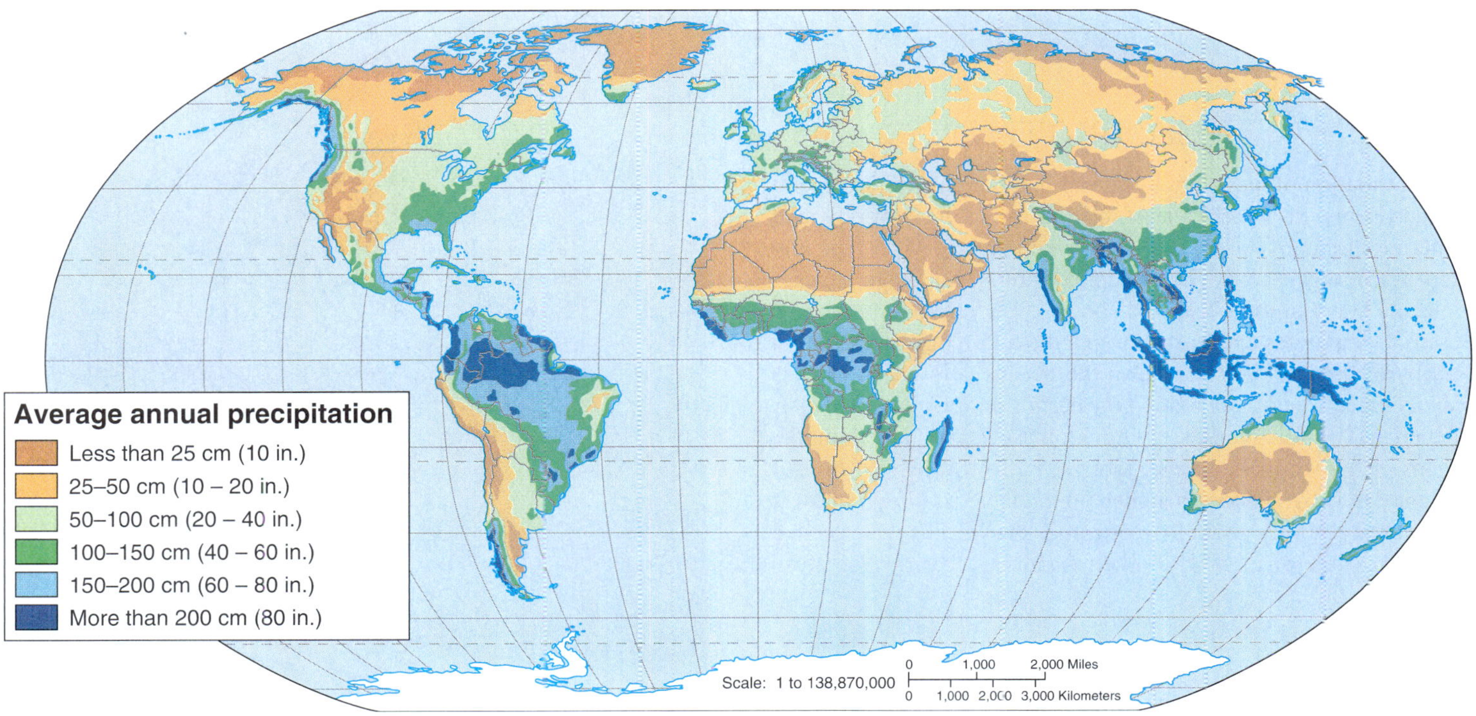

FIGURE 10.2 *Average annual precipitation. Note wet areas that support tropical rainforests occur along the equator, while the major world deserts occur in zones of dry, descending air between 20° and 40° north and south.*

TABLE 10.2 Earth's Water Compartments

COMPARTMENT	VOLUME (1,000 km^3)	PERCENT OF TOTAL WATER	AVERAGE RESIDENCE TIME
Total	1,386,000	100	2,800 years
Oceans	1,338,000	96.5	3,000 to 30,000 years*
Ice and snow	24,364	1.76	1 to 100,000 years*
Saline groundwater	12,870	0.93	Days to thousands of years*
Fresh groundwater	10,530	0.76	Days to thousands of years*
Fresh lakes	91	0.007	1 to 500 years*
Saline lakes	85	0.006	1 to 1,000 years*
Soil moisture	16.5	0.001	2 weeks to 1 year*
Atmosphere	12.9	0.001	1 week
Marshes, wetlands	11.5	0.001	Months to years
Rivers, streams	2.12	0.0002	1 week to 1 month
Living organisms	1.12	0.0001	1 week

Source: Data from UNEP, 2002.
*Depends on depth and other factors.

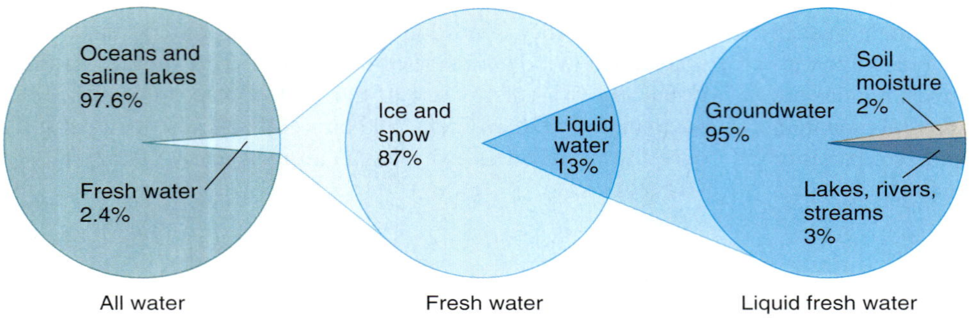

FIGURE 10.3 *The easily accessible water in lakes, rivers, and streams represents only 3 percent of all liquid fresh water, which is 13 percent of all fresh water, which is 2.4 percent of all water on the earth.*

MAJOR WATER COMPARTMENTS

The distribution of water often is described in terms of interacting compartments in which water resides, sometimes briefly and sometimes for eons (table 10.2). The length of time water typically stays in a compartment is its **residence time.** On average, a water molecule stays in the ocean for about 3,000 years, for example, before it evaporates and starts through the hydrologic cycle again. Nearly all the world's water is in the oceans (fig. 10.3). Oceans play a crucial role in moderating the earth's temperature, and over 90 percent of the world's living biomass is contained in the oceans. What we mainly need, though, is fresh water. Of the 2.4 percent that is fresh, most is locked up in glaciers or in groundwater. Amazingly, only about 0.1 percent of the world's water is in a form accessible to us and to other organisms that rely on fresh water (fig. 10.4).

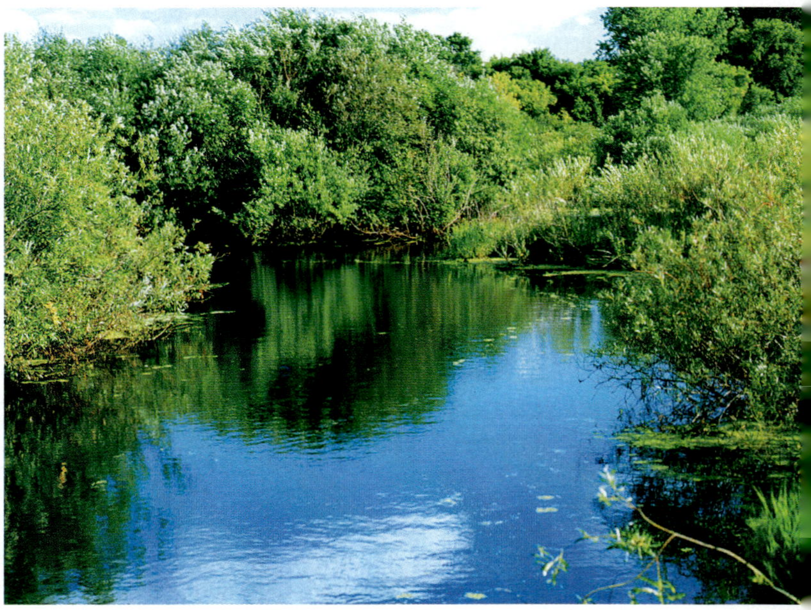

FIGURE 10.4 *Water is essential for life, yet only about 0.1 percent of the world's supply is accessible, fresh, liquid water.*

Groundwater

Groundwater is one of our most important freshwater resources. Originating as precipitation that percolates into layers of soil and rock, groundwater makes up the largest compartment of liquid, fresh water. The groundwater within 1 km of the surface is more than 100 times the volume of all the freshwater lakes, rivers, and reservoirs combined.

Plants get moisture from a relatively shallow layer of soil containing both air and water, known as the *zone of aeration* (fig. 10.5). Depending on rainfall amount, soil type, and surface topography, the zone of aeration may be a few centimeters or many meters deep. Lower soil layers, where all soil pores are filled with water, make up the *zone of saturation,* the source of water in most wells; the top of this zone is the **water table.**

Geologic layers that contain water are known as **aquifers.** Aquifers may consist of porous layers of sand or gravel or of cracked or porous rock. Below an aquifer, relatively impermeable layers of rock or clay keep water from seeping out at the bottom. Instead, water seeps more or less horizontally through the porous layer. Depending on geology, it can take from a few hours to several years for water to move a few hundred meters through an aquifer. If impermeable layers lie above an aquifer, pressure can develop within the water-bearing layer. A well or conduit puncturing the aquifer flows freely at the surface and is called an *artesian well* or spring.

Areas where surface water filters into an aquifer are **recharge zones** (fig. 10.6). Most aquifers recharge extremely slowly, and road and house construction or water use at the surface can further slow recharge rates. Contaminants can also enter aquifers through recharge zones. Urban or agricultural runoff in recharge zones is often a serious problem. About 2 billion people—approximately one-third of the world's population—depend on groundwater for drinking and other uses. Every year 700 km^3 are withdrawn by humans, mostly from shallow, easily polluted aquifers.

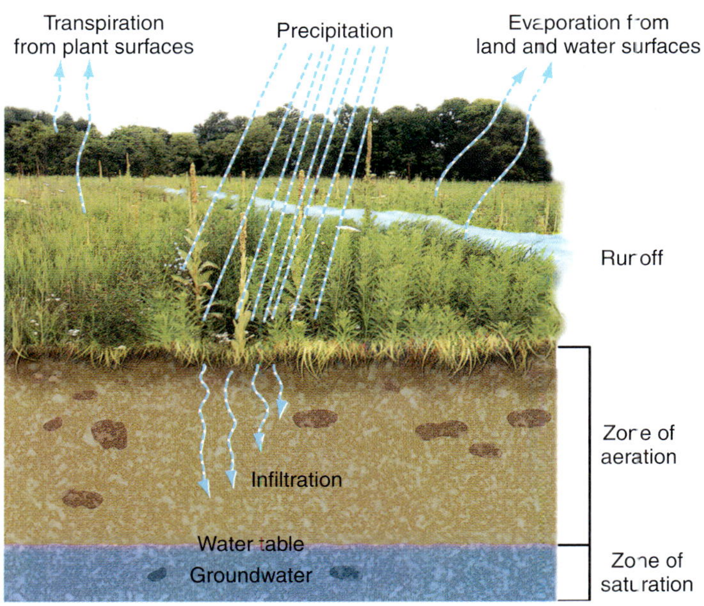

FIGURE 10.5 *Precipitation that does not evaporate or run off over the surface percolates through the soil in a process called infiltration. The upper layers of soil hold droplets of moisture between air-filled spaces. Lower layers, where all spaces are filled with water, make up the zone of saturation, or groundwater.*

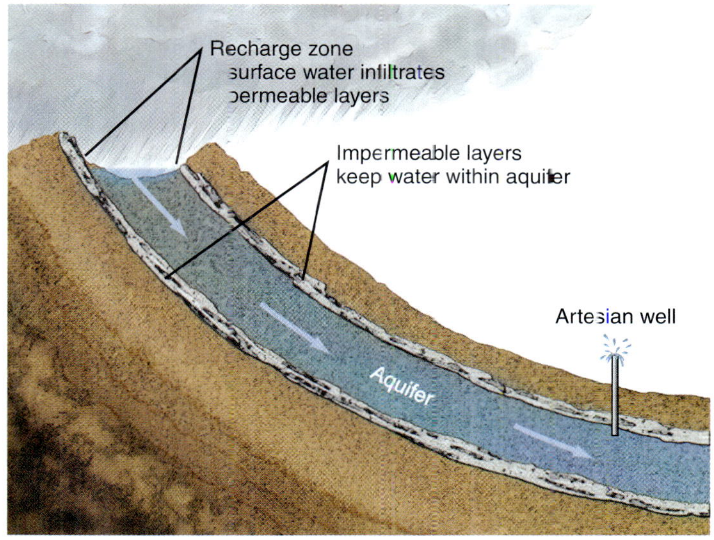

FIGURE 10.6 *An aquifer is a porous, water-bearing layer of sand, gravel, or rock. This aquifer is confined between layers of rock or clay and bent by geologic forces, creating hydrostatic pressure. A break in the overlying layer creates an artesian well or spring.*

Rivers, Lakes, and Wetlands

Fresh, flowing surface water is one of our most precious resources. Rivers contain a minute amount of water at any one time. Most rivers would begin to dry up in weeks or days if they were not constantly replenished by precipitation, snowmelt, or groundwater seepage.

The volume of water carried by a river is its **discharge,** or the amount of water that passes a fixed point in a given amount of time. This is usually expressed as liters or cubic feet of water per second. The 16 largest rivers in the world carry nearly half of all surface runoff on the earth, and a large fraction of that occurs in a single river, the Amazon, which carries 10 times as much water as the Mississippi (table 10.3).

Lakes contain nearly 100 times as much water as all rivers and streams combined, but much of this water is in a few of the world's largest lakes. Lake Baikal in Siberia, the Great Lakes of North America, the Great Rift Lakes of Africa, and a few other lakes contain vast amounts of water, not all of it fresh. Worldwide, lakes are almost as important as rivers in terms of water supplies, food, transportation, and settlement.

Wetlands—bogs, swamps, wet meadows, and marshes—play a vital and often unappreciated role in the hydrologic cycle. Their lush plant growth stabilizes soil and holds back surface runoff, allowing time for infiltration into aquifers and producing even, year-long stream flow. When wetlands are disturbed, their natural water-absorbing capacity is reduced, and surface waters run off quickly, resulting in floods and erosion during the rainy season and low stream flow the rest of the year.

TABLE 10.3 World's Ten Largest Rivers

RIVER	LOCATION	ANNUAL DISCHARGE (m^3/SECOND)*
Amazon	Brazil, Peru	175,000
Orinoco	Venezuela, Colombia	45,300
Congo	Congo	39,200
Yangtze	Tibet, China	28,000
Brahmaputra	South Asia	19,000
Mississippi	United States	18,400
Mekong	Southeast Asia	18,300
Paraná	Paraguay, Argentina	18,000
Yenisey	Russia	17,200
Lena	Russia	16,000

Source: Data from World Resource Institute.
*1 m^3 = 264 gal.

The Atmosphere

The atmosphere contains only 0.001 percent of the total water supply, but it is the most important mechanism for redistributing water around the world. An individual water molecule resides in the atmosphere for about ten days, on average. Some water evaporates and falls within hours. Water can also travel halfway around the world before it falls, replenishing streams and aquifers on land.

WATER AVAILABILITY AND USE

Clean, fresh water is essential for nearly every human endeavor (fig. 10.7). Collectively, we now appropriate more than half of all the freshwater in the world. Perhaps more than any other environmental factor, the availability of water determines the location and activities of humans on the earth. **Renewable water supplies** are resources that are replenished regularly—mainly surface water and shallow groundwater. Renewable water is most plentiful in the tropics, where rainfall is heavy, followed by midlatitudes, where rainfall is regular.

Water-Rich and Water-Poor Countries

Water availability is usually measured in terms of renewable water per capita, so population density, as well as total water volumes, dictate renewable supplies for human use. The highest per capita water supplies generally occur in countries with moist climates and low population densities. Iceland, for example, has about 160 million gal per person per year. In contrast, Kuwait, where temperatures are extremely high and rain almost never falls, has less than 3,000 gal per person per year from renewable natural sources. Almost all of Kuwait's water comes from imports and desalinized seawater. In countries such as Libya and Israel, where water is one of the most crucial environmental resources, renewable supplies do not meet basic needs. These countries manage by "mining" groundwater, depleting sources that are probably unrenewable on a human time scale.

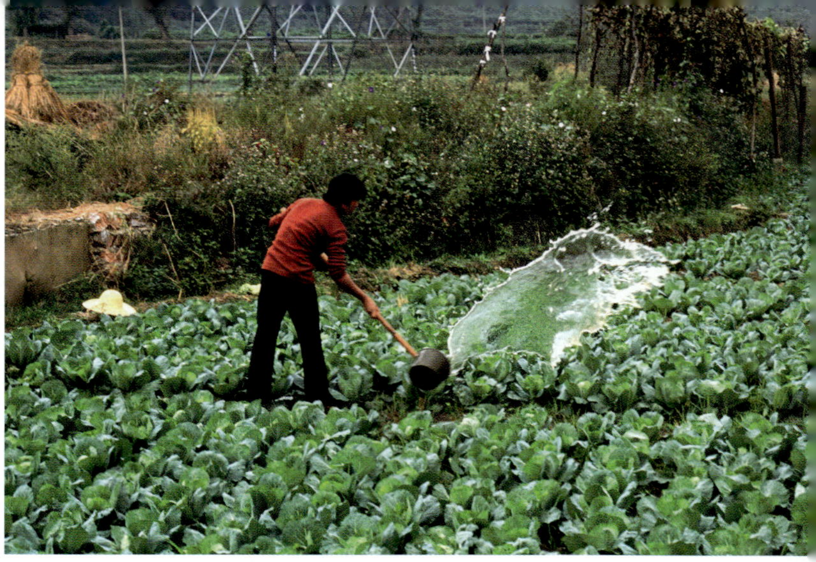

FIGURE 10.7 *We depend on fresh water in many ways, but for billions of people, water shortages are a brutal fact of life.*

APPLICATION: Mapping the Water-Rich and Water-Poor Countries

The top ten water-rich countries, in terms of water availability per capita, and the ten most water-poor countries are listed below. Locate these countries on the political map (page 000). Describe the patterns. Where are the water-rich countries concentrated? (Hint: does latitude matter?) Where are the water-poor countries most concentrated?

Water-rich countries: Iceland, Surinam, Guyana, Papua New Guinea, Gabon, Solomon Islands, Canada, Norway, Panama, Brazil

Water-poor countries: Kuwait, Egypt, United Arab Emirates, Malta, Jordan, Saudi Arabia, Singapore, Moldavia, Israel, Oman

Answers: Water-rich countries (per capita) are either in the far north, where populations and evaporation are low, or in the tropics. Water-poor countries are in the desert belt at about 15° to 25° latitude or are densely populated island nations (e.g., Malta, Singapore).

Much of the western United States has insufficient water to meet all the demands placed on this vital resource. The U.S. Department of the Interior warns that by 2025 many western states will face water crises (fig. 10.8). After five years of severe drought, flow in the Colorado River has decreased so much that Lake Powell has lost 60 percent of its volume and the lake surface has dropped more than 33 m (100 ft). Electric generation could cease in four years, if current conditions continue, and the reservoir may never refill. Serious suggestions have been made to remove the dam and let the river run free.

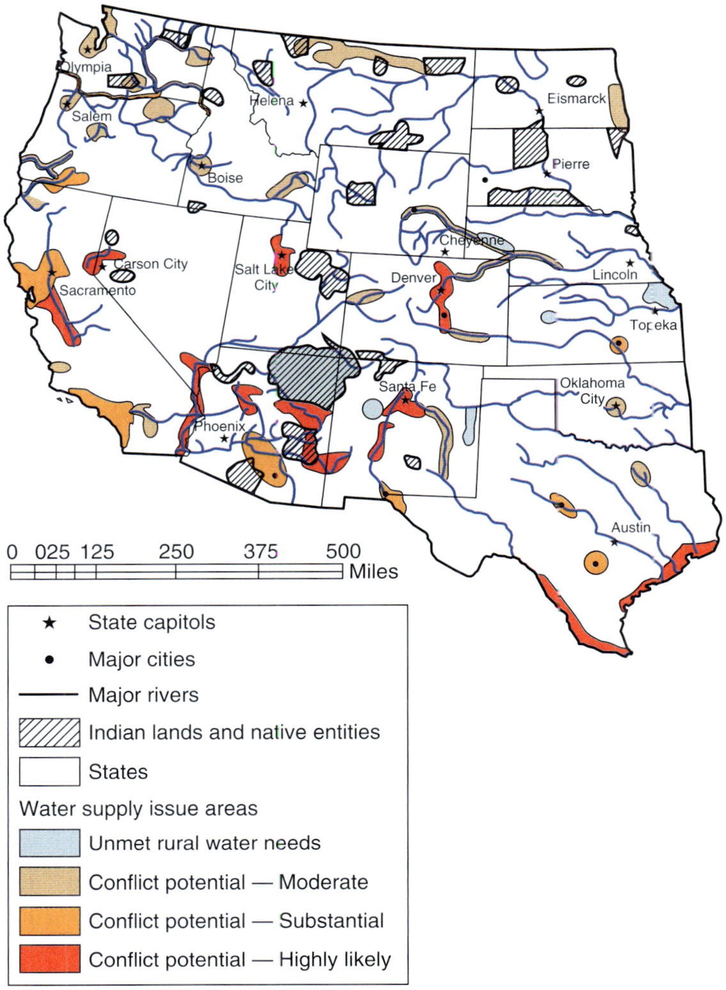

FIGURE 10.8 *Rapidly growing populations in arid regions are straining available water supplies. By 2025, the Department of the Interior warns, shortages could cause conflicts in many areas.*
Source: Data from U.S. Department of Interior.

As you can see, interannual variability in rainfall is an important issue in water availability. In the African Sahel region, like the American southwest, abundant rainfall occurs some years but not others. Usually natural ecosystems can survive these changes, but human societies, and ecosystems greatly altered by grazing, farming, or urban development, can be badly destabilized by rainfall fluctuations. Some of the world's earliest civilizations, such as the Sumerians and Babylonians of Mesopotamia, were based on communal efforts to divert floods during wet seasons or wet years and to store water in dry years. Many climatologists now worry that the greenhouse effect (see chapter 9) will bring about more serious or frequent droughts in dry parts of the world.

Water Use

In contrast to energy resources, which usually are consumed when used, water can be used over and over if it is not too badly contaminated. Water **withdrawal** is the total amount of water taken from a water body. Much of this water could be returned to circulation in a reusable form. Water **consumption,** on the other hand, is loss of water due to evaporation, absorption, or contamination.

The natural cleansing and renewing functions of the hydrologic cycle replace the water we need if natural systems are not overloaded or damaged. Water is a renewable resource, but renewal takes time. The rate at which many of us now use water may make it necessary to conscientiously protect, conserve, and replenish our water supply.

Quantities of Water Used

Water use has been increasing about twice as fast as population growth over the past century. Water withdrawals are expected to continue to grow as more land is irrigated to feed an expanding population (fig. 10.9). Conflicts increase as different countries, economic sectors, and other stakeholders compete for the same, limited water supply. Water wars may well be the major source of hostilities in the twenty-first century.

Worldwide, agriculture claims about 70 percent of total water withdrawal, ranging from 93 percent of all water used in India to only 4 percent in Kuwait, which cannot afford to spend its limited water on crops. In many developing countries and in parts of the United States, the most common type of irrigation is to simply flood the whole field or run water in rows between crops. As much as half the water can be lost through evaporation or seepage from unlined irrigation canals bringing water to fields. Sprinklers are more efficient in distributing water, but they are more costly and energy intensive (fig. 10.10). Water-efficient drip irrigation can save significant amounts of water but currently is used on only about 1 percent of the world's croplands (fig. 10.11).

Industry uses about one-fourth of water withdrawals worldwide. Some European countries use 70 percent of water for industry; less-industrialized countries use as little as 5 percent. Cooling water for power plants is by far the largest single industrial use of water, typically accounting for 50 to 75 percent of industrial withdrawal.

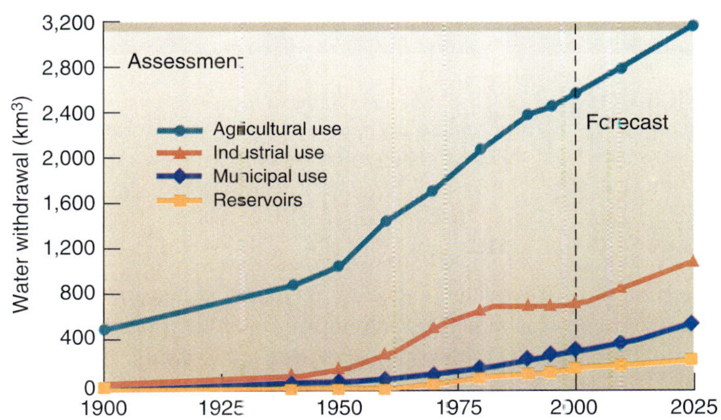

FIGURE 10.9 *Global water withdrawals have increased more than seven-fold over the past century and are expected to continue to rise in the future.*
Source: Data from UNESCO, 2001.

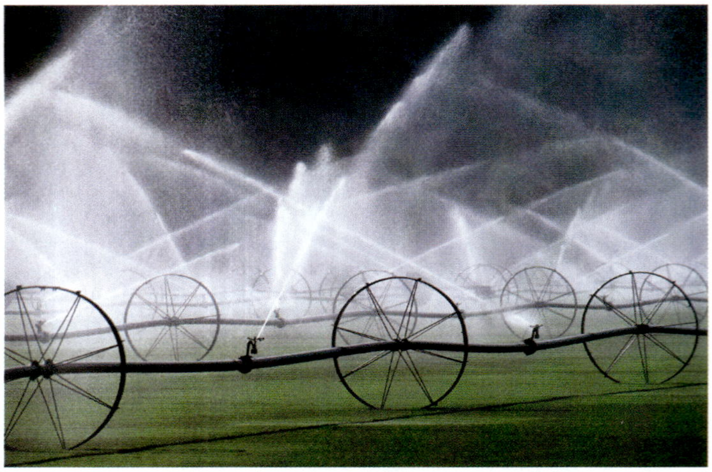

FIGURE 10.10 *Rolling sprinklers allow farmers to irrigate crops on uneven terrain. In some areas, irrigation consumes 90 percent of all available water.*

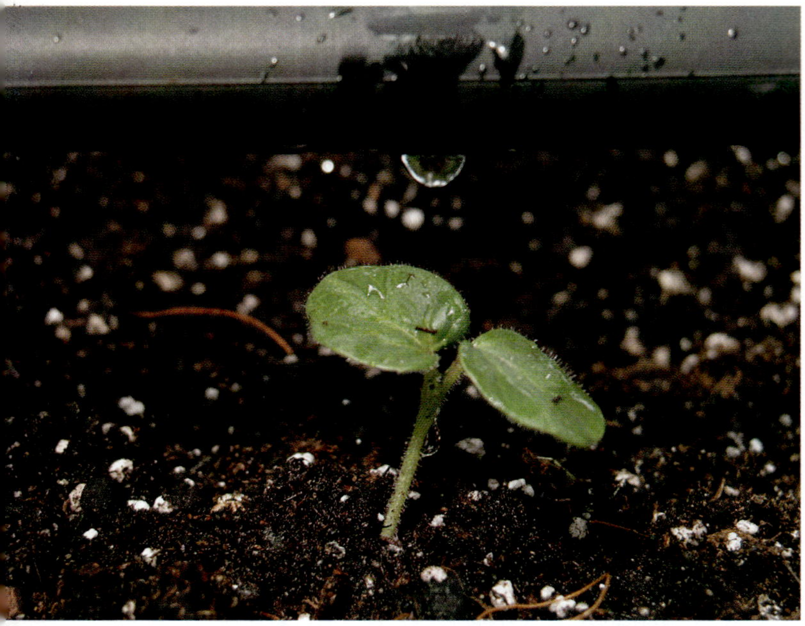

FIGURE 10.11 *Drip irrigation delivers measured amounts of water exactly where the plants need and can use it. This technique can save up to 90 percent of irrigation water usage and reduces salt buildup. It also is an efficient way to deliver soluble nutrients.*

Domestic, or household, water use accounts for only about 6 percent of world water use. This includes water for drinking, cooking, and washing. The amount of water used per household varies enormously, however, depending on a country's wealth. The United Nations reports that people in developed countries consume on average, about ten times more water daily than those in developing nations. Poorer counries can't afford the infrastructure to obtain and deliver water to citizens. Inadequate water supplies, on the other hand, prevent agriculture, industry, sanitation, and other devleopments that reduce poverty.

FRESHWATER SHORTAGES

Clean drinking water and basic sanitation are necessary to prevent communicable diseases and to maintain a healthy life. For many of the world's poorest people, one of the greatest environmental threats to health remains the continued use of polluted water. In 2004 the United Nations estimated that at least 1.5 billion people lacked access to safe drinking water and 3 billion didn't have adequate sanitation. These deficiencies result in hundreds of millions of cases of water-related illness and more than 5 million deaths every year. As populations grow, more people move into cities, and agriculture and industry compete for increasingly scarce water supplies, water shortages are expected to become even worse. By 2025 two-thirds of the world's people will be living in water-stressed countries—defined by the United Nations as consumption of more than 10 percent of renewable freshwater resources. One of the highest priorities announced at the UN World Summit in Johannesburg in 2002 was to reduce by one-half the proportion of people without reliable access to clean water and improved sanitation.

A Precious Resource

The World Health Organization considers an average of 1,000 m^3 (264,000 gal) per person per year to be a necessary amount of water for modern domestic, industrial, and agricultural uses. Some 45 countries, most of them in Africa or the Middle East, cannot meet the minimum essential water needs of all their citizens. In some countries, the problem is access to *clean* water. In Mali, for example, 88 percent of the population lacks clean water; in Ethiopia, it is 94 percent. Rural people often have less access to clean water than do city dwellers. Causes of water shortages include natural deficits, overconsumption by agriculture or industry, and inadequate funds for purifying and delivering good water.

More than two-thirds of the world's households have to fetch water from outside the home (fig. 10.12). This is heavy work, done mainly by women and children and sometimes taking several hours a day. Improved public systems bring many benefits to these poor families.

Availability does not always mean affordability. A typical poor family in Lima, Peru, for instance, uses one-sixth as much water as a middle-class American family but pays three times as much for it. If they followed government recommendations to boil all water to prevent cholera, up to one-third of the poor family's income could be used just in acquiring and purifying water.

Investments in rural development have brought significant improvements in recent years. Since 1990, nearly 800 million people—about 13 percent of the world's population—have gained access to clean water. The percentage of rural families with safe drinking water has risen from less than 10 percent to nearly 75 percent.

Depleting Groundwater

Groundwater provides nearly 40 percent of the fresh water for agricultural and domestic use in the United States. Nearly half of all Americans and about 95 percent of the rural population depend on groundwater for drinking and other domestic purposes. Overuse of these supplies dries up wells, natural springs, and even groundwater-fed wetlands, rivers, and lakes. Pollution of aquifers through dumping of contaminants on recharge zones, leaks through abandoned wells, or deliberate injection of toxic wastes can make this valuable resource unfit for use.

In many areas of the United States, groundwater is being withdrawn from aquifers faster than natural recharge can replace it. On a local level, this causes a cone of depression in the water table (fig. 10.13). On a broader scale, heavy pumping can deplete a whole aquifer. The Ogallala Aquifer underlies eight Great Plains states from Texas to North Dakota. This porous bed of sand, gravel, and sandstone once held more water than all the freshwater lakes, streams, and rivers on the earth. Excessive pumping for irrigation has removed so much water that wells have dried up in many places, and farms, ranches, even whole towns are being abandoned. Recharging many such aquifers will take thousands of years. Using "fossil" water like this is essentially water mining. For all practical purposes, these aquifers are nonrenewable resources.

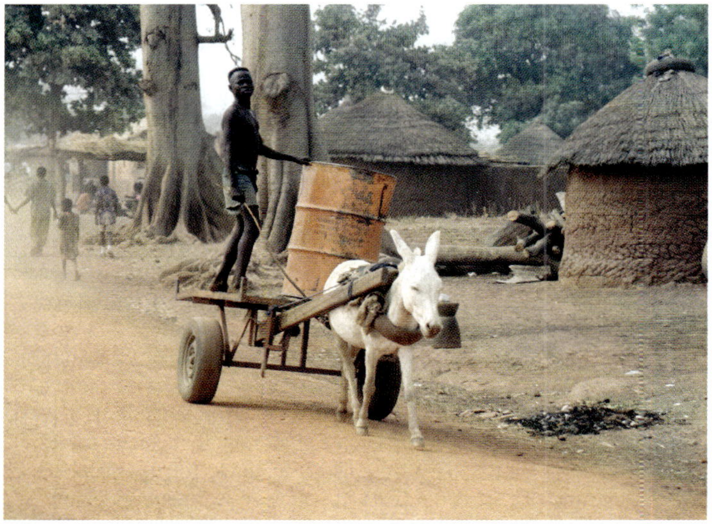

FIGURE 10.12 *Village water supplies in Ghana.*

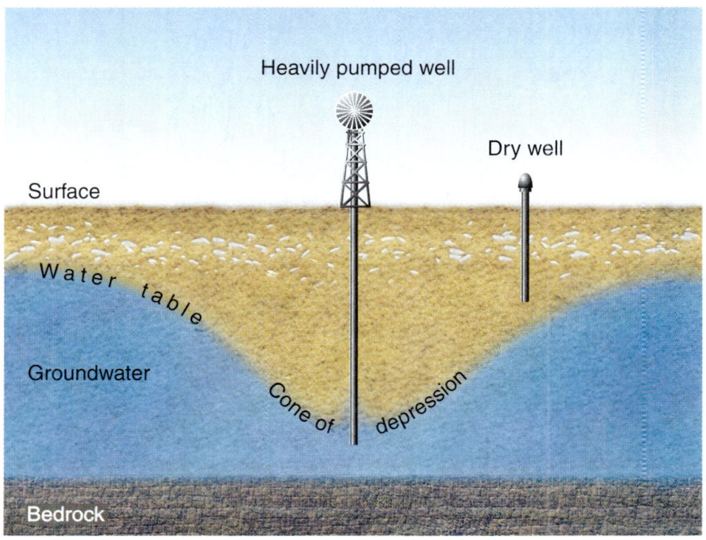

FIGURE 10.13 *A cone of depression forms in the water table under a heavily pumped well. This may dry up nearby shallow wells or make pumping so expensive that it becomes impractical.*

Water withdrawal also allows aquifers to collapse. Subsidence, or sinking of the ground surface, follows. The San Joaquin Valley in California has sunk more than 10 m in the past 50 years because of excessive groundwater pumping. Where aquifers become compressed, recharge becomes impossible.

Another consequence of aquifer depletion is saltwater intrusion. Along coastlines and in areas where saltwater deposits are left from ancient oceans, overuse of freshwater reservoirs often allows saltwater to intrude into aquifers used for domestic and agricultural purposes.

Can We Increase Water Supplies?

On a human time scale, the amount of water on the earth is fixed. Many efforts have been made to redistribute water resources, however. Towing icebergs from Antarctica has been proposed, and creating rain in dry regions has been accomplished, with mixed success, by cloud seeding—distributing condensation nuclei in humid air to help form raindrops. Desalination is locally important: in the arid Middle East, where energy and money are available but water is scarce, desalination is sometimes the principal source of water. Most efforts, however, have involved dams, canals, water diversions, and desalination. We will discuss some of the benefits and negative consequences of these projects next.

Dams, Reservoirs, and Canals

Dams and canals are a fundamental basis of civilization; they can also be a source of environmental disaster and injustice. Some of the great civilizations (Sumeria, Egypt, China, and the Incan culture of South America) were organized around the large-scale redistribution of water from rivers to irrigated farm fields. More than half the world's 227 largest rivers have been blocked by dams or diversion structures with adverse effects on freshwater ecosystems. Of the 50,000 large dams in the world, 90 percent were built in the twentieth century, and half of those are in China. Economically speaking, at least one-third of those dams should never have been built (see related story "South Water North" at www.mhhe.com/cases).

Dams and Justice

While many people benefit from the water and hydroelectricity provided by dams and diversion projects, other stakeholders, including wildlife and ecosystems, suffer. Towns and farms have been starved by the huge dams and diversions. Fishing enthusiasts, whitewater boaters, and others mourn the loss of rivers drowned in reservoirs or dried up by diversion projects. These projects also have been criticized for using public funds to increase the value of privately held farmland and for encouraging agricultural development and urban growth in arid lands, where other uses might be more appropriate (see Case Study, p. 238).

CASE STUDY

WATER WARS ON THE KLAMATH

Until a century ago, the Klamath River was the third most productive salmon fishery south of the Canadian border. The 35-km (22-mi)-long Upper Klamath Lake, the largest lake in the Pacific Northwest, once contained great schools of C'wam and Qapdo (Lost River and shortnose suckers). Millions of hectares of marshes, lakes, and dry steppe in the Klamath Basin teemed with waterfowl and wildlife. At least 80 percent of the birds following the Pacific Flyway stopped to feed in the area. Native American tribes, including the Klamath and Paiute in the upper basin and the Yurok and Hupa downstream, depended on the abundant fish and wildlife for their survival.

In 1905 the newly formed United States Bureau of Reclamation was directed to "reclaim the sunbaked prairies and worthless swamps" in the upper Klamath Basin. Spending $50 million, the bureau built 7 dams, 45 pumping stations, and more than 1,600 km (1,000 mi) of canals and ditches. The project drained three-quarters of the wetlands in the upper basin and provided irrigation water to 90,000 ha (220,000 acres) of cropland. Promises of cheap land and subsidized water lured some 1,400 farmers to the valley to grow potatoes, alfalfa, sugar beets, mint, onions, and cattle. In the 1990s, irrigators in the Klamath Basin used almost 1 million acre-feet (325 billion gallons, or 1.2 trillion liters) of surface water per year.

These water diversions left salmon stranded in dried-up streams, while oxygen-depleted lake water was contaminated with agricultural runoff and clogged with algae. Downstream, Native American tribes and commercial fishermen, who once had brought in about 500,000 kg (roughly a million pounds) of salmon per year, saw their catches decline by as much as 90 percent. More than 7,000 jobs were lost when the fisheries collapsed. In 1997 the C'wam and Qapdo were declared endangered, and Coho salmon were listed as threatened. A coalition of commercial and sports fishermen, environmentalists, and native people sued the government for damaging fish and wildlife resources. A federal judge agreed and ordered the Bureau of Reclamation to reduce irrigation flow and to maintain minimum water levels in rivers and lakes.

A severe drought in 2001 precipitated a crisis. For the first time in its history, the bureau closed the gates on its irrigation canals and cut off water to the farmers. Outraged at being denied the water they had come to believe was their inalienable right, angry farmers broke open headgate locks and let water flow to their drying fields. News media flocked to the site to film the confrontation. Conservative politicians condemned government actions and pledged to uphold property rights and to eliminate the Endangered Species Act. Progressives supported fishing and tribal rights. And environmentalists called for more water for the Lower Klamath Wildlife Refuge, the first in the United States established to protect migratory waterfowl and home to the largest population of wintering bald eagles in the lower 48 states.

Sympathizing with the farmers, Interior Secretary Gale Norton went to Upper Klamath Lake and personally opened the gates to give them more water. Favoring a market-based approach, she suggested a "water bank," in which farmers could voluntarily sell surplus water to Indian tribes or the Fish and Wildlife Service. The tribes and others objected that, while this approach might work when water was abundant, there probably wouldn't be any surplus in dry years. In 2002 more than 30,000 salmon died when the river dried to a string of warm, stagnant pools. Unfortunately, no surplus water was available to rescue them.

Conservationists argue that two-thirds of Klamath County's irrigated acreage is watered with inefficient flood irrigation in which about half the water is lost to evaporation. Farmers could save water by installing efficient drip or sprinkler systems, or they could abandon water-demanding crops, such as alfalfa and potatoes, and convert to dryland agriculture. Farmers demanded compensation for the "taking" of water they considered promised to them in perpetuity.

This case illustrates some of the complexity and importance of water resources. With growing demands on dwindling supplies, it becomes increasingly difficult to satisfy all the needs we have for this precious commodity. If you were secretary of the interior, how would you weigh the competing claims for water in the Klamath Basin?

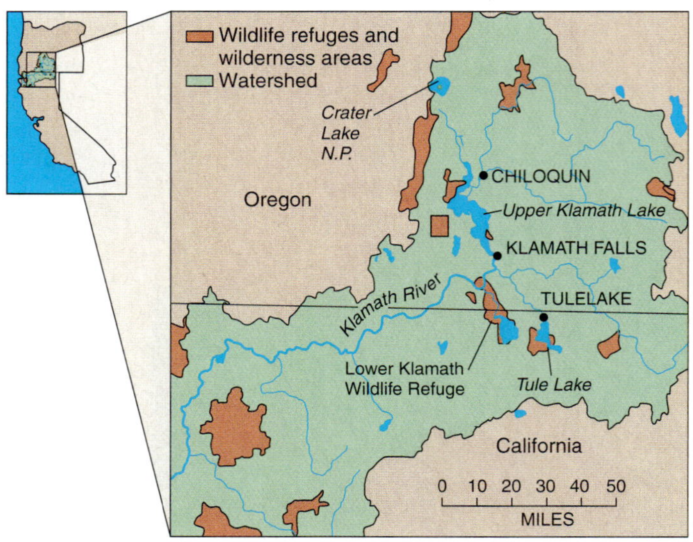

The Klamath River rises in the Cascade Mountains and flows about 400 km (250 mi) across Oregon and Washington to the Pacific Ocean.

Worldwide, large dams often flood towns and farmlands, raising international outcry. In India, the Sardar Sarovar Dam on the sacred Narmada River has been the focus of decades of protest. Many of the 1 million villagers and tribal people being displaced by this project have engaged in mass resistance and civil disobedience, while police have tried to remove them forcibly. In Nepal, construction of the 240-m (850-ft)-high Tehri Dam on the Bhagirathi River has stirred fears that a strong earthquake in this active seismic region might cause the dam to collapse and cause a catastrophic flood downstream. This dam is only one of 17 high dams that Nepal and India plan for the Himalaya Mountains. Similar fears of earthquakes and floods of biblical proportions have plagued China's Three Gorges Dam on the Yangtze River (see related story "Three Gorges" at www.mhhe.com/cases).

Canada's James Bay project built by Hydro-Quebec has diverted three major rivers flowing west into Hudson Bay and has flooded more than 10,000 km^2 (4,000 mi^2) of forest and tundra to generate 26,000 megawatts of electrical power. In 1984 10,000 caribou drowned while trying to follow ancient migration routes across the newly flooded land. The loss of traditional hunting and fishing sites has been culturally devastating for native Cree people. In addition, mercury leeched out of rocks in newly submerged lands has entered the food chain, and many residents show signs of mercury poisoning.

Environmental Costs of Dams

Dams ensure a year-round water supply, but they also waste tremendous amounts of water from evaporation and through seepage into porous rock beds. Some dams built in the western United States lose more water than they make available. Evaporative losses from Lake Mead and Lake Powell on the Colorado River are about 1 km^3 (264 billion gal) per year (fig. 10.14). The salts left behind by evaporation and agricultural runoff nearly double the salinity of the river. Mexico had to sue the United States to force construction of a $350 million desalination plant at Yuma, Arizona, to make the water partially usable again.

Dams also collect silt, decreasing the effectiveness of reservoirs and starving streambeds and sandbars downstream. As the turbulent Colorado River slows in the reservoirs created by Glen Canyon and Boulder Dams, it drops its load of suspended material. More than 10 million metric tons of silt per year collect behind these dams. Imagine a line of 20,000 dump trucks backed up to Lake Mead and Lake Powell every day, dumping dirt into the water. Within as little as 100 years, these reservoirs could be full of silt and useless for either water storage or hydroelectric generation (fig. 10.15).

In Egypt, the Aswân High Dam was built to irrigate thousands of hectares of farmland, but the dam loses much of the Nile's river to evaporation. Without the annual floods that carried rich silt to farmlands for thousands of years, many farming areas are becoming infertile, and the famous Nile Delta—and its rich fisheries—are disappearing.

Dams and river channelization also drown or destroy free-flowing rivers. One of the first and most divisive battles over this loss was in the Hetch Hetchy Valley in Yosemite National Park. In the early 1900s, San Francisco wanted to dam the Tuolumne River

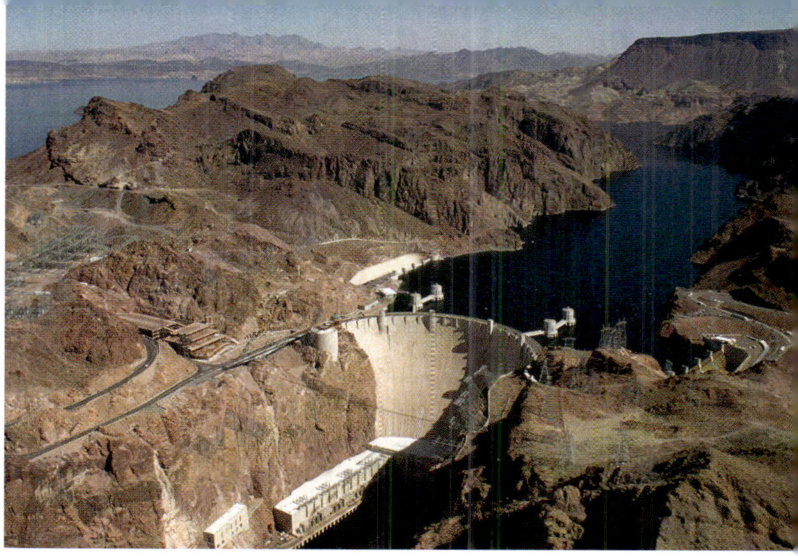

FIGURE 10.14 *Hoover Dam provides valuable electric power to Nevada and California but Lake Mead, behind the dam, loses about 1.3 billion m^3 of water per year to evaporation.*

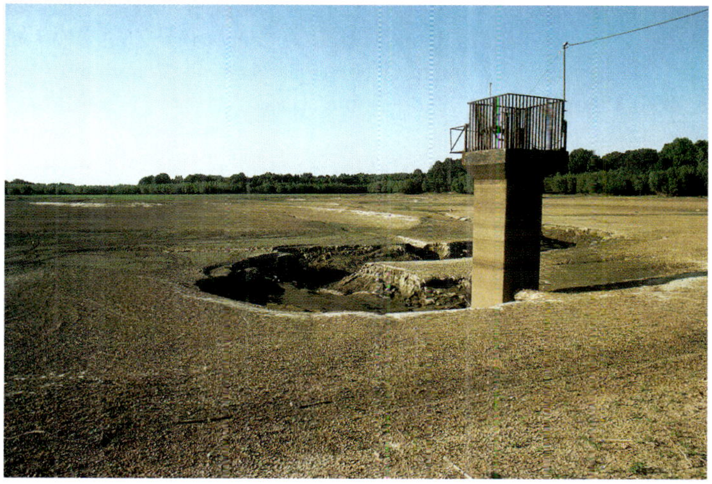

FIGURE 10.15 *This dam is now useless because its reservoir has filled with silt and sediment.*

to produce hydroelectric power and provide water for the city water system. This project was supported by many prominent San Francisco citizens because it represented an opportunity for both clean water and municipal power. John Muir, founder of the Sierra Club and protector of Yosemite Park, said, "These temple destroyers, devotees of ravaging commercialism, seem to have perfect contempt for Nature, and, instead of lifting their eyes to the God of the mountains, lift them to the Almighty Dollar. Dam Hetch Hetchy! As well dam for water-tanks the people's cathedrals and churches, for no holier temple has ever been consecrated by the heart of man." After a prolonged and bitter fight, the developers won, and the dam was built.

Price Mechanisms and Water Policy

Throughout most of U.S. history, water policies generally worked against conservation. In the well-watered eastern United States, water policy was based on riparian use rights: those who lived along a river bank had the right to use as much water as they liked, as long as they didn't interfere with its quality or availability to neighbors downstream. In the drier western regions, where water is often a limiting resource, water law is based primarily on the Spanish system of prior appropriation rights, or "first in time are first in right." But the appropriated water has to be put to "beneficial" use by being consumed. This creates a policy of "use it or lose it." Water left in a stream, even if essential for recreation, aesthetic enjoyment, or to sustain ecological communities, is not being appropriated or put to "beneficial" (that is, economic) use. Under this system, water rights can be bought and sold, but water owners frequently are reluctant to conserve water for fear of losing their rights.

In most federal "reclamation" projects, customers have been charged only for the immediate costs of water delivery. The costs of building dams and distribution systems have been subsidized, and the potential value of competing uses has been routinely ignored. Farmers in California's Central Valley, for instance, for many years paid only about one-tenth of what it cost the government to supply water to them. This didn't encourage conservation. Subsidies created by underpriced water amounted to as much as \$500,000 per farm per year in some areas.

WATER MANAGEMENT AND CONSERVATION

Watershed management and conservation are often more economical and environmentally sound ways to prevent flood damage and store water for future use than building huge dams and reservoirs. A **watershed,** or catchment, is all the land drained by a stream or river. It has long been recognized that retaining vegetation and groundcover in a watershed helps hold back rainwater and lessens downstream floods. In 1998 Chinese officials acknowledged that unregulated timber cutting upstream on the Yangtze contributed to massive floods that killed 30,000 people. Similarly, after disastrous floods in the upper Mississippi Valley in 1993, it was suggested that, rather than allowing residential, commercial, or industrial development on floodplains, these areas should be reserved for water storage, aquifer recharge, wildlife habitat, and agriculture. Further discussion of flooding hazards can be found in chapter 11.

Sound farming and forestry practices can reduce runoff. Retaining crop residue on fields reduces flooding, and minimizing plowing and forest cutting on steep slopes protects watersheds. Effects of deforestation on weather and water supplies are discussed in chapter 6. Wetlands conservation preserves natural water storage capacity and aquifer recharge zones. A river fed by marshes and wet meadows tends to run consistently clear and steady, rather than in violent floods.

A series of small dams on tributary streams can hold back water before it becomes a great flood. Ponds formed by these dams provide useful wildlife habitat and stock-watering facilities. They also catch soil where it could be returned to the fields. Small dams can be built with simple equipment and local labor, eliminating the need for massive construction projects and huge dams.

In 1998 U.S. Forest Service chief, Mike Dombeck, announced a major shift in his agency's priorities. "Water," he said, "is the most valuable and least appreciated resource the national forests provide. More than 60 million people in 33 states obtain their drinking water from national forest lands. Protecting watersheds is far more economically important than logging or mining, and will be given the highest priority in forest planning."

You Can Make a Difference: Domestic Conservation

We could probably save as much as half of the water we now use for domestic purposes without great sacrifice or serious changes in our lifestyles. Simple steps, such as taking shorter showers, fixing leaks, and washing cars, dishes, and clothes as efficiently as possible, can go a long way toward forestalling the water shortages that many authorities predict. Isn't it better to adapt to more conservative uses now when we have a choice than to be forced to do it by scarcity in the future?

Conserving appliances, such as low-volume shower heads and efficient dishwashers, can reduce water consumption greatly (see What Can You Do? p. 241). If you live in an arid part of the country, you might consider whether you really need a lush, green lawn that requires constant watering, feeding, and care. Planting native groundcover in a "natural lawn" or developing a rock garden or landscape in harmony with the surrounding ecosystem can be both ecologically sound and aesthetically pleasing (fig. 10.16). Cultivated lawns, golf courses, and parks in the United States use more water, fertilizer, and pesticides per hectare than any other kind of land.

Toilets are our greatest water user (fig. 10.17). Usually each flush uses several gallons of water to dispose of a few ounces of waste. Each person in the United States uses about 50,000 l (13,000 gal) of drinking-quality water annually to flush toilets. Low-flush toilets and composting toilets can drastically reduce

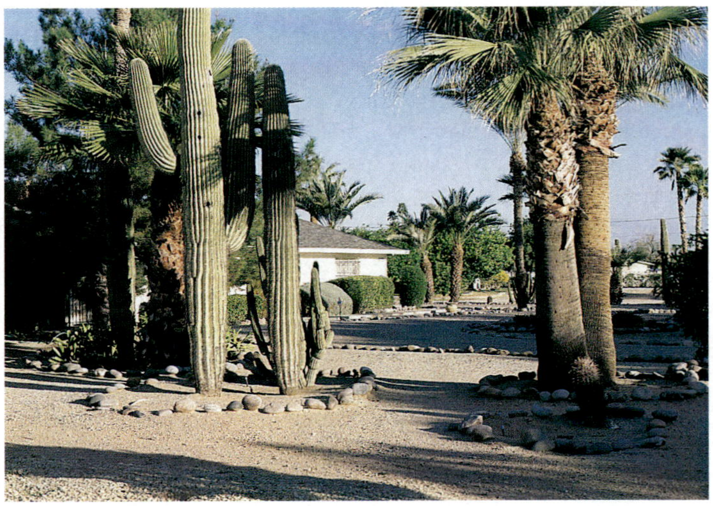

FIGURE 10.16 *By using native plants in a natural setting, residents of Phoenix save water and fit into the surrounding landscape.*

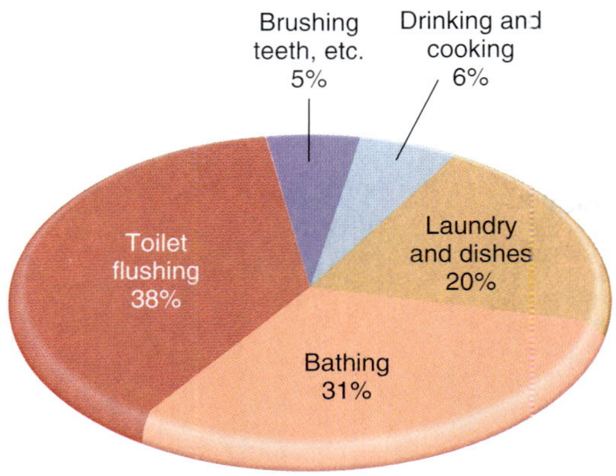

FIGURE 10.17 *Typical household water use in the United States.*
Source: Data from U.S. Environmental Protection Agency, 2004.

this water use. Low-flow shower heads can reduce our second-largest household water use.

These steps are so important that a number of cities (including Los Angeles, Orlando, Austin, and Phoenix) ordered that water-saving toilets, showers, and faucets be installed in all new buildings. The motivation was two-fold: to relieve overburdened sewer systems and to conserve water.

Significant amounts of water also can be reclaimed and recycled (see the section "Sewage Treatment"). California uses more than 555 million m^3 (450,000 acre-feet) of recycled water annually. That's equivalent to about two-thirds of the water consumed by Los Angeles every year.

Signs of Progress

Growing recognition that water is a precious and finite resource has changed policies and encouraged conservation across the United States. Despite a growing population, the United States is now saving some 144 million l (38 million gal) per day—a tenth the volume of Lake Erie—compared with per capita consumption rates of 20 years ago. With 37 million more people in the United States now than in 1980, we get by with 10 percent less water. New requirements for water-efficient fixtures and low-flush toilets in many cities help conserve water on the home front. More efficient irrigation methods on farms also are a major reason for the downward trend. New sprinkler systems have small spray heads just a foot or so above the plant tops and apply water much more directly. Even better is drip irrigation, which applies water directly to plant roots (see fig. 10.10). California and Florida farmers currently water about 500,000 ha with this technique.

Charging a higher proportion of real costs to users of public water projects has helped encourage conservation, and so have water marketing policies that allow prospective users to bid on water rights. Both the United States and Australia have had effective water pricing and allocation policies that encourage the most socially beneficial uses and discourage wasteful water uses. It will be important, as water markets develop, to be sure that environmental, recreational, and wildlife values are not sacrificed to the lure of high-bidding industrial and domestic users.

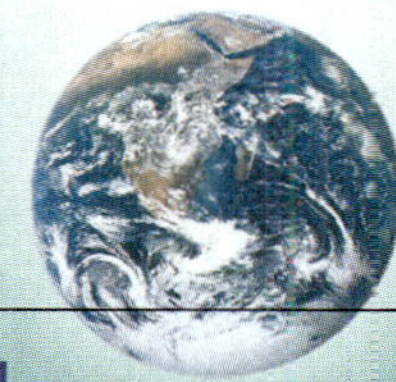

what can you do?

Saving Water and Preventing Pollution

Each of us can conserve much of the water we use and avoid water pollution in many simple ways.

- Don't flush every time you use the toilet. Take shorter showers, and shower instead of taking baths.
- Don't let the faucet run while brushing your teeth or washing dishes. Draw a basin of water for washing and another for rinsing dishes. Don't run the dishwasher when it's half full.
- Use water-conserving appliances: low-flow showers, low-flush toilets, and aerated faucets.
- Fix leaking faucets, tubs, and toilets. A leaky toilet can waste 50 gal per day. To check your toilet, add a few drops of dark food coloring to the tank and wait 15 minutes. If the tank is leaking, the water in the bowl will change color.
- Put a brick or full water bottle in your toilet tank to reduce the volume of water in each flush.
- Dispose of used motor oil, household hazardous waste, batteries, and so on responsibly. Don't dump anything down a storm sewer that you wouldn't want to drink.
- Avoid using toxic or hazardous chemicals for simple cleaning or plumbing jobs. A plunger or plumber's snake will often unclog a drain just as well as caustic acids or lye. Hot water and soap can accomplish most cleaning tasks.
- If you have a lawn, or know someone who does, use water, fertilizer, and pesticides sparingly. Plant native, low-maintenance plants that have low water needs.
- Use recycled (gray) water for lawns, house plants, and car washing.

WATER POLLUTION

Any physical, biological, or chemical change in water quality that adversely affects living organisms or makes water unsuitable for desired uses can be considered pollution. There are natural sources of water contamination, such as poison springs, oil seeps, and sedimentation from erosion, but here we will focus primarily on human-caused changes that affect water quality or usability.

Point and Nonpoint Source Pollution

Pollution control standards and regulations usually distinguish between point and nonpoint pollution sources. Factories, power plants, sewage treatment plants, underground coal mines, and oil wells are classified as **point sources** because they discharge pollution from specific locations, such as drain pipes, ditches, or sewer outfalls (fig. 10.18). These sources are discrete and identifiable, so they are relatively easy to monitor and regulate. It is generally

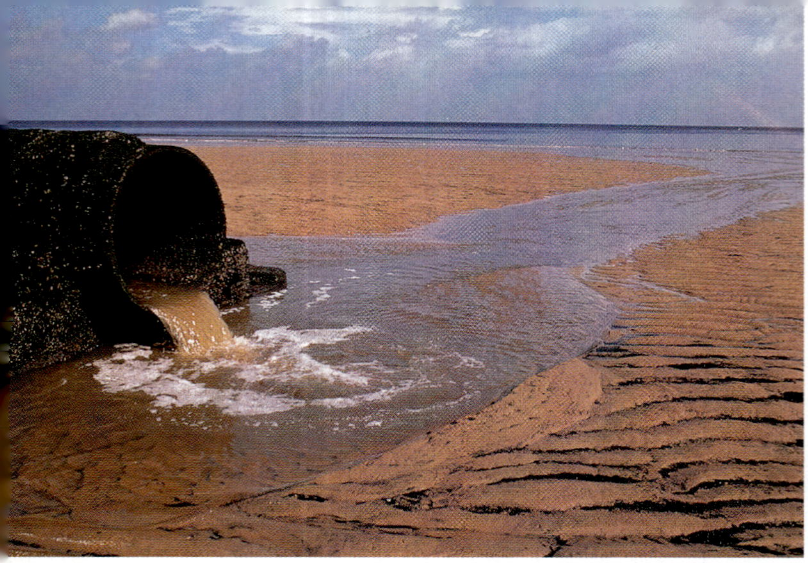

FIGURE 10.18 *Sewer outfalls, industrial effluent pipes, acid draining out of abandoned mines, and other point sources of pollution are generally easy to recognize.*

possible to divert effluent from the waste streams of these sources and treat it before it enters the environment.

In contrast, **nonpoint sources** of water pollution are diffuse, having no specific location where they discharge into a particular body of water. They are much harder to monitor and regulate than point sources because their sources are hard to identify. Nonpoint sources include runoff from farm fields and feedlots, golf courses, lawns and gardens, construction sites, logging areas, roads, streets, and parking lots (fig. 10.19). While point sources may be fairly uniform and predictable throughout the year, nonpoint sources are often highly episodic. The first heavy rainfall after a dry period may flush high concentrations of gasoline, lead, oil, and rubber residues off city streets, for instance, while subsequent runoff may be much cleaner.

Perhaps the ultimate in diffuse, nonpoint pollution is atmospheric deposition of contaminants carried by air currents and precipitated into watersheds or directly onto surface waters as rain, snow, or dry particles. The Great Lakes, for example, have been found to be accumulating industrial chemicals, such as PCBs (polychlorinated biphenyls) and dioxins, as well as agricultural toxins, such as the insecticide toxaphene, that cannot be accounted for by local sources alone. The nearest sources for many of these chemicals are sometimes thousands of kilometers away.

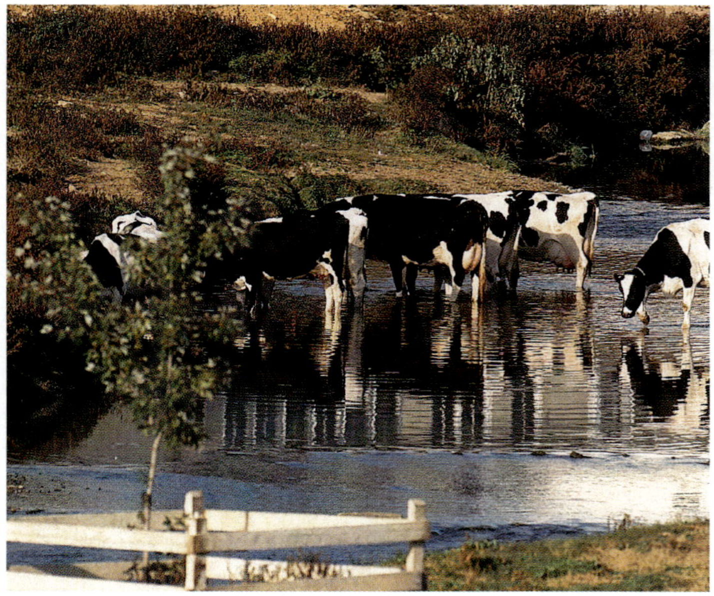

FIGURE 10.19 *This bucolic scene looks peaceful and idyllic, but allowing cows to trample stream banks is a major cause of bank erosion and water pollution. Nonpoint sources such as this have become the leading unresolved cause of stream and lake pollution in the United States.*

Biological Pollution

Although the types, sources, and effects of water pollutants are often interrelated, it is convenient to divide them into major categories for discussion (table 10.4). Here, we look at some of the important sources and effects of different pollutants.

TABLE 10.4 Major Categories of Water Pollutants

CATEGORY	EXAMPLES	SOURCES
CAUSE HEALTH PROBLEMS		
1. Infectious agents	Bacteria, viruses, parasites	Human and animal excreta
2. Organic chemicals	Pesticides, plastics, detergents, oil, gasoline	Industrial, household, and farm use
3. Inorganic chemicals	Acids, caustics, salts, metals	Industrial effluents, household cleansers, surface runoff
4. Radioactive materials	Uranium, thorium, cesium, iodine, radon	Mining and processing of ores, power plants, weapons production, natural sources
CAUSE ECOSYSTEM DISRUPTION		
1. Sediment	Soil, silt	Land erosion
2. Plant nutrients	Nitrates, phosphates, ammonium	Agricultural and urban fertilizers, sewage, manure
3. Oxygen-demanding wastes	Animal manure, plant residues	Sewage, agricultural runoff, paper mills, food processing
4. Thermal changes	Heat	Power plants, industrial cooling

Infectious Agents

The most serious water pollutants in terms of human health worldwide are pathogenic organisms (see chapter 8). Among the most important waterborne diseases are typhoid, cholera, bacterial and amoebic dysentery, enteritis, polio, infectious hepatitis, and schistosomiasis. Malaria, yellow fever, and filariasis are transmitted by insects that have aquatic larvae. Altogether, at least 25 million deaths each year are blamed on these water-related diseases. Nearly two-thirds of the mortalities of children under 5 years old are associated with waterborne diseases.

The main source of these pathogens is untreated or improperly treated human wastes. Animal wastes from feedlots or fields near waterways and food processing factories with inadequate waste treatment facilities also are sources of disease-causing organisms.

In developed countries, sewage treatment plants and other pollution-control techniques have reduced or eliminated most of the worst sources of pathogens in inland surface waters. Furthermore, drinking water is generally disinfected by chlorination, so epidemics of waterborne diseases are rare in these countries. The United Nations estimates that 90 percent of the people in developed countries have adequate (safe) sewage disposal, and 95 percent have clean drinking water.

The situation is quite different in less-developed countries, where billions of people lack adequate sanitation and access to clean drinking water. Conditions are especially bad in remote, rural areas, where sewage treatment is usually primitive or nonexistent and purified water is either unavailable or too expensive to obtain. The World Health Organization estimates that 80 percent of all sickness and disease in less-developed countries can be attributed to waterborne infectious agents and inadequate sanitation.

Fecal Coliform Bacteria and Oxygen Demand

Detecting specific pathogens in water is difficult, time-consuming, and costly, so water quality is usually described in terms of concentrations of **coliform bacteria**—any of the many types that live in the colon, or intestines, of humans and other animals. The most common of these is *Escherichia coli* (or *E. coli*), which lives symbiotically in many animals, but other bacteria, such as *Shigella, Salmonella,* or *Listeria,* can also cause fatal diseases. If any coliform bacteria are present in a water sample, infectious pathogens are usually assumed to be present also. Therefore, the Environmental Protection Agency (EPA) considers water with any coliform bacteria at all to be unsafe for drinking.

The amount of oxygen dissolved in water is a good indicator of water quality and of the kinds of life it will support. An oxygen content above 6 parts per million (ppm) will support game fish and other desirable forms of aquatic life. At oxygen levels below 2 ppm, water will support mainly worms, bacteria, fungi, and other detritus feeders and decomposers. Oxygen is added to water by diffusion from the air, especially when turbulence and mixing rates are high, and by photosynthesis of green plants, algae, and cyanobacteria. Therefore, turbulent, rapidly flowing water is constantly aerated, so it often recovers quickly from oxygen-depleting processes. Oxygen is removed from water by respiration and chemical processes that consume oxygen.

Adding organic materials, such as sewage or paper pulp, to water stimulates activity and oxygen consumption by decomposers. Consequently, **biochemical oxygen demand (BOD),** or the amount of dissolved oxygen consumed by aquatic microorganisms, is a standard measure of water contamination. Alternatively, chemical oxygen demand (COD) is a measure of all organic matter in water. In addition, **dissolved oxygen (DO) content** can be measured directly, with high DO levels indicating good-quality water.

Downstream from a point source, such as a municipal sewage plant discharge, a characteristic decline and restoration of water quality can be detected either by measuring DO content or by observing the types of flora and fauna that live in successive sections of the river. The oxygen decline downstream is called the **oxygen sag** (fig. 10.20). Upstream from the pollution source, oxygen levels support normal populations of clean-water organisms. Immediately below the source of pollution, oxygen levels begin to fall as decomposers metabolize waste materials. Trash fish, such as carp, bullheads, and gar, are able to survive in this oxygen-poor environment, where they eat both decomposer organisms and the waste itself.

Farther downstream, the water may become so oxygen depleted that only the most resistant microorganisms and invertebrates can survive. Eventually, most of the nutrients are used up, decomposer populations are smaller, and the water becomes oxygenated once again. Depending on the volumes and flow rates of the effluent plume and the river receiving it, normal communities may not appear for several miles downstream.

Plant Nutrients and Cultural Eutrophication

Water clarity (transparency) is affected by sediments, chemicals, and the abundance of plankton organisms; clarity is a useful measure of water quality and water pollution. Rivers and lakes that have clear water and low biological productivity are said to be **oligotrophic** (*oligo* = little + *trophic* = nutrition). By contrast, **eutrophic** (*eu* + *trophic* = well-nourished) waters are rich in organisms and organic materials. Eutrophication, an increase in nutrient levels and biological productivity, often accompanies successional changes (see chapter 5) in lakes. Tributary streams bring in sediments and nutrients that stimulate plant growth. Over time, ponds and lakes often fill in, becoming marshes or even terrestrial biomes. The rate of eutrophication depends on water chemistry and depth, volume of inflow, mineral content of the surrounding watershed, and biota of the lake itself.

Human activities can greatly accelerate eutrophication, an effect called **cultural eutrophication.** Cultural eutrophication is mainly caused by increased nutrient input into a water body. Increased productivity in an aquatic system sometimes can be beneficial. Fish and other desirable species may grow faster, providing a welcome food source. Often, however, eutrophication produces "blooms" of algae or thick growths of aquatic plants stimulated by elevated phosphorus or nitrogen levels (fig. 10.21). Bacterial populations then increase, fed by larger amounts of organic matter. The water often becomes cloudy, or turbid, and has unpleasant tastes and odors. Cultural eutrophication can accelerate the "aging" of a water body enormously over natural rates. Lakes

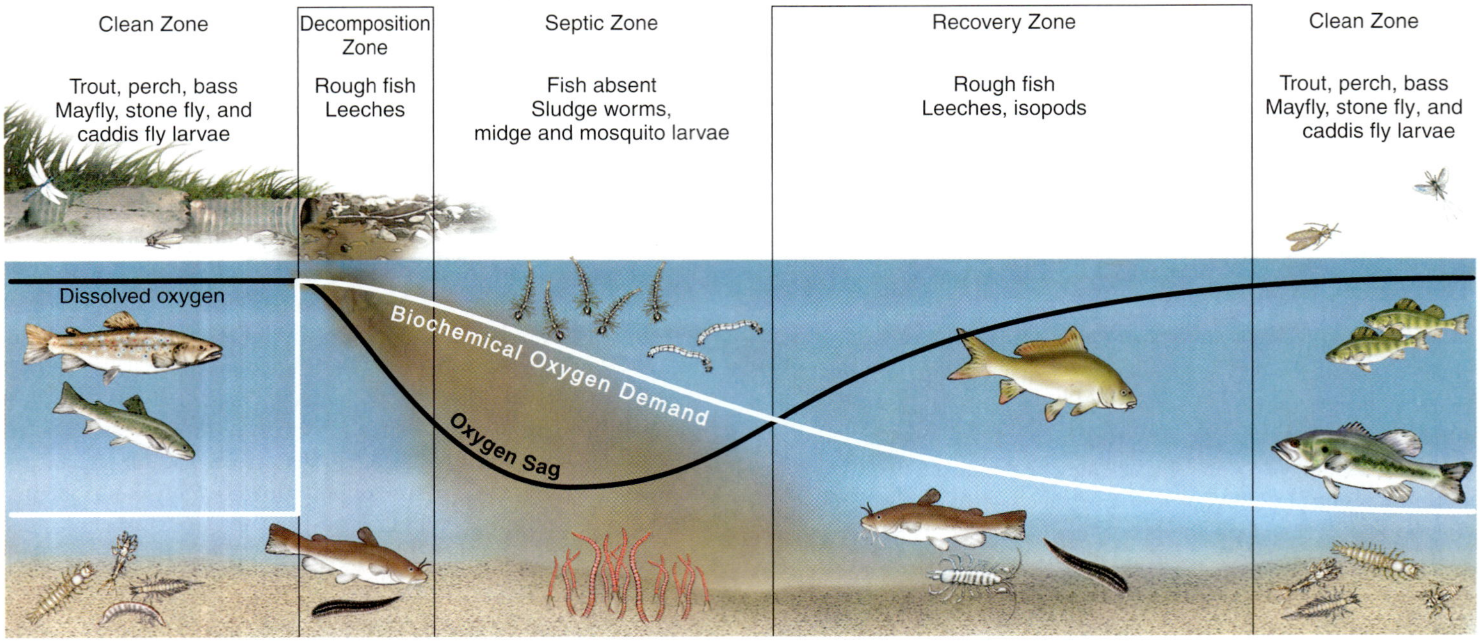

FIGURE 10.20 *Oxygen sag downstream of an organic source. A great deal of time and distance may be required for the stream and its inhabitants to recover.*

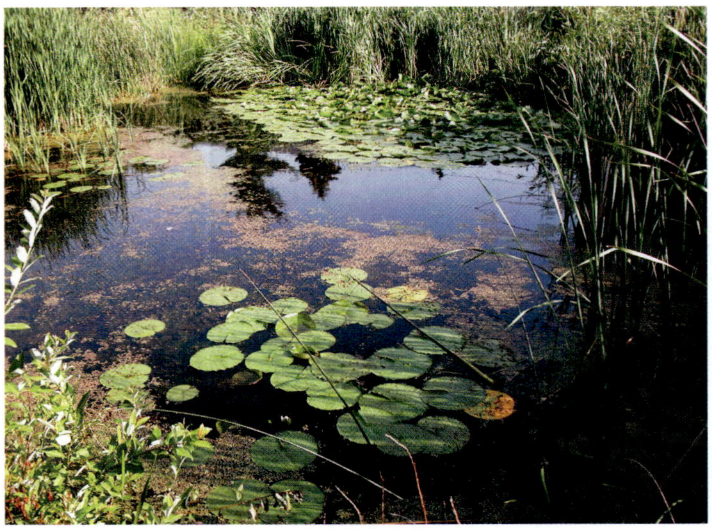

FIGURE 10.21 *Eutrophic lake. Nutrients from agriculture and domestic sources have stimulated growth of algae and aquatic plants. This reduces water quality, alters species composition, and lowers the lake's recreational and aesthetic values.*

and reservoirs that normally might exist for hundreds or thousands of years can be filled in a matter of decades.

Eutrophication also occurs in marine ecosystems, especially in nearshore waters and partially enclosed bays or estuaries. Partially enclosed seas, such as the Black, Baltic, and Mediterranean Seas, tend to be in especially critical condition. During the tourist season, the coastal population of the Mediterranean, for example, swells to 200 million people. Eighty-five percent of the effluents from large cities go untreated into the sea. Beach pollution, fish kills, and contaminated shellfish result. Extensive "dead zones" often form where rivers dump nutrients into estuaries and shallow seas. The largest in the world occurs during summer months in the Gulf of Mexico at the mouth of the Mississippi River. This hypoxic (oxygen-depleted) zone can cover 21,000 km^2, or about the area of New Hampshire. A federal study of the condition of U.S. coastal waters announced in 2004 that 28 percent of estuaries are impaired for aquatic life, and 80 percent of all coastal water is in fair to poor condition.

Toxic Tides

Excessive nutrients support blooms of deadly aquatic microorganisms in polluted nearshore waters. Red tides—and other colors, depending on the species involved—have become increasingly common where nutrients and wastes wash down rivers.

One of the most feared of these organisms is *Pfiesteria piscicida,* an extraordinarily poisonous dinoflagellate that only recently has been recognized as a killer of fish and shellfish in polluted rivers and estuaries. In North Carolina's Pamlico Sound, *Pfiesteria* kills hundreds of thousands to millions of fish annually. Dinoflagellates are peculiar organisms with complex life cycles and many different shapes. *Pfiesteria* can change into at least two dozen distinct forms and sizes, depending on water temperature, turbulence, and food supply. The right conditions can cause a population explosion. If fish blunder into this profuse swarm, *Pfiesteria* quickly turn into a toxic, swimming form that attacks with soluble poisons. These toxins produce skin lesions and paralyze fish, so they can't escape. The predatory *Pfiesteria* feed on both the flesh and the oozing sores.

Humans are harmed if they eat contaminated seafood or even if they breathe airborne *Pfiesteria* cells or secretions. Symptoms of *Pfiesteria* poisoning include headaches, blurred vision, aching joints, difficulty breathing, memory loss, and long-term damage to the brain, liver, and other organs. (See related story "A Flood of Pigs" at www.mhhe.com/cases.)

Inorganic Pollutants

Some toxic inorganic chemicals are naturally released into water from rocks by weathering processes (see chapter 11). Humans accelerate the transfer rates in these cycles thousands of times above natural background levels by mining, processing, using, and discarding minerals.

Among the chemicals of greatest concern are heavy metals, such as mercury, lead, tin, and cadmium. Supertoxic elements, such as selenium and arsenic, also have reached hazardous levels in some waters. Other inorganic materials, such as acids, salts, nitrates, and chlorine, that are nontoxic at low concentrations may become concentrated enough to lower water quality and adversely affect biological communities.

Metals

Many metals, such as mercury, lead, cadmium, and nickel, are highly toxic in minute concentrations. Because metals are highly persistent, they accumulate in food chains and have a cumulative effect in humans.

Currently the most widespread toxic metal contamination in North America is mercury released from incinerators and coal-burning power plants. Transported through the air, mercury precipitates in water supplies, where it bioconcentrates in food webs to reach dangerous levels in top predators. As a general rule, Americans are warned not to eat more than one meal of fish per week. Top marine predators, such as shark, swordfish, bluefin tuna, and king mackerel, tend to have especially high mercury content. Pregnant women and small children should avoid these species entirely. Public health officials estimate that 600,000 American children now have mercury levels in their bodies high enough to cause mental and developmental problems, while one woman in six in the United States has blood-mercury concentrations that would endanger a fetus.

Mine drainage and leaching of mining wastes are serious sources of metal pollution in water. A survey of water quality in eastern Tennessee found that 43 percent of all surface streams and lakes and more than half of all groundwater used for drinking supplies were contaminated by acids and metals from mine drainage. In some cases, metal levels were 200 times higher than what is considered safe for drinking water.

Nonmetallic Salts

Some soils contain high concentrations of soluble salts, including toxic selenium and arsenic (see Case Study, p. 246). You have probably heard of poison springs and seeps in the desert, where percolating groundwater brings these compounds to the surface. Irrigation and drainage of desert soils can mobilize these materials on a larger scale and result in serious pollution problems, as in Kesterson Marsh in California, where selenium poisoning killed thousands of migratory birds in the 1980s.

Salts, such as sodium chloride (table salt), that are nontoxic at low concentrations also can be mobilized by irrigation and concentrated by evaporation, reaching levels that are toxic for plants and animals. Salinity levels in the Colorado River and surrounding farm fields have become so high in recent years that millions of hectares of valuable croplands have had to be abandoned. In northern states, millions of tons of sodium chloride and calcium chloride are used to melt road ice in the winter. Leaching of road salts into surface waters has a devastating effect on some aquatic ecosystems.

Acids and Bases

Acids are released as by-products of industrial processes, such as leather tanning, metal smelting and plating, petroleum distillation, and organic chemical synthesis. Coal mining is an especially important source of acid water pollution. Sulfur compounds in coal react with oxygen and water to make sulfuric acid. Thousands of kilometers of streams in the United States have been acidified by acid mine drainage, some so severely that they are essentially lifeless.

Acid precipitation (see chapter 9) also acidifies surface-water systems. In addition to damaging living organisms directly, these acids leach aluminum and other elements from soil and rock, further destabilizing ecosystems.

Organic Chemicals

Thousands of different natural and synthetic organic chemicals are used in the chemical industry to make pesticides, plastics, pharmaceuticals, pigments, and other products that we use in everyday life. Many of these chemicals are highly toxic (see chapter 8). Exposure to very low concentrations (perhaps even parts per quadrillion, in the case of dioxins) can cause birth defects, genetic disorders, and cancer. Some can persist in the environment because they are resistant to degradation and toxic to organisms that ingest them.

The two principal sources of toxic organic chemicals in water are (1) improper disposal of industrial and household wastes and (2) pesticide runoff from farm fields, forests, roadsides, golf courses, and private lawns. The EPA estimates that about 500,000 metric tons of pesticides are used in the United States each year. Much of this material washes into the nearest waterway, where it passes through ecosystems and may accumulate in high levels in nontarget organisms. The bioaccumulation of DDT in aquatic ecosystems was one of the first of these pathways to be understood (see chapter 3). Dioxins and other chlorinated hydrocarbons (hydrocarbon molecules that contain chlorine atoms) have been shown to accumulate to dangerous levels in the fat of salmon, fish-eating birds, and humans and to cause health problems similar to those resulting from toxic metal compounds.

Hundreds of millions of tons of hazardous organic wastes are thought to be stored in dumps, landfills, lagoons, and underground

CASE STUDY

ARSENIC IN DRINKING WATER

When we think of water pollution, we usually visualize sewage or industrial effluents pouring out of a discharge pipe, but there are natural toxins that threaten us as well. One of these is arsenic, a common contaminate in drinking water that may be poisoning millions of people around the world. Arsenic has been known since the fourth century B.C. to be a potent poison. It has been used for centuries as a rodenticide, insecticide, and weed killer, as well as a way of assassinating enemies. Because it isn't metabolized or excreted from the body, arsenic accumulates in hair and fingernails, where it can be detected long after death. Napoleon Bonaparte was recently found to have high enough levels of arsenic in his body to suggest he was poisoned.

Perhaps the largest population to be threatened by naturally occurring groundwater contamination by arsenic is in West Bengal, India, and adjacent areas of Bangladesh. Arsenic occurs naturally in the sediments that make up the Ganges River delta (see map). Rapid population growth, industrialization, and intensification of agricultural irrigation, however, have put increasing stresses on the limited surface-water supplies. Most surface water is too contaminated to drink, so groundwater has all but replaced other water sources for most people in this region.

In the 1960s, thousands of deep tube wells were sunk throughout the region to improve water supplies. Much of this humanitarian effort was financed by loans from the World Bank. At first, villagers were suspicious of well water, regarding it as unnatural and possibly evil. But as surface-water supplies diminished and populations grew, Bengal and Bangladesh became more and more dependent on this new source of supposedly fresh, clean water. By the late 1980s, health workers had become aware of widespread signs of chronic arsenic poisoning among villagers. Symptoms include watery and inflamed eyes, gastrointestinal cramps, gradual loss of strength, scaly skin and skin tumors, anemia, confusion, and eventually death.

Why is arsenic poisoning appearing now? Part of the reason is increased dependence on well water, but some villages have had wells for centuries with no problem. One theory is that excessive withdrawals now lower the water table during the dry season, exposing arsenic-bearing minerals to air, which converts normally insoluble salts to soluble oxides. When aquifers are refilled during the next rainy season, dissolved arsenic can be pumped out. Health workers estimate that the total number of potential victims in India and Bangladesh may exceed 200 million people. But with no other source of easily accessible or affordable water, few of the poorest people have much choice.

There are worries that millions of Americans also are exposed to dangerously high levels of arsenic. In 1942 the U.S. government set the acceptable level of arsenic in drinking water at 50 ppb. A 1999 study by the National Academy of Sciences found a 1 in 100 risk for cancer from drinking water with that level of arsenic for a lifetime. This is 10,000 times the normally accepted risk level. Following years of heated debate, the U.S. limit was revised in 2002 to meet the World Health Organization standard of 10 ppb. Local officials and private water supply owners argued that it would cost too much to upgrade their systems.

In the end, public outrage over tainted water, combined with the enormous public health costs of chronic arsenic poisoning, convinced the federal government to enforce stricter standards.

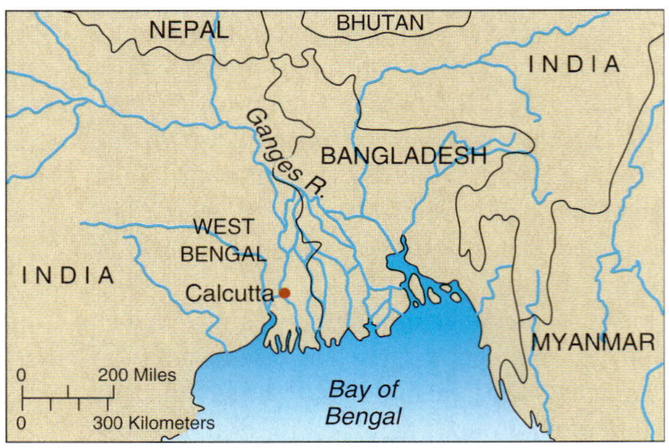

West Bengal and adjoining areas of Bangladesh have hundreds of millions of people who may be exposed to dangerous arsenic levels in well water.

tanks in the United States (see chapter 13). Many, perhaps most, of these sites have leaked toxic chemicals into surface waters, groundwater, or both. The EPA estimates that about 26,000 hazardous waste sites will require cleanup because they pose an imminent threat to public health, mostly through water pollution.

Sediment and Thermal Pollution

Sediment is a natural and necessary part of river systems. Sediment fertilizes floodplains and creates fertile deltas. But human activities, chiefly farming and urbanization, greatly accelerate erosion and increase sediment loads in rivers. Silt and sediment are considered the largest source of water pollution in the United States, being responsible for 40 percent of the impaired river miles in EPA water quality surveys. Cropland erosion contributes about 25 billion metric tons of soil, sediment, and suspended solids to world surface waters each year. Forest disturbance, road building, urban construction sites, and other sources add at least 50 billion additional tons.

This sediment fills lakes and reservoirs, obstructs shipping channels, clogs hydroelectric turbines, and makes purification of drinking water more costly. Sediments smother gravel beds in which insects take refuge and fish lay their eggs. Sunlight is blocked, so that plants cannot carry out photosynthesis, and oxygen levels decline. Murky, cloudy water also is less attractive for swimming, boating, fishing, and other recreational uses (fig. 10.22). Sediment washed into the ocean clogs estuaries and coral reefs.

Thermal pollution, usually effluent from cooling systems of power plants or other industries, alters water temperature. Raising or lowering water temperatures from normal levels can adversely affect water quality and aquatic life. Water temperatures are usually much more stable than air temperatures, so aquatic organisms tend to be poorly adapted to rapid temperature changes. Lowering the temperature of tropical oceans by even 1° can be lethal to some corals and other reef species. Raising water temperatures can have similar devastating effects on sensitive organisms. Oxygen solubility in water decreases as temperatures increase, so species requiring high oxygen levels are adversely affected by warming water.

Humans also cause thermal pollution by altering vegetation cover and runoff patterns. Reducing water flow, clearing streamside trees, and adding sediment all make water warmer and alter the ecosystems in a lake or stream.

Warm-water plumes from power plants often attract fish and birds, which find food and refuge there, especially in cold weather. This artificial environment can be a fatal trap, however. Florida's manatees, an endangered mammal, are attracted to the abundant food supply and warm water in power plant thermal plumes. Often they are enticed into spending the winter much farther north than they normally would. On several occasions, a midwinter power plant breakdown has exposed a dozen or more of these rare animals to a sudden, deadly thermal shock.

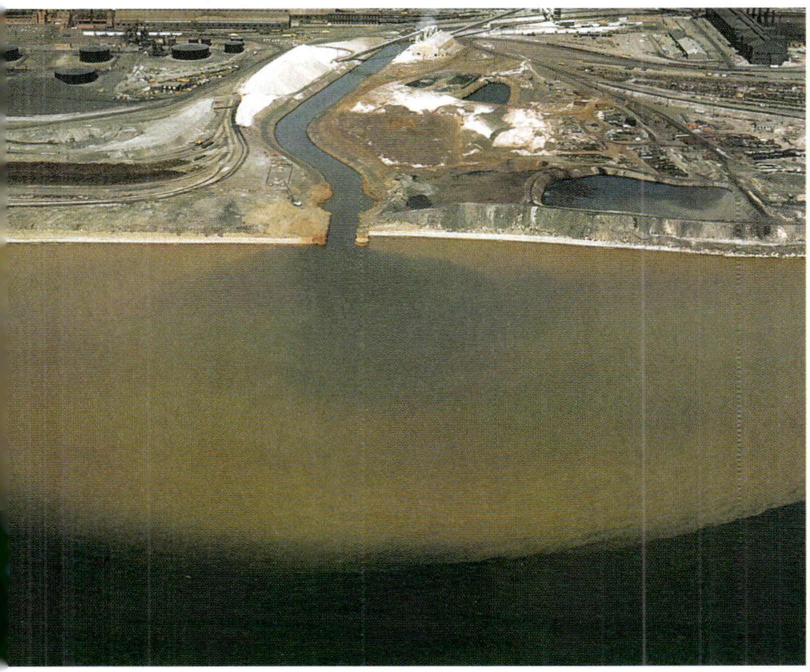

FIGURE 10.22 *Sediment and industrial waste flow from this drainage canal into Lake Erie.*

WATER QUALITY TODAY

Surface-water pollution is often both highly visible and one of the most common threats to environmental quality. In more developed countries, reducing water pollution has been a high priority over the past few decades. Billions of dollars have been spent on control programs, and considerable progress has been made. Still, much remains to be done.

Surface Waters in the United States and Canada

Like most developed countries, the United States and Canada have made encouraging progress in protecting and restoring water quality in rivers and lakes over the past 40 years. In 1948 only about one-third of Americans were served by municipal sewage systems, and most of those systems discharged sewage without any treatment or with only primary treatment (the bigger lumps of waste are removed). Most people depended on cesspools and septic systems to dispose of domestic wastes.

Areas of Progress

The 1972 Clean Water Act established a National Pollution Discharge Elimination System (NPDES), which requires an easily revoked permit for any industry, municipality, or other entity dumping wastes in surface waters. The permit requires disclosure of what is being dumped and gives regulators valuable data and evidence for litigation. As a consequence, only about 10 percent of our water pollution now comes from industrial and municipal point sources. One of the biggest improvements has been in sewage treatment.

Since the Clean Water Act was passed in 1972, the United States has spent more than $180 billion in public funds and perhaps ten times as much in private investments on water pollution control. Most of that effort has been aimed at point sources, especially to build or upgrade thousands of municipal sewage treatment plants. As a result, nearly everyone in urban areas is now served by municipal sewage systems, and no major city discharges raw sewage into a river or lake except as overflow during heavy rainstorms.

This campaign has led to significant improvements in surface-water quality in many places. Fish and aquatic insects have returned to waters that formerly were depleted of life-giving oxygen. Swimming and other water-contact sports are again permitted in rivers, in lakes, and at ocean beaches that once were closed by health officials.

The Clean Water Act goal of making all U.S. surface waters "fishable and swimmable" has not been fully met, but in 2003 the EPA reported that 91 percent of all monitored river miles and 88 percent of all assessed lake acres are suitable for their designated uses. This sounds good, but you have to remember that not all water bodies are monitored. Furthermore, the designated goal for some rivers and lakes is merely to be "boatable." Water quality doesn't have to be very high to be able to put a boat on it. Even in "fishable" rivers and lakes, there isn't a guarantee that you can catch anything other than rough fish, such as carp or bullheads, nor can you be sure that what you catch is safe to eat. Even with billions of dollars of investment in sewage treatment plants, elimination of much of the industrial dumping and other gross sources of pollutants, and a general improvement in water quality, the EPA reports that 21,000 water bodies still do not meet their designated uses. According to the EPA, an overwhelming majority of the American people—almost 218 million—live within 16 km (10 mi) of an impaired water body.

In 1998 a new regulatory approach to water quality assurance was instituted by the EPA. Rather than issue standards on a river by river approach or factory-by-factory permit discharge, the focus was changed to watershed-level monitoring and protection. Some 4,000 watersheds are now monitored for water quality (fig. 10.23). You can find information about your watershed at www.epa.gov/owow/tmdl/. The intention of this program is to give the public more and better information about the health of their watersheds. In addition, states can have greater flexibility as they identify impaired water bodies and set priorities, and new tools can be used to achieve goals. States are required to identify waters not meeting water quality goals and to develop **total maximum daily loads (TMDL)** for each pollutant and each listed water body. A TMDL is the amount of a particular pollutant that a water body can receive from both point and nonpoint sources. It considers seasonal variation and includes a margin of safety.

By 1999, all 56 U.S. states and territories had submitted TMDL lists, and the EPA had approved most of them. Of the 5.6 million km of rivers monitored, only 480,000 km fail to meet their clean water goals. Similarly, of 40 million lake ha, only 12.5 percent (in about 20,000 lakes) fail to meet their goal. To give states more flexibility in planning, the EPA has proposed new rules that include allowances for reasonably foreseeable increases in pollutant loadings to encourage "Smart Growth." In the future, TMDLs also will include load allocations from all nonpoint sources, including air deposition and natural background levels.

An encouraging example of improved water quality is seen in Lake Erie. Although widely regarded as "dead" in the 1960s, the lake today is promoted as the "walleye capital of the world." Bacteria counts and algae blooms have decreased more than 90 percent since 1962. Water that once was murky brown is now clear. Interestingly, part of the improved water quality is due to immense numbers of exotic zebra mussels, which filter the lake water very efficiently. Swimming is now officially safe along 96 percent of the lake's shoreline. Nearly 40,000 nesting pairs of double-crested cormorants nest in the Great Lakes region, up from only about 100 in the 1970s.

Canada's 1970 Water Act has produced comparable results. Seventy percent of all Canadians in towns over 1,000 population are now served by some form of municipal sewage treatment. In Ontario, the vast majority of those systems include tertiary treatment. After ten years of controls, phosphorus levels in the Bay of Quinte in the northeast corner of Lake Ontario have dropped nearly by half, and algal blooms that once turned waters green are less frequent and less intense than they once were. Elimination of mercury discharges from a pulp and paper mill on the Wabigoon-English River system in western Ontario has resulted in a dramatic decrease in mercury contamination. Twenty years ago this mercury contamination was causing developmental retardation in local residents. Extensive flooding associated with hydropower projects has raised mercury levels in fish to dangerous levels elsewhere, however.

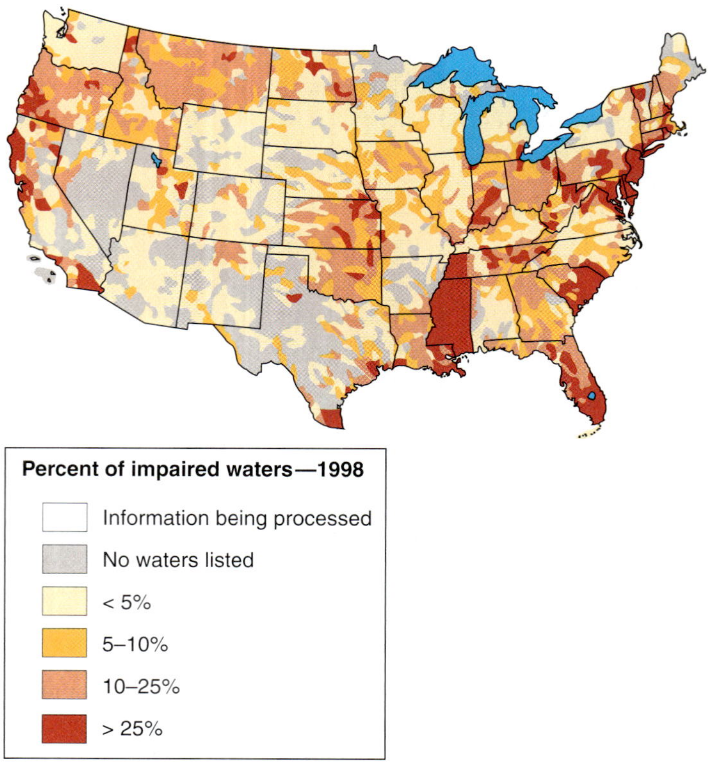

FIGURE 10.23 *Percent of impaired U.S. rivers in the contiguous 48 states by watershed in 1998.*
Source: Data from U.S. Environmental Protection Agency, 1999.

Remaining Problems

The greatest impediments to achieving national goals in water quality in both the United States and Canada are sediment, nutrients, and pathogens, especially from nonpoint discharges of pollutants. These sources are harder to identify and to reduce or treat than are specific point sources. About three-fourths of the water pollution in the United States comes from soil erosion, fallout of air pollutants, and surface runoff from urban areas, farm fields, and feedlots. In the United States, as much as 25 percent of the

46,800,000 metric tons (52 million tons) of fertilizer spread on farmland each year is carried away by runoff (fig. 10.24).

Cattle in feedlots produce some 129,600,000 metric tons (144 million tons) of manure each year, and the runoff from these sites is rich in viruses, bacteria, nitrates, phosphates, and other contaminants. A single cow produces about 30 kg (66 lbs) of manure per day, or about as much as that produced by ten people. Some feedlots have 100,000 animals with no provision for capturing or treating runoff water. Imagine drawing your drinking water downstream from such a facility. Pets also can be a problem. It is estimated that the wastes from about a half million dogs in New York City are disposed of primarily through storm sewers and therefore do not go through sewage treatment.

Loading of both nitrates and phosphates in surface water have decreased from point sources but have increased about fourfold since 1972 from nonpoint sources. Fossil fuel combustion has become a major source of nitrates, sulfates, arsenic, cadmium, mercury, and other toxic pollutants that find their way into water. Carried to remote areas by atmospheric transport, these combustion products now are found nearly everywhere in the world. Toxic organic compounds, such as DDT, PCBs, and dioxins, also are transported long distances by wind currents.

Surface Waters in Other Countries

Japan, Australia, and most of Western Europe also have improved surface-water quality in recent years. Sewage treatment in the wealthier countries of Europe generally equals or surpasses that in the United States. Sweden, for instance, serves 98 percent of its population with at least secondary sewage treatment (compared with 70 percent in the United States), and the other 2 percent have primary treatment. Poorer countries have much less to spend on sanitation. Spain serves only 18 percent of its population with even primary sewage treatment. In Ireland, it is only 11 percent, and in Greece, less than 1 percent of the people have even primary treatment. Most of the sewage, both domestic and industrial, is dumped directly into the ocean.

The fall of the "iron curtain" in 1989 revealed appalling environmental conditions in much of the former Soviet Union and its satellite states in Eastern and central Europe. The countries closest geographically and socially to Western Europe, the Czech Republic, Hungary, former East Germany, and Poland, have made massive investments and encouraging progress toward cleaning up environmental problems. Parts of Russia itself, however, along with former socialist states in the Balkans and central Asia, remain some of the most polluted places on earth. In Russia, for example, only about half the tap water is fit to drink. In cities such as St. Petersburg, even boiling and filtering aren't enough to make municipal water safe. About one-third of all Russians live in regions where air pollution levels are ten times higher than World Health Organization safety standards. Life expectancies for Russian men have plummeted from about 72 years in 1980 to 59 years in 2003. Deaths now exceed births in Russia by about 1 million per year. Only about one-quarter of all Russian children are considered healthy. In heavily industrialized cities, such as Magnitogorsk, a steel-manufacturing center in the Ural Mountains, nine out of ten children suffer from pollution-related illnesses and birth defects.

High levels of radioactivity from the Chernobyl nuclear power plant accident in 1986 remain in many former Eastern Bloc countries. The Danube River, which originates in Bavaria and Austria and flows through Slovakia, Poland, Hungary, Serbia, Romania, and Bulgaria before emptying into the Black Sea, illustrates some of the problems besetting the area. Draining a landscape with a long history of unregulated mining and heavy industry, the Danube carries chrome, copper, mercury, lead, zinc, and oil to the Black Sea at 20 times the levels these materials flow into the North Sea. Just one city, Bratislava, the capital of Slovakia, dumps 73 million m^3 (about 2 billion gal) of industrial and municipal wastes into the river each year. With a population of about 100 million people in its catchment area, the beautiful blue Danube isn't blue anymore. Bombing in Serbia during the Kosovo War in 1999 further exacerbated the situation by releasing oil, industrial chemicals, agricultural fertilizers, pesticides, and other toxic materials into the Danube.

However, there are some encouraging pollution-control stories. In 1997 Minamata Bay in Japan, long synonymous with mercury poisoning, was declared officially clean again. Another important success is found in Europe, where one of its most important rivers has been cleaned up significantly through international cooperation. The Rhine, which starts in the rugged Swiss Alps and winds 1,320 km through five countries before emptying through a Dutch delta into the North Sea, has long been a major commercial artery into the heart of Europe. More than 50 million

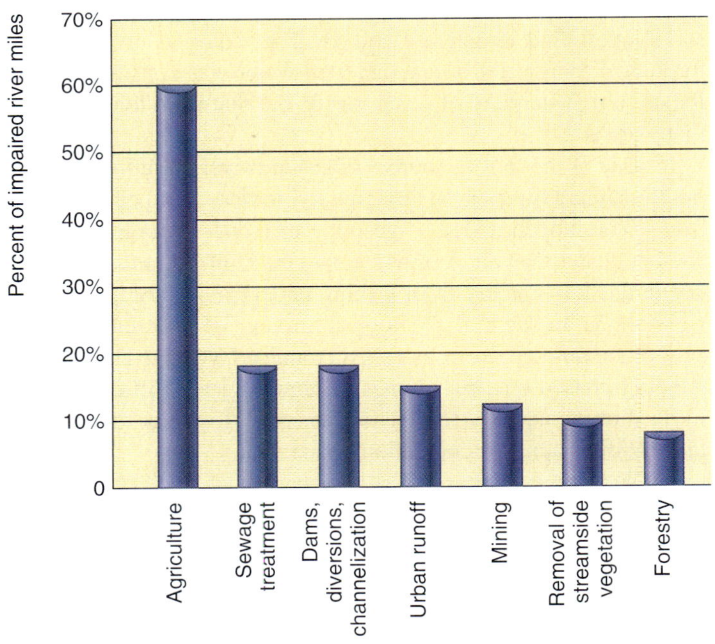

FIGURE 10.24 *Percentage of impaired river miles in the United States by source of damage. Totals add up to more than 100 percent because one river can be affected by many sources.*

Source: Data from USDA and Natural Resources Conservation Service, *America's Private Land: A Geography of Hope*, USDA, 1996.

people live in its catchment basin, and nearly 20 million get their drinking water from the river or its tributaries. By the 1970s, the Rhine had become so polluted that dozens of fish species disappeared and swimming was discouraged along most of its length.

Efforts to clean up this historic and economically important waterway began in the 1950s, but a disastrous fire at a chemical warehouse near Basel, Switzerland, in 1986 provided the impetus for major changes. Through a long and sometimes painful series of international conventions and compromises, land-use practices, waste disposal, urban runoff, and industrial dumping have been changed and water quality has significantly improved. Oxygen concentrations have gone up five-fold since 1970 (from less than 2 mg/l to nearly 10 mg/l, or about 90 percent of saturation) in long stretches of the river. Chemical oxygen demand has fallen five-fold during the same period, and organochlorine levels have decreased as much as ten-fold. Many species of fish and aquatic invertebrates have returned to the river. In 1992, for the first time in decades, mature salmon were caught in the Rhine.

The less-developed countries of South America, Africa, and Asia have even worse water quality than do the poorer countries of Europe. Sewage treatment is usually either totally lacking or woefully inadequate. In urban areas, 95 percent of all sewage is discharged untreated into rivers, lakes, or the ocean. Low technological capabilities and little money for pollution control are made even worse by burgeoning populations, rapid urbanization, and the shift of much heavy industry (especially the dirtier ones) from developed countries where pollution laws are strict to less-developed countries where regulations are more lenient.

Appalling environmental conditions often result from these combined factors (fig. 10.25). Two-thirds of India's surface waters are contaminated sufficiently to be considered dangerous to human health. The Yamuna River in New Delhi has 7,500 coliform bacteria per 100 ml (37 times the level considered safe for swimming in the United States) *before* entering the city. The coliform count increases to an incredible 24 *million* cells per 100 ml as the river leaves the city! At the same time, the river picks up some 20 million liters of industrial effluents every day from New Delhi. It's no wonder that disease rates are high and life expectancy is low in this area. Only 1 percent of India's towns and cities have any sewage treatment, and only eight cities have anything beyond primary treatment.

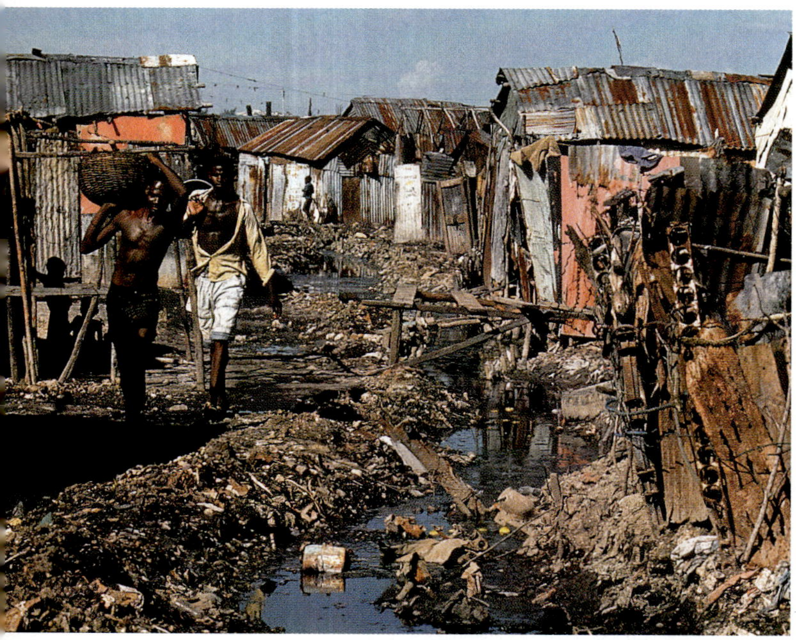

FIGURE 10.25 *Ditches in this Haitian slum serve as open sewers, into which all manner of refuse and waste are dumped. The health risks of living under these conditions are severe.*

In Malaysia, 42 of 50 major rivers are reported to be "ecological disasters." Residues from palm oil and rubber manufacturing, along with heavy erosion from logging of tropical rainforests, have destroyed all higher forms of life in most of these rivers. In the Philippines, domestic sewage makes up 60 to 70 percent of the total volume of Manila's Pasig River. Thousands of people use the river not only for bathing and washing clothes but also as their source of drinking and cooking water. China treats only 2 percent of its sewage. Of 78 monitored rivers in China, 54 are reported to be seriously polluted. Of 44 major cities in China, 41 use "contaminated" water supplies, and few do more than rudimentary treatment before it is delivered to the public.

Groundwater and Drinking-Water Supplies

About half the people in the United States, including 95 percent of those in rural areas, depend on underground aquifers for their drinking water. This vital resource is threatened in many areas by overuse and pollution and by a wide variety of industrial, agricultural, and domestic contaminants. For decades it was widely assumed that groundwater was impervious to pollution because soil would bind chemicals and cleanse water as it percolated through. Springwater or artesian well water was considered to be the definitive standard of water purity, but that is no longer true in many areas.

One of the serious sources of groundwater pollution throughout the United States is MTBE (methyl tertiary butyl ether), a suspected carcinogen added to gasoline to reduce carbon monoxide and ozone in urban air. Aquifers across the United States have been contaminated—mainly from leaking underground storage tanks at gas stations. In one U.S. Geological Survey (USGS) study, 27 percent of shallow urban wells tested contained MTBE. The additive is being phased out, but plumes of tainted water will continue to move through aquifers for decades to come. Liability for this contamination is a highly contentious issue.

The EPA estimates that every day some 4.5 trillion l (1.2 trillion gal) of contaminated water seep into the ground in the United States from septic tanks, cesspools, municipal and industrial landfills and waste disposal sites, surface impoundments, agricultural fields, forests, and wells (fig. 10.26). The most toxic of these are probably waste disposal sites. Agricultural chemicals and wastes are responsible for the largest total volume of pollutants and area affected. Because deep underground aquifers often have residence times of thousands of years, many contaminants are extremely stable once underground. It is possible, but expensive, to pump water out of aquifers, clean it, and then pump it back.

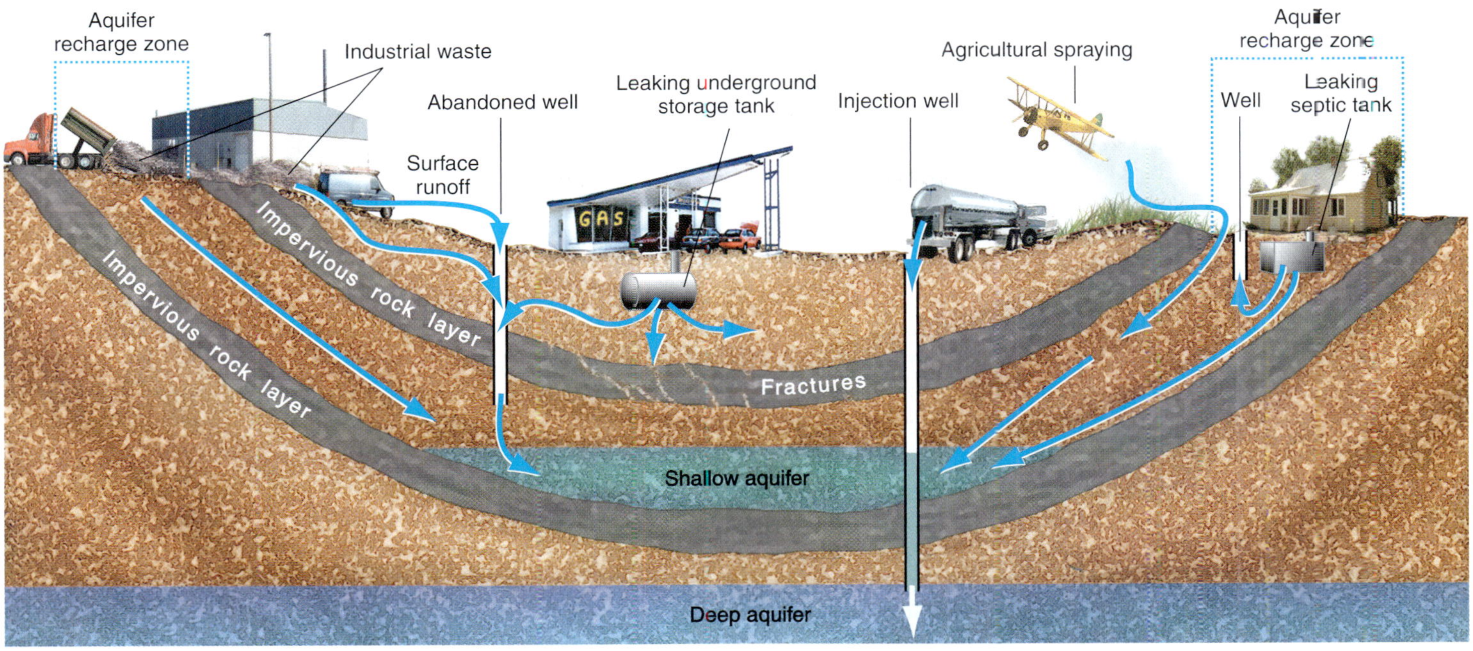

FIGURE 10.26 *Sources of groundwater pollution. Septic systems, landfills, and industrial activities on aquifer recharge zones leach contaminants into aquifers. Wells provide a direct route for injection of pollutants into aquifers.*

In farm country, especially in the Midwest's corn belt, fertilizers and pesticides commonly contaminate aquifers and wells. Herbicides such as atrazine and alachlor are widely used on corn and soybeans and show up in about half of all wells in Iowa, for example. Nitrates from fertilizers often exceed safety standards in rural drinking water. These high nitrate levels are dangerous to infants (nitrates combine with hemoglobin in the blood and result in "blue-baby" syndrome).

Every year, epidemiologists estimate that around 1.5 million Americans fall ill from infections caused by fecal contamination. In 1993, for instance, a pathogen called cryptosporidium got into the Milwaukee public water system, making 400,000 people sick and killing at least 100 people. The total costs of these diseases amount to billions of dollars per year. Preventative measures, such as protecting water sources and aquifer recharge zones and updating treatment and distribution systems, would cost far less.

Ocean Pollution

Although we don't use ocean waters directly, ocean pollution is serious and one of the fastest-growing water pollution problems. Coastal bays, estuaries, shoals, and reefs are often overwhelmed by pollution. Dead zones and poisonous algal blooms are increasingly widespread. Toxic chemicals, heavy metals, oil, sediment, and plastic refuse affect some of the most attractive and productive ocean regions. The potential losses caused by this pollution amount to billions of dollars each year. In terms of quality of life, the costs are incalculable.

Discarded plastic flotsam and jetsam are becoming a ubiquitous mark of human impact on the oceans. Since plastic is lightweight and nonbiodegradable, it is carried thousands of miles on ocean currents and lasts for years. Even the most remote beaches of distant islands are likely to have bits of polystyrene foam containers or polyethylene packing material that were discarded half a world away. It has been estimated that 6 million metric tons of plastic bottles, packaging material, and other litter are tossed from ships every year into the ocean, where they ensnare and choke seabirds, mammals, and even fish (fig. 10.27).

Oil pollution affects beaches and open seas around the world. Oceanographers estimate that between 3 million and 6 million

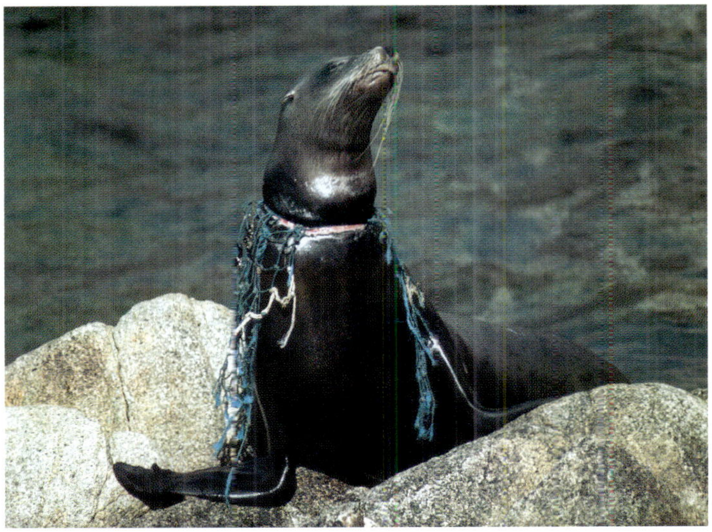

FIGURE 10.27 *A deadly necklace. Marine biologists estimate that cast-off nets, plastic beverage yokes, and other packing residue kill hundreds of thousands of birds, mammals, and fish each year.*

metric tons of oil are discharged into the world's oceans each year from oil tankers, fuel leaks, intentional discharges of fuel oil, and coastal industries. About half of this amount is due to maritime transport. Of this portion, most is not from dramatic, headline-making accidents such as the 1989 *Exxon Valdez* spill in Alaska but, rather, from routine, open-sea bilge pumping and tank cleaning. These activities are illegal but very common.

The transport of huge quantities of oil creates opportunities for major oil spills through a combination of human and natural hazards. Military conflict in the Middle East destabilizes shipping routes. More important, drilling and transport in stormy seas cause spills. Plans to drill for oil along the seismically active California and Alaska coasts have been controversial because of the damage that spills could cause to these biologically rich coastal ecosystems.

Fortunately, awareness of ocean pollution is growing. Oil spill cleanup technologies and response teams are improving, although most oil is eventually decomposed by natural bacteria. Efforts are growing to control waste plastic. Sixteen states now require that six-pack yokes be made of biodegradable or photodegradable plastic, limiting their longevity as potential killers. International concern about ocean ship waste is increasing, and some shipping companies have been prosecuted and fined for dumping fuel oil. Beach pollution—mainly plastic debris, but also sewage waste, oil, and chemical contaminants—is becoming more common, but it is also more frequently reported in the mainstream media. Volunteer efforts are helping to reduce beach pollution locally: in one day, volunteers in Texas gathered more than 300 tons of plastic refuse from Gulf Coast beaches.

POLLUTION CONTROL

The cheapest and most effective way to reduce pollution is to avoid producing it or releasing it in the first place. Eliminating lead from gasoline has resulted in a widespread and significant decrease in the amount of lead in U.S. surface waters. Studies have shown that as much as 90 percent less road deicing salt can be used in many areas without significantly affecting the safety of winter roads. Careful handling of oil and petroleum products can greatly reduce the amount of water pollution caused by these materials. Although we still have problems with persistent chlorinated hydrocarbons spread widely in the environment, the banning of DDT and PCBs in the 1970s has resulted in significant reductions in levels in wildlife.

Industry can reduce pollution by recycling or reclaiming materials that otherwise might be discarded in the waste stream. These approaches usually have economic as well as environmental benefits. Companies can extract valuable metals and chemicals and sell them, instead of releasing them as toxic contaminants into the water system. Both markets and reclamation technologies are improving as awareness of these opportunities grows. In addition, modifying land use is an important component of reducing pollution.

Nonpoint Sources and Land Management

Farmers have long contributed a huge share of water pollution, especially in the developed world. Increasingly, though, farmers are finding ways to save money and water quality at the same time. Soil conservation practices on farmlands (see chapter 7) maintain soil fertility, as well as protect water quality. Precise application of fertilizer, irrigation water, and pesticides saves money and reduces water contamination. Preserving wetlands that act as natural processing facilities for removing sediment and contaminants helps protect surface and groundwaters.

In urban areas, reducing waste that enters storm sewers is essential. It is getting easier for city residents to recycle waste oil and to properly dispose of paint and other household chemicals that they once dumped into storm sewers or the garbage. Urbanites can also minimize use of fertilizers and pesticides. Regular street sweeping greatly reduces nutrient loads (from decomposing leaves and debris) in rivers and lakes. Runoff can also be diverted away from streams and lakes. Many cities are separating storm sewers and municipal sewage lines to avoid overflow during storms.

A good example of the problems of watershed management is seen in Chesapeake Bay, America's largest estuary. Once fabled for its abundant oysters, crabs, shad, striped bass, and other valuable fisheries, the bay had deteriorated seriously by the early 1970s. Citizens' groups, local communities, state legislatures, and the federal government together established an innovative pollution-control program that made the bay the first estuary in America targeted for protection and restoration.

Among the principal objectives of this plan is reducing nutrient loading through land-use regulations in the bay's six watershed states to control agricultural and urban runoff. Pollution-prevention measures, such as banning phosphate detergents, also are important, as are upgrading wastewater treatment plants and improving compliance with discharge and filling permits. Efforts are underway to replant thousands of hectares of sea grasses and to restore wetlands that filter out pollutants. Since the 1980s, annual phosphorous discharges into Chesapeake Bay have dropped 40 percent. Nitrogen levels, however, have remained constant or have even risen in some tributaries. Although progress has been made, the goals of reducing both nitrogen and phosphate levels by 40 percent and restoring viable fish and shellfish populations are still decades away. Still, as EPA Administrator Carol Browner says, it demonstrates the "power of cooperation" in environmental protection. (See related story "Watershed Protection in the Catskills" at www.mhhe.com/cases.)

Sewage Treatment

As we have already seen, human and animal wastes usually create the most serious health-related water pollution problems. More than 500 types of disease-causing (pathogenic) bacteria, viruses, and parasites can travel from human or animal excrement through water.

Natural Processes

In the poorer countries of the world, most rural people simply go out into the fields and forests to relieve themselves, as they have always done. Where population densities are low, natural processes eliminate wastes quickly, making this an effective method of sanitation. The high population densities of cities, however, make this practice unworkable. Even major cities of many less-developed countries are often littered with human waste that has been left for rains to wash away or for pigs, dogs, flies, beetles, or other scavengers to consume. This is a major cause of disease, as well as being extremely unpleasant. Studies have shown that a significant portion of the airborne dust in Mexico City is actually dried, pulverized human feces.

Where intensive agriculture is practiced—especially in wet rice paddy farming in Asia—it has long been customary to collect "night soil" (human and animal waste) to be spread on the fields as fertilizer. This waste is a valuable source of plant nutrients, but it is also a source of disease-causing pathogens in the food supply.

Until about 50 years ago, most rural American families and quite a few residents of towns and small cities depended on a pit toilet, or "outhouse," for waste disposal. Untreated wastes tended to seep into the ground, however, and pathogens sometimes contaminated drinking water. The development of septic tanks and properly constructed drain fields represented a considerable improvement in public health. Septic systems allow solids to settle in a tank, where bacteria decompose them; liquids percolate through soil, where soil bacteria presumably purify them. Where population densities are not too high, this can be an effective method of waste disposal. With urban sprawl, however, groundwater pollution often becomes a problem.

Municipal Sewage Treatment

Over the past 100 years, sanitary engineers have developed ingenious and effective municipal wastewater treatment systems to protect human health, ecosystem stability, and water quality. This topic is an important part of pollution control, and is a principal responsibility of every municipal government.

Primary treatment physically separates large solids from the waste stream with screens and settling tanks (fig. 10.28a). Settling tanks allow grit and some dissolved (suspended) organic solids to fall out as sludge. Water drained from the top of settling

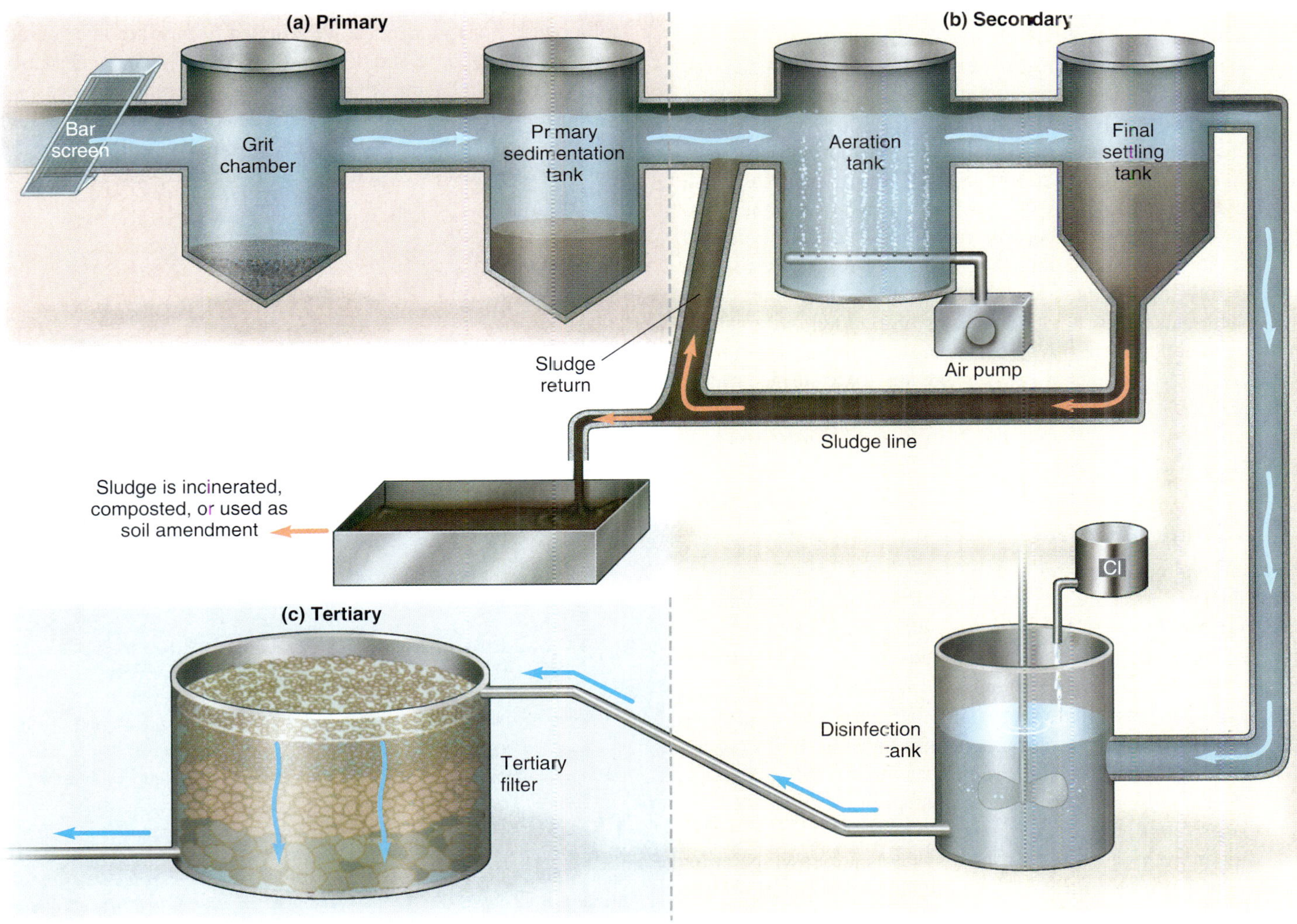

FIGURE 10.28 *Activated sludge wastewater treatment.* (a) *Primary treatment removes only solids and suspended sediment.* (b) *Secondary treatment, through aeration of activated sludge, followed by sludge removal and chlorination of effluent, kills pathogens and removes most organic material.* (c) *During tertiary treatment, passage through a trickling bed evaporator and/or a tertiary filter further removes inorganic nutrients, oxidizes any remaining organics, and reduces effluent volume.*

tanks still carries up to 75 percent of the organic matter, including many pathogens. These are treated by **secondary treatment,** in which aerobic bacteria break down dissolved organic compounds. In secondary treatment, effluent is aerated, often with sprayers or in an aeration tank, in which air is pumped through the microorganism-rich slurry (fig. 10.28b). Fluids can also be stored in a sewage lagoon, where sunlight, algae, and air process waste more cheaply but more slowly. Effluent from secondary treatment processes is usually disinfected with chlorine, UV light, or ozone to kill harmful bacteria before it is released to a nearby waterway.

Tertiary treatment removes dissolved metals and nutrients, especially nitrates and phosphates, from the secondary effluent. Although wastewater is usually free of pathogens and organic material after secondary treatment, it still contains high levels of these inorganic nutrients. If discharged into surface waters, these nutrients stimulate algal blooms and eutrophication. Allowing effluent to flow through a wetland or lagoon can remove nitrates and phosphates. Alternatively, chemicals often are used to bind and precipitate nutrients (fig. 10.28c).

Sewage sludge would be valuable fertilizer if it were not contaminated by metals, toxic chemicals, and pathogenic organisms. The toxic content of most sewer sludge necessitates disposal by burial in a landfill or incineration. Sludge disposal is a major cost in most municipal sewer budgets.

In many American cities, sanitary sewers are connected to storm sewers, which carry runoff from streets and parking lots. Storm sewers are routed to the treatment plant rather than discharged into surface waters because runoff from streets, yards, and industrial sites generally contains a variety of refuse, fertilizers, pesticides, oils, rubber, tars, lead (from gasoline), and other undesirable chemicals. Unfortunately heavy storms often overload the system, especially where the system is old and already overtaxed. As a result, large volumes of raw sewage and toxic surface runoff are dumped directly into receiving waters. To prevent this overflow, cities are spending hundreds of millions of dollars to separate storm and sanitary sewers.

Low-Cost Waste Treatment

A number of alternative treatment systems have been developed. One of the most attractive is using natural or artificial wetlands to process wastes. Arcata, California, for instance, needed an expensive sewer plant upgrade. Instead, the city transformed a 65-ha garbage dump into a series of ponds and marshes that serve as a simple, low-cost, waste treatment facility. Arcata saved millions of dollars and improved the environment simultaneously. The marsh is a haven for wildlife and has become a prized recreation area for the city. Eventually, the purified water flows into Humboldt Bay, where marine life flourishes.

Similar wetland waste treatment systems are now operating in many developing countries. Effluent from these operations can be used to irrigate crops or raise fish for human consumption if care is taken first to destroy pathogens. Usually 20 to 30 days of exposure to sun, air, and aquatic plants is enough to make the water safe. These systems make an important contribution to human food supplies. A 2,500-ha waste-fed aquaculture facility in Calcutta, for example, supplies about 7,000 metric tons of fish annually to local markets.

The World Bank estimates that more than 3 billion people will be without sanitation services by the year 2030 under a business-as-usual scenario (fig. 10.29). With investments in innovative programs, however, sanitation could be provided to about half those people, and a great deal of misery and suffering could be avoided.

Remediation

Just as there are many sources of water contamination, there are many ways to clean it up. New developments in environmental engineering are providing promising solutions to many water pollution problems. Containment methods keep dirty water from spreading. Chemicals can be added to toxic wastewater to precipitate, immobilize, or solidify contaminants. Many pollutants can be destroyed or detoxified by chemical reactions that oxidize, reduce, neutralize, hydrolyze, precipitate, or otherwise change their chemical composition. Where chemical techniques are ineffective, physical methods may work. Solvents and other volatile organic compounds, for instance, can be stripped from solution by aeration and then burned in an incinerator. (See related story "International Accord to Clean Up the Rhine River" at www.mhhe.com/cases.)

Often, living organisms can clean contaminated water effectively and inexpensively. We call this **bioremediation.** Restored wetlands, for instance, along stream banks or lake margins can

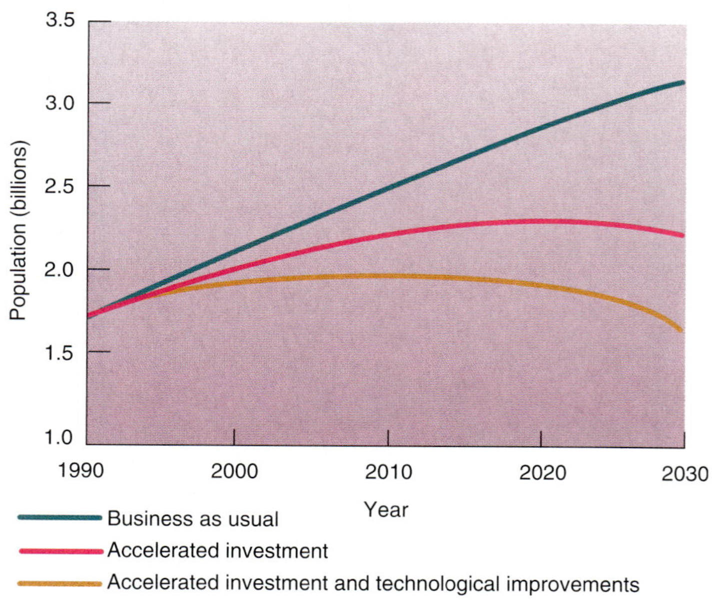

FIGURE 10.29 *World population without adequate sanitation—three scenarios in the year 2030. If business as usual continues, more than 3 billion people will lack safe sanitation. Accelerated investment in sanitation services could lower this number. Higher investment, coupled with technological development, could keep the number of people without adequate sanitation from growing, even though the total population increases.*

Source: World Bank estimates based on research paper by Dennis Anderson and William Cavendish, "Efficiency and Substitution in Pollution Abatement: Simulation Studies in Three Sectors."

effectively filter out sediment and remove pollutants. They generally cost far less than mechanical water treatment facilities and provide wildlife habitat.

Lowly duckweed (*Lemna* sp.), the green scum you often see covering the surface of eutrophic ponds, grows fast and can remove large amounts of organic nutrients from water. Large duckweed lagoons are being used as inexpensive, low-tech, sewage treatment plants in developing countries. The duckweed can also be harvested and used as feed, fuel, or fertilizer. Up to 35 percent of its dry mass is protein—about twice as much as alfalfa, a popular animal feed.

Ocean Arks International in Falmouth, Massachusetts, has been developing holistic systems for water purification that are combinations of different plants and animals, including algae, rooted aquatic plants, clams, snails, and fish, each chosen to provide a particular service in a contained environment. Technically, the water that has flowed through such a system is drinkable, although few people feel comfortable doing so. More often, the final effluent is used to flush toilets or for irrigation. Called ecological engineering, this novel approach can save resources and money, and it can serve as a valuable educational tool (fig. 10.30).

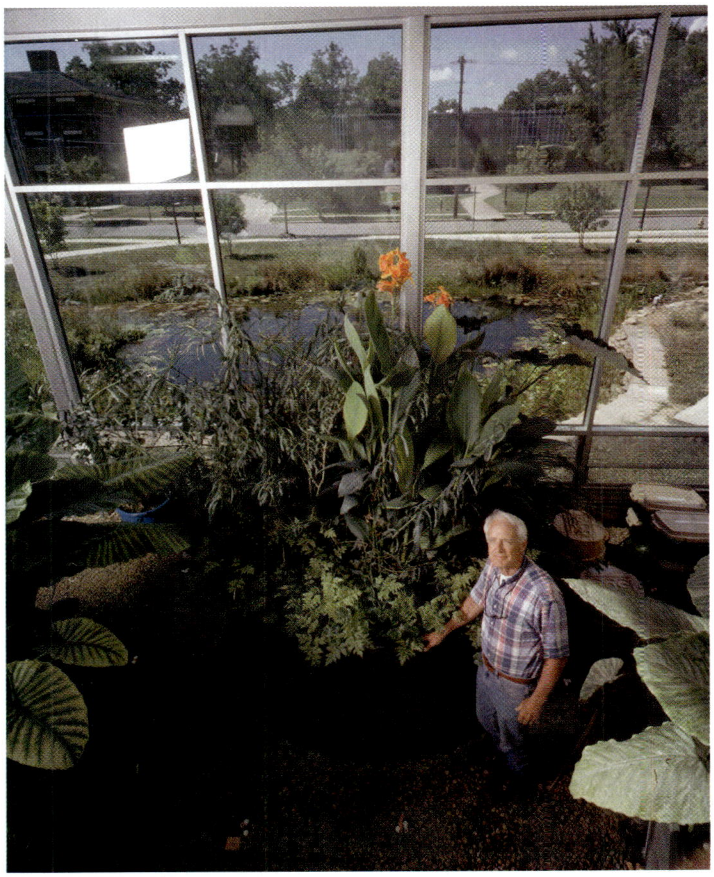

FIGURE 10.30 *In-house wastewater treatment in Oberlin College's Environmental Studies building. Constructed wetlands outside, and tanks inside, allow plants to filter water and remove nutrients.*

WATER LEGISLATION

Water pollution control has been among the most broadly popular and effective of all environmental legislation in the United States. It has not been without controversy, however. Table 10.5 describes some of the most important water legislation in the United States.

The Clean Water Act

Passage of the U.S. Clean Water Act of 1972 was a bold, bipartisan step that made clean water a national priority. Along with the Endangered Species Act and the Clean Air Act, this is one of the most significant and effective pieces of environmental legislation ever passed by the U.S. Congress. It also is an immense and complex law, with more than 500 sections regulating everything from urban runoff, industrial discharges, and municipal sewage treatment to land-use practices and wetland drainage.

The ambitious goal of the Clean Water Act was to return all U.S. surface waters to "fishable and swimmable" conditions. For point sources, the act requires discharge permits and use of the best practicable control technology (BPT). For toxic substances,

TABLE 10.5 Some Important U.S. Water Quality Legislation

1. *Federal Water Pollution Control Act (1972).* Establishes uniform nationwide controls for each category of major polluting industries.
2. *Marine Protection Research and Sanctuaries Act (1972).* Regulates ocean dumping and established sanctuaries for protection of endangered marine species.
3. *Ports and Waterways Safety Act (1972).* Regulates oil transport and the operation of oil-handling facilities.
4. *Safe Drinking Water Act (1974).* Requires minimum safety standards for every community water supply. Among the contaminants regulated are bacteria, nitrates, arsenic, barium, cadmium, chromium, fluoride, lead, mercury, silver, and pesticides; radioactivity and turbidity also are regulated. This act also contains provisions to protect groundwater aquifers.
5. *Resource Conservation and Recovery Act (RCRA) (1976).* Regulates the storage, shipping, processing, and disposal of hazardous wastes and sets limits on the sewering of toxic chemicals.
6. *Toxic Substances Control Act (TOSCA) (1976).* Categorizes toxic and hazardous substances, establishes a research program, and regulates the use and disposal of poisonous chemicals.
7. *Comprehensive Environmental Response, Compensation, and Liability Act (CERCLA) (1980) and Superfund Amendments and Reauthorization Act (SARA) (1984).* Provide for sealing, excavation, or remediation of toxic and hazardous waste dumps.
8. *Clean Water Act (1985) (amending the 1972 Water Pollution Control Act).* Sets as a national goal the attainment of "fishable and swimmable" quality for all surface waters in the United States.
9. *London Dumping Convention (1990).* Calls for an end to all ocean dumping of industrial wastes, tank-washing effluents, and plastic trash. The United States is a signatory to this international convention.

the act sets national goals of best available, economically achievable technology (BAT) and zero discharge goals for 126 priority toxic pollutants. As discussed earlier, these regulations have had a positive effect on water quality. While not yet swimmable or fishable everywhere, surface-water quality in the United States has significantly improved on average over the past quarter century. Perhaps the most important result of the act has been investment of $54 billion in federal funds and more than $128 billion in state and local funds for municipal sewage treatment facilities.

Opponents of federal regulation have tried repeatedly to weaken or eliminate the Clean Water Act. They regard restriction of their "right" to dump toxic chemicals and wastes into wetlands and waterways to be an undue loss of freedom. They resent being forced to clean up municipal water supplies and call for cost/benefit analysis that places greater weight on economic interests in all environmental planning.

Supporters of the Clean Water Act would like to see a shift away from an "end-of-the-pipe" focus on effluent removal and more attention to changing industrial processes, so that toxic substances aren't produced in the first place. Environmentalists also would like to see stricter enforcement of existing regulations, mandatory minimum penalties for violations, more effective community right-to-know provisions, and increased powers for citizen lawsuits against polluters.

SUMMARY

- The hydrologic cycle constantly purifies and redistributes fresh water, providing an endlessly renewable resource. More than 97 percent of all water in the world is salty ocean water. Lakes, rivers, and other surface freshwater bodies make up less than 0.01 percent of all the water in the world, but they provide more than half of all water for human use and for habitat and nourishment for aquatic ecosystems that play a vital role in the chain of life.
- In the United States, about one-tenth of the water we withdraw from our resources is for direct personal use. Our two largest water uses are agricultural irrigation and industrial cooling. Only about half the water we withdraw is consumed or degraded so that it is unsuitable for other purposes; much could be reused or recycled. Water conservation and recycling would have both economic and environmental benefits.
- Water shortages in many parts of the world result from rising demand, unequal distribution, and increased contamination. Water storage and transfer projects are a response to flooding and water shortages. Giant dams and diversion projects can have environmental and social costs far above the benefits they provide. Among the problems they pose are evaporation and infiltration losses, siltation of reservoirs, and loss of recreation and wildlife habitat. Many conservationists prefer watershed management and small dams as means of flood control and water storage.
- Any physical, biological, or chemical change in water quality that adversely affects living organisms or makes water unsuitable for desired uses can be considered pollution. Worldwide, the most serious water pollutants for human health are pathogenic organisms from human and animal wastes. We have traditionally taken advantage of the capacity of ecosystems to destroy these organisms, but as population density has grown, these systems have become overloaded and ineffective.
- In industrialized nations, toxic chemical wastes have become an increasing problem. Agricultural and industrial chemicals have been released or spilled into surface waters and are seeping into groundwater supplies. The extent of this problem is probably not yet fully appreciated.
- Pollution levels in the ocean are increasing. Major causes of ocean pollution are oil spills from tanker bilge pumping or accidents, as well as oil well blowouts. Surface runoff and sewage outfalls discharge fertilizers, pesticides, organic nutrients, and toxic chemicals that have a variety of deleterious effects on marine ecosystems.
- Silt and sediment make up the greatest quantity of water pollutants. Biomass production by aquatic organisms, land erosion, and refuse discharge all contribute to this problem. Salts and metals from highway and farm runoff and industrial activities also damage water quality. In some areas, drainage from mines and tailings piles delivers sediment and toxic materials to rivers and lakes.
- Appropriate land-use practices and careful disposal of industrial, domestic, and agricultural wastes are essential for control of water pollution. Natural processes and living organisms have a high capacity to remove or destroy water pollutants, but these systems become overloaded and ineffective when pollution levels are too high. Reducing pollution sources is often the best solution to our pollution problems.

QUESTIONS FOR REVIEW

1. Describe the path a molecule of water might follow through the hydrologic cycle from the ocean to land and back again.
2. Define *aquifer*. How does water get into an aquifer?
3. What fraction of the world's water is fresh?
4. What is drip irrigation, and what are its benefits?
5. Describe some problems associated with dam building and water diversion projects.
6. Define *water pollution*.
7. Describe eight major sources of water pollution in the United States. What pollution problems are associated with each source?
8. What is eutrophication? What causes it?
9. What is an impaired river mile? What percentage of U.S. river miles are impaired?
10. Describe primary, secondary, and tertiary processes for sewage treatment. What is the quality of the effluent from each of these processes?
11. Describe remediation techniques and how they work.

THINKING SCIENTIFICALLY

1. What changes might occur in the hydrologic cycle if our climate were to warm or cool significantly?
2. Why does it take so long for deep ocean waters to circulate through the hydrologic cycle? What happens to substances that contaminate deep ocean water or deep aquifers in the ground?
3. How precise do you think the estimate is that 1.5 billion people lack access to safe drinking water? If, in 2025, two-thirds of the world's population live in countries with severe water shortages, what might be the number of people who lack access to clean water? Why is this number ambiguous?
4. Do you think that water pollution is worse now than it was in the past? What considerations go into a judgment such as this? How do your personal experiences influence your opinion?
5. What additional information would you need to make a judgment about whether conditions are getting better or worse? How would you weigh different sources, types, and effects of water pollution?
6. Under what conditions might sediment in water or cultural eutrophication be beneficial? How should we balance positive and negative effects?
7. Suppose that part of the silt in a river is natural and part is human-caused. How might you evaluate what proportion of the silt is caused by humans?

KEY TERMS

aquifers 233
biochemical oxygen demand (BOD) 243
bioremediation 254
coliform bacteria 243
consumption 235
cultural eutrophication 243
discharge 233
dissolved oxygen (DO) content 243
eutrophic 243
hydrologic cycle 231
nonpoint sources 242
oligotrophic 243
oxygen sag 243
point sources 241
primary treatment 253
recharge zones 233
renewable water supplies 234
residence time 232
secondary treatment 254
tertiary treatment 254
thermal pollution 247
total maximum daily loads (TMDL) 248
watershed 240
water table 233
withdrawal 235

SUGGESTED READINGS

Ayres, Gene. 2003. "Rocket Fuel in Our Food." *Worldwatch* 16(6):12–20.

Baron, J. S., et al. 2002. "Meeting ecological and societal needs for freshwater." *Ecological Applications* 12(5):1247–60.

Gleick, Peter H. 2003. "Global freshwater resources: soft-path solutions for the 21st century." *Science* 302:1524–28.

Glennon, Robert. 2003. *Water Follies*. Island Press.

Grenoble, Penelope. 2003. "Yangtze Farewell." *Orion* 22(6):26–33.

Katsoyiannis, I. A., and A. I. Zouboulis. 2004. "Application of biological processes for the removal of arsenic from groundwaters." *Water Research* 38(1):17–26.

Olmstead, Sheila M. 2003. "Water Supply and Poor Communities: What's Price Got To Do With It?" *Environment* 45(10):22–35.

Pestana, M. H. D., and M. L. L. Formoso. 2003. "Mercury contamination in Lavras do Sul, south Brazil: a legacy from past and recent gold mining." *The Science of the Total Environment* 307(1–3):125–40.

Postel, Sandra. 2001. "Growing Food with Less Water." *Scientific American* 284(2):46–51.

Reisner, Marc. 1993. *Cadillac Desert: The American West and Its Disappearing Water.* Penguin Books.

Shiva, Vandana. 2002. *Water Wars: Privatization, Pollution and Profit.* South End Press.

Yang, Shinwoo, and Kenneth Carlson. 2003. "Evolution of antibiotic occurrence in a river through pristine, urban and agricultural landscapes." *Water Research* 37(19):4645–56.

Welcome to McGraw-Hill's Online Learning Center

http://www.mhhe.com/cunningham3e

WEB EXERCISES

Stream Flow Data

Stream gauging stations, which keep records of water flow in streams for many years, are one of the most important tools we have for understanding water resources. Stream gauge records are used to estimate water availability for drinking and for irrigation, pollution levels, and many other types of information. In the United States, the U.S. Geological Survey maintains a vast network of stream gauges.

Go to http://water.usgs.gov/realtime.html. This page shows a map of today's water flow compared with normal conditions for this time of year. Each dot represents a gauging station. Look at the map explanation below the map. Which colors represent unusually high flow rates? Which color represents approximately normal flow rates (25th to 75th percentile)? Which colors represent low flow rates? Which colors predominate in your area today?

Click on your state. (If your state is below freezing or very dry this month, use a different state.) This will lead you to a map of colored dots for the state you chose. When the state map loads, click on a colored dot near you on the map. (If any information is missing for questions 1–4, try selecting another site.)

1. When you click on a dot, you will get information on stream flow for that station. The first graph is stream flow—the amount of water in the stream today, in cubic feet per second. Note the numbers on the vertical axis. Is the stream flowing in tens of cubic feet per second? Hundreds? Thousands? How does today's flow compare with the median flow (blue triangles)? Has the flow been high or low for the past month?
2. The second graph is stage, the water level. (Why is this not exactly the same as flow rate?) How high is today's water level, compared with the past month?
3. In some states, most sites have a third graph showing rainfall. If your site does, look at the second and third graphs together. Are there any rainfall events (spikes in the rainfall graph) that help explain highs in the stage graph? Based on the rainfall graph, does most of the water in the stream at this gauging point come from rainfall here or somewhere upstream?
4. Now hit the "Back" button to go back to the state map, and look at several different gauging stations (colored dots) in different areas of your state. Which part of your state is driest? Which region is wettest? Are the numbers in different regions similar, or is flow at some sites several times greater than at other sites? Do most sites have fairly constant flow, or do some have dramatic peaks and valleys? What generalizations can you make about surface-water availability in the state?

Surf Your Watershed

What are the water sources like where you live? Go to the EPA's water quality website, "Surf Your Watershed," at http://cfpub.epa.gov/surf/locate/index.cfm and enter your zip code below the map image. When one or more watershed ID numbers are returned to you, select one, and look at the information about your area. What are water quality conditions like in your area? What are some of the threats to water quality?

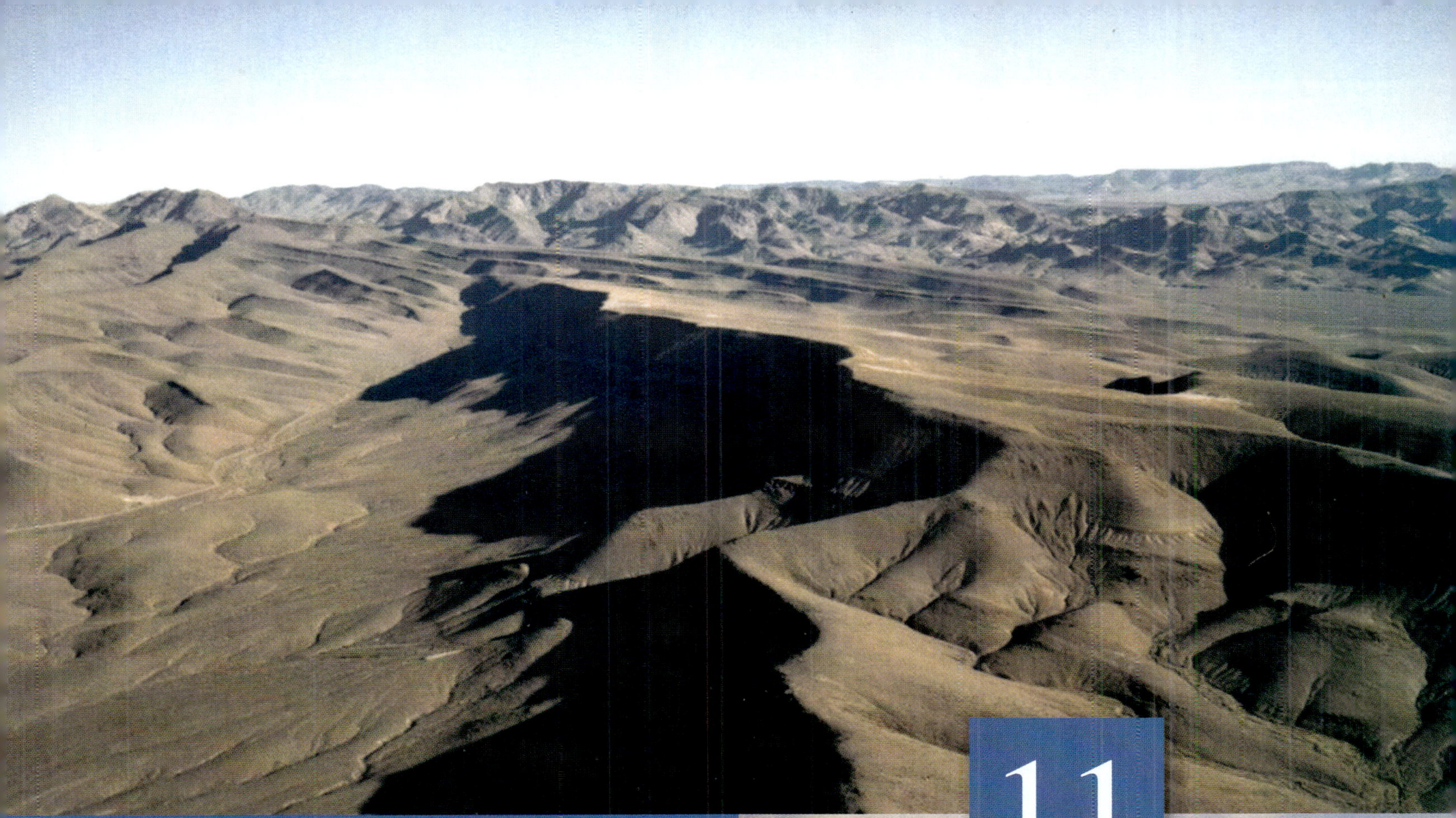

Yucca Mountain, Nevada (long ridge in center of photo) *has been chosen as the United States' first permanent high-level nuclear waste storage site.*

11

Environmental Geology and Earth Resources

When we heal the earth, we heal ourselves.

–David Orr

Welcome to McGraw-Hill's Online Learning Center

http://www.mhhe.com/cunningham3e

LEARNING ONLINE

Visit our webpage at www.mhhe.com/cunningham3e for data sources, further readings, additional case studies, current environmental news, and regional examples within the Online Learning Center to help you understand the material in this chapter. You'll also find active links to information pertaining to this chapter, including

USGS
Basic geology
Earthquakes
Volcanoes
Mining and minerals
Landslides and geologic hazards

OBJECTIVES

After studying this chapter, you should be able to

- understand some basic geologic principles, including how plate-tectonic movements affect conditions for life on the earth.
- explain how the three major rock types form and how the rock cycle works.
- summarize economic mineralogy and strategic minerals.
- discuss the environmental effects of mining and mineral processing.
- recognize the geologic hazards of earthquakes, volcanoes, floods, and erosion.

Radioactive Waste Disposal at Yucca Mountain

In July 2002 the U.S. Senate voted to designate Yucca Mountain, Nevada, as the permanent resting place for 77,000 metric tons of high-level nuclear waste, most of it spent fuel from the nation's 107 nuclear power plants (fig. 11.1). Nuclear power proponents celebrated: after twenty years of research and lobbying, the site was finally approved. With a repository on the horizon, plans for new nuclear plants could proceed, and existing plants could look forward to clearing out 50,000 tons of spent nuclear fuel currently in temporary, sometimes inadequate, storage at reactor sites. The state of Nevada, meanwhile, immediately filed a lawsuit to stop the plan. Nevada Governor Kenny Guinn charged that the Department of Energy (DOE) had lowered its scientific standards for evaluating the geologic integrity of the site. Opponents charged that heavy-handed eastern politics, not sound geology, was behind the decision to put the entire nation's nuclear waste in Nevada.

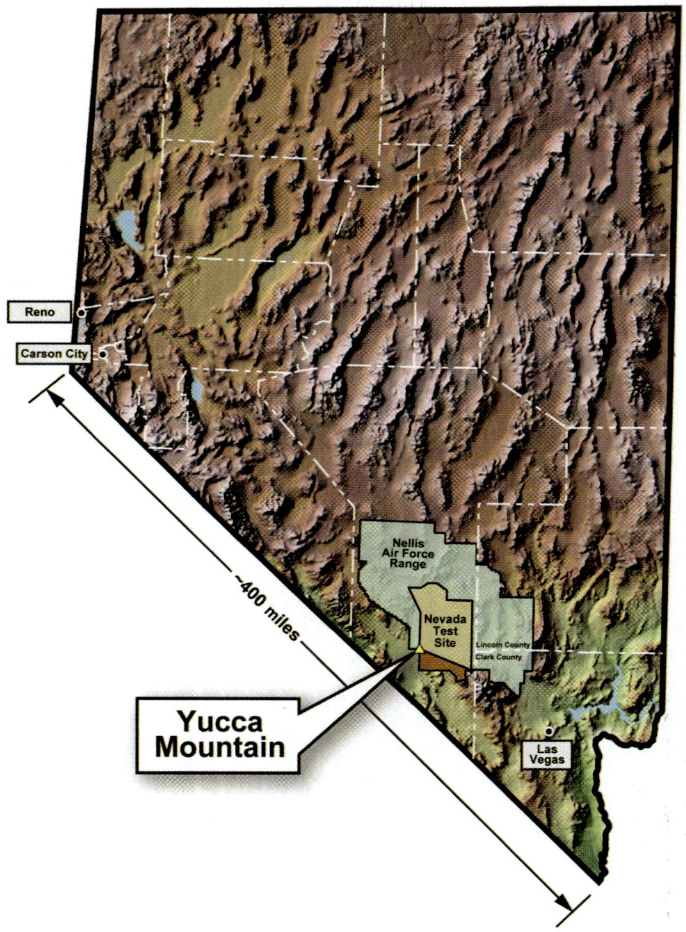

FIGURE 11.1 *Yucca Mountain, Nevada, is the designated storage site for high-level radioactive waste.*

The stakes at Yucca Mountain are high. The DOE and the nuclear power industry have invested more than $4 billion in research, testing, and promotion of the site. The lack of permanent storage has been an obstacle to construction of nuclear power plants since the 1980s. Further, cleanup is beginning at old military installations, such as Hanford, Washington, and Rocky Flats, Colorado. These are some of the nation's worst toxic waste sites, and permanent storage is needed for their radioactive materials.

Geology is key to siting a waste repository of any kind. For high-level radioactive wastes, the DOE needed to find a site where a labyrinth of deep tunnels could keep extremely dangerous materials isolated and secure for 10,000 years, more than twice the length of recorded human history. (The waste will remain highly radioactive for more than 500,000 years, but the DOE considers itself unlikely to be responsible for the site for that long.) This time span requires a geologically stable area—no active faults like those in California, no volcanoes like those in Washington and Oregon. Bedrock needs to be relatively impermeable, not riddled with underground channels and sinkholes, as in Florida and parts of Texas. There must be no groundwater, which would soak storage casks and mobilize radioactive materials, possibly allowing tainted water to reach the surface. This rules out the central Great Plains and most of the eastern United States, where plentiful rainfall keeps water tables high and aquifers full.

Yucca Mountain fits these requirements better than most places in the United States. But there is conflicting evidence, and conflicting interpretations of evidence, about whether even Yucca Mountain is good enough. DOE geologists insist that the only aquifers in the area are 300 m below the site; other geologists say there is evidence in the rocks that aquifers have risen in the past, suggesting that they might rise again to the level of the repository tunnels. Critics of the site point out that the area has more than 30 known faults. Geologists disagree on how long these faults have been dormant, and on how long it will be before they shift again. In addition, there are seven dormant volcanoes in the area. While these are likely to remain dormant for 10,000 years, their activity in several hundred thousand years is hard to predict. Opponents of the site also worry about the potential dangers of shipping waste, potentially 28,000 truckloads and 10,000 rail cars over the site's 30-year life span. Defenders point out that high-level waste is currently stored at more than 130 temporary sites, and those sites are clearly unsafe for the long term.

Unless you live along an earthquake fault or near a volcano, you might think of the earth as solid, stable, and unchanging. The extraordinary difficulty of finding a nuclear waste repository reminds us that, in fact, the earth is constantly shifting and changing—although usually on a time scale much slower than we can perceive. The Yucca Mountain controversy also highlights the importance of understanding geologic processes and forces if we are to solve environmental, policy, and energy problems. In this chapter, we'll look at how rocks are formed, where mineral resources are found, how the earth moves, and how these forces affect us all.

A DYNAMIC PLANET

Although we think of the ground under our feet as solid and stable, the earth is a dynamic and constantly changing structure. Titanic forces stir inside the earth, causing continents to split, move apart, and then crash into each other in slow but inexorable collisions. In this section, we will look at the structure of our planet and some of the forces that shape it.

A Layered Sphere

The **core,** or interior of the earth is composed of a dense, intensely hot mass of metal—mostly iron—thousands of kilometers in diameter (fig. 11.2). Solid in the center but more fluid in the outer core, this immense mass generates the magnetic field that envelops the earth.

Surrounding the molten outer core is a hot, pliable layer of rock called the **mantle.** The mantle is much less dense than the core because it contains a high concentration of lighter elements, such as oxygen, silicon, and magnesium.

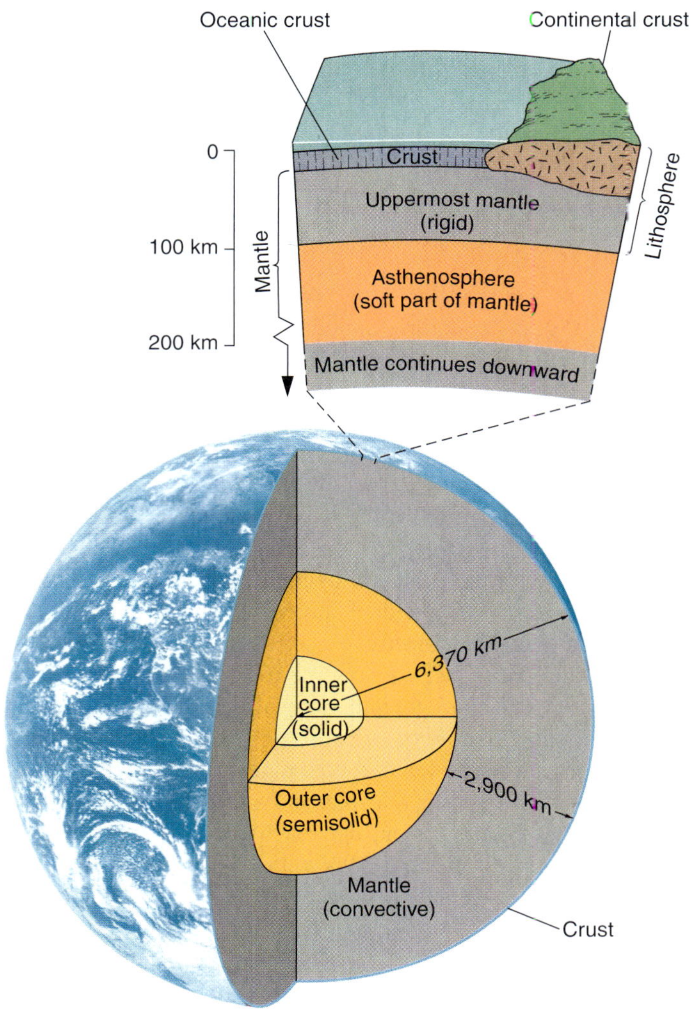

FIGURE 11.2 *Earth's cross section. Slow convection in the mantle causes the thin, brittle crust to move.*

The outermost layer of the earth is the cool, lightweight, brittle rock **crust.** The crust below oceans is relatively thin (8–15 km), dense, and young (less than 200 million years old) because of constant recycling. Crust under continents is relatively thick (25–75 km), light, and as old as 3.8 billion years because additional material is continually being added. It also is predominantly granitic, while oceanic crust is mainly dense basaltic rock. Table 11.1 compares the composition of the whole earth (dominated by the dense core) and the crust.

Tectonic Processes and Shifting Continents

The huge convection currents in the mantle are thought to break the overlying crust into a mosaic of huge blocks called **tectonic plates** (fig. 11.3). These plates slide slowly across the earth's surface like immense icebergs, in some places breaking up into smaller pieces, in other places crashing ponderously into each other to create new, larger landmasses. Ocean basins form where continents crack and pull apart. The Atlantic Ocean, for example, is growing slowly as Europe and Africa move away from the Americas. **Magma** (molten rock) forced up through the cracks forms new oceanic crust that piles up underwater in **midocean ridges.** Creating the largest mountain range in the world, these ridges wind around the earth for 74,000 km (46,000 mi) (see fig. 11.3). Although concealed from our view, this jagged range boasts higher peaks, deeper canyons, and sheerer cliffs than any continental mountains. Slowly spreading from these fracture zones, ocean plates push against continental plates.

Earthquakes are caused by grinding and jerking as plates slide past each other. Mountain ranges like those on the west coast of North America and in Japan are pushed up at the margins of colliding continental plates. The Himalayas are still rising as the Indian subcontinent grinds slowly into Asia. Southern California is slowly sailing north toward Alaska. In about 30 million years, Los Angeles will pass San Francisco, if both still exist by then.

When an oceanic plate collides with a continental landmass, the continental plate usually rides up over the seafloor, while the

TABLE 11.1 Eight Most Common Chemical Elements (Percent) in Whole Earth and Crust

WHOLE EARTH		CRUST	
Iron	33.3	Oxygen	45.2
Oxygen	29.8	Silicon	27.2
Silicon	15.6	Aluminum	8.2
Magnesium	13.9	Iron	5.8
Nickel	2.0	Calcium	5.1
Calcium	1.8	Magnesium	2.8
Aluminum	1.5	Sodium	2.3
Sodium	0.2	Potassium	1.7

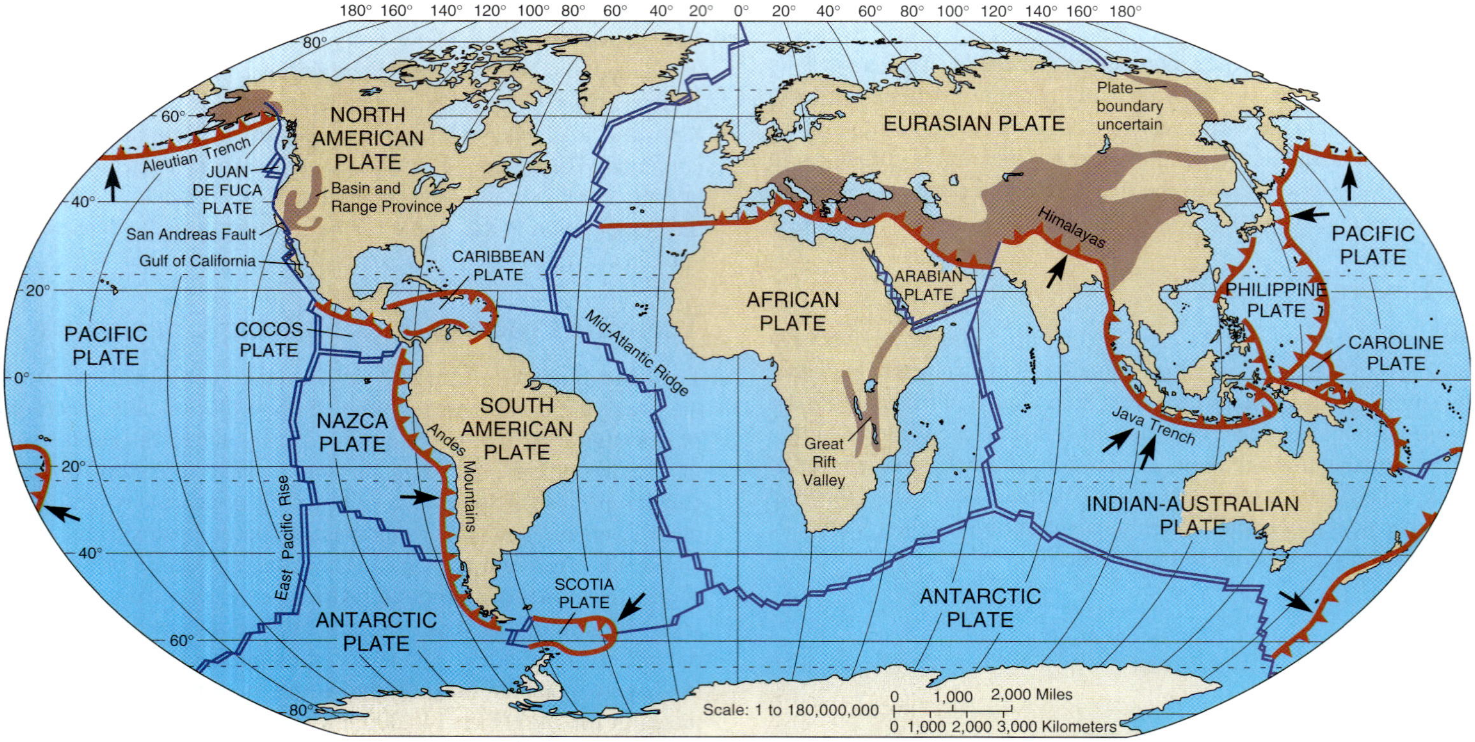

FIGURE 11.3 *Map of tectonic plates. Plate boundaries are dynamic zones, characterized by earthquakes, volcanism, and the formation of great rifts and mountain ranges. Arrows indicate direction of subduction where one plate is diving beneath another. These zones are sites of deep trenches in the ocean floor and high levels of seismic and volcanic activity.*
Sources: Data from U.S. Department of the Interior, U.S. Geological Survey.

oceanic plate is **subducted,** or pushed down into the mantle, where it melts and rises back to the surface as magma (fig. 11.4). Deep ocean trenches mark these subduction zones, and volcanoes form where the magma erupts through vents and fissures in the overlying crust. Trenches and volcanic mountains ring the Pacific Ocean rim from Indonesia to Japan to Alaska and down the west coast of the Americas, forming a so-called ring of fire where oceanic plates are being subducted under the continental plates. This ring is the source of more earthquakes and volcanic activity than any other region on the earth.

Over millions of years, continents can drift long distances. Antarctica and Australia once were connected to Africa, for instance, somewhere near the equator and supported luxuriant forests. Geologists suggest that several times in the earth's history most or all of the continents have gathered to form supercontinents, which have ruptured and re-formed over hundreds of millions of years (fig. 11.5). The redistribution of continents has profound effects on the earth's climate and may help explain the periodic mass extinctions of organisms marking the divisions between many major geologic periods (fig. 11.6).

MINERALS AND ROCKS

A **mineral** is a naturally occurring, inorganic solid with a definite chemical composition and a specific internal crystal structure. A mineral is solid; therefore, ice is a mineral (with a distinct composition and crystal structure), but liquid water is not. Similarly molten lava is not crystalline, although it generally hardens to create distinct minerals. Metals (such as iron, copper, aluminum, or gold) come from mineral ores, but once purified, metals are no longer natural and thus are not minerals. Depending on the conditions in which they were formed, mineral crystals can be microscopically small, such as asbestos fibers, or huge, such as the tree-size selenite crystals recently discovered in a Chihuahua, Mexico mine.

A **rock** is a solid, cohesive aggregate of one or more minerals. Within the rock, individual mineral crystals (or grains) are mixed together and held firmly in a solid mass. The grains may be large or small, depending on how the rock was formed, but each grain retains its own unique mineral qualities. Each rock type has a characteristic mixture of minerals, grain sizes, and ways in which the grains are mixed and held together. Granite, for example, is a mixture of quartz, feldspar, and mica crystals. Rocks with a granite-like mineral content but much finer crystals are called rhyolite; chemically similar rocks with large crystals are called pegmatite.

Rock Types and How They Are Formed

Although rocks appear hard and permanent, they are part of a relentless cycle of formation and destruction. They are crushed, folded, melted, and recrystallized by dynamic processes related to

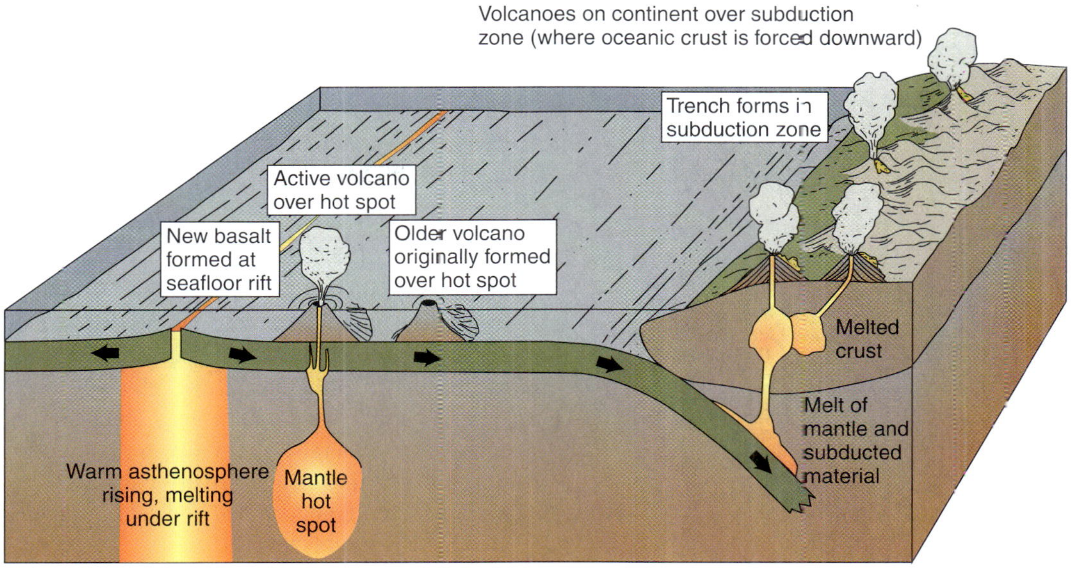

FIGURE 11.4 *Plate tectonic movement. Where thin, oceanic plates diverge, upwelling magma forms midocean ridges. A chain of volcanoes, such as the Hawaiian Islands, may form as plates pass over a hot spot. Where plates converge, melting can cause volcanoes, such as the Cascades.*

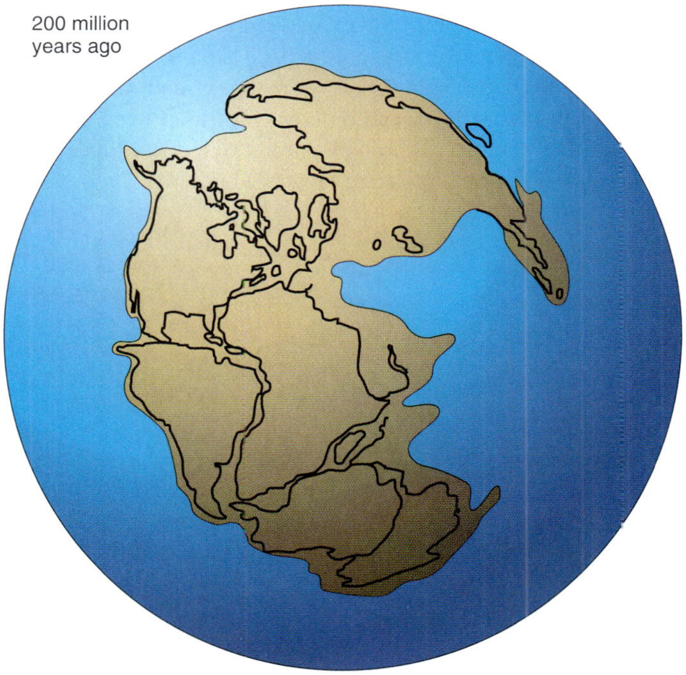

FIGURE 11.5 *Pangaea, the ancient supercontinent of 200 million years ago, combined all the world's continents in a single landmass.*

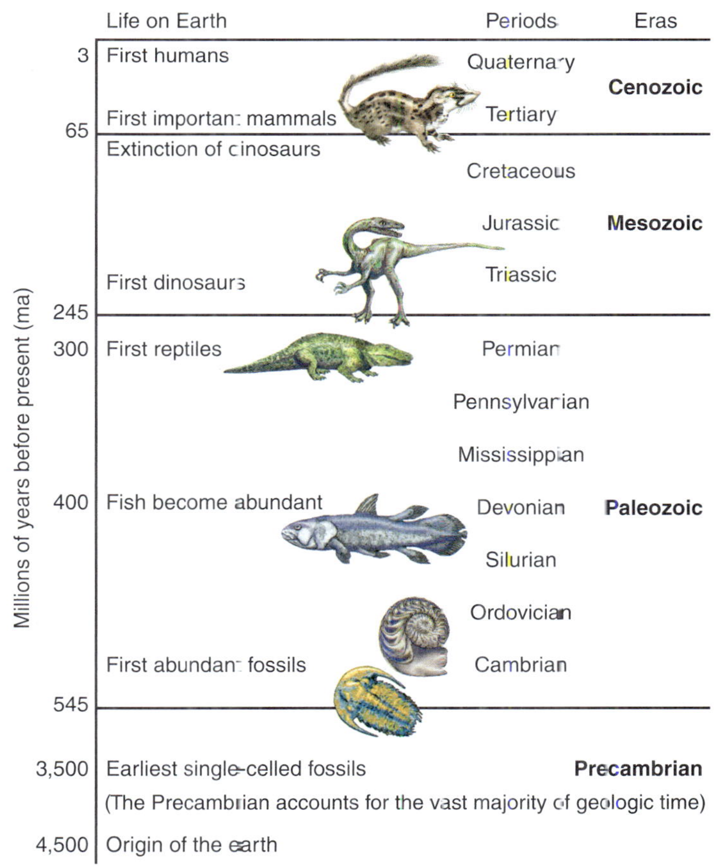

FIGURE 11.6 *Periods and eras in geologic time, and major life-forms that mark some periods.*

those that shape the large-scale features of the earth's crust. We call this cycle of creation, destruction, and metamorphosis the **rock cycle** (fig. 11.7). Understanding something of how this cycle works helps explain the origin and characteristics of different types of rocks.

There are three major rock classifications: igneous, metamorphic, and sedimentary. **Igneous rocks** (from *igni,* the Latin

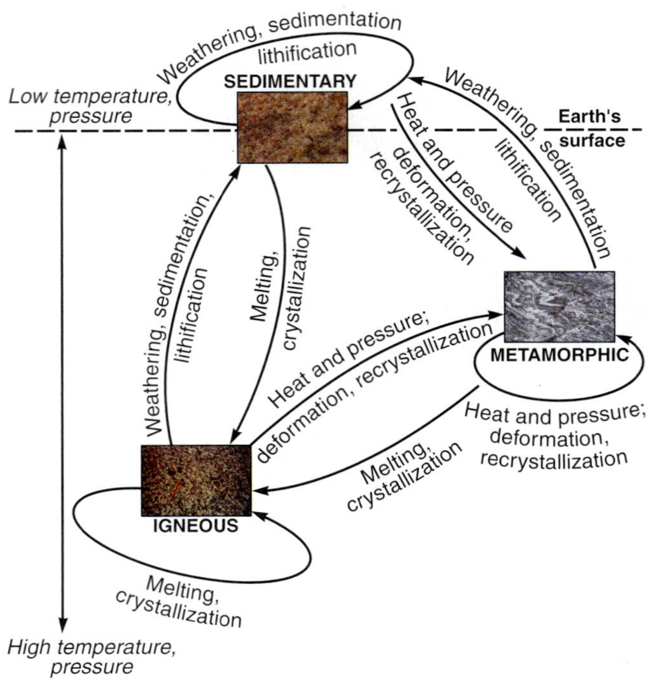

FIGURE 11.7 *The rock cycle includes a variety of geologic processes that can transform any rock.*

word for fire) are solidified from hot, molten magma or lava. Most rock in the earth's crust is igneous. Magma extruded to the surface from volcanic vents cools quickly to make finely crystalline rocks, such as basalt, rhyolite, or andesite. Magma that cools slowly in subsurface chambers or is intruded between overlying layers makes coarsely crystalline rocks, such as gabbro (rich in iron and silica) or granite (rich in aluminum and silica), depending on the chemical composition of the magma.

Metamorphic rocks form from the melting, contorting, and recrystallizing of other rocks. Deep in the ground, tectonic forces squeeze, fold, heat, and recrystallize solid rock. Under these conditions, chemical reactions can alter both the composition and the structure of the component minerals. Metamorphic rocks are classified by their chemical composition and by the degree of recrystallization: some minerals form only under extreme pressure and heat (diamonds or jade, for example); others form under more moderate conditions (graphite or talc). Some common metamorphic rocks are marble (from limestone), quartzite (from sandstone), and slate (from mudstone and shale). Metamorphic rocks often have swirling patterns left by the twisting and folding that created them.

Sedimentary rocks are formed when loose grains of other rocks are consolidated by time and pressure. Sandstone, for example, is solidified from layers of sand, and mudstone consists of extremely hardened mud and clay. Tuff is formed from volcanic ash, and conglomerates are aggregates of sand and gravel. Some sedimentary rocks develop from crystals that precipitate out of extremely salty water. Rock salt, made of the mineral halite, is ground up to produce ordinary table salt (sodium chloride). Salt deposits often form when a body of saltwater dries up, leaving salt crystals behind. Limestone is a rock composed of cemented remains of marine organisms. You can often see the shapes of shells and corals in a piece of limestone. Sedimentary formations often have distinctive layers that show different conditions when they were laid down. Erosion can reveal these layers and inform us of their history (fig. 11.8).

Weathering and Sedimentation

Most crystalline rocks are extremely hard and durable, but exposure to air, water, changing temperatures, and reactive chemical agents slowly breaks them down in a process called **weathering.** Mechanical weathering is the physical breakup of rocks into smaller particles without a change in chemical composition of the constituent minerals. You have probably seen mountain valleys scraped by glaciers, or river and shoreline pebbles that are rounded from being rubbed against one another as they are tumbled by waves and currents.

Chemical weathering is the selective removal or alteration of specific minerals in rocks. This alteration leads to weakening and disintegration of rock. Among the more important chemical weathering processes are oxidation (combination of oxygen with an element to form an oxide or a hydroxide mineral) and hydrolysis (hydrogen atoms from water molecules combine with other chemicals to form acids). The products of these reactions are more susceptible to both mechanical weathering and dissolving in water. For instance, when carbonic acid (formed when rainwater absorbs CO_2) percolates through porous limestone layers in the ground, it dissolves the rock and creates caves.

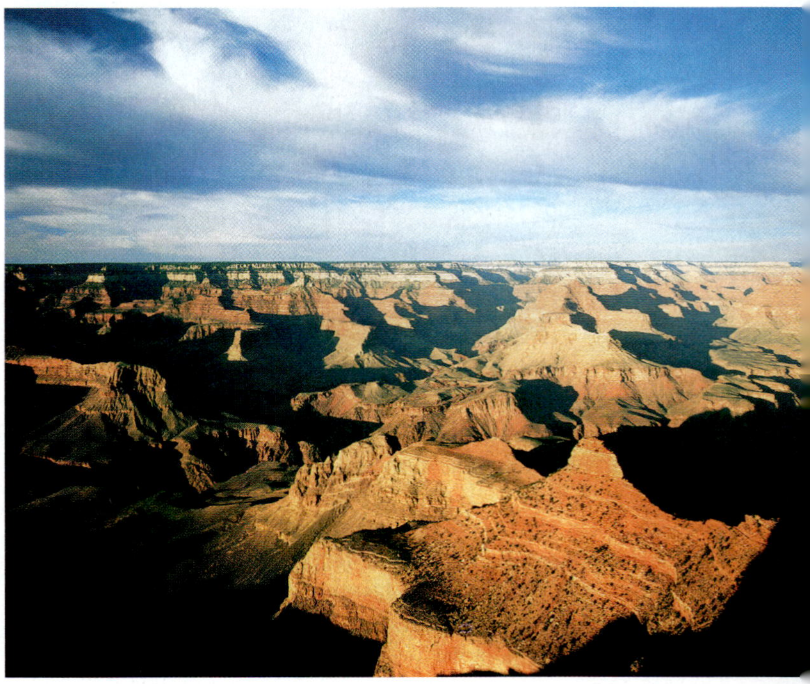

FIGURE 11.8 *Arizona's Grand Canyon is a collosal example of erosion that reveals millions of years of geologic history.*

Particles of rock loosened by wind, water, ice, and other weathering forces are carried downhill, downwind, or downstream until they come to rest again in a new location. The deposition of these materials is called **sedimentation.** Water, wind, and glaciers deposit particles of sand, clay, and silt far from their source. Much of the American Midwest, for instance, is covered with hundreds of meters of sedimentary material left by glaciers (till, or rock debris deposited by glacial ice), wind (loess, or fine dust deposits), river deposits of sand and gravel, and ocean deposits of sand, silt, clay, and limestone.

ECONOMIC GEOLOGY AND MINERALOGY

Economic mineralogy is the study of minerals that are valuable for manufacturing and trade. Most economic minerals are metal ores, minerals with unusually high concentrations of metals. Lead, for example, often comes from the mineral galena (PbS), and copper comes from sulfide ores, such as bornite (Cu_5FeS_4). Nonmetallic geologic resources include graphite, feldspar, quartz crystals, diamonds, and other crystals that are valued for their usefulness or beauty. Metals have been so important in human affairs that major epochs of human history are commonly known by the dominant materials and the technology to use them (Stone Age, Bronze Age, Iron Age, etc.). The mining, processing, and distribution of these materials have broad implications for both our culture and our environment. Most economically valuable crustal resources exist everywhere in small amounts; the important thing is to find them concentrated in economically recoverable levels.

Public policy in the United States has encouraged mining on public lands as a way of boosting the economy and utilizing natural resources. Today these policies are controversial, and there are efforts to recover public revenue from these publicly owned resources. (See related story "Should We Revise the 1872 Mining Law?" at www.mhhe.com/cases.)

Metals

Metals are malleable substances that are useful and valuable because they are strong, relatively light, and can be reshaped for many purposes. The availability of metals and the methods to extract and use them have determined technological developments, as well as economic and political power for individuals and nations.

The metals consumed in greatest quantity by world industry include iron (740 million metric tons annually), aluminum (40 million metric tons), manganese (22.4 million metric tons), copper and chromium (8 million metric tons each), and nickel (0.7 million metric tons). Most of these metals are consumed in the United States, Western Europe, Japan, and China. They are produced primarily in South America, South Africa, and Russia (fig. 11.9). It is easy to see how these facts contribute to a worldwide mineral trade network that has become crucially important to the economic and social stability of all nations involved. Table 11.2 shows the primary uses of these metals.

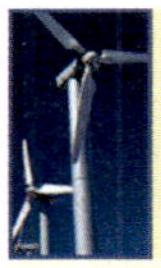

TABLE 11.2 Primary Uses of Some Major Metals Consumed in the United States

METAL	USE
Aluminum	Packaging foods and beverages (38%), transportation, electronics
Chromium	High-strength steel alloys
Copper	Building construction, electric and electronic industries
Iron	Heavy machinery, steel production
Lead	Leaded gasoline, car batteries, paints, ammunition
Manganese	High-strength, heat-resistant steel alloys
Nickel	Chemical industry, steel alloys
Platinum group	Automobile catalytic converters, electronics, medical uses
Gold	Medical, aerospace, electronic uses; accumulation as monetary standard
Silver	Photography, electronics, jewelry

Nonmetal Mineral Resources

Nonmetal minerals constitute a broad class that covers resources from gemstones to sand, gravel, salts, limestone, and soils. Sand and gravel production for road and building construction comprise by far the greatest volume and dollar value of all nonmetal mineral resources and a far greater volume than all metal ores. Sand and gravel are used mainly in brick and concrete construction, in paving, as loose road filler, and for sandblasting. High-purity silica sand is our source of glass. These materials usually are retrieved from surface pit mines and quarries, where they were deposited by glaciers, winds, or ancient oceans.

Limestone, like sand and gravel, is mined and quarried for concrete and crushed for road rock. It also is cut for building stone, pulverized for use as an agricultural soil additive that neutralizes acidic soil, and roasted in lime kilns and cement plants to make plaster (hydrated lime) and cement.

Evaporites (materials deposited by evaporation of chemical solutions) are mined for halite, gypsum, and potash. These are often found at or above 97 percent purity. Halite, or rock salt, is used for water softening and ice melting on winter roads in some northern areas. Refined, it is a source of table salt. Gypsum (calcium sulfate) now makes our plaster wallboard, but it has been used to cover walls ever since the Egyptians plastered their frescoed tombs along the Nile River some 5,000 years ago. Potash is an evaporite composed of a variety of potassium chlorides and potassium sulfates. These highly soluble potassium salts have long been used as a soil fertilizer.

Sulfur deposits are mined mainly for sulfuric acid production. In the United States, sulfuric acid use amounts to more than 200 lbs per person per year, mostly because of its use in industry, car batteries, and some medicinal products.

Durable, highly valuable, and easily portable, gemstones and precious metals have long been a way to store and transport

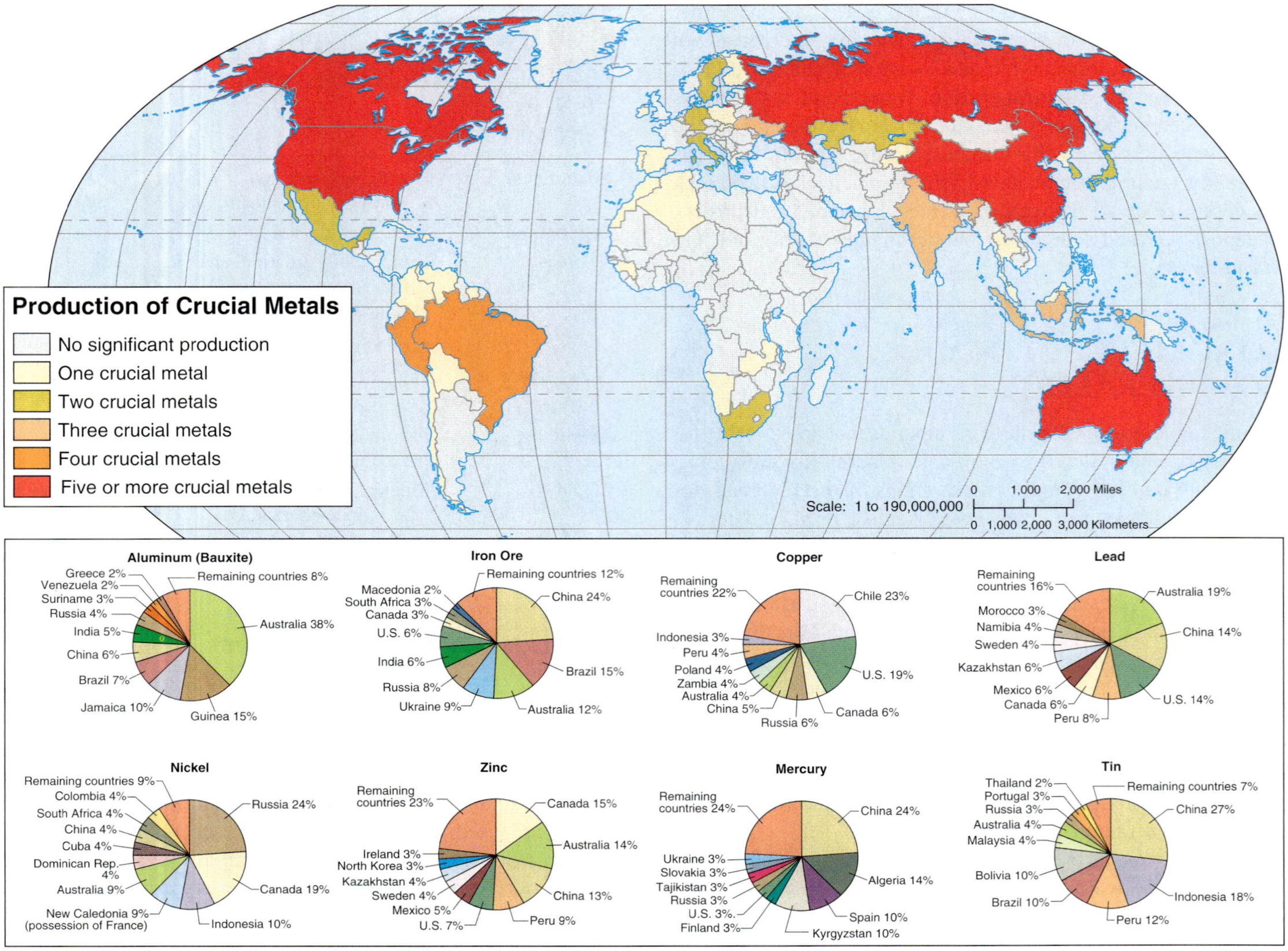

FIGURE 11.9 *World production of metals most essential for an industrial economy. Principal consumers are the United States, Western Europe, Japan, and China.*

wealth. Unfortunately, these valuable materials also have bankrolled despots, criminal gangs, and terrorism in many countries. In recent years, brutal civil wars in Africa have been financed—and often motivated by—gold, diamonds, tantalum ore, and other high-priced commodities. In 2004 investigators discovered that members of the terrorist group Al Qaida used diamonds purchased in Liberia to finance the September 11, 2001 attacks in the United States. Much of this illegal trade ends up in the $100 billion per year global jewelry trade, two-thirds of which sells in the United States. Many people who treasure a diamond ring or a gold wedding band as a symbol of love and devotion are unaware that it may have been obtained through slave labor, torture, and environmentally destructive mining and processing methods. Civil rights organizations are campaigning to require better documentation of the origins of gems and precious metals to prevent their use as financing for crimes against humanity (see related story "Conflict Diamonds" at www.mhhe.com/cases).

In 2004 a group of Nobel Peace Laureates called on the World Bank to overhaul its policies on lending for resource extractive industries. "War, poverty, climate change, and ongoing violations of human rights—all of these scourges are all too often linked to the oil and mining industries," wrote Archbishop Desmond Tutu, winner of the 1984 Nobel Peace Prize for helping eliminate apartheid in South Africa. In response, the World Bank appointed an Extractive Industries Review headed by former Indonesian Environment Minister Emil Salim. Its final report, which was still under discussion at the time of this writing, is said to embrace many concerns raised by environmental and community organizations.

Fuels: Oil, Coal, and Uranium

Modern society functions largely on energy produced from geologic deposits of oil, coal, and natural gas. Nuclear energy, which

APPLICATION: What Geologic Resources Are You Using Right Now?

Make a list of the geologic materials used in some of the objects you are using right now. For example, the computer used to write this chapter is made largely of plastic (from oil), silicon chips (sand), and copper wire, and it runs on energy from coal- and uranium-powered electric plants.

Start your list with some of the following items: glasses, chair, table, pencil, lightbulb, window, building, wristwatch, coffee cup, tooth fillings.

runs on uranium, makes up a large portion of our electricity resources. Energy production from these sources is discussed in chapter 12. Oil, coal, and gas are organic, created over millions of years as extreme heat and pressure transformed the remains of ancient organisms. They are not minerals, because they have no crystalline structure, but they can be considered part of economic mineralogy because they are such important geologic resources. In addition to providing energy, oil is the source material for plastics, and natural gas is used to make agricultural fertilizers.

The search for these organic deposits is one of the most important parts of economic mineralogy. Debates over exploitation and ownership of these resources play important roles in national and international politics. The Persian Gulf War of 1990 was fought over control of vast underground oil deposits, as has been Russia's war in Chechnya. Debates over exploiting potential oil reserves in the Alaskan National Wildlife Refuge (ANWR) have raged in the United States for decades. (See related stories "Exploiting Oil in ANWR" and "Oil and the War in Chechnya?" at www.mhhe.com/cases.) Recently, Canada's oil shale and tar sands have become another source of oil (see chapter 12).

ENVIRONMENTAL EFFECTS OF RESOURCE EXTRACTION

Each of us depends daily on geologic resources mined or pumped from sites around the world. We use scores of metals and minerals, many of which we've never even heard of, in our lights, computers, watches, fertilizers, and cars. Extracting and purifying these resources can have severe environmental and social consequences. The most obvious effect of mining and well drilling is often the disturbance or removal of the land surface. Farther-reaching effects, though, include air and water pollution. The EPA lists more than 100 toxic air pollutants, from acetone to xylene, released from U.S. mines and wells every year. Nearly 80,000 metric tons of particulate matter (dust) and 11,000 tons of sulfur dioxide are released from nonmetal mining alone. Chemical- and sediment-runoff pollution is a major problem in many local watersheds (see What Do You Think? p. 268).

Gold and other metals are often found in sulfide ores that produce sulfuric acid when exposed to air and water. In addition,

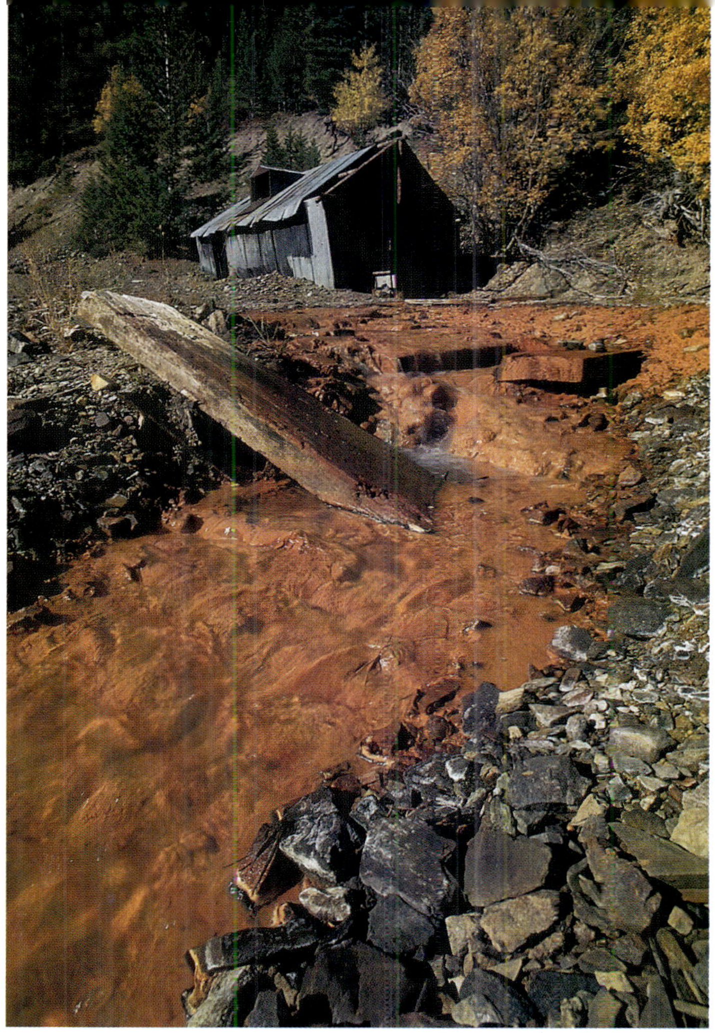

FIGURE 11.10 *Thousands of abandoned mines on public lands poison streams and groundwater with acid, metal-laced drainage. This old mine in Montana drains into the Blackfoot River, the trout stream featured in Norman Maclean's book* A River Runs through It.

metal elements often occur in very low concentrations—10 to 20 parts per billion may be economically extractable for gold, platinum, and other metals. Consequently, vast quantities of ore must be crushed and washed to extract metals. Cyanide, mercury, and other toxic substances are used to chemically separate metals from the minerals that contain them, and these substances can easily contaminate lakes and streams. Further, a great deal of water is used in washing crushed ore with cyanide and other solutions. In arid Nevada, the USGS estimates that mining consumes about 230,000 m^3 (60 million gal) per day. After use in ore processing, much of this water contains sulfuric acid, arsenic, heavy metals, and other contaminants. Mine runoff leaking into lakes and streams can damage or destroy aquatic ecosystems (fig. 11.10).

Mining

There are many techniques for extracting geologic materials. The most common methods are open-pit mining, strip-mining, and underground mining. An ancient method of accumulating gold, diamonds, and coal is placer mining, in which pure nuggets are

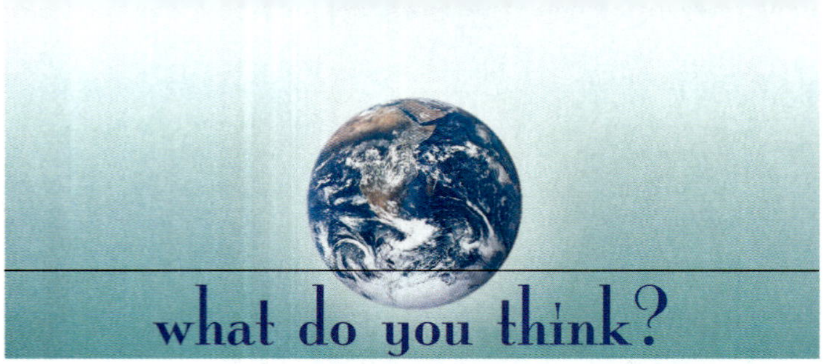

Coal-Bed Methane

Vast deposits of coal, oil, and gas lie under the sage scrub and arid steppe of North America's intermountain West. Geologists estimate that at least 346 trillion ft^3 of "technically recoverable" natural gas and 62 billion barrels of petroleum liquids occur in five intermountain basins stretching from Montana to New Mexico. These deposits would provide a 15-year supply of gas at present usage rates, and at least four times as much oil as the most optimistic estimates for the Arctic National Wildlife Refuge. About half of that gas and oil is in or around relatively shallow coal seams, which makes it vastly cheaper to extract than most other gas supplies. Drilling a typical offshore gas well costs tens of millions of dollars, and a deep conventional gas well costs several million dollars, but a coal-bed methane well is generally less than $100,000. The total value of the methane and petroleum liquids from the Rocky Mountains could be as much as $200 billion over the next decade.

Most coal-bed methane is held in place by pressure from overlying aquifers. Pumping the water out these aquifers releases the gas but creates phenomenal quantities of effluent, which often is contaminated with salt and other minerals. A typical coal-bed well produces 75,000 liters of water per day. Dumping it on the surface can poison fields and pastures, erode stream banks, contaminate rivers, and harm fish and wildlife. Drawing down aquifers depletes the wells on which many ranches depend and dries up natural springs and wetlands essential for wildlife. Ranchers complain that livestock and wildlife are killed by traffic and poisoned by discarded toxic waste around well sites. "It may be a clean fuel," says one rancher, "but it's a dirty business."

Another objection to coal-bed methane extraction is simply the enormous scope of the enterprise. In Wyoming's Powder River Basin, energy companies have already installed 12,000 wells and have proposed 39,000 more. Eventually, this area could contain as many as 140,000 wells, together with the sprawling network of roads, pipelines, compressor stations, and wastewater pits necessary for such a gargantuan undertaking. The Green River Basin and the San Juan Basin, with three to five times as much potential gas and oil as Powder River, have even greater probability for environmental damage.

In 2002 the U.S. Environmental Protection Agency (EPA) gave its worst possible rating to the Environmental Impact Statement (EIS) for the proposed Powder River wells because of concerns over wastewater disposal. Nevertheless, the Bush administration approved the plan and ordered federal land managers across the Rockies to look for ways to remove or reduce environmental restrictions on gas drilling. This order came in spite of a federal study finding that 63 percent of the natural gas in the five basins was completely open to drilling, 25 percent had some restrictions, and only 12 percent of the gas was totally protected, which was about what conservationists had been saying.

An unlikely coalition of ranchers, hunters, anglers, conservationists, water users, and renewable energy activists have banded together to fight against coal-bed gas extraction, calling on Congress to protect private property rights, preserve water quality, and conserve sensitive public lands. Lifelong Republicans, who once looked with suspicion and disgust at environmentalists, suddenly find themselves banding together with tree-huggers and off-the-grid hippie communes to protect their way of life.

On the other side, producers argue that they are helping preserve the American way of life. If we want to be independent of foreign energy sources, they point out, we need to develop our own energy sources. A decade ago, environmentalists were promoting natural gas as a clean energy alternative because it produces far less carbon dioxide and air pollutants, such as particulates and sulfur oxides, than does burning coal. Disagreeable as gas well effluents may be, they aren't nearly as toxic and long-lasting as nuclear waste.

What do you think? Does having access to cleaner fuels justify the social and environmental costs of their extraction? If you had a vote in this issue, what restrictions would you impose on the companies carrying out these projects? Could renewable energy sources, such as wind or solar, substitute for coal-bed methane?

Ethical Issues

What responsibility do those of us who consume fuel have for the way it's produced? How would you weigh the rights of a minority (a few thousand ranchers) against the needs of tens of millions of urban residents who would benefit from cheaper energy prices and cleaner air? Much of the land involved is arid and appears barren to those of us used to more verdant landscapes, yet it is loved and treasured by those who live there. How would you set a value on the solitude, history, and harsh beauty of these places?

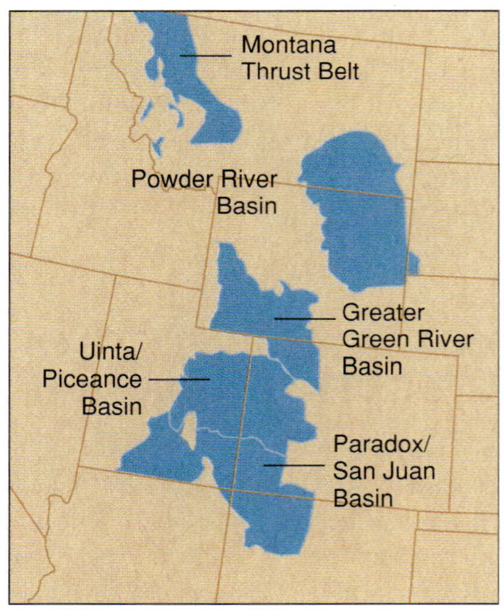

Coal-bed methane deposits occur in five intermountain basins in the western United States.

washed from stream sediments. Since the California gold rush of 1849, placer miners have used water cannons to blast away hillsides. This method, which chokes stream ecosystems with sediment, is still used in Alaska, Canada, and many other regions. Another ancient, and much more dangerous, method is underground mining. Ancient Roman, European, and Chinese miners tunneled deep into tin, lead, copper, coal, and other mineral seams. Mine tunnels occasionally collapse, and natural gas in coal mines can explode. Water seeping into mine shafts also dissolves toxic minerals. Contaminated water seeps into groundwater; it is also pumped to the surface, where it enters streams and lakes.

In underground coal mines, another major environmental risk is fires. Hundreds of coal mines smolder in the United States, China, Russia, India, South Africa, and Europe. The inaccessibility and size of these fires make many impossible to extinguish or control. One mine fire in Centralia, Pennsylvania, has been burning since 1962; control efforts have cost at least $40 million, but the fire continues to expand. China, which depends on coal for much of its heating and electricity, has hundreds of smoldering mine fires; one has been burning for 400 years. According to a recent study from the International Institute for Aerospace Survey in the Netherlands, these fires consume up to 200 million tons of coal every year and emit as much carbon dioxide as all the cars in the United States. Toxic fumes containing mercury, arsenic, selenium, radon, and other hazardous emissions are also released from these fires.

Open-pit mines are used to extract massive beds of metal ores and other minerals. The size of modern open pits can be hard to comprehend. The Bingham Canyon mine, near Salt Lake City, Utah, is 800 m (2,640 ft) deep and nearly 4 km (2.5 mi) wide at the top. More than 5 billion tons of copper ore and waste material have been removed from the hole since 1906. A chief environmental challenge of open-pit mining is that groundwater accumulates in the pit. In metal mines, a toxic soup results. No one yet knows how to detoxify these lakes, which endanger wildlife and nearby watersheds. (See related story "Death in a Mine Pit" at www.mhhe.com/cases.)

Half the coal used in the United States comes from strip mines. Since coal is often found in expansive, horizontal beds, the entire land surface can be stripped away to cheaply and quickly expose the coal. The overburden, or surface material, is placed back into the mine, but usually in long ridges called spoil banks. Spoil banks are very susceptible to erosion and chemical weathering. Since the spoil banks have no topsoil (the complex organic mixture that supports vegetation—see chapter 7), revegetation occurs very slowly.

The 1977 federal Surface Mining Control and Reclamation Act (SMCRA) requires better restoration of strip-mined lands, especially where mines replaced prime farmland. Since then, the record of strip-mine reclamation has improved substantially. Complete mine restoration is expensive, often more than $10,000 per hectare. Restoration is also difficult because the developing soil is usually acidic and compacted by the heavy machinery used to reshape the land surface.

Bitter controversy has grown recently over mountaintop removal, a coal mining method practiced mainly in Appalachia. Long, sinuous ridge-tops are removed by giant, 20-story-tall shovels to expose horizontal beds of coal (fig. 11.11). Up to 215 m (700 ft) of ridge-top is pulverized and dumped into adjacent river valleys. The debris can be laden with selenium, arsenic, coal, and other toxic substances. At least 900 km (560 mi) of streams have been buried in West Virginia alone. Environmental lawyers have sued to stop the destruction of streams, arguing that it violates the Clean Water Act (chapter 10). In response, the Bush administration

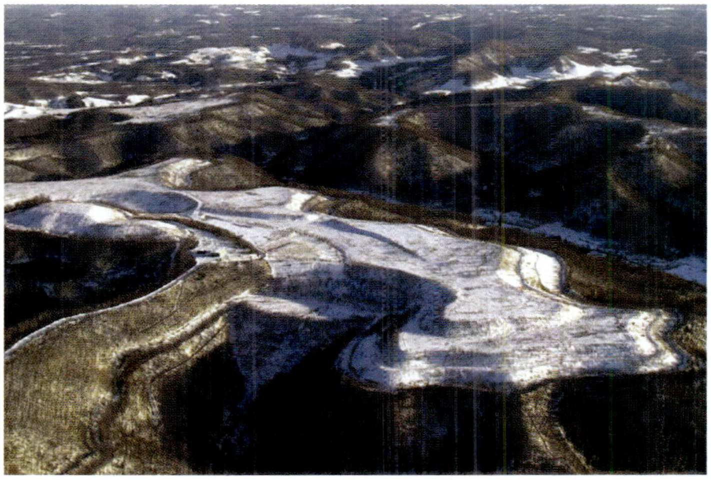

FIGURE 11.11 *Mountaintop removal mining is a relatively new, and deeply controversial, method of extracting Appalachian coal.*

issued a "clarification" of the Clean Water Act, rewriting the law to allow stream filling by any sort of mining or industrial debris, rather than forbidding any stream destruction. Environmentalists charge that the new wording subverts the Clean Water Act, giving a green light to all sorts of stream destruction. West Virginians are deeply divided about mountaintop removal because they live in affected stream valleys but also depend on a coal economy.

The Mineral Policy Center in Washington, D.C., estimates that 19,000 km (12,000 mi) of rivers and streams in the United States are contaminated by mine drainage. The EPA estimates that cleaning up impaired streams, along with 550,000 abandoned mines in the United States, may cost $70 billion. Worldwide, mine closing and rehabilitation costs are estimated in the trillions of dollars. Because of the volatile prices of metals and coal, many mining companies have gone bankrupt before restoring mine sites, leaving the public responsible for cleanup. In 2002 more than 500 leading mine executives and their critics convened at the Global Mining Initiative, a meeting in Toronto aimed at improving the sustainability of mining. Executives acknowledged that in the future they will increasingly be held liable for environmental damages, and they said they were seeking ways to improve the industry's social and environmental record. Jay Hair, secretary general of the International Council on Mining and Metals, stated that "environmental protection and social responsibility are important" and that mining companies were interested in participating in sustainable development. Mine executives also recognized that, increasingly, big cleanup bills will cut into company values and stock prices. Finding creative ways to keep mines cleaner from the start will make good economic sense, even if it's not easy to do.

Processing

Metals are extracted from ores by heating or by using chemical solvents. Both processes release large quantities of toxic materials that can be even more environmentally hazardous than mining.

Smelting—roasting ore to release metals—is a major source of air pollution. One of the most notorious examples of ecological devastation from smelting is a wasteland near Ducktown, Tennessee. In the mid-1800s, mining companies began excavating the rich copper deposits in the area. To extract copper from the ore, they built huge, open-air wood fires, using timber from the surrounding forest. Dense clouds of sulfur dioxide released from sulfide ores poisoned the vegetation and acidified the soil over a 50-mi^2 (13,000-ha) area. Rains washed the soil off the denuded land, creating a barren moonscape.

Sulfur emissions from Ducktown smelters were reduced in 1907 after Georgia sued Tennessee over air pollution. In the 1930s the Tennessee Valley Authority (TVA) began treating the soil and replanting trees to cut down on erosion. Recently, upwards of $250,000 per year has been spent on this effort. While the trees and other plants are still spindly and feeble, more than two-thirds of the area is considered "adequately" covered with vegetation. Similarly, smelting of copper-nickel ore in Sudbury, Ontario, a century ago caused widespread ecological destruction that is slowly being repaired following pollution-control measures (see fig. 9.26).

Chemical extraction is used to dissolve or mobilize pulverized ore, but it uses and pollutes a great deal of water. A widely used method is **heap-leach extraction,** which involves piling crushed ore in huge heaps and spraying it with a dilute alkaline-cyanide solution (fig. 11.12). The solution percolates through the pile and dissolves gold. The gold-containing solution is then pumped to a processing plant that removes the gold by electrolysis. A thick clay pad and plastic liner beneath the ore heap is supposed to keep the poisonous cyanide solution from contaminating surface or groundwater, but leaks are common.

Once all the gold is recovered, mine operators may simply walk away from the operation, leaving vast amounts of toxic effluent in open ponds behind earthen dams. A case in point is the Summitville Mine near Alamosa, Colorado. After extracting $98 million in gold, the absentee owners declared bankruptcy in 1992, abandoning millions of tons of mine waste and huge, leaking ponds of cyanide. The Environmental Protection Agency may spend more than $100 million trying to clean up the mess and keep the cyanide pool from spilling into the Alamosa River.

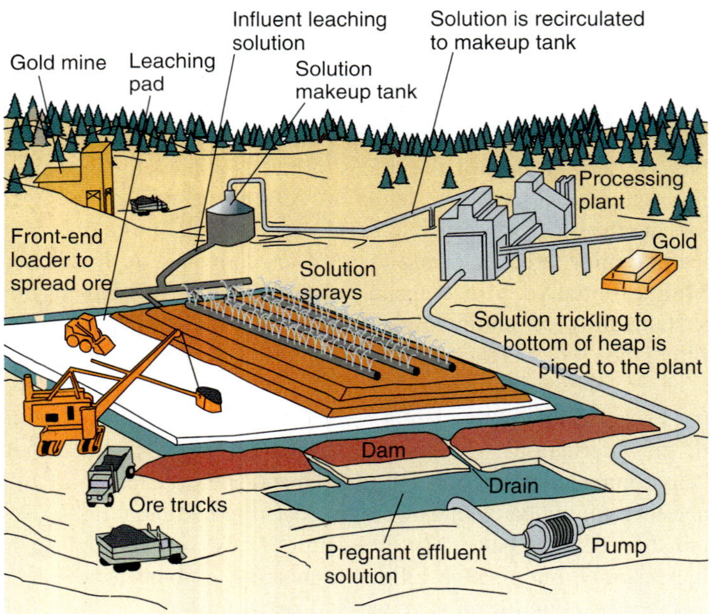

FIGURE 11.12 *In a heap-leach operation, huge piles of low-grade ore are heaped on an impervious pad and sprayed continuously with a cyanide solution. As the leaching solution trickles through the crushed ore, it extracts gold and other precious metals. The "pregnant" effluent solution is then pumped to a processing plant, where metals are extracted and purified. This technique is highly profitable but carries large environmental risks.*
Source: Data from George Laycock, *Audubon Magazine,* vol. 91(7), July 1989.

CONSERVING GEOLOGIC RESOURCES

Conservation offers great potential for extending our supplies of economic minerals and reducing the effects of mining and processing. The advantages of conservation are significant: less waste to dispose of, less land lost to mining, and less consumption of money, energy, and water resources.

Recycling

Some waste products already are being exploited, especially for scarce or valuable metals. Aluminum, for instance, must be extracted from bauxite by electrolysis, an expensive, energy-intensive process. Recycling waste aluminum, such as beverage cans, on the other hand, consumes one-twentieth of the energy of extracting new aluminum. Today, nearly two-thirds of all aluminum beverage cans in the United States are recycled, up from only 15 percent 20 years ago. The high value of aluminum scrap ($650 a ton versus $60 for steel, $200 for plastic, $50 for glass, and $30 for paperboard) gives consumers plenty of incentive to deliver their cans for collection. Recycling is so rapid and effective that half of all the aluminum cans now on a grocer's shelf will be made into another can within two months. Table 11.3 shows the energy cost of extracting other materials.

Platinum, the catalyst in automobile catalytic exhaust converters, is valuable enough to be regularly retrieved and recycled from used cars (fig. 11.13). Other commonly recycled metals are gold, silver, copper, lead, iron, and steel. The last four are readily available in a pure and massive form, including copper pipes, lead batteries, and steel and iron auto parts. Gold and silver are valuable enough to warrant recovery, even through more difficult means.

Steel and Iron Recycling: Minimills

While total U.S. steel production has fallen in recent decades—largely because of inexpensive supplies from new and efficient Japanese steel mills—a new type of mill subsisting entirely on a readily available supply of scrap/waste steel and iron is a growing industry. Minimills, which remelt and reshape scrap iron and steel, are smaller and cheaper to operate than traditional integrated mills that perform every process from preparing raw ore to finishing

TABLE 11.3 Energy Requirements in Producing Various Materials from Ore and Raw Source Materials

	ENERGY REQUIREMENT (MJ/kg)[1]	
PRODUCT	NEW	FROM SCRAP
Glass	25	25
Steel	50	26
Plastics	162	n.a.[2]
Aluminum	250	8
Titanium	400	n.a.[2]
Copper	60	7
Paper	24	15

Source: Data from E. T. Hayes, *Implications of Materials Processing,* 1997.

[1]Megajoules per kilogram.

[2]Not available.

iron and steel products. Minimills produce steel at between $225 and $480 per metric ton, while steel from integrated mills costs $1,425 to $2,250 per metric ton, on average. The energy cost is also lower in minimills: 5.3 million BTU/ton of steel, compared with 16.08 million BTU/ton in integrated mill furnaces. Minimills now produce about half of all U.S. steel. Recycling is slowly increasing as raw materials become more scarce and wastes become more plentiful.

Substituting New Materials for Old

Mineral and metal consumption can be reduced by new materials or new technologies developed to replace traditional uses. This is a long-standing tradition; for example, bronze replaced stone technology, and iron replaced bronze. More recently, the introduction of plastic pipe has decreased our consumption of copper, lead, and steel pipes. In the same way, the development of fiber-optic technology and satellite communication reduces the need for copper telephone wires.

Iron and steel have been the backbone of heavy industry, but we are now moving toward other materials. One of our primary uses for iron and steel has been machinery and vehicle parts. In automobile production, steel is being replaced by polymers (long-chain organic molecules similar to plastics), aluminum, ceramics, and new high-technology alloys. All of these reduce vehicle weight and cost, while increasing fuel efficiency. Some of the newer alloys that combine steel with titanium, vanadium, or other metals wear much better than traditional steel. Ceramic engine parts provide heat insulation around pistons, bearings, and cylinders, keeping the rest of the engine cool and operating efficiently. Plastics and glass fiber–reinforced polymers are used in body parts and some engine components.

Electronics and communications (telephone) technology, once major consumers of copper and aluminum, now use ultra-

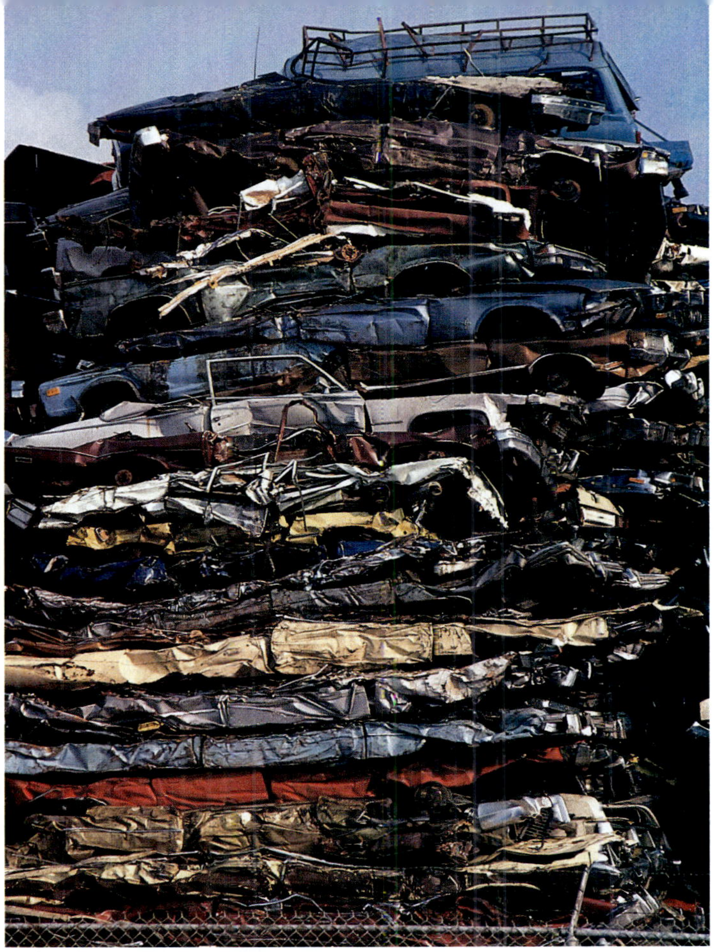

FIGURE 11.13 *The richest metal source we have—our mountains of scrapped cars—offers a rich, inexpensive, and ecologically beneficial resource that can be "mined" for a number of metals.*

high-purity glass cables to transmit pulses of light, instead of metal wires carrying electron pulses. Once again, this technology has been developed for its greater efficiency and lower cost, but it also affects consumption of our most basic metals.

GEOLOGIC HAZARDS

Earthquakes, volcanoes, floods, and landslides are normal earth processes, events that have made our earth what it is today. However, when they affect human populations, their consequences can be among the worst and most feared disasters that befall us.

Earthquakes

Earthquakes are sudden movements in the earth's crust that occur along faults (planes of weakness), where one rock mass slides past another one. When movement along faults occurs gradually and relatively smoothly, it is called creep or seismic slip and may be undetectable to the casual observer. When friction prevents rocks from slipping easily, stress builds up until it is finally released with a sudden jerk. The point on a fault at which the first movement occurs during an earthquake is called the epicenter.

Earthquakes have always seemed mysterious, sudden, and violent, coming without warning and leaving ruined cities and dislocated landscapes in their wake. Cities such as Kobe, Japan, or Mexico City, parts of which are built on soft landfill or poorly consolidated soil, usually suffer the greatest damage from earthquakes (fig. 11.14). Water-saturated soil can liquify when shaken. Buildings sometimes sink out of sight or fall down like a row of dominoes under these conditions (see related stories on earthquakes at www.mhhe.com/cases).

Earthquakes frequently occur along the edges of tectonic plates, especially where one plate is being subducted, or pushed down, beneath another. Earthquakes also occur in the centers of continents, however. In fact, one of the largest earthquakes ever recorded in North America was one of an estimated magnitude 8.8 that struck the area around New Madrid, Missouri, in 1812. Fortunately, few people lived there at the time, and the damage was minimal.

Modern contractors in earthquake zones attempt to prevent damage and casualties by constructing buildings that can withstand tremors. The primary methods used are heavily reinforced structures, strategically placed weak spots in the building that can absorb vibration from the rest of the building, and pads or floats beneath the building on which it can shift harmlessly with ground motion.

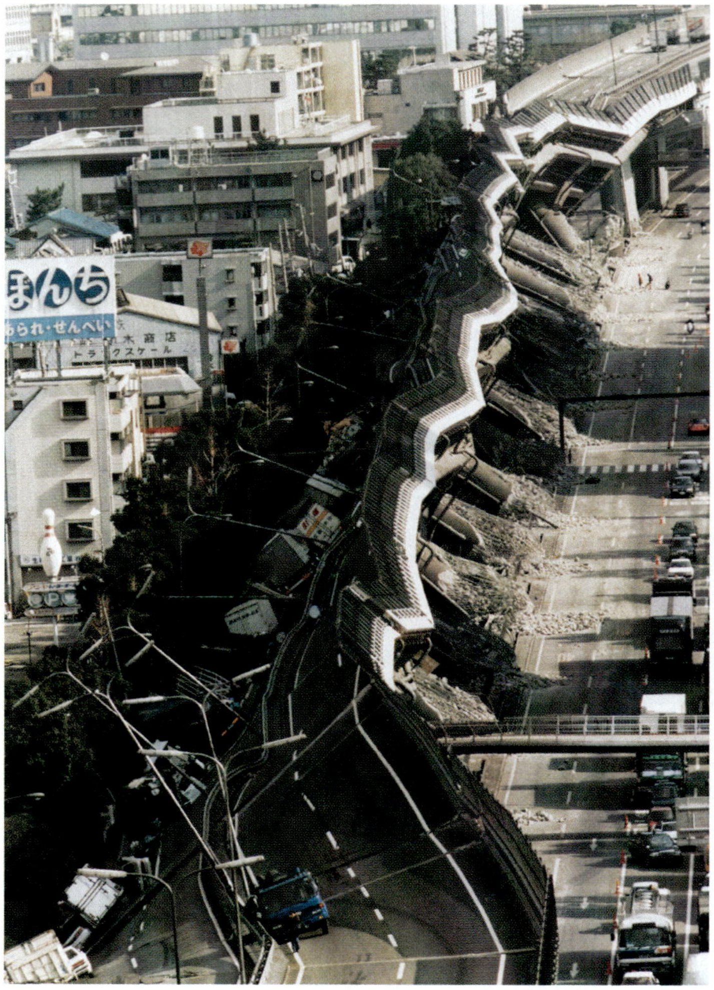

FIGURE 11.14 *An elevated freeway buckled and collapsed as a result of the 1995 earthquake in Kobe, Japan.*

One of the most notorious effects of earthquakes is the tsunami. These giant sea swells (sometimes improperly called tidal waves) can move at 1,000 km/h (600 mph), or faster, away from the center of an earthquake. When these swells approach the shore, they can create breakers as high as 65 m (nearly 200 ft). Tsunamis also can be caused by underwater volcanic explosions or massive seafloor slumping. In 2004, an undersea earthquake of magnitude 9.0 hit northern Indonesia. The resulting tsunami killed at least 114,000 people and left millions homeless from Thailand to Kenya.

Volcanoes

Volcanoes and undersea magma vents are the sources of most of the earth's crust. Over hundreds of millions of years, gaseous emissions from these sources formed the earth's earliest oceans and atmosphere. Many of the world's fertile soils are weathered volcanic materials. Volcanoes have also been an ever present threat to human populations (fig. 11.15). One of the most famous historic volcanic eruptions was that of Mount Vesuvius in southern Italy, which buried the cities of Herculaneum and Pompeii in A.D. 79. The mountain had been showing signs of activity before it erupted, but many citizens chose to stay and take a chance on survival. On August 24, the mountain buried the two towns in ash. Thousands were killed by the dense, hot, toxic gases that accompanied the ash flowing down from the volcano's mouth. It continues to erupt from time to time.

Nuees ardentes (French for "glowing clouds") are deadly, denser-than-air mixtures of hot gases and ash like those that inundated Pompeii and Herculaneum. Temperatures in these clouds may exceed 1,000°C, and they move at more than 100 km/h (60 mph). *Nuees ardentes* destroyed the town of St. Pierre on the Caribbean island of Martinique on May 8, 1902. Mount Pelee released a cloud of *nuees ardentes* that rolled down through the town, killing between 25,000 and 40,000 people within a few minutes. All of

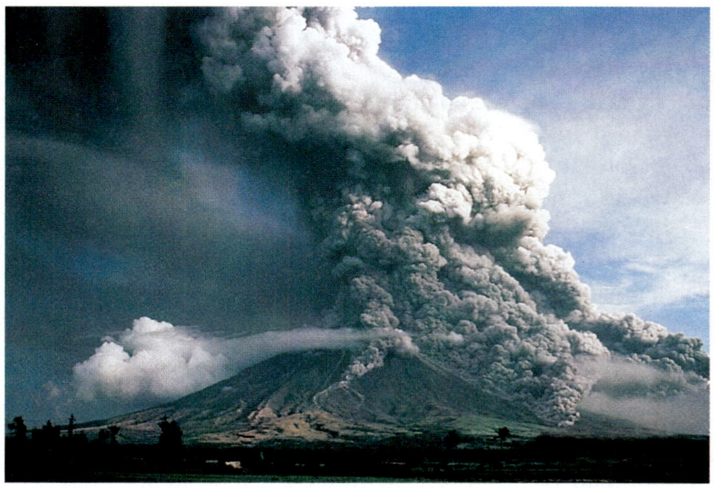

FIGURE 11.15 *Lava and ash flow spill down the slopes of Mayon volcano in the Philippines in this September 23, 1984, image. Because more than 73,000 people evacuated danger zones, this eruption caused no casualties.*

the town's residents died except for a single prisoner being held in the town dungeon.

Mudslides are also disasters sometimes associated with volcanoes. The 1985 eruption of Nevado del Ruíz, 130 km (85 mi) northwest of Bogotá, Colombia, caused mudslides that buried most of the town of Armero and devastated the town of Chinchina. An estimated 25,000 people were killed. Heavy mudslides also accompanied the eruption of Mount St. Helens in Washington in 1980. Sediments mixed with melted snow destroyed roads, bridges, and property, but because of sufficient advance warning, there were few casualties. Geologists worry that similar mudflows from an eruption at Mount Rainier would threaten much larger populations (fig. 11.16).

Volcanic eruptions often release large volumes of ash and dust into the air. Mount St. Helens expelled 3 km^3 of dust and ash, causing ash fall across much of North America. This was only a minor eruption. An eruption in a bigger class of volcanoes was that of Tambora in Indonesia in 1815, which expelled 175 km^3 of dust and ash, more than 58 times that of Mount St. Helens. These dust clouds circled the globe and reduced sunlight and air temperatures enough so that 1815 was known as the year without a summer.

It is not just a volcano's dust that blocks sunlight. Sulfur emissions from volcanic eruptions combine with rain and atmospheric moisture to produce sulfuric acid (H_2SO_4). Droplets of H_2SO_4 interfere with solar radiation and can significantly cool the world climate. In 1991 Mount Pinatubo in the Philippines emitted 20 million tons of sulfur dioxide aerosols, which remained in the stratosphere for two years. This thin haze cooled the entire earth by 1°C for about two years. It also caused a 10 to 15 percent reduction in stratospheric ozone, allowing increased ultraviolet light to reach the earth's surface.

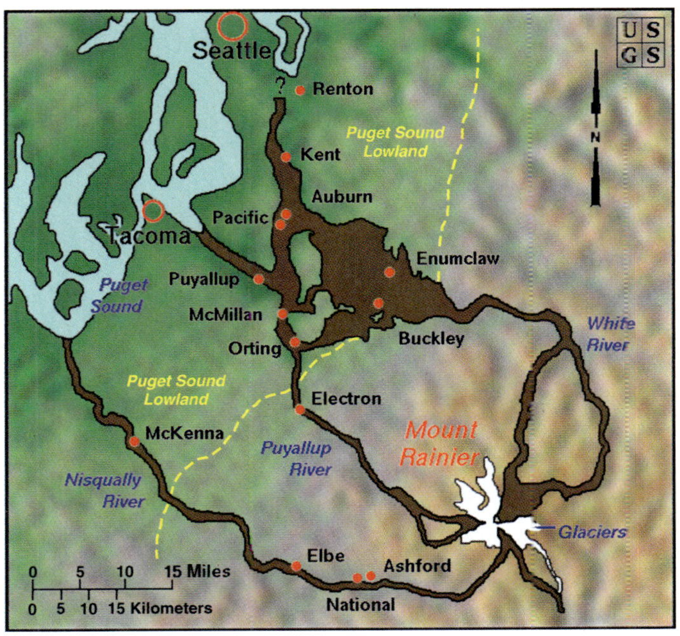

FIGURE 11.16 *Volcanic activity at Mount Rainier has produced at least 12 large mudflows in the past 6,000 years* (brown areas). *Future flows could threaten large populations now in the area.*
Source: Data from T. W. Sisson, USGS Open File Report 95-642.

Floods

In most moderately humid climates, stream channels adjust to accommodate average maximum stream flows. Much of the year, the water level may be well below the stream bank height, but heavy rains or sudden snow melt can deliver more water than the stream can carry. Excess water that overflows stream banks and covers adjacent land is considered a **flood.** The severity of floods can be described by the depth of water above the normal stream banks or by how frequently a similar event normally occurs—on average—for a given area. Note that these are statistical averages over long time periods. A "10-year flood" would be expected to occur once in every ten years; a "100-year flood" would be expected to occur once every century. But two 100-year floods can occur in successive years or even in the same year.

The biggest economic loss from floods is usually not the buildings and property they carry away but, rather, the contamination they cause. Virtually everything floodwaters touch in a house—carpets, furniture, drapes, electronics, even drywall and insulation—must be removed and discarded. Although floods usually don't take as many lives as some other natural disasters, they are among the most costly because they occur relatively frequently and in populated river corridors.

Many human activities increase both the severity and frequency of floods. Paving roads and parking lots reduces water infiltration into the soil and speeds the rate of runoff into streams and lakes. Clearing forests for agriculture and filling cities with buildings similarly increase both the volume and rate of water discharge after a storm.

Under normal conditions, floods are mitigated by **floodplains**—low land that is periodically inundated during normal floods. However, floodplains are usually fertile, flat, and easily farmed. They are convenient for building and close to the river. In much of the developed world, floodplains are widely farmed, developed with cities and houses, and cleared of vegetation. Floodplains have lost much of their ability to absorb floodwaters.

Even more than development, though, flood-control structures have separated floodplains from rivers. Levees and flood walls are built to contain water within riverbanks, and river channels are dredged and deepened to allow water to recede faster. Every flood-control structure simply transfers the problem downstream, however. The water has to go somewhere. If it doesn't soak into the ground upstream, it will simply exacerbate floods somewhere downstream—leading to more levee development, and then to more flooding farther downstream, and so on.

Flood Control

More than $25 billion of river-control systems have been built on the Mississippi and its tributaries. These systems have protected many communities over the past century. In the major floods of 1993, however, this elaborate system helped turn a large flood into a major disaster. Deprived of the ability to spill out over floodplains, the river is pushed downstream to create faster currents and deeper floods until eventually a levee gives way somewhere. Hydrologists calculate that the floods of 1993 were about 3 m (10 ft) higher than they would have been, given the same rainfall in 1900 before the flood-control structures were in place (fig. 11.17).

Under current rules, the government is obligated to finance most levees and flood-control structures. Many people think that it would be much better to spend this money to restore wetlands, replace groundcover on water courses, build check dams on small streams, move buildings off the floodplain, and undertake other nonstructural ways of reducing flood danger. According to this view, floodplains should be used for wildlife habitat, parks, recreation areas, and other uses not susceptible to flood damage.

The National Flood Insurance Program administered by the Federal Emergency Management Agency (FEMA) was intended to aid people who cannot buy insurance at reasonable rates, but its effects have been to encourage building on the floodplains by making people feel that, whatever happens, the government will take care of them. Many people would like to relocate homes and businesses out of harm's way after the recent floods or to improve them so they will be less susceptible to flooding, but owners of damaged property can collect only if they rebuild in the same place and in the same way as before. This perpetuates problems rather than solves them.

Erosion

Gravity constantly pulls downward on every material everywhere on earth. Hillsides, beaches, even relatively flat farm fields can lose material to erosion. Often water helps mobilize loose material, and catastrophic slumping, beach erosion, and gully development can occur in a storm. Where houses are built on erodible surfaces, enormous loss of property can result.

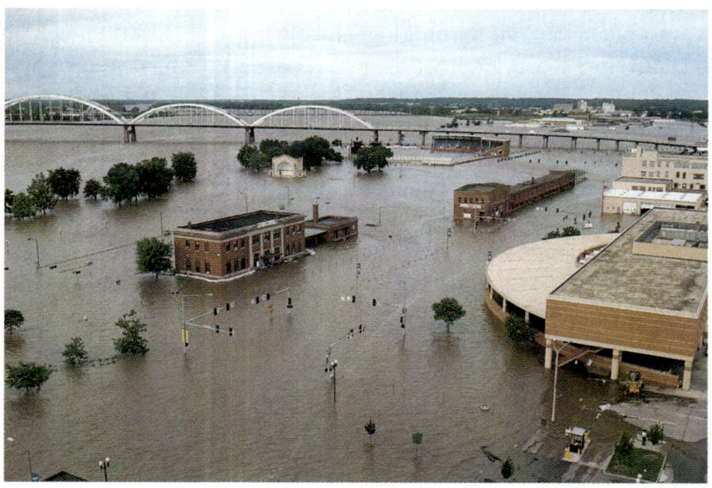

FIGURE 11.17 *The Mississippi River inundated downtown Davenport, Iowa, during the summer floods of 1993. Although sympathetic with the heartbreak and economic losses caused by this flooding, many people argue that floodplains such as this never should have been settled in the first place.*

Landslides, also called mass wasting or mass movement, occur when masses of material move downslope. Slow and subtle landslips are common, but rockslides, mudslides, and slumping can be swift and dangerous. In the United States alone, landslides and related mass wasting cause over $1 billion in property damage every year. When unconsolidated sediments on a hillside are saturated by a storm or exposed by logging, road building, or house construction, slopes are especially susceptible to sudden landslides.

Often people are unaware of the risks they face by locating on or under unstable hillsides. Sometimes they simply ignore clear and obvious danger. In southern California, where land prices are high, people often build expensive houses on steep hills and in narrow canyons. Most of the time, this dry environment appears quite stable, but the chaparral vegetation burns frequently and fiercely. When fires expose the soil in late summer, heavy winter rains cause mudslides and debris flows that destroy whole neighborhoods (fig. 11.18).

Gullying is the development of deep trenches on relatively flat ground. Especially on farm fields, which have a great deal of

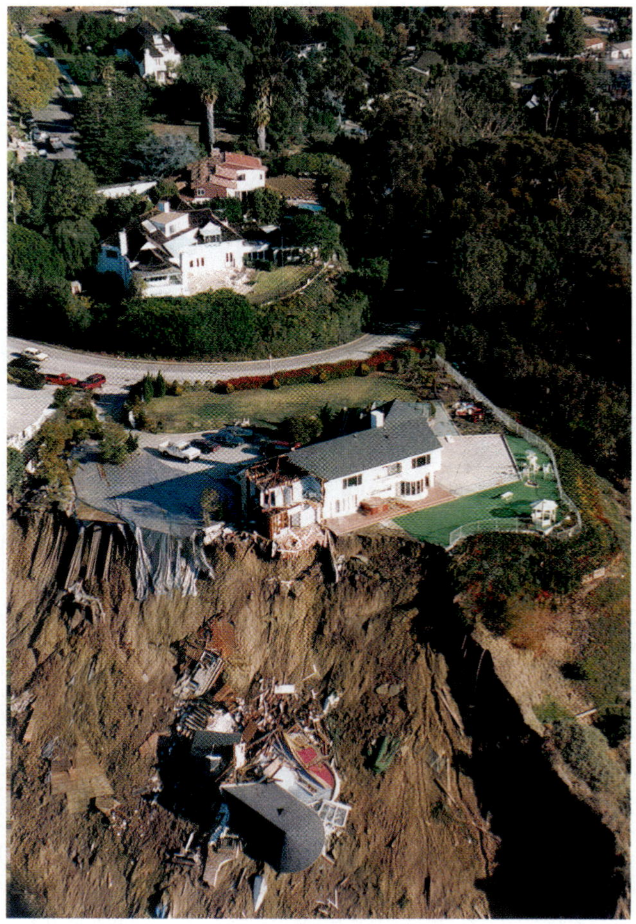

FIGURE 11.18 *Parts of an expensive house slide down the hillside in Pacific Palisades, California. Building at the edge of steep slopes made of unconsolidated sediment in an earthquake-prone region is a risky venture.*

loose soil unprotected by plant roots, rainwater running across the surface can dig deep gullies. Sometimes land becomes useless for farming because gullying is so severe and because erosion has removed the fertile topsoil. Agricultural soil erosion has been described as an invisible crisis. Erosion has reduced the fertility of millions of acres of prime farmland in the United States alone.

Beach erosion occurs on all sandy shorelines because the motion of the waves is constantly redistributing sand and other sediments. One of the world's longest and most spectacular sand beaches runs down the Atlantic coast of North America from New England to Florida and around the Gulf of Mexico. Much of this beach lies on some 350 long, thin **barrier islands** that stand between the mainland and the open sea. Behind these barrier islands lie shallow bays or brackish lagoons fringed by marshes or swamps.

Early inhabitants recognized that the shore was a hazardous place to live and settled on the bay side of barrier islands or as far upstream on coastal rivers as was practical. Modern residents, however, place a high value on living where they have an ocean view and ready access to the beach. And they assume that modern technology makes them immune to natural forces. The most valuable and prestigious property is closest to the shore. Over the past 50 years, more than 1 million acres of estuaries and coastal marshes have been filled to make way for housing or recreational developments.

Construction directly on beaches and barrier islands can cause irreparable damage to the whole ecosystem. Normally fragile vegetative cover holds the shifting sand in place. Damaging this vegetation with construction, building roads, and breaching dunes with roads can destabilize barrier islands. Storms then wash away beaches or even whole islands. A single severe storm in 1962 caused $300 million in property damage along the east coast of the United States and left hundreds of beach homes tottering into the sea (fig. 11.19). FEMA estimates that 25 percent of all coastal homes in the United States will have the ground washed out from under them by 2060.

Cities and individual property owners often spend millions of dollars to protect beaches from erosion. Sand is dredged from the ocean floor or hauled in by the truckload, only to wash away again in the next storm. Building artificial barriers, such as groins or jetties, can trap migrating sand and build beaches in one area, but they often starve downstream beaches and make erosion there even worse (fig. 11.20).

As is the case for inland floodplains, government policies often encourage people to build where they probably shouldn't. Subsidies for road building and bridges, support for water and sewer projects, tax exemptions for second homes, flood insurance, and disaster relief are all good for the real estate and construction businesses but invite people to build in risky places. Flood insurance typically costs $300 per year for $80,000 of coverage. In 1998 FEMA paid out $40 billion in claims, 80 percent of which were flood-related. Settlement usually requires that structures be rebuilt exactly where and as they were before. There is no restriction on how many claims can be made, and policies are rarely canceled, no matter what the risk. Some beach houses have been rebuilt—at public expense—three times in a decade. The General Accounting Office found that 2 percent of federal flood policies were responsible for 30 percent of the claims.

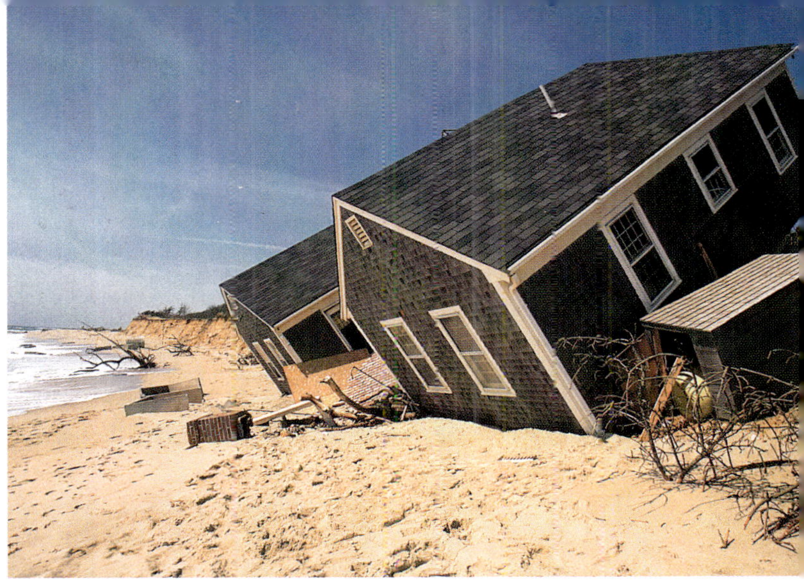

FIGURE 11.19 *Winter storms have eroded the beach and undermined the foundations of homes on this barrier island. Breaking through protective dunes to build such houses damages sensitive plant communities and exposes the whole island to storm sand erosion. Coastal zone management attempts to limit development on fragile sites.*

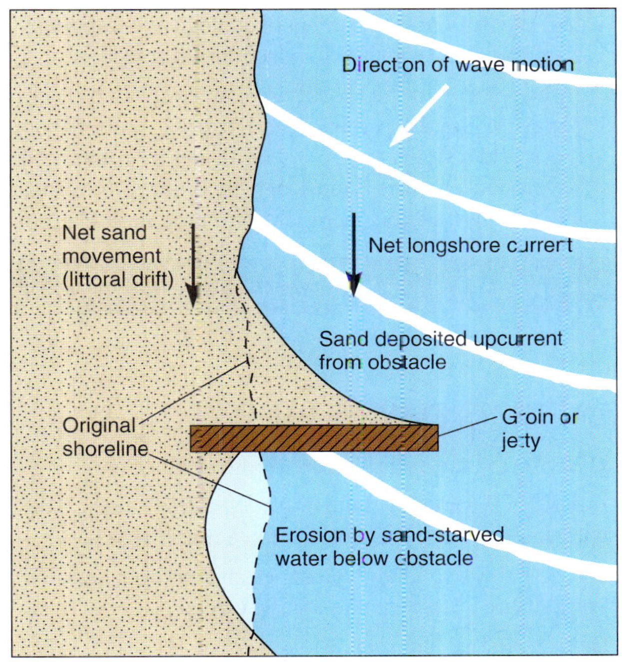

FIGURE 11.20 *Groins are structures built perpendicular to a beach to slow erosion and trap sand. They build up beaches toward prevailing wind and wave direction but starve beaches and increase erosion downstream. Dashed line indicates original shoreline.*

The Coastal Barrier Resources Act of 1982 prohibited federal support, including flood insurance, for development on sensitive islands and beaches. In 1992, however, the U.S. Supreme Court ruled that ordinances forbidding floodplain development amount to an unconstitutional "taking," or confiscation, of private property.

SUMMARY

- The earth is a complex, dynamic system. Although it seems stable and permanent to us, the crust is in constant motion. Huge blocks called tectonic plates slide over the surface of the ductile mantle. They crash into each other in ponderous slow motion, crumpling their margins into mountain ranges and causing earthquakes. Often one plate slides under another, carrying rock layers down into the mantle, where they melt and flow back toward the surface to form new rocks.
- Rocks are classified according to composition, structure, and origin. The three basic types of rock are igneous, metamorphic, and sedimentary. These rock types can be transformed from one to another by way of the rock cycle, a continuous process of weathering, transport, burial in sediments, metamorphism, melting, and recrystallization.
- During the cooling and crystallization process that forms rock from magma, minerals and metals can become concentrated enough to become economically important reserves if they are close enough to the surface to be reached by mining. Having a reliable supply of strategically important minerals and metals is vital in industrialized societies.
- A few places in the world are especially rich in mineral deposits. Southern Africa and Russia contain some of the world's richest supplies of strategic minerals. Less-developed countries, most of which are in the tropics or the Southern Hemisphere, are often the largest producers of iron, aluminum, copper, gold, and other metals on which the industrialized world depends. The major consumers of these resources are the industrialized countries.
- Both extraction and processing of metals and mineral resources can have negative environmental effects. Mine drainage has polluted thousands of kilometers of streams and rivers. Fumes from smelters kill forests and spread pollution over large areas. Surface mining results in removal of natural ecosystems, soil disruption, creation of trenches or open pits, and tailings accumulations. It is now required that strip-mined areas be recontoured, but revegetation is often difficult and limited in species composition. Smelting and chemical extraction processes also create pollution problems.
- Worldwide, only a small percentage of metals are recycled, although it is not a difficult process technically. Recycling saves energy and reduces environmental damage caused by mining and smelting. It reduces waste production and makes our metal supplies last much longer. Substitution of materials usually occurs when mineral supplies become so scarce that prices are driven up.
- Earthquakes, volcanoes, floods, and erosion are natural geologic processes. When they affect human lives and property, however, they become some of the worst "natural disasters" known. Some of these natural disasters, especially floods and erosion, are made more serious by human activities and land-use decisions.

QUESTIONS FOR REVIEW

1. Describe the layered structure of the earth.
2. Figure 11.3 shows subduction and rifting zones. Describe what happens at these tectonic plate margins.
3. Why are there so many volcanoes and earthquakes along the "ring of fire" that rims the Pacific Ocean?
4. Define *mineral* and *rock*.
5. Describe the rock cycle, and name the three main rock types that it produces.
6. Give some examples of nonmetal mineral resources, and describe how they are used.
7. What are some environmental hazards associated with mineral extraction?
8. Describe some ways we can reduce our consumption of new mineral resources.
9. Describe some of the leading geologic hazards and their effects.
10. Why is home building on beaches and barrier islands risky?

THINKING SCIENTIFICALLY

1. Understanding and solving the environmental problems of mining are basically geologic problems, but geologists need information from a variety of environmental and scientific fields. What are some of the other sciences (or disciplines) that could contribute to solving mine contamination problems?
2. Geologists are responsible for identifying and mapping mineral resources. But mineral resources are buried below the soil and covered with vegetation. How do you suppose geologists in the field find clues about the distribution of rock types?
3. If you had an igneous rock with very fine crystals and one with very large crystals, which would you expect to have formed deep in the ground, and why?
4. Heat and pressure tend to help concentrate metal ores. Explain why such ores might often occur in mountains such as the Andes in South America.
5. The idea of tectonic plates shifting across the earth's surface is central to explanations of geologic processes. Why is this idea still called the "theory" of plate tectonic movement?

6. Geologic evidence from fossils and sediments provided important evidence for past climate change. What sorts of evidence in the rocks and landscape around you suggest that the place where you live once looked much different than it does today?

KEY TERMS

barrier islands 275
core 261
crust 261
earthquakes 271
flood 273
floodplains 273
heap-leach extraction 270
igneous rocks 263
landslides 274
magma 261
mantle 261
metamorphic rocks 264
midocean ridges 261
mineral 262
rock 262
rock cycle 263
sedimentary rocks 264
sedimentation 265
smelting 270
subducted 262
tectonic plates 261
volcanoes 272
weathering 264

SUGGESTED READINGS

Bawden, G. W., et al. 2001. Tectonic contraction across Los Angeles after removal of groundwater pumping effects. *Nature* 412:812–15.

Gould, Stephen Jay. *Wonderful Life: The Burgess Shale and the Nature of History.* W. W. Norton.

Kennedy, Danny. 1997. U.S. mine gouges for gold. *Earth Island Journal* 12(2):24.

Knoo, Andrew H. 2003. *When Life Nearly Died: The Greatest Mass Extinction of All Time.* Thames & Hudson.

McPhee, John. 2000. *Annals of a Former World.* Farrar Strauss Giroux.

Rudwick, Martin J. S. 1995. *Scenes from Deep Time: Early Pictorial Representations of the Prehistoric World.* University of Chicago Press.

Winchester, Simon. 2002. *The Map That Changed the World: William Smith and the Birth of Modern Geology.* Perennial Press.

Welcome to McGraw-Hill's Online Learning Center

http://www.mhhe.com/cunningham3e

WEB EXERCISES

Exploring Recent Earthquakes

Go to the World Data Center for Seismology at http://neic.usgs.gov/. Click on "Current earthquake information"; then choose "Current earthquake maps" (the second item in the list) to see the location of recent earthquakes.

1. Where was the largest earthquake in the world in the past month? Where was the most recent one? Click on the map location of the most recent earthquake, and record the following information. When did it occur? Where was it exactly? How deep was it? What was its magnitude?
2. One of the largest earthquakes in recent years was one of magnitude 8.4 off the coast of South America in 2001. Where and when did this occur? How much damage did it cause? Why was the damage less than it otherwise might have been? Hint: look first for "Large/Significant Earthquakes" by year at http://neic.usgs.gov/current_seismicity.html; then click on 2001 to find the largest. A brief summary is presented under "Large/Noteworthy Earthquakes in 2001." A more detailed analysis is given under "Significant Earthquakes of the World in 2001."

For another view of recent earthquakes, go to www.crustal.ucsb.edu/ics/understanding/ and click on the rotating globe. If you have a broadband connection, increase the speed of rotation to get a smoother motion. Does information given on this page agree with your answer to question 1?

Understanding Volcanoes

USGS Hawaii Volcano Observatory is one of the most important places for studying and understanding volcanoes. Visit the observatory's website at http://hvo.wr.usgs.gov/.

1. Which of the volcanoes discussed at this website is the largest in the world? Which is the most active?
2. Why are earthquakes discussed on this volcano website?
3. What are the major hazards to people from these volcanoes?

For a good collection of volcano images, go to the USGS Cascades Volcano Observatory at http://vulcan.wr.usgs.gov/Photo/framework.html.

Evaluating Erosion on Farmland

The Natural Resources Conservation Service (NRCS), part of the U.S. Department of Agriculture, is the agency that monitors agricultural resources and conditions. Among its data-gathering efforts, the NRCS produces a Natural Resources Inventory (NRI), with maps of farmland conditions across the mainland United States. Visit the NRCS/NRI website at www.nrcs.usda.gov/technical/land/erosion.html.

Find the list of erosion maps. Look at several of the maps. First identify the meaning of the colors. Then identify the major concentration of high and low erosion rates.

1. Where is wind erosion worst? Where is water erosion worst?
2. Where are the most acres of highly erodible cropland? What kind of physical features might occur there?

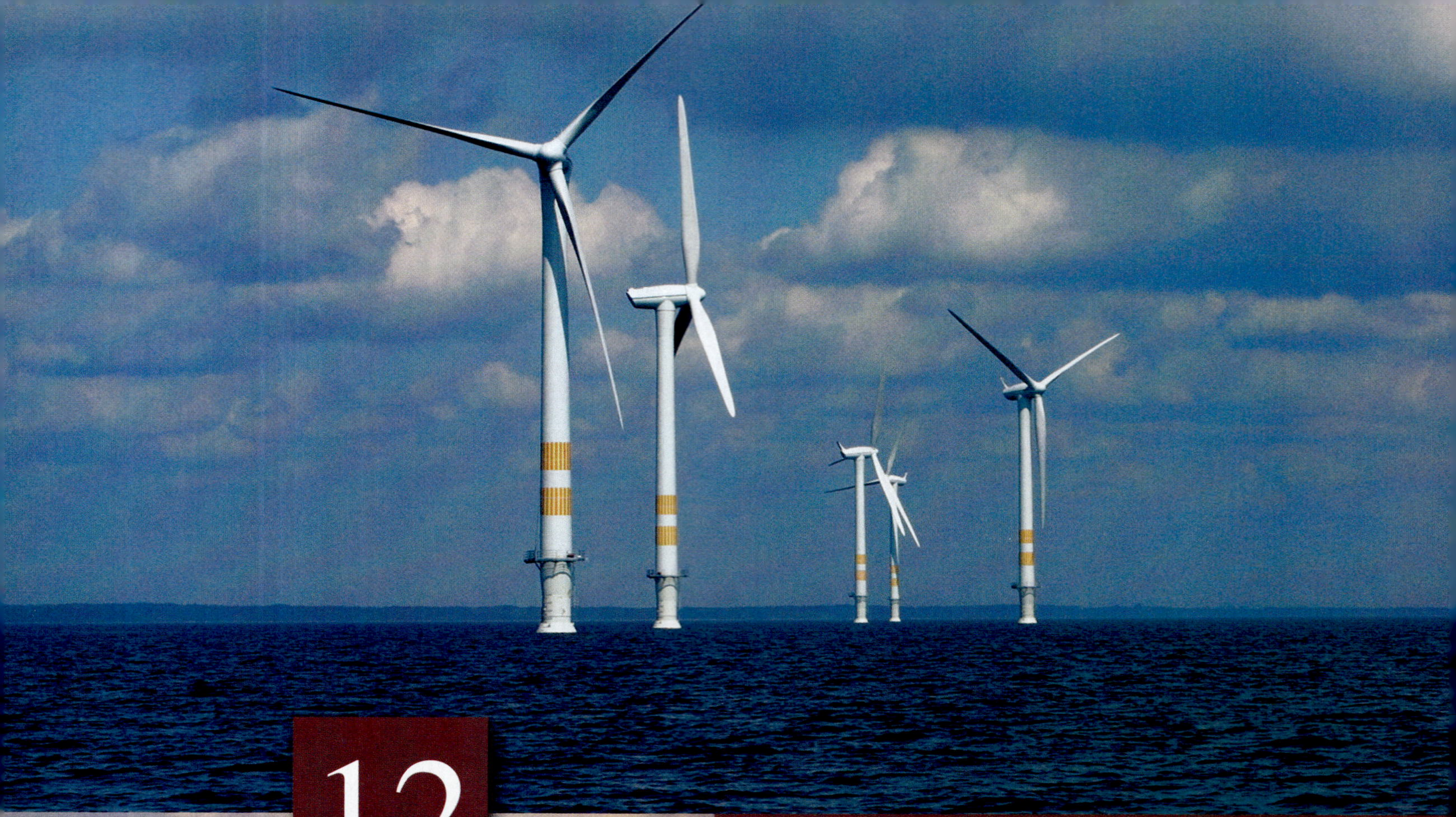

12 Energy

My father rode a camel. I drive a car. My son flies a jet airplane. His son will ride a camel.

–Saudi saying

Windmills, each taller than the Statue of Liberty, stand on a shoal off the Swedish coast.

Welcome to McGraw-Hill's Online Learning Center

http://www.mhhe.com/cunningham3e

LEARNING ONLINE

Visit our webpage at www.mhhe.com/cunningham3e for data sources, further readings, additional case studies, current environmental news, and regional examples within the Online Learning Center to help you understand the material in this chapter. You'll also find active links to information pertaining to this chapter, including:

Fossil fuels: oil/coal/gas
Nuclear power
Sustainable energy
Efficiency and energy conservation
Solar energy
Wind power
Fuel cells and hydrogen economy
Hydro and geothermal energy

OBJECTIVES

After studying this chapter, you should be able to

- summarize our current energy sources, and explain briefly how our energy compares with that of other people in the world.
- analyze the resources and reserves of fossil fuels in the world.
- evaluate the costs and benefits of using coal, oil, and natural gas.
- understand how nuclear reactors work, why they are dangerous, and how they might be made safer.
- appreciate the opportunities for energy conservation available to us.
- understand how active and passive systems capture solar energy and how photovoltaic collectors generate electricity.
- comprehend the promise and problems of using biomass as an energy source.
- explain how hydropower, wind, and other energy from the earth's forces can contribute to our energy supply.

Sea Power

In 2003 British Prime Minister Tony Blair and Swedish Prime Minister Goran Persson surprised the world (and many of their constituents) by pledging to reduce carbon dioxide emissions by 60 percent by 2050. Calling climate change "unquestionably the most urgent environmental challenge we face," Blair said that issues of global poverty and environmental degradation—especially global warming—are just as devastating in their potential impact as terrorism or weapons of mass destruction." Noting that his country is "well on the way" to meeting its greenhouse gas reduction target of 12.5 percent under the United Nations Kyoto Protocol, Blair said that this goal is not enough to avert global warming. He said that, "to stop further damage to the climate, we need a reduction of 60 percent worldwide." Furthermore, he said, "I believe we can achieve that target at reasonable cost."

To reach this ambitious goal, both the United Kingdom and Sweden are moving away from fossil fuels and promoting a portfolio of conservation and renewable energy projects, including windmills, fuel cells, wave power, solar energy, and cogeneration (combined production of heat and electricity). Together, it is hoped, these alternative sources will produce at least 20 percent of each country's electricity by 2020.

Of the new energy sources, offshore wind power is likely to be the largest for these countries. Coinciding with Blair's promise for greenhouse gas reductions, the British government began a new round of licensing seabed locations for thousands of giant windmills. Noting that the U.K. has among the best wind resources in Europe and great expertise in offshore development from North Sea oil, the Minister of Trade predicted that wind could provide up to half of Britain's renewable energy, while providing up to 20,000 jobs. The U.K. could become a net energy exporter in 2010 for the first time in 30 years, rather than importing 75 percent of its supply, as is predicted under a business-as-usual scenario.

Offshore wind projects already underway in the U.K. are expected to provide as much electricity as six large nuclear power plants. Some people object to the visual impact of windmills up to 127 meters tall (417 ft) from the water line to the tip of the blades. Others, however, see these wind farms as welcome alternatives to our present energy sources. As American author Bill McKibben says, "The choice is not between windmills and untouched nature. It's between windmills and the destruction of the planet's biology." A spokesperson for Greenpeace U.K. said, "For 30 years Greenpeace has opposed the pollution of our oceans but can today fully support this massive commitment to harness wind power at sea."

Wind energy is the fastest-growing generation source in the world (although admittedly it's growing from a small base). Worldwide, wind power now exceeds 35,000 MW of installed capacity, generating enough electricity to power 3.5 million average American homes or twice that many in Europe. Over the next five years, this capacity is expected to double. Europe has the fastest growth in wind power, with installations up 33 percent in 2002. Germany and Denmark currently lead in wind power, already obtaining about 20 percent of their electricity from wind. And Spain—the home of Don Quixote—increased its wind power capacity 44 percent in 2002.

This example illustrates both the need for, and promise of, renewable energy sources if we are to live in a sustainable world. In this chapter we'll look at both the fossil fuel and nuclear power that provide most of our energy supply currently, as well as the options for conservation and environmentally friendly renewable energy supplies.

ENERGY SOURCES AND USES

Being able to utilize external energy to do useful work is one of the most unique characteristics of humans. Access to a source of high-quality energy is essential for continuation of the current way of life. But what do these terms mean? **Work** is the application of force through a distance. **Energy** is the capacity to do work. **Power** is the rate of flow of energy, or the rate at which work is done. The energy we use to move our muscles, to think, and to carry out metabolic functions comes from stored chemical energy (or potential energy) in our food. Food energy is generally measured in calories (cal). One cal is the amount of energy to heat 1 g of water 1°C. A kilocalorie (or food Calorie) is 1,000 cal. In physics, the basic metric unit of force is a newton, which is the force necessary to accelerate 1 kilogram 1 meter per second. A **joule (J)** is the amount of work done when a force of 1 newton is exerted over 1 meter, or 1 amp per second flows through 1 ohm. One J equals 0.238 cal. Some other common energy units are presented in table 12.1.

TABLE 12.1 Some Energy Units

1 joule (J) = the force exerted by a current of 1 amp per second flowing through a resistance of 1 ohm

1 watt (W) = 1 joule (J) per second

1 kilowatt-hour (kwh) = 1 thousand (10^3) watts exerted for 1 hour

1 megawatt (MW) = 1 million (10^6) watts

1 gigawatt (GW) = 1 billion (10^9) watts

1 petajoule (PJ) = 1 quadrillion (10^{15}) joules

1 British thermal unit (BTU) = energy to heat 1 lb of water 1°F

1 PJ = 947 billion Btu, or 278 million kwh

1 standard barrel (bbl) of oil = 42 gal (160 liters) or 5.8 million Btu

1 metric ton of standard coal = 27.8 million Btu or 4.8 bbl oil

Current Energy Sources

Fossil fuels (petroleum, natural gas, and coal) now provide about 86 percent of all commercial energy in the world (fig. 12.1). Renewable sources—solar, wind, geothermal, and hydroelectricity—make up about 9.5 percent of our commercial power (but hydro accounts for most of that). Although not included in these data, private systems (individual houses, businesses, industries) may capture nearly as much renewable energy (excluding hydropower) as that reported in commercial transactions. This summary probably also underrepresents the importance of biomass because these fuels often are gathered by the people using them, or they are sold in the informal economy and not reported internationally. In many poorer countries, such as Haiti, Bhutan, and Malawi, biomass supplies more than 90 percent of the energy used for heating and cooking. This is an important energy source for poor people but can be a serious cause of forest destruction (see chapter 6).

Nuclear power is roughly equal to hydroelectricity worldwide (about 6.5 percent of all commercial energy), but it makes up about 20 percent of all electric power in more-developed countries, such as Canada and the United States. We have enough nuclear fuel to produce power for a long time, and it has the benefit of not contributing to global warming (see chapter 9), but as we discuss later in this chapter, safety concerns make this option unacceptable to most people.

Per Capita Consumption

Perhaps the most important facts about fossil fuel consumption are that we in the 20 richest countries consume nearly 80 percent of the natural gas, 65 percent of the oil, and 50 percent of the coal produced each year. Although we make up less than one-fifth of the world's population, we use more than one-half of the commercial energy supply. The United States and Canada, for instance, constitute only 5 percent of the world's population but consume about one-quarter of the available energy. To be fair, however, some of that energy goes to grow crops or manufacture goods that are later shipped to developing countries.

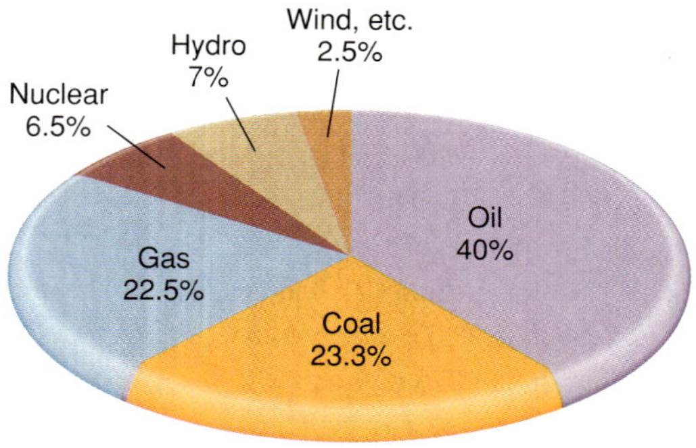

FIGURE 12.1 *Worldwide commercial energy consumption. This does not include energy collected for personal use or traded in informal markets.*
Source: Data from British Petroleum, 2003.

How much energy do you use every year? Most of us don't think about it much, but maintaining the lifestyle we enjoy requires an enormous energy input. On average, each person in the United States and Canada uses more than 300 gigajoules (GJ) (equivalent to about 60 barrels of oil) per year. By contrast, in some of the poorest countries of the world, such as Ethiopia, Nepal, and Bhutan, each person generally consumes less than 1 GJ per year. This means that each of us consumes, on average, almost as much energy in a single day as a person in one of these countries consumes in a year.

Clearly, energy consumption is linked to the comfort and convenience of our lives (fig. 12.2). Those of us in the richer countries enjoy many amenities not available to most people in the world. The link is not absolute, however. Several European countries, including Sweden, Denmark, and Switzerland, have higher standards of living than does the United States by almost any measure but use about half as much energy. These countries have had effective energy conservation programs for many years. Japan also has a far lower energy consumption rate than might be expected for its industrial base and income level. Because Japan has few energy resources of its own, it has developed very efficient energy conservation measures.

How We Use Energy

The largest share (32.6 percent) of the energy used in the United States is consumed by industry (fig. 12.3). Mining, milling, smelting, and forging of primary metals consume about one-quarter of

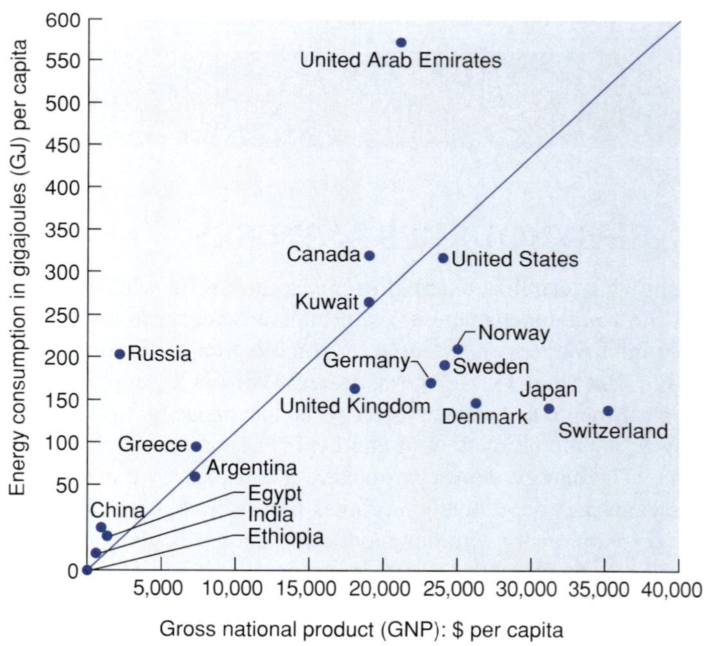

FIGURE 12.2 *Per capita energy use and GNP. In general, higher energy use correlates with a higher standard of living. Denmark and Switzerland, however, use about half as much energy as the United States does and have a higher standard of living by most measures.*
Source: Data from World Resources Institute, 1996–97.

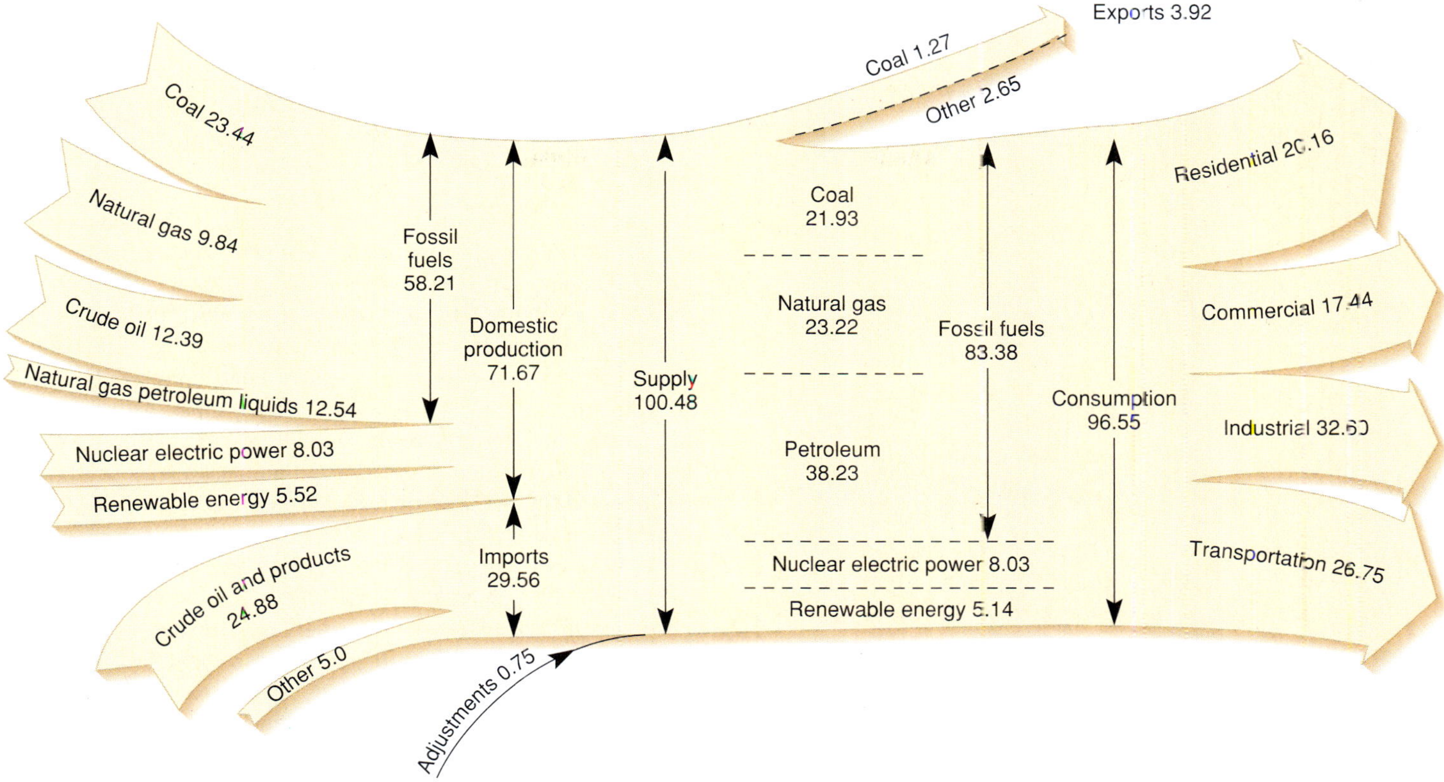

FIGURE 12.5 *U.S. energy flow, 2002. Quantities are in quadrillion Btu (quads).*
Source: Data from U.S. Energy Flow, U.S. Department of Energy, 2003.

the industrial energy share. The chemical industry is the second largest industrial user of fossil fuels, but only half of its use is for energy generation. The remainder is raw material for plastics, fertilizers, solvents, lubricants, and hundreds of thousands of organic chemicals in commercial use. The manufacture of cement, glass, bricks, tile, paper, and processed foods also consumes large amounts of energy. Residential and commercial buildings use roughly 37.6 percent of the primary energy consumed in the United States, mostly for space heating, air conditioning, lighting, and water heating. Small motors and electronic equipment take an increasing share of residential and commercial energy. In many office buildings, computers, copy machines, lights, and human bodies liberate enough waste heat that a supplementary source is not required, even in the winter.

Transportation consumes about 26 percent of all energy used in the United States each year. About 98 percent of that energy comes from petroleum products refined into liquid fuels, and the remaining 2 percent is provided by natural gas and electricity. Almost three-quarters of all transport energy is used by motor vehicles. Nearly 3 trillion passenger miles and 600 billion ton miles of freight are carried annually by motor vehicles in the United States. About 75 percent of all freight traffic in the United States is carried by trains, barges, ships, and pipelines, but because they are very efficient, they use only 12 percent of all transportation fuel.

Finally, analysis of how energy is used has to take into account waste and loss of potential energy. About half of all the energy in primary fuels is lost during conversion to more useful forms, while being shipped to the site of end use, or during use. Electricity, for instance, is generally promoted as a clean, efficient source of energy because, when it is used to run a resistance heater or an electrical appliance, almost 100 percent of its energy is converted to useful work and no pollution is given off. What happens before then, however? We often forget that huge amounts of pollution are released during mining and burning of the coal that fires power plants. Furthermore, nearly two-thirds of the energy in the coal that generated that electricity was lost in thermal conversion in the power plant. About 10 percent more is lost during transmission and stepping down to household voltages. Similarly, about 75 percent of the original energy in crude oil is lost during distillation into liquid fuels, transportation of that fuel to market, storage, marketing, and combustion in vehicles.

Natural gas is our most efficient fuel. Only 10 percent of its energy content is lost in shipping and processing, since it moves by pipelines and usually needs very little refining. Ordinary gas-burning furnaces are about 75 percent efficient, and high-economy furnaces can be as much as 95 percent efficient. Because natural gas has more hydrogen per carbon atom than oil or coal, it produces about half as much carbon dioxide—and therefore contributes half as much to global warming—per unit of energy.

APPLICATION: Energy Calculations

Most college students either already own or are likely to buy an automobile and a computer sometime soon. How do these items compare in energy usage? Suppose that you were debating between a high-mileage car, such as the Honda Insight, or a sport utility vehicle, such as a Ford Excursion. How do the energy requirements of these two purchases measure up? To put it another way, how long could you run a computer on the energy you would save by buying an Insight rather than an Excursion? (See What Do You Think, p. 290, for more information about hybrids.)

Here are some numbers you need to know. The Insight gets about 75 mpg, while the Excursion gets about 12 mpg. A typical American drives about 15,000 mi per year. A gallon of regular, unleaded gasoline contains about 115,000 Btu on average. Most computers use about 100 watts of electricity. One kilowatt-hour (kwh) = 3,413 Btu.

1. How much energy does the computer use if it is left on continuously? (You really should turn it off at night or when it isn't in use, but we'll simplify the calculations.)

   100 watt/h × 24 h/day × 365 days/yr = _______ kwh/yr
2. How much gasoline would you save in an Insight, compared with an Excursion?
   a. Excursion:
      15,000 mi/yr ÷ 12 mpg = _______ gal/yr
   b. Insight:
      15,000 mi/yr ÷ 75 mpg = _______ gal/yr
   c. Gasoline savings (*a* – *b*) = _______ gal/yr
   d. Energy savings:
      (gal × 115,000 Btu) = _______ Btu/yr
   e. Converting Btu to kwh:
      (Btu × 0.00029 Btu/kwh) = _______ kwh/yr saved
3. How long would the energy saved run your computer?

   kwh/yr saved by Insight ÷ kwh/yr consumed by computer = _______

Answers: 1. The computer consumes 876 kwh/yr if run continuously. *2.* The Excursion consumes 1,250 gal/yr; the Insight uses 200 gal/yr. Savings are 1,050 gal/yr = 120 million BTU/yr, or 35,000 kwh/yr. *3.* 40 years.

FOSSIL FUELS

Fossil fuels are organic chemicals created by living organisms millions of years ago and buried in sediments, where high pressures and temperatures concentrated and transformed them into energy-rich compounds. Coal is solid, petroleum (crude oil) is liquid, oil shales and tar sands are semisolid tars trapped in rock, and natural gas (methane and other gaseous hydrocarbons) is, as its name suggests, a gas. Most of these fuels were laid down during the Carboniferous period (286 million to 360 million years ago), when the earth's climate was warmer and wetter than it is now, but some are thought to date as far back as Precambrian times, perhaps a billion years ago. Because fossil fuels take so long to form, they are essentially nonrenewable resources.

Coal

World coal deposits are vast, ten times greater than conventional oil and gas resources combined. Coal seams can be 100 m thick and can extend across tens of thousands of square kilometers that were vast, swampy forests in prehistoric times. The total resource is estimated to be 10 trillion metric tons. If all this coal could be extracted, and if coal consumption continued at present levels, this would amount to several thousand years' supply. At present rates of consumption, these **proven-in-place reserves**—those explored and mapped but not necessarily economic at today's prices—will last about 200 years. Proven reserves are generally a small fraction of a total resource (fig. 12.4).

Where are these coal deposits located? They are not evenly distributed throughout the world (fig. 12.5). North America has about one-fourth of all proven reserves. China and Russia have nearly as much. Eastern and Western Europe have fairly large coal supplies in spite of their relatively small size. Africa and Latin America have very little coal despite their large size. Antarctica is thought to have large coal deposits, but they would be difficult, expensive, and ecologically damaging to mine.

It would seem that the abundance of coal deposits is a favorable situation. But do we really want to use all of the coal? Coal mining is a dirty, dangerous activity. Underground mines are notorious for cave-ins, explosions, and lung diseases, such as black-lung suffered by miners. Surface mines (called strip mines, where large machines strip off overlying sediment to expose coal seams)

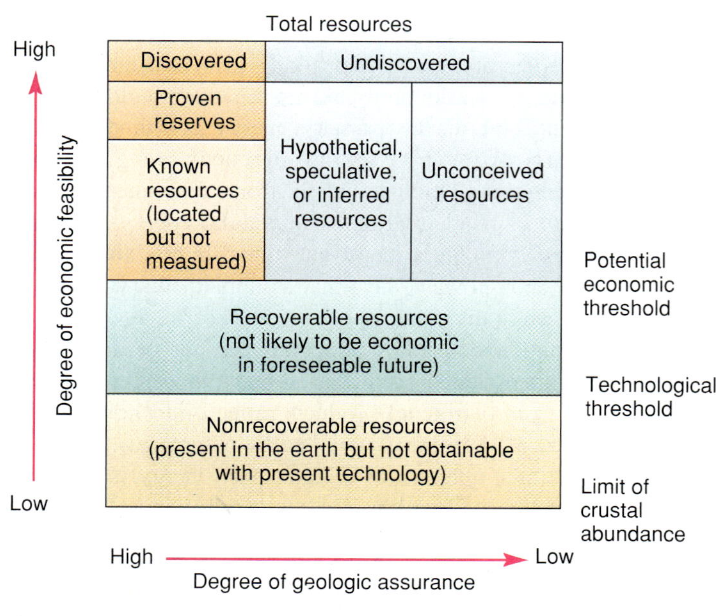

FIGURE 12.4 *Categories of natural resources according to economic and technological feasibility, as well as geologic assurance.*

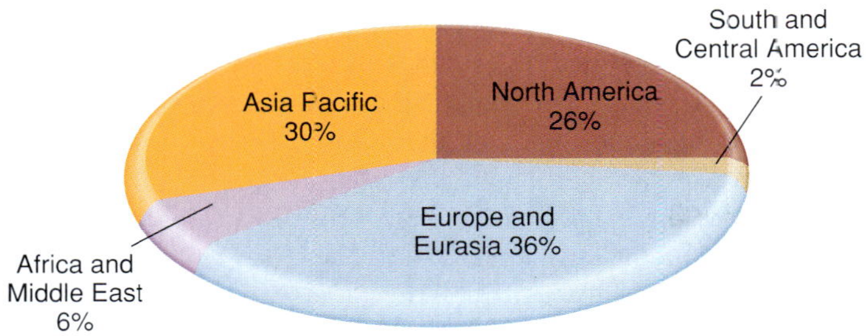

FIGURE 12.5 *Proven-in-place coal reserves by region, 2002.*
Source: World Energy Council 2002.

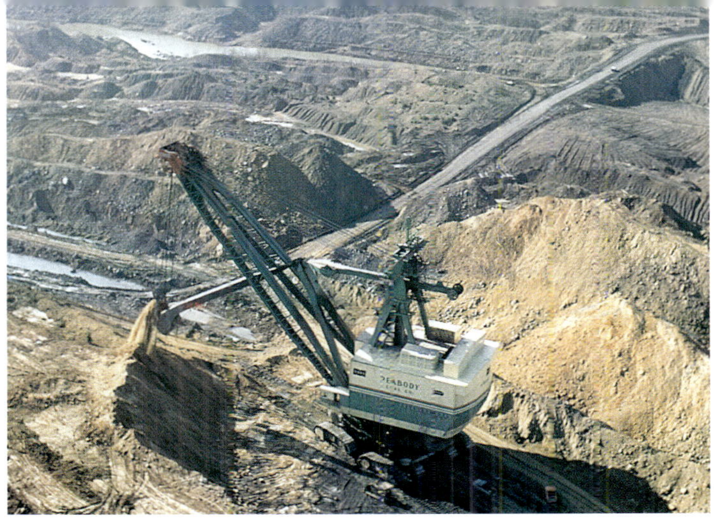

FIGURE 12.6 *Some giant mining machines stand as tall as a 20-story building and can scoop up thousands of cubic meters of rock per hour. Note the pick-up trucks in the machine's shadow.*

are cheaper and generally safer for workers than tunneling, but leave huge holes where coal has been removed and vast piles of discarded rock and soil (fig. 12.6). An especially damaging technique employed in Appalachia is called mountaintop removal. Typically, the whole top of a mountain ridge is scraped off to access buried coal. The waste rock pushed down into the nearest valley buries forests, streams, houses, and farms (see chapter 11 for further discussion of this issue). Mine reclamation is now mandated in the United States, but efforts often are only partially successful.

Coal comes in a variety of forms with varying chemical composition, harness, and energy content. Lignite, the softest of this family, is not much more concentrated than peat and has about 4,000 BTU/lb. It can have very low sulfur content (0.06 to 0.4 percent by weight) but is high in ash. Subbituminous and bituminous coal have energy contents between 8,000 and 15,000 BTU/lb and generally have 1 to 5 percent sulfur content. Anthracite, which is the hardest coal, can be 96 percent carbon and have more than 15,000 BTU/lb. Coal can also have dangerous concentrations of toxic minerals, such as mercury, arsenic, chromium, and lead. The United States uses about one-third of the total world coal production, mainly for generating electricity.

Coal burning releases large amounts of air pollution. Every year the roughly one billion tons of coal burned in the United States (83 percent for electric power generation) releases 18 million metric tons of sodium dioxide (SO_2), 5 million metric tons of nitrogen oxides (NO_x), 4 million metric tons of airborne particulates, 600,000 metric tons of hydrocarbons and carbon monoxide, 40 tons of mercury, and close to a trillion metric tons of carbon dioxide (CO_2). This is about three-quarters of the SO_2, one-third of the NO_x, and about half of the industrial CO_2 released in the United States each year. As described in chapter 9, sulfur and nitrogen oxides combine with water in the air to form sulfuric and nitric acid, making coal burning the largest single source of acid rain in many areas. These air pollutants have many deleterious effects, including human health costs, injury to domestic and wild plants and animals, and damage to buildings and property. Total losses from air pollution are estimated to be between \$5 billion and \$10 billion per year in the United States alone. By some accounts, at least 5,000 excess human deaths per year can be attributed to coal production and burning.

Oil

The total amount of oil in the world is estimated to be about 4 trillion bbl (600 billion metric tons), half of which is thought to be ultimately recoverable. Some 465 billion bbl of oil already have been consumed. In 2004 the proven reserves were roughly 1 trillion bbl, enough to last only 40 years at the current consumption rate of 25 billion bbl per year. It is estimated that another 800 billion bbl either remain to be discovered or are not recoverable at current prices with present technology. Many geologists expect that within a decade or so world oil production will peak and then begin to decline. As this happens, oil prices will rise, which will make other energy sources more economically attractive. Dr. M. King Hubbert, a Shell geophysicist, first predicted in the 1940s a bell-shaped curve for U.S. oil production, peaking in the 1970s, which it did. So far, world oil production seems to be following a similar path (fig. 12.7). These estimates don't take into account the very large

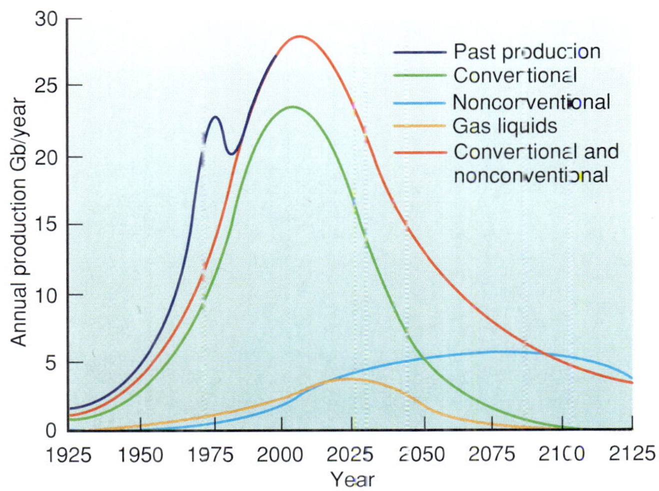

FIGURE 12.7 *Worldwide production of crude oil with predicted Hubbert production. Gb = billion barrels.*
Source: Jean Laherrère, www.hubbertpeak.org.

potential from unconventional semiliquid hydrocarbon resources, such as shale oil and tar sands, which might double the total reserve if they can be mined with acceptable social, economic, and environmental impacts.

By far the largest supply of proven-in-place oil is in Saudi Arabia, which has 250 billion bbl, about one-fourth of the total proven world reserve (fig. 12.8). Altogether, the countries of the Middle East control nearly two-thirds of all known oil reserves—a fact that explains a great deal about American foreign policy in recent years. Among the places considered most likely to contain undiscovered oil, in addition to the Middle East, are the northeast Greenland Shelf, the western Siberian and Caspian areas, and the Niger and Congo delta areas of Africa. Sediments under and around the Caspian Sea have been estimated to hold 200 billion bbl of oil. If this is true, this region is second only to Saudi Arabia in size of oil reserves.

The United States has already used more than half of its original recoverable petroleum resource. Of the 120 billion bbl thought to remain, about 58 billion bbl are proven-in-place. If we stopped importing oil and depended exclusively on indigenous supplies, our proven reserves would last only ten years at current rates of consumption. The regions of North America with the greatest potential for substantial new oil discoveries are portions of the continental shelf along the California coast, the Arctic Ocean, and the Grand Banks, all of which are prime wildlife areas. Proposals to do exploratory drilling in these areas have been strongly opposed by many people concerned about the potential for long-term environmental damage from drilling activities and oil spills like that of the *Exxon Valdez* in Prince William Sound. Other people argue that having an inexpensive, plentiful energy supply, even if only for a few decades, is worth the social and environmental costs (see related story "Oil Drilling in the Arctic" at www.mhhe.com/cases).

Like coal, petroleum often contains high sulfur levels. Because it is highly corrosive, the sulfur in oil is usually stripped out before the fuel is shipped to market and thus doesn't end up in urban air nearly as often as that from coal. Oil is used primarily for transportation (the gasoline in your car or truck) and heating.

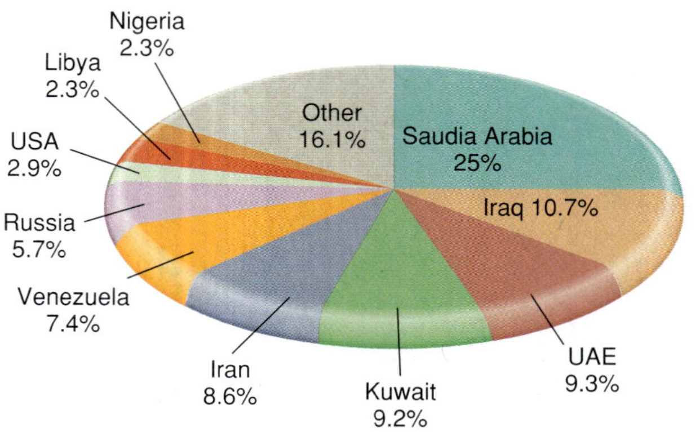

FIGURE 12.8 *Proven oil reserves. Ten countries account for nearly 84 percent of all known recoverable oil.*
Source: Data from British Petroleum, 2003.

Because about one-quarter of all energy used in the United States fuels transportation, and oil provides more than 90 percent of that transportation energy, oil combustion is responsible for between one-quarter and two-thirds of the volatile organic compounds, nitrogen oxides, and carbon monoxide emitted each year.

Oil drilling is far less destructive to the earth's surface than coal mining, but the huge amounts of oil shipped around the world and used as lubricants and fuels result in very serious soil and water pollution. Oceanographers estimate that between 3 million and 6 million metric tons of oil are discharged into the world's rivers and oceans every year. About half of this comes from oil tanker accidents and dumping of ballast water. The rest is mostly deliberate dumping of used motor oil. Many people believe that a storm sewer is a good place to discard waste oil and don't realize that the sewer probably leads directly into a lake, river, or seashore.

Oil Shales and Tar Sands

Estimates of our recoverable oil supplies usually don't account for the very large potential from unconventional resources. The World Energy Council estimates that oil shales, tar sands, and other unconventional deposits contain ten times as much oil as liquid petroleum reserves. **Tar sands** are composed of sand and shale particles coated with bitumen, a viscous mixture of long-chain hydrocarbons. Shallow tar sands are excavated and mixed with hot water and steam to extract the bitumen, then fractionated to make useful products. For deeper deposits, superheated steam is injected to melt the bitumen, which can then be pumped to the surface, like liquid crude. Once the oil has been retrieved, it still must be cleaned and refined to be useful.

Canada and Venezuela have the world's largest and most accessible tar sand resources. Canadian deposits in northern Alberta are estimated to be equivalent to 300 billion bbl of oil, or nearly as much as Saudi Arabian oil reserves. Current Alberta production is about 1 billion bbl per day, or more than the output of Alaska's North Slope. By 2010 Alberta is expected to increase its flow to 2 billion bbl per day, or twice the maximum projected output of the Arctic National Wildlife Refuge (ANWR). Furthermore, because Alberta tar sand beds are 20 times larger and closer to the surface than ANWR oil, the Canadian resource will last longer and may be cheaper to extract. Canada is already the largest supplier of oil to the United States, having surpassed Saudi Arabia in 2000.

There are severe environmental costs, however, in producing this oil. A typical plant producing 125,000 bbl of oil per day creates about 15 million m^3 of toxic sludge, releases 5,000 tons of greenhouse gases, and consumes or contaminates billions of liters of water each year. Surface mining could destroy millions of hectares of boreal forest. Native Cree, Chipewyan, and Metis people worry about effects on traditional ways of life if forests are destroyed and wildlife and water are contaminated. Many Canadians dislike becoming an energy colony for the United States, and environmentalists argue that investing billions of dollars to extract this resource simply makes us more dependent on fossil fuels.

Oil shales are fine-grained sedimentary rock rich in solid organic material called kerogen. Like tar sands, the kerogen can be heated, liquefied, and pumped out like liquid crude oil. Oil shale beds up to 600 m (1,800 ft) thick underlie much of Colorado, Utah, and Wyoming. If these deposits could be extracted at a reasonable price and with acceptable environmental impacts, they might yield the equivalent of several trillion barrels of oil. Mining and extraction of oil shale use vast amounts of water (a scarce resource in the arid western United States) and create enormous quantities of waste. The rock matrix expands when heated, resulting in twice or three times the volume of waste as was dug out of the ground. Billions of dollars were spent in the 1980s on pilot projects to produce synthetic oil. When oil prices dropped, these schemes were abandoned. Should we explore these unconventional resources further?

Natural Gas

Natural gas is the world's third largest commercial fuel, making up 23 percent of global energy consumption. Because natural gas produces only half as much CO_2 as an equivalent amount of coal, substitution could help reduce global warming (see chapter 9). Natural gas is difficult to ship across oceans, however, and to store in large quantities. North America is fortunate to have an abundant, easily available supply of gas and a pipeline network to deliver it to market. Many countries cannot afford such a pipeline network, and much of the natural gas produced in conjunction with oil pumping in remote areas is simply burned (flared off), an unfortunate waste of a valuable resource (fig. 12.9).

Russia has 31 percent of known natural gas reserves (mostly in Siberia and the Central Asian republics) and account for about 40 percent of all global production. Both Eastern and Western Europe buy substantial quantities of gas from these wells. Figure 12.10 shows the distribution of proven natural gas reserves in the world.

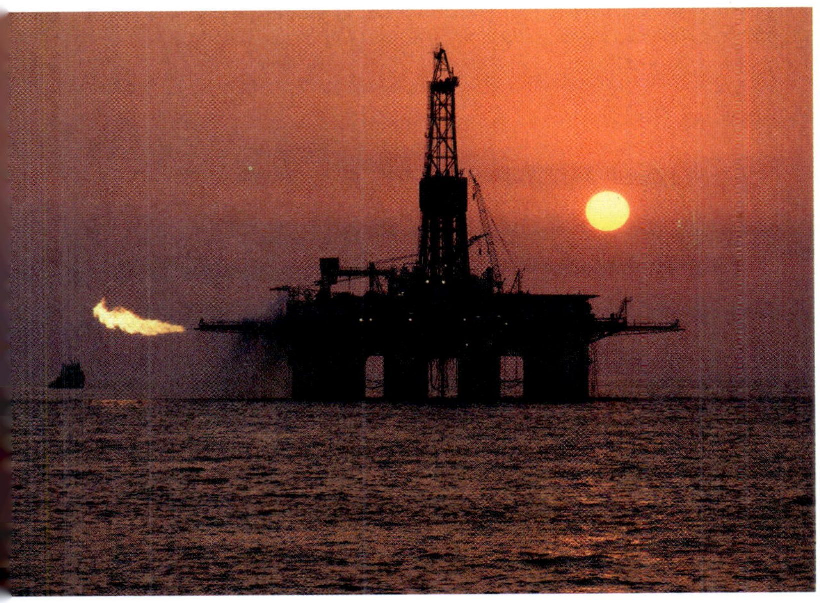

FIGURE 12.9 *Natural gas is difficult to store and ship. In remote locations such as this offshore platform, it often is flared off.*

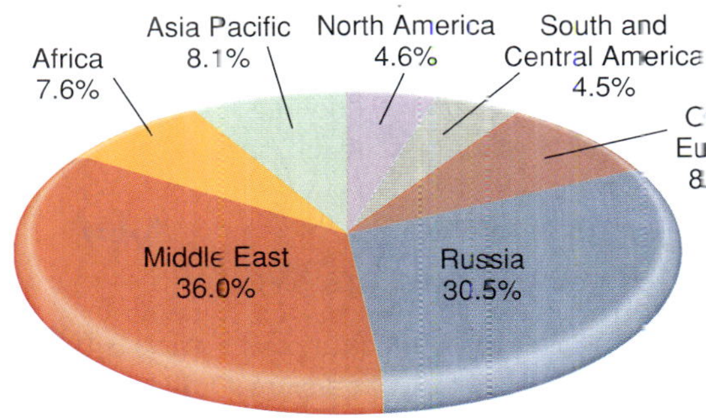

FIGURE 12.10 *Proven natural gas reserves by region, 2002.*
Source: Data from British Petroleum, 2003.

The total ultimately recoverable natural gas resources in the world are estimated to be 10,000 trillion ft^3, corresponding to about 80 percent as much energy as the recoverable reserves of crude oil. The proven world reserves of natural gas are 5,500 trillion ft^3 (125,000 million metric tons). Because gas consumption rates are only about half of those for oil, current gas reserves represent roughly a 60-year supply at present usage rates. Proven reserves in the United States are about 250 trillion ft^3, or 4.6 percent of the world total. This is a ten-year supply at current rates of consumption. Known reserves are more than twice as large.

Large amounts of methane are released from coal deposits. The Rocky Mountain front in Colorado, Wyoming, and Montana could have 10 percent of the total world methane supply. Proposals for up to 140,000 coal-bed methane wells in Wyoming's Power River Basin, for example, have raised concerns about water pollution and land damage (see What Do You Think? p. 268). Other states could face similar problems.

NUCLEAR POWER

In 1953 President Dwight Eisenhower presented his "Atoms for Peace" speech to the United Nations. He announced that the United States would build nuclear-powered electrical generators to provide clean, abundant energy. He predicted that nuclear energy would fill the deficit caused by predicted shortages of oil and natural gas. It would provide power "too cheap to meter" for continued industrial expansion of both the developed and the developing world. It would be a supreme example of "beating swords into plowshares." Technology and engineering would tame the evil genie of atomic energy and use its enormous power to do useful work.

However, rapidly increasing construction costs, declining demand for electric power, and safety fears have made nuclear energy much less attractive than promoters expected. Of the 140 reactors on order in 1975, 100 were subsequently canceled. Nuclear power now produces less than 8 percent of the U.S. energy supply (2 percent more than the world average). All of it is used to generate electricity.

The nuclear power industry has been campaigning for greater acceptance, arguing that reactors don't release greenhouse gases that cause global warming. About half the existing nuclear reactors in the United States have had their licenses renewed for an additionl 20 years beyond their original 40-year design, and several new plants are now on the drawing board. However, worries about susceptiblity to terrorist attacks make many people fearful of this power source (fig. 12.11).

How Do Nuclear Reactors Work?

The most commonly used fuel in nuclear power plants is U^{235}, a naturally occurring radioactive isotope of uranium. Ordinarily, U^{235} makes up only about 0.7 percent of uranium ore—too little to sustain a chain reaction in most reactors. It must be purified and concentrated by mechanical or chemical procedures. When the U^{235} concentration reaches about 3 percent, the uranium is formed into cylindrical pellets slightly thicker than a pencil and about 1.5 cm long. Although small, these pellets pack an amazing amount of energy. Each 8.5-g pellet is equivalent to a ton of coal or 4 bbl of crude oil.

The pellets are stacked in hollow metal rods approximately 4 m long. About 100 of these rods are bundled together to make a **fuel assembly.** Thousands of fuel assemblies containing about 100 tons of uranium are bundled in a heavy steel vessel called the reactor core. Radioactive uranium atoms are unstable—that is, when struck by a high-energy subatomic particle called a neutron, they undergo **nuclear fission** (splitting), releasing energy and more neutrons. When uranium is packed tightly in the reactor core, the neutrons released by one atom will trigger the fission of another uranium atom and the release of still more neutrons (fig. 12.12). Thus, a self-sustaining **chain reaction** is set in motion, and vast amounts of energy are released.

The chain reaction is moderated (slowed) in a power plant by a neutron-absorbing cooling solution that circulates between the fuel rods. In addition, **control rods** of neutron-absorbing material, such as cadmium or boron, are inserted into spaces between fuel assemblies to shut down the fission reaction or are withdrawn to allow it to proceed. Water or some other coolant is circulated between the fuel rods to remove excess heat. The greatest danger in one of these complex machines is a cooling system failure. If the pumps fail or pipes break during operation, the nuclear fuel quickly overheats, and a "meltdown" can result that releases deadly radioactive material. Although nuclear power plants cannot explode like a nuclear bomb, the radioactive releases from a worst-case disaster, such as the meltdown of the Chernobyl reactor in the Soviet Ukraine in 1986, are just as devastating as a bomb. (See related story on Chernobyl at www.mhhe.com/cases.)

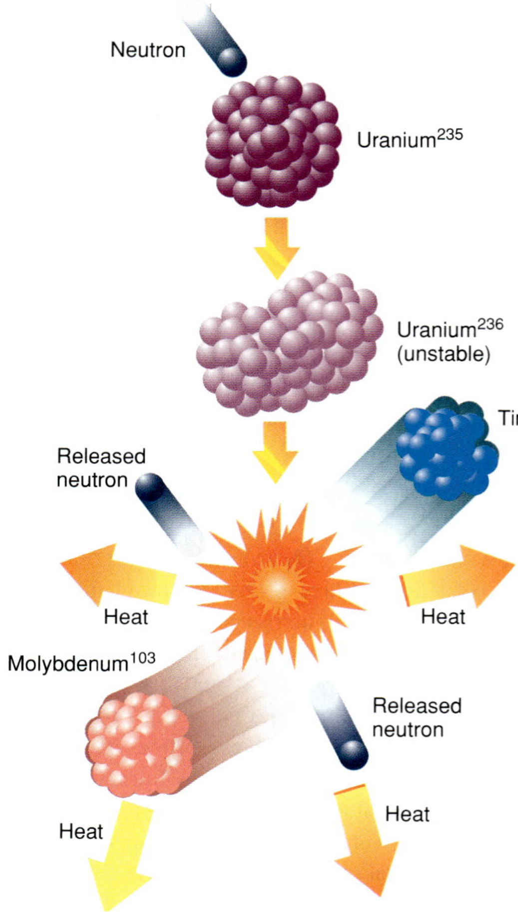

FIGURE 12.12 *The process of nuclear fission is carried out in the core of a nuclear reactor. In the sequence shown here, the unstable isotope uranium-235 absorbs a neutron and splits to form tin-131 and molybdenum-103. Two or three neutrons are released per fission event and continue the chain reaction. The total mass of the reaction product is slightly less than the starting material. The residual mass is converted to energy (mostly heat).*

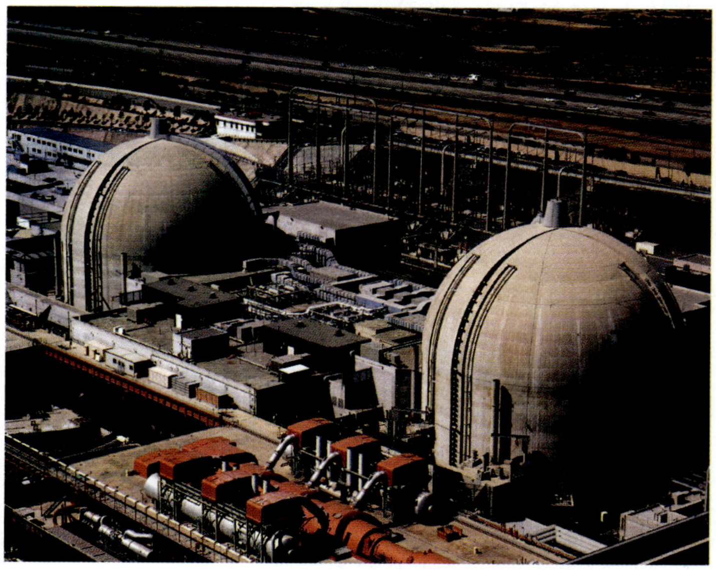

FIGURE 12.11 *Two nuclear reactors (domes) at the San Onofre Nuclear Generating Station sit between the beach and Interstate 5, the major route between Los Angeles and San Diego.*

Nuclear Reactor Design

Seventy percent of the world's nuclear plants are pressurized water reactors (PWR). Water circulates through the core, absorbing heat as it cools the fuel rods (fig. 12.13). This primary cooling water is heated to 317°C (600°F) and reaches a pressure of 2,235 psi. It then is pumped to a steam generator, where it heats a secondary water-cooling loop. Steam from the secondary loop drives a high-speed turbine generator that produces electricity. Both the reactor vessel and the steam generator are contained in a thick-walled, concrete-and-steel containment building that prevents radiation from escaping and is designed to withstand high pressures and temperatures in case of accidents. Engineers operate the plant from a complex, sophisticated control room containing many gauges and meters that indicate how the plant is running.

Overlapping layers of safety mechanisms are designed to prevent accidents, but these fail-safe controls make reactors very expensive and very complex. A typical nuclear power plant has 40,000 valves, compared with only 4,000 in a fossil fuel–fired plant of similar size. In some cases, the controls are so complex that they confuse operators and cause accidents, rather than prevent them. Under normal operating conditions, a PWR releases very little radioactivity and is probably less dangerous for nearby residents than a coal-fired power plant.

In Britain, France, and the former Soviet Union, a common reactor design uses graphite, both as a moderator and as the structural material for the reactor core. In the British MAGNOX design (named after the magnesium alloy used for its fuel rods), gaseous carbon dioxide is blown through the core to cool the fuel assemblies and carry heat to the steam generators. In the Soviet design, called RBMK (the Russian initials for a graphite-moderated, water-cooled reactor), low-pressure cooling water circulates through the core in thousands of small metal tubes.

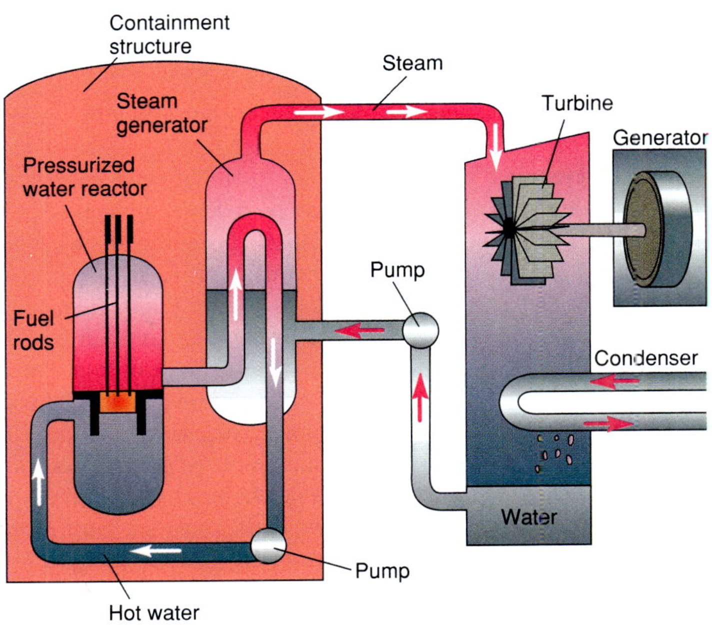

FIGURE 12.13 *Pressurized water nuclear reactor. Water is superheated and pressurized as it flows through the reactor core. Heat is transferred to nonpressurized water in the steam generator. The steam drives the turbogenerator to produce electricity.*

These designs were originally thought to be very safe because graphite has a high capacity for both capturing neutrons and dissipating heat. Designers claimed that these reactors could not possibly run out of control; unfortunately, they were proven wrong. The small cooling tubes are quickly blocked by steam if the cooling system fails, and the graphite core burns when exposed to air. Burning graphite in the Chernobyl nuclear plant made the fire much more difficult to control than it might have been in another reactor design.

Nuclear Wastes

One of the most difficult problems associated with nuclear power is the disposal of wastes produced during mining, fuel production, and reactor operation. How these wastes are managed may ultimately be the overriding obstacle to nuclear power.

Enormous piles of mine wastes and abandoned mill tailings in uranium-producing countries represent another serious waste disposal problem. Production of 1,000 tons of uranium fuel typically generates 100,000 tons of tailings and 3.5 million liters of liquid waste. There now are approximately 200 million tons of radioactive waste in piles around mines and processing plants in the United States. This material is carried by the wind or washes into streams, contaminating areas far from its original source. Canada has even more radioactive mine waste on the surface than does the United States.

In addition to the leftovers from fuel production, there are about 100,000 tons of low-level waste (contaminated tools, clothing, building materials, etc.) and about 15,000 tons of high-level (very radioactive) wastes in the United States. The high-level wastes consist mainly of spent fuel rods from commercial nuclear power plants and assorted wastes from nuclear weapons production. For the past 20 years, spent fuel assemblies from commercial reactors have been stored in deep, water-filled pools at the power plants. These pools were originally intended only as temporary storage until the wastes were shipped to reprocessing centers or permanent disposal sites.

With internal waste storage pools now full but neither reprocessing nor permanent storage available, a number of utility companies are beginning to store nuclear waste in large, metal dry casks placed outside power plants (fig. 12.14). These projects are meeting with fierce opposition from local residents, who fear the casks will leak. Most nuclear power plants are built near rivers, lakes, or seacoasts. Extremely toxic radioactive materials could spread quickly over large areas if leaks occur. A hydrogen gas explosion and fire in 1997 in a dry storage cask at Wisconsin's Point Beach nuclear plant intensified opponents' suspicions about this form of waste storage.

In 1987 the U.S. Department of Energy announced plans to build the first high-level waste repository on a barren desert ridge near Yucca Mountain, Nevada. After 15 years of research and $4 billion in exploratory drilling, it still isn't certain that the site is safe (see chapter 11). Nevertheless, Congress approved the project in 2002, and President Bush signed the bill. Intensely radioactive wastes are to be buried deep in the ground, where it is hoped that they will remain unexposed to groundwater and earthquakes for

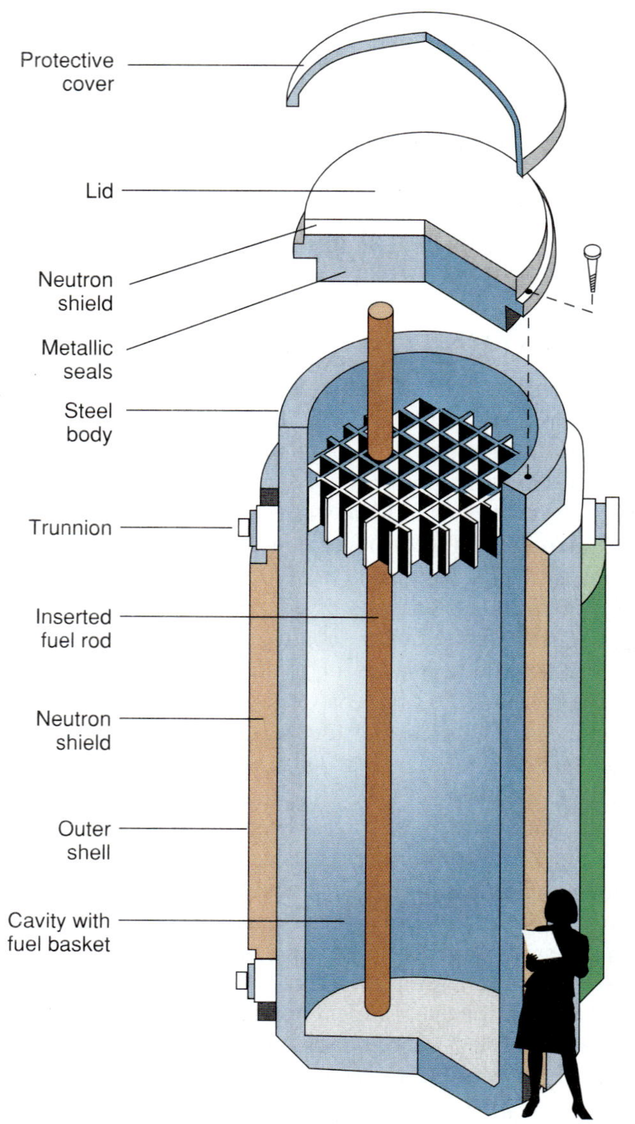

FIGURE 12.14 *Dry cask storage for nuclear waste. Each cask is 17 ft tall and 8.5 ft in diameter, has steel walls 10 in. thick, and weighs 122 tons when fully loaded with 40 fuel assemblies. The casks are expected to last 40 years and cost $700,000 each. Critics worry that the casks will leak, but proponents point out that they can be monitored easily and replaced if necessary.*

the thousands of years required for the radioactive materials to decay to a safe level. Although the area is very dry now, we can't be sure that it will always remain that way. Total costs now are expected to be at least $35 billion. Although the facility was supposed to open in 1998, the earliest possible date is now 2010.

Some nuclear experts believe that **monitored, retrievable storage** would be a much better way to handle wastes. This method involves holding wastes in underground mines or secure surface facilities where they can be watched. If canisters begin to leak, they could be removed for repacking. Safeguarding the wastes would be expensive, and the sites might be susceptible to wars and terrorist attacks. We might need a perpetual priesthood of nuclear guardians to ensure that the wastes are never released into the environment.

ENERGY CONSERVATION

One of the best ways to avoid energy shortages and to relieve environmental and health effects of our current energy technologies is simply to use less. (See What Can You Do? p. 289.) Conservation offers many benefits both to society and to the environment.

Using Energy More Efficiently

Much of the energy we consume is wasted. This statement is not a simple admonishment to turn off lights and turn down furnace thermostats in winter; it is a technological challenge. Our ways of using energy are so inefficient that most potential energy in fuel is lost as waste heat, becoming a form of environmental pollution. More efficient and less energy-intensive industry, transportation, and domestic practices could save large amounts of energy. In response to federal regulations and high gasoline prices, automobile gas-mileage averages in the United States more than doubled from 13 mpg in 1975 to 28.8 mpg in 1988. Unfortunately, the oil glut and falling fuel prices of the 1990s discouraged further conservation. By 2004 the average slipped to only 20.4 mpg.

Much more could be done. High-efficiency automobiles are already available. Both Honda and Toyota have low-emission, hybrid gas-electric vehicles that get up to 30.3 km/liter (72 mpg) on the highway (see What Do You Think? p. 290). Amory B. Lovins of the Rocky Mountain Institute in Colorado estimates that raising the average fuel efficiency of the U.S. car and light-truck fleet by 1 mpg would cut oil consumption about 295,000 bbl per day. In one year, this would equal the total amount the U.S. Department of the Interior hopes to extract from the Arctic National Wildlife Refuge in Alaska.

Many improvements in domestic energy efficiency have occurred in the past decade. Today's average new home uses one-half the fuel required in a house built in 1974, but much more can be done. Household energy losses can be reduced by one-half to three-fourths by using better insulation, installing double- or triple-glazed windows, purchasing thermally efficient curtains or window coverings, and sealing cracks and loose joints. Reducing air infiltration is usually the cheapest, quickest, and most effective way of saving energy because it is the largest source of losses in a typical house. It doesn't take much skill or investment to caulk around doors, windows, foundation joints, electrical outlets, and other sources of air leakage. Mechanical ventilation is needed to prevent moisture buildup in tightly sealed homes.

For even greater savings, new houses can be built with extra-thick, superinsulated walls; air-to-air heat exchangers to warm incoming air; and even double-walled sections that create a "house within a house." The R-2000 program in Canada details how energy conservation can be built into homes. Special double-glazed windows that have internal reflective coatings and that are filled with an inert gas (argon or xenon) have an insulation factor of R11, the same as a standard 4-inch-thick insulated wall, or ten

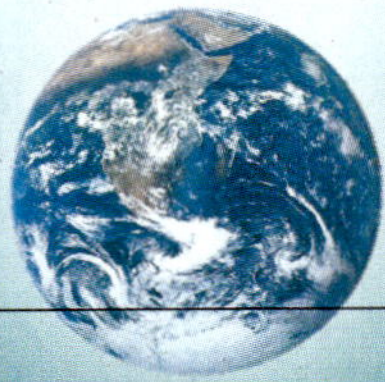

what can you do?

Some Things You Can Do to Save Energy

1. Drive less: make fewer trips, use telecommunications and mail instead of going places in person.
2. Use public transportation, walk, or ride a bicycle.
3. Use stairs instead of elevators.
4. Join a car pool or drive a smaller, more efficient car; reduce speeds.
5. Insulate your house or add more insulation to the existing amount.
6. Turn thermostats down in the winter and up in the summer.
7. Weatherstrip and caulk around windows and doors.
8. Add storm windows or plastic sheets over windows.
9. Create a windbreak on the north side of your house; plant deciduous trees or vines on the south side.
10. During the winter, close windows and drapes at night; during summer days, close windows and drapes if using air conditioning.
11. Turn off lights, television sets, and computers when not in use.
12. Stop faucet leaks, especially hot water.
13. Take shorter, cooler showers; install water-saving faucets and showerheads.
14. Recycle glass, metals, and paper; compost organic wastes.
15. Eat locally grown food in season.
16. Buy locally made, long-lasting materials.

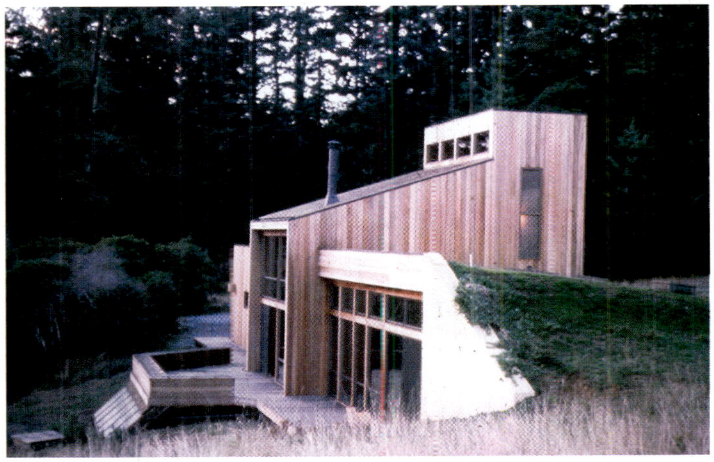

FIGURE 12.15 *Earth-sheltered homes take advantage of the stable temperatures and insulating qualities of the earth. This house has south-facing windows for maximum solar gain and high clerestory windows that give light to the back of the house as well as summer ventilation.*
Courtesy National Renewable Energy Laboratory/NREL/PIX.

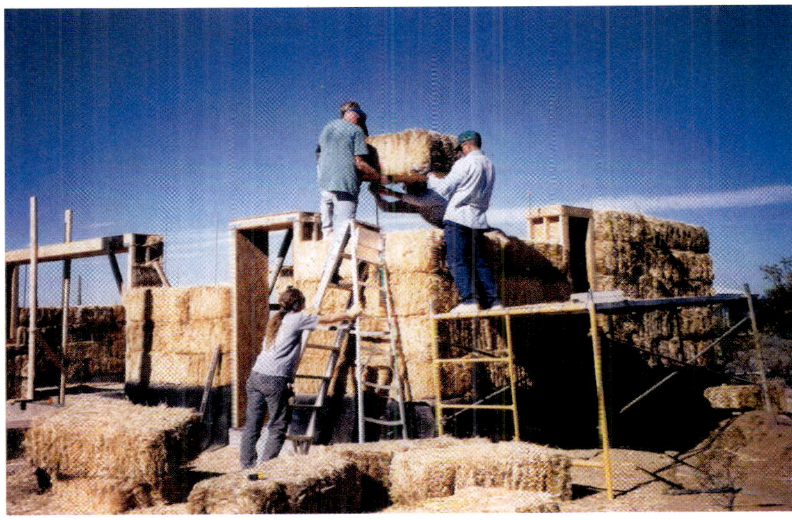

FIGURE 12.16 *Carolyn Roberts and her sons build a straw bale house near Tucson, AZ.*
Courtesy Carolyn Roberts/A House of Straw.

times as efficient as a single-pane window. Superinsulated houses now being built in Sweden require 90 percent less energy for heating and cooling than the average American home.

Orienting homes so that living spaces have passive solar gain in the winter and are shaded by trees or roof overhang in the summer also helps conserve energy. Earth-sheltered homes built into the south-facing side of a slope or protected on three sides by an earth berm are exceptionally efficient energy savers because they maintain relatively constant subsurface temperatures (fig. 12.15). Sod roofs provide good insulation, prevent rain runoff, and last longer than asphalt shingles. Because they are heavier, however, they need stronger supports.

Straw-bale construction offers both high insulating qualities and a renewable, inexpensive building material that can be assembled by amateurs (fig. 12.16). This isn't a new technique. Settlers on the Great Plains built straw-bale houses a century ago because they didn't have wood. Some of those houses are still standing. The bales are strong and will support the roof without any additional timber framing. They must be thoroughly waterproofed, however, with stucco, adobe, or plaster both inside and out so the straw doesn't decay. It's also important to seal them so mice and other vermin can't take up residence. The thick walls are terrific sound insulators as well as highly energy-efficient. The cost can be far less than a conventionally built home.

One of the most direct and immediate ways that individuals can save energy is to turn off appliances. Few of us realize how much electricity is used by appliances in a standby mode. You may think you've turned off your TV, DVD player, cable box, or printer, but they're really continuing to draw power in an "instant-on" mode. For the average home, standby appliances can represent up to 25 percent of the monthly electric bill. Home office equipment, including computers, printers, cable modems, and copiers, usually

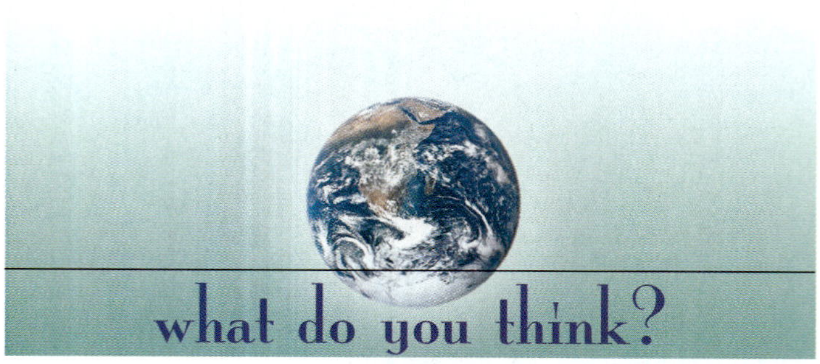

Hybrid Automobile Engines

In 1990 the California Air Resources Board shocked the automobile industry by ordering it to start producing emission-free vehicles or face stiff penalties. It's not surprising that California was the first state to get tough on automobile emissions. Auto exhaust counts for 90 percent of the state's carbon monoxide, 77 percent of its nitrogen oxides, and 55 percent of its smog-producing hydrocarbons. At the time this order was issued, however, only battery-powered electric vehicles were available. Although several manufacturers built all-electric autos, the batteries were heavy and expensive, and they required more frequent recharging than customers would accept. Even though 90 percent of all daily commutes are less than 80 km (50 mi), most people want the ability to take a long road trip of several hundred kilometers without needing to stop for fuel or recharging.

An alternative that appears to have much more customer appeal is the hybrid gas-electric vehicle. The first of these hybrid cars to be marketed in the United States is the two-seat Honda Insight. Its 3-cylinder, 1.0-liter gas engine is the main power source. A 7-hp electric motor helps during acceleration and hill climbing. When the small battery pack begins to run down, it is recharged by the gas engine, so that the vehicle never needs to be plugged in. More electricity is captured during "regenerative" braking, further increasing efficiency. With a streamlined, lightweight plastic and aluminum body, the Insight gets 72 mpg (30.3 km/liter) in highway driving and has low enough emissions to satisfy California requirements. Quick acceleration and nimble handling make the Insight fun to drive.

Both Toyota and Honda have also introduced five-passenger hybrids. The Toyota is called a Prius, and the Honda is a Civic hybrid. During most city driving, they depend only on a quiet, emission-free, battery-powered electric motor. The 1.5-liter gas engine kicks in to help accelerate or when the batteries need recharging. Some drivers are unnerved by the noiseless electric motor of hybrids. Sitting at a stoplight, it makes no sound at all. You might think it's dead, but when the light changes, you glide off silently and smoothly. Both the hybrid Civic and Prius sell for about $20,000 and qualify currently for a $2,000 Federal Clean-Fuel Vehicle tax deduction. The Sierra Club estimates that, in 160,000 km (100,000 mi), a Prius will generate 27 tons of CO_2, a Ford Taurus will generate 64 tons, and the Ford Excursion SUV will produce 134 tons. In 1999 the Sierra Club awarded both the Insight and the Prius an "excellence in engineering" award, the first time this organization has ever endorsed commercial products.

The 2004 Prius has more interior space, better performance, and more distinctive styling than its predecessor. A more aerodynamic shape, better batteries, and higher voltage give the Prius II excellent fuel efficiency. The EPA rates the Prius at 60 mpg (25 km/l) in city driving and 51 mpg (22 km/l) on the highway. Although Toyota also has an experimental fuel cell car, it expects hybrids to be the best automobile choice for the next 20 years at least. Toyota is also working on a diesel hybrid for the European market.

Most American automobile makers are skeptical of hybrid designs and are putting most of their research into fuel cells, which may be years from commercial use but have the promise of being truly zero-emission. Ford and General Motors have prototype hybrid vehicles with 42-V generators (versus 500 V in the Prius). These "mild" hybrids use the electrical system primarily to run CD players, dashboard computers, extra lights, and other accessories. Mileage is improved very little.

What do you think? Would you buy a vehicle with a hybrid engine system? Would you take a chance on this new technology to get a quiet, clean, efficient, environmentally friendly means of transportation? Do you think that automobile makers are wise to wait for fuel cells, or should they be producing hybrid vehicles as well?

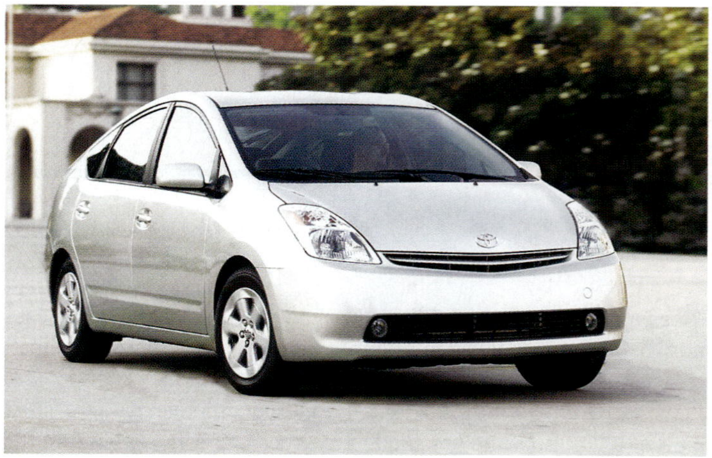

The hybrid gas-electric Toyota Prius seats five adults and gets 60 mpg (25 km/l) in city driving while meeting super-low emission standards.

are the biggest energy consumers (fig. 12.17). Putting your computer to sleep saves about 90 percent of the energy it uses when fully on, but turning it completely off is even better.

Industrial energy savings are another important part of our national energy budget. More efficient electric motors and pumps, new sensors and control devices, advanced heat-recovery systems, and material recycling have reduced industrial energy requirements significantly. In the early 1980s, U.S. businesses saved $160 billion per year through conservation. When oil prices collapsed, however, many businesses returned to wasteful ways.

Cogeneration

One of the fastest growing sources of new energy is **cogeneration,** the simultaneous production of both electricity and steam or hot water in the same plant. By producing two kinds of useful energy in the same facility, the net energy yield from the primary fuel is increased from 30–35 percent to 80–90 percent. In 1900 half the electricity generated in the United States came from plants that also provided industrial steam or district heating. As power plants became larger, dirtier, and less acceptable as neighbors, they were

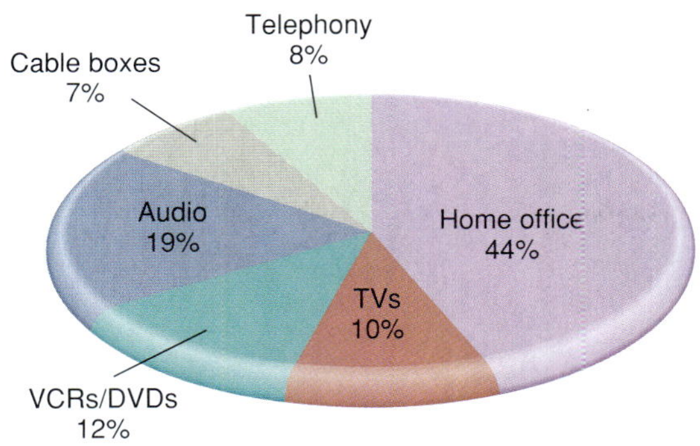

FIGURE 12.17 *Typical standby energy consumption by household electrical appliances.*
Source: Data from U.S. Department of Energy.

forced to move away from their customers. Waste heat from the turbine generators became an unwanted pollutant to be disposed of in the environment. Furthermore, long transmission lines, which are unsightly and lose up to 20 percent of the electricity they carry, became necessary.

By the 1970s, cogeneration had fallen to less than 5 percent of our power supplies, but interest in this technology is being renewed. The capacity for cogeneration more than doubled in the 1980s to about 30,000 megawatts. District heating systems are being rejuvenated, and plants that burn municipal wastes are being studied. New combined-cycle coal-gasification plants, or "mini-nukes," offer high efficiency and clean operation that may be compatible with urban locations. Small neighborhood- or apartment building–sized power-generating units are being built that burn methane (from biomass digestion), natural gas, diesel fuel, or coal (fig. 12.18). The Fiat Motor Company makes a small generator for about $10,000 that produces enough electricity and heat for four or five energy-efficient houses. These units are especially valuable for facilities, such as hospitals or computer centers, that can't afford power outages.

SOLAR ENERGY

The sun is a giant nuclear furnace in space, constantly bathing our planet with a free energy supply. Solar heat drives winds and the hydrologic cycle. All biomass, as well as fossil fuels and our food (both of which are derived from biomass), results from conversion of light energy (photons) into chemical bond energy by photosynthetic bacteria, algae, and plants.

The average amount of solar energy arriving at the top of the atmosphere is 1,330 watts m^2. About half of this energy is absorbed or reflected by the atmosphere (more at high latitudes than at the equator), but the amount reaching the earth's surface is some 10,000 times all the commercial energy used each year. However, this tremendous infusion of energy comes in a form that, until recently, has been too diffuse and low in intensity to be used except for environmental heating and photosynthesis. Figure 12.19 shows solar energy levels over the United States for typical summer and winter days.

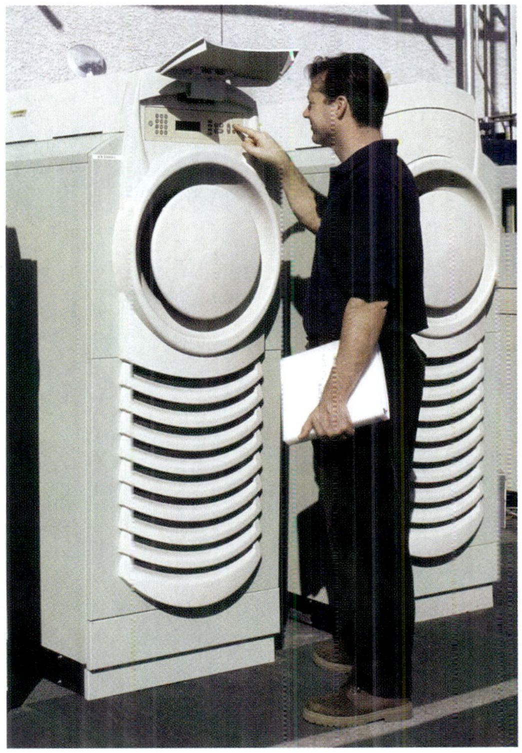

FIGURE 12.18 *A technician adjusts a gas microturbine that produces on-site heat and electricity for businesses, industry, or multiple housing units.*
Source: Courtesy Capstone Micro Turbines.

Passive Solar Heat

Our simplest and oldest use of solar energy is **passive heat absorption,** using natural materials or absorptive structures with no moving parts to simply gather and hold heat. For thousands of years, people have built thick-walled stone and adobe dwellings that slowly collect heat during the day and gradually release it at night. After cooling at night, these massive building materials maintain a comfortable daytime temperature within the house, even as they absorb external warmth (fig. 12.20).

A modern adaptation of this principle is a glass-walled "sunspace," or greenhouse, on the south side of a building. Massive energy-storing materials, such as brick walls, stone floors, or barrels of heat-absorbing water, incorporated into buildings collect heat that is released slowly at night. An interior, heat-absorbing wall called a Trombe wall is an effective passive heat collector. Some Trombe walls are built of glass blocks enclosing a water-filled space or water-filled circulation tubes so heat from solar rays can be absorbed and stored, while light passes through to inside rooms.

Active Solar Heat

Active solar systems generally pump a heat-absorbing fluid medium (air, water, or an antifreeze solution) through a relatively small collector, rather than passively collecting heat in a stationary

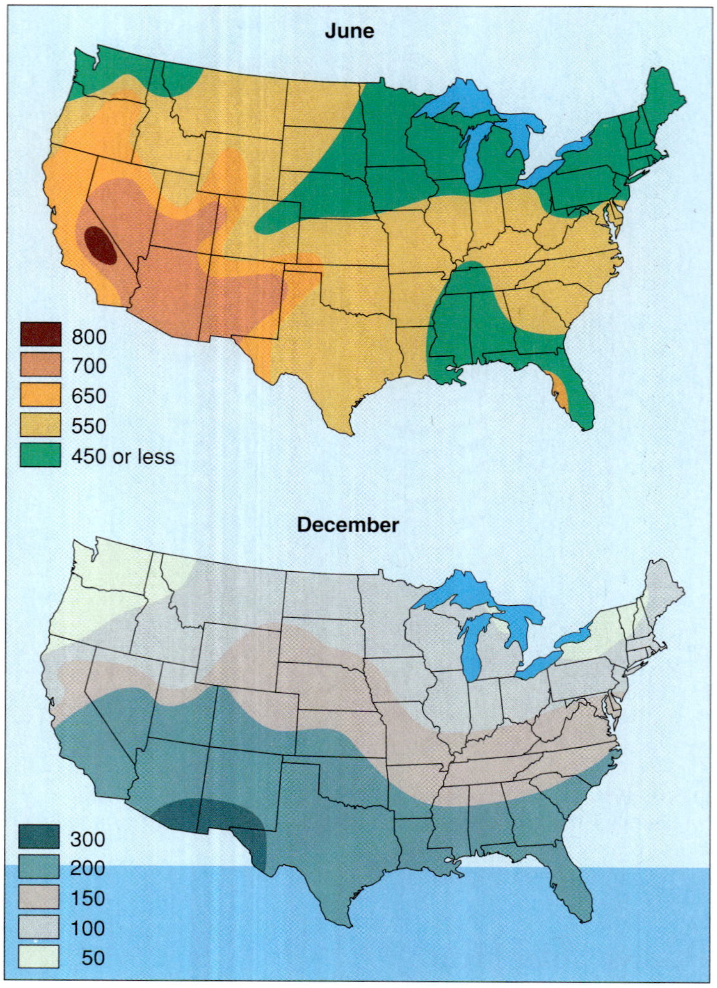

FIGURE 12.19 *Average daily solar radiation in the United States in June and December. One langley, the unit for solar radiation, equals 1 cal/cm^2 of earth surface (3.69 Btu/ft^2).*
Source: Data from National Weather Bureau, U.S. Department of Commerce.

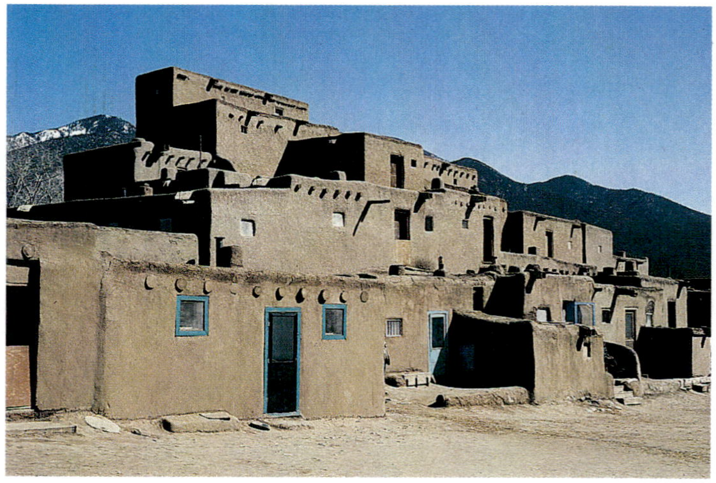

FIGURE 12.20 *Taos Pueblo in northern New Mexico uses adobe construction to keep warm at night and cool during the day.*

medium, such as masonry. Active collectors can be located adjacent to or on top of buildings, rather than being built into the structure.

A flat, black surface sealed with a double layer of glass makes a good solar collector. A fan circulates air over the hot surface and into the house through ductwork of the type used in standard forced-air heating. Alternatively, water can be pumped through the collector to pick up heat for space heating or to provide hot water. Water heating consumes 15 percent of the U.S. domestic energy budget, so savings in this area alone can be significant. A simple, flat panel with about 5 m^2 of surface can reach 95°C (200°F) and can provide enough hot water for an average family of four almost anywhere in the United States. In California, 650,000 homes now heat water with solar collectors. In Greece, Italy, Israel, and other countries where fuels are very expensive, up to 70 percent of domestic hot water comes from solar collectors.

Sunshine doesn't reach us all the time, of course. How can solar energy be stored for times when it is needed? A number of options are available. In a climate where sunless days are rare and seasonal variations are small, a small, insulated water tank is a good solar energy storage system. In areas where clouds block the sun for days at a time or where energy must be stored for winter use, a large, insulated bin containing a heat-storing mass, such as stone, water, or clay, provides solar energy storage. During the summer months, a fan blows the heated air from the collector into the storage medium. In the winter, a similar fan at the opposite end of the bin blows the warm air into the house. During the summer, the storage mass is cooler than the outside air, and it helps cool the house by absorbing heat. During the winter, it is warmer and acts as a heat source by radiating stored heat. In many areas, six or seven months' worth of thermal energy can be stored in 10,000 gal of water or 40 tons of gravel, about the amount of water in a small swimming pool or the gravel in two average-size dump trucks.

High-Temperature Solar Energy

Parabolic mirrors are curved reflecting surfaces that collect light and focus it into a concentrated point. There are two ways to use mirrors to collect solar energy to generate high temperatures. One technique uses long, curved mirrors focused on a central tube containing a heat-absorbing fluid (fig. 12.21). Fluid flowing through the tubes reaches much higher temperatures than possible in a basic flat-panel collector. Another high-temperature system uses thousands of smaller mirrors arranged in concentric rings around a tall, central tower. The mirrors, driven by electric motors, track the sun and focus its light on a heat absorber at the top of the "power tower," where molten salt is heated to temperatures as high as 500°C (1,000°F), which then drives a steam-turbine electric generator.

Under optimum conditions, a 50-ha (130-acre) mirror array should be able to generate 100 MW of clean, renewable power. The only power tower in the United States is Southern California Edison's Solar II plant in the Mojave Desert east of Los Angeles. Its 2,000 mirrors focused on a 100-m (300-ft)-tall tower generate 10 MW, or enough electricity for 5,000 homes at an operating cost far below

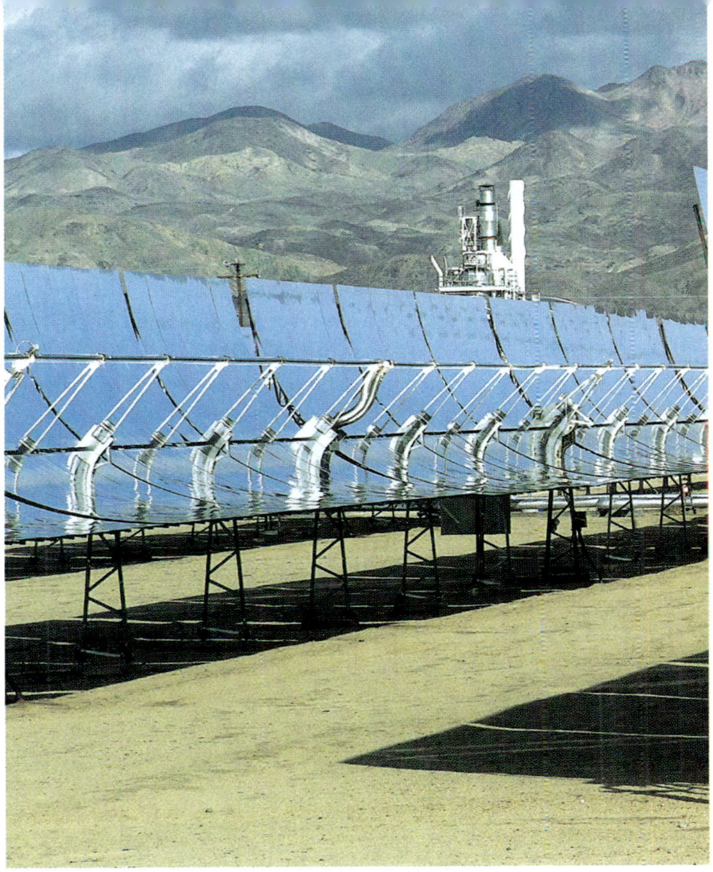

FIGURE 12.21 *Parabolic mirrors focus sunlight on steam-generating tubes at this power plant in the California desert.*

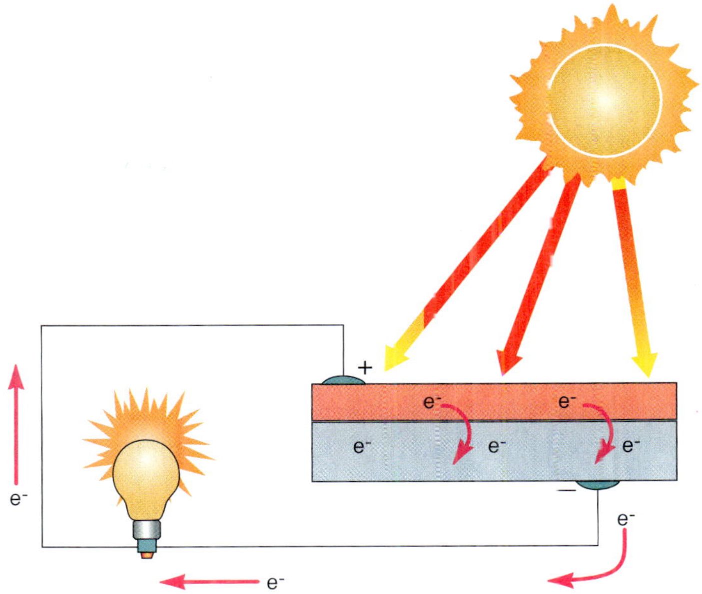

FIGURE 12.22 *The operation of a photovoltaic cell. Boron impurities incorporated into the upper silicon crystal layers cause electrons (e-) to be released when solar radiation hits the cell. The released electrons move into the lower layer of the cell, thus creating a shortage of electrons, or a positive charge, in the upper layer and an oversupply of electrons, or negative charge, in the lower layer. The difference in charge creates an electric current in a wire connecting the two layers.*

that of nuclear power or oil. We haven't had enough experience with these facilities to know how reliable the mirrors, motors, heat absorbers, and other equipment will be over the long run.

Photovoltaic Energy

The **photovoltaic cell** offers an exciting potential for capturing solar energy in a way that will provide clean, versatile, renewable energy. This simple device has no moving parts and negligible maintenance costs, produces no pollution, and has a lifetime equal to that of a conventional fossil fuel or nuclear power plant.

Photovoltaic cells capture solar energy and convert it directly to electrical current by separating electrons from their parent atoms and accelerating them across a one-way electrostatic barrier formed by the junction between two different types of semiconductor material (fig. 12.22). The photovoltaic effect, which is the basis of these devices, was first observed in 1839 by French physicist Alexandre-Edmond Becquerel, who also discovered radioactivity. His discovery didn't lead to any useful applications until 1954, when researchers at Bell Laboratories in New Jersey learned how to carefully introduce impurities into single crystals of silicon.

These handcrafted, single-crystal cells were much too expensive for any practical use until the advent of the U.S. space program. In 1958, when *Vanguard I* went into orbit, its radio was powered by six palm-sized photovoltaic cells that cost $2,000 per peak watt of output, more than 2,000 times as much as conventional energy at the time. Since then, prices have fallen dramatically. In 1970 they cost $100 per watt; in 2002 they were about $5 per watt. This makes solar energy cost-competitive with other sources in some areas. A photovoltaic array of about 30–40m^2 will generate enough electricity for an efficient house (fig. 12.23).

By 2020 photovoltaic cells could be less than $1 per watt of generating capacity. With 15 percent efficiency and a 30-year life, they should be able to produce electricity for around 6¢ per kilowatt hour. At that time, coal-fired steam power will probably cost about half again as much, and nuclear power will likely cost twice as much as photovoltaic energy.

During the past 25 years, the efficiency of energy captured by photovoltaic cells has increased from less than 1 percent of incident light to more than 10 percent under field conditions and over 75 percent in the laboratory. Promising experiments are underway using exotic metal alloys, such as gallium arsenide, and semiconducting polymers of polyvinyl alcohol, which are more efficient in energy conversion than silicon crystals. Every year college students from all over North America race solar-powered cars across the country to test solar technology and publicize its potential. Perhaps you and your classmates would like to build a solar car and enter the race.

One of the most promising developments in photovoltaic cell technology in recent years is the invention of amorphous silicon collectors. First described in 1968 by Stanford Ovshinky, a self-taught inventor from Detroit, these noncrystalline silicon semiconductors can be made into lightweight, paper-thin sheets

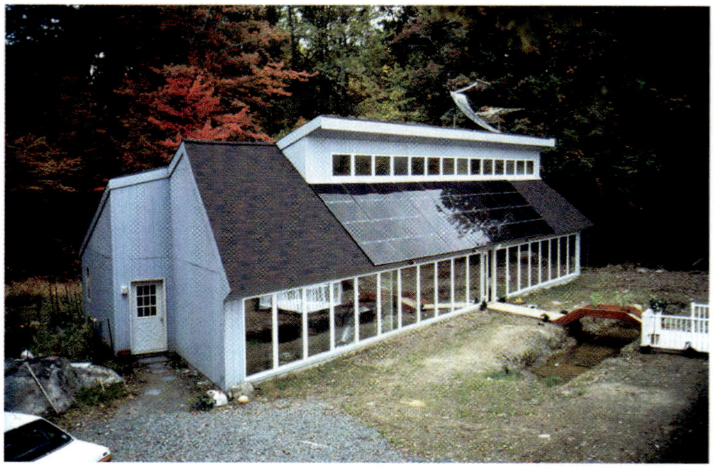

FIGURE 12.23 *Solar roof tiles* (shiny area) *can generate enough electricity for a house full of efficient appliances. On sunny days, this array can produce a surplus to sell back to the utility company, making it even more cost-efficient.*
Courtesy National Renewable Energy Laboratory/NREL/PIX.

APPLICATION: Payback Times

It currently costs about $20,000 for enough photovoltaic cells, batteries, and inverters to run all the appliances, lights, and other electrical services of a modern house. If you live in a place with reliable, sustained winds of at least 15 mph (on average) year-round, you could buy a wind generator for about half as much. By contrast, purchasing electricity from a public utility would cost about $600 to $1,200 per year for comparable consumption levels in most parts of the United States or Canada.

1. What would be the payback time for installing solar or wind power under these conditions?
2. What payback would you consider acceptable?
3. How would you factor in our responsibilities to future generations or the value of clean air and clear water in your decision?

Answers: ***1.*** Solar = 33.3 or 16.6 years; wind = 16.6 or 8.3 years. ***2.*** and ***3.*** Depends on your values and beliefs.

that require much less material than conventional photovoltaic cells. They also are vastly cheaper to manufacture and can be made in a variety of shapes and sizes, permitting ingenious applications. Roof tiles with photovoltaic collectors layered on their surface already are available. Even flexible films can be coated with amorphous silicon collectors. Silicon collectors already are providing power to places where conventional power is unavailable, such as lighthouses, mountaintop microwave repeater stations, villages on remote islands, and ranches in the Australian outback.

You probably already use amorphous silicon photovoltaic cells. They are being built into solar-powered calculators, watches, toys, photosensitive switches, and a variety of other consumer products. Japanese electronic companies presently lead in this field, having foreseen the opportunity for developing a market for photovoltaic cells. This market is already more than $100 million per year. Japanese companies now have home-roof arrays capable of providing all the electricity needed for a typical home at prices in some areas competitive with power purchased from a utility.

Think about how solar power could affect your future energy independence. Imagine the benefits of being able to build a house anywhere and having a cheap, reliable, clean, quiet source of energy with no moving parts to wear out, no fuel to purchase, and little equipment to maintain. You could have all the energy you need without commercial utility wires or monthly energy bills. Coupled with modern telecommunications and information technology, an independent energy source would make it possible to live in the countryside and yet have many of the employment and entertainment opportunities and modern conveniences available in a metropolitan area.

Transporting and Storing Electrical Energy

Electrical energy is difficult and expensive to store or to transport over long distances. If we come to depend on solar, wind, or other renewable energy sources, we may need many more high-voltage power lines to transport electricity to distant markets (fig. 12.24). Many property owners resist having power lines cross their land because they are unsightly and may create hazardous electromagnetic fields. The Bush administration has proposed giving eminent

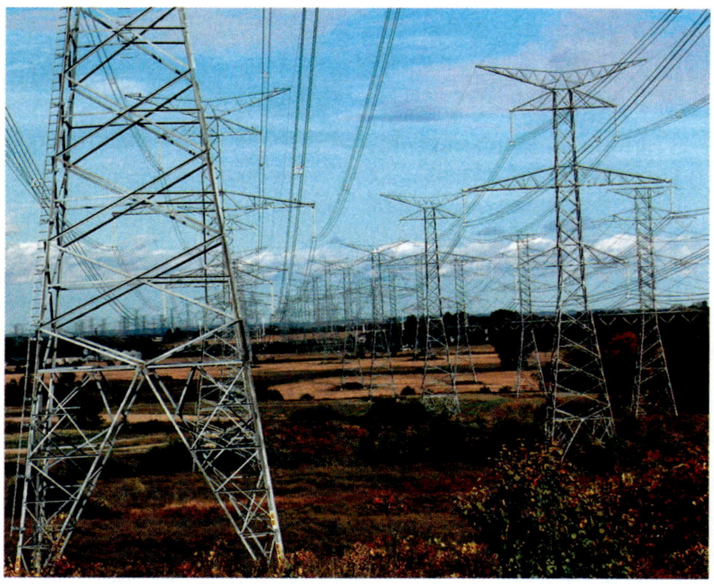

FIGURE 12.24 *As we come to depend more on wind, solar, and hydropower energy, we will probably need more transmission lines to get that energy to market.*

domain to utilities to expedite transmission-line siting. An alternative would be to use electricity at remote sites to electrolyze water, then ship hydrogen through buried pipelines. Hydrogen is the ideal fuel for fuel cells, discussed later in this chapter.

Storage is a problem for photovoltaic generation as well as other sources of electric power. Traditional lead-acid batteries are heavy and have low energy densities; that is, they can store only moderate amounts of energy per unit mass or volume. Acid from batteries is hazardous, and lead from smelters or battery manufacturing is a serious health hazard for workers who handle these materials. A typical lead-acid battery array sufficient to store several days of electricity for an average home would cost about $5,000 and weigh 3 or 4 tons. All the components for an electric car are readily available, but as mentioned earlier in What Do You Think? (p. 290), battery technology limits how far they can go between charges.

Another strategy is to store energy in a form that can be turned back into electricity when needed. Pumped-hydro storage involves pumping water to an elevated reservoir at times when excess electricity is available. The water is released to flow back down through turbine generators when extra energy is needed. Using a similar principle, pressurized air can be pumped into such reservoirs as natural caves, depleted oil and gas fields, abandoned mines, or special tanks. An Alabama power company uses off-peak electricity to pump air at night into a deep salt mine. By day, the air flows back to the surface through turbines, driving a generator that produces electricity. Cool night air is heated to 1,600°F by compression plus geothermal energy, increasing pressure and energy yield.

Flywheels also are the subject of current experimentation for energy storage. Massive, high-speed flywheels, spinning in a nearly friction-free environment, store large amounts of mechanical energy in a small area. This energy is easily convertible to electrical energy. It is difficult, however, to find materials strong enough to hold together when spinning at high speed. Flywheels have a disconcerting tendency to fail explosively and unexpectedly, sending shrapnel in all directions.

Promoting Renewable Energy

Utility restructuring currently being planned in the United States could include policies to encourage conservation and alternative energy sources. Among the proposed policies are (1) "distributional surcharges" in which a small per kilowatt-hour charge is levied on all utility customers to help finance renewable energy research and development, (2) "renewables portfolio" standards to require power suppliers to obtain a minimum percentage of their energy from sustainable sources, and (3) **green pricing** that allows utilities to profit from conservation programs and charge premium prices for energy from renewable sources.

Some states already are pursuing these policies. For example, Iowa has a Revolving Loan Fund supported by a surcharge on investor-owned gas and electric utilities. This fund provides low-interest loans for renewable energy and conservation. Several states have initiated green pricing programs as a way to encourage a transition to sustainable energy. One of the first is in Colorado, where 1,000 customers have agreed to pay $2.50 per month above their regular electric rates to help finance a 10-MW wind farm being built on the Colorado-Wyoming border. Buying a 100-kW "block" of wind power provides the same environmental benefits as planting a half acre of trees or not driving an automobile 4,000 km (2,500 mi) per year. Not all green pricing plans are as straightforward as this, however. Some utilities collect the premium rates for facilities that already exist or for renewable energy bought from other utilities at much lower prices.

FUEL CELLS

Rather than store and transport energy, another alternative is to generate it locally, on demand. **Fuel cells** are devices that use ongoing electrochemical reactions to produce an electrical current. They are very similar to batteries except that, rather than recharging them with an electrical current, you add more fuel for the chemical reaction.

All fuel cells consist of a positive electrode (the cathode) and a negative electrode (the anode) separated by an electrolyte, a material that allows the passage of charged atoms, called ions, but is impermeable to electrons (fig. 12.25). In the most common systems, hydrogen or a hydrogen-containing fuel is passed over the anode, while oxygen is passed over the cathode. At the anode, a reactive catalyst, such as platinum, strips an electron from each hydrogen atom, creating a positively charged hydrogen ion (a proton). The hydrogen ion can migrate through the electrolyte to the cathode, but the electron is excluded. Electrons flow through an external circuit, and the electrical current generated by their passage can be used to do useful work. At the cathode, the electrons and protons are reunited and combined with oxygen to make water.

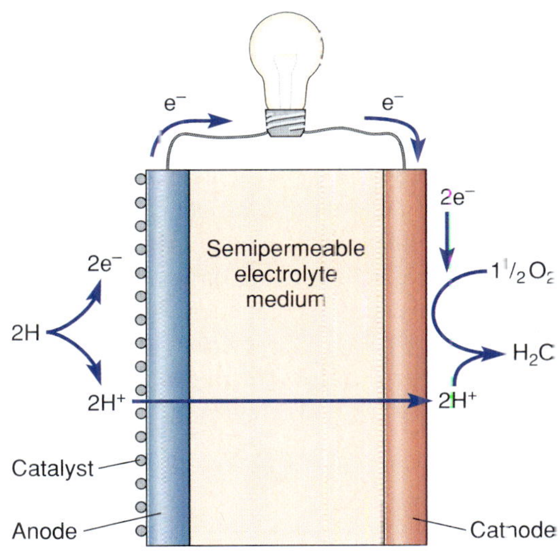

FIGURE 12.25 *Fuel cell operation. Electrons are removed from hydrogen atoms at the anode to produce hydrogen ions (protons) that migrate through a semipermeable electrolyte medium to the cathode, where they reunite with electrons from an external circuit and oxygen atoms to make water. Electrons flowing through the circuit connecting the electrodes create useful electrical current.*

Fuel cells provide direct-current electricity as long as they are supplied with hydrogen and oxygen. For most uses, oxygen is provided by ambient air. Hydrogen can be supplied as a pure gas, but storing hydrogen gas is difficult and dangerous because of its explosive nature. Liquid hydrogen takes far less space than the gas but must be kept below –250°C (–400°F), not a trivial task for most mobile applications. The alternative is a device called a **reformer** or converter that strips hydrogen from fuels such as natural gas, methanol, ammonia, gasoline, ethanol, or even vegetable oil. Many of these fuels can be derived from sustainable biomass crops. Even methane effluents from landfills and wastewater treatment plants can be used as a fuel source. Where a fuel cell can be hooked permanently to a gas line, hydrogen can be provided by solar, wind, or geothermal facilities that use electricity to hydrolyze water.

A fuel cell run on pure oxygen and hydrogen produces no waste products except drinkable water and radiant heat. When a reformer is coupled to the fuel cell, some pollutants are released (most commonly carbon dioxide), but the levels are typically far less than conventional fossil fuel combustion in a power plant or an automobile engine. Although the theoretical efficiency of electrical generation of a fuel cell can be as high as 70 percent, the actual yield is closer to 40 or 45 percent. This is not much better than a very good fossil fuel power plant or a gas turbine electrical generator. On the other hand, the quiet, clean operation and variable size of fuel cells make them useful in buildings where waste heat can be captured for water heating or space heating. A 45-story office building at 4 Times Square, for example, has two 200-kW fuel cells on its fourth floor that provide both electricity and heat. The same building has photovoltaic panels on its façade, natural lighting, fresh-air intakes to reduce air conditioning, and a number of other energy conservation features.

Fuel cells would be ideal zero-emission power sources for vehicles. Fuel cell buses are being tested in Canada, and Honda introduced an experimental fuel cell automobile in California in 2002.

The current from a fuel cell is proportional to the size (area) of the electrodes, while the voltage is limited to about 1.23 volts per cell. A number of cells can be stacked together until the desired power level is reached. A fuel cell stack that provides almost all of the electricity needed by a typical home (along with hot water and space heating) would be about the size of a refrigerator. A 200-kW unit fills a medium-size room and provides enough energy for 20 houses or a small factory. Tiny fuel cells running on methanol might soon be used in cell phones, pagers, toys, computers, videocameras, and other appliances now run by batteries. Rather than buy new batteries or spend hours recharging spent ones, you might just add an eyedropper of methanol every few weeks to keep your gadgets operating.

BIOMASS

Wood fires have been a primary source of heating and cooking for thousands of years (fig. 12.26). As recently as 1850, wood supplied 90 percent of the fuel used in the United States. Wood now provides less than 1 percent of the energy in the United States, but in many of the poorer countries of the world, wood and other biomass fuels still provide up to 95 percent of all energy used. The 1,500 million m^3 of fuelwood collected in the world each year is about half of all wood harvested.

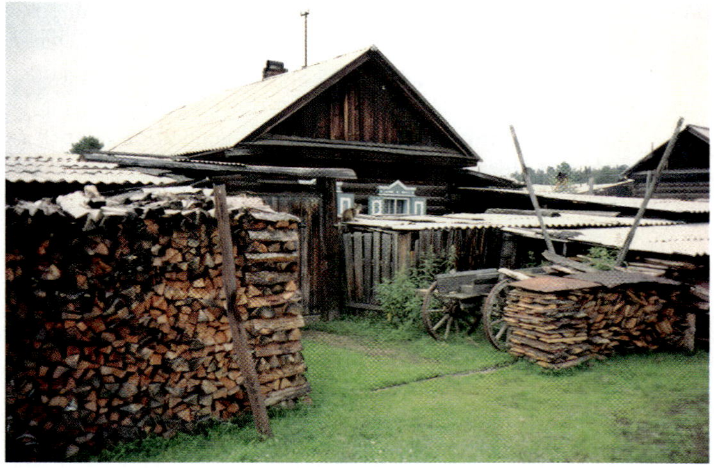

FIGURE 12.26 *Firewood is an important resource in this Siberian village near Lake Baikal.*

In northern industrialized countries, wood burning has increased since 1975 in an effort to avoid rising oil, coal, and gas prices. Most northern areas have adequate wood supplies to meet demands at current levels, but problems associated with wood burning may limit further expansion of this use. Inefficient and incomplete burning of wood in fireplaces and stoves produces smoke laden with fine ash and soot and hazardous amounts of carbon monoxide and hydrocarbons. In valleys where inversion layers trap air pollutants, the effluent from wood fires can be a major source of air quality degradation and health risk. Polycyclic aromatic compounds produced by burning are especially worrisome because they are carcinogenic (cancer-causing). Some communities have passed ordinances limiting the use of woodstoves.

Wood chips, sawdust, wood residue, and other plant materials are being used in some places in the United States and Europe as fuel in industrial boilers (fig. 12.27). In Vermont, for instance, where fossil fuels are expensive and 80 percent of the land is covered by forest, 250,000 cords of unmarketable cull wood are burned annually to fuel a 50-MW power plant in Burlington. Pollution-control equipment is easier to install and maintain in a central power plant than in individual home units. Wood burning also contributes less to acid precipitation than does coal. Because wood has little sulfur, it produces few sulfur gases. And because it burns at lower temperatures than coal, it also produces fewer nitrogen oxides. Burning wood as a renewable crop doesn't produce any net increase in atmospheric carbon dioxide (and, therefore, doesn't add to global warming) because all the carbon released by burning biomass was taken up from the atmosphere when the biomass was grown.

Fuelwood Crisis in Less-Developed Countries

Two billion people—about 40 percent of the total world population—depend on firewood and charcoal as their primary energy source.

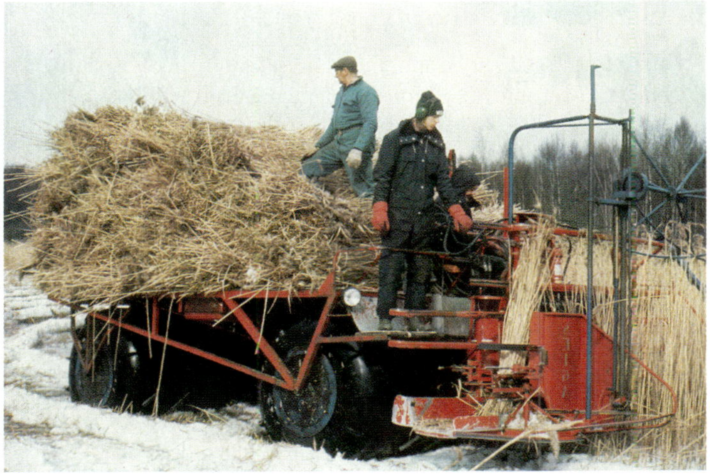

FIGURE 12.27 *Harvesting marsh reeds (*Phragmites *sp.) in Sweden as a source of biomass fuel. In some places, biomass from wood chips, animal manure, food-processing wastes, peat, marsh plants, shrubs, and other kinds of organic material make a valuable contribution to energy supplies. Care must be taken, however, to avoid environmental damage in sensitive areas.*

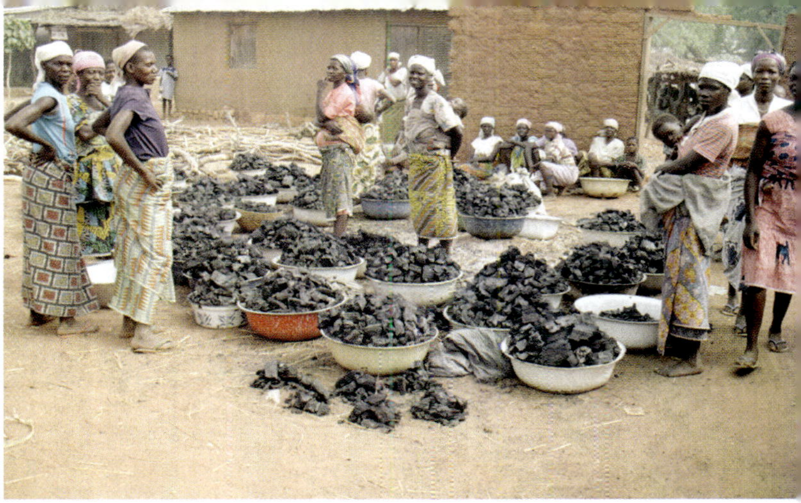

FIGURE 12.28 *A charcoal market in Ghana. Firewood and charcoal provide the main fuel for billions of people. Forest destruction results in wildlife extinction, erosion, and water loss.*
Courtesy National Renewable Energy Laboratory/NREL/PIX.

Of these people, three-quarters (1.5 billion) do not have an adequate, affordable supply. Many people in the less-developed countries face a daily struggle to find enough fuel to warm their homes and cook their food. The problem is intensifying because rapidly growing populations in many developing countries create increasing demands for firewood and charcoal from a diminishing supply (fig. 12.28).

As firewood becomes increasingly scarce, women and children, who do most of the domestic labor in many cultures, spend more and more hours searching for fuel. In some places, it now takes eight hours or more just to walk to the nearest fuelwood supply and even longer to walk back with a load of sticks and branches that will last only a few days.

Currently, about half of all wood harvested each year worldwide is used as fuel. Eighty-five percent of that fuel is harvested in developing countries, whereas three-quarters of all industrial roundwood (lumber, poles, beams, and building materials) is harvested and consumed in developed countries. The poorest countries, such as Ethiopia, Bhutan, Burundi, and Bangladesh, depend on biomass for 90 percent of their energy. Often the harvest is sustainable, consisting of deadwood, branches, trimmings, and shrubs. In Pakistan, for example, some 4.4 million tons of twigs and branches and 7.7 million tons of shrubs and crop residue are consumed as fuel each year with destruction of very few living trees.

In other countries, however, desperate people often chop down anything that will burn. In Haiti, for instance, more than 90 percent of the once forested land has been almost completely denuded, and people cut down even valuable fruit trees to make charcoal they can sell in the marketplace. It is estimated that the 1,700 million tons of fuelwood now harvested each year globally is at least 500 million tons less than is needed. By 2025 the worldwide demand for fuelwood is expected to be about twice current harvest rates, while supplies will not have expanded much beyond current levels. Some places will be much worse than this average. In some African countries, such as Mauritania, Rwanda, and the Sudan, firewood demand already is ten times the sustainable yield. Reforestation projects, agroforestry, community woodlots, and inexpensive, efficient, locally produced woodstoves could help alleviate expected fuelwood shortages in many places.

Dung and Methane as Fuels

Where wood and other fuels are in short supply, people often dry and burn animal manure. This may seem like a logical use of waste biomass, but it can intensify food shortages in poorer countries. Not putting this manure back on the land as fertilizer reduces crop production and food supplies. In India, for example, where fuelwood supplies have been chronically short for many years, a limited manure supply must fertilize crops and provide household fuel. Cows in India produce more than 800 million tons of dung per year, more than half of which is dried and burned in cooking fires. If that dung were applied to fields as fertilizer, it could boost crop production of edible grains by 20 million tons per year, enough to feed about 40 million people.

When cow dung is burned in open fires, more than 90 percent of the potential heat and most of the nutrients are lost. Compare that with the efficiency of using dung to produce methane gas, an excellent fuel. In the 1950s, simple, cheap methane digesters were designed for villages and homes, but they were not widely used. In China, 6 million households use biogas for cooking and lighting. Two large municipal facilities in Nanyang will soon provide fuel for more than 20,000 families. Perhaps other countries will follow China's lead.

Methane gas, the main component of natural gas, is produced by anaerobic decomposition (digestion by anaerobic [oxygen-free] bacteria) of any moist organic material. Many people are familiar with the fact that swamp gas is explosive. Swamps are simply large methane digesters, basins of wet plant and animal wastes sealed from the air by a layer of water. Under these conditions, organic materials are decomposed by anaerobic rather than aerobic (oxygen-using) bacteria, producing flammable gases instead of carbon dioxide. The same process can be reproduced artificially by placing organic wastes in a container and providing warmth and water (fig. 12.29). Bacteria are ubiquitous enough to start the culture spontaneously.

Burning methane produced from manure provides more heat than burning the dung itself, and the sludge left over from bacterial digestion is a rich fertilizer, containing bacterial biomass as well as most of the nutrients originally in the dung. Whether the manure is of livestock or human origin, airtight digestion also eliminates some health hazards associated with direct use of dung, such as exposure to fecal pathogens and parasites.

How feasible is methane—from manure or from municipal sewage—as a fuel resource in developed countries? Methane is a clean fuel that burns efficiently. It is produced in a low-technology, low-capital process from any kind of organic waste material: livestock manure, kitchen and garden scraps, and even municipal garbage and sewage. In fact, municipal landfills are active sites of methane production, contributing as much as 20 percent of the annual output of methane to the atmosphere. This is a waste of a valuable resource and a threat to the environment because methane absorbs infrared radiation and contributes to the greenhouse effect (see chapter 9). Some municipalities are drilling gas wells into landfills and garbage dumps. Cattle feedlots and chicken farms in the United States are a tremendous potential fuel source. Collectible crop residues and feedlot wastes each year contain 4.8 billion GJ (4.6 quadrillion Btu) of energy, more than all the nation's farmers use. Municipal sewage treatment plants routinely use anaerobic digestion as a part of their treatment process, and many facilities collect the methane they produce and use it to generate heat or electricity for their operations. Although this technology is well developed, its utilization could be much more widespread.

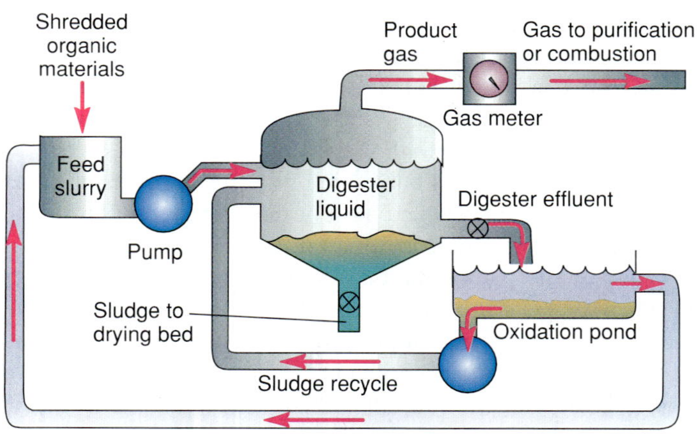

FIGURE 12.29 *Continuous unit for converting organic material to methane by anaerobic fermentation. One kilogram of dry organic matter will produce 1–1.5 m^3 of methane, or 2,500–3,600 million cal per metric ton.*

Source: Solar Energy as a National Energy Resource, NSF/NASA Solar Energy Panel, National Science Foundation, December 1972.

Fuels from Biomass

Ethanol (grain alcohol) and methanol (wood alcohol) are produced by anaerobic digestion of plant materials with high sugar content, mainly grain and sugarcane. Ethanol can be burned directly in automobile engines adapted to use this fuel, or it can be mixed with gasoline (up to about 10 percent) to be used in any normal automobile engine. A mixture of gasoline and ethanol is often called **gasohol.** Engines can also be adapted to burn E85 fuel, which is 85 percent ethanol. Diesel engines can burn plant oils (such as corn, soybean, or sunflower oil), which are sometimes called biodiesel.

Ethanol in gasohol raises octane ratings and is a good substitute for lead antiknock agents, the major cause of lead pollution. It also helps reduce carbon monoxide emissions in automobile exhaust. Gas stations in U.S. cities that exceed EPA air quality standards have been ordered to sell so-called oxygenated fuels containing ethanol or methanol.

Ethanol production could be a solution to grain surpluses and bring a higher price for grain crops than the food market offers. Given our current methods of farming, however, it may take more energy for petroleum-based fertilizer, pesticides, vehicle fuel, and manufacturing processes than is produced in ethanol. Industry claims that corn-based ethanol using state-of-the-art technology produces about 150 percent as much net energy as totoal inputs. Cellulose-based procsses may be slightly more efficient. Although the 2004 Farm Bill granted $3 billion in support of ethanol production, this is more a subsidy for grain farmers than a step toward energy independence.

Methanol might have many advantages as a motor vehicle fuel. Since it burns at a lower temperature than gasoline or diesel, the bulky, heavy radiator might be eliminated, making automobiles sleeker and more efficient. With some combination of flywheel-energy storage, intermittent burning engines, turbochargers, and other high-tech devices, we might be able to have personal transportation that is both energy efficient and less polluting. Both methanol and ethanol make good fuels for fuel cells. Methanol can be produced from woody crops that require less petroleum-based inputs than grain-based ethanol.

ENERGY FROM THE EARTH'S FORCES

The winds, waves, tides, ocean thermal gradients, and geothermal areas are renewable energy sources. Although available only in selected locations, these sources could make valuable contributions to our total energy supply.

Hydropower

Falling water has been used as an energy source since ancient times. The invention of water turbines in the nineteenth century greatly increased the efficiency of hydropower dams. By 1925 falling water generated 40 percent of the world's electric power. Since then, hydroelectric production capacity has grown 15-fold, but fossil fuel use has risen so rapidly that water power is now only one-quarter of total electrical generation. Still, many coun-

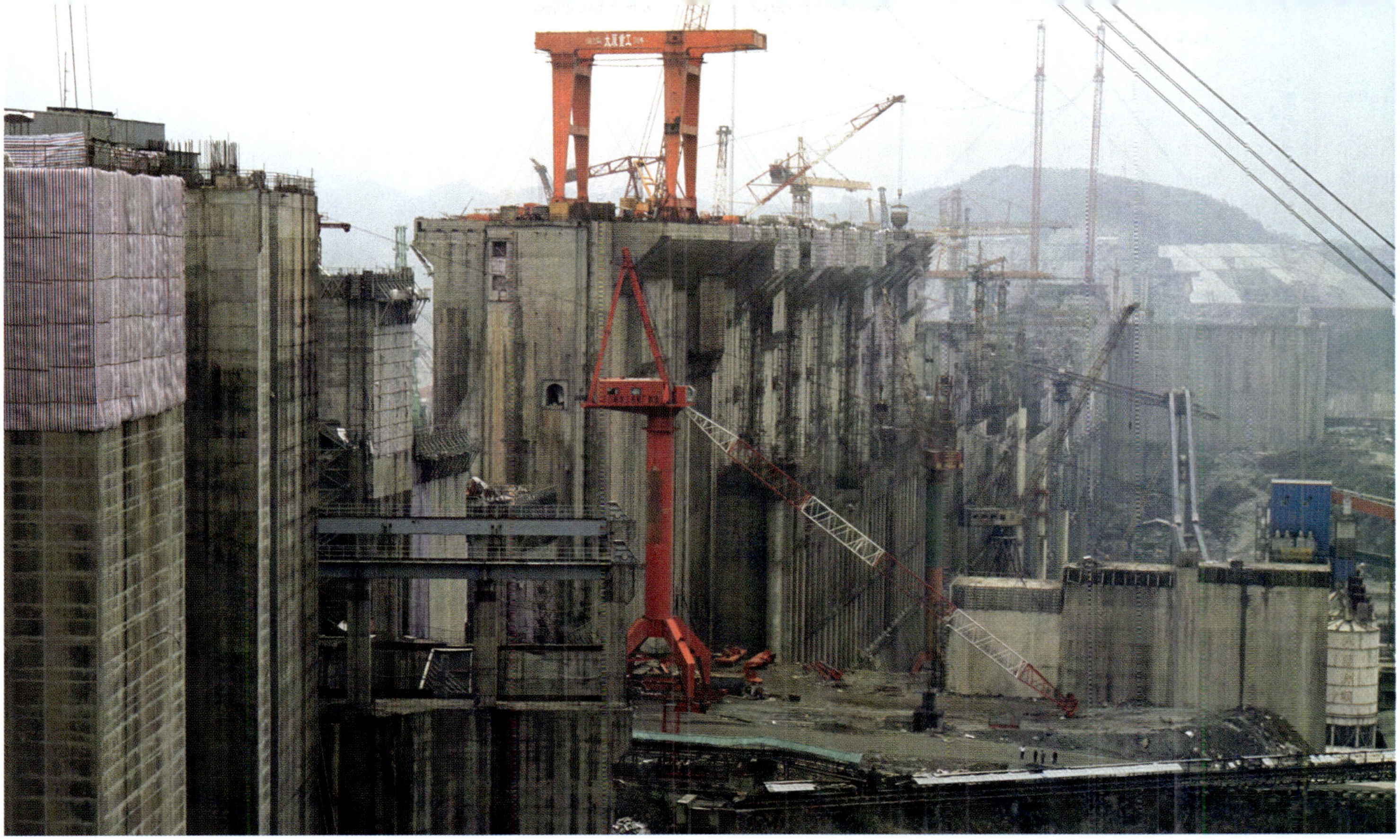

FIGURE 12.30 *The Three Gorges Dam on China's Yangtze River will be the largest in the world when completed in 2009.*

tries produce most of their electricity from falling water. Norway, for instance, depends on hydropower for 99 percent of its electricity; Brazil, New Zealand, and Switzerland all produce at least three-quarters of their electricity with water power. Canada is the world's leading producer of hydroelectricity, running 400 power stations with a combined capacity exceeding 60,000 MW. First Nations people protest that their rivers are being diverted and lands flooded to generate electricity, most of which is sold to the United States.

The total world potential for hydropower is estimated to be about 3 million MW. If all of this capacity were put to use, the available water supply could provide between 8 and 10 terrawatt hours (1,012 watt-hours) of electrical energy. Currently, we use only about 10 percent of the potential hydropower supply. The energy derived from this source in 1994 was equivalent to about 500 million tons of oil, or 8 percent of the total world commercial energy consumption.

Much of the hydropower development in recent years has been in enormous dams. There is a certain efficiency of scale in giant dams, and they bring pride and prestige to the countries that build them, but they can have unwanted social and environmental effects that spark protests in many countries. China's Three Gorges Dam on the Yangtze River will span 2.0 km (1.2 mi) and will be 185 m (600 ft) tall when completed in 2009 (fig. 12.30). The reservoir it creates will be 644 km (400 mi) long and will displace more than 1 million people (see related story Three Gorges Dam at ww.mhhe.com/cases).

In tropical climates, large reservoirs often suffer enormous water losses. Lake Nasser, formed by the Aswan High Dam in Egypt, loses 15 billion m^3 each year to evaporation and seepage. Unlined canals lose another 1.5 billion m^3. Together, these losses represent one-half of the Nile River flow, or enough water to irrigate 2 million ha of land. The silt trapped by the Aswan High Dam formerly fertilized farmland during seasonal flooding and provided nutrients that supported a rich fishery in the delta region. Farmers now must buy expensive chemical fertilizers, and the fish catch has dropped almost to zero. Schistosomiasis, spread by snails that flourish in the reservoir, is an increasingly serious problem.

Wind Energy

The air surrounding the earth has been called a 20-billion-km^3 storage battery for solar energy. The World Meteorological Organization has estimated that 20 million MW of wind power could be commercially tapped worldwide, not including contributions from windmill clusters at sea. This is about 50 times the total present world nuclear generating capacity. Wind power has advantages and disadvantages, as do other nontraditional technologies. Like solar power and hydropower, wind power taps a natural physical force. Like solar power (its ultimate source), wind power is an abundant, nonpolluting resource, and it causes minimal environmental disruption. Also like solar power, however, it requires expensive storage during peak production times to offset nonwindy periods.

As the world's conventional fuel prices rise, interest in wind energy is growing rapidly. In the 1980s the United States was a world leader in wind technology, and California hosted 90 percent of all existing wind power generators. Some 17,000 windmills marched across windy mountain ridges at Altamont, Tehachapi, and San Gorgino Passes. Poor management, technical flaws, and overdependence on subsidies, however, led to bankruptcy of major corporations, including Kenetech, once the largest turbine producer in the United States. Now Danish, German, and Japanese wind machines are capturing the rapidly growing world market. Wind technology is now Denmark's second-largest export, employing 20,000 people and bringing in about $1 billion (U.S.) per year.

The 30,000 MW of installed wind power currently in operation worldwide demonstrates the economy of wind turbines. Theoretically up to 60 percent efficient, windmills typically produce about 35 percent efficiency under field conditions. Where conditions are favorable, wind power is now cheaper than any other new energy source, with electric prices typically between 4¢ and 5¢ per kilowatt-hour in places with steady winds averaging at least 24 km/h (15 mph). Large areas of western North America meet this requirement (fig. 12.31).

The World Energy Council predicts that wind could account for 200,000 MW of electricity by 2020, depending on how seriously politicians take global warming and how many uneconomical nuclear reactors go offline. One thousand MW meets the energy needs of about 50,000 typical U.S. households or is equivalent to about 6 million bbl of oil. Shell Oil suggests that half of all the world's energy could be wind and solar generated by the middle of this century.

The standard modern wind turbine uses only two or three propeller blades. More blades on a windmill provide more torque in low-speed winds, so that the traditional midwestern windmill, with 20 or 30 blades, was most appropriate for small-scale use in less reliable wind fields. Fewer blades operate better in high-speed winds, providing more energy for less material cost at wind speeds of 25 to 40 km/h (15 to 25 mph). A two-blade propeller can extract most of the available energy from a large vertical area and has less material to weaken and break in a storm. Three-bladed propellers often are preferred because they are easier to balance and spin more smoothly (fig. 12.32).

Wind farms are large concentrations of wind generators producing commercial electricity. California continues to lead the United States in wind power, with 2,043 MW installed capacity in 2004, or about one-third of the U.S. total. Texas with 1,294 MW is second in installed capacity. Minnesota, Iowa, Oregon, Washington, Wyoming, Colorado, and New Mexico all have between 200 and 600 MW of installed wind power. Construction of wind farms is not limited to mountain ridges, as the opening story in this chap-

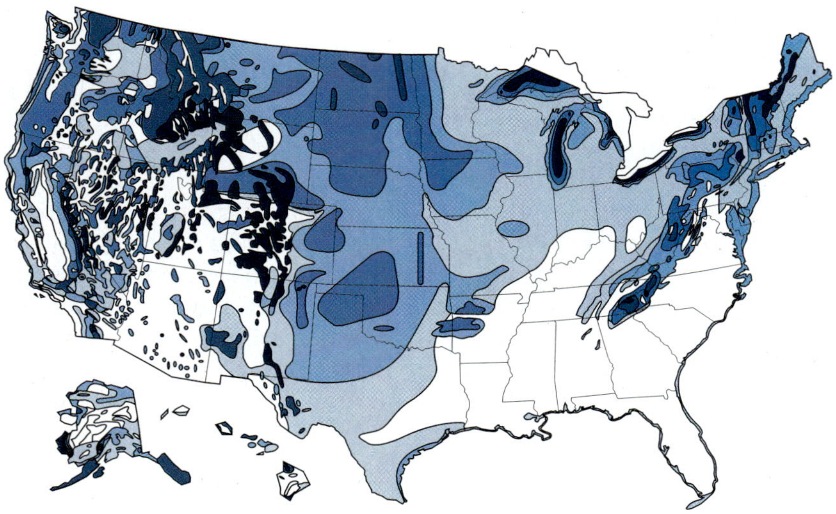

Wind Power Classification

Wind Power Class	Resource Potential	Wind Power Density at 50m W/m^2	Wind Power at 50m m/s	Wind Speed at 50m mph
2	Marginal	200 — 300	5.6 — 6.4	12.5 — 14.3
3	Fair	300 — 400	6.4 — 7.0	14.3 — 15.7
4	Good	400 — 500	7.0 — 7.5	15.7 — 16.8
5	Excellent	500 — 600	7.5 — 8.0	16.8 — 17.9
6	Outstanding	600 — 800	8.0 — 8.8	17.9 — 19.7
7	Superb	800 — 1600	8.8 — 11.1	19.7 — 24.8

FIGURE 12.31 *United States wind resource map. Mountain ranges and areas of the high plains have the highest wind potential, but much of the country has a fair to good wind supply.*
Source: Data from U.S. Department of Energy.

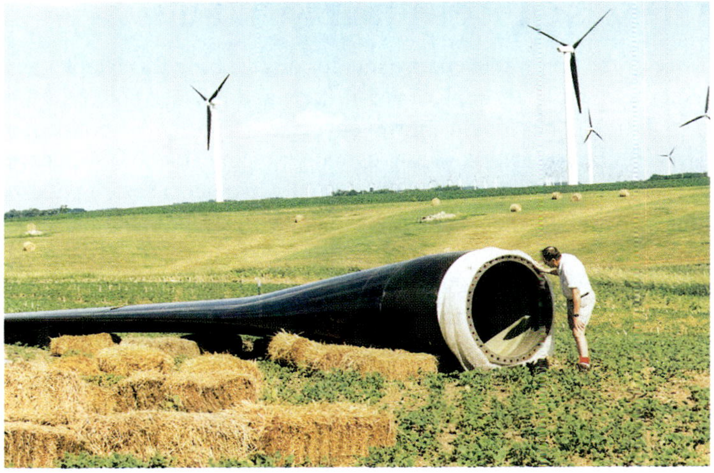

FIGURE 12.32 *A 23-meter-long, 1.6-meter-wide fiberglass blade waits to be attached to a new wind generator.*

TABLE 12.2 Jobs and Land Required for Alternative Energy Sources

TECHNOLOGY	LAND USE (m^2 PER GIGAWATT-HOUR FOR 30 YEARS)	JOBS (PER TERAWATT-HOUR PER YEAR)
Coal	3,642	116
Photovoltaic	3,237	175
Solar thermal	3,561	248
Wind	1,335	542

Source: Data from Lester R. Brown et al., *Saving the Planet,* 1991. W. W. Norton & Co., Inc.

ter shows. In addition to Britain and Sweden, Denmark, Spain, and the Netherlands have large offshore wind farms. Germany leads the world in wind power, with 10,000 MW currently installed, and plans to build 22,000 MW by 2010.

Do wind farms have any negative impacts? They generally occupy places with wind and weather too severe for residential or other development. Most wind farms are too far from residential areas to be heard or seen. But they do interrupt the view in remote, isolated places and destroy the sense of isolation and natural beauty. Bird kills have been a problem for some California wind farms. Careful placement outside of migration corridors and the addition of warning devices can reduce mortality greatly.

Wouldn't wind power take up a huge land area if we were to depend on it for a major part of our energy supply? As table 12.2 shows, the actual space taken up by towers, roads, and other structures on a wind farm is only about one-third as much as would be consumed by a coal-fired power plant or solar thermal energy system to generate the same amount of energy over a 30-year period. Furthermore, the land under windmills is more easily used for grazing or farming than is a strip-mined coal field or land under solar panels. Farmers are finding wind energy to be a lucrative corp. A single tower sitting on 0.1 ha (0.25 acre) can pay $100,000 per year.

When a home owner or community invests independently in wind generation, the same question arises as with solar energy: what should be done about energy storage when electricity production exceeds use? Besides the storage methods mentioned earlier, many private electricity producers believe the best use for excess electricity is to sell it to the public utility grid. In states that allow net energy pricing, you sell excess power from wind or solar systems back to a local utility. Ideally, the utility pays you something close to its average wholesale price. The 1978 Public Utilities Regulatory Policies Act required utilities to buy power generated by small hydro, wind, cogeneration (simultaneous production of useful heat and electricity), and other privately owned technologies at a fair price. Not all utilities yet comply, but some—notably in California, Oregon, Maine, and Vermont—are purchasing significant amounts of private energy.

Geothermal, Tidal, and Wave Energy

The earth's internal temperature can provide a useful source of energy in some places. High-pressure, high-temperature steam fields exist below the earth's surface. Around the edges of continental plates or where the earth's crust overlays magma (molten rock) pools close to the surface, this energy is expressed in the form of hot springs, geysers, and fumaroles. Yellowstone National Park is the largest geothermal region in the United States. Iceland, Japan, and New Zealand also have high concentrations of geothermal springs and vents. Depending on the shape, heat content, and access to groundwater, these sources produce wet steam, dry steam, or hot water.

While few places have geothermal steam, the earth's warmth can help reduce energy costs nearly everywhere. Pumping water through deeply buried pipes can extract enough heat so that a heat pump will operate more efficiently. Similarly, the relatively uniform temperature of the ground can be used to augment air conditioning in the summer (fig. 12.33).

Ocean tides and waves contain enormous amounts of energy that can be harnessed to do useful work. A tidal station works like a hydropower dam, with its turbines spinning as the tide flows through them. A high-tide/low-tide differential of several meters is required to spin the turbines. Unfortunately, variable tidal periods often cause problems in integrating this energy source into the electric utility grid. Nevertheless, demand has kept some plants running for many decades.

The first North American tidal generator, producing 20 MW, was completed in 1984 at Annapolis Royal, Nova Scotia. A much larger project has been proposed to dam the Bay of Fundy and produce 5,000 MW of power on the bay's 17-m tides. The total flow at each tide through the Bay of Fundy theoretically could generate energy equivalent to the output of 250 large nuclear power plants. The environmental consequences of such a gargantuan project,

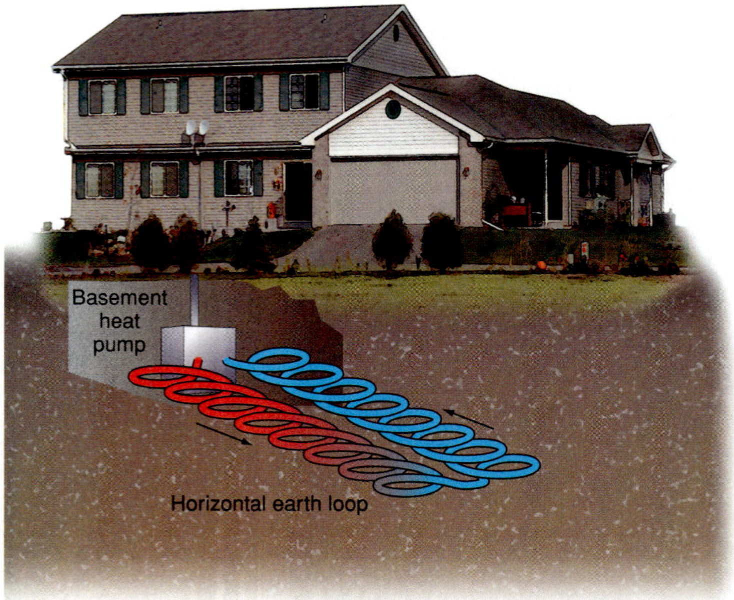

FIGURE 12.33 *Geothermal energy can cut heating and cooling costs by half in many areas. In summer (shown here), warm water is pumped through buried tubing (earth loops), where it is cooled by constant underground temperatures. In winter, the system reverses and the relatively warm soil helps heat the house. Where space is limited, earth loops can be vertical. If more space is available, the tubing can be laid in shallow horizontal trenches, as shown here.*

however, may prevent its ever being built. The main worries are saltwater flooding of freshwater aquifers when seawater levels rise behind the dam and the flooding and destruction of rich shoals and salt flats, breeding grounds for aquatic species and a vital food source for millions of migrating shorebirds. There also would be heavy siltation, as well as scouring of the seafloor, as water shoots through the dam.

Ocean wave energy can easily be seen and felt on any seashore. The energy that waves expend as millions of tons of water are picked up and hurled against the land, over and over, day after day, can far exceed the combined energy budget for both insolation (solar energy) and wind power in localized areas. Captured and turned into useful forms, that energy could make a substantial contribution to meeting local energy needs.

Numerous attempts have been made to use wave energy to drive electrical generators. Generally, these take the form of a floating bar that moves up and down as the wave passes. When coupled to a dynamo, this mechanical energy can be converted to electricity in the same way that a waterwheel or steam turbine works. England, with a long coastline facing the stormy North Sea, plans to build an extensive system of wave-energy platforms. Unfortunately for developers of this energy source, the stormy coasts where waves are strongest are usually far from major population centers that need the power. In addition, the storms that bring this energy destroy the equipment intended to exploit it.

WHAT'S OUR ENERGY FUTURE?

None of the renewable energy sources discussed in this chapter are likely to completely replace fossil fuels and nuclear power in the near future. They could, however, make a substantial collective contribution toward providing us with the conveniences we crave in a sustainable, environmentally friendly manner. They could also make us energy independent and balance our international payment deficit.

The World Energy Council projects that renewables could provide about 40 percent of world cumulative energy consumption under an idealized "ecological" scenario assuming that political leaders take global warming seriously and pass taxes to encourage conservation and protect the environment (fig. 12.34). This scenario also envisions measures to shift wealth from the north to the south and to enhance economic equity. By the end of the twenty-first century, renewable sources could provide all our energy needs if we take the necessary steps to make this happen.

Environmentalists point to the dangers of air pollution, global climate change, and other environmental problems associated with burning fossil fuels. Businesses stress the importance of a reliable energy supply for economic growth. While both call for a new policy, they disagree on what it should contain. Conservatives tend to favor increasing production and easing regulations on power plant operation and transmission-line siting, rather than limiting demand. Progressives, on the other hand, prefer conservation measures, such as forcing automakers to increase average fuel efficiency of cars and light trucks and providing heating bill assistance for low-income households.

The Republican-sponsored Energy Bill, based largely on the recommendations of a secret task force headed by Vice President Dick Cheney, and made up entirely of oil, coal, gas and nuclear company representatives, calls for $30 billion in subsidies for traditional energy, but only $5 billion for conservation or renewables. At the time of this writing, the Energy Bill had passed several times in the House of Representatives but was blocked in the Senate. Ask your instructor what has happened to this act.

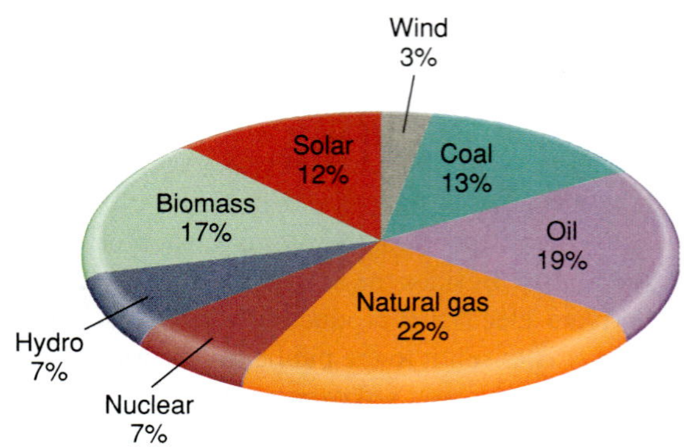

FIGURE 12.34 *Idealized "ecological" scenario for cumulative world energy consumption, 2000 to 2100.*
Source: Data from World Energy Council, 2002.

Speaking for his task force, Mr. Cheney said that oil, coal, and natural gas would remain the United States' primary energy resources for "years down the road." He strongly supported the use of nuclear power and claimed that the United States needs to build one large electric-generating plant each week for the next 20 years. He dismissed as 1970s-era thinking the notion that "we could simply conserve or ration our way out" of an energy crisis. "Conservation," he said, "may be a sign of personal virtue, but it is not a sufficient basis for a sound, comprehensive energy policy."

In light of what you've read in this chapter about current and potential sources, what sort of energy policy would you suggest if you were invited to advise government officials? How much conservation is it realistic or fair to ask people to adopt? What's a reasonable percentage of our energy that might come from renewable sources in 20 or 50 years? If you wanted to move toward the "ecological scenario" described by the World Energy Council, how would you go about implementing that plan? What government actions do you think would be most effective in accomplishing these goals?

SUMMARY

- Energy is the capacity to do work. Power is the rate of doing work. Globally, about 86 percent of all commercial energy is generated by fossil fuels, with about 40 percent coming from petroleum. Coal produces 23 percent, and natural gas (methane) accounts for 22.5 percent of our commercial supply.
- Petroleum and natural gas were not used in large quantities until the beginning of the twentieth century, but there already are worries about supplies being depleted. Coal supplies will last several more centuries at present rates of usage, but it appears that the fossil fuel age will have been a rather short episode in the total history of humans. Nuclear power provides about 7 percent of commercial energy worldwide.
- The environmental damage caused by mining, shipping, processing, and using fossil fuels may necessitate cutting back on our use of these energy sources. Coal is an especially dirty and dangerous fuel, at least as we currently obtain and use it. Coal combustion is a major source of acid precipitation, which is suspected of being a significant cause of environmental damage in many areas. We now recognize that carbon dioxide buildup in the atmosphere has the potential to trap heat and raise the earth's temperature to catastrophic levels.
- The greatest worry about nuclear power is the danger that accidents or terrorist attacks could release hazardous radioactive materials into the environment. Several accidents, most notably the "meltdown" at the Chernobyl plant in the Soviet Ukraine in 1986, have convinced many people that this technology is too risky to pursue.
- Other major worries about nuclear power include where to put the waste products of the nuclear fuel cycle and how to ensure that the wastes will remain safely contained for the thousands of years required for "decay" of the radioisotopes to nonhazardous levels. Yucca Mountain, Nevada, has been chosen for a high-level waste repository, but many experts believe that burying these toxic residues in nonretrievable storage is a mistake.
- Several sustainable energy sources could reduce or eliminate our dependence on fossil fuels and nuclear energy. Some of these sources have been used for centuries but have been neglected since fossil fuels came into widespread use. Passive solar heat, fuelwood, windmills, and waterwheels, for instance, once supplied a major part of the external energy for human activities. With increased concern about the dangers and costs associated with conventional commercial energy, these ancient energy sources are being reexamined as part of a more sustainable future for humankind.
- Exciting new technologies have been invented to use renewable energy sources. Active solar air and water heating, for instance, require less material and function more quickly than passive solar collection. Parabolic mirrors collect solar energy to produce temperatures high enough to be used as process heat in manufacturing. Wind is now the cheapest form of new energy in many places. It has potential to supply one-third or more of our energy requirements.
- Fuel cells use catalysts and semipermeable electrolytes to extract energy from fuels such as hydrogen or methanol at high efficiency and with very low emissions. Ocean thermal electric conversion and tidal and wave power can produce useful amounts of energy in some localities. The relatively constant temperature of the ground can be used by heat pumps to augment heating and cooling nearly everywhere.

- One of the most promising technologies is direct electricity generation by photovoltaic cells. Since solar energy is available everywhere, photovoltaic collectors could provide clean, inexpensive, nonpolluting, renewable energy, independent of central power grids or fuel supply systems.
- Biomass also may have some modern applications. In addition to direct combustion, biomass can be converted into methane or ethanol, which are clean-burning, easily storable, and transportable fuels. These alternative uses of biomass also allow nutrients to be returned to the soil and help reduce our reliance on expensive, energy-consuming artificial fertilizers.

QUESTIONS FOR REVIEW

1. What is energy? What is power?
2. What are the major sources of commercial energy worldwide and in the United States?
3. How does our energy use compare with that of people in other countries?
4. How much coal, oil, and natural gas are in proven reserves worldwide? Where are those reserves located?
5. What are the most important health and environmental consequences of our use of fossil fuels?
6. Describe how nuclear reactors work and why they are dangerous.
7. Describe methods proposed for storing and disposing of nuclear wastes.
8. What is the difference between active and passive solar energy?
9. How do photovoltaic cells work?
10. What is a fuel cell, and how does it work?
11. Describe some problems with wood burning in both industrialized nations and developing nations.
12. What are some advantages and disadvantages of wind power?

THINKING SCIENTIFICALLY

1. If you were considering an alternative energy source for your region and climate, what factors would you need to take into account? Where might you get this information, or how would you measure it yourself?
2. If you were the energy czar of your state or country, where would you invest your budget? Why?
3. What are the advantages and disadvantages of being disconnected from central utility power?
4. Consumers are reluctant to invest in new, sustainable-energy technology because they don't know how it will hold up in the long run. How would you assess the long-term reliability and efficiency of these alternative energy sources?
5. We have discussed a number of different energy sources and energy technologies in this chapter. Each has advantages and disadvantages. If you were an energy policy analyst, how would you compare such different problems as the risk of a nuclear accident versus air pollution effects from burning coal?
6. If your local utility company were going to build a new power plant in your community, what kind would you prefer? Why?
7. The nuclear industry is placing ads in popular magazines and newspapers, claiming that nuclear power is environmentally friendly, since it doesn't contribute to the greenhouse effect. How do you respond to that claim?
8. Our energy policy effectively treats some strip-mined lands as national sacrifice areas, since we know that they will never be restored to their original state when mining is finished. How do we decide who wins and who loses in this transaction?
9. Storing nuclear wastes in dry casks outside nuclear power plants is highly controversial. Opponents claim the casks will inevitably leak. Proponents claim the casks can be designed to be safe. What evidence would you consider adequate or necessary to choose between these two positions?
10. Although we have used vast amounts of energy resources in the process of industrialization and development, some would say that it was a necessary investment to get to a point at which we can use energy more efficiently and sustainably. Do you agree? Might we have followed a different path?

KEY TERMS

active solar systems 291
chain reaction 286
cogeneration 290
control rods 286
energy 279
fossil fuels 280
fuel assembly 286
fuel cells 295
gasohol 298
green pricing 295
joule (J) 279
monitored, retrievable storage 288
nuclear fission 286
oil shales 284
passive heat absorption 291
photovoltaic cell 293
power 279
proven-in-place reserves 282
reformer 296
tar sands 284
wind farms 300
work 279

SUGGESTED READINGS

Banerjee, Subhankar. 2003. *Arctic National Wildlife Refuge: Seasons of Life and Land.* Mountaineers Books.

Blair, Tony. 2003. "Meeting the Sustainable Development Challenge." *Environment* 45(4):20–28.

Chow, J. R., et al. 2003. "Energy resources and global development." *Science* 302 1528–31.

Deffeyes, Kenneth S. 2001. *Hubbert's Peak: The Impending World Oil Shortage.* Princeton University Press.

Freeze, Barbara. 2003. *Coal: A Human History*. Perseus.

Gipe, Paul. 1999. *Wind Energy Basics: A Guide to Small and Micro Wind Systems.* Real Goods Solar Living Books.

Renner, Michael. 2001. "Employment in Wind Power." *World Watch* 14(1):22–30.

Roberts, Carolyn. 2002. *A House of Straw.* Chelsea Green.

Vaitheeswaran, Vijay. 2003. *Power to the People: How the Coming Energy Revolution Will Transform an Industry, Change Our Lives, and Maybe Even Save the Planet.* Farrar, Straus and Giroux.

Wald, Matthew L. 2003. "Dismantling nuclear reactors." *Scientific American* 288(3):60–70.

Welcome to McGraw-Hill's Online Learning Center

http://www.mhhe.com/cunningham3e

WEB EXERCISES

Fossil Fuel Supplies

Go to http://greenwood.cr.usgs.gov/energy/WorldEnergy/DDS-60/. Click on the world maps link and look at the "World Petroleum Assessment 2000 Regions with Geologic Provinces" (the first map listed).

1. Where are the major petroleum reserves?
2. Why are most of them along coastlines?
3. What might be the environmental risks of oil drilling and shipping in these regions?
4. Where is there no oil? Why might this be? Find the "Executive Summary" on this page.
5. How many barrels of oil and gas are reported to be in world reserves?
6. Where are the greatest volumes of undiscovered oil expected to be found?
7. Why might we not have explored these places already?

You can also find energy information at http://energy.cr.usgs.gov/energy/WorldEnergy/WEnergy.html.

Solar Photovoltaics

Go to www.eere.energy.gov, the home page of the Energy Efficiency and Renewable Energy Program within the U.S. Department of Energy. Click on "Solar" and then "Photovoltaics" to get detailed information about this exciting new technology. For more basic information, click on the box labeled "Solar Cell Animation" in the upper right-hand corner of the Solar page to see a brief but informative movie about photovoltaics (PV). (Hint: the url is www.eere.energy.gov/pv/video.html, if you want to go there directly or you get lost in the previous pages.) This is a gateway to a wealth of basic information about how photovoltaics work. Look at the index and answer the following questions:

1. What is amorphous silicon?
2. What are the environmental concerns about PV?
3. Who discovered the PV effect? When?
4. How does a PV cell work?
5. Give one example of a success story involving PV systems

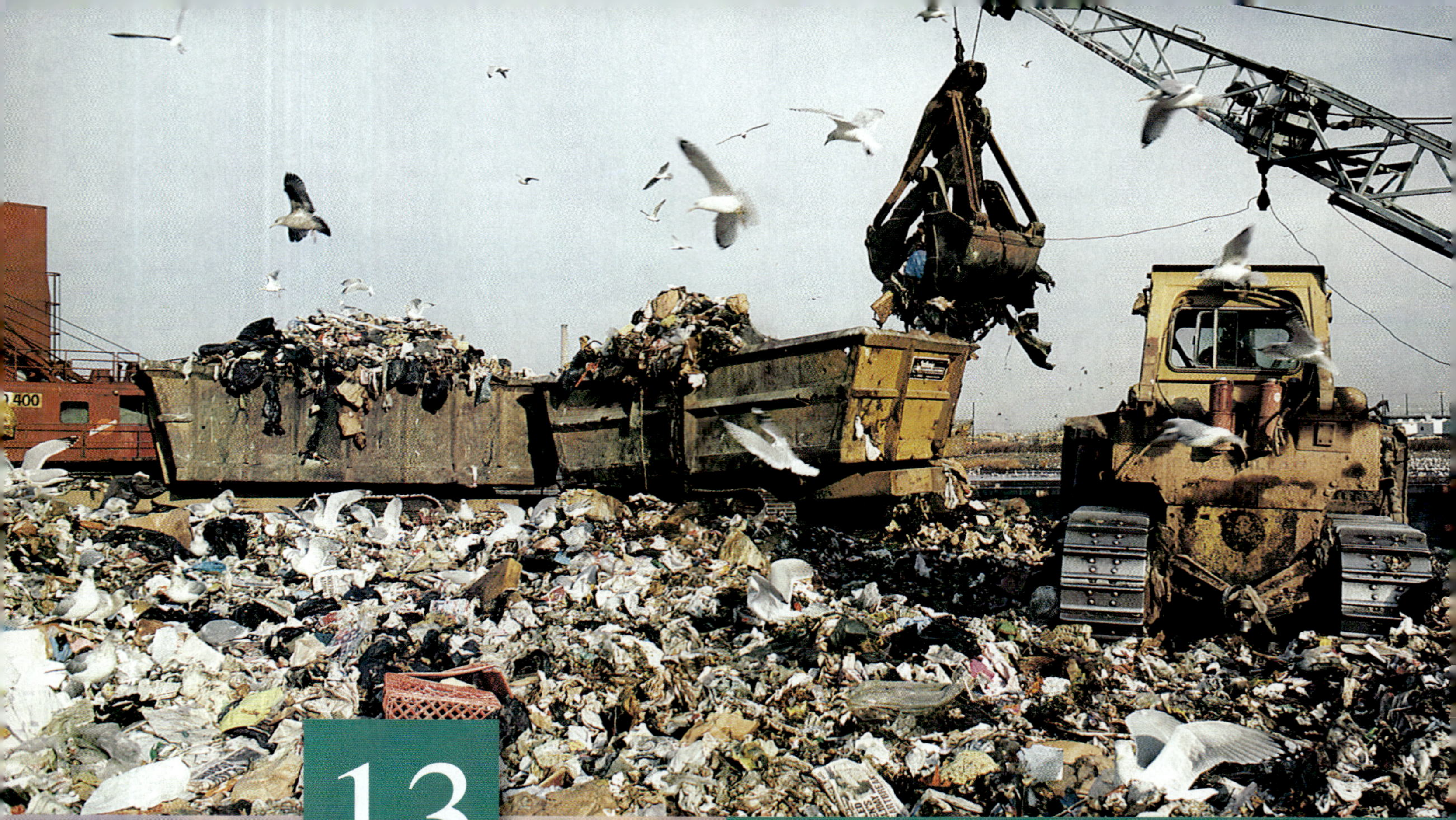

A crane unloads a garbage barge at Fresh Kills on Staten Island, the world's largest landfill before it closed in 2001.

13

Solid and Hazardous Waste

There's always an easy solution to every human problem—neat, plausible, and wrong.

–H. L. Mencken

Welcome to McGraw-Hill's Online Learning Center

http://www.mhhe.com/cunningham3e

LEARNING ONLINE

Visit our webpage at www.mhhe.com/cunningham3e for data sources, further readings, additional case studies, current environmental news, and regional examples within the Online Learning Center to help you understand the material in this chapter. You'll also find active links to information pertaining to this chapter, including

Superfund sites
Toxic stubstances and disease
Persistent organic pollutants (POPs)
Environmental justice
Consumer recycling
Hazardous waste
Composting

OBJECTIVES

After studying this chapter, you should be able to

- identify the major components of the waste stream, and describe how wastes have been—and are being—disposed of in North America and around the world.
- explain the differences between dumps, sanitary landfills, and modern, secure landfills.
- summarize the benefits, problems, and potential of recycling and reusing wastes.
- analyze some alternatives for reducing the waste we generate.
- understand what hazardous and toxic wastes are and how we dispose of them.
- evaluate the options for hazardous waste management.
- outline some ways we can destroy or permanently store hazardous wastes.

Garbology: The Science of Trash

What can the stuff we throw away every day tell us about our society—and ourselves? That's an interesting question addressed by Professor William Rathje, his colleagues, and his students at the University of Arizona. Trained in classical archeology, Rathje decided to use his scientific tools to study contemporary society, rather than ancient ones. Most archeological digs, he reasoned, no matter how dignified or scholarly they seem, are essentially organized trash picking. The broken pottery shards or stone tools carefully dug out of old midden heaps or fire pits by archeologists are really nothing more than the discards of somebody else's daily life. Why not, he reasoned, look at modern garbage in the same way?

Starting in the early 1970s, Rathje and his coworkers systematically collected garbage bags from homes in Tucson and Phoenix, Arizona. Trash was painstakingly sorted, classified, weighed, and recorded. To protect individual privacy, records were kept only by census tracks, rather than by specific households.

After several years of intercepting garbage headed for the landfill, Rathje decided to turn to excavations to look at older refuse. Digging trenches and boring holes as much as 90 ft deep in more than a dozen municipal dumps, Rathje's team has recovered trash dating back to the 1940s. In addition to sorting and classifying larger objects by type, brand, size, material, and condition, the team also washes and filters small items through decreasing mesh–size screens to analyze the composition of "fines" created in tightly packed landfills.

This analysis of what we throw away reveals some interesting things about how modern Americans live. Packaging now makes up about half of all the garbage we discard. Paper bags, metal cans, glass bottles, wrapping paper, and a wide variety of plastic products fall in this category. Some materials, on the other hand, are less prevalent than you might imagine. While some people believe that disposable diapers account for up to 30 percent of all landfill volume, Rathje and his coworkers found that diapers make up only about 1 percent of contemporary trash.

Often, objective research can reveal interesting differences between what people say they do and their actual behavior. In one study in Phoenix, four out of five households claimed that they recycled conscientiously. Researchers found, however, that the garbage of nine out of ten of those houses contained aluminum cans, glass bottles, newsprint, and other easily recyclable materials. Extrapolating to the whole city, Rathje estimated that $2 million in valuable materials were being buried in landfills every year. Newsprint makes up the largest single item in our trash, accounting for 16 percent of what's discarded in a typical city. Together with cardboard, office paper, and other related products, paper accounts for about 38 percent of our waste stream.

One of the biggest surprises from Rathje's work is how well most materials are preserved in landfills. We imagine that landfills are giant compost piles, where everything organic decomposes and disappears in a few months. Quite to the contrary, landfill digs have found newspapers dating from the 1950s that are just as legible today as when they were printed. In one case, pork chops buried for 40 years still looked edible. Because the trash is packed tightly in the landfill and protected from air, water, and sunlight, it is preserved almost perfectly. We feel good about using biodegradable materials as a way of protecting our environment, but when they go into a landfill, they will probably last for centuries.

So what does garbology show us about modern life? We throw away a tremendous amount of stuff. Much of what we discard could be used again or recycled in other useful products if we would only take the time to sort it and send it to a recycling center, rather than just dump it in the trash. But we too often take the easy course, rather than the more environmentally responsible one. In this chapter we'll look further at what we throw away, where it goes, and what some of our options are for reducing the material we discard.

WASTE

Waste is everyone's business. We all produce unwanted by-products and residues in nearly everything we do. According to the Environmental Protection Agency (EPA), the United States produces 11 billion tons of solid waste each year. Nearly half of that amount consists of agricultural waste, such as crop residues and animal manure, which are generally recycled into the soil on the farms where they are produced. They represent a valuable resource as groundcover to reduce erosion and as fertilizer to nourish new crops, but they also constitute the single largest source of nonpoint air and water pollution in the country. About one-third of all solid wastes are mine tailings, overburden from strip mines, smelter slag, and other residues produced by mining and primary metal processing. Much of this material is stored in or near its source of production and isn't mixed with other kinds of wastes. Improper disposal practices, however, can result in serious and widespread pollution.

Industrial waste—other than mining and mineral production—amounts to some 400 million metric tons per year in the United States. Most of this material is recycled, converted to other forms, destroyed, or disposed of in private landfills or deep injection wells. About 60 million metric tons of industrial waste fall in a special category of hazardous and toxic waste, which we will discuss later in this chapter.

Municipal waste—a combination of household and commercial refuse—amounts to about 230 million metric tons per year in the United States. That's just over 2 kg (4.6 lbs) per person per day—twice as much per capita as Europe or Japan, and five to ten times as much as most developing countries (fig. 13.1).

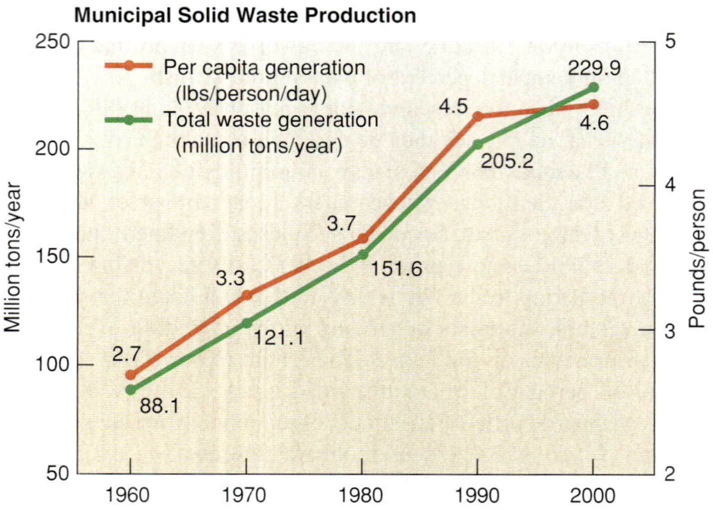

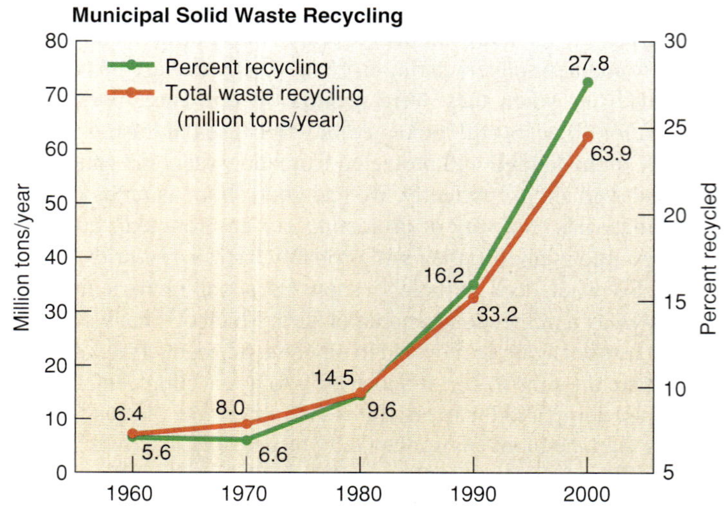

FIGURE 13.1 *Bad news and good news in U. S. solid waste production. Per capita waste has risen steadily to more than 2 kg per person per day. Recycling rates are also rising, however.*
Source: Data from Environmental Protection Agency, 2001.

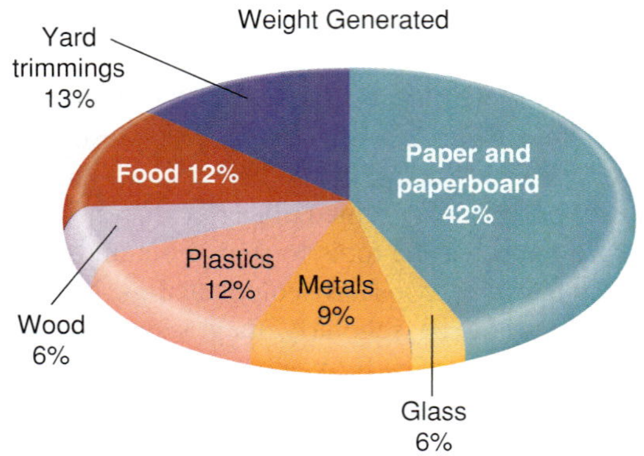

FIGURE 13.2 *Municipal solid waste composition in the United States by weight before recycling.*
Source: Data from Environmental Protection Agency Office of Solid Waste Management, 2000.

The Waste Stream

Does it surprise you to learn that you generate that much garbage? Think for a moment about how much we discard every year. There are organic materials, such as yard and garden wastes, food wastes, and sewage sludge from treatment plants; junked cars; worn-out furniture; and consumer products of all types. Newspapers, magazines, advertisements, and office refuse make paper one of our major wastes (fig. 13.2). In spite of recent progress in recycling, many of the 200 billion metal, glass, and plastic food and beverage containers used every year in the United States end up in the trash. Although plastic makes up only about 10 percent of our waste by weight, it comprises about 20 percent by volume. Wood, concrete, bricks, and glass come from construction and demolition sites, dust and rubble from landscaping and road building. All of this varied and voluminous waste has to arrive at a final resting place somewhere.

The **waste stream** is a term that describes the steady flow of varied wastes that we all produce, from domestic garbage and yard wastes to industrial, commercial, and construction refuse. Many of the materials in our waste stream would be valuable resources if they were not mixed with other garbage. Unfortunately, our collecting and dumping processes mix and crush everything together, making separation an expensive and sometimes impossible task. In a dump or incinerator, much of the value of recyclable materials is lost.

Another problem with refuse mixing is that hazardous materials in the waste stream get dispersed through thousands of tons of miscellaneous garbage. This mixing makes the disposal or burning of what might have been rather innocuous stuff a difficult, expensive, and risky business. Spray-paint cans, pesticides, batteries (zinc, lead, or mercury), cleaning solvents, smoke detectors containing radioactive material, and plastics that produce dioxins and PCBs (polychlorinated biphenyls) when burned are mixed willy-nilly with paper, table scraps, and other nontoxic materials. The best thing to do with household toxic and hazardous materials is to separate them for safe disposal or recycling, as we will see later in this chapter.

WASTE DISPOSAL METHODS

Where do our wastes go now? In this section, we will examine some historic methods of waste disposal, as well as some future options. Notice that our presentation begins with the least desirable—but most commonly used—measures and proceeds to discuss some preferable options. Keep in mind as you read this that modern waste management reverses this order and stresses the "three Rs" of reduction, reuse, and recycling before destruction or, finally, secure storage of wastes.

Open Dumps

Often, the way people dispose of waste is to simply drop it someplace. Open, unregulated dumps are still the predominant method of waste disposal in most developing countries. The giant Third World megacities have enormous garbage problems. Mexico City, the largest city in the world, generates some 10,000 tons of trash each day. Until recently, most of this torrent of waste was left in giant piles, exposed to the wind and rain, as well as rats, flies, and other vermin. Manila, in the Philippines, has at least ten huge open dumps. The most notorious is called "Smoky Mountain" because of its constant smoldering fires (fig. 13.3). Thousands of people live and work on this 30-m-high heap of refuse. They spend their days sorting through the garbage for edible or recyclable materials. Health conditions are abysmal, but these people have nowhere else to go. The government would like to close these dumps, but how will the residents be housed and fed? Where else will the city put its garbage?

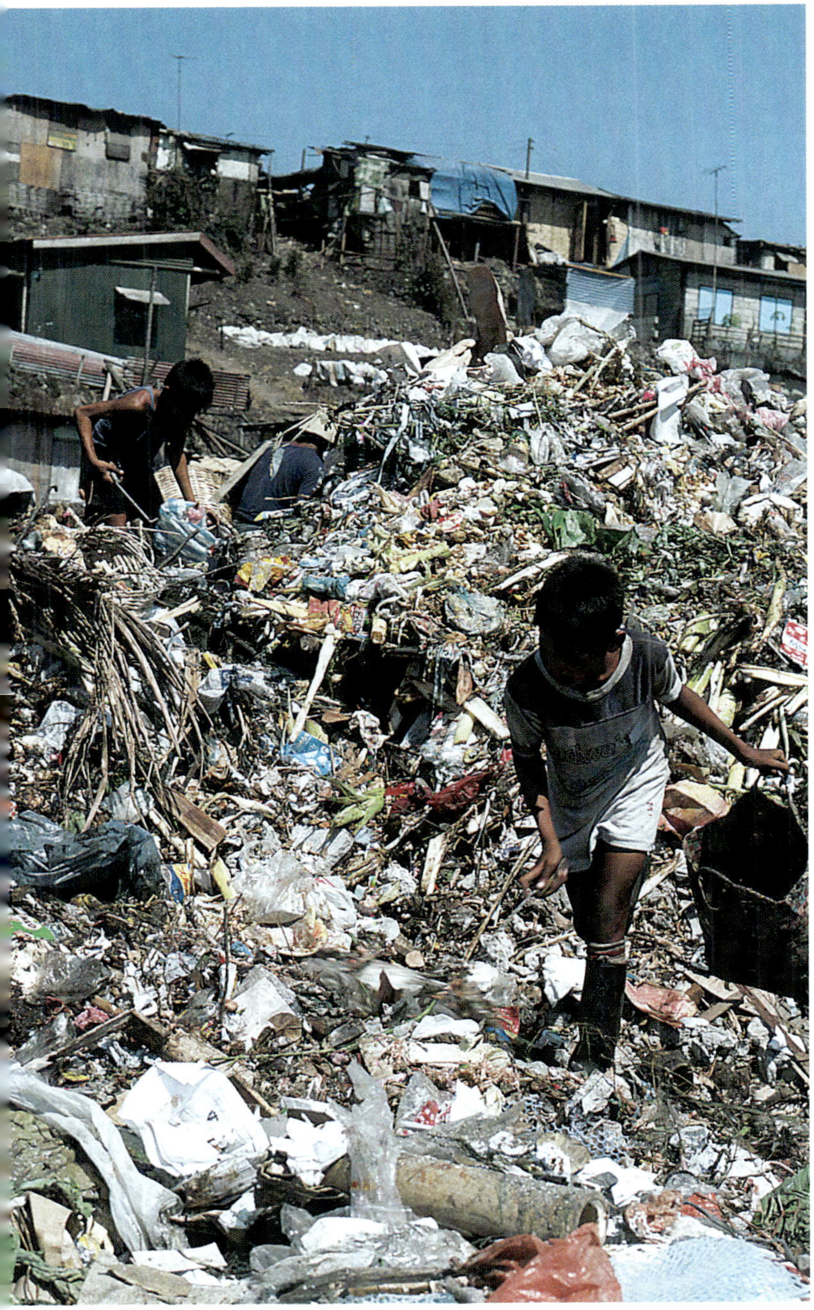

FIGURE 13.3 *Scavengers sort through the trash at "Smoky Mountain," one of the huge metropolitan dumps in Manila, Philippines. Some 20,000 people live and work on these enormous garbage dumps. The health effects are tragic.*

Most developed countries forbid open dumping at least in metropolitan areas, but illegal dumping is still a problem. You have undoubtedly seen trash accumulating along roadsides and in vacant, weedy lots in the poorer sections of cities. Is this just a question of aesthetics? Consider the problem of waste oil and solvents. An estimated 200 million liters of waste motor oil are poured into the sewers or allowed to soak into the ground every year in the United States. This is about five times as much as was spilled by the *Exxon Valdez* in Alaska in 1989! No one knows the volume of solvents and other chemicals disposed of by similar methods.

Increasingly, these toxic chemicals are showing up in the groundwater supplies on which nearly half the people in America depend for drinking (see chapter 10). An alarmingly small amount of oil or other solvents can pollute large quantities of drinking or irrigation water. One liter of gasoline, for instance, can make a million liters of water undrinkable. The problem of illegal dumping is likely to become worse as acceptable sites for waste disposal become more scarce and costs for legal dumping escalate. We clearly need better enforcement of antilittering laws, as well as a change in our attitudes and behavior.

Ocean Dumping

The oceans are vast, but not so large that we can continue to treat them as carelessly as has been our habit. Every year some 25,000 metric tons (55 million lbs) of packaging, including half a million bottles, cans, and plastic containers, are dumped at sea. Beaches, even in remote regions, are littered with the nondegradable flotsam and jetsam of industrial society (fig. 13.4). About 150,000 tons (330 million lbs) of fishing gear—including more than 1,000 km (660 mi) of nets—are lost or discarded at sea each year. Environmental groups estimate that 50,000 northern fur seals are entangled in this refuse and drown or starve to death every year in the North Pacific alone.

Until recently, many cities in the United States dumped municipal refuse, industrial waste, sewage, and sewage sludge into the ocean. Federal legislation now prohibits this dumping. New York City, the last to stop offshore sewage sludge disposal, finally ended this practice in 1992. Still, 60 million to 80 million m^3 of dredge spoil—much of it highly contaminated—are disposed of at sea. Some people claim that the deep abyssal ocean plain is the most remote, stable, and innocuous place to dump our wastes. Others argue that we know too little about the values of these remote places or the rare species that live there to smother them with sludge and debris.

Landfills

Over the past 50 years, most American and European cities have recognized the health and environmental hazards of open dumps. Increasingly, cities have turned to **sanitary landfills,** where solid waste disposal is regulated and controlled. To decrease smells and

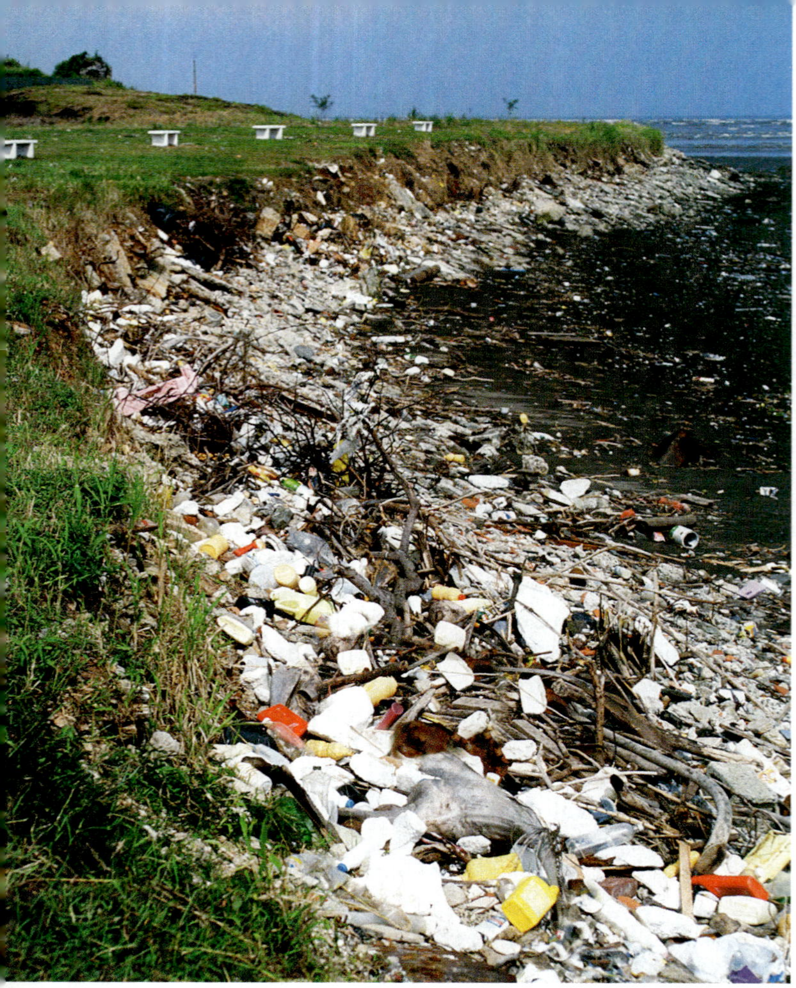

FIGURE 13.4 *Dumping of trash at sea is a global problem. Even on the most remote islands, beaches are covered with plastic flotsam and jetsam.*

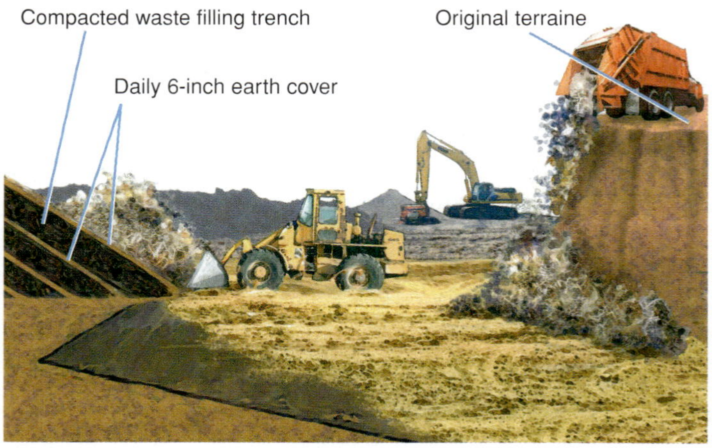

FIGURE 13.5 *In a sanitary landfill, trash and garbage are crushed and covered each day to prevent accumulation of vermin and spread of disease. A waterproof lining is now required to prevent leaching of chemicals into underground aquifers.*

litter and to discourage insect and rodent populations, landfill operators are required to compact the refuse and cover it every day with a layer of dirt (fig. 13.5). This method helps control pollution, but the dirt fill also takes up as much as 20 percent of landfill space. Since 1994, all operating landfills in the United States have been required to control such hazardous substances as oil, chemical compounds, toxic metals, and contaminated rainwater that seep through piles of waste. An impermeable clay and/or plastic lining underlies and encloses the storage area. Drainage systems are installed in and around the liner to catch drainage and to help monitor chemicals that may be leaking. Modern municipal solid waste landfills now have many of the safeguards of hazardous waste repositories described later in this chapter.

More careful attention is now paid to the siting of new landfills. Sites located on highly permeable or faulted rock formations are passed over in favor of sites with less leaky geologic foundations. Landfills are being built away from rivers, lakes, floodplains, and aquifer recharge zones, rather than near them, as was often done in the past. More care is being given to a landfill's long-term effects, so that costly cleanups and rehabilitation can be avoided.

APPLICATION: How Much Waste Do You Create?

Collect all the dry trash (excluding food waste) that you discard in a typical day or week. Sort it into major categories: packaging material, junk mail, etc., as well as material type: paper, cardboard, glass, metal, plastic.

1. What is the total weight and volume of your trash?
2. Which categories and materials make up the largest amount?
3. How much of what you discard could be reused or recycled?
4. Are there ways that you could reduce your trash generation?

Historically, landfills have been a convenient and relatively inexpensive waste-disposal option in most places, but this situation is changing rapidly. Rising land prices and shipping costs, as well as increasingly demanding landfill construction and maintenance requirements, are making this a more expensive disposal method. The cost of disposing of a ton of solid waste in Philadelphia went from $20 in 1980 to more than $100 in 1990. Union County, New York, experienced an even steeper price rise. In 1987, it paid $70 to get rid of a ton of waste; a year later, the same ton cost $420, or about $10 for a typical garbage bag. The United States now spends about $10 billion per year to dispose of trash. A decade from now, it may cost us $100 billion per year to dispose of our trash and garbage.

Currently, 55 percent of all municipal solid waste in the United States is landfilled, 30 percent is recycled, and 15 percent is incinerated. Suitable places for waste disposal are becoming scarce in many areas. Other uses compete for open space. Citizens have become more concerned and vocal about health hazards, as well as aesthetics. It is difficult to find a neighborhood or community willing to accept a new landfill. Since 1984, when stricter financial and environmental protection requirements for landfills took effect, about three-quarters of all existing landfills in the United States have closed. In many cases, this means that old, small, uneconomical landfills closed, while larger, more modern ones took over. Nevertheless, many major cities are running out of local landfill space. They export their trash, at enormous expense, to neighboring communities and even other states. More than half the solid waste from New Jersey goes out of state, some of it up to 800 km (500 mi) away.

Exporting Waste

Although most industrialized nations in the world have agreed to stop shipping hazardous and toxic waste to less-developed countries, the practice still continues. In 1999, for example, 3,000 tons of incinerator waste from a plastics factory in Taiwan were unloaded from a ship in the middle of the night and dumped in a field near the small coastal Cambodian village of Bet Trang. The village residents thought they had been blessed with a windfall. They emptied out chunks of crumbling residue so they could use the white, plastic shipping bags as bedding and roofing material. They rinsed out bags to use for rice storage, and they ripped them open with their teeth to get string to use as clotheslines and lashing for their oxcarts. Children played happily on the big pile of dusty, white material.

In the following weeks, unfortunately, the villagers discovered that, rather than a treasure, they had a calamity. The first sign of trouble was when one of the dock workers who unloaded the waste died and five others were hospitalized with symptoms of nerve damage and respiratory distress. Villagers also began to complain of a variety of illnesses. The village was evacuated, and about 1,000 residents of the nearby city of Sihanoukville fled in panic. Subsequent analysis found high levels of mercury and other toxic metals in the residue. The Formosa Plastics Corporation, which shipped the waste, admitted paying a $3 million bribe to Cambodian officials to permit its dumping. They said they couldn't dispose of the waste in Taiwan because of a threat of public protest. Following an international uproar, the plastics company agreed to go back and pick up the waste. But the villagers who handled the toxic wastes face an uncertain future. Is it safe to reinhabit their homes? Is it wise to have children? Will they suffer long-term health effects from exposure to this material? (See related story "The Voyage of the Khian Sea" at www.mhhe.com/cases.) The United Nations' "Basel Convention," signed by 148 countries in 1989, prohibits transboundary shipping of hazardous wastes. Still, "toxic traders" find loopholes and illegal avenues to continue this business.

As we will discuss later in this chapter, "garbage imperialism" also operates within richer countries as well. Poor neighborhoods and minority populations are much more likely than richer ones to be the recipients of dumps, waste incinerators, and other locally unwanted land uses (LULUs). In recent years, attention has turned, in the United States, to Indian reservations, which are exempt from some state and federal regulations concerning waste disposal. Virtually every tribe in America has been approached with schemes to store wastes on their reservation (see Investigating Our Environment p. 312).

Another method of disposing of toxic wastes is to "recycle" them as asphalt or concrete filler for building highways. This is considered a beneficial use, but what happens to the toxins as the roadway is slowly worn away by traffic? Similar waste products are "land farmed," or sold as fertilizer and soil amendments. There are no safety standards for fertilizer composition because it's not intended for human consumption, but much of it is used on crops that humans will eat or that will be fed to livestock that are part of our food chain. For example, Florida has about a billion cubic meters of phosphogypsum, a waste product of phosphate mining, that producers want to market as a soil amendment. While it's true that phosphate is an essential plant nutrient, this particular product is also radioactive. In another case in Oregon, metal-rich dust and ash from steel mills is classified as hazardous waste when it leaves the mill. After being mixed with other minerals, however, it becomes fertilizer that will be spread on farm fields. Manufacturers are required to report the "active" ingredient—such things as nitrogen, phosphorus, and phosphate—content of their product, but much can go unreported as "inert" matter.

Incineration and Resource Recovery

Landfilling is still the disposal method for the majority of municipal waste in the United States. Faced with growing piles of garbage and a lack of available landfills at any price, however, public officials are investigating other disposal methods. The method to which they frequently turn is burning. Another term commonly used for this technology is **energy recovery,** or waste-to-energy, because the heat derived from incinerated refuse is a useful resource. Burning garbage can produce steam used directly for heating buildings or generating electricity. Internationally, well over 1,000 waste-to-energy plants in Brazil, Japan, and Western Europe generate much-needed energy while reducing the amount that needs to be landfilled. In the United States more than 110 waste incinerators burn 45,000 metric tons of garbage daily. Some of these are simple incinerators; others produce steam and/or electricity.

Types of Incinerators

Municipal incinerators are specially designed burning plants capable of burning thousands of tons of waste per day. In some plants, refuse is sorted as it comes in to remove unburnable or recyclable materials before combustion. This is called **refuse-derived fuel** because the enriched burnable fraction has a higher energy content than the raw trash. Another approach, called **mass burn,** is to dump everything smaller than sofas and refrigerators into a giant furnace and burn as much as possible (fig. 13.6). This technique avoids the expensive and unpleasant job of sorting through the garbage for nonburnable materials, but it often causes greater problems with air pollution and corrosion of burner grates and chimneys.

INVESTIGATING Our Environment

Environmental Justice

When a new landfill, petrochemical factory, incinerator, or other unwanted industrial facility is proposed for a minority neighborhood, charges of environmental racism often are raised by those who oppose this siting. Everyday experiences tell us that minority neighborhoods are much more likely to have high pollution levels and facilities that you wouldn't want to live near than are middle- or upper-class white neighborhoods. But does this prove that land-use decisions are racist or just that minorities are less politically powerful than middle- or upper-class residents? Could it be that land prices are simply cheaper and public resistance to locating a polluting facility in a place that's already polluted is less than putting it in a cleaner environment? Or does this distinction matter? Perhaps showing that a disproportionate number of minorities live in dirtier places is evidence enough of racism. How would you decide?

One of the first systematic studies showing this inequitable distribution of environmental hazards based on race in the United States was conducted by Robert D. Bullard in 1978. Asked for help by a predominantly black community in Houston that was slated for a waste incinerator, Bullard discovered that all five of the city's existing landfills and six of eight incinerators were located in African-American neighborhoods. In a book entitled *Dumping on Dixie,* Bullard showed that this pattern of risk exposure in minority communities is common throughout the United States. Among his findings are:

- Three of the five largest commercial hazardous waste landfills, accounting for about 40 percent of all hazardous waste disposal in the United States, are located in predominantly African-American or Hispanic communities.
- Sixty percent of African Americans and Latinos and nearly half of all Asians, Pacific Islanders, and Native Americans live in communities with uncontrolled toxic waste sites.
- The average percentage of the population made up by minorities in communities without a hazardous waste facility is 12 percent. By contrast, communities with one hazardous waste facility have, on average, twice as high (24 percent) a minority population, while those with two or more such facilities average three times as high a minority population (38 percent) as those without one.

But does this prove that race, not class or income, is the strongest determinant of who is exposed to environmental hazards? What additional information might you look for to make this distinction? One of the lines of evidence Dr. Bullard raises is the fact that the discrepancy between the pollution exposure of middle-class blacks and that of middle-class whites is even greater than the difference between poorer whites and blacks. While upper-class whites can "vote with their feet" and move out of polluted and dangerous neighborhoods, Bullard argues, minorities are restricted by color barriers and prejudice to less desirable locations.

Some additional evidence uncovered by this research is variation in the way toxic waste sites are cleaned up and how polluters are punished in different neighborhoods. White communities see faster responses and get better results once toxic wastes are discovered than do minority communities. For instance, the EPA takes 20 percent longer to place a hazardous waste site in a minority community on the Superfund National Priority List than it does for one in a white community. Penalties assessed against polluters of white communities average six times higher than those against polluters of minority communities. Cleanup is more thorough in white communities as well. Most toxic wastes in white communities are treated—that is, removed or destroyed. By contrast, waste sites in minority neighborhoods are generally only "contained" by putting a cap over them, leaving contaminants in place to potentially resurface or leak into groundwater at a later date.

How would you evaluate these findings? Do they convince you that racism is at work, or do you think that other explanations might be equally likely? Which of these arguments do you find most persuasive, or what other evidence would you need to make a reasoned judgment about whether or not environmental racism is a factor in determining who gets exposed to pollution and who enjoys a cleaner, more pleasant environment?

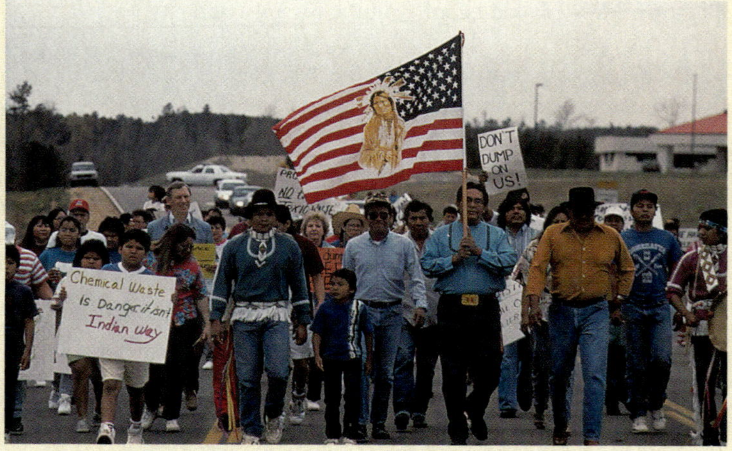
DON'T DUMP ON US!
Chemical Waste is Dangr it isn't Indian Way

Native Americans march in protest of toxic waste dumping on tribal lands.

In either case, residual ash and unburnable residues representing 10 to 20 percent of the original volume are usually taken to a landfill for disposal. Because the volume of burned garbage is reduced by 80 to 90 percent, disposal is a smaller task. However, the residual ash usually contains a variety of toxic components that make it an environmental hazard if not disposed of properly. Ironically, one worry about incinerators is whether enough garbage will be available to feed them. Some communities in which recycling has been really successful have had to buy garbage from neighbors to meet contractual obligations to waste-to-energy facilities. In other places, fears that this might happen have discouraged recycling efforts.

Incinerator Cost and Safety

The cost-effectiveness of garbage incinerators is the subject of heated debates. Initial construction costs are high—usually between $100 million and $300 million for a typical municipal

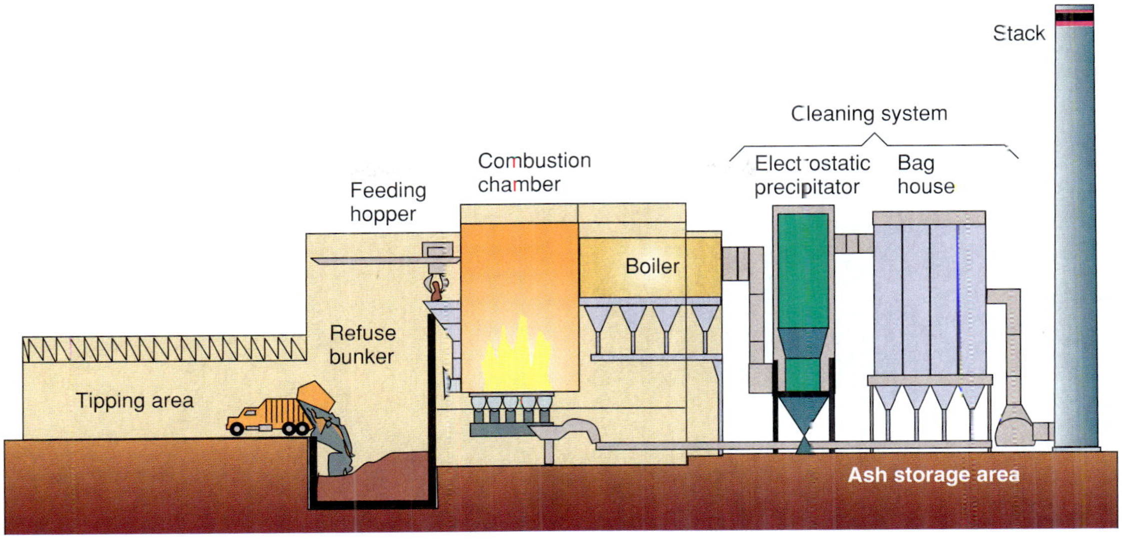

FIGURE 13.6 *A municipal mass burn garbage incinerator. Steam produced in the boiler can be used to generate electricity or to heat nearby buildings.*

facility. Tipping fees at an incinerator (the fee charged to haulers for each ton of garbage dumped) are often much higher than those at a landfill. As landfill space near metropolitan areas becomes more scarce and more expensive, however, landfill rates are certain to rise. It may pay in the long run to incinerate refuse so that the lifetime of existing landfills will be extended.

Environmental safety of incinerators is another point of concern. The EPA has found alarmingly high levels of dioxins, furans, lead, and cadmium in incinerator ash. These toxic materials are more concentrated in the fly ash (lighter, airborne particles capable of penetrating deep into the lungs) than in heavy bottom ash. Dioxin levels can be as high as 780 ppb (parts per billion). One part per billion of TCDD, the most toxic dioxin, is considered a health concern. All of the incinerators studied exceeded cadmium standards, and 80 percent exceeded lead standards. Proponents of incineration argue that, if they are run properly and equipped with appropriate pollution-control devices, incinerators are safe for the general public. Opponents counter that neither public officials nor pollution-control equipment can be trusted to keep the air clean. They argue that recycling and source reduction efforts are better ways to deal with waste problems.

The EPA, which generally supports incineration, acknowledges the health threat of incinerator emissions but holds that the danger is very slight. The EPA estimates that dioxin emissions from a typical municipal incinerator may cause one death per million people in 70 years of operation. Critics of incineration claim that a more accurate estimate is 250 deaths per million in 70 years.

One way to reduce these dangerous emissions is to remove batteries containing heavy metals and plastics containing chlorine before wastes are burned. Bremen, Germany, is one of several European cities now trying to control dioxin emissions by keeping all plastics out of incinerator waste. Bremen is requiring households to separate plastics from other garbage. This is expected to eliminate nearly all dioxins and other combustion by-products and prevent the expense of installing costly pollution-control equipment that otherwise would be necessary to keep the burners operating. Minneapolis has initiated a recycling program for the small "button" batteries used in hearing aids, watches, and calculators in an attempt to lower mercury emissions from its incinerator.

SHRINKING THE WASTE STREAM

Having less waste to discard is obviously better than struggling with disposal methods, all of which have disadvantages and drawbacks. In this section we will explore some of our options for recycling, reuse, and reduction of the wastes we produce.

Recycling

The term *recycling* has two meanings in common usage. Sometimes we say we are recycling when we really are reusing something, such as refillable beverage containers. In terms of solid waste management, however, **recycling** is the reprocessing of discarded materials into new, useful products (fig. 13.7). Some recycling processes reuse materials for the same purposes; for instance, old aluminum cans and glass bottles are usually melted and recast into new cans and bottles. Other recycling processes turn old materials into entirely new products. Old tires, for instance, are shredded and turned into rubberized road surfacing. Newspapers become cellulose insulation, kitchen wastes become a valuable soil amendment, and steel cans become new automobiles and construction materials.

There have been some dramatic successes in recycling in recent years. New Jersey, for instance, now claims a 60 percent recycling rate, something thought unattainable a decade ago. The high value of aluminum scrap (as much as $1,200 per ton in recent years) has spurred a large percentage of aluminum recycling nearly everywhere. About two-thirds of all aluminum cans are

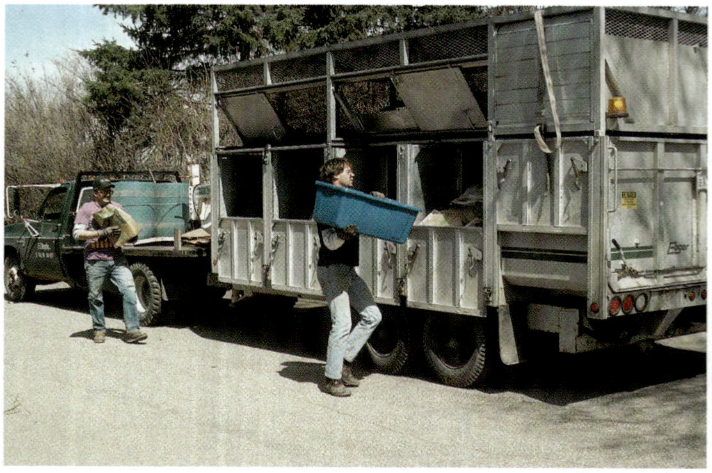

FIGURE 13.7 *Trucks with multiple compartments pick up residential recyclables at curbside, greatly reducing the amount of waste that needs to be buried or burned.*

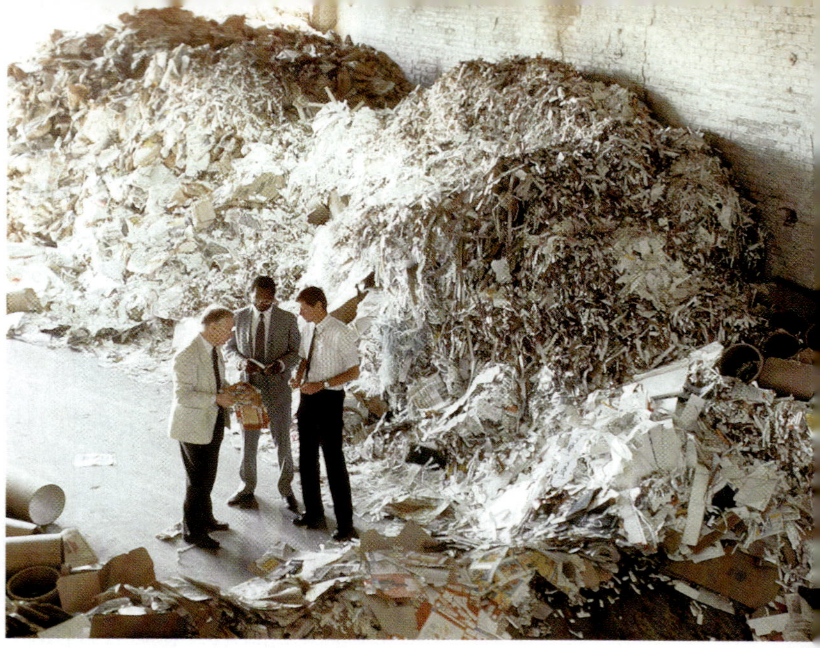

FIGURE 13.8 *Creating a stable, economically viable market for recycled products often is harder than collecting materials.*

now recycled, up from only 15 percent 20 years ago. This recycling is so rapid that half of all the aluminum cans now on grocery shelves will be made into another can within two months.

Recycling Challenges

Despite encouraging gains in recycling rates, major challenges exist. Despite the value of aluminum, Americans still throw away nearly 350,000 metric tons of aluminum beverage containers each year. That is enough to make 3,800 Boeing 747 airplanes. Plastics recyclers have developed innovative methods and products, but the low price of virgin plastic, made from oil, is usually less than the cost of transporting and storing used plastics. Consequently, less than 5 percent of the United States' 24 million tons of plastic waste is recycled each year.

Wild fluctuations in commodity prices make it still harder to develop a market for recycled materials. Newsprint, for example, cost $160 a ton in 1995; by 1999 it dropped to just $42 per ton (fig. 13.8).

Contamination is a major obstacle in plastics recycling. Most of the 24 billion plastic soft drink bottles sold every year in the United States are made of PET (polyethylene terphthalate), which can be remanufactured into carpet, fleece clothing, plastic strapping, and nonfood packaging. However, even a trace of vinyl—a single PVC (polyvinyl chloride) bottle in a truckload, for example—can make PET useless. Although most bottles are now marked with a recycling number, it's hard for consumers to remember which is which. Because single-use beverage containers are so costly to recycle, they have been outlawed in Denmark and Finland. A looming worry is the prospect of single-use plastic beer bottles. Already being test-marketed, these bottles are made of PET but are amber colored to block sunlight and have a special chemical coating to keep out oxygen, which would ruin the beer. The special color, interior coating, and vinyl cap lining will make these bottles incompatible with regular PET, and it will probably cost more to remove them from the waste stream than the reclaimed plastic is worth. Plastic recycling already is down 50 percent from a decade ago because so many soft drink bottles are sold and consumed on the go, and never make it into recycling bins. Throw-away beer bottles could badly set back recycling programs.

Benefits of Recycling

Recycling is usually a better alternative to either dumping or burning wastes. It saves money, energy, raw materials, and land space, while also reducing pollution. Recycling also encourages individual awareness and responsibility for the refuse produced (fig. 13.9). Curbside pickup of recyclables costs around $35 per ton, as opposed to the $80 paid to dispose of them at an average metropolitan landfill. Many recycling programs cover their own expenses with materials sales and may even bring revenue to the community.

Recycling drastically reduces pressure on landfills and incinerators. Philadelphia is investing in neighborhood collection centers that will recycle 600 tons a day, enough to eliminate the need for a previously planned, high-priced incinerator. New York City, down to one available landfill but still producing 27,000 tons of garbage a day, set a target of 50 percent waste reduction to be accomplished by recycling office paper and household and commercial waste. In 2002 Mayor Michael Bloomberg discontinued most recycling, arguing that the program was too expensive. The city quickly found that disposing of waste was more expensive than recycling, and most programs were reinstated.

Japan probably has the most successful recycling program in the world. Half of all household and commercial wastes in Japan are recycled, while the rest are about equally incinerated or landfilled. Japan has also instituted a new law requiring that restaurants and food producers and distributors recycle at least 20 percent of food waste by 2006.

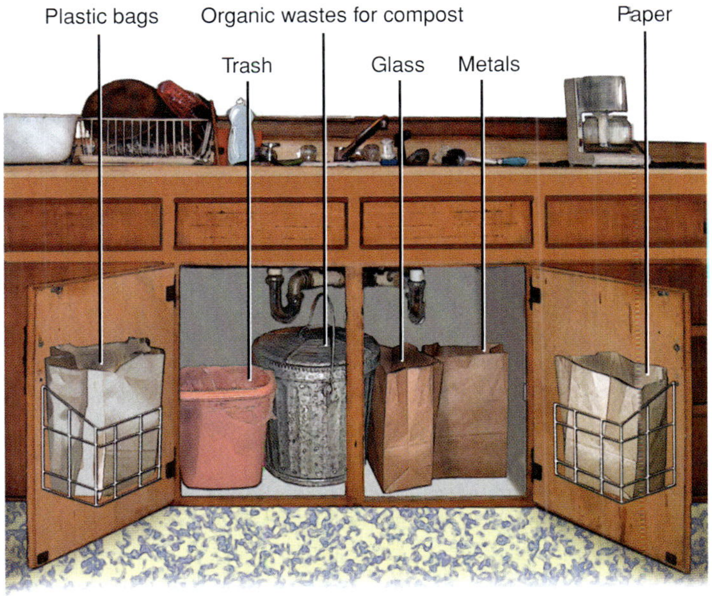

FIGURE 13.9 *Source separation in the kitchen—the first step in a strong recycling program.*

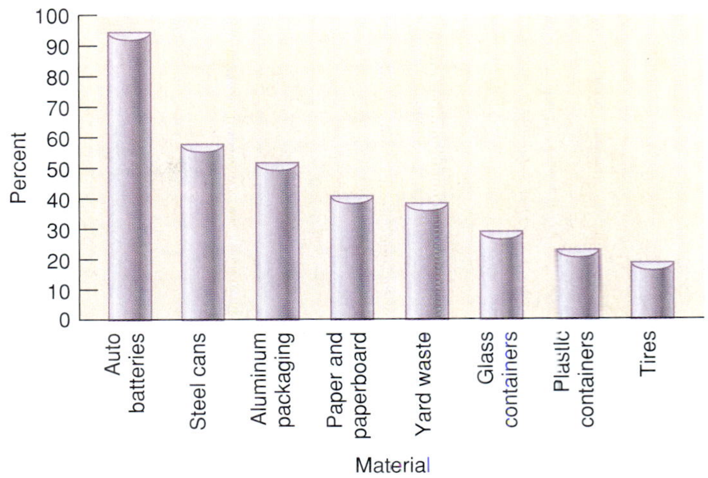

FIGURE 13.10 *Recycling rates of selected materials in the United States.*
Source: Data from Environmental Protection Agency, 2003.

Recycling lowers our demands for raw resources (fig. 13.10). In the United States we cut down 2 million trees every day to produce newsprint and paper products, a heavy drain on our forests. Recycling the print run of a single Sunday issue of the *New York Times* would spare 75,000 trees. Every piece of plastic we make reduces the reserve supply of petroleum and makes us more dependent on foreign oil. Recycling 1 ton of aluminum saves 4 tons of bauxite (aluminum ore) and 700 kg of petroleum coke and pitch, as well as keeping 35 kg of aluminum fluoride out of the air.

Recycling also reduces energy consumption and air pollution. Plastic bottle recycling could save 50 to 60 percent of the energy needed to make new ones. Making new steel from old scrap offers up to 75 percent energy savings. Producing aluminum from scrap instead of bauxite ore cuts energy use by 95 percent, yet we still throw away more than a million tons of aluminum every year. If aluminum recovery were doubled worldwide, more than a million tons of air pollutants would be eliminated every year.

Reducing litter is an important benefit of recycling. Ever since disposable paper, glass, metal, foam, and plastic packaging began to accompany nearly everything we buy, these discarded wrappings have collected on our roadsides and in our lakes, rivers, and oceans. Litter is a costly as well as unsightly problem. We pay an estimated 32¢ for each piece of litter picked up by crews along state highways, which adds up to $500 million every year. "Bottle bills" requiring deposits on bottles and cans have reduced littering in many states.

Creating Incentives for Recycling

In many communities, citizens have done such a good job of collecting recyclables that a glut has developed. In some cities, mountains of some waste materials accumulate in warehouses because there are no markets for them. Too often, wastes that we carefully separate for recycling end up being mixed together and dumped in a landfill or incinerator.

Our present public policies often tend to favor extraction of new raw materials. Energy, water, and raw materials are often sold to industries below their real cost to create jobs and stimulate the economy. For instance, in 1999 a pound of recycled clear PET, the material in most soft-drink bottles, sold for about 40¢. By contrast, a pound of off-grade, virgin PET cost 25¢. Setting the prices of natural resources at their real cost would tend to encourage efficiency and recycling. State, local, and national statutes requiring government agencies to purchase a minimum amount of recycled material have helped create a market for used materials. Each of us can play a role in creating markets as well. If we buy things made from recycled materials—or ask for them if they aren't available—we will help recycling programs succeed.

Composting

Pressed for landfill space, many cities have banned yard waste from municipal garbage. Rather than bury this valuable organic material, they are turning it into a useful product through **composting:** biological degradation or breakdown of organic matter under aerobic (oxygen-rich) conditions. The organic compost resulting from this process makes a nutrient-rich soil amendment that aids water retention, slows soil erosion, and improves crop yields. A home compost pile is an easy and inexpensive way to dispose of organic waste in an interesting and environmentally friendly way. All you need to do is to pile up lawn clippings, vegetable waste, fallen leaves, wood chips, or other organic matter in an out-of-the way place keep it moist, and turn it over every week or so (fig. 13.11). Within a few months, naturally occurring microorganisms will decompose the organic material into a rich, pleasant-smelling compost that you can use as a soil amendment.

Some cities and counties have developed successful composting programs. Residents pay a small amount to drop off yard waste, and they can buy back rich, inexpensive fertilizer.

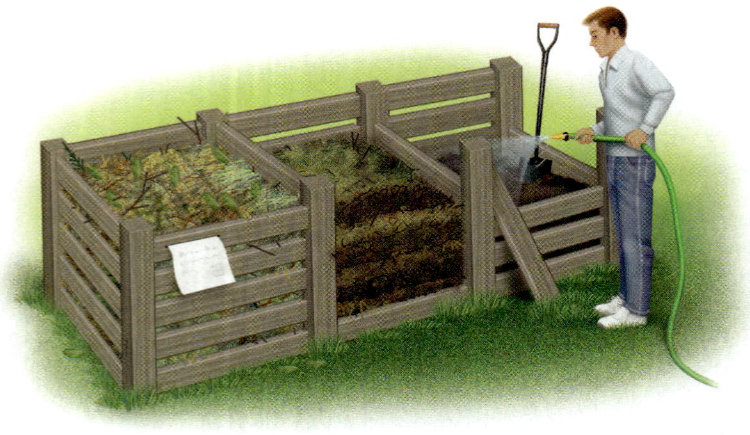

FIGURE 13.11 *Composting is a good way to convert yard waste, vegetable scraps, and other organic materials into useful garden mulch. Mix everything together, keep it moist and well aerated, and in a few weeks, you will have a rich, odor-free mulch. This three-bin system allows you to have batches in different stages.*

Energy from Waste

Every year we throw away the energy equivalent of 80 million barrels of oil in organic waste in the United States. In developing countries up to 85 percent of the waste stream is food, textiles, vegetable matter, and other biodegradable materials. Worldwide, at least one-fifth of municipal waste is organic kitchen and garden refuse. In a landfill, much of this matter is decomposed by microorganisms generating billions of cubic meters of methane ("natural gas"), which contributes to global warming if allowed to escape into the atmosphere (see chapter 9). Many cities are drilling methane wells in their landfills to capture this valuable resource. Fuel cells are a good way to use this methane (see chapter 12).

This valuable organic material can be burned in an incinerator rather than buried in landfills, but there are worries about air pollution from incineration. Organic wastes also can be decomposed in large, oxygen-free digesters to produce methane under more controlled conditions than in a landfill and with less air pollution than mass garbage burning.

Anaerobic digestion also can be done on a small scale. Millions of household methane generators provide fuel for cooking and lighting for homes in China and India (see chapter 12). In the United States some farmers produce all the fuel they need to run their farms—both for heating and for running trucks and tractors—by generating methane from animal manure.

Demanufacturing

Demanufacturing is the disassembly and recycling of obsolete consumer products, such as television sets, computers, telephones, refrigerators, washing machines, and air conditioners. There are at least two billion televisions and personal computers in use globally. Televisions often are discarded after only about five years, and computers, play-stations, cellular telepones, and other electronics become obsolete even faster. Stoves, refrigerators, and other "white goods" have a much longer lifetime—typically about 12 years—but the EPA estimates that Americans dispose of 54 million of these household appliances every year. Many of these consumer products contain both valuable materials and toxins that must be kept out of the environment. Older refrigerators and air conditioners, for example, have chloroflurocarbons (CFCs) that destroy stratospheric ozone and cannot be released into the air. Because new production has been banned, recycled CFCs are worth about $100 per pound. For both reasons, it pays to recycle them.

Computers and other electronic equipment contain both toxic metals (mercury, lead, gallium, germanium, nickel, palladium, beryllium, selenium, arsenic) and valuable scrap, such as gold, silver, copper, and steel. The United States now discards 50 million computers per year, or one per person every three and a half years. It's estimated that 90 percent of the cadmium, lead, and mercury contamination in our solid waste stream comes from consumer electronics.

Unfortunately, the cheapest way to demanufacture used electronics is often to ship them to developing countries. The majority of electronic products collected in the United States goes to China, where poor villages, including young children, break them apart to retrieve copper, silver, gold, lead, and other metals. Effects on workers handling toxic materials may be severe, especially for growing children. Soil, groundwater, and surface water contamination at these sites has been found to be as much as 200 times the World Health Organization's standards. An estimated 100,000 workers demanufacture electronics in southeastern China alone (fig. 13.12).

In response to such problems, the European Union now requires that recycling fees be built into the purchase price of many electronics. This adds about $20 to the purchase price, less than 1 percent for many computers. Increasingly, local governments are requiring electronics recycling. Massachusetts is the first state to require that both households and businesses recycle used computer parts. Recycling companies in the United States are beginning to develop comprehensive electronics recycling systems, and these offer growing alternatives to shipping our hazardous waste overseas.

Reuse

Even better than recycling or composting is cleaning and reusing materials in their present form, thus saving the cost and energy of remaking them into something else. We do this already with some specialized items. Auto parts are regularly sold from junkyards, especially for older car models. In some areas stained-glass windows, brass fittings, fine woodwork, and bricks salvaged from old houses bring high prices. Some communities sort and reuse a variety of materials received in their dumps (fig. 13.13).

In many cities, glass and plastic bottles are routinely returned to beverage producers for washing and refilling. The reusable, refillable bottle is the most efficient beverage container we have. It is better for the environment than remelting and more profitable for local communities. A reusable glass container makes an average of 15 round-trips between factory and customer before

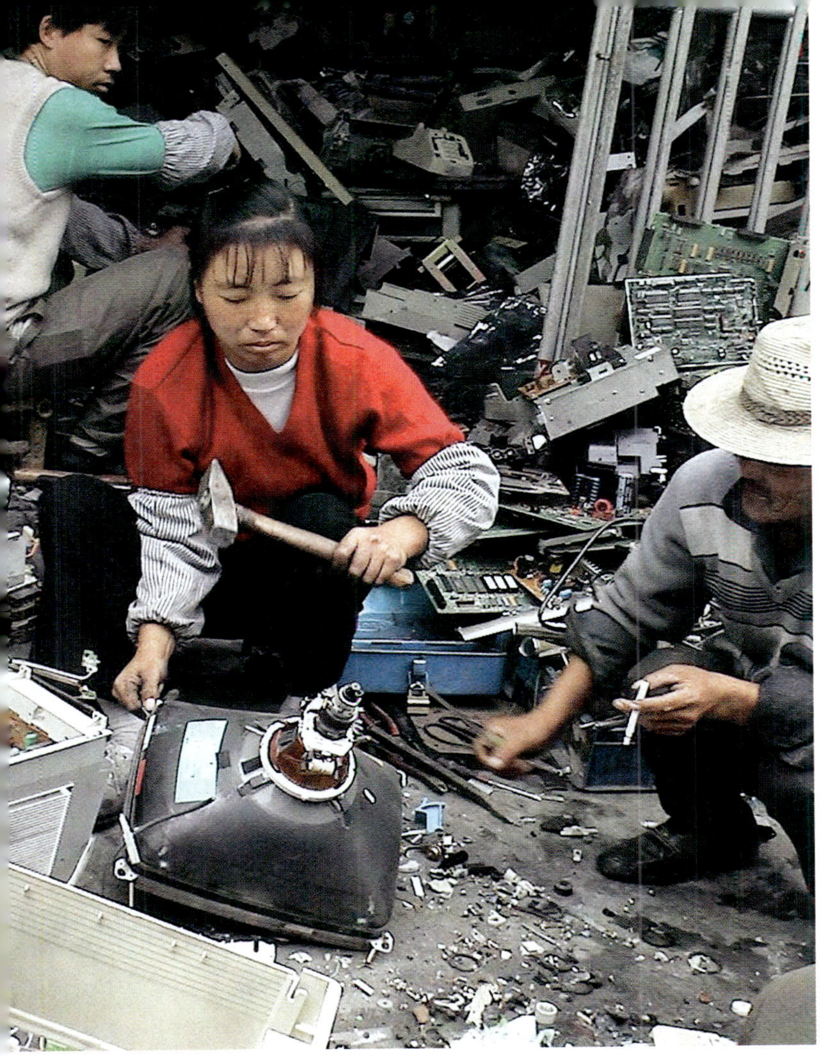

FIGURE 13.12 *A Chinese woman smashes a cathode ray tube from a computer monitor in order to remove valuable metals. This kind of unprotected demanufacturing is highly hazardous to both workers and the environment.*

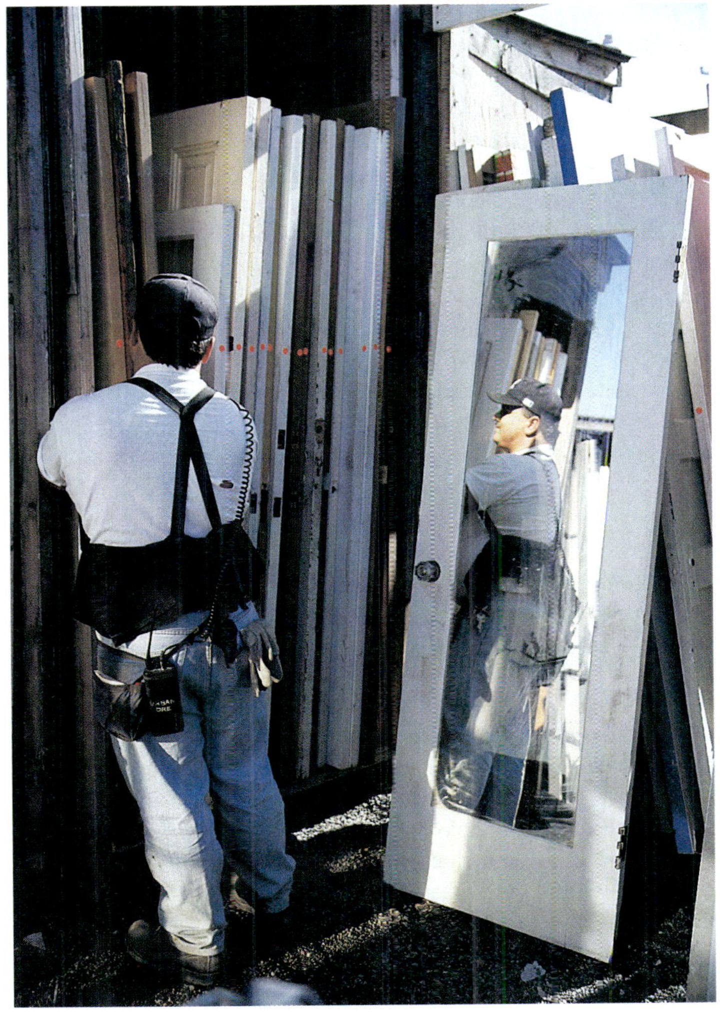

FIGURE 13.13 *Reusing discarded products is a creative and efficient way to reduce wastes. This recycling center in Berkeley, California, is a valuable source of used building supplies and a money saver for the whole community.*

it becomes so scratched and chipped that it has to be recycled. Reusable containers also favor local bottling companies and help preserve regional differences.

Since the advent of cheap, lightweight, disposable food and beverage containers, many small, local breweries, canneries, and bottling companies have been forced out of business by huge national conglomerates. These big companies can afford to ship food and beverages great distances, as long as it is a one-way trip. If they had to collect their containers and reuse them, canning and bottling factories serving large regions would be uneconomical. Consequently, the national companies favor recycling rather than refilling because they prefer fewer, larger plants and don't want to be responsible for collecting and reusing containers. In some circumstances, life-cycle assessment shows that washing and decontaminating containers takes as much energy and produces as much air and water pollution as manufacturing new ones.

In many less affluent nations, reuse of all sorts of manufactured goods is an established tradition. Where most manufactured products are expensive and labor is cheap, it pays to salvage, clean, and repair products. Cairo, Manila, Mexico City, and many other cities have large populations of poor people who make a living by scavenging. Entire ethnic populations may survive on scavenging, sorting, and reprocessing scraps from city dumps. Eliminating waste shipments can reduce pollution but may threaten livelihoods. How can we resolve this dilemma?

Producing Less Waste

Even better than reusing materials is generating less waste in the first place. The What Can You Do? on p. 318 describes some contributions you can make to reduce the volume of our waste stream. Industry also can play an important role in source reduction. In Minnesota, the 3M Company has saved over $500 million since 1975 by changing manufacturing processes, finding uses for waste products, and listening to employees' suggestions. What is waste to one division is a treasure to another.

Excess packaging of food and consumer products is one of our greatest sources of unnecessary waste. Paper, plastic, glass, and metal packaging material makes up 50 percent of our domestic trash by volume (see related story "South Africa's National Flower?" at www.mhe.com/cases). Much of that packaging is primarily for marketing and has little to do with product protection (fig. 13.14). Manufacturers and retailers might be persuaded to reduce these wasteful practices if consumers ask for products without excess packaging. Canada's National Packaging Protocol (NPP) recommends that packaging minimize depletion of virgin resources and production of toxins in manufacturing. The preferred hierarchy is (1) no packaging, (2) minimal packaging, (3) reusable packaging, and (4) recyclable packaging. This plan sets an ambitious target of 50 percent reduction in excess packaging.

Where disposable packaging is necessary, we still can reduce the volume of waste in our landfills by using materials that are compostable or degradable. **Photodegradable plastics** break down when exposed to ultraviolet radiation. **Biodegradable plastics** incorporate such materials as cornstarch that microorganisms can decompose. Several states have introduced legislation requiring biodegradable or photodegradable six-pack beverage yokes, fast-food packaging, and disposable diapers. These degradable plastics often don't decompose completely; they only break down to small particles that remain in the environment. In doing so, they can release toxic chemicals. And in modern, lined landfills, they don't decompose at all. Furthermore, they make recycling less feasible and may lead people to believe that littering is okay.

Some environmental groups are beginning to worry that we have put too much emphasis on recycling. Many people believe that, if they recycle aluminum cans and newspapers, they are doing everything they can for the environment. While recycling is an important part of waste management, we have to remember that it is actually the third "R" in the waste hierarchy. The two preferred methods—reduction and reuse—get lost in our enthusiasm for recycling.

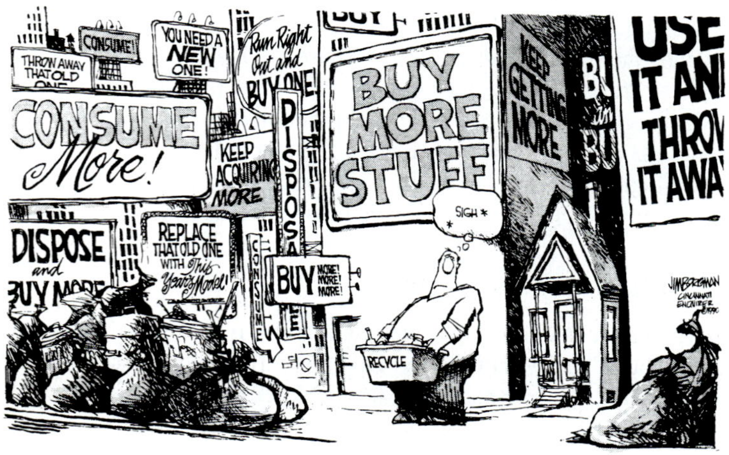

THROW AWAY THAT OLD
CONSUME!
YOU NEED A NEW ONE!
Run Right Out and BUY ONE!
CONSUME More!
KEEP ACQUIRING MORE
DISPOSA
BUY MORE STUFF
KEEP GETTING MORE
USE IT AN THROW IT AWA
SIGH
DISPOSE and
REPLACE THAT OLD ONE WITH This Year's Model!
CONSUME
BUY MORE! MORE! MORE!
RECYCLE

FIGURE 13.14 *How much more do we need? Where will we put what we already have?*
Reprinted with special permission of King Features Syndicate.

what can you do?

Reducing Waste

1. Buy foods that come with less packaging; shop at farmers' markets or co-ops, using your own containers.
2. Take your own washable, refillable beverage container to meetings or convenience stores.
3. When you have a choice at the grocery store among plastic, glass, or metal containers for the same food, buy the reusable or easier-to-recycle glass or metal.
4. Separate your cans, bottles, papers, and plastics for recycling.
5. Wash and reuse bottles, aluminum foil, plastic bags, and so on for your personal use.
6. Compost yard and garden wastes, leaves, and grass clippings.
7. Help your school develop responsible systems for disposing of electronics and other waste.
8. Write to your senators and representatives, and urge them to vote for container deposits, recycling, and safe incinerators or landfills.

Source: Data from Minnesota Pollution Control Agency.

HAZARDOUS AND TOXIC WASTES

The most dangerous aspect of the waste stream is that it often contains highly toxic and hazardous materials that are injurious to both human health and environmental quality (fig. 13.15). We now produce and use a vast array of flammable, explosive, caustic, acidic, and highly toxic chemical substances for industrial, agricultural, and domestic purposes. According to the EPA, U.S. industries generate about 265 million metric tons of officially classified hazardous wastes each year, slightly more than 1 ton for each person in the country. In addition, considerably more toxic and hazardous waste material is generated by industries or processes not regulated by the EPA. Shockingly, at least 40 million metric tons (22 billion lbs) of toxic and hazardous wastes are released into the air, water, and land in the United States each year. The biggest sources of these toxins are the chemical and petroleum industries (fig. 13.16).

What Is Hazardous Waste?

Legally, a **hazardous waste** is any discarded material, liquid or solid, that contains substances known to be (1) fatal to humans or laboratory animals in low doses; (2) toxic, carcinogenic, mutagenic, or teratogenic to humans or other life-forms; (3) ignitable with a flash point less than 60°C; (4) corrosive; or (5) explosive or

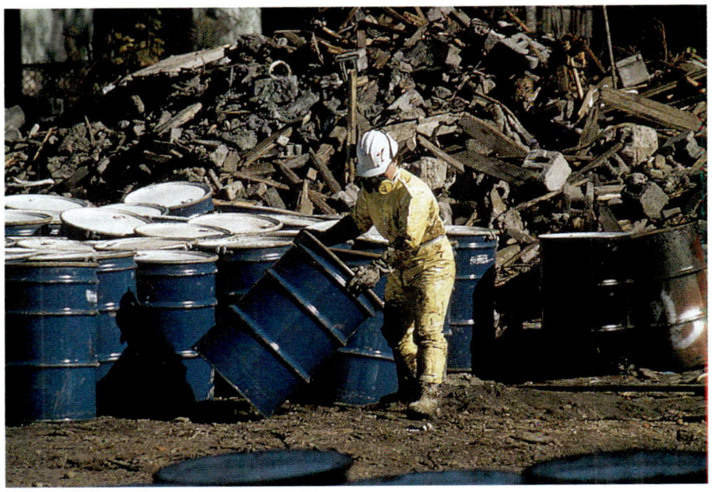

FIGURE 13.15 *Modern society produces large amounts of toxic and hazardous waste.*

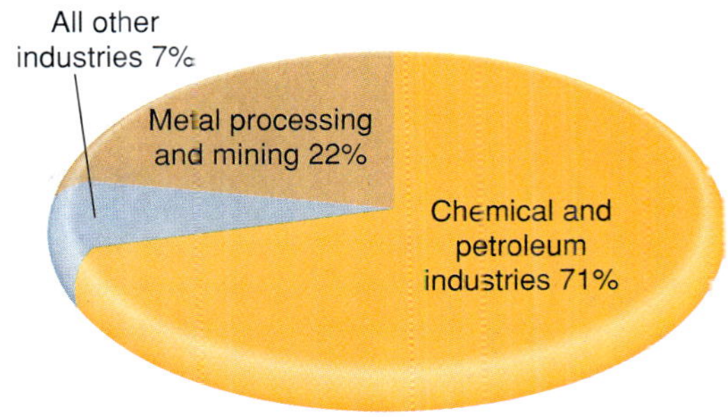

FIGURE 13.16 *Producers of hazardous wastes in the United States.*
Source: Data from the U.S. EPA, 2002.

highly reactive (undergoes violent chemical reactions either by itself or when mixed with other materials). Notice that this definition includes both toxic and hazardous materials, as defined in chapter 8. Certain compounds are exempt from regulation as hazardous waste if they are accumulated in less than 1 kg (2.2 lbs) of commercial chemicals or 100 kg of contaminated soil, water, or debris. Even larger amounts (up to 1,000 kg) are exempt when stored at an approved waste treatment facility for the purpose of being beneficially used, recycled, reclaimed, detoxified, or destroyed.

Hazardous Waste Disposal

Most hazardous waste is recycled, converted to nonhazardous forms, stored, or otherwise disposed of on-site by the generators—chemical companies, petroleum refiners, and other large industrial facilities—so that it doesn't become a public problem. Still, the hazardous waste that does enter the waste stream or the environment represents a serious environmental problem. And orphan wastes left behind by abandoned industries remain a serious threat to both environmental quality and human health. For years little attention was paid to this material. Wastes stored on private property, buried, or allowed to soak into the ground were considered of little concern to the public. An estimated 5 billion metric tons of highly poisonous chemicals were improperly disposed of in the United States between 1950 and 1975 before regulatory controls became more stringent.

Federal Legislation

Two important federal laws regulate hazardous waste management and disposal in the United States. The Resource Conservation and Recovery Act (RCRA, pronounced "rickra") of 1976 is a comprehensive program that requires rigorous testing and management of toxic and hazardous substances. A complex set of rules requires generators, shippers, users, and disposers of these materials to keep meticulous account of everything they handle and what happens to it from generation (cradle) to ultimate disposal (grave) (fig. 13.17).

The Comprehensive Environmental Response, Compensation, and Liability Act (CERCLA or Superfund Act), passed in 1980 and modified in 1984 by the Superfund Amendments and Reauthorization Act (SARA), is aimed at rapid containment, cleanup, or remediation of abandoned toxic waste sites. This statute authorizes the EPA to undertake emergency actions when a threat exists that toxic material will leak into the environment. The EPA is empowered to bring suit for the recovery of its costs from potentially responsible parties, such as site owners, operators, waste generators, or transporters.

SARA also established (under title III) a community right to know and state emergency response plans that give citizens access to information about what is present in their communities. One of the most useful tools in this respect is the **Toxic Release Inventory,** which requires 20,000 manufacturing facilities to report annually on releases of more than 300 toxic materials. You can find specific information in the inventory about what is in your neighborhood.

The government does not have to prove that anyone violated a law or what role he or she played in a Superfund site. Rather, liability under CERCLA is "strict, joint, and several," meaning that anyone associated with a site can be held responsible for the entire cost of cleaning it up, no matter how much of the mess they made.

APPLICATION: A Personal Hazardous Waste Inventory

Make a survey of your house or apartment to see how many toxic materials you can identify. If you live in a dorm, you may need to survey your parents' house. Read the cautionary labels. Which of the products are considered hazardous? When you use them, do you usually follow all the safety procedures recommended? Where is the nearest hazardous waste collection site for disposal of unwanted household products? If you don't know, call your city administrator or mayor's office to find out.

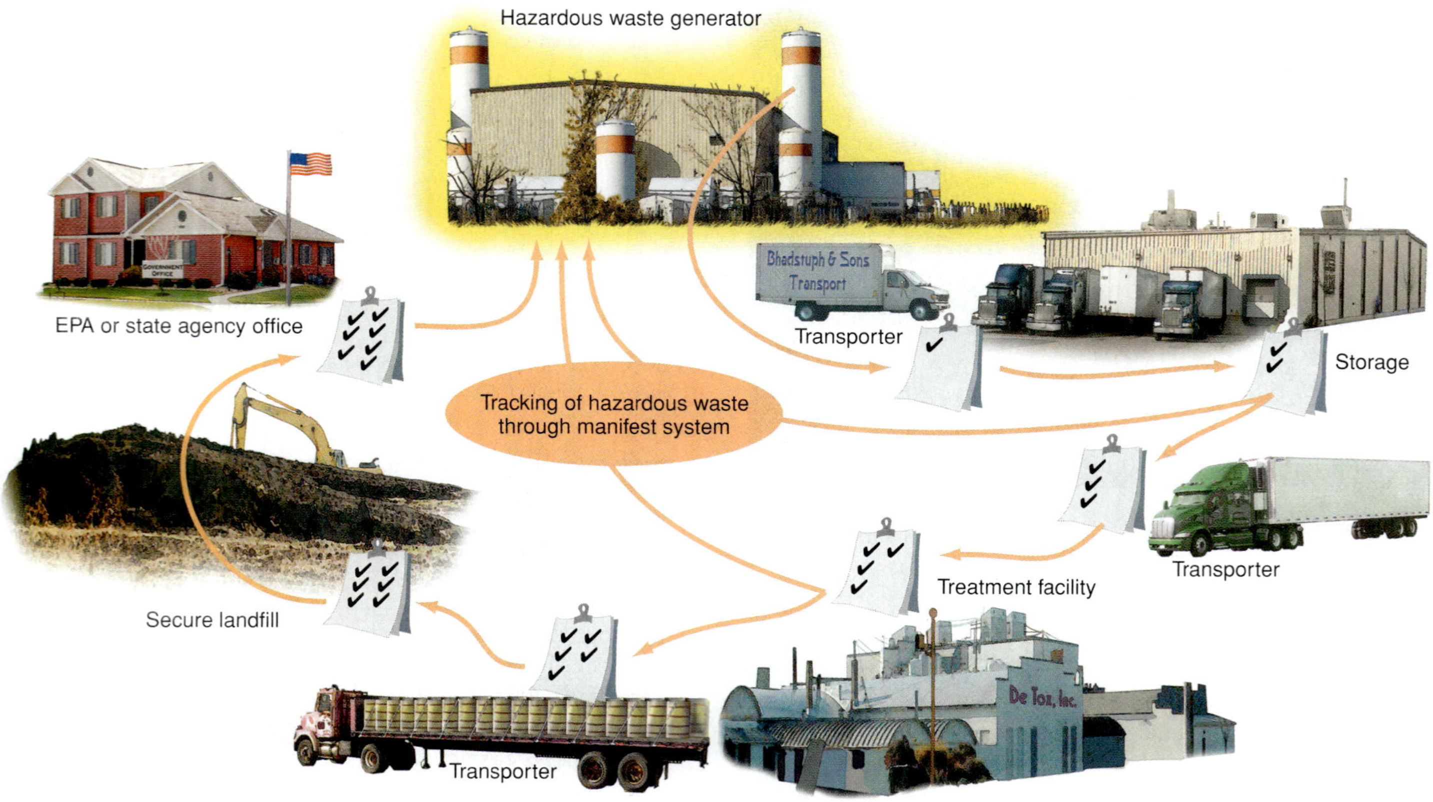

FIGURE 13.17 *Toxic and hazardous wastes must be tracked from "cradle to grave" by detailed shipping manifests.*

In some cases property owners have been assessed millions of dollars for removal of wastes left there years earlier by previous owners. This strict liability has been a headache for the real estate and insurance businesses.

CERCLA was amended in 1995 to make some of its provisions less onerous. In cases where treatment is unavailable or too costly and it is likely that a less costly remedy will become available within a reasonable time, interim containment is now allowed. The EPA also now has the discretion to set site-specific cleanup levels, rather than adhere to rigid national standards.

Superfund Sites

The EPA estimates that there are at least 36,000 seriously contaminated sites in the United States. The General Accounting Office (GAO) places the number much higher, perhaps more than 400,000 when all are identified. By 2004, some 1,671 sites had been placed on the National Priority List (NPL) for cleanup with financing from the federal Superfund program. The **Superfund** is a revolving pool designed to (1) provide an immediate response to emergency situations that pose imminent hazards and (2) to clean up or remediate abandoned or inactive sites. Without this fund, sites would languish for years or decades while the courts decided who was responsible for paying for the cleanup. Originally a $1.6 billion pool, the fund peaked at $3.6 billion. From its inception, the fund was financed by taxes on producers of toxic and hazardous wastes. Industries opposed this "polluter pays" tax, because current manufacturers are often not the ones responsible for the original contamination. In 1995 Congress agreed to let the tax expire. Since then the Superfund has dwindled, and the public has picked up an increasing share of the bill. In the 1980s the public covered less than 20 percent of the Superfund. In 2004, however, general revenues paid the entire cost off a greatly reduced program, and the industry share was zero.

Total costs for hazardous waste cleanup in the United States are estimated to be between $370 billion and $1.7 trillion, depending on how clean sites must be and what methods are used. For years, Superfund money was spent mostly on lawyers and consultants, and cleanup efforts were often bogged down in disputes over liability and best cleanup methods. During the 1990s, however, progress improved substantially, with a combination of rule adjustments and administrative commitment to cleanup. From 1993 to 2000, the number of completed NPL cleanups jumped from 155 to 757, just over half the then listed sites (fig. 13.18). Since 2000 progress has slowed again, due to underfunding and a lower priority among administrators.

What qualifies a site for the NPL? These sites are considered to be especially hazardous to human health and environmental quality because they are known to be leaking or have a potential for leaking supertoxic, carcinogenic, teratogenic, or mutagenic materials (see chapter 8). The ten substances of greatest concern or most commonly detected at Superfund sites are lead, trichloroethylene, toluene, benzene, PCBs, chloroform, phenol, arsenic, cad-

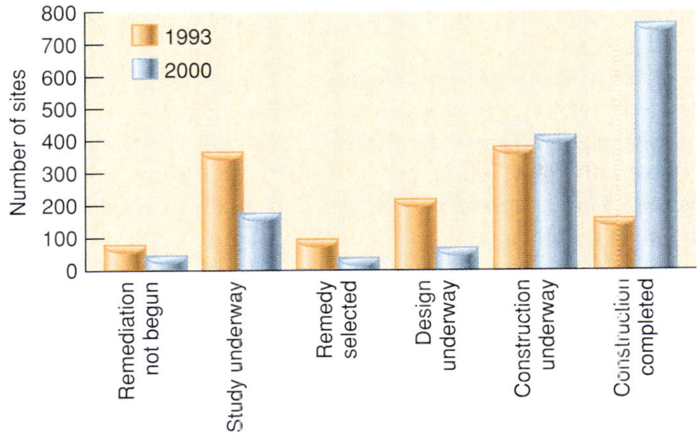

FIGURE 13.18 *Progress on Superfund National Priority List (NPL) sites. After years of little progress, the number of completed sites jumped from 155 in 1993 to 757 in 2000. Over 90 percent of the currently listed NPL sites are under construction or completed.*
Source: Data from Environmental Protection Agency, 2001.

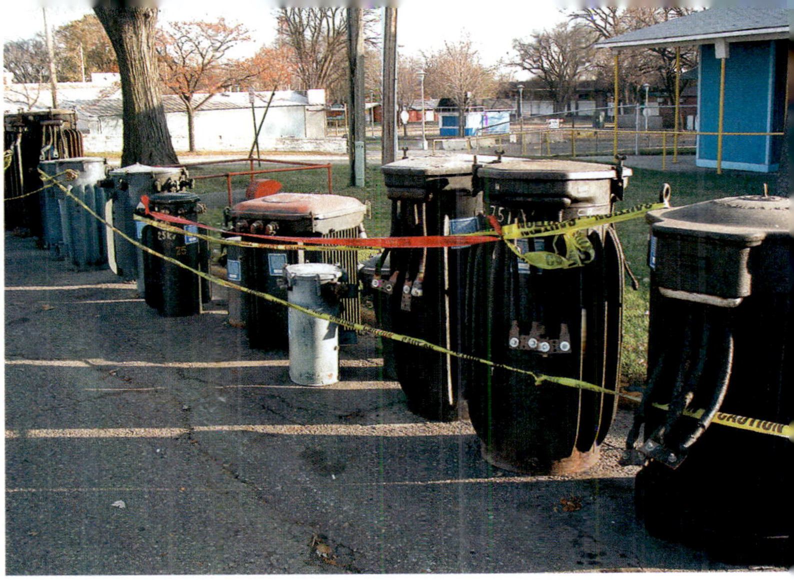

FIGURE 13.19 *Old electrical transformers filled with PCBs await disposal. If they leak, it could be a million-dollar problem.*

mium, and chromium. These and other hazardous or toxic materials are known to have contaminated groundwater at 75 percent of the sites now on the NPL. In addition, 56 percent of these sites have contaminated surface waters, and airborne materials are found at 20 percent of the sites. Seventy million Americans, including 10 million children, live within 6 km of a Superfund site.

Where are these thousands of hazardous waste sites, and how did they get contaminated? Old industrial facilities, such as smelters, mills, petroleum refineries, and chemical manufacturing plants, are highly likely to have been sources of toxic wastes. Regions of the country with high concentrations of aging factories, such as the "rust belt" around the Great Lakes or the Gulf Coast petrochemical centers, have large numbers of Superfund sites. Mining districts also are prime sources of toxic and hazardous waste. Within cities, factories and places such as railroad yards, bus repair barns, and filling stations, where solvents, gasoline, oil, and other petrochemicals were spilled or dumped on the ground, often are highly contaminated.

Some of the most infamous toxic waste sites were old dumps where many different materials were mixed together indiscriminately. For instance, Love Canal in Niagara Falls, New York, was an open dump that both the city and nearby chemical factories used as a disposal site. More than 20,000 tons of toxic chemical waste were buried under what later became a housing development. Another infamous example occurred in Hardeman County, Tennessee, where about a quarter of a million barrels of chemical waste were buried in shallow pits that subsequently leaked toxins into the groundwater.

How Clean Is Clean?

Among the biggest problems in cleaning up hazardous waste sites are questions of liability and the degree of purity required (fig. 13.19). In many cities, these problems have created large areas of contaminated properties, known as **brownfields,** that have been abandoned or are not being used to their potential because of real or suspected pollution. Up to one-third of all commercial and industrial sites in the urban core of many big cities fall in this category. In heavy industrial corridors the percentage typically is higher.

For years no one was interested in redeveloping brownfields because of liability risks. Who would buy a property, knowing that they might be forced to spend years in litigation and negotiations and be forced to pay millions of dollars for pollution they didn't create? Even if a site has been cleaned to current standards, there is a worry that additional pollution might be found in the future or that more stringent standards might be applied.

In many cases, property owners complain that unreasonably high levels of purity are demanded in remediation programs. Consider the case of Columbia, Mississippi. For many years a 35-ha (81-acre) site in Columbia was used for turpentine and pine tar manufacturing. Soil tests showed concentrations of phenols and other toxic organic compounds exceeding federal safety standards. The site was added to the Superfund NPL, and remediation was ordered. Some experts recommended that the best solution was to simply cover the surface with clean soil and enclose the property with a fence to keep people out. The total costs would have been about $1 million. Instead, the EPA ordered Reichhold Chemical, the last known property owner, to excavate more than 12,500 tons of soil and haul it to a commercial hazardous waste dump in Louisiana at a cost of some $4 million. The intention is to make the site safe enough to be used for any purpose, including housing—even though no one has proposed building anything there. According to the EPA, the dirt must be clean enough for children to play in—even eat every day for 70 years— without risk.

Similarly, in places where contaminants have seeped into groundwater, the EPA generally demands that cleanup be carried to drinking-water standards. Many critics believe that these pristine standards are unreasonable. Former Congressman Jim Florio, a principal author of the original Superfund Act, says, "It doesn't make any sense to clean up a rail yard in downtown Newark so it can be used as a drinking water reservoir." Depending on where the site is, what else is around it, and what its intended uses are, much less stringent standards may be perfectly acceptable.

Brownfield redevelopment is increasingly seen as an opportunity for rebuilding cities, creating jobs, increasing the tax base, and preventing needless destruction of open space at urban margins. In 2002 the EPA established a new brownfields revitalization fund designed to encourage restoration of more sites, as well as more kinds of sites. In some communities former brownfields are being turned into "eco-industrial parks" that feature environmentally friendly businesses and bring in much-needed jobs to innercity neighborhoods (see chapter 14).

Options for Hazardous Waste Management

What shall we do with toxic and hazardous wastes? In our homes, we can reduce waste generation and choose less toxic materials. Buy only what you need for the job at hand. Use up the last little bit, or share leftovers with a friend or neighbor. Many common materials that you probably already have make excellent alternatives to commercial products.

Produce Less Waste

As with other wastes, the safest and least expensive way to avoid hazardous waste problems is to avoid creating the wastes in the first place. Manufacturing processes can be modified to reduce or eliminate waste production. In Minnesota, the 3M Company reformulated products and redesigned manufacturing processes to eliminate more than 140,000 metric tons of solid and hazardous wastes, 4 billion liters (1 billion gal) of wastewater, and 80,000 metric tons of air pollution each year. It frequently found that these new processes not only spared the environment but also saved money by using less energy and fewer raw materials.

Recycling and reusing materials also eliminates hazardous wastes and pollution. Many waste products of one process or industry are valuable commodities in another. Already, about 10 percent of the wastes that would otherwise enter the waste stream in the United States are sent to surplus material exchanges, where they are sold as raw materials for use by other industries. This figure could probably be raised substantially with better waste management. In Europe at least one-third of all industrial wastes are exchanged through clearinghouses, where beneficial uses are found. This represents a double savings: the generator doesn't have to pay for disposal, and the recipient pays little, if anything, for raw materials.

Convert to Less Hazardous Substances

Several processes are available to make hazardous materials less toxic. *Physical treatments* tie up or isolate substances. Charcoal or resin filters absorb toxins. Distillation separates hazardous components from aqueous solutions. Precipitation and immobilization in ceramics, glass, or cement isolate toxins from the environment, so that they become essentially nonhazardous. One of the few ways to dispose of metals and radioactive substances is to fuse them in silica at high temperatures to make a stable, impermeable glass that is suitable for long-term storage. Plants, bacteria, and fungi can also concentrate or detoxify contaminants (see Investigating Our Environment p. 323).

Incineration is applicable to mixtures of wastes. A permanent solution to many problems, it is quick and relatively easy, but not necessarily cheap—nor always clean—unless done correctly. Wastes must be heated to over 1,000°C (2,000°F) for a sufficient period of time to complete destruction. The ash resulting from thorough incineration is reduced in volume up to 90 percent and often is safer to store in a landfill or another disposal site than the original wastes. Nevertheless, incineration remains highly controversial (fig. 13.20).

Chemical processing can transform materials so they become nontoxic. Included in this category are neutralization, removal of metals or halogens (chlorine, bromine, etc.), and oxidation. The Sunohio Corporation of Canton, Ohio, for instance, has developed a process called PCBx, in which chlorine in such molecules as PCBs is replaced with other ions that render the compounds less toxic. A portable unit can be moved to the location of the hazardous wastes, eliminating the need for shipping them.

Store Permanently

Inevitably, there will be some materials that we can't destroy, make into something else, or otherwise cause to vanish. We will have to store them out of harm's way. There are differing opinions about how best to do this.

Retrievable Storage Dumping wastes in the ocean or burying them in the ground generally means that we have lost control of them. If we learn later that our disposal technique was a mistake, it is difficult, if not impossible, to go back and recover the wastes. For many supertoxic materials, the best way to store them may be in **permanent retrievable storage.** This means placing waste storage containers in a secure building, salt mine, or bedrock cavern,

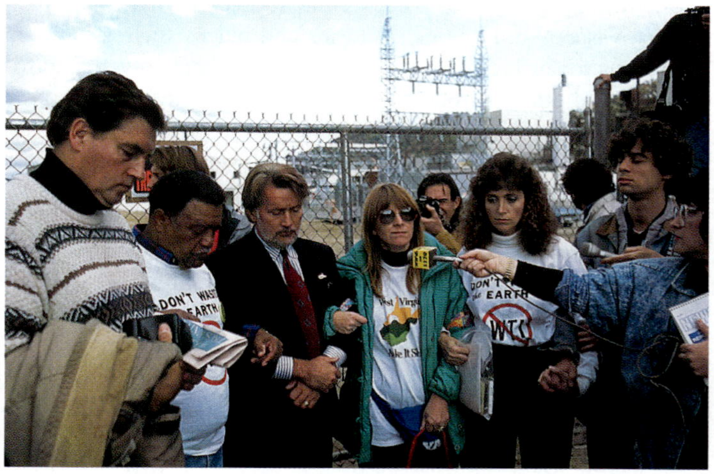

FIGURE 13.20 *Actor Martin Sheen joins local activists in a protest in East Liverpool, Ohio, site of the largest hazardous waste incinerator in the United States. About 1,000 people marched to the plant to pray, sing, and express their opposition. Involving celebrities draws attention to your cause. A peaceful, well-planned rally builds support and acceptance in the broader community.*

INVESTIGATING Our Environment

Bioremediation

Cleaning up the thousands of hazardous waste sites at factories, farms, and gas stations is an expensive project. In the United States alone, waste cleanup is projected to cost at least $700 billion. Usually hazardous waste remediation (cleanup) involves digging up soil and incinerating it, potentially releasing toxins into the air, or trucking it to a secure landfill. Contaminated groundwater is frequently pumped out of the ground; hopefully, contaminants are retrieved at the same time.

A promising alternative to these methods involves **bioremediation,** or biological waste treatment. Microscopic bacteria and fungi can absorb, accumulate, and detoxify a remarkable variety of toxic compounds. They can also accumulate heavy metals, and some have been developed that can metabolize (break down) PCBs. Aquatic plants such as water hyacinths and cattails can also be used to purify contaminated effluent.

Recently, an increasing variety of plants have been used in phytoremediation (cleanup using plants). Some types of mustard can extract lead, arsenic, zinc, and other metals from contaminated soil. Radioactive strontium and cesium have been extracted from soil near the Chernobyl nuclear power plant using common sunflowers. Poplar trees can absorb and break down toxic organic chemicals. Natural bacteria in groundwater, when provided with plenty of oxygen, can neutralize contaminants in aquifers. Experiments have shown that pumping air *into* groundwater can be a more effective cleanup method than pumping water *out*.

How do plants, bacteria, and fungi do all this? Many of the biophysical details are poorly understood, but in general, plant roots are designed to efficiently extract nutrients, water, and trace minerals from soil and groundwater. The mechanisms involved may aid extraction of metallic and organic contaminants. Some plants also use toxic elements as a defense against herbivores: locoweed, for example, selectively absorbs elements such as selenium, concentrating toxic levels in its leaves. Absorption can be extremely effective. Bracken fern growing in Florida has been found to contain arsenic at concentrations more than 200 times higher than in the soil in which it was growing.

Genetically modified plants are also being developed to process toxins. Poplars have been developed to process toxins, using a gene borrowed from bacteria that transforms a toxic compound of mercury into a safer form. In another experiment, a gene for producing mammalian liver enzymes, which specialize in breaking down toxic organic compounds, was inserted into tobacco plants. The plants succeeded in producing the liver enzymes and breaking down toxins absorbed through their roots.

These remediation methods are not without risks. Insects could consume leaves containing concentrated substances, allowing contaminants to enter the food chain. Some absorbed contaminants are volatilized, or emitted in gaseous form, through pores in plant leaves. Once contaminants are absorbed into plants, the plants themselves are usually toxic and must be landfilled. But the cost of phytoremediation can be less than half the cost of landfilling or treating toxic soil, and the volume of plant material requiring secure storage is a fraction of the volume of the contaminated dirt.

Cleaning up hazardous and toxic waste sites will be a big business for the foreseeable future, in North America and around the world. Innovations such as bioremediation offer promising prospects for business development, as well as for environmental health and saving taxpayer money.

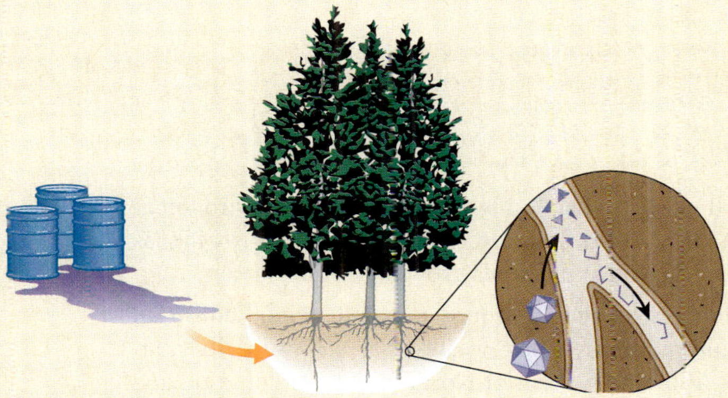

Fast-growing poplar trees have been developed that can absorb and break down toxic compounds.

where they can be inspected periodically and retrieved, if necessary, for repacking or for transfer if a better means of disposal is developed. This technique is more expensive than burial in a landfill because the storage area must be guarded and monitored continuously to prevent leakage, vandalism, or other dispersal of toxic materials. Remedial measures are much cheaper with this technique, however, and it may be the best system in the long run.

Secure Landfills One of the most popular solutions for hazardous waste disposal has been landfilling. Although, as we saw earlier in this chapter, many such landfills have been environmental disasters, newer techniques make it possible to create safe, modern **secure landfills** that are acceptable for disposing of many hazardous wastes. The first line of defense in a secure landfill is a thick bottom cushion of compacted clay that surrounds the pit like a bathtub (fig. 13.21). Moist clay is flexible and resists cracking if the ground shifts. It is impermeable to groundwater and will safely contain wastes. A layer of gravel is spread over the clay liner, and perforated drainpipes are laid in a grid to collect any seepage that escapes from the stored material. A thick polyethylene liner, protected from punctures by soft padding materials, covers the gravel bed. A layer of soil or absorbent sand cushions the inner liner, and the wastes are packed in drums, which then are placed into the pit, separated into small units by thick berms of soil or packing material.

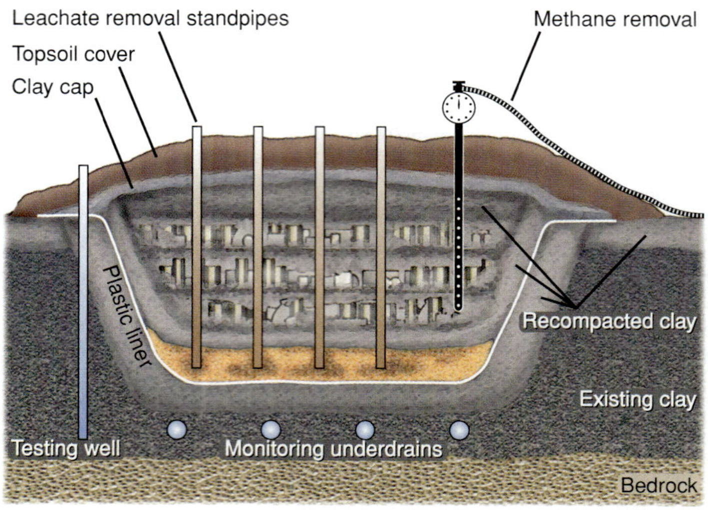

FIGURE 13.21 *A secure landfill for toxic waste. A thick plastic liner and two or more layers of impervious compacted clay enclose the landfill. A gravel bed between the clay layers collects any leachate, which can then be pumped out and treated. Well samples are tested for escaping contaminants and methane is collected for combustion.*

When the landfill has reached its maximum capacity, a cover much like the bottom sandwich of clay, plastic, and soil—in that order—caps the site. Vegetation stabilizes the surface and improves its appearance. Sump pumps collect any liquids that filter through the landfill, either from rainwater or leaking drums. This leachate is treated and purified before being released. Monitoring wells check groundwater around the site to ensure that no toxins have escaped.

Most landfills are buried below ground level to be less conspicuous; however, in areas where the groundwater table is close to the surface, it is safer to build above-ground storage. The same protective construction techniques are used as in a buried pit. An advantage to such a facility is that leakage is easier to monitor because the bottom is at ground level.

Transportation of hazardous wastes to disposal sites is of concern because of the risk of accidents. Emergency-preparedness officials conclude that the greatest risk in most urban areas is not nuclear war or natural disaster but crashes involving trucks or trains carrying hazardous chemicals through densely packed urban corridors. Another worry is who will bear financial responsibility for abandoned waste sites. Hazardous wastes remain toxic long after the businesses that created them are gone. As is the case with nuclear wastes (see chapter 12), we may need new institutions for perpetual care of these wastes.

SUMMARY

- Global waste production is a critical issue in environmental quality. Global waste production is rapidly growing, as nonbiodegradable materials grow in a waste stream.
- Solid waste includes domestic, commercial, industrial, agricultural, and mining wastes that are primarily nontoxic. About 60 percent of North American domestic and industrial wastes are deposited in landfills; most of the rest is incinerated or recycled. Old landfills were often leaky and messy and an important source of groundwater contamination. Modern landfills must have impermeable liners that prevent seepage to groundwater, and they must be covered with soil and monitored for gas emissions and water contamination.
- Incineration is our second most important method of waste disposal. Incineration can destroy organic compounds, and it can be used to produce energy. Airborne contaminants can result from burning, however, especially if incinerators are not operated at optimal temperatures or if toxic substances are burned.
- Recycling and composting (of yard waste and other organic materials) are growing in North America and globally. The growing cost of waste disposal makes collection increasingly cost-effective, and the rapid depletion of landfill space makes recycling attractive. A principal obstacle to recycling is weak or unstable markets for recycled plastic, paper, and other materials. The growing use of disposable plastic beverage containers poses another important barrier to widespread recycling. Japan is a world leader in recycling, with about 60 percent of domestic waste being recycled.
- Reusing, demanufacturing, and reducing material consumption are important additional strategies for reducing the waste stream.
- Hazardous and toxic wastes are waste materials that cause health problems, including birth defects, neurological disorders, reduced resistance to infection, and cancer. Environmental costs of hazardous and toxic waste include contamination of water supplies, poisoning of soil, and destruction of habitat.
- The major categories of hazardous wastes are ignitable, corrosive, reactive, explosive, and toxic materials. Some materials of greatest concern are heavy metals, solvents, and synthetic organic chemicals, such as pesticides and herbicides.

- Disposal practices for solid and hazardous wastes have often been unsatisfactory. Thousands of abandoned, often unknown waste disposal sites still leak toxic materials into the environment. Techniques for controlling hazardous wastes include not making the material in the first place; incineration; secure landfills; and physical, chemical, or biological treatment to detoxify or immobilize wastes.
- The Superfund is a revolving fund to finance cleanup of some of our worst hazardous waste sites. The Superfund was established by the Comprehensive Environmental Response, Compensation, and Liability Act (CERCLA) of 1980. Many sites on the Superfund's National Priority List are abandoned factories or dumps.
- Dangerous wastes are often removed from wealthy countries or neighborhoods to poorer ones, and cleanup efforts may be faster and more complete in wealthier areas. Proponents of environmental justice try to identify these patterns and rectify them.
- People often resist having transfer facilities, storage sites, disposal operations, or transportation of hazardous materials (often referred to as Locally Unwanted Land Uses, or LULUs) near where they live. Safe handling and liability remain unanswered in solid and hazardous waste disposal.

QUESTIONS FOR REVIEW

1. What are solid wastes and hazardous wastes? What is the difference between them?
2. Describe the difference between an open dump, a sanitary landfill, and a modern, secure, hazardous waste disposal site.
3. Why are landfill sites becoming limited around most major urban centers in the United States? What steps are being taken to solve this problem?
4. Describe some concerns about waste incineration.
5. List some benefits and drawbacks of recycling wastes. What are the major types of materials recycled from municipal waste, and how are they used?
6. What is composting, and how does it fit into solid waste disposal?
7. Describe some ways that we can reduce the waste stream to avoid or reduce disposal problems.
8. What materials are most recycled in the United States?
9. What societal problems are associated with waste disposal? Why do people object to waste handling in their neighborhoods?
10. What are brownfields, and why do cities want to redevelop them?

THINKING SCIENTIFICALLY

1. If you were planning an archeological dig of a modern garbage dump, would you record weight or volume of the objects uncovered? Why would this matter?
2. A toxic waste disposal site has been proposed for the Pine Ridge Indian Reservation in South Dakota. Many tribal members oppose this plan, but some favor it because of the jobs and income it will bring to an area with 70 percent unemployment. If local people choose immediate survival over long-term health, should we object or intervene?
3. Should industry officials be held responsible for dumping chemicals that were legal when they did it but are now known to be extremely dangerous? At what point can we argue that they should have known about the hazards involved?
4. Suppose that your brother or sister has decided to buy a house next to a toxic waste dump because it costs $20,000 less than a comparable house elsewhere. What do you say to him or her?
5. Is there a fundamental difference between incinerating municipal, medical, or toxic industrial waste? Would you oppose an incinerator in your neighborhood for one type of waste but not others? Why or why not?
6. The Netherlands incinerates much of its toxic waste at sea by a shipborne incinerator. Would you support this as a way to dispose of our wastes as well? What are the critical considerations for or against this approach?
7. Some scientists argue that permanent retrievable storage of toxic and hazardous wastes is preferable to burial. How can we be sure that material that will be dangerous for thousands of years will remain secure? If you were designing such a repository, how would you address this question?

KEY TERMS

biodegradable plastics 318
bioremediation 323
brownfields 321
composting 315
demanufacturing 316
energy recovery 311
hazardous waste 318
mass burn 311
permanent retrievable storage 322
photodegradable plastics 318
recycling 313
refuse-derived fuel 311
sanitary landfills 309
secure landfills 323
Superfund 320
Toxic Release Inventory 319
waste stream 308

SUGGESTED READINGS

Bergman, B. J. 1999. "The hidden life of computers." *Sierra* 84(4): 32–33.

Blumberg, Louis, and Robert Gottlieb. 1989. *War on Waste: Can America Win Its Battle with Garbage?* Island Press.

Kazuhiro, Ueta, and Harumi Koizumi. 2001. "Reducing household waste: Japan learns from Germany." *Environment* 43(9):20–32.

McDonough, William, and Michael Braungart. 2002. *Cradle to Cradle: Remaking the Way We Make Things.* North Point Press.

Rathje, William, and Cullen Murphy. 1992. *Rubbish! The Archaeology of Garbage.* HarperCollins.

Taylor, David. 1999. "Talking trash: The economic and environmental issues of landfills." *Environmental Health Perspectives* 107(8):A404–A409.

Warren-Rhodes, Kimberley, and Albert Koenig. 2001. "Escalating trends in the urban metabolism of Hong Kong: 1971–1997." *AMBIO: A Journal of the Human Environment* 30(7):429–38.

Welcome to McGraw-Hill's Online Learning Center

http://www.mhhe.com/cunningham3e

WEB EXERCISES

Recycling Challenge

The Internet Consumer Recycling Guide, www.idiom.com/~bryce/recycle/, provides a detailed list of recyclable materials and where to send them. Before you look at this website, take five minutes and write down at least 25 different types of items in the room around you. These items can be small (paper clips, hair clips, books, food packaging, etc.) or large (carpets, furniture, computers, light fixtures, plumbing, etc.). Once you have made the list, mark all those that are recyclable and note how you would recycle them.

Now look at the Recycling Guide webpage. Look at all three "guide" pages—The World's Shortest Comprehensive Recycling Guide, the Guide to Recycling Common Materials, and Guide to Hard-to-Recycle Materials. How many additional items on your list can be recycled, according to these guides? How many could be recycled in principle but would be hard to recycle in your community? Why? What recycled products could be made by recycling the materials on your list?

How many of the items on your list might be available with recycled content? How many of them could you have avoided acquiring in the first place?

Mapping Superfund Sites

The National Priority List (NPL) is a list of contaminated sites scheduled for cleanup using money from the so-called Superfund. To be placed on this list, sites must be nominated and studied. A final decision can take years. Remediation can take many years more. How many Superfund sites are in your state (or any state you choose)? Go to www.epa.gov/superfund/sites/npl/npl.htm, where you'll find a map of the United States. Click on a state to see a state map. How many sites are there in your state, or in the one you chose? As you look at the state map, can you identify whether sites are clustered on a river, on a coastline, or on some other natural features? Can you think of any reasons sites are placed as they are?

Click on the site nearest you, and you'll see a list of sites in that state. Click on the name of the site, and you should go to a description of the facility, its dates, and the types of contamination. Have you heard of this site? What type of site is it? Has it been cleaned up?

Click on several of the sites in your state. What is the approximate range of ages of these sites? How many were polluted before you were born? Do you think you should be responsible for cleaning them up? If not you, then who?

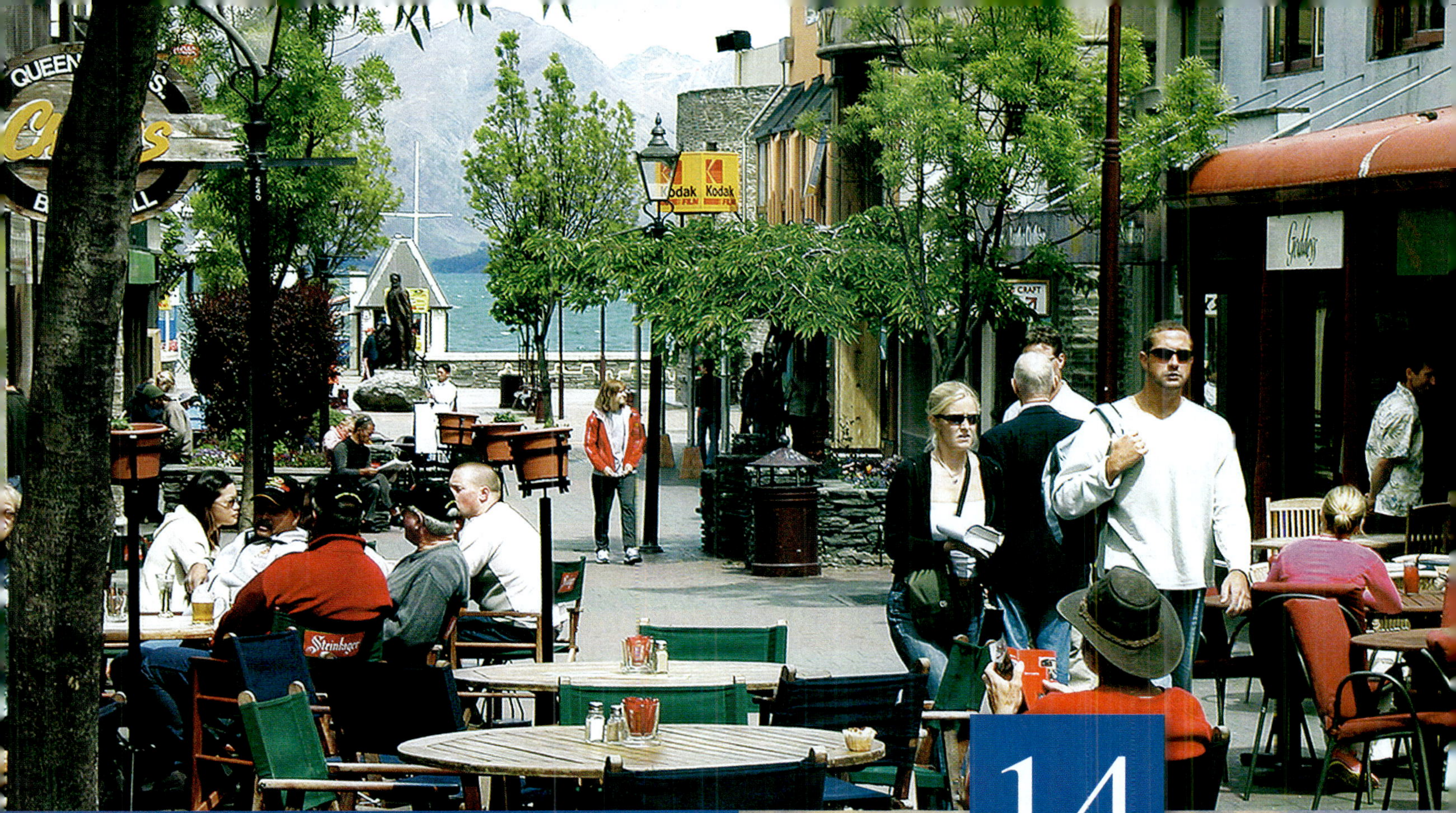

This walking street in Queenstown, NZ, provides opportunities for shopping, dining, and socializing in a pleasant outdoor setting.

14

Sustainability and Human Development

A world where some live in comfort and plenty, while half of the human race lives on less than $2 a day, is neither just, nor stable.

–G. W. Bush

Welcome to McGraw-Hill's Online Learning Center

http://www.mhhe.com/cunningham3e

LEARNING ONLINE

Visit our webpage at www.mhhe.com/cunningham3e for data sources, further readings, additional case studies, current environmental news, and regional examples within the Online Learning Center to help you understand the material in this chapter. You'll also find active links to information pertaining to this chapter, including

Ecological economics
Ecological design
Sustainable city
Sustainable development
Trade and the environment
Urban ecology
Urban sprawl

OBJECTIVES

After studying this chapter, you should be able to

- explain the difference between neoclassical and ecological economics, and how each discipline views ecological processes and natural resources.
- distinguish between different types and categories of resources.
- discuss internal and external costs, market approaches to pollution control, and cost-benefit analysis.
- analyze the role of business and some possible strategies for achieving future sustainability.
- recognize the push-and-pull factors that lead to urban growth.
- appreciate how cities fail to be sustainable and how they might become more sustainable.
- understand the causes and consequences of sprawl, and how smart growth could solve some urban problems.
- see the connection between sustainable economic development, social justice, and the solution of urban problems.

Curitiba: An Environmental Showcase

A few decades ago Curitiba, Brazil, was like many cities in developing countries: growing rapidly, with increasing air pollution and traffic congestion and deteriorating and inadequate roads, water systems, housing, and waste disposal systems. Looking at the gradual decay and corruption of other Brazilian cities, Jaime Lerner, a landscape architect and former student activist, ran for mayor in 1969. For the next 20 years Lerner motivated and organized a campaign of civic action that turned around the city's decline. Curitiba, with a population of about 2 million, has become an outstanding example of sustainable urban development. Environmentally and socially healthy by any country's standards, Curitiba has a worldwide reputation for its innovative urban planning and environmental protection policies.

The heart of Curitiba's environmental plan is education for both children and adults. Signs posted along roadways proclaim "50 kg of paper equals one tree" and "Recycle; it pays." School children study ecology along with Portuguese and math. With the assistance of children who encourage their parents, the city has successfully instituted a complex recycling plan that requires careful separation of different kinds of materials. The city calculates that 1,200 trees per day are saved by paper recycled in this program. "Imagine if the whole of Brazil did this," Lerner exclaims. "We could save 26 million trees per year!" More than 70 percent of the residents now recycle. Food and bus coupons are given out in exchange for recyclables, providing an alternative to welfare while also protecting the environment.

Another area in which Curitiba is setting an example is transportation. Faced with a population that tripled in two decades, bringing increasing levels of traffic congestion and air pollution, Curitiba had a transportation dilemma. The choices were either to bulldoze freeways through the historic heart of the city or to institute mass transit. The city chose mass transit. The system has special buses, elevated bus stops, and a network of smaller feeder routes that work quickly and efficiently. Now more than three-quarters of the city's population leave their cars at home every day. The system is so successful that ridership has increased from 25,000 passengers a day 20 years ago to more than 1.5 million per day now, or 70 percent of all trips in the city. The result is not only less congestion and pollution but also major energy savings.

Other measures to clear the air and reduce congestion include a limit on building height and construction of an industrial park outside city boundaries. Maximum use is made of all materials and buildings. Water and energy conservation are practiced widely. Even litter—a ubiquitous component of most Brazilian cities—is absent in Curitiba. The city has more green space per capita than most American cities. To further beautify their city, civic volunteers have planted 1.5 million trees—more than any other place in Brazil.

Although many residents initially were skeptical of this environmental plan, now a remarkable 99 percent of the city's inhabitants would not want to live anywhere else. The World Bank uses Curitiba as an example of what can be done through civic leadership and public participation to clean up the urban environment. Even in a developing country without a great deal of wealth and resources, Curitiba has demonstrated that a remarkable level of sustainability can be achieved. Some people claim that Curitiba, with its cool climate and high percentage of European immigrants, may be a special case among Brazilian cities. Lerner claims that Curitiba has no special features except concern, creativity, and communal efforts to care for its environment.

Curitiba's example illustrates some of the ingredients of sustainable development. In this chapter we will look at sustainability—efforts to reduce our impacts on the environment and improve human well-being at the same time. And we will discuss additional opportunities for, and obstacles to, sustainable resource use.

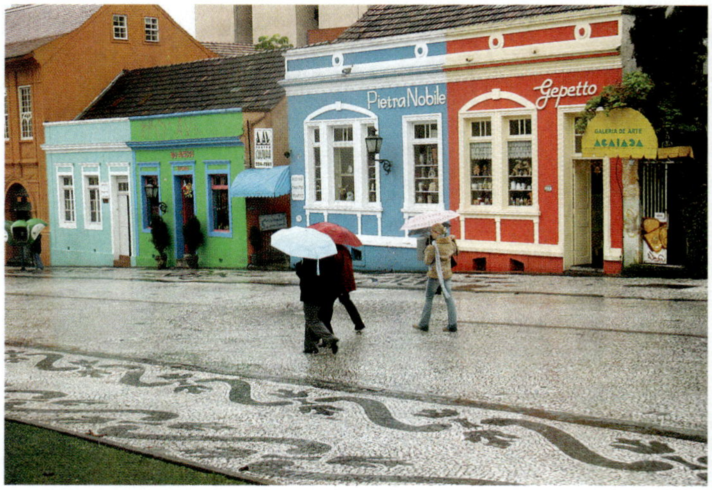

In Curitiba, Brazil, much of the city center has been converted to pedestrian shopping streets while historic buildings have been converted to new uses.

SUSTAINABILITY AND RESOURCES

Sustainability has become a central theme of environmental science and of human development and resource use. Although the idea of sustainability has many facets, the central idea is that we should use **resources** (anything that is useful for creating wealth or improving our lives) in ways that do not diminish them. Resources and natural amenities, including wildlife, natural beauty, and open space, should be preserved, so that future generations can have lifestyles at least as healthy and happy as ours—or perhaps better.

Can sustainability be achieved and, if so, how? This is one of the core questions in environmental science because human impacts will continue to damage our environment unless we find intelligent alternatives and solutions. Key problems of unsustainability have been woven through much of this book. In this chapter we will look at a few of the root problems of unsustainability and some promising steps toward sustainable use of our environment and sustainable development of human communities.

Sustainable Development

By now it is clear that security and living standards for the world's poorest people are inextricably linked to environmental protection. One of the most important questions in environmental science is how we can continue improvements in human welfare within the limits of the earth's natural resources. A possible solution to this dilemma is **sustainable development,** a term popularized in a 1987 report of the World Commission on Environment and Development called *Our Common Future.* In the words of this report, *sustainable development* means "meeting the needs of the present without compromising the ability of future generations to meet their own needs." *Development* means improving people's lives. Sustainable development means extending progress, without exhausting resources, beyond the foreseeable future.

Many people argue that endlessly continuing development, continually improving the lives of more and more people, requires constantly increased resource exploitation. Consequently, the very notion of sustainable development should be impossible. Many of our resources are nonrenewable, and the capacity of the biosphere to absorb our wastes is limited. As we will discuss in the following section, the possibility of sustainable development depends partly on how you define resources, your theories about resource use, and your views on the possibility of extending the use of the resources we have.

To be truly enduring, the benefits of sustainable development must be available to all humans, rather than to just the members of a privileged group. Many of the world's people live in poverty and in unhealthy conditions. By 2050, demographers predict, at least two-thirds of the world's population will live in urban areas. These cities have an extraordinary impact on their surrounding environments. But they also are powerful engines for cultural, economic, and political change. It is probably in cities that the struggle to achieve sustainability will be won or lost. Because cities are so important in our struggle for environmental, social, and economic sustainabilty, they are the focus of the second half of this chapter.

Does sustainable development mean raising all the world's people to the same level of consumption that North Americans and Europeans have? No. It does mean trying to raise the level of health, security, political stability, and quality of life around the world, however. Many places, such as Curitiba, have demonstrated that healthy, satisfying lives are possible without the extravagant resource use we currently have in the wealthiest nations.

Can Development Be Sustainable?

While economic growth makes possible a more comfortable lifestyle, it doesn't automatically result in a cleaner environment. People will purchase clean water and sanitation if they can afford to do so. For low-income people, however, more money tends to result in higher air pollution because they can afford to burn more fuel for transportation and heating. Given enough money, people will be able to afford both convenience and clean air. Some environmental problems, such as waste generation and carbon dioxide emissions, continue to rise sharply with increasing wealth because we are slow to notice and curb their effects. If we are able to sustain economic growth, we will need to develop personal restraint or social institutions to deal with these problems.

Sometimes development has caused environmental, economic, and social disasters. Large-scale hydropower projects, such as the Three Gorges Dam in China (see related story at www.mhhe.com/cases), that are intended to generate valuable electrical power also displace local residents, destroy wildlife, and accumulate water pollutants. Similarly, introduction of "miracle" crop varieties in Asia and huge grazing projects in Africa financed by international lending agencies have crowded out wildlife, diminished the diversity of traditional crops, and destroyed markets for small-scale farmers.

Other development projects, however, work more closely with both nature and local social systems. Socially conscious businesses and environmental, nongovernmental organizations sponsor ventures that allow people in developing countries to grow or make high-value products—often using traditional techniques and designs—that can be sold on world markets for good prices. "Fair trade" coffee importers, for instance, provide a market for sustainably grown coffee, and for small coffee growers, at a fair price. This is an example of economic development that raises incomes in rural Central America and also rewards farmers for treating their environment with care.

Resources in Classical Economics

To understand the problems and promise of sustainability, you need to understand the different kinds of resources we use. The way we treat resources depends largely on how we view and define them. *Classical economics,* developed in the 1700s by philosophers such as Adam Smith (1723–1790) and Thomas Malthus (1766–1834), assumes that resources are finite—that resources such as iron, gold, water, and land exist in fixed amounts. According to this view, as populations grow, scarcity of these resources reduces quality of life, increases competition, and ultimately causes populations to fall again. In a free market, where fully informed buyers and sellers make free, independent decisions to buy and sell, the price of a pound of butter depends on the supply of available butter (it is cheap when plenty is available) and the demand for butter (buyers pay more when they must compete to get the resource, fig. 14.1).

This price mechanism has been modified by the idea of *marginal costs.* Buyers and sellers evaluate the added return for buying (or making and selling) slightly more of a product, or the marginal cost of slightly greater production or purchase. If the return is greater than the marginal cost, then a sale is made.

The nineteenth-century economist John Stuart Mill assumed that most resources are finite, but he developed the idea of a

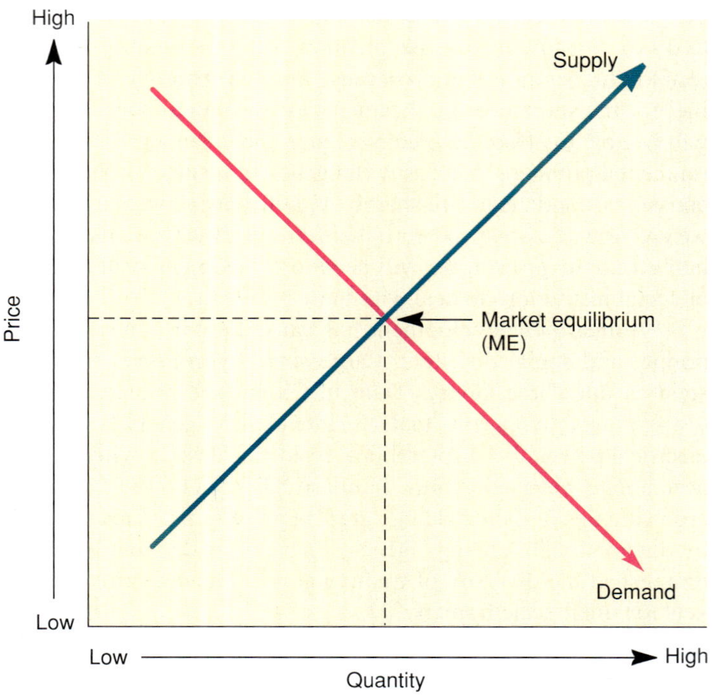

FIGURE 14.1 *Classic supply/demand curves. When price is low, supply is low and demand is high. As prices rise, supply increases but demand falls. Market equilibrium is the price at which supply and demand are equal.*

steady-state economy. Rather than boom-and-bust cycles of population and resource use, as envisioned by Malthus, Mill proposed that economies can achieve an equilibrium of resource use and production. Intellectual and moral development continues, he argued, once this stable, secure state is achieved.

Neoclassical Economics

Neoclassical economics, developed in the nineteenth century, expanded the idea of resources to include labor, knowledge, and capital. Labor and knowledge are resources because they are necessary to create goods and services; they are not finite because every new person can add more labor and energy to an economy. **Capital** is any form of wealth that contributes to the production of more wealth. Money can be invested to produce more money. Mineral resources can be developed and manufactured into goods that return more money. Economists distinguish several kinds of capital:

1. Natural capital: goods and services provided by nature
2. Human capital: knowledge, experience, human enterprise
3. Manufactured (built) capital: tools, buildings, roads, technology

To this list some social theorists would add social capital, the shared values, trust, cooperation, and organization that can develop in a group of people but cannot exist in one individual alone.

Because the point of capital is the production of more capital (that is, wealth), neoclassical economics emphasizes the idea of growth. Growth results from the flow of resources, goods, and services (fig. 14.2). Continued growth is always necessary for continued prosperity, according to this view. Natural resources contribute to production and growth, but they are not critical supplies that limit growth. They are not limiting because resources are considered to be interchangeable and substitutable. As one resource becomes scarce, neoclassical economics predicts that a substitute will be found.

Since production of wealth is central to neoclassical economics, an important measure of growth and wealth is consumption. If a society consumes more oil, more minerals, and more food, it is presumably becoming wealthier. This idea has extended to the idea of *throughput,* the amount of resources a society uses and discards. More throughput is a measure of greater consumption and greater wealth, according to this view. Throughput is commonly measured in terms of **gross national product (GNP),** the sum of all products bought and sold in an economy.

Natural resource economics extends the neoclassical viewpoint to treat natural resources as important waste sinks (absorbers), as well as sources of raw materials. Natural capital (resources) is considered more abundant, and therefore cheaper, than built or human-made capital.

Ecological Economics

Ecological economics, developed in recent decades, applies ecological ideas of system functions and recycling to the definition of resources. Ecological economics also recognizes efficiency in nature, and it acknowledges the importance of ecosystem functions for the continuation of human economies and cultures. In nature, one species' waste is another's food, so that nothing is wasted. We need an economy that recycles materials and uses

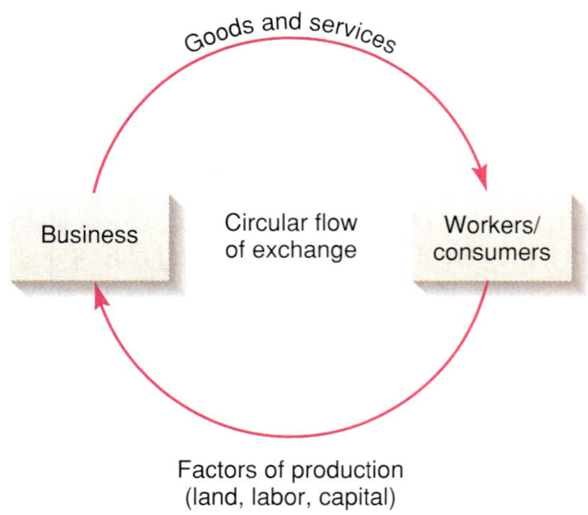

FIGURE 14.2 *The neoclassical model of the economy focuses on the flow of goods, services, and factors of production (land, labor, capital) between business and individual workers/consumers. The social and environmental consequences of these relationships are irrelevant in this view.*

energy efficiently, much as a biological community does. Ecological economics also treats the natural environment as part of our economy, so that natural capital becomes a key consideration in economic calculations. Ecological functions, such as absorbing and purifying wastewater, processing air pollution, providing clean water, carrying out photosynthesis, and creating soil, are known as **ecological services** (table 14.1). These services are free: we don't pay for them directly (although we often pay indirectly when we suffer from their absence). Therefore, they are often excluded from conventional economic accounting, a situation that ecological economists attempt to rectify (fig. 14.3).

Many ecological economists also promote the idea of a steady-state economy. As with John Stuart Mill's original conception of steady states, these economists argue that economic health can be maintained without constantly growing consumption and throughput. Instead, efficiency and recycling of resources can allow steady prosperity where there is little or no population growth. Low birth rates and death rates (like *K*-adapted species, see chapter 3), political and social stability, and reliance on renewable energy would characterize such a steady-state economy. Like Mill, these economists argue that human and social capital—knowledge, happiness, art, life expectancies, and cooperation—can continue to grow even without constant expansion of resource use.

Both ecological economics and neoclassical economics distinguish between renewable and nonrenewable resources. **Nonrenewable resources** exist in finite amounts: minerals, fossil fuels, and also groundwater that recharges extremely slowly are all fixed, at least on a human timescale. **Renewable resources** are naturally replenished and recycled at a fairly steady rate. Fresh water, living organisms, air, and food resources are all renewable (fig. 14.4).

These categories are important, but they are not as deterministic as you might think. Nonrenewable resources, such as iron and gold, can be extended through more efficient use: cars now use less steel than they once did, and gold is mixed in alloys to extend its use. Substitution also reduces demand for these resources: car parts once made of iron are now made of plastic and ceramics; copper wire, once stockpiled to provide phone lines, is now being replaced with cheap, lightweight fiber-optic cables made from silica (sand). Recycling also extends supplies of nonrenewable resources. Aluminum, platinum, gold, silver, and many other valuable metals are routinely recycled now, further reducing the demand for extracting new sources. The only limit to recycling is usually the relative costs of extracting new resources compared with collecting used materials. Recoverable sources of nonrenewable resources are also

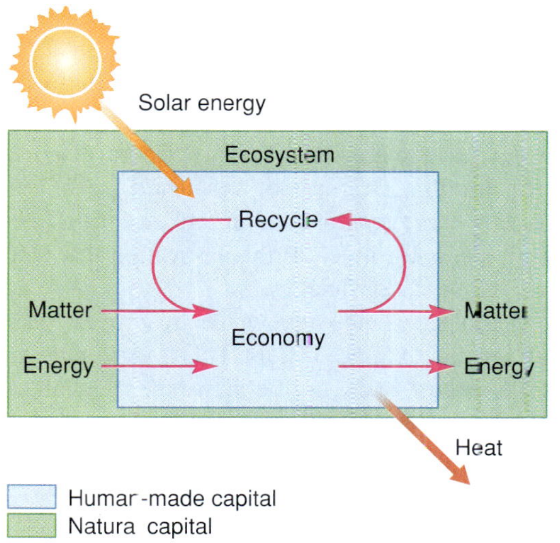

FIGURE 14.3 *An ecological economics view considers natural capital and recycling integral to the economy. Human-made capital is created using limited supplies of natural capital.*
Source: Data from Herman Daly in A. M. Jansson et al., *Investing in Natural Capital,* ISEE.

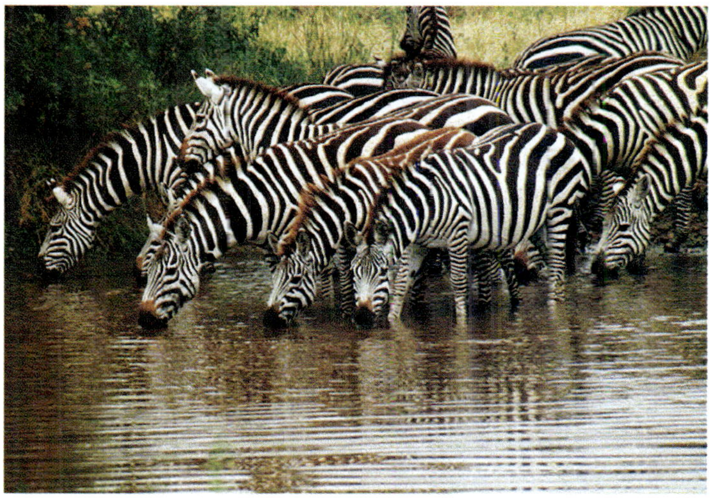

FIGURE 14.4 *Biological resources are renewable in that they replace themselves by reproduction, but if overused or misused, populations die. If a species is lost, it cannot be re-created. It is permanently lost as a component of its ecosystem and as a resource to humans.*

TABLE 14.1 Important Ecological Services

We depend on our environment to continually provide

1. A regulated global energy balance and climate; chemical composition of the atmosphere and oceans; water catchment and groundwater recharge; production, and recycling of organic and inorganic materials; maintenance of biological diversity.
2. Space and suitable substrates for human habitation, crop cultivation, energy conversion, recreation, and nature protection.
3. Oxygen, fresh water, food, medicine, fuel, fodder, fertilizer, building materials, and industrial inputs.
4. Aesthetic, spiritual, historic, cultural, artistic, scientific, and educational opportunities and information.

Source: Data from R. S. de Groot, *Investing in Natural Capital,* 1994.

expanded by technological improvements. New methods make it possible to mine very dilute metal ores, for example. Gold ore of extremely low concentrations is now economically recoverable—that is, you can make money on it—even though the price of gold has fallen because of greater efficiency, more discoveries, and resource substitution. Scarcity of resources, seen by classical economists as the trigger for conflict and suffering, can actually provide the impetus for much of the innovation that leads to substitution, recycling, and efficiency.

On the other hand, renewable resources can become exhausted if they are managed badly. This is especially apparent in biological resources, such as the passenger pigeon, American bison, and Atlantic cod. All these species once existed in extraordinary numbers, but within a few years, each was brought to the brink of extinction (or eliminated entirely) by overharvesting.

Scarcity and Limits to Growth

Are we about to run out of essential natural resources? It stands to reason that, if we consume a fixed supply of nonrenewable resources at a constant rate, we'll eventually use up all the economically recoverable reserves. There are many warnings in the environmental literature that our extravagant depletion of nonrenewable resources sooner or later will result in catastrophe, misery, and social decay. Models for exploitation rates of nonrenewable resources—called Hubbert curves after Stanley Hubbert, who developed them—often closely match historic experience for natural resource depletion (fig. 14.5).

Many economists, however, contend that human ingenuity and enterprise often allow us to respond to scarcity in ways that postpone or alleviate dire effects of resource use. The question of whether this view is right has to do with the important theme of **limits to growth.**

In the early 1970s an influential study of resource limitations was funded by the Club of Rome, an organization of wealthy business owners and influential politicians. The study was carried out by a team of scientists, from the Massachusetts Institute of Technology, headed by Donnela Meadows. The results of this study were published in the 1972 book *Limits to Growth.* A complex computer model of the world economy was used to examine various scenarios of different resource depletion rates, growing population, pollution, and industrial output. Given the Malthusian assumptions built into this model, catastrophic social and environmental collapse seemed inescapable.

Figure 14.6 shows one example of the world model. Food supplies and industrial output rise as population grows and resources are consumed. Once past the carrying capacity of the environment, however, a crash occurs as population, food production, and industrial output all decline precipitously. Pollution continues to grow as society decays and people die, but eventually it also falls. Notice the similarity between this set of curves and the "boom-and-bust" population cycles described in chapter 3.

Many economists criticized this model because it underestimated technological development and factors that might mitigate the effects of scarcity. In 1992 the Meadows group published updated computer models in *Beyond the Limits* that include technological progress, pollution abatement, population stabilization, and new public policies that work for a sustainable future. If we adopt these changes sooner rather than later, the models show an outcome like that in figure 14.7, in which all factors stabilize sometime in this century at an improved standard of living for everyone. Of course, none of these computer models shows what will happen, only what some possible outcomes might be, depending on the choices we make.

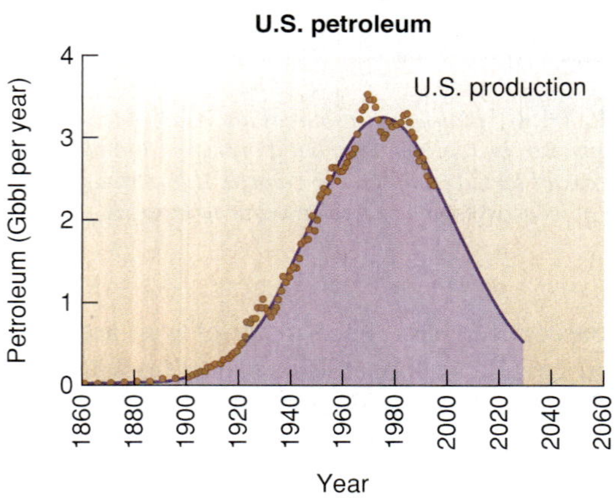

FIGURE 14.5 *U.S. petroleum production. Dots indicate actual production. The bell-shaped curve is a theoretical Hubbert curve for a nonrenewable resource. The shaded area under the curve, representing 220 Gbbl (Gbbl = Gigabarrels or billions of standard 42-gal barrels), is an estimate of the total economically recoverable resource.*

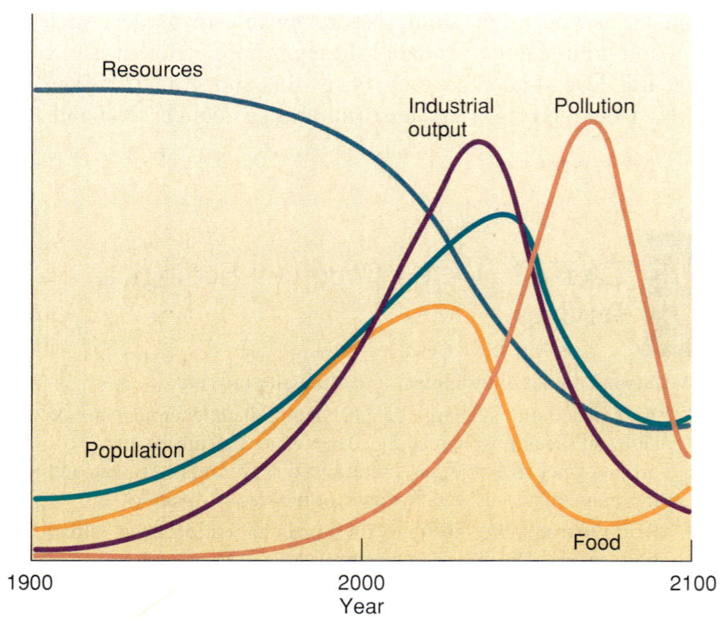

FIGURE 14.6 *A run of one of the world models in* Limits to Growth. *This model assumes business-as-usual for as long as possible until Malthusian limits cause industrial society to crash. Notice that pollution continues to increase well after industrial output, food supplies, and population have all plummeted.*

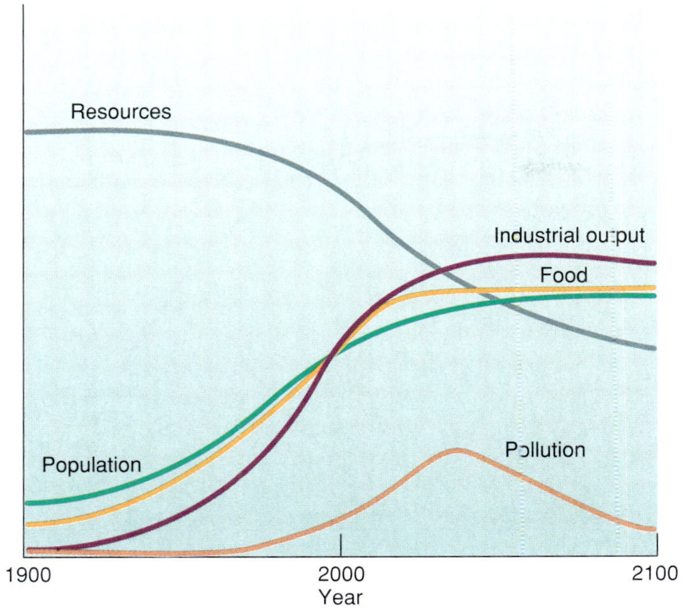

FIGURE 14.7 *A run of the world model from* Beyond the Limits. *This model assumes that population and consumption are curbed, new technologies are introduced, and sustainable environmental policies are embraced immediately, rather than after resources are exhausted.*

Communal Property and the Tragedy of the Commons

One of the difficulties of economics and resource management is that there are many resources we all share but nobody owns. Clean air, fish in the ocean, clean water, wildlife, and open space are all natural amenities that we exploit but that nobody clearly controls.

In 1968 biologist Garret Hardin wrote **"The Tragedy of the Commons,"** an article describing how commonly held resources are degraded and destroyed by self-interest. Using the metaphor of the "commons," or community pastures in colonial New England villages, Hardin theorized that it behooves each villager to put more cows on the pasture. Each cow brings more wealth to the individual farmer, but the costs of overgrazing are shared by the entire community. The individual farmer, then, suffers only part of the cost, but gets to keep all the profits from the extra cows s/he put on the pasture. Consequently, the commons becomes overgrazed, exhausted, and depleted. This dilemma is also known as the "free rider problem." The best solution, Hardin argued, is to give coercive power to the government or to privatize resources so that a single owner controls resource use.

This metaphor has been applied to many resources, especially to human population growth. It benefits every poor villager to produce a few more children, but collectively these children consume all the resources available, making us all poorer in the end. The same argument has been applied to many resource overuse problems, such as depletion of ocean fisheries, pollution, African famines, and urban crime.

Recent critics have pointed out that what Hardin was really describing was not a commons, or collectively owned and managed resource, but an **open access system,** in which there are no rules to manage resource use. In fact, many common resources have been managed successfully for centuries by cooperative agreements among users. Native American management of wild rice beds, Swiss village-owned mountain forests and pastures, Maine lobster fisheries, and communal irrigation systems in Spain, Bali, Laos, and many other countries have all remained viable under communal management.

Each of these "commons," or **communal resource management systems,** shares a number of features: (1) community members have lived on the land or used the resource for a long time and anticipate that their children and grandchildren will as well, thus giving them a strong interest in sustaining the resource and maintaining bonds with their neighbors; (2) the resource has clearly defined boundaries; (3) the community group size is known and enforced; (4) the resource is relatively scarce and highly variable, so that the community is forced to be interdependent; (5) the management strategies appropriate for local conditions have evolved over time and are collectively enforced; that is, those affected by the rules have a say in them; (6) the resource and its use are actively monitored, discouraging anyone from cheating or taking too much; (7) conflict resolution mechanisms reduce discord; and (8) incentives encourage compliance with rules, while sanctions for noncompliance keep community members in line.

Rather than being the only workable solution to problems in common pool resources, privatization and increasing external controls often prove to be disastrous. Where small villages have owned and operated local jointly held forests and fishing grounds for generations, nationalization and commodification of resources generally have led to rapid destruction of both society and ecosystems. Where communal systems once enforced restraint over harvesting, privatization encouraged narrow self-interest and allowed outsiders to take advantage of the weakest members of the community.

COST-BENEFIT ANALYSIS AND NATURAL RESOURCE ACCOUNTING

Decision making about sustainable resource use often entails **cost-benefit analysis (CBA),** the process of accounting and comparing the costs of a project and its benefits. Ideally, this process assigns values to social and environmental effects of a given undertaking, as well as the value of the resources consumed or produced. However, the results of CBA often depend on how resources are accounted for and measured in the first place. CBA is one of the main conceptual frameworks of resource economics, and it is used by decision makers around the world as a way of justifying the building of dams, roads, and airports, as well as in considering what to do about biodiversity loss, air pollution, and global climate change. CBA is a useful way of rational decision making about these projects. It is also widely disputed because it tends to discount the value of natural resources, ecological services, and human communities, and it is used to justify projects that jeopardize all these resources.

APPLICATION: Costs and Benefits

Figure 14.8 shows an example of the relative costs and benefits of reducing air pollution in Poland.

1. For the first 30 percent of reduction (on the X axis), benefits rise rapidly. What are some of the economic benefits that might be represented by this rising curve?
2. What might be some of the nearly free pollution reduction steps represented by the "costs" curve in the first 30 percent reduction?
3. If you were planning a budget, you would want to maximize benefits and minimize costs. For what percentage of pollution reduction would you aim? At what point would you redirect your budget to other priorities?

Answers: *1.* Benefits include improved health; less damage to buildings, crops, and materials; and improved quality of life. *2.* Conservation, improved planning and efficiency in transportation, buildings, and energy production; replacing old, inefficient industrial plants and vehicles. *3.* At any reduction up to 70 percent, benefits outweigh costs.

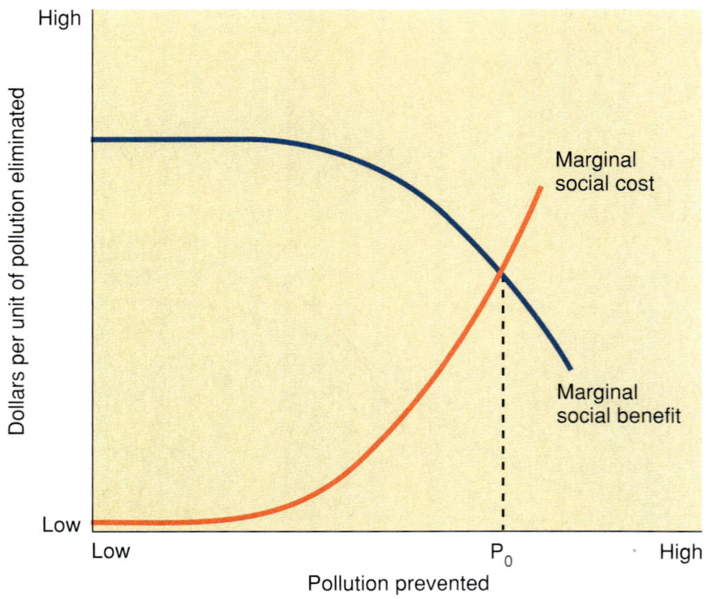

FIGURE 14.8 *To achieve maximum economic efficiency, regulations should require pollution prevention up to the optimum point (P_0) at which the costs of eliminating pollution just equal the social benefits of doing so.*

In CBA the monetary value of all benefits of a project are counted up and compared with the monetary costs of the project. Usually, the direct expenses of a project are easy to ascertain: how much will you have to pay for land, materials, and labor? The monetary worth of lost opportunities—to swim or fish in a river or to see birds in a forest—on the other hand, is much harder to appraise, as are inherent values of the existence of wild species or wild rivers. What is a bug or a bird worth, for instance, or the opportunity for solitude or inspiration? Eventually, the decision maker compares all the costs and benefits to see whether the project is justified or whether an alternative action might bring greater benefit at less cost.

Critics of CBA point out its absence of standards, inadequate attention to alternatives, and the placing of monetary values on intangible and diffuse or distant costs and benefits. Who judges how costs and benefits will be estimated? How can we compare things as different as the economic gain from cheap power with loss of biodiversity or the beauty of a free-flowing river? Critics claim that placing monetary values on everything could lead to a belief that only money and profits count and that any behavior is acceptable as long as you can pay for it. Sometimes speculative or even hypothetical results are given specific numerical values in CBA and then treated as if they were hard facts.

Figure 14.8 shows an example of a cost-benefit analysis for reducing particulate air pollution (soot) in Poland. As you can see, removing the highest 40 percent of particulates is highly cost effective. Approaching 70 percent particulate removal, however, the costs may exceed benefits. Data such as these can be useful to decision makers. On the other hand, this same study showed that controlling sulfur emissions had high costs and negligible benefits. Might this conclusion result from the ways "benefits" were evaluated?

Accounting for Nonmonetary Resources

Values such as wildlife, nonhuman ecological systems, and ecological services can be incorporated with natural resource accounting. In theory this accounting contributes to sustainable resource use because it can put a value on long-term or intangible goods that are necessary but often disregarded in economic decision making. One important part of natural resource accounting is assigning a value to ecological services (table 14.2). Another is using alternative measures of wealth and development. As mentioned earlier, GNP is a widely used measure of wealth that is based on rates of consumption and throughput. GNP doesn't account for natural resource depletion or ecosystem damage, however. The World Resources Institute, for example, estimates that soil erosion in Indonesia reduces the value of crop production about 40 percent per year. If natural capital were taken into account, Indonesian GNP would be reduced by at least 20 percent annually. Similarly, Costa Rica experienced impressive increases in timber, beef, and banana production between 1970 and 1990. But decreased natural capital during this period, represented by soil erosion, forest destruction, biodiversity losses, and accelerated water runoff, added up to at least $4 billion, or about 25 percent of annual GNP.

Measuring Real Progress

A number of systems have been proposed as alternatives to GNP that reflect genuine progress and social welfare. In their 1989 book, Herman Daly and John Cobb proposed a **genuine progress index (GPI),** which takes into account real per capita income,

TABLE 14.2 Estimated Annual Value of Ecological Services

ECOSYSTEM SERVICES	VALUE (TRILLION $ U.S.)
Soil formation	17.1
Recreation	3.0
Nutrient cycling	2.3
Water regulation and supply	2.3
Climate regulation (temperature and precipitation)	1.8
Habitat	1.4
Flood and storm protection	1.1
Food and raw materials production	0.8
Genetic resources	0.8
Atmospheric gas balance	0.7
Pollination	0.4
All other services	1.6
Total value of ecosystem services	33.3

Source: Adapted from R. Costanza et al., "The Value of the World's Ecosystem Services and Natural Capital," in *Nature*, vol. 387, 1997.

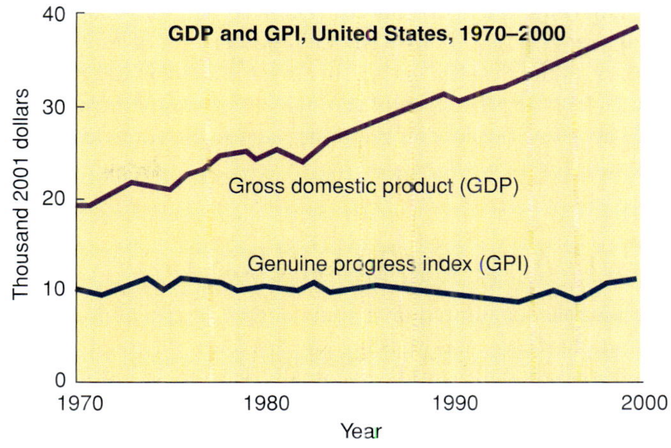

FIGURE 14.9 *Although per capita GDP in the United States nearly doubled between 1970 and 2000 in inflation-adjusted dollars, a genuine progress index that takes into account natural resource depletion, environmental damage, and options for future generations hardly increased at all.*
Source: Data from *Redefining Progress*, 2001.

quality of life, distributional equity, natural resource depletion, environmental damage, and the value of unpaid labor. They point out that, while per capita GDP in the United States nearly doubled between 1970 and 2000, per capita GPI increased only 4 percent (fig. 14.9). Some social service organizations would add to this index the costs of social breakdown and crime, which would decrease real progress even further over this time span.

The United Nations Development Program (UNDP) uses a benchmark called the human development index (HDI) to track social progress. HDI incorporates life expectancy, educational attainment, and standard of living as critical measures of development. Gender issues are accounted for in the gender development index (GDI), which is simply HDI adjusted or discounted for inequality or achievement between men and women.

In its annual Human Development Report, the UNDP compares country-by-country progress. As you might expect, the highest development levels are generally found in North America, Europe, and Japan. In 2003 Norway ranked first in the world in both HDI and GDI. The United States ranked seventh and Canada was eighth, although subtracting the HDI rank from GDP index placed Canada first in the world on an equity-adjusted basis. The 25 countries with the lowest HDI in 2003 were all in Africa. Haiti ranked the lowest in the Western Hemisphere.

Although poverty remains widespread in many places, encouraging news also can be found in development statistics. Poverty has fallen more in the past 50 years, the UNDP reports, than in the previous 500 years. Child death rates in developing countries as a whole have been more than halved. Average life expectancy has increased by 30 percent, while malnutrition rates have declined by almost a third. The proportion of children who lack primary school has fallen from more than half to less than a quarter. And the share of rural families without access to safe water has fallen from nine-tenths to about one-quarter.

Some of the greatest progress has been made in Asia. China and a dozen other countries with populations that add up to more than 1.6 billion have decreased the proportion of their people living below the poverty line by half. Still, in the 1990s the number of people with incomes less than $1 (U.S.) per day increased by almost 100 million to 1.3 billion—and the number appears to be growing in every region except Southeast Asia and the Pacific. Even in industrial countries, more than 100 million people live below the poverty line and 37 million are chronically unemployed.

Internal and External Costs

One of the factors that can make resource-exploiting enterprises look good in cost-benefit analysis is externalizing costs. **Externalizing costs** is the act of disregarding or discounting resources or goods that contribute to producing something but for which the producer does not actually pay. Usually, external costs are diffuse and difficult to quantify. Generally, they belong to society at large, not to the individual user. When a farmer harvests a crop in the fall, for example, the value of seeds, fertilizer, and the sale of the crop is tabulated; the value of soil lost to erosion, water quality lost to nonpoint-source pollution, and depleted fish populations is not accounted for. These are most often costs shared by the whole society, rather than borne by the resource user. They are external to the accounting system, and they are generally ignored in cost-benefit analysis—or when the farmer evaluates whether the year was profitable. Larger enterprises, such as dam building, logging, and road building, generally externalize the cost of ecological services lost along the way.

One way to use the market system to optimize resource use is to make sure that those who reap the benefits of resource use also bear all the external costs. This is referred to as **internalizing costs.** Calculating the value of ecological services or diffuse pollution is not easy, but it is an important step in sustainable resource accounting.

TRADE AND DEVELOPMENT

A sustainable society requires some degree of equitable resource distribution: if most wealth is held by just a few people, the misery and poverty of the majority eventually lead to social instability and instability of resource supplies. Accordingly, wealthy industrial nations have worked harder in recent decades to assist in developing the economies in poorer countries.

International Trade

Expanding trade relations has been promoted as a way to distribute wealth, stimulate economies around the world, and at the same time satisfy the desires of consumers in wealthy countries. According to the economic theory of *comparative advantage,* each place has some sort of goods or services it can sell cheaper, or better, than others can. International trade allows us to take advantage of all the best or cheapest products from around the world. If Egypt can produce cotton cheaper than Texas, then we should buy our cotton from Egypt. If Malaysia can manufacture athletic shoes with labor that costs a few cents an hour, then we should buy our shoes from Malaysia. Building factories in Malaysia also stimulates the Malaysian economy, even though workers earn only a small fraction of what a worker in a wealthy country would earn.

A problem with international trade is that it externalizes costs on a grand scale. Tropical hardwood products can be sold extremely cheaply in the United States—as lumber, plywood, shipping pallets, and so on. The environmental costs of producing those hardwood products occur far from the consumer who buys a piece of cheap Brazilian plywood. Making matters worse, the environmental costs of the plywood are usually exported to places where there are few legal controls on pollution and resource extraction. A factory in the United States, for example, is legally bound to minimize its production of air and water pollution. Pollution control can be expensive, and internalizing this cost makes a factory less profitable. A similar factory in Mexico might have far less responsibility for pollution control, making it cheaper, at least in the short term, to produce goods there than in the United States. Ongoing protests in the United States and elsewhere around the world against the World Trade Organization (WTO) and other forces of globalization have been largely about such exporting and externalizing of environmental and social costs of production. (See related story "The Battle in Seattle" at www.mhhe.com/cases.)

Another criticism of international trade is that the international banking systems that finance it are set up by and for the wealthy countries. The WTO and the General Agreement on Tariffs and Trade (GATT), for example, regulate 90 percent of all international trade. The WTO and GATT are both made up of relationships and agreements between corporations in a few very wealthy countries. Representatives of less powerful countries often charge that these agreements trap poorer regions into the role of suppliers of natural resources—timber, mineral ores, fruit, and cheap labor. These countries are forced to mine their natural capital for only small returns in wealth.

International Development and the World Bank

The World Bank has more influence on the financing and policies of developing countries than any other institution. Of some $25 billion loaned each year for Third World projects by multinational development banks, about two-thirds comes from the World Bank. This institution was founded in 1945 to provide aid to war-torn Europe and Japan. In the 1950s its emphasis shifted to development aid for Third World countries. This aid was justified on humanitarian grounds, but it also conveniently provided markets and political support for growing American and European multinational corporations.

The World Bank is jointly owned by 150 countries, but one-third of its support comes from the United States. Its president has always been an American. The bulk of its $66.8 billion capital comes from private investors. The bank makes loans for development projects, and the investors hope to make a profit on the investment, usually from interest paid on the loans.

Many World Bank projects have been environmentally destructive and highly controversial. In Botswana, for example, $18 million was provided to increase beef production for export by 20 percent, despite already severe overgrazing on fragile grasslands. The project failed, as had two previous beef production projects in the same area. In Ethiopia, rich floodplains in the Awash River Valley were flooded to provide electric power and irrigation water for cash export crops. More than 150,000 subsistence farmers were displaced, and food production was seriously reduced.

Recently, the World Bank has begun to attempt some environmental and social review of its loans. In part this change comes from demands from the U.S. Congress that projects be environmentally and socially benign. Whether this will improve the World Bank's track record remains to be seen.

Microlending

The World Bank deals in huge loans for massive projects. These are impressive to investors and to the countries that borrow the money. They are also a huge economic gamble, and on average the economic return on large loans has been quite low.

Recently, smaller, local lending programs have begun to develop. These are aimed at small-scale, widespread development, and their results have been very promising. The first of these was Bangladesh's Grammeen (village) Bank network. These banks make small loans, averaging just $67, to help poor people buy a sewing machine, a bicycle, a loom, a cow, or some other commodity that will help them start, or improve, a home business (fig. 14.10). Ninety percent of the customers are women, usually with no collateral or

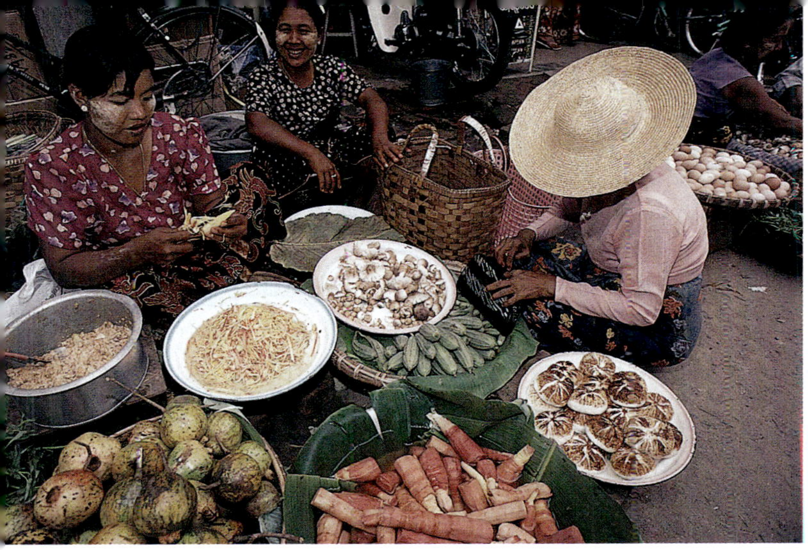

FIGURE 14.10 *A small loan can help start a business like this Indonesian woman's food stand.*

TABLE 14.3 Goals for an Eco-Efficient Economy

- Introduce no hazardous materials into the air, water, or soil.
- Measure prosperity by how much natural capital we can accrue in productive ways.
- Measure productivity by how many people are gainfully and meaningfully employed.
- Measure progress by how many buildings have no smokestacks or dangerous effluents.
- Make the thousands of complex governmental rules that now regulate toxic or hazardous materials unnecessary.
- Produce nothing that will require constant vigilance from future generations.
- Celebrate the abundance of biological and cultural diversity.
- Live on renewable solar income rather than fossil fuels.

steady income. Still, loan repayment rates are 98 percent—compared with only 30 percent at a conventional bank. This program enhances dignity, respect, and cooperation in a village community, and it teaches individual responsibility and enterprise.

Comparable programs have now sprung up around the world. In the United States, more than a hundred organizations have begun providing microloans and small grants for training. The Women's Self-Employment Project in Chicago, for instance, teaches job skills to single mothers in housing projects. Similarly, "tribal circle" banks on Native American reservations successfully finance microscale economic development projects.

GREEN BUSINESS AND GREEN DESIGN

Businesspeople and consumers are increasingly aware of the unsustainability of producing the goods we use every day. Recently, a number of business innovators have tried to develop green businesses, which produce environmentally and socially sound products. Environmentally conscious, or "green," companies, such as the Body Shop, Patagonia, Aveda, Malden Mills, Johnson and Johnson, and others, have shown that operating according to the principles of sustainable development and environmental protection can be good for public relations, employee morale, and sales (table 14.3).

Green business works because consumers are becoming aware of the ecological consequences of their purchases. Increasing interest in environmental and social sustainability has caused an explosive growth of green products. The *National Green Pages* published by Co-Op America currently lists more than 2,000 green companies. You can find eco-travel agencies, telephone companies that donate profits to environmental groups, entrepreneurs selling organic foods, shade-grown coffee, straw-bale houses, paint thinner made from orange peels, sandals made from recycled auto tires, and a plethora of hemp products, including burgers, ale, clothing, shoes, rugs, and shampoo. Although these eco-entrepreneurs represent a tiny sliver of the $7 trillion per year U.S. economy, they often are pioneers in developing new technologies and offering innovative services. Markets also grow over time: organic food marketing has grown from a few funky local co-ops to a $7 billion market segment. Most supermarket chains now carry some organic food choices. Similarly, natural-care health and beauty products reached $2.8 billion in sales in 1999 out of a $33 billion industry. By supporting these products, you can ensure that they will continue to be available and, perhaps, even help expand their penetration into the market.

Corporations committed to eco-efficiency and clean production include such big names as Monsanto, 3M, DuPont, and Duracell. Applying the famous three *R*s—reduce, reuse, recycle—these firms have saved money and gotten welcome publicity (see related story "Eco-Efficient Carpeting" at www.mhhe.com/cases). Savings can be substantial. Pollution-prevention programs at 3M, for example, have saved $857 million over the past 25 years. In a major public relations achievement, DuPont has cut its emissions of airborne cancer-causing chemicals almost 75 percent since 1987. Small operations can benefit as well. Stanley Selengut, owner of three eco-tourist resorts in the U.S. Virgin Islands, attributes $5 million worth of business to free press coverage about the resorts' green building features and sustainable operating practices.

Design for the Environment

Architects are starting to get on board the green bandwagon, too. Acknowledging that heating, cooling, lighting, and operating buildings is one of our biggest uses of energy and resources, architects such as William McDonough are designing "green office" projects. Among McDonough's projects are the Environmental Defense Fund headquarters in New York City; the Environmental Studies Center at Oberlin College in Ohio; the European headquarters for Nike in Hilversum, the Netherlands, and the Gap corporate offices in San Bruno, California (fig. 14.11). Each uses a combination of energy-efficient designs and technologies, including natural lighting and efficient water systems. The Gap office

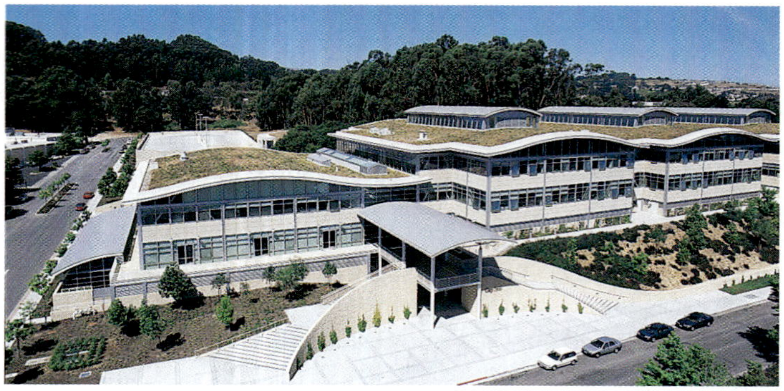

FIGURE 14.11 *The award-winning Gap, Inc. corporate offices in San Bruno, California, demonstrate some of the best features of environmental design. A roof covered with native grasses provides insulation and reduces runoff. Natural lighting, an open design, and careful relation to its surroundings make this a pleasant place to work.*

what can you do?

Personally Responsible Consumerism

Each of us can do many things to lower our ecological impacts and support "green" businesses through responsible consumerism and ecological economics.

- Practice living simply. Ask yourself if you really need more material goods to make your life happy and fulfilled.
- Rent, borrow, or barter when you can. Can you reduce the amount of stuff you consume by renting, instead of buying, machines and equipment you actually use only rarely?
- Recycle or reuse building materials: doors, windows, cabinets, appliances. Shop at salvage yards, thrift stores, yard sales, or other sources of used clothes, dishes, appliances, etc.
- Consult the *National Green Pages* from Co-Op America for a list of eco-friendly businesses. Write to companies from which you buy goods or services, and ask them what they are doing about environmental protection and human rights.
- Buy green products. Look for efficient, high-quality materials that will last and that are produced in the most environmentally friendly manner possible. Subscribe to clean-energy programs if they are available in your area. Contact your local utility and ask that it provide this option if it doesn't now.
- Buy locally grown or locally made products made under humane conditions by workers who receive a fair wage.
- Think about the total life-cycle costs of the things you buy, especially big purchases, such as cars. Try to account for the environmental impacts, energy use, and disposal costs, as well as initial purchase price.
- Stop junk mail. Demand that your name be removed from mass-mailing lists.
- Invest in socially and environmentally responsible mutual funds or "green" businesses when you have money for investment.

building, for example, is intended to promote employee well-being and productivity, as well as efficiency. It has high ceilings, abundant skylights, windows that open, a full-service fitness center (including pool), and a landscaped atrium for each office bay that brings the outside in. The roof is covered with native grasses. Warm interior tones and natural wood surfaces (all wood used in the building was harvested by certified sustainable methods) give a friendly feeling. Paints, adhesives, and floor coverings are low-toxicity, and the building is one-third more energy-efficient than strict California laws require. The pleasant environment helps improve employee effectiveness and retention. Gap, Inc., estimates that the increased energy and operational efficiency will have a four- to eight-year payback.

Jobs and the Environment

For years business leaders and politicians have portrayed environmental protection and jobs as mutually exclusive. They claim that pollution control, protection of natural areas and endangered species, and limits on use of nonrenewable resources will strangle the economy and throw people out of work. Ecological economists dispute this claim, however. Their studies show that only 0.1 percent of all large-scale layoffs in the United States in recent years were due to government regulations (fig. 14.12). Environmental protection, they argue, is not only necessary for a healthy economic system; it actually creates jobs and stimulates business.

Japan, already a leader in efficiency and environmental technology, has recognized the multibillion-dollar economic potential of "green" business. The Japanese government is investing $4 billion per year on research and development, and now it is selling about $12 billion worth of equipment and services per year worldwide. It is already marketing advanced waste incinerators, pollution-control equipment, alternative energy sources, and water treatment systems. The superefficient "hybrid" gas-electric cars only recently introduced to the U.S. market have been available in Japan for several years. Unfortunately, the United States has been resisting international pollution-control conventions, rather than recognizing the potential for economic growth and environmental protection in the field of "green" business.

URBAN DEVELOPMENT AND SUSTAINABLE CITIES

Understanding sustainable resource use and sustainable development requires paying some attention to cities. Cities are where most of our consumed resources end up (fig. 14.13). Nearly half the people in the world now live in urban areas, and in a century, 80 to 90 percent of us are expected to live in urban agglomerations. Cities have extraordinary, often disastrous impacts on the environment. They can also have beneficial environmental effects:

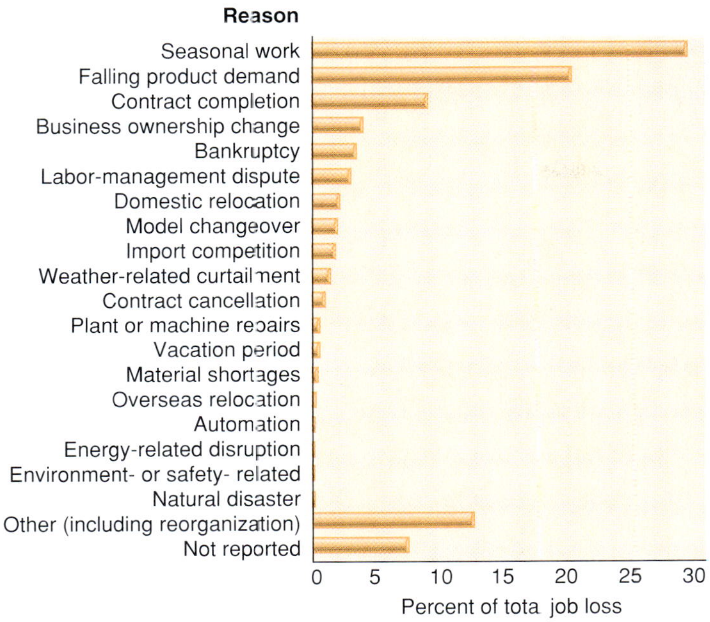

FIGURE 14.12 *Although opponents of environmental regulation often claim that protecting the environment costs jobs, studies by economist E. S. Goodstein show that only 0.1 percent of all large-scale layoffs in the United States were the result of environmental laws.*
Source: Data from E. S. Goodstein, Economic Policy Institute, Washington, D.C.

resource use is more efficient where people can share goods and services; less energy is spent in transportation and production when people don't have to travel too far. Some of the greatest promise for innovative improvements also comes from cities, where people are close enough together to share ideas and resources, to teach each other new methods of doing things, and to recognize the need for cooperative, collaborative environmental problem solving. In this section we will explore the ways that cities fail to be sustainable and look at some of the ways they might contribute to sustainability.

Urban Growth

Until recently, the vast majority of humanity has always lived in rural areas, where farming, fishing, hunting, timber harvesting, animal herding, mining, or other natural resource–based occupations were the main form of economic activity. Cities—where people live in high enough densities to have specialized professions—have always been the center of most political organization, economic power, and learning, but relatively few people have actually lived in cities.

Since the beginning of the industrial revolution some 300 years ago, however, cities have grown rapidly in both size and power. In every developing country, the transition from an agrarian society to an industrial one has been accompanied by **urbanization,** an increasing concentration of the population in cities and a transformation of land use and society to a metropolitan pattern of organization.

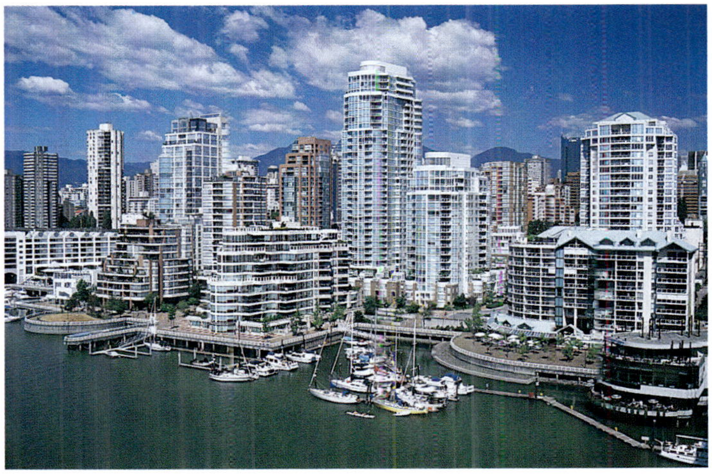

FIGURE 14.13 *For 6,000 years, cities have been centers of education, religion, politics, and economics. With industrialization and globalization, cities are now growing rapidly especially in the developing world. If present trends continue, most people will live in urban areas in a few decades.*

How big are cities? Some have only a few thousand people, but more and more cities are growing to extraordinary size (table 14.4). Many of the world's large cities have expanded until they merged with their neighbors to form giant urban complexes, also known as **megacities** or megalopolises. In the United States, urban areas between Boston and Washington, D.C., have merged into a nearly continuous megacity (sometimes called Bos-Wash), containing

TABLE 14.4 The World's Largest Urban Areas (Populations in Millions)

1900		2015**	
London, England	6.6	Tokyo, Japan	31.0
New York, USA	4.2	New York, USA	29.9
Paris, France	3.3	Mexico City	21.0
Berlin, Germany	2.4	Seoul, Korea	19.8
Chicago, USA	1.7	São Paolo, Brazil	18.5
Vienna, Austria	1.6	Osaka, Japan	17.6
Tokyo, Japan	1.5	Jakarta, Indonesia	17.4
St. Petersburg, Russia	1.4	Delhi, India	16.7
Philadelphia, USA	1.4	Los Angeles, USA	16.6
Manchester, England	1.3	Beijing, China	16.0
Birmingham, England	1.2	Cairo, Egypt	15.5
Moscow, Russia	1.1	Manila, Philippines	13.5
Peking, China*	1.1	Buenos Aires, Brazil	12.9

Source: Data from T. Chandler, *Three Thousand Years of Urban Growth,* 1974, Academic Press; and *World Gazetter,* 2003.
*Now spelled Beijing.
**Projected.

about 35 million people (fig. 14.14). The Tokyo-Yokohama-Osaka-Kobe corridor (referred to as Toko-hama) contains nearly 50 million people.

The United States underwent a dramatic rural-to-urban shift in the nineteenth and early twentieth centuries. In 1850 more than 90 percent of Americans lived in rural areas. A century later, only about one-third of the U.S. population was rural, and less than 5 percent were farmers. Now, many developing countries are experiencing a similar demographic movement. In 1850 only about 2 percent of the world's population lived in cities. By 2002 half the people in the world were urban. Only Africa and South Asia remain predominantly rural, but people there are swarming into cities in ever increasing numbers. About three-fourths of the people in Europe, North America, and Latin America already live in cities (table 14.5). Some urbanologists predict that by 2100 the whole world will be urbanized to the levels now seen in developed countries.

TABLE 14.5 Urban Share of Total Population (Percentage)

	1950	2000	2030*
Africa	18.4	40.6	57.0
Asia	19.3	43.8	59.3
Europe	56.0	75.0	81.5
Latin America	40.0	70.3	79.7
North America	63.9	77.4	84.5
Oceania	32.0	49.5	60.7
World	38.3	59.4	70.5

*Projected.
Source: Data from United Nations Population Division, 2003.

Cities in Developing Countries

Recent urban growth has been particularly dramatic in the large cities of the developing world. In 1900 13 cities had populations over 1 million; all except Tokyo and Peking were in Europe or North America (see table 14.4). By 1995 there were 235 metropolitan areas of more than 1 million people, but only 3 of the largest cities were in developed countries. Cities such as Mumbai, Jakarta, Manila, Cairo, and Mexico City receive thousands of new immigrants *every day.* Many of these large cities are expected to grow by 50 percent in just the next 25 years (fig. 14.15).

Ninety percent of the population growth over the next 25 years is expected to occur in the less-developed countries of the world (fig. 14.16). Most of that growth will be in the already overcrowded cities of the least affluent countries, such as India, China, Mexico, and Brazil. The combined population of these cities is expected to jump from its present 6 billion to more than 8 billion by the year 2025. Meanwhile, rural populations in these countries are expected to remain constant or even decline somewhat as rural people migrate into the cities.

Can cities function with 20 or 25 million people? Can they supply the public services necessary to sustain a civilized life? Adding 750,000 new people annually to Mexico City amounts to building a new city the size of Baltimore or San Francisco every year. This growth is occurring, as is most urban growth in the world, in a country with a sagging economy, an unstable government, and a high foreign debt load.

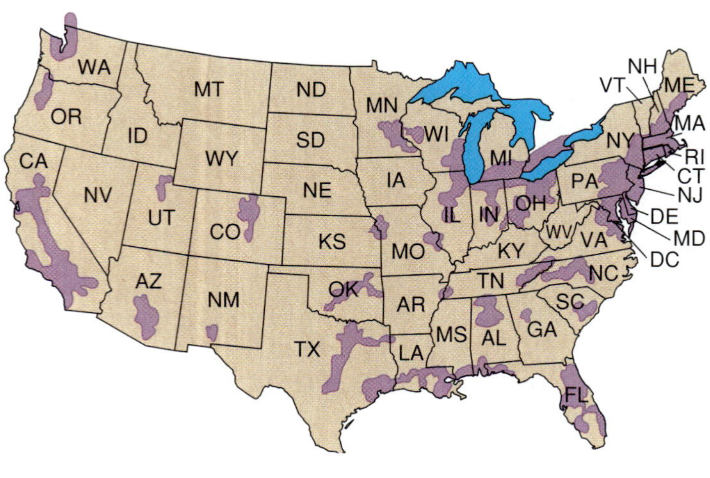

FIGURE 14.14 *Urban core agglomerations* (lavender areas) *are forming megalopolises in many areas. While open space remains in these areas, the flow of information, capital, labor, goods, and services links each into an interacting system.*
Source: Data from U.S. Census Bureau, 1998.

Causes of Urban Growth

Urban populations grow in two ways: by natural increase (more births than deaths) and by immigration. Natural increase is fueled by improved food supplies, better sanitation, and advances in medical care that reduce death rates and cause populations to grow both within cities and in the rural areas around them (see chapter 4). In Latin America and East Asia natural increase is responsible for two-thirds of urban population growth. In Africa and West Asia immigration is the largest source of urban growth. Immigration to cities can be caused both by **push factors** that force people out of the country and by **pull factors** that draw them into the city.

Immigration Push-and-Pull Factors

People migrate to cities for many reasons. In some areas the countryside is overpopulated and simply can't support more people. The "surplus" population is forced to migrate to cities in search of jobs, food, and housing. In some places economic forces or political, racial, or religious conflicts drive people out of their homes. Recent wars in Sierra Leone and the Congo, for example, depopulated the countryside and drove people into cities. The United Nations estimated that in 1992 at least 40 or 50 million people were displaced by political, economic, or social instability. Many

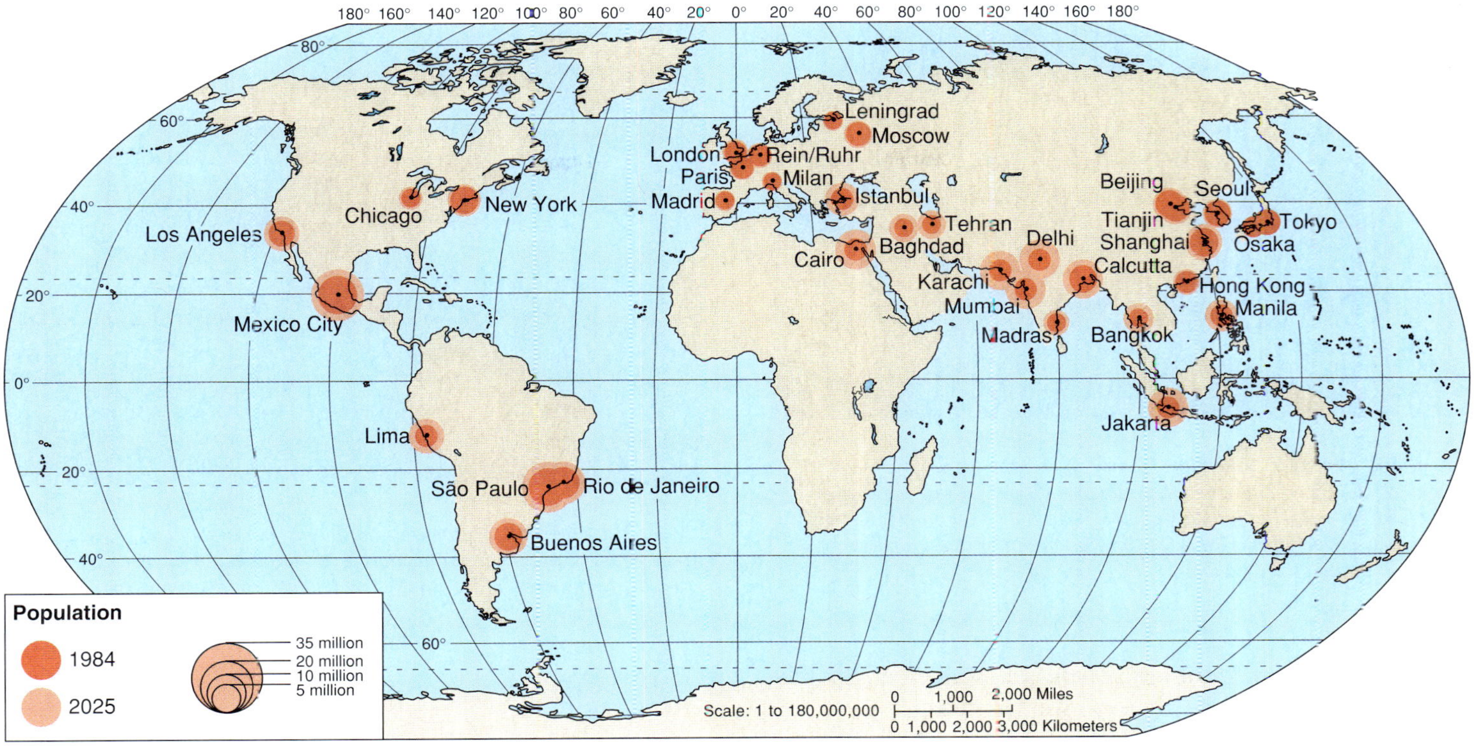

FIGURE 14.15 *By 2025 at least 400 cities will have populations of 1 million or more, and 93 supercities will have populations above 5 million. Three-fourths of the world's largest cities will be in developing countries that already have trouble housing, feeding, and employing their people.*

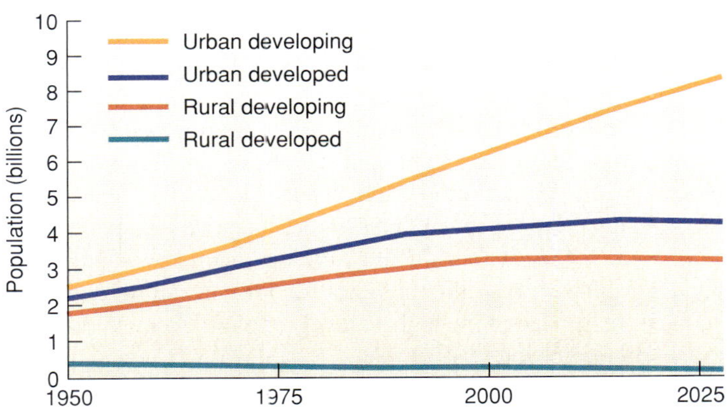

FIGURE 14.16 *Urban and rural growth in developed and developing countries.*

Source: Data from United Nations (UN) Population Division, *World Urbanization Prospects (The 1996 Revision),* on diskette (UN, New York, 1996).

of these refugees end up in the already overcrowded megacities of the developing world. Changes in agriculture also push people to cities. In the United States, mechanization of agriculture made much farm labor obsolete early in the twentieth century. The same forces displace people from the land in other countries today. Where farmland is owned by a minority of wealthy landlords, as is the case in many developing countries, peasants are often ejected when new cash crops or cattle grazing become economically viable.

Many people also move to the city because of the opportunities there. Cities offer jobs, housing, entertainment, and freedom from the constraints of village traditions. Possibilities exist in the city for upward social mobility, prestige, and power not ordinarily available in the country. Cities support specialization in arts, crafts, and professions for which markets don't exist elsewhere.

Modern communications also draw people to cities by broadcasting images of luxury and opportunity. An estimated 90 percent of the people in Egypt, for instance, have access to a television set. The immediacy of television makes city life seem more familiar and attainable than ever before (fig. 14.17). We generally assume that poor people in the streets of teeming Third World cities have no place else to go, but in spite of what appear to be dismal conditions, life in the city may be preferable to what the country had to offer.

Government Policies

Government policies often favor urban over rural areas in ways that both push and pull people into the cities. Developing countries commonly spend most of their budgets on improving urban areas (especially around the capital city, where leaders live). This gives the major cities a virtual monopoly on new jobs, housing, education, and opportunities, all of which bring in rural people searching for a better life. Lima, for example, has only 20 percent of Peru's population, but has 50 percent of the national wealth, 60 percent of the manufacturing, 65 percent of

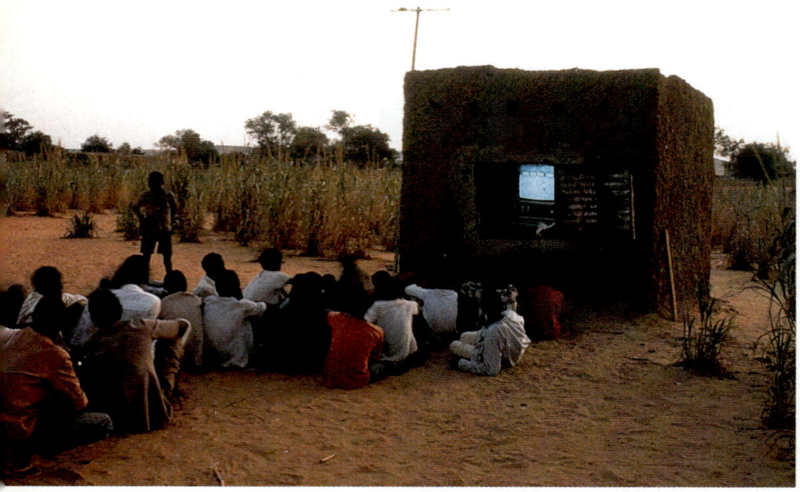

FIGURE 14.17 *Nine out of ten people in the world now have access to television. There may be only one TV per village, as in this scene from Nigeria, but it opens a window to the wider world. Most of what everyone watches is made in the United States and glorifies consumerism and materialism.*

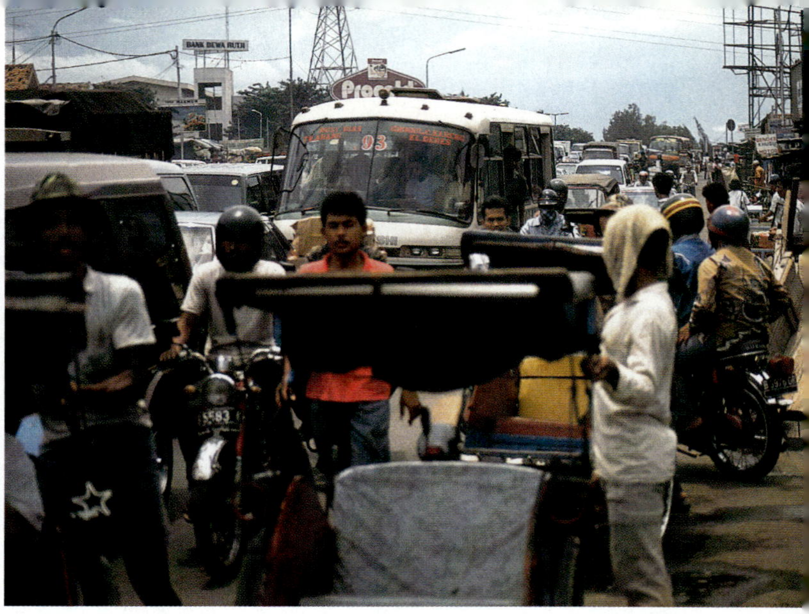

FIGURE 14.18 *Motorized rickshaws, motor scooters, bicycles, street vendors, and pedestrians all vie for space on the crowded streets of Jakarta. The heat, noise, smells, and sights are overpowering. In spite of the difficulties of living here, people work hard and have hope for the future.*

the retail trade, 73 percent of the industrial wages, and 90 percent of all banking in the country. Similar statistics pertain to São Paulo, Mexico City, Manila, Cairo, Lagos, Bogotá, and a host of other cities.

Governments often manipulate exchange rates and food prices for the benefit of more politically powerful urban populations, but at the expense of rural people. Importing lower-priced food pleases city residents, but local farmers then find it uneconomical to grow crops. As a result, an increased number of people leave rural areas to become part of a large urban workforce, keeping wages down and industrial production high. Zambia, for instance, sets maize prices below the cost of local production to discourage farming and to maintain a large pool of workers for the mines. Keeping the currency exchange rate high stimulates export trade but makes it difficult for small farmers to buy the fuels, machinery, fertilizers, and seeds they need. This depresses rural employment and rural income while stimulating the urban economy. The effect is to transfer wealth from the country to the city.

URBAN PROBLEMS IN DEVELOPING COUNTRIES

Cities in the developing world often lack the infrastructure, organization, stability, and political will to supply adequate food, water, housing, jobs, and basic services for their residents. Much of the problem arises from unplanned and uncontrollable growth, with which city governments cannot hope to keep up. A first-time visitor to a supercity—particularly in a less-developed country—is often overwhelmed by the immense crush of pedestrians and vehicles of all sorts that clog the streets. Jakarta, for instance, is one of the most densely populated cities in the world (fig. 14.18). Traffic is chaotic almost all the time. People often spend three or four hours each way commuting to work from outlying areas.

Air and Water Pollution

The dense traffic (commonly old, poorly maintained vehicles), smoky factories, and use of wood or coal fires for cooking and heating often create a thick pall of air pollution in Third World cities. Lenient pollution laws, corrupt officials, inadequate testing equipment, ignorance about the sources and effects of pollution, and lack of funds to correct dangerous situations usually exacerbate the problem. What is its human toll? An estimated 60 percent of Calcutta's residents are thought to suffer from respiratory diseases linked to air pollution. Lung cancer mortality in Shanghai is reported to be four to seven times higher than rates in the countryside. Mexico City, which sits in a high mountain bowl with abundant sunshine, little rain, high traffic levels, and frequent air stagnation, has one of the highest levels of photochemical smog in the world (see chapter 9).

Few cities in developing countries can afford to build modern waste treatment systems for their rapidly growing populations. The World Bank estimates that only 35 percent of urban residents in developing countries have satisfactory sanitation services. The situation is especially desperate in Latin America, where only 2 percent of urban sewage receives any treatment. In Egypt, Cairo's sewer system was built about 50 years ago to serve a population of 2 million people. It is now being overwhelmed by more than 10 million people. Less than one-tenth of India's 3,000 towns and cities have even partial sewage systems and water treatment facilities. Some 150 million of India's urban residents lack access to sanitary sewer systems. In Colombia, the Bogotá River, 200 km (125 mi) downstream from Bogotá's 5 million residents, still has an average fecal bacteria count of 7.3 million cells per liter, more than 700,000 times the safe drinking level and 3,500 times higher than the safe limit for swimming.

INVESTIGATING Our Environment

Urban Ecology

Traditionally, most ecologists have studied pristine, natural ecosystems, trying to understand how nature works without human disturbance. In recent years, however, we have come to recognize that cities are ecological systems, too. If ecology is the relationship among organisms and their environment, what could be more ecological than studying the organism (humans) with the greatest impact on other species and our environment? As the human population becomes increasingly urbanized, perhaps the most important place to study human ecology is in cities. Rather than merely seeing humans as disturbing factors, some scientists are beginning to gather data on how urban ecosystems work.

Urban areas share many characteristics with natural ecosystems. Energy flows into and out of the city, and is degraded and dispersed as it is used to do work. Materials are used to create structures, some living and some nonliving. Species compete for shelter, food, habitat, and other resources. The most successful species flourish and proliferate; less fit ones dwindle and eventually vanish. Every day, a typical American city of a million people consumes roughly 1 million metric tons (roughly 2 billion lbs) of raw materials. This urban material flow includes 500,000 m^3 (1.3 million gal) of water, the energy equivalent of about 20,000 metric tons of fossil fuels, 13,000 metric tons of other minerals (including food packaging and construction materials), 12,000 metric tons of farm products, and 10,000 metric tons of wood and paper products.

To remove municipal waste from this city of a million residents, about 1,000 fully loaded garbage trucks travel every day to rural areas carrying the discarded remnants of this urban metabolism. In addition, the city's municipal wastewater treatment plants discharge somewhat more than 500,000 m^3 of water (that lost to evaporation is offset by precipitation and solids added to the wastewater stream). You may remember from chapter 2 that most natural ecosystems recycle materials. Recycling and reuse also occur in urban ecology, although rarely with the speed and efficiency of natural systems.

Urban biodiversity and wildlife also can be important. While many biologists have tended to assume that cities are devoid of life other than humans and our domesticated companion animals and plants, we are now beginning to appreciate that urban open space can be essential refuges for wild creatures as well. As cities grow, it's not uncommon for consolidated urban areas to be more than 100 miles (160 km) across. This would present an insurmountable barrier to many migrating animals if the city consists of nothing but concrete, glass, and metal. Urban parks, forests, corridors along rivers, and even ordinary yards, if managed properly, can provide a refuge for migrating wildlife and can sustain local populations that contribute significantly to overall biodiversity. Planting native vegetation and designing landscapes to provide maximum food and shelter are important steps in protecting and promoting urban biodiversity.

Long-term ecological research (LTER) sites are ecologically significant sites identified and funded by the National Science Foundation to allow long-term, in-depth research on ecological problems and questions. Although most of the LTER sites are in remote locations, where nature has minimal human interference, two LTER sites were set up in Phoenix and Baltimore. Funded by the National Science Foundation for an initial period of six years at nearly a million dollars per year, but with an understanding that the research will go on much beyond that, these projects use modern technology to study every aspect of urban ecology. How does the city shape its own weather? What plants and animals live in the city, and where, and how? What ecological processes cycle materials and energy? How do human activities influence those processes?

One of the first things that scientists are discovering is that cities are not homogenous; like other ecosystems, they have shifting patches of contrasting conditions. Using computer models and sophisticated mapping techniques, ecologists can explore how patches change in space and time. Elsewhere, environmental scientists have investigated important problems of pollution and environmental health in cities. Where are toxic and hazardous materials generated, stored, and released in the city? How do they move around and where do they accumulate?

In Detroit, a group of students worked with experts to map data on more than 5,000 children with elevated blood lead levels. Not surprisingly, they found a correlation between low incomes, old housing, incidence of poisoning, and concentration of special-education students. Sometimes public awareness of a problem is one of the best outcomes of this research. Another large group of students in the Detroit area used geographic information systems (digital maps) together with chemical and biological analysis to prepare a detailed study of water quality and ecosystem health in the Rouge River. Perhaps students at your school could organize a similar study of the urban ecology in your area.

Worldwide, clean water is more available to urban people than to rural people, but access to good water is a major problem. Available water is often unsafe, and diarrhea, dysentery, typhoid, and other waterborne diseases are common. Many rivers and streams in Third World countries are little more than open sewers, yet they are all that poor people have for washing clothes, bathing, cooking, and—in the worst cases—drinking.

Housing

The United Nations estimates that at least 1 billion people—20 percent of the world's population—live in crowded, unsanitary slums of the central cities and in the vast shantytowns and squatter settlements that ring the outskirts of most Third World cities. Around 100 million people have no home at all. In Mumbai, India, for example, it is estimated that a half million people sleep on the streets, sidewalks, and traffic circles because they can find no other place to live (fig 14.19).

Slums provide housing to large populations. These are generally legal but inadequate multifamily tenements or rooming houses, often converted from some other use. Families live crowded in small rooms with inadequate ventilation and sanitation. Often, the structures are rickety and unsafe.

Shantytowns, with shacks built of corrugated metal, discarded packing crates, brush, plastic sheets, and other scavenged materials, develop on the outskirts of most large Third World cities. Shantytowns are illegal, but they quickly fill in the unoccupied edges of town, where squatters (illegal residents) can build shelters close to jobs in the city. Many governments try to clean out illegal settlements by bulldozing the huts and sending riot

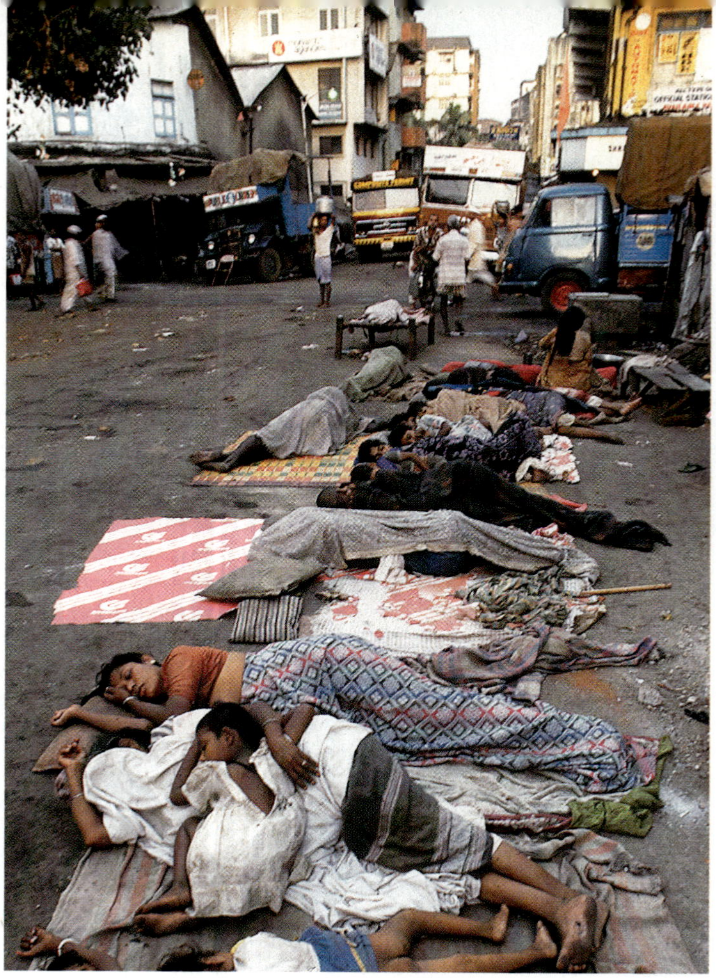

FIGURE 14.19 *In Mumbai, India, as many as half a million people sleep on the streets because they have no other place to live. Ten times as many live in crowded, dangerous slums and shantytowns throughout the city.*

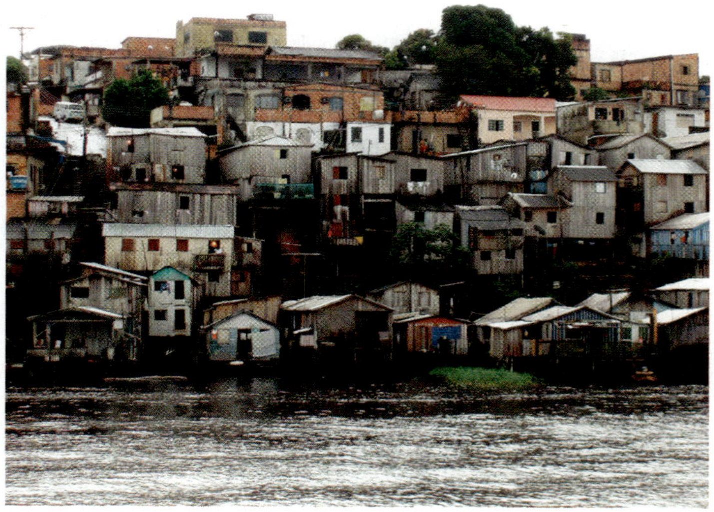

FIGURE 14.20 *Shantytowns called* favelas *perch on hillsides above the Amazon in Manaus, Brazil.*

police to drive out the settlers, but the people either move back in or relocate to another shantytown. Two-thirds of the population of Calcutta live in unplanned squatter settlements, and nearly half of the 20 million people in Mexico City live in uncontrolled, unauthorized shantytowns. Often, shantytowns occupy dangerous ground: in Bhopal, India, and Mexico City, for example, squatter settlements were built next to deadly industrial sites. In Brazil shantytowns called *favelas* perch on steep hillsides unwanted for other building (fig. 14.20). As desperate and inhumane as conditions are in these slums and shantytowns, many people do more than merely survive there. They keep themselves clean, raise families, educate their children, find jobs, and save a little money to send home to their parents.

Many of the worst urban environmental problems of the more-developed countries have been substantially reduced in recent years. Improved sanitation and medical care have reduced or totally eliminated many of the communicable diseases that once afflicted urban residents. Air and water quality have improved dramatically as heavy industry, such as steel smelting and chemical manufacturing, have moved to developing countries. In consumer and information economies, workers no longer need to be concentrated in central cities. They can live and work in dispersed sites. Automobiles now make it possible for the working class to enjoy amenities such as single-family houses, yards, and access to recreation that once were available only to the elite.

In the United States, some of the most rapidly growing metropolitan areas—such as Phoenix, Arizona; Princeton, New Jersey; Orlando, Florida; Montgomery County, Maryland; and San Jose, California—are centers for high-technology companies located in landscaped suburban office parks. These cities often lack a recognizable downtown, being organized instead around low-density housing developments, national-chain shopping malls, and extensive freeway networks. For many high-tech companies, being located near industrial centers and shipping hubs is less important than a good climate, ready access to air travel, and amenities such as natural beauty and open space.

Old manufacturing cities, such as Philadelphia and Detroit, have suffered declining populations and infrastructure as their industrial base fades away (fig. 14.21). In some "rust belt" cities, up to half of inner-city housing and commercial property is abandoned and derelict. This presents an opportunity for redevelopment of brownfields (polluted industrial areas) and construction of new housing and urban parks, but financing these projects is difficult as tax revenues decline.

Urban Sprawl

While the move to suburbs and rural areas has brought many benefits to the average citizen, it also has caused numerous urban problems. Cities that once were compact now spread over the landscape, consuming open space and wasting resources. This pattern of urban growth is known as **sprawl.** While there is no universally accepted definition of the term, sprawl generally includes the characteristics outlined in table 14.6.

In most American metropolitan areas, the bulk of new housing is in large, tract developments that leapfrog out beyond the

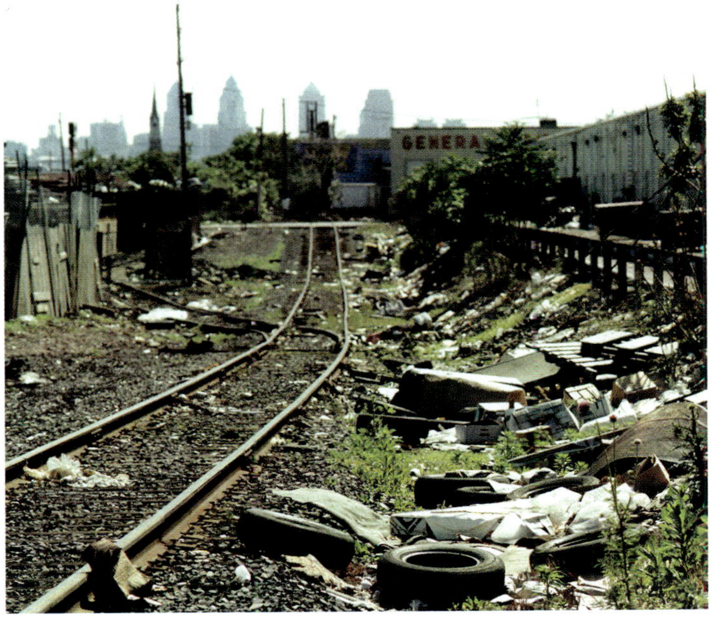

FIGURE 14.21 *In many older American cities, flight to the suburbs has left large areas of pollution and urban decay in the inner city.*

TABLE 14.6 Characteristics of Urban Sprawl

1. Unlimited outward extension
2. Low-density residential and commercial development
3. Leapfrog development that consumes farmland and natural areas
4. Fragmentation of power among many small units of government
5. Dominance of freeways and private automobiles
6. No centralized planning or control of land uses
7. Widespread strip-malls and "big-box" shopping centers
8. Great fiscal disparities among localities
9. Reliance on deteriorating older neighborhoods for low-income housing
10. Decaying city centers as new development occurs in previously rural areas

Source: Data from PlannersWeb, Burlington, Vermont, 2001.

edge of the city in a search for inexpensive rural land with few restrictions on land use or building practices (fig. 14.22). The U.S. Department of Housing and Urban Development estimates that urban sprawl consumes some 200,000 ha (roughly 500,000 acres) of farmland each year. With planning authority divided among many small, local jurisdictions, most metropolitan areas have no way to regulate growth or provide for rational, efficient resource use. Small towns and township or county officials generally welcome this growth because it profits local landowners and businesses. Although the initial price of tract homes often is less than comparable urban property, there are external costs in the form of new roads, sewers, water mains, power lines, schools, shopping centers, and other infrastructure required by this low-density development. Ironically, people who move out to rural areas to escape from urban problems such as congestion, crime, and pollution often find that they have simply brought those problems with them. A neighborhood that seemed tranquil and remote when they first moved in soon becomes just as crowded, noisy, and difficult as the city they left behind as more people join them in their rural retreat.

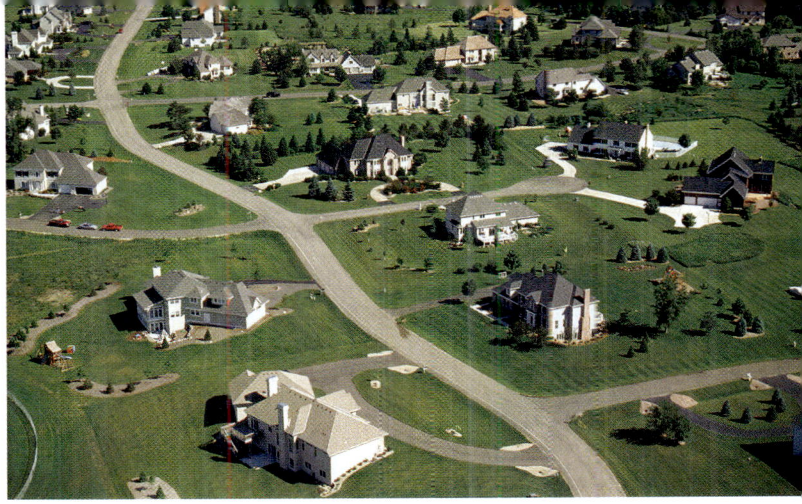

FIGURE 14.22 *Huge houses on sprawling lots consume land, alienate us from our neighbors, and make us ever more dependent on automobiles.*

Because many Americans live far from where they work, shop, and recreate, they consider it essential to own a private automobile. The average U.S. driver spends about 443 hours per year behind a steering wheel. This means that, for most people, the equivalent of one full 8-hour day per week is spent sitting in an automobile. Building the roads, parking lots, filling stations, and other facilities needed for an automobile-centered society takes a vast amount of space and resources. In some metropolitan areas, one-third of all land is devoted to the automobile. To make it easier for suburban residents to get from their homes to jobs and shopping, we provide an amazing network of freeways and highways. At a cost of several trillion dollars to build, the interstate highway system was designed to allow us to drive at high speeds from source to destination without ever having to stop.

As more and more drivers clog the highways, the reality is far different. In Los Angeles, for example, which has the worst congestion in the United States, the average speed in 1982 was 58 mph (93 km/hr) and the average driver spent less than 4 hours per year in traffic jams. In 2002 the average speed in Los Angeles was half that of 20 years earlier, and the typical driver spent 136 hours per year in bumper-to-bumper traffic. Although new automobiles are much more efficient and cleaner-operating than those of a few decades ago, the fact that we drive so much farther today and spend so much more time idling in stalled traffic means that we burn more fuel and produce more pollution than ever before.

Altogether, traffic congestion costs the United States $78 billion per year in wasted time and fuel. Some people argue that the existence of traffic jams in cities shows that more freeways are needed. Often, however, building more traffic lanes simply encourages more people to drive farther than before. Rather than ease congestion and save fuel, more freeways can exacerbate the problem (fig. 14.23).

Smart Growth

Are there alternatives to unplanned sprawl and wasteful resource use? One option proposed by many urban planners is **smart growth,** which makes effective use of land resources and existing infrastructure by encouraging in-fill development that avoids costly duplication of services and inefficient land use (table 14.7). Smart growth aims to provide a mix of land uses to create a variety of affordable housing choices and opportunities. It also attempts to provide a variety of transportation choices, including pedestrian-friendly neighborhoods. This approach to planning also seeks to maintain a unique sense of place by respecting local cultural and natural features.

By making land-use planning open and democratic, smart growth makes urban expansion fair, predictable, and cost-effective.

TABLE 14.7 Goals for Smart Growth

1. Create a positive self-image for the community.
2. Make the downtown vital and livable.
3. Alleviate substandard housing.
4. Solve problems with air, water, toxic waste, and noise pollution.
5. Improve communication between groups.
6. Improve community member access to the arts.

Source: Data from Vision 2000, Chattanooga, Tennessee.

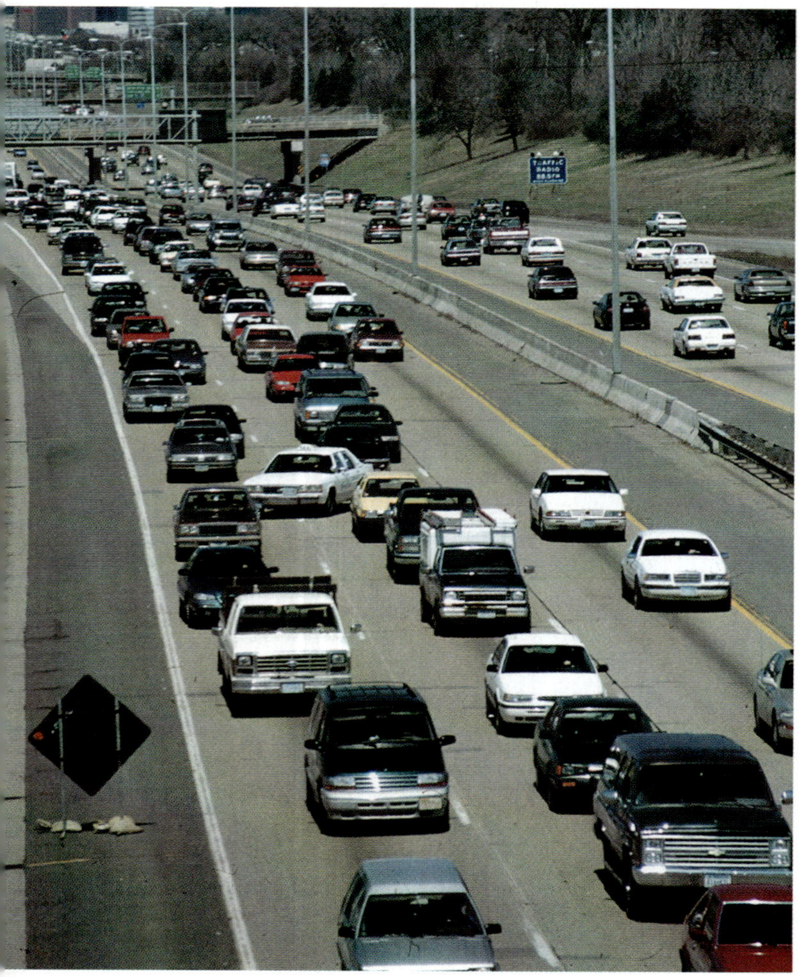

FIGURE 14.23 *Building freeways to reduce congestion is like trying to diet by loosening your belt.*

All stakeholders are encouraged to participate in creating a vision for the city and to collaborate with rather than confront each other. Goals are established for staged and managed growth in urban transition areas with compact development patterns. This approach is not opposed to growth. It recognizes that the goal is not to block growth but to channel it to areas where it can be sustained over the long term. Smart growth strives to enhance access to equitable public and private resources for everyone and to promote the safety, livability, and revitalization of existing urban and rural communities.

Smart growth protects environmental quality. It tries to reduce traffic and to conserve farmlands, wetlands, and open space. As cities grow and transportation and communications enable more community interaction, the need for regional planning becomes greater and more pressing. Community and business leaders must make decisions based on a clear understanding of regional growth needs and how infrastructure can be built most efficiently and for the greatest good.

One of the best examples of successful urban land-use planning in the United States is Portland, Oregon, which has rigorously enforced a boundary on its outward expansion, requiring instead that development be focused on in-filling unused space within the city limits. Because of its many urban amenities, Portland is considered one of the best cities in America. Between 1970 and 1990 the Portland population grew by 50 percent, but its total land area grew only 2 percent. During this time, Portland property taxes decreased 29 percent and vehicle miles traveled increased only 2 percent. By contrast, Atlanta, which had similar population growth, experienced an explosion of urban sprawl that increased its land area three-fold, drove up property taxes 22 percent, and increased traffic miles by 17 percent. A result of this expanding traffic and increasing congestion was that Atlanta's air pollution increased by 5 percent, while Portland, which has one of the best public transit systems in the nation, saw a decrease of 86 percent.

Urban Sustainability in the Developed World

Rather than abandon the cultural history and infrastructure investment in existing cities, a group of architects and urban planners is attempting to redesign metropolitan areas to make them more appealing, efficient, and livable. European cities such as Stockholm, Sweden; Helsinki, Finland; Leichester, England; and Neerlands, the Netherlands, have a long history of innovative urban planning. In the United States, Andres Duany, Elizabeth Plater-Zyberk, Peter Calthorpe, and Sym Van Der Ryn have been leaders in this movement. Using what is sometimes called a neo-traditionalist approach, these designers attempt to recapture some of the best features of small towns and livable cities of the past. They are designing urban neighborhoods that integrate houses, offices, shops, and civic buildings. Ideally, no house should be more than a five-minute walk from a neighborhood center with a convenience store, a coffee shop, a bus stop, and other amenities. A mix of apartments, townhouses, and detached houses in a variety of price ranges ensures that neighborhoods will include a diversity of ages and income levels (fig. 14.24). Some design principles of this movement include

- Limit city size or organize cities in modules of 30,000 to 50,000 people—large enough to be a complete city but small enough to be a community.
- Maintain greenbelts in and around cities. These provide recreational space and promote efficient land use, as well as help ameliorate air and water pollution.
- Determine in advance where development will take place. This protects property values and prevents chaotic development. Planning can also protect historical sites, agricultural resources, and ecological services of wetlands, clean rivers, and groundwater replenishment.
- Locate everyday shopping and services so people can meet daily needs with greater convenience, less stress, less automobile dependency, and less use of time and energy. This might be accomplished by encouraging small-scale commercial development in or close to residential areas.
- Encourage walking or the use of small, low-speed, energy-efficient vehicles (microcars, motorized tricycles, bicycles, etc.) for many local trips now performed in full-size automobiles. Creating special traffic lanes, reducing the number or size of parking spaces, and closing shopping streets to big cars might encourage such alternatives.
- Promote more diverse, flexible housing as an alternative to conventional detached, single-family houses. In-fill building between existing houses saves energy, reduces land costs, and might help provide a variety of living arrangements. Allowing single-parent families or groups of unrelated adults to share housing and to use facilities cooperatively also provides alternatives to those not living in a traditional nuclear family.
- Make cities more self-sustainable by growing food locally, recycling wastes and water, using renewable energy sources, reducing noise and pollution, and creating a cleaner, safer environment. Encourage community gardening. Reclaimed inner-city space or a greenbelt of agricultural and forestland around the city provides food and open space, and also contributes valuable ecological services, such as purifying air, supplying clean water, and protecting wildlife habitat and recreation land.
- Invite public participation in decision making. Emphasize local history, culture, and environment to create a sense of community and identity. Create local networks in which residents take responsibility for crime prevention fire protection, and home care of children and the elderly, sick, and disabled. Coordinate regional planning through metropolitan boards that cooperate with but do not supplant local governments.
- Plan cluster housing, or open-space zoning, which preserves at least half of a subdivision as natural areas, farmland, or other forms of open space. Studies have shown that people who move to the country don't necessarily want to live miles from the nearest neighbor; what most desire is long views across an interesting landscape and an opportunity to see wildlife. By carefully clustering houses on smaller lots, a conservation subdivision can provide the same number of buildable lots as a conventional subdivision and still preserve 50 to 70 percent of the land as open space (fig. 14.25, right). This not only reduces development costs (less distance to build roads, lay telephone lines, sewers, power cables, etc.) but also helps to foster a greater sense of community among new residents.
- Preserve urban habitat. It can make a significant contribution toward saving biodiversity as well as improving mental health and giving us access to nature.

These planning principles aren't just a matter of esthetics. Dr. Richard Jackson, former director of the National Center for Environmental Health in Atlanta, points out a strong association between urban design and our mental and physical health. As our cities have become ever more spread out and impersonal, we have fewer opportunities for healthful exercise and socializing. Chronic diseases, such as cardiovascular diseases, asthma, diabetes, obesity, and depression, are becoming the predominant health concerns in the United States.

"Despite common knowledge that exercise is healthful," Dr. Jackson says, "fewer than 40% of adults are regularly active, and

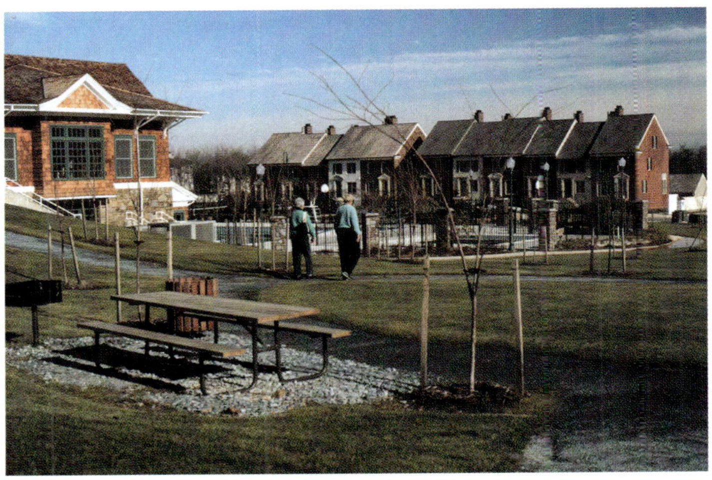

FIGURE 14.24 *By clustering buildings together, Kentlands, Maryland, has maintained a high percentage of open space as public commons.*

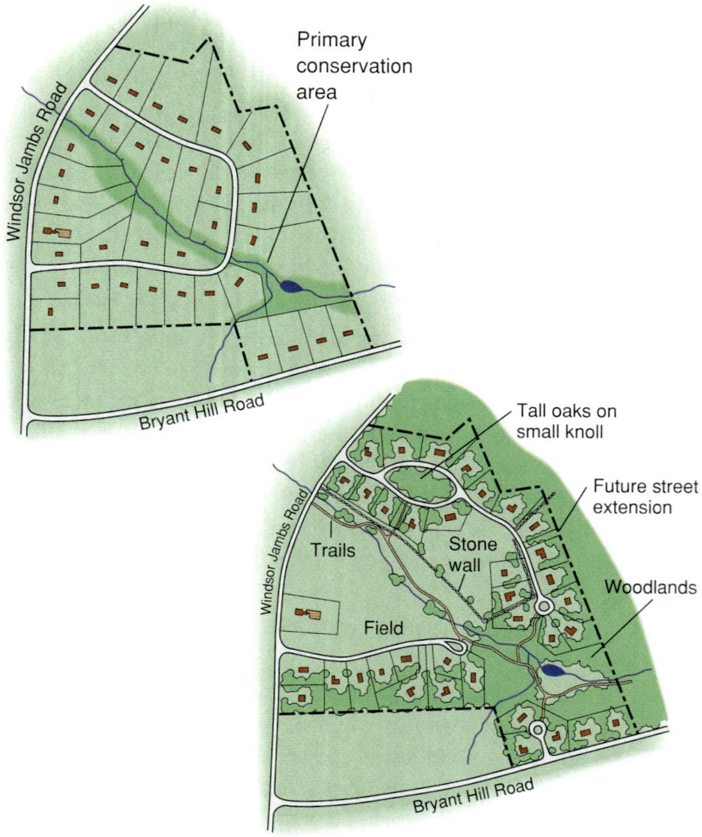

FIGURE 14.25 *Conventional subdivision* (left) *and an open-space plan* (right). *Although both plans provide 36 home sites, the conventional development allows for no open space. Cluster housing on smaller lots in the open-space design preserves at least half of the area as woods, prairie, wetlands, farms, or other conservation lands, while providing residents with more attractive vistas and recreational opportunities than a checkerboard development.*

25% do no physical activity at all. The way we design our communities makes us increasingly dependent on automobiles for the shortest trip, and recreation has become not physical but observational." Long commutes and a lack of reliable mass transit and walkable neighborhoods mean that we spend more and more time in stressful road congestion. "Road rage" isn't imaginary. Every commuter can describe unpleasant encounters with rude drivers. Urban design that offers the benefits of more walking, more social contact, and surroundings that include water and vegetation can provide healthful physical exercise and psychic respite.

Sustainable Development in the Third World

What can be done to improve conditions in Third World cities? Curitiba, Brazil (described at the beginning of this chapter), is an outstanding example of what can be done, even in relatively undeveloped countries, to improve transportation, protect central cities, and create a sense of civic pride. Other cities have far to go, however, to reach this standard. Among the immediate needs are housing, clean water, sanitation, food, education, health care, and basic transportation for their residents. The World Bank estimates that improved living conditions in urban households in the developing world could vastly increase health and productivity worldwide.

Some countries, recognizing the need to use vacant urban land, are redistributing unproductive land or closing their eyes to illegal land invasions. Indonesia, Peru, Tanzania, Zambia, and Pakistan have learned that squatter settlements make a valuable contribution to meeting national housing needs. Squatters' rights are being upheld in some cases, and such services as water, sewers, schools, and electricity are being provided to the settlements (fig. 14.26). Some countries intervene directly in land distribution and land prices. Tunisia, for instance, has a "rolling land bank" to buy and sell land. This strong and effective program controls urban land prices and reduces speculation and unproductive land ownership.

Many planners argue that social justice and sustainable economic development are answers to the urban problems discussed in this chapter. If people have the opportunity and money to buy better housing, adequate food, clean water, sanitation, and other things they need for a decent life, they will do so. Democracy, security, and improved economic conditions help in slowing population growth and reducing rural-to-city movement. An even more important measure of progress may be institution of a social welfare safety net guaranteeing that old or sick people will not be abandoned and alone.

Some countries have accomplished these goals even without industrialization and high incomes. Sri Lanka, for instance, has lessened the disparity between the core and periphery of the country. Giving all people equal access to food, shelter, education, and health care eliminates many incentives for interregional migration. Both population growth and city growth have been stabilized, even though the per capita income is only $800 (U.S.) per year. China has done something similar on a per capita income of around $300 (U.S.) per year.

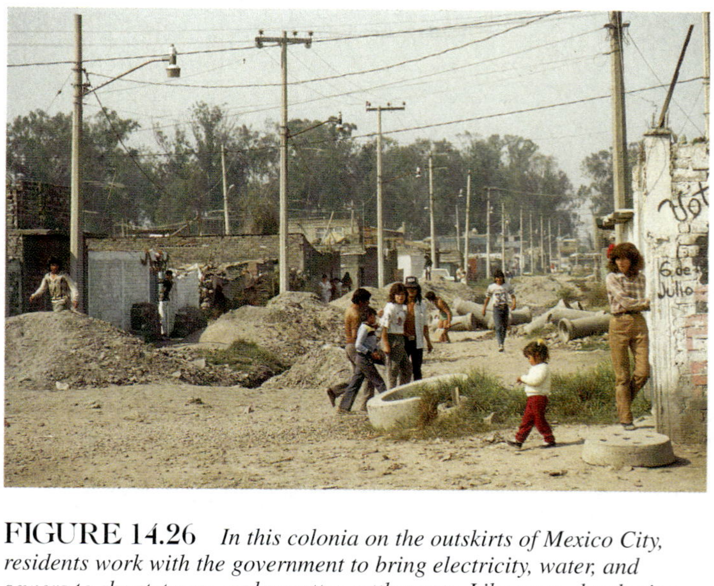

FIGURE 14.26 *In this colonia on the outskirts of Mexico City, residents work with the government to bring electricity, water, and sewers to shantytowns and squatter settlements. Like many developing countries, Mexico recognizes that helping people help themselves is the best way to improve urban living.*

CASE STUDY

A MODEL SUSTAINABLE CITY

Chattanooga, Tennessee, is nestled in the Tennessee River Valley, at the foot of the Cumberland Plateau. This medium-size industrial city provides an inspiring example of participatory city planning that has produced a clean urban environment, a vibrant economy, and strong social capital. Twenty-five years ago, the U.S. Department of Health, Education, and Welfare named Chattanooga America's dirtiest city. Factory smoke trapped between the mountains gave city air the highest particulate count in the nation—dirtier, even, than Los Angeles. Per capita tuberculosis rates were three times the national average. Chattanooga Creek was so polluted by toxic waste from coke ovens and steel mills that the Environmental Protection Agency designated 4 km (2.5 mi) of it a Superfund site.

Social conditions declined along with environmental quality. As industries moved out and the upper class fled to the suburbs, the city was left with abandoned factories, boarded-up buildings, a declining tax base, unemployment, crime, and despair. The worst conditions were concentrated in the poorest neighborhoods, producing further frustration and social division.

In 1984 the city council, led by David Crockett—the great nephew of the famous frontiersman—started a series of town meetings to get residents talking about the city and its future. More than 1,700 people brainstormed ways to achieve clean air and water, jobs, affordable housing, personal safety, a place to fish, and somewhere to walk along the river. By giving everyone a voice, the process built community spirit and a broad base of support. Suddenly, people with energy and good ideas from every part of the city got involved.

Public-private partnerships led to nearly $800 million in investments (two-thirds from the private sector) and created 8,000 new permanent and temporary jobs. The Chattanooga Neighborhood Enterprise Corporation invested $60 million in affordable housing. More than 1,000 first-time home buyers obtained low-interest loans, while other residents got home-improvement help. By 1990 Chattanooga was in compliance with national air quality standards. Public transport is now widely used and efficient. The riverfront has been cleaned up. A 35-km (22-mi)-long riverfront park with walking and bike trails has been built along both sides of the river through downtown. Fountains, flowers, shade trees, street musicians, and outdoor festivals now fill the park. Property values have shot up, and people are moving back to the center city to take advantage of the recreational and cultural opportunities.

Using principles of urban ecology, the city has created a livable environment, a strong sense of community, and a flourishing economy. As David Crockett says, it is "a city that is cleaner, greener, and safer; that values human and natural resources; and that provides an economic system that will keep our children here."

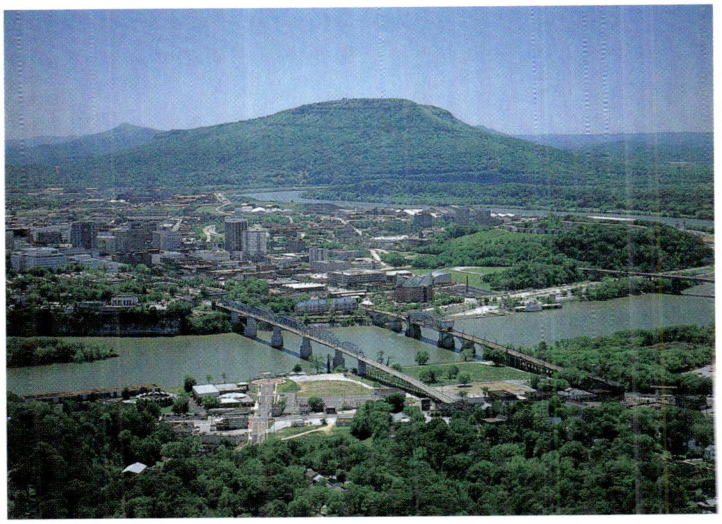

Chattanooga's waterfront has been cleaned up and has become an asset rather than a liability.

Whether sustained, environmentally sound economic development is possible for a majority of the world's population remains one of the most important and most difficult questions in environmental science. The unequal relationship between the richer "northern" countries and their impoverished "southern" neighbors is a major part of this dilemma. Some people argue that the best hope for developing countries may be to "delink" themselves from the established international economic systems and develop direct south-south trade based on local self-sufficiency, regional cooperation, barter, and other forms of nontraditional exchange that are not biased in favor of the richer countries.

SUMMARY

- Sustainable futures depend on how we use and conserve our resources and our environment. Our definitions of *resources* shape the ways we identify and use them, as well as the ways we theorize their future use.
- Ecological economics brings the insights of ecology into more traditional economic analysis. It calls for consideration of the role of natural capital and ecological services in planning and accounting. A resource is anything with potential use for creating wealth or giving satisfaction. Minerals and fossil fuels are examples of nonrenewable resources. Biological organisms and ecological processes are renewable and self-reproducing but can be exhausted by overuse.
- Questions about the scarcity of resources and their effects on economic development are important in determining what kind of society we have. Open-access systems encourage narrow self-interests and resource exploitation. In communal property resource systems, self-governing, locally based community management has successfully sustained natural resources for centuries in many cases.
- Cost-benefit analysis can be a useful tool in environmental management. Ultimately, our aim should be to internalize costs that are now treated as externalities. GNP is used as a measure of economic progress, but new measures for human well-being and environmental health, such as the Human Development Index, are needed.
- Green business and green design are efforts to reduce the environmental and social costs of the things we buy and use. These efforts are important contributors to sustainability, and they have proven profitable for businesses that use them.
- Cities are where almost half of us live and where many of our resources are used. Cities are growing worldwide, especially in developing countries. Only Africa and South Asia remain predominantly rural, and cities are growing rapidly there as well. A variety of push-and-pull factors contribute to this urban growth.
- The consequences of urbanization in many developing areas include overstressed infrastructure, pollution, and crowding. Among the worst problems faced in these cities are traffic congestion, air pollution, inadequate or nonexistent sewers and waste disposal systems, water pollution, and housing shortages. Millions of people live in appalling slums and shantytowns, yet these people raise families, educate their children, learn new jobs and new ways of living, and have hope for the future.
- In wealthier countries, problems of cities include urban decay and sprawl, as well as inefficiency and pollution associated with our reliance on cars and on low-density suburban development patterns. Planners propose a variety of strategies that may help make cities in both the developed and the developing worlds healthier, safer, and more environmentally sound and sustainable environments.

QUESTIONS FOR REVIEW

1. Identify the ways resources are defined by classical, neoclassical, and ecological economics.
2. Explain the difference between renewable and nonrenewable resources. Are nonrenewable resources always limiting factors in economic productivity?
3. Explain how scarcity and technological progress can extend resource availability and the carrying capacity of the environment.
4. Why does the marketplace sometimes fail to optimally allocate natural resource values?
5. What are some ways of accounting for environmental resources and including them in cost-benefit analysis?
6. Worldwide, how many people now live in cities, and how many live in rural areas?
7. What changes in urbanization are predicted to occur in the next 50 years, and where will those changes occur?
8. Where is most urban growth going on? What are the environmental and social costs of urbanization?
9. Why are urban areas in some U.S. cities decaying? What can be done about this?
10. Describe some aspects of a sustainable city.

THINKING SCIENTIFICALLY

1. When an ecologist warns that we are using up irreplaceable natural resources and an economist rejoins that ingenuity and enterprise will find substitutes for most resources, what underlying premises and definitions shape their arguments?
2. What would be the effect on the developing countries of the world if we were to change to a steady-state economic system? How could we achieve a just distribution of resource benefits while still protecting environmental quality and future resource use?
3. If you were doing a cost-benefit study, how would you assign a value to the opportunity for good health or the existence of

rare and endangered species in faraway places? Is there a danger or cost in simply saying some things are immeasurable and priceless and therefore off limits to discussion?

4. If natural capitalism, or eco-efficiency, has been so good for some entrepreneurs, why haven't all businesses moved in this direction?
5. What relationships can you draw between principles of thermodynamics and principles of ecological economics?
6. A city could be considered an ecosystem. Using what you learned in chapters 2 and 3, describe the structure and function of a city in ecological terms.
7. Look at the major urban area(s) in your state. Why were they built where they are? Are those features now a benefit or drawback?
8. Boulder, Colorado, has been a leader in controlling urban growth. One consequence is that housing costs have skyrocketed, and poor people have been driven out. If you lived in Boulder, would you vote for additional population limits? What do you think is an optimum city size?
9. This chapter presents a number of proposals for suburban redesign. Which of them would be appropriate or useful for your community? Try drawing up a plan for the ideal design of your neighborhood.

KEY TERMS

capital 330
communal resource management systems 333
cost-benefit analysis (CBA) 333
ecological economics 330
ecological services 331
externalizing costs 335
genuine progress index (GPI) 334
gross national product (GNP) 330
internalizing costs 336
limits to growth 332
megacities 339
nonrenewable resources 331
open access system 333
pull factors 340
push factors 340
renewable resources 331
resources 328
smart growth 346
sprawl 344
steady-state economy 330
sustainable development 329
"The Tragedy of the Commons" 333
urbanization 339

SUGGESTED READINGS

Antrop, M. 2004. "Landscape change and the urbanization process in Europe." *Landscape and Urban Planning* 67(1–4):9–26.

Arendt, R. 1999. *Growing Greener: Putting Conservation into Local Plans and Ordinances.* Island Press.

Ayres, Ed. 2004. "The hidden shame of the global industrial economy." *WorldWatch* 17(1):20–29.

Calthorpe, Peter, and William Fulton. 2000. *The Regional City: Planning for the End of Sprawl.* Island Press.

Costanza, Robert, et al. 1997. "The Value of the World's Ecosystem Services and Natural Capital." *Nature* 387:253–60.

Daley, Herman E., and Joshua Farley. 2004. *Ecological Economics: Principles and Applications.* Island Press.

Duany, Andres, Jeff Speck, and Elizabeth Plater-Zyberk. 2002. *Smart Growth Manual.* McGraw-Hill.

Lele, Sharachchandra M., and Richard B. Norgaard. 1996. "Sustainability and the Scientist's Burden." *Conservation Biology* 10(2):354–65.

McDonough, William, and Michael Braungart. 2002. *Cradle to Cradle.* North Point Press.

Mumford, Lewis. 1968. *The City in History.* Harvard Books.

Welcome to McGraw-Hill's Online Learning Center

http://www.mhhe.com/cunningham3e

WEB EXERCISES

Calculating Your Ecological Footprint

One way of assessing the resource consumption patterns of communities and individuals is to calculate an ecological footprint. To learn about this concept and how it is done, go to www.rprogress.org/, the webpage of Redefining Progress. You can find information there about individual consumption levels and those of whole nations as well as an interesting discussion of genuine progress indicators and real measures of satisfaction. For a quick calculation of your ecological footprint, go to www.earthday.net/footprint/info.asp. By answering 14 simple questions, you can find out how much land it takes to support your present lifestyle. Suggestions are given for average consumption rates of residents of Canada and the United States. At the end, you are asked how much space should be reserved for other species. This shows you how many earths it would take to support the whole human population at your level of consumption. For more detailed information on how ecological footprints are calculated, go to www.rprogress.org/programs/sustainability/ef/methods/calculating.html.

Smart Growth

To learn more about smart growth, go to the website of the Smart Growth Network at www.smartgrowth.org/about/default.asp. Choose one of the topics under either Principles or Issues, such as "Create walkable neighborhoods." Summarize the issue, in your own words, and look at the case studies to find a positive example of how this problem can be addressed. Could these solutions work in your city or neighborhood? Why or why not? What special characteristics might have contributed to successful implementation of smart growth principles in the example you've studied?

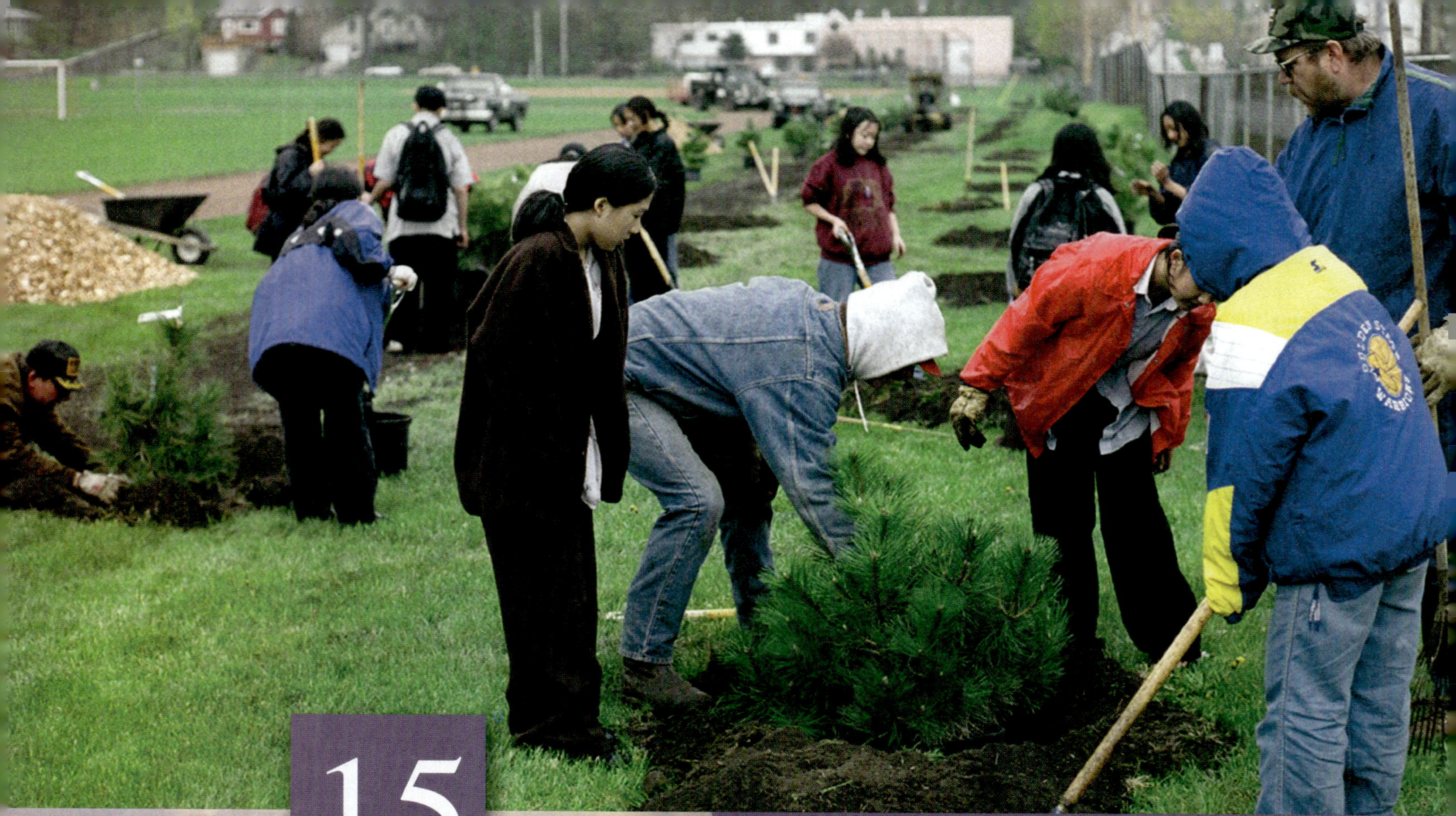

Student volunteers plant trees in a campus-greening project.

15 Environmental Science and Policy

You must be the change you wish to see in the world.
–Mahatma Gandhi

LEARNING ONLINE

Visit our webpage at www.mhhe.com/cunningham3e for data sources, further readings, additional case studies, current environmental news, and regional examples within the Online Learning Center to help you understand the material in this chapter. You'll also find active links to information pertaining to this chapter, including

Environmental policy
Legislative watch
Earth justice
Environmental law
Earthwatch: citizen science
Union of Concerned Scientists
Student Environmental Action Coalition
Simple living

OBJECTIVES

After studying this chapter, you should be able to

- understand how adaptive and precautionary principles can help us make decisions in "wicked" problems where scientific evidence is incomplete or contradictory.
- be aware of the goals and opportunities in environmental education and environmental careers.
- summarize the cycle by which policy is established.
- describe the path of a bill through the legislature.
- recognize the differences among civil, criminal, and administrative law.
- judge the effectiveness of litigation in environmental issues.
- consider the reasons that international treaties have or have not been successful.
- scrutinize collaborative, community-based planning methods.
- compare radical and mainline environmental groups and the tactics they employ to bring about social change.

River Watch

Would you like to help protect your environment, participate in important scientific research, and have fun, all at the same time? If so, River Watch may have a program for you. River Watch is a citizen science organization that trains people in community-based watershed monitoring and assessment. Over half a million people across America participate every year in gathering and interpreting data on the health of their watersheds and their communities. These programs create opportunities for people to learn science through hands-on projects and gather information that helps community leaders identify and solve problems. And they track ecological and human health trends to assess whether protection and restoration efforts are working.

River Watch works with schools, nonprofit organizations, government agencies, and Native American tribes. It provides guidance and support to help groups plan and carry out programs. The River Network maintains a national directory of river and watershed conservation organizations. It can help you find a group in your area; if there isn't one, it will give advice on how to organize an effective group. It can also provide training and expert assistance to help you learn biomonitoring techniques.

Community-based monitoring programs help citizens and policymakers understand the natural forces that shape watersheds and make them unique. Participants assess how clean and healthy their rivers and streams are and identify watershed problems and sources. Citizens take stock of the social, political, and economic contexts for their work and evaluate the effectiveness of watershed protection and restoration activities. Data collected from such widespread, coordinated projects provide a valuable information source for scientific research.

Through its Healthy Waters/Healthy Communities program, River Watch works with people to investigate links between community health problems and pollution. Teams identify hazards and exposure routes, monitor contamination levels, research the known health effects of contaminants, and conduct health surveys. Finally, citizens are encouraged to use their information to develop action plans and lobby officials for remediation and environmental restoration.

Although River Watch uses a variety of methods to assess ecosystem health, a favorite technique is to sample aquatic macroinvertebrates, including insects—such as mayflies, stoneflies, caddisflies, midges, and beetles—crustaceans (e.g., crayfish), worms, clams, and snails (fig. 15.1). Rivers are living communities. The organisms that make up this community can tell us a great deal about what's happening in the ecosystem. Stresses caused by pollution, sedimentation, changes in stream flow, or introduction of invasive species all have lasting effects on aquatic communities. Assessing who lives in a water body gives us useful data on its health and can suggest steps to remediate damage.

River Watch is only one example of how we can learn about our environment and help shape environmental policy. Many other organizations sponsor citizen-science programs and offer opportunities for informed activism. We'll look at a variety of environmental groups in this chapter. We'll also look at governmental policies that affect our environment, as well as how science and a well-educated public can help protect environmental quality.

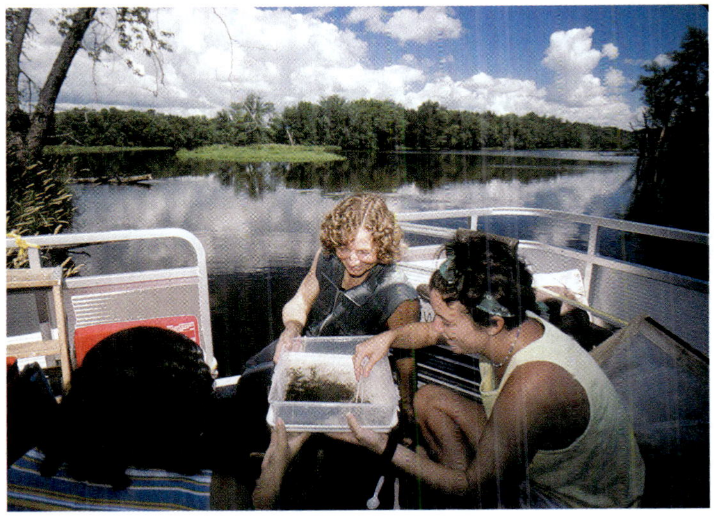

FIGURE 15.1 *Sampling benthic (bottom-dwelling) aquatic macroinvertebrates can tell you a lot about the health of the ecosystem.*

MAKING DECISIONS IN AN UNCERTAIN WORLD

Once you understand the environmental processes and problems we've seen in this book, what do you do next? One thing you can do is to put your knowledge to work helping society make good decisions and rules, or policies, that affect your environment and your community. But first it is important to know something about how policies are made and how decisions can be formed in the face of uncertainty and competing interests.

Throughout this book, we've looked at difficult environmental problems. You have read that global carbon dioxide emissions are about four times what they were in 1950 and that up to one-fourth of all tropical species might go extinct if the worst-case climate change scenarios come true. You have learned that exposure to toxic and hazardous chemicals can cause birth defects, cancer, and chronic ailments. More than 20 percent of the world's people lack access to adequate food, basic sanitation, and clean water (fig. 15.2). Both science and policy can help solve these problems. Table 15.1 summarizes some of the most important

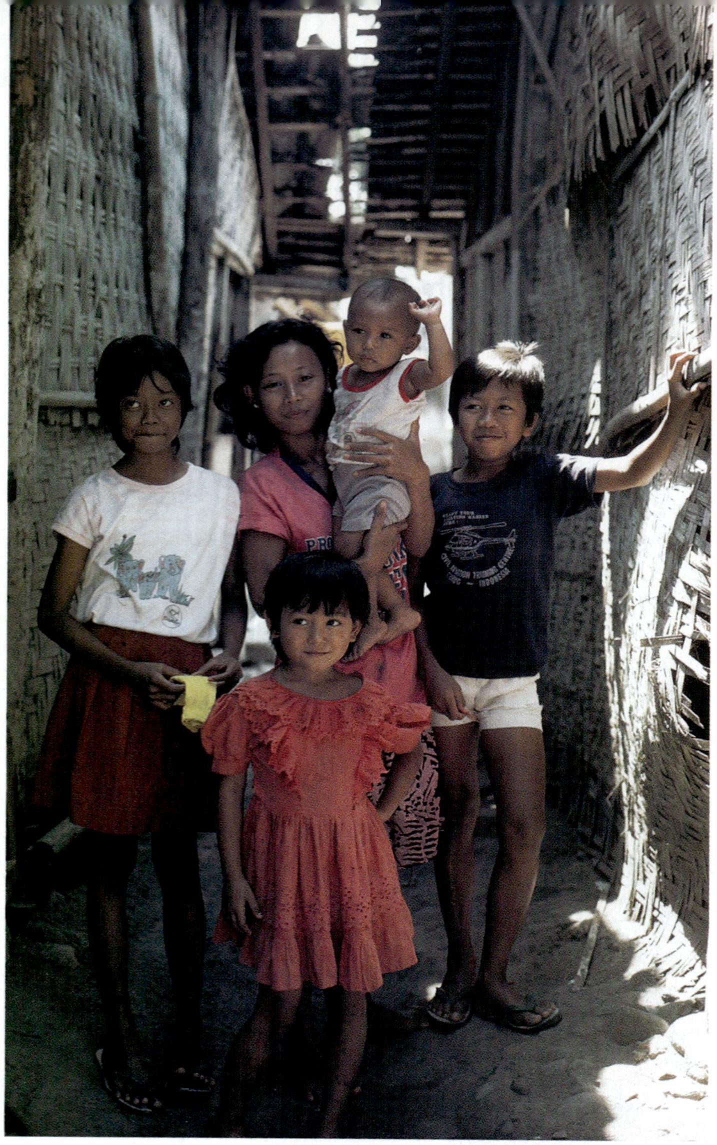

FIGURE 15.2 *More than 1 billion people—such as this Indonesian family—live in acute poverty, lacking access to secure food supplies, safe drinking water, housing, education, health services, and decent jobs.*

TABLE 15.1 Some Important Current Questions in Environmental Science

1. What effects will global climate change have, and what can we do to prevent or mitigate adverse effects of these changes?
2. How and where can we best prevent habitat and biodiversity losses?
3. Where will freshwater shortages be most severe, and how can we conserve and extend our water supplies?
4. What are the most important sources of air and water pollution, and how can we reduce them?
5. How can we encourage energy conservation and a switch to renewable energy sources?
6. What are the effects of large-scale, chemical-intensive agriculture, and what are the barriers to sustainable, regenerative farming?
7. What can we do to encourage a demographic shift to balanced population growth?
8. How can we move toward an ecologically sustainable, socially just economy?
9. What health risks are associated with environmental factors, and how can we reduce those risks?
10. What are our ethical responsibilities toward nature, and how can we foster an ethic of environmental stewardship and sustainability?

questions on which environmental scientists are currently working. In this chapter, we'll consider how answers provided by science can help establish public policy. We'll also look at ways you can get involved in this process.

In chapter 1 we defined science as a way of exploring and explaining the world around us. Ideally, science provides an orderly, methodical approach to collecting and analyzing information. The core of modern science is formulating hypotheses and then testing them in an objective, impartial, controlled manner. One of the most important things for you to understand about science is that hypotheses can be falsified—shown to be wrong—but they almost never can be shown to be unquestionably correct. Therefore, theories and explanations based on scientific data are always conditional. An overwhelming body of evidence currently may support a particular scientific interpretation, but we always have to be aware that the next investigation or experiment could provide evidence that completely overturns all our previous understanding of a particular topic. This may sound frustrating, but think of it as an ongoing process that gets us closer and closer to an understanding of the world around us.

Adaptive Management

How can we make decisions in the face of this scientific uncertainty? The answer is that our plans generally have to be conditional and contextual. Scientific information can help us understand environmental issues, but the policies we create based on this understanding will always depend on further study and more confirming evidence. An approach currently favored by many natural resource managers is called **adaptive management,** or "learning by doing." In adaptive management, policies are designed from the outset to use scientific principles to examine alternatives and assess outcomes. Rather than assume that what seems the best initial policy option will always remain so, adaptive management sets up scientific experiments to monitor how conditions are changing, and what effects our actions (or inactions) are having on both target and nontarget elements of the system. The goal of adaptive management is to enable us to live with the unexpected. It aims to yield understanding as much as to produce answers or solutions (table 15.2).

As an example of adaptive management, suppose that a forest supervisor is debating whether clear-cutting or selective harvesting is the best option for forest harvesting. Using adaptive management principles, she or he would set up a series of care-

TABLE 15.2 Institutional Conditions for Adaptive Management

1. There is a mandate to take action in the face of uncertainty.
2. Decision makers are aware they are experimenting, anyway.
3. Decision makers care about improving outcomes over biological time scales.
4. Preservation of pristine environments is no longer an option, and human intervention cannot produce desired outcomes predictably.
5. Resources are sufficient to measure ecosystem-scale behavior.
6. Theory, models, and field methods are available to estimate and infer ecosystem-scale behavior.
7. Hypotheses can be formulated.
8. Organizational culture encourages learning from experience.
9. There is sufficient stability to measure long-term outcomes; institutional patience is essential.

Source: From *Compass and Gyroscope* by Kai N. Lee. Copyright © 1993 by the author. Reproduced by permission of Island Press, Washington, D.C.

fully planned experiments to study the effects of projects as they are carried out. As information becomes available, management plans—and the monitoring programs that assess them—can constantly be adapted to changing conditions and interpretations. If the original hypothesis is confirmed, the management techniques may be applied on a wider scale or in a new situation. If unexpected results are discovered, new approaches can be tested. Another important aspect of adaptive design is that it tends to be broader and more holistic than the single-resource focus of previous management approaches. Ecological, social, and economic impacts of our actions are considered equally important with the sheer availability or market cost of a commodity.

"Wicked" Problems

One reason that plans need to be conditional and why management should incorporate scientific experiments is that many environmental problems have no simple answer. Questions such as "What does ecosystem health mean?" or "How clean is clean?" don't have clear right or wrong answers. They depend on your worldview and how you define these terms. Different people come to different conclusions, even if they share the same information.

Environmental scientists describe these issues as being **"wicked" problems,** not in the sense of having malicious intent but, rather, as obstinate or intractable dilemmas. These problems often are nested within other sets of interlocking issues. The definition of both the problem and its solutions differ for various stakeholders. There are no value-free, objective answers for these puzzles, only choices that are better or worse, depending on your viewpoint. "Wicked" problems are important and have serious consequences. They also are complex, and those who bear the costs often are different from those who would benefit from proposed solutions (fig. 15.3). These problems usually can't be solved by simple regulations, more research, or appeals to ethics. Often the best solution comes from community-based planning and consensus building. Inherent uncertainty gives these questions no clear end point. You cannot know when all possible solutions have been explored.

Recent advancements in understanding how ecological systems work give us some insight into many "wicked" problems. Like biological organisms, social problems often change and evolve over time. Their history unfolds in complex ways, depending on chance interactions and unpredictable events. Like ecological systems, many environmental issues may never reach a stable equilibrium. Each involves an assemblage of issues and actors that are unique in time and place. They can't be standardized. There are no good precedents from previous experience. The solutions are unique, and what may work today may not be applicable tomorrow.

The Precautionary Principle

The fact that many of the dilemmas we face are ambiguous doesn't mean that we can avoid decisions while we study the situation forever. In many cases if we wait until we have an absolutely certain solution, it may be too late to act. We need the best information available to make an informed decision, but sometimes we need to take a courageous, but modest, stand that chooses among the best possible policy options. We need to recognize that science doesn't have all the answers. We may need to modify our position as we learn more (see related story "Reasoned Judgment" at www.mhhe.com/cases).

Drawing on studies of ecological systems, many conservation biologists advocate a **precautionary principle** that says we should plan a margin of safety for error or surprises in natural systems. This approach says that when human health or the environment are threatened, precautionary measures should be taken even

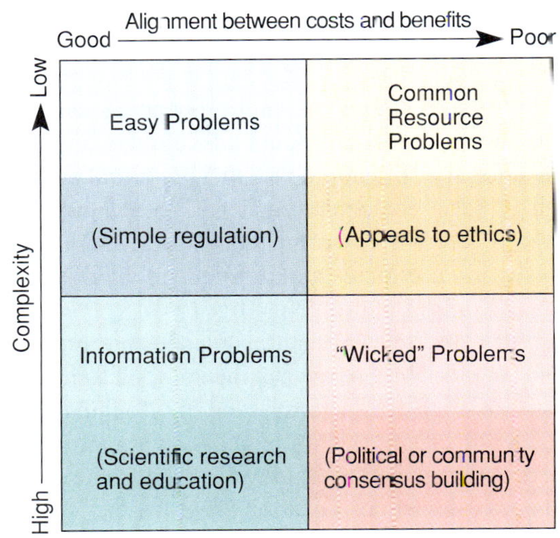

FIGURE 15.3 *The difficulty of environmental decision making increases as problems become more complex and the congruence between those who bear costs and enjoy benefits decreases. Solutions are shown in parentheses.*

if some cause-and-effect relationships are not fully established scientifically. There are four basic tenets of precautionary action:

- People have a duty to take anticipatory steps to prevent harm. If you have a reasonable suspicion that something bad might happen, you have an obligation to try to stop it.
- The burden of proof of carelessness of a new technology, process, activity, or chemical lies with the proponents, not with the general public.
- Before using a new technology, process, or chemical or starting a new activity, people have an obligation to examine a full range of alternatives, including the alternative of not using it.
- Decisions applying the precautionary principle must be open, informed, and democratic and must include the affected parties.

The European Union has effectively adopted the precautionary principle by shifting the burden to industry to prove that products are safe, rather than requiring regulators to prove they are dangerous. Opponents of this approach claim that it could prevent us from doing anything productive or innovative. What do you think? Is this principle just common sense or an invitation to decision paralysis?

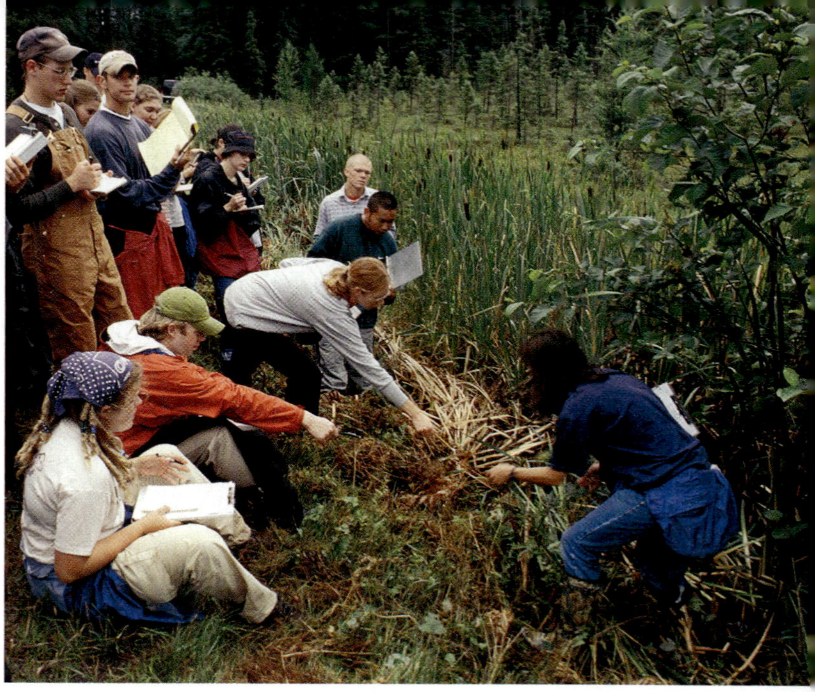

FIGURE 15.4 *Environmental education helps develop awareness and appreciation of ecological systems and how they work.*

ENVIRONMENTAL EDUCATION

We've defined environmental science in this book as a systematic study of our environment and our place in it. A relatively new field, environmental science is highly interdisciplinary; it integrates information from many fields of study to understand how the world works and how we should behave as environmental citizens. We also have described environmental science as mission-oriented, implying that we all have a responsibility to get involved to do something about the problems we have created. What can each of us do to fulfill that responsibility?

The National Environmental Education Act sets two broad goals: (1) to improve understanding among the general public of natural and built environments and the relationships between humans and their environment, including global aspects of environmental problems, and (2) to encourage postsecondary students to pursue careers related to the environment. Specific objectives proposed to meet these goals include developing an awareness of and appreciation for our natural and social/cultural environment, a knowledge of basic ecological concepts, an acquaintance with a broad range of current environmental issues, and experience in using investigative, critical-thinking, and problem-solving skills in solving environmental problems (fig. 15.4).

Outdoor activities and natural sciences are important components of this mission, but environmental topics such as responsible consumerism, waste disposal, and environmental ethics can and should be incorporated into reading, writing, arithmetic, and every other part of education. Table 15.3 presents one set of guidelines for an environmental education program.

TABLE 15.3 Outcomes from Environmental Education

1. *The natural context:* An environmentally educated person understands the scientific concepts and facts that underlie environmental issues and the interrelationships that shape nature.
2. *The social context:* An environmentally educated person understands how human society is influencing the environment, as well as the economic, legal, and political mechanisms that provide avenues for addressing issues and situations.
3. *The valuing context:* An environmentally educated person explores his or her values in relation to environmental issues; from an understanding of the natural and social contexts, the person decides whether to keep or change those values.
4. *The action context:* An environmentally educated person becomes involved in activities to improve, maintain, or restore natural resources and environmental quality for all.

Source: A Greenprint for Minnesota, Minnesota Office of Environmental Education, 1993.

Environmental Literacy

Speaking to the first broad goals of the National Environmental Education Act, former Environmental Protection Agency (EPA) administrator William K. Reilly called for broad **environmental literacy,** in which every citizen is fluent in the principles of ecology and has a "working knowledge of the basic grammar and underlying syntax of environmental wisdom." Environmental literacy, according to Reilly, can help create a stewardship ethic—a sense of duty to care for and manage wisely our natural endowment and our productive resources for the long haul. "Environmental education," he said, "boils down to one profoundly important imperative: preparing ourselves for life in the next century. As it is now the twenty-first century, it will not be enough for a few specialists to know what is going on while the rest of us wander about in ignorance."

While you've made a great start toward learning about your environment by reading this book and taking a class in environmental science, we hope you will continue to read and expand your horizons after your class is finished. A large body of environmental literature can help you in this quest. Some of the most influential environmental books of all time are listed in table 15.4. To this list, we would add some personal favorites: *The Singing Wilderness* by Sigurd F. Olson, *My First Summer in the Sierra* by John Muir, and *Remaking Society: Pathways to a Green Future* by Murray Bookchin.

Environmental Careers

The need for both environmental educators and environmental professionals opens up many job opportunities in environmental fields. The EPA estimates, for example, that 100,000 new professionals will be needed in the United States in the next five years alone to deal with hazardous waste problems (fig. 15.5). Scientists are needed to understand the natural world and the effects of human activity on the environment. Lawyers and other specialists are central to developing government and industry policy, laws, and regulations to protect the environment. Engineers are in demand to develop technologies and products to clean up pollution and to prevent its production in the first place. Economists, geographers, and social scientists are key in evaluating the costs of pollution and resource depletion and in developing solutions that are socially, culturally, politically, and economically appropriate for different parts of the world. In addition, business will be looking for a new class of environmentally literate and responsible leaders who appreciate how products sold and services rendered affect our environment.

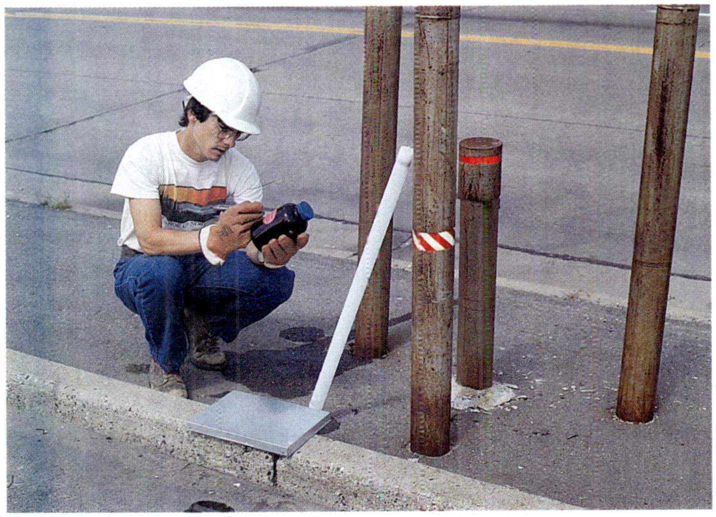

FIGURE 15.5 *Many interesting, well-paid jobs are opening up in environmental fields. Here, a technician takes a well sample to test for water contamination.*

TABLE 15.4 The Environmentalist's Bookshelf

What are some of the most influential and popular environmental books? In a survey[1] of environmental experts and leaders around the world on the best books on nature and the environment, the top ten were

A Sand County Almanac by Aldo Leopold (100)[2]
Silent Spring by Rachel Carson (81)
State of the World by Lester Brown and the Worldwatch Institute (31)
The Population Bomb by Paul Ehrlich (28)
Walden by Henry David Thoreau (28)
Wilderness and the American Mind by Roderick Nash (21)
Small Is Beautiful: Economics as If People Mattered by E. F. Schumacher (21)
Desert Solitaire: A Season in the Wilderness by Edward Abbey (20)
The Closing Circle: Nature, Man, and Technology by Barry Commoner (18)
The Limits to Growth: A Report for the Club of Rome's Project on the Predicament of Mankind by Donella H. Meadows et al. (17)

[1]Robert Merideth, 1992, G. K. Hall/Macmillan, Inc.
[2]Indicates number of votes for each book. Because the preponderance of respondents were from the United States (82 percent), American books are probably overrepresented.

Trained people are essential in these professions at every level, from technical and clerical support staff to top managers. Perhaps the biggest national demand over the next few years will be for environmental educators to help train an environmentally literate populace. We urgently need many more teachers at every level who are trained in environmental education.

Can environmental protection and resource conservation—a so-called green perspective—be a strategic advantage in business? Many companies think so. An increasing number are jumping on the environmental bandwagon, and most large corporations now have an environmental department. A few are beginning to explore integrated programs to design products and manufacturing processes that minimize environmental impacts. Often called "design for the environment," this approach is intended to avoid problems at the beginning, rather than deal with them later on a case-by-case basis. In the long run, executives believe this will save money and make their businesses more competitive in future markets. The alternative is to face increasing pollution-control and waste disposal costs—now estimated to be more than $100 billion per year for all American businesses—as well as to be tied up in expensive litigation and administrative proceedings.

The market for pollution-control technology and know-how is also expected to be huge. Cleaning up the former East Germany alone is expected to cost some $200 billion. Many companies are positioning themselves to cash in on this enormous market. Germany and Japan appear to be ahead of America in the pollution control field because they have had more stringent laws for many years, giving them more experience in reducing effluents.

How can you prepare yourself to enter this market? The best bet is to get some technical training: environmental engineering, analytical chemistry, microbiology, ecology, limnology, groundwater hydrology, and computer science all have great potential. Currently, a chemical engineer with a graduate degree and some experience in an environmental field can practically name his or her salary. Some other very good possibilities are environmental law and business administration, both rapidly expanding fields.

For those who aren't inclined toward technical fields, there are still many opportunities for environmental careers. A good liberal arts education will help you develop skills, such as communication, critical thinking, balance, vision, flexibility, and caring, that should serve you well. Writers, editors, graphic arts professionals, and others who can communicate with the public have an important role to play in most environmental issues. Environmental attorneys, political scientists, anthropologists, and sociologists, among others, can help resolve environmental problems.

Citizen Science

While university classes often tend to be theoretical and abstract, many students are discovering they can also learn via hands-on experience and undergraduate research programs. Internships in agencies or environmental organizations are one way of doing this. Another is to get involved in organized **citizen science** projects in which ordinary people work with established scientists to answer real scientific questions. Community-based research was pioneered in the Netherlands, where several dozen research centers now study environmental issues, ranging from water quality in the Rhine River, cancer rates by geographic area, and substitutes for harmful organic solvents. In each project, students and neighborhood groups team with scientists and university personnel to collect data. Their results have been incorporated into official government policies.

Similar research opportunities exist in the United States and Canada. In addition to River Watch, described at the beginning of this chapter, there are many other citizen-science projects in which you could participate (fig. 15.6). The Cornell University Bird Lab coordinates more than a dozen volunteer research projects dealing with birds, ranging from census of rare and endangered species, to the spread of exotic birds, to disease outbreaks. (See related story at www.mhhe.com/cases.) Earthwatch offers a much smaller but more intense opportunity to take part in research. Every year hundreds of Earthwatch projects field a team of a dozen or so volunteers who spend a week or two working on issues ranging from loon nesting behavior to archaeological digs. The Student Conservation Association places students in internships in which you can learn valuable job skills while also doing valuable resource work. You might be able to get academic credit as well as helpful practical experience in one of these research experiences.

ENVIRONMENTAL POLICY

A policy is a rule or decision about how to act or deal with problems. On a personal, informal level, you might have a policy always to get your homework in on time. On a national, formal level, we have policies such as the Clean Air Act, a set of rules, agreed upon by a majority of the U.S. Congress, restricting air pollutants and setting fines for those who exceed legal limits. There are international policies as well: the 1987 Montreal Protocol set agreed-upon limits to the production of ozone-depleting chemicals (chapter 9), and the Convention on International Trade in Endangered Species (CITES) is an international agreement to restrict trade in endangered species (chapter 5).

In this chapter, **environmental policy** will refer to official rules and regulations concerning the environment that are adopted, implemented, and enforced by some government agency, as well as to general public opinion about environmental issues. National policies are established through negotiation and compromise in a democratic society. Sometimes this wrangling can take decades. Theoretically, it allows all voices to be heard, and the resulting policy serves the interest of the majority.

Making policy isn't necessarily a clean process, though. Rules can seem harsh and unfair to minorities (fig. 15.7). The

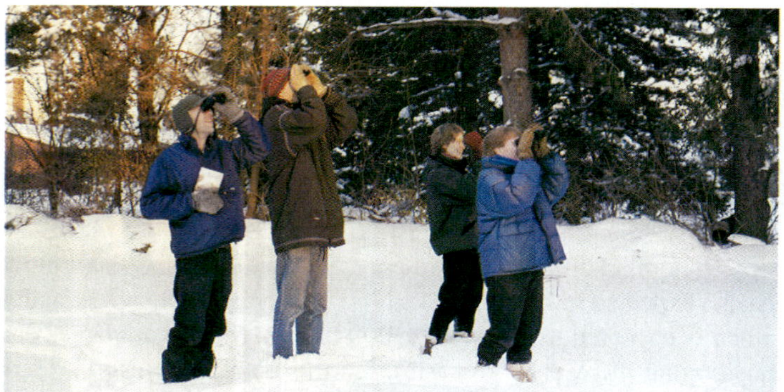

FIGURE 15.6 *Participating in citizen-science projects is a good way to learn about science and your local environment.*

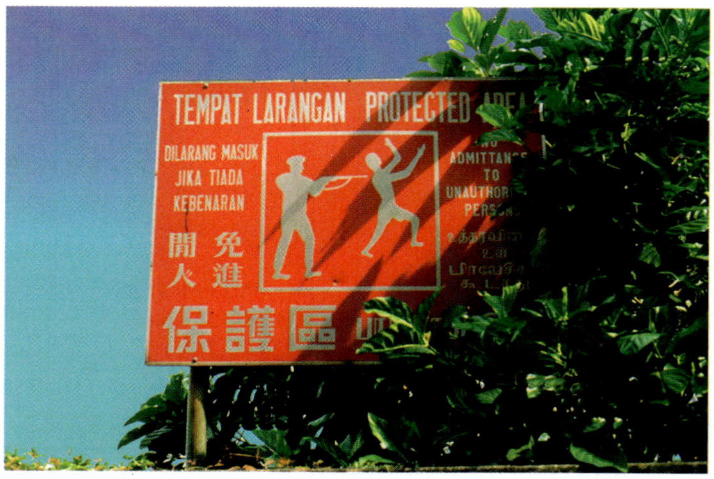

FIGURE 15.7 *What level of force is justified in environmental protection? This park in Singapore takes a draconian stance.*

unfair influence of money and power in government also can be discouraging to voters. But sound policy for the public good can be formed—especially when the public is active and vocal in defending its interests. In the sections that follow, we will discuss the formation of rules and laws in general. Events don't always follow principles. The best way to make sure they do is to develop an informed and involved populace.

The Policy Cycle

How do policy issues and options make their way onto the stage of public debate? Problems are identified and acted upon in a **policy cycle** that acts to continually define and refine the public agenda (fig. 15.8). The first stage in this process is problem identification. Sometimes the government identifies issues for groups that have no voice or don't recognize problems themselves. In other cases, the public identifies a problem, such as loss of biodiversity or health effects of exposure to toxic waste, and demands redress by the government. In either case, proponents describe the issue—either privately or publicly—and characterize the risks and benefits of their preferred course of action.

Seizing the initiative in issue identification often allows a group to define terms, set the agenda, organize stakeholders, choose tactics, aggregate related issues, and legitimate (or delegitimate) issues and actors. It can be a great advantage to set the format or choose the location of a debate. Next, stakeholders develop proposals for preferred policy options, often in the form of legislative proposals or administrative rules. Proponents build support for their position through media campaigns, public education, and personal lobbying of decision makers. By following the legislative or administrative process through its many steps, interest groups ensure that their proposals finally get enacted into law or established as a rule or regulation.

The next step is implementation. Ideally, government agencies faithfully carry out policy directives as they organize bureaucracies, provide services, and enforce rules and regulations, but often it takes continued monitoring to make sure the system works as it should. Evaluating the results of policy decisions is as important as establishing them in the first place. Measuring impacts on target and nontarget populations shows us whether the intended goals, principles, and course of action are being attained. Finally, suggested changes or adjustments are considered that will make the policy fairer or more effective.

There are different routes by which this cycle is carried out. Special economic interest groups, such as industry associations, labor unions, or wealthy and powerful individuals, don't need (or often want) much public attention or support for their policy initiatives. They generally carry out the steps of issue identification, agenda setting, and proposal development privately because they can influence legislative or administrative processes directly through their contacts with decision makers. Public interest groups, on the other hand, often lack direct access to corridors of power and need to rally broad general support to legitimate their proposals.

An important method for getting public interest on the table is to attract media attention. Organizing a dramatic protest or media event can generate a lot of free publicity (fig. 15.9). Announcing a dire threat or sensational claim is a good way to gain attention. The problem is that it takes ever increasing levels of hysteria and hyperbole to get yourself heard in the flood of shocking news with which we are bombarded every day. Ironically, many groups that bemoan the overload of rhetorical overstatement that engulfs us contribute to it to be heard above the din. Nevertheless, an overwhelming majority of Americans believe that environmental protection is an important priority (fig. 15.10).

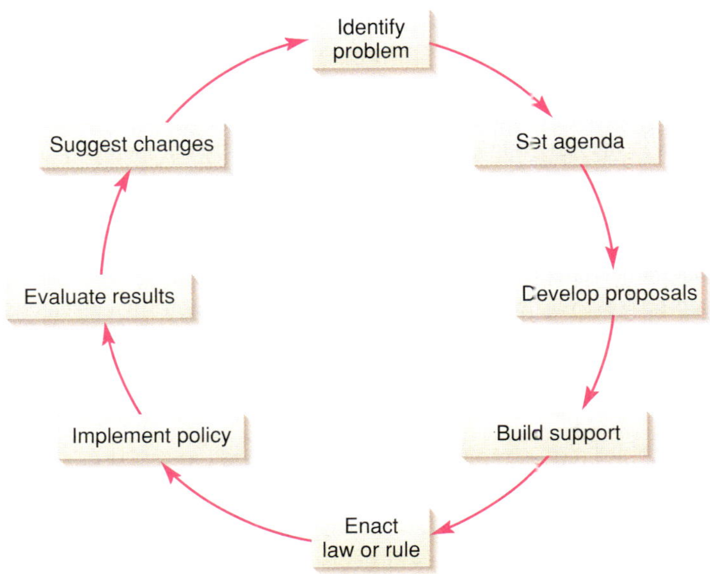

FIGURE 15.8 *The policy cycle.*

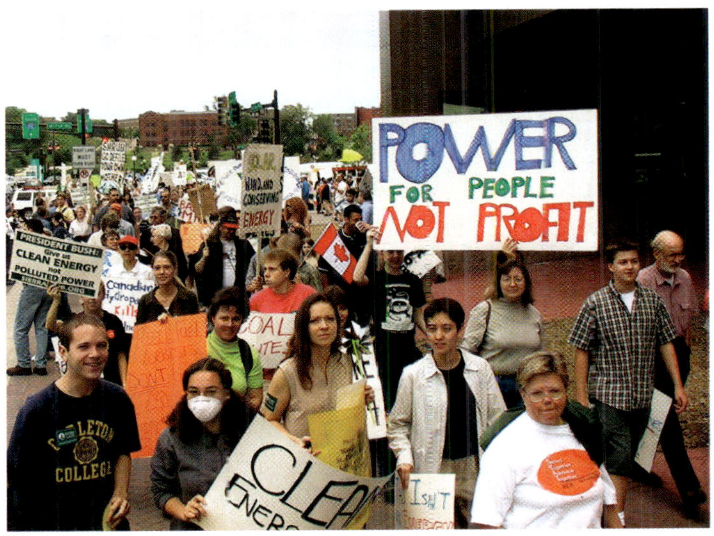

FIGURE 15.9 *Protestors demonstrate against monetary policies and international institutions that threaten livelihoods and environmental quality.*

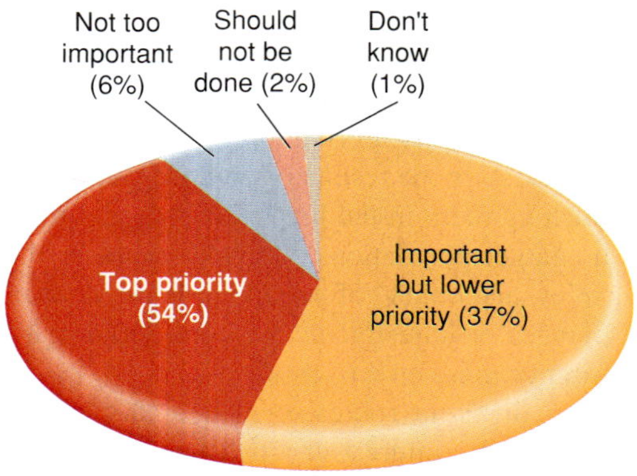

FIGURE 15.10 *More than half the respondents in a Princeton University survey in 2000 said that environmental protection should be a top priority for the president and congress.*

Political Decision Making

The policies we establish depend to a great extent on the system within which they operate. For many of us, the ideal political system is one that is open, honest, transparent, and reaches the best possible decisions to maximize benefits to everyone. In a pluralistic, democratic society, we aim to give everyone an equal voice in policy making. Ideally, many separate interests put forward their solutions to public problems that are discussed, debated, and evaluated fairly and equally. Facts and access are open to everyone. Policy choices are made democratically but compassionately; implementation is reasonable, fair, and productive. Unfortunately, this isn't always the way our system works. Our political system usually gives those with the most power and money the greatest voice in public affairs. Still, there have been altruistic movements in the past to ensure human rights and environmental protection that reveal an impulse for generosity and goodwill among the general public.

Another model for public decision making is rational choice and science-based management. Politicians call for "sound science" to be used in policy making, but with no generally accepted definition of the term, it often merely means studies validating a particular interest or ideology (see related story "Sound Science" at www.mhhe.com/cases). In this utilitarian approach, no policy should have greater total costs than benefits. In choosing among policy alternatives, we should always prefer those with the greatest cumulative welfare and the least negative impacts. Professional administrators would weigh various options and make an objective, methodical decision that would bring maximum social gain. There are many reasons, however, that rational choice doesn't always work in the public arena.

- Many conflicting values and needs cannot be compared because they aren't comparable or we don't have perfect information.
- There are few generally agreed-upon broad societal goals, but rather, benefits to specific groups and individuals, many of which are in conflict.
- Policymakers generally aren't motivated to make decisions on the basis of societal goals, but rather to maximize their own rewards: power, status, money, or reelection.
- Large investments in existing programs and policies create "path dependence" and "sunken costs" that prevent policymakers from considering good alternatives foreclosed by previous decisions.
- Uncertainty about the consequences of various policy options compels decision makers to stick as closely as possible to previous policies to reduce the likelihood of adverse, calamitous, unanticipated consequences.
- Policymakers, even if well meaning, don't have sufficient intelligence or adequate data or models to calculate accurate costs and benefits when large numbers of diverse political, social, economic, and cultural values are at stake.
- The segmented nature of policy making in large bureaucracies makes coordinating decision making difficult.

NEPA and EIS

The **National Environmental Policy Act (NEPA)** forms the cornerstone of U.S. environmental policy. Signed into law by President Nixon in 1970, NEPA does three important things: (1) it authorizes the Council on Environmental Quality (CEQ), the oversight board for general environmental conditions; (2) it directs federal agencies to take environmental consequences into account in decision making; and (3) it requires an Environmental Impact Statement (EIS) for every major federal project having a significant impact on the quality of the human environment. When NEPA was being debated, there were suggestions that it should be a constitutional amendment guaranteeing the right of a clean environment to everyone. Difficulties in defining what "clean" means, along with worries about how we could achieve this ambitious goal, limited NEPA to a statute with more limited, but still important, powers than a constitutional amendment. What do you think? Does everyone have an inherent right to a clean environment? How would you define "clean"?

The EIS process has proven to be one of the most powerful tools in the environmental arsenal. It requires more open and environmentally sensitive planning in both the agencies themselves and in private corporations seeking to do business with the government. An EIS can bring to light adverse aspects of a project that might otherwise remain hidden. It can provide valuable information about a proposal to opponents who can't afford to do their own research.

An EIS doesn't forbid environmentally destructive activities if they comply otherwise with relevant laws, but it demands that we admit what we're really doing. Once embarrassing information is revealed, however, few agencies will bulldoze ahead, ignoring public opinion. Consequently, NEPA is hated by many who view it as a threat to business and property rights. In recent years, these forces have received a sympathetic hearing in federal and state agencies. A series of decisions have significantly weakened this important law (see related story "Is NEPA an Impediment?" at www.mhhe.com/cases).

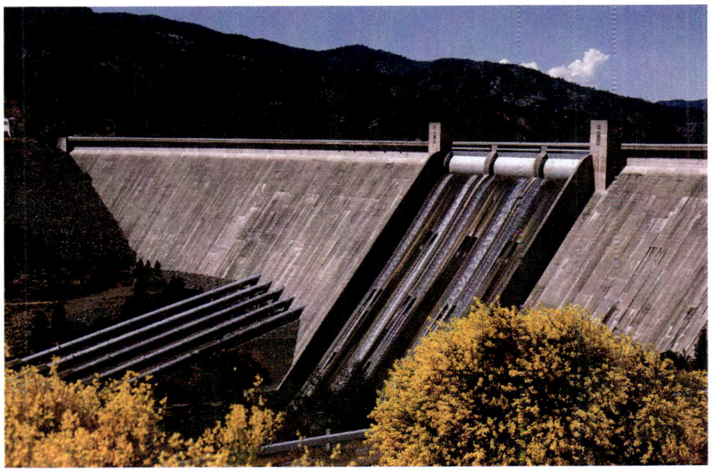

FIGURE 15.11 *Every major federal project in the United States must be preceded by an Environmental Impact Statement.*

What kinds of projects require an EIS? The activity must be federal and it must be major, with a significant impact on the human environment (fig. 15.11). Evaluations are always somewhat subjective as to whether specific activities meet these characteristics. Each case is unique and depends on context, geography, the balance of beneficial versus harmful effects, and whether any areas of cultural, scientific, or historical importance might be affected. To do a complete EIS for a project is usually time-consuming and costly. The final document is often hundreds of pages long and generally takes six to nine months to prepare. Sometimes just requesting an EIS is enough to sideline a questionable project. In other cases it gives adversaries time to rally public opposition and to research information with which to criticize what's being proposed. If agencies don't agree to prepare an EIS voluntarily, environmentalists can petition the courts to force them to do so.

Every EIS must contain the following elements: (1) purpose and need for the project, (2) alternatives to the proposed action (including taking no action), and (3) a statement of positive and negative environmental impacts of the proposed activities. In addition, an EIS should make clear the relationship between short-term resources and long-term productivity, as well as any irreversible commitment of resources resulting from project implementation.

ENVIRONMENTAL LAW

Laws are rules set by authority, society, or custom. Church laws, social mores, administrative regulations, and a variety of other codes of behavior can be considered laws if they are backed by some enforcement power. **Environmental law** includes official rules, decisions, and actions concerning environmental quality, natural resources, and ecological sustainability. In the United States a wide variety of environmental laws are promulgated at both the local and national levels. Because every country has different legislative and legal processes, this chapter will focus primarily on the U.S. system in the interest of simplicity and space. Environmental law can be established or modified in each of the three branches of government: legislative, judicial, and executive—statutory, case, and administrative law, respectively. Understanding how these systems work is an important step in becoming an environmentally literate person.

APPLICATION: Environment, Science, and Policy in Your Community

Take several minutes with your classmates and make a list of five current, environment-related policy issues in your community or state. (Hint: consider energy, economic developments, population changes, traffic congestion, water and air quality, or public health issues in the news.) Discuss which branch of government—legislative, executive, or judicial—you think should take the lead in addressing each issue. Why did you designate these authorities as you did?

Select one issue from your list, and discuss the following: What are some of the sources of uncertainty involved in the decision-making process? How could scientific research help identify or solve this policy issue? Where in the rule-making process could scientific data help inform decision makers?

Statutory Law: The Legislative Branch

Establishing laws at either the state or the federal level is one of the most important ways of protecting our environment. Many environmental groups spend a good deal of their time and resources trying to influence the legislative process. In this section we'll look at how that system works.

Federal laws (statutes) are enacted by Congress and must be signed by the president. They originate as legislative proposals called bills, which are usually drafted by the congressional staff, often in consultation with representatives of various interest groups. Thousands of bills are introduced every year in Congress. Some are very narrow, providing funds to build a specific section of road or to help a particular person, for instance. Others are extremely broad, perhaps overhauling the Social Security system or changing the entire tax code. Similarly, environmental legislation might deal with a very specific local problem or a national or international issue. Often a number of competing bills on a single issue may be introduced as proponents from different sides attempt to incorporate their views into law. A bill may have a single sponsor if it is the pet project of a particular legislator, or it may have 100 or more co-authors if it is an issue of national importance.

A Convoluted Path

After introduction, each bill is referred to a committee or subcommittee with jurisdiction over the issue for hearings and debate. Most hearings take place in Washington, D.C., but if the bill is controversial or legislators want to attract publicity for themselves or the issue, they may conduct field hearings closer to the site of the controversy. The public often has an opportunity to give testimony at field hearings (fig. 15.12). Although it's not likely that you will change the opinions of many legislators, no matter how fervent or cogent your testimony, these events can be a good place to gain attention and educate the public about a topic. Hearings and debates also build a record of legislative intent that can be valuable in later interpretation and implementation of laws by courts and administrative agencies.

If a bill has sufficient support within the subcommittee, its language will be "marked up" or revised and modified to be more widely acceptable and to improve its chances of passage. At this stage several competing bills might be combined into a single compromise version and forwarded to the full committee for more hearings, debate, and a vote. If it fails in the full committee, the bill is sent back to the subcommittee for more work and further compromise. A bill that succeeds in the full committee is reported to the full House or Senate for a floor debate. Often, opponents of a bill will attempt to amend it during each of these stages to lessen its impact or to make it so unpalatable that even the original authors can no longer support it. Some amendments add completely unrelated material or even reverse the bill's intent. As bills move along this convoluted pathway, interested parties can follow their progress in the *Congressional Quarterly Weekly,* a publication both in print and online that tracks proposed legislation. Many environmental groups also maintain websites with up-to-date information on events in Congress.

By the time an issue has passed through both the House and Senate, the versions approved by the two bodies are likely to be different. They go then to conference committee to iron out any differences between them. After going back to the House and Senate for confirmation, the final bill goes to the president, who may either sign it into law or veto it. If the president vetoes the bill, it may still become law if two-thirds of the House and Senate vote to override the veto. If the president takes no action within 10 days of receiving a bill from Congress, the bill becomes law without his signature. One exception to this procedure is that, if Congress adjourns before the 10-day period elapses, the bill does not become law. The president, by doing nothing, is said to have exercised a "pocket veto."

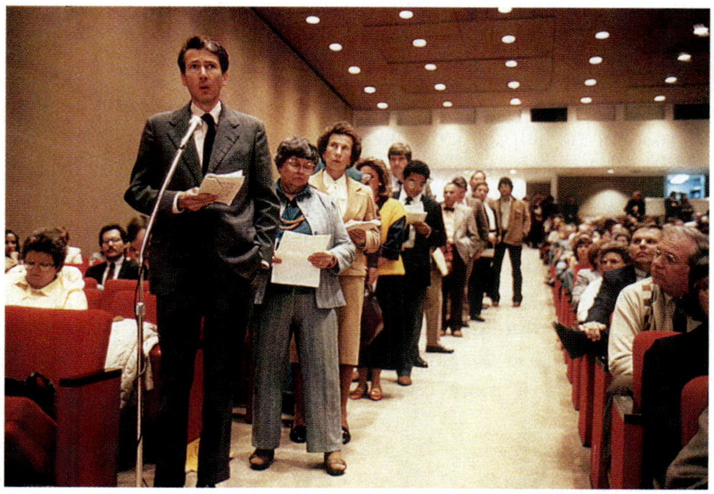

FIGURE 15.12 *Citizens line up to testify at a legislative hearing. By getting involved in the legislative process, you can be informed and have an impact on government policy.*

The Thomas website, maintained by Congress, also has current information about the progress of legislation. You can find out how your senators and representative voted on critical environmental issues by consulting The League of Conservation Voters, which ranks each member of Congress on his or her voting record. Several environmental organizations have regular email environmental news bulletins with up-to-date information about what's happening in Washington, D.C. Table 15.5 lists some of the most important recent U.S. environmental legislation.

Lobbying

Groups or individuals with an interest in pending legislation can often influence outcomes by **lobbying,** or using personal contacts, public pressure, and political action to persuade legislators to vote in their favor. Most major environmental organizations maintain offices in Washington, D.C., from which they monitor legislative and administrative programs and policies. Hundreds of professional environmental lobbyists and volunteer activists attend hearings, meet with legislators and agency personnel, draft proposed legislation and administrative rules, and work to shape the national environmental agenda.

In a survey of professional lobbyists, a majority agreed that personal contacts are the most effective way to influence decision makers. Your own senator or representative is more likely to be interested in your views than someone with whom you have no connection. Even if you aren't rich, illustrious, or politically connected, you can often get a fair hearing from legislative staff—if not their bosses—if you have a persuasive case concerning an important topic.

Being involved in local election campaigns can greatly increase your access to legislators. Writing letters or making telephone calls also are highly effective ways to get your message across. All legislators now have email addresses, but letters and phone calls are usually taken more seriously. Getting media attention can sway the opinions of decision makers. Organizing protests, marches, demonstrations, or other kinds of public events can call attention to your issue (fig. 15.13). Public education campaigns, press conferences, TV ads, and a host of other activities can be helpful. Joining together with other like-minded groups can greatly increase your clout and ability to get things done. It's hard for a single individual or even a small group to have much impact, but if you can organize a mass movement, you may be very effective in influencing public policy.

Case Law: The Judicial Branch

Over the past 30 years, appeals to the judicial system have often been the most effective ways for seeking redress for environmental damage and forcing changes in how things are done. Activist

TABLE 15.5 Major U.S. Environmental Laws

LEGISLATION	PROVISIONS
National Environmental Policy Act of 1969	Declared national environmental policy, required Environmental Impact Statements, created Council on Environmental Quality.
Clean Air Act of 1970	Established national primary and secondary air quality standards. Required states to develop implementation plans. Major amendments in 1977 and 1990.
Clean Water Act of 1972	Set national water quality goals and created pollutant discharge permits. Major amendments in 1977 and 1996.
Federal Pesticides Control Act of 1972	Required registration of all pesticides in U.S. commerce. Major modifications in 1996.
Marine Protection Act of 1972	Regulated dumping of waste into oceans and coastal waters.
Coastal Zone Management Act of 1972	Provided funds for state planning and management of coastal areas.
Endangered Species Act of 1973	Protected threatened and endangered species. Directed FWS to prepare recovery plans.
Safe Drinking-Water Act of 1974	Set standards for safety of public drinking-water supplies and to safeguard groundwater. Major changes made in 1986 and 1996.
Toxic Substances Control Act of 1976	Authorized EPA to ban or regulate chemicals deemed a risk to health or the environment.
Federal Land Policy and Management Act of 1976	Charged the BLM with long-term management of public lands. Ended homesteading and most sales of public lands.
Resource Conservation and Recovery Act of 1976	Regulated hazardous-waste storage, treatment, transportation, and disposal. Major amendments in 1984.
National Forest Management Act of 1976	Gave statutory permanence to national forests. Directed USFS to manage forests for "multiple use."
Surface Mining Control and Reclamation Act of 1977	Limited strip-mining on farmland and steep slopes. Required restoration of land to original contours.
Alaska National Interest Lands Act of 1980	Protected 40 million ha (100 million acres) of parks, wilderness, and wildlife refuges.
Comprehensive Environmental Response, Compensation and Liability Act of 1980	Created \$1.6 billion "Superfund" for emergency response, spill prevention, and site remediation for toxic wastes. Established liability for cleanup costs.
Superfund Amendments and Reauthorization Act of 1994	Increased Superfund to \$8.5 billion. Shared responsibility for cleanup among potentially responsible parties. Emphasized remediation and public "right to know."

Source: Data from N. Vig and M. Kraft, *Environmental Policy in the 1990s*, 3rd Congressional Quarterly Press.

judges and sympathetic juries in both federal and state court systems have been willing to take a stand where legislatures have been too timid or conservative to do so. Many groups spend a great deal of their time and energy bringing lawsuits that will shape environmental policy and law. The Environmental Defense Fund, for example, operates primarily in this arena.

The judicial branch of government establishes environmental law by ruling on the constitutionality of statutes and interpreting their meaning. We describe the body of legal opinions built up by many court cases as **case law.** Often legislation is written in vague and general terms so as to make it widely enough accepted to gain passage. Congress, especially in the environmental area, often leaves it to the courts to "fill in the gaps." When trying to interpret a law, the courts depend on the legislative record from hearings and debates to determine congressional intent. What was a particular statute meant to do by those who wrote and passed it?

Legal Standing

Before a trial can start, the litigants must satisfy certain threshold requirements. The first of these is **legal standing**, or whether the participants have a right to initiate an action. The main criterion for standing is a valid interest in the case. Plaintiffs must show that they are materially affected by the situation they petition the court to redress. This is an important point in environmental cases. Groups or individuals often want to sue a person or corporation for degrading the environment. Unless they can show that they personally suffer from the degradation, however, courts are likely to deny standing. In a landmark 1969 case, for example, the Sierra Club challenged a decision of the U.S. Forest Service and the Department of the Interior to lease public land in California to Walt Disney Enterprises for a ski resort. The land in question was a beautiful valley that cut into the southern boundary of Sequoia National Park (fig. 15.14). Building a road into the valley would have necessitated cutting through a grove of giant redwood trees within the park. The Sierra Club argued that it should be granted standing in the case to represent the trees, animals, rocks, and mountains that couldn't defend their own interests in court. After all, the club pointed out, corporations such as Walt Disney Enterprises are treated as persons and represented by attorneys in the courts. Why not grant trees the same rights? The case went all the way to the U.S. Supreme Court, which ruled that the Sierra Club failed to show that it or any of its members would be materially

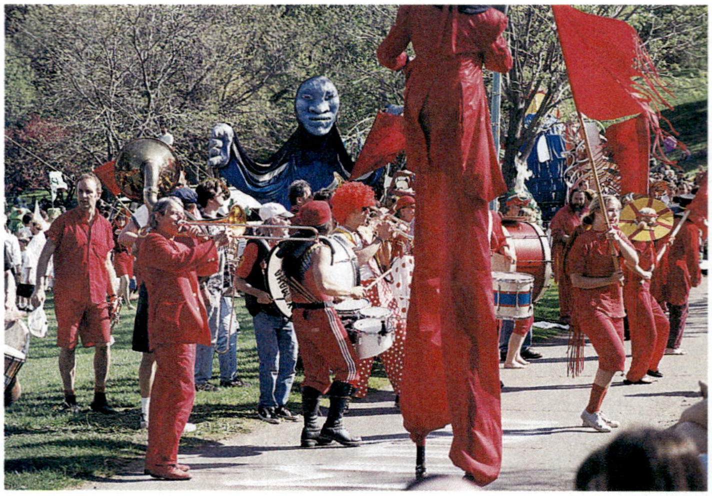

FIGURE 15.13 *Making a ruckus on behalf of environmental protection can attract attention to your cause.*

affected by the development. It turned out that the valley had too many avalanches to be safe for a resort. Still, the question of standing remains an important one.

Criminal Law

Criminal law derives from those federal and state statutes that prohibit wrongs against the state or society. Serious crimes, like murder or rape, that are punishable by long jail terms or heavy fines are called felonies. Lesser crimes, such as shoplifting or vandalism, that result in smaller fines or shorter sentences in a county or city jail are labeled misdemeanors. A criminal case is always initiated by a government prosecutor. Guilt or innocence of the defendant is determined by a jury of peers, but the sentence is imposed, often in consultation with the jury, by the judge. The judge is responsible for keeping order in the hearings and for determining points of law. The jury acts as a fact-finding body that weighs the truth and reliability of the witnesses and evidence.

Violation of many environmental statutes constitutes a criminal offense. In 1975 the U.S. Supreme Court ruled that corporate officers can be held criminally liable for violations of environmental laws if they were grossly negligent, or the illegal actions can be considered willful and knowing violations. In 1982 the EPA created an Office for Criminal Investigation. Recently, as many as 592 criminal prosecutions per year have been brought to court for environmental crimes, but the enthusiasm for prosecuting these cases varies with different administrations (fig. 15.15). In one of the toughest criminal sentences imposed so far, the president of a Colorado company was sentenced in 1999 to 14 years in prison for knowingly dumping chlorinated solvents that contaminated the water table.

In 2003 the Colonial Pipeline Company was fined $34 million for oil spills, the largest civil penalty ever under the EPA. Also in 2003 Monsanto and its subsidiaries agreed to an out-of-court settlement of $700 million for dumping PCBs in Anniston, Alabama. Altogether, the EPA forced polluters to pay $3.9 billion in 2003 for pollution controls and cleanup. Too often international environmental crimes go unpunished because of jurisdictional complications. The European Union has called for a Global Environmental Crime Intelligence Unit, much like the renowned Interpol, to investigate illegal logging, waste dumping, and other transborder crimes.

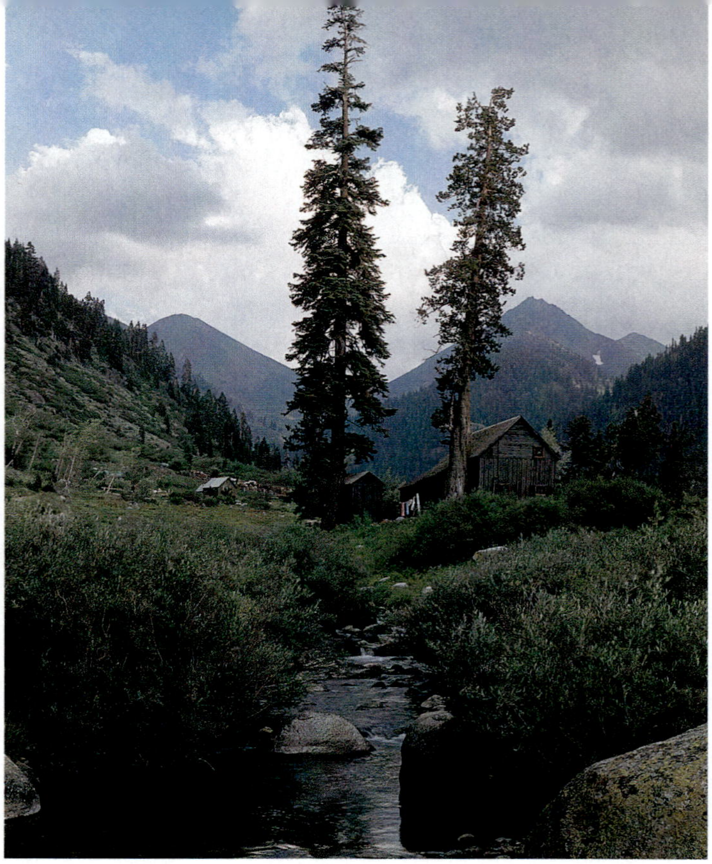

FIGURE 15.14 *Mineral King Valley at the southern border of Sequoia National Park was the focus of an important environmental law case in 1969. The Disney Corporation wanted to build a ski resort there, but the Sierra Club sued on behalf of the trees, rocks, and native wildlife to protect the valley.*

Civil Law

Civil law is defined as a body of laws regulating relations between individuals or between individuals and corporations. Issues such as property rights and personal dignity and freedom are protected by civil law. The defendant in a civil case has a right to be tried by a jury, but in highly technical issues, this right often is waived and the case is heard only by the judge. Being found guilty of a civil offense can result in financial penalties but not jail time.

In contrast to a criminal case, where the burden of proof lies with the prosecution and defendants are considered innocent until proven guilty, civil cases can be decided on a "preponderance of evidence." This makes civil cases considerably easier to win than criminal cases when evidence is ambiguous. A number of mitigating factors also are taken into account in determining guilt and assigning penalties in civil cases. Guilt or innocence is based on

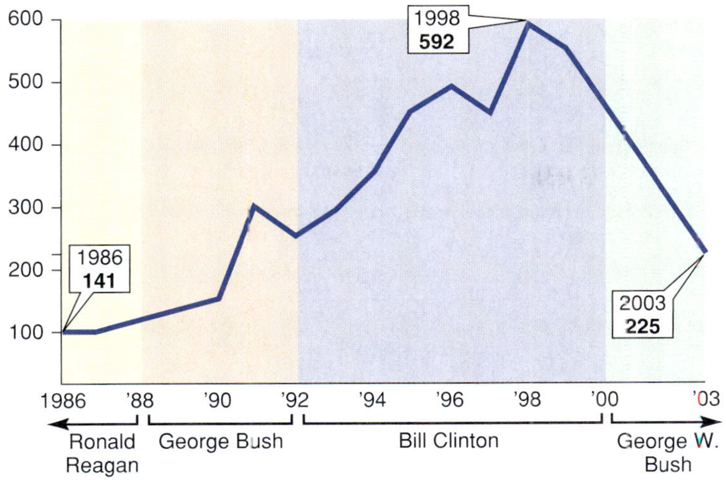

FIGURE 15.15 *The number of criminal cases referred each year for prosecution by the EPA has varied with the political climate in Washington.*
Source: U.S. EPA, 2003.

whether the defendant could reasonably have anticipated and avoided the offense. A "good faith effort" to comply or solve the problem can be a factor. The compliance history is important. Is this a first-time offender or a habitual repeater? Finally, is there evidence of economic benefit to the perpetrator? That is, did the violator gain personally from the action? If so, it is more likely that willful intent was involved.

Civil cases can be brought in both state and federal court. In 1999 the Atlanta-based Colonial Pipeline Company was ordered to pay over $20 million in damages to local landowners and the state of South Carolina for spilling about 3.5 million liters (nearly a million gallons) of diesel fuel into the Reedy River near Simpsonville, South Carolina. And in 2000 the Koch Oil Company, one of the largest pipeline and refinery operators in the United States, agreed to pay $35 million in fines and penalties to state and federal authorities for negligence in more than 300 oil spills in Texas, Oklahoma, Kansas, Alabama, Louisiana, and Missouri over the previous decade. Koch also agreed to spend more than $1 billion on cleanup and improved operations.

Sometimes the purpose of a civil suit is to seek an injunction or some other protection from the actions of an individual, a corporation, or a governmental agency. You might ask the courts, for example, to order the government to cease and desist from activities that are in violation of either the spirit or the letter of the law. This sort of civil action is heard only by a judge; no jury is present. Environmental groups have been very successful in asking courts to stop logging and mining operations, to enforce implementation of the Endangered Species Act, to require agencies to enforce air and water pollution laws, and a host of other efforts to protect the environment and conserve natural resources. Often, rather than sue a corporation directly for environmental damage, it is more effective to sue the government for not enforcing laws that would have prevented the damage. A big corporation with deep pockets may have the resources and incentive to tie up litigation for years with motions and countersuits. Federal or state agencies may be more inclined to agree that you are right and be willing to settle the matter quickly.

SLAPP Suits

Because defending a lawsuit is so expensive, the mere threat of litigation can be a chilling deterrent. Increasingly, environmental activists are being harassed with **Strategic Lawsuits against Political Participation (SLAPP).** Citizens who criticize businesses that pollute or government agencies that are derelict in their duty to protect the environment are often sued in retaliation. While most of these preemptive strikes are groundless and ultimately dismissed, defending yourself against them can be exorbitantly expensive and take up time that might have been spent working on the original issue. Public interest groups and individual activists—many of whom have little money to defend themselves—often are intimidated from taking on polluters. For example, a West Virginia farmer wrote an article about a coal company's pollution of the Buckhannon River. The company sued him for $200,000 for defamation. Similarly, citizen groups fighting a proposed incinerator in upstate New York were sued for $1.5 million by their own county governments. After a Texas woman called a nearby landfill a dump, her husband was named in a $5 million suit for failing to "control his wife." Of course, these suits also are expensive for the company or agency that initiates them, but they may be far cheaper than paying a fine or losing a big project.

Administrative Law: The Executive Branch

More than 100 federal agencies and thousands of state and local boards and commissions have environmental oversight. They usually have power to set rules, adjudicate disputes, and investigate misconduct. Federal agencies often delegate power to a matching state agency to decentralize authority. The enabling legislation to create each agency is called an "organic" act because it establishes a basic unit of governmental organization. In the federal government most executive agencies come under the jurisdiction of cabinet-level departments, such as Agriculture, Interior, or Justice (fig. 15.16).

Agency rule-making and standard-setting can be either formal or informal. In an informal case, notice and background for proposed rules are published in the *Federal Register.* All interested parties have opportunities to submit comments. This is often an important way for environmentally concerned citizens and public interest groups to have an impact on environmental policy. In formal rule-making, a public hearing is held, with witnesses and testimony much like a civil trial. Witnesses can be cross-examined. A complete transcript is made, and final findings are published in the public record. It is generally more difficult for individuals to intervene in a formal hearing, although sometimes, there is an opportunity to submit written comments.

Rule-making is often a complex, highly technical process that is difficult for citizen groups to understand and monitor. The proceedings are usually less dramatic and colorful than criminal trials, and yet can be very important for environmental protection. The

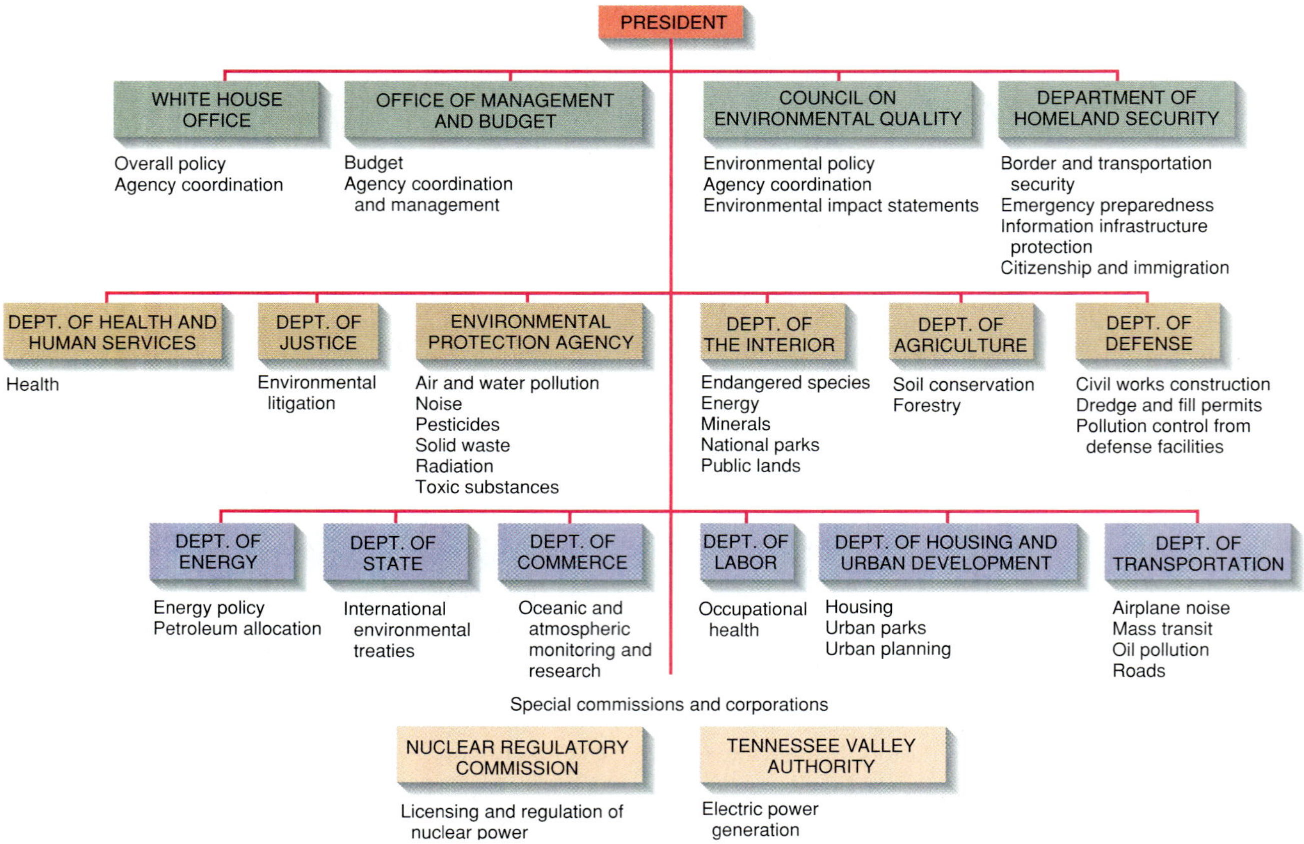

FIGURE 15.16 *Major agencies of the executive branch of the U.S. federal government with responsibility for resource management and environmental protection.*
Source: Data from U.S. General Accounting Office.

Bush administration has made profound changes in U.S. environmental policy through rule-making that avoids open debate or public scrutiny.

Regulatory Agencies

The EPA is the primary agency with responsibility for protecting environmental quality in the United States. Created in 1970 at the same time as NEPA, the EPA has more than 18,000 employees and ten regional offices. Often in conflict with Congress, other agencies of the executive branch, and environmental groups, the EPA has to balance many competing interests and conflicting opinions. Greatly influenced by politics, the agency changes dramatically, depending on which party is in power and what attitudes toward the environment prevail at any given time.

The Departments of the Interior and Agriculture are to natural resources what the EPA is to pollution. Interior is home to the National Park Service, which is responsible for more than 376 national parks, monuments, historic sites, and recreational areas. It also houses the Bureau of Land Management (BLM), which administers some 140 million ha (350 million acres) of land, mostly in the western United States. In addition, Interior is home to the U.S. Fish and Wildlife Service, which operates more than 500 national wildlife refuges and administers endangered species protection.

The Department of Agriculture is home to the U.S. Forest Service, which manages about 175 national forests and grasslands, totaling some 78 million ha (193 million acres). With 39,000 employees, the Forest Service is nearly twice as large as the EPA (fig. 15.17). The Department of Labor houses the Occupational Safety and Health Administration (OSHA), which oversees workplace safety. Research that forms the basis for OSHA standards is carried out by the National Institute for Occupational Safety and Health (NIOSH). In addition, several independent agencies that are not tied to any specific department also play a role in environmental protection and public health. The Consumer Products Safety Commission passes and enforces regulations to protect consumers, and the Food and Drug Administration is responsible for the purity and wholesomeness of food and drugs.

All of these agencies have a tendency to be "captured" by the industries they are supposed to be regulating. Many of the people with expertise to regulate specific areas came from the industry or sector of society that their agency oversees. Furthermore, the people with whom they work most closely and often develop friendships are those they are supposed to watch. And when they leave the agency to return to private life—as many do when the administration changes—they are likely to go back to the same industry or sector where their experience and expertise lies. The

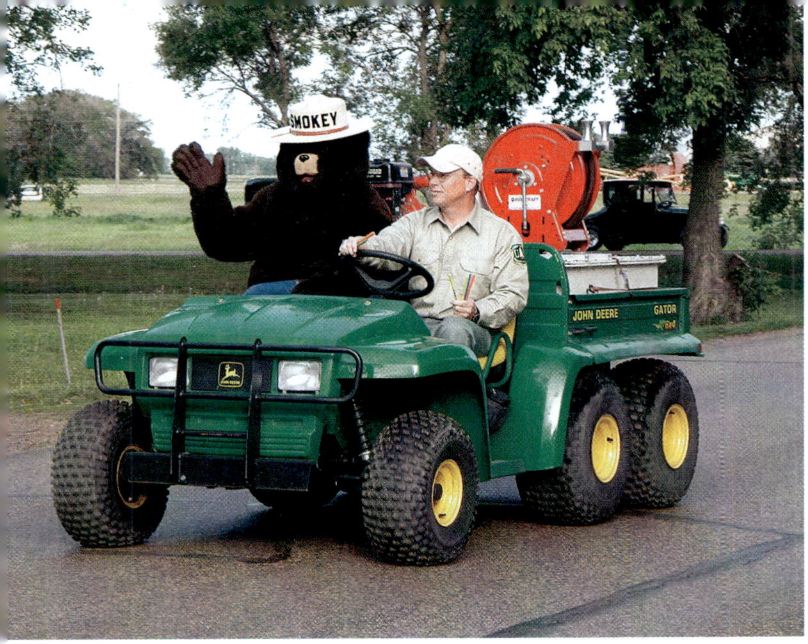

FIGURE 15.17 *Smokey Bear symbolizes the Forest Service's role in extinguishing forest fires.*

effect is often what's called a "revolving door," where workers move back and forth between industry and government. As a result, regulators often become overly sympathetic with and protective of the industry they should be overseeing.

INTERNATIONAL TREATIES AND CONVENTIONS

As recognition of the interconnections in our global environment has advanced, the willingness of nations to enter into protective **international treaties and conventions** has grown (table 15.6). The earliest of these conventions had no nations as participants; they were negotiated entirely by panels of experts. Not only the number of parties taking part in these negotiations has grown, but the rate at which parties are signing on and the speed at which agreements take force also have increased rapidly (fig. 15.18). The Convention on International Trade in Endangered Species (CITES), for example, was not enforced until 14 years after ratification, but the Convention on Biological Diversity was enforceable after just one year and had 160 signatories only four years after introduction. Over the past 25 years, more than 170 treaties and conventions have been negotiated to protect our global environment. Designed to regulate activities ranging from intercontinental shipping of hazardous waste, to deforestation, overfishing, trade in endangered species, global warming, and wetland protection, these agreements theoretically cover almost every aspect of human impacts on the environment.

Unfortunately, many of these environmental treaties constitute little more than vague good intentions. Even though we often call them laws, there is no body that can legislate or enforce international environmental protection. The United Nations and a variety of regional organizations bring stakeholders together to negotiate solutions to a variety of problems, but the agreed-upon solutions generally rely on moral persuasion and public embarrassment for compliance. Most nations are unwilling to give up sovereignty. There is an international court, but it has no enforcement power. Nevertheless, there are creative ways to strengthen international environmental protection.

One of the principal problems with most international agreements is the tradition that they must be passed by unanimous consent. A single recalcitrant nation effectively has veto power over the wishes of the vast majority. For instance, more than 100 countries at the UN Conference on Environment and Development (UNCED), held in Rio de Janeiro in 1992, agreed to restrictions on the release of greenhouse gases. At the insistence of U.S. negotiators, however, the climate convention was reworded so that it only urged—but did not require—nations to stabilize their emissions.

As a way of avoiding this problem, some treaties incorporate innovative voting mechanisms. When a consensus cannot be reached, they allow a qualified majority to add stronger measures in the form of amendments that do not need ratification. All members are legally bound to the whole document unless they expressly

TABLE 15.6 Some Major International Treaties and Conventions

DATE	TITLE	COVERS
1971	Convention on Wetlands of International Importance (Ramsar)	Protects wetlands, especially as waterfowl habitat
1972	Convention to Protect World Cultural and Natural Heritage	Protects cultural sites and natural resources
1973	Convention on International Trade in Endangered Species (CITES)	Restricts trade in endangered plants and animals
1979	Convention on Migratory Species (CMS)	Protects migratory species, especially birds
1982	United Nations Law of the Sea (UNCLOS)	Declares the oceans international commons
1985	Protocol on Substances That Deplete the Ozone Layer (Ozone)	Initiates phaseout of chlorofluorocarbons
1989	Convention on the Transboundary Movements of Hazardous Waste (Basel)	Bans shipment of hazardous waste
1992	Convention on Biodiversity (CBD)	Protects biodiversity as national resources
1992	United Nations Framework Convention on Climate Change (UNFCCC)	Rolls back carbon dioxide production in industrialized countries
1994	Convention to Combat Desertification (CCD)	Provides assistance to fight desertification, especially in Africa

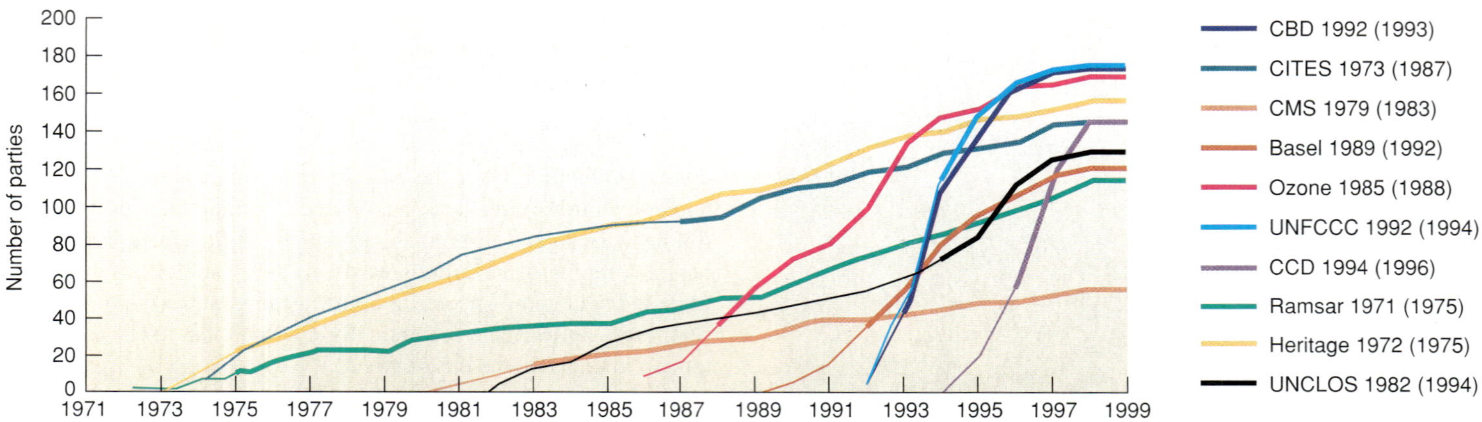

FIGURE 15.18 *Additions of participating parties to some major international environmental treaties. The thick portion of each line shows when the agreement went into effect* (date in parentheses). *See table 15.6 for complete treaty names.*
Source: Data from United Nations Environment Programme from Global Environment Outlook–2000.

object. This approach was used in the Montreal Protocol, passed in 1987 to halt the destruction of stratospheric ozone by chlorofluorocarbons (CFCs). The agreement allowed a vote of two-thirds of the 140 participating nations to amend the protocol. Although initially the protocol called for only a 50 percent reduction in CFC production, subsequent research showed that ozone was being depleted faster than previously thought (see chapter 9). The protocol was strengthened by amendment to an outright ban on CFC production, in spite of the objection of a few countries.

When strong accords with meaningful sanctions cannot be passed, sometimes the pressure of world opinion generated by revealing the sources of pollution can be effective. Activists can use this information to expose violators. For example, the environmental group Greenpeace discovered monitoring data in 1990 showing that Britain was disposing of coal ash in the North Sea. Although not explicitly forbidden by the Oslo Convention on ocean dumping, this evidence proved to be an embarrassment, and the practice was halted.

Trade sanctions can be an effective tool to compel compliance with international treaties. The Montreal Protocol, for example, bound signatory nations not to purchase CFCs or products made using them from countries that refused to ratify the treaty. Because many products employed CFCs in their manufacture, this stipulation proved to be very effective. On the other hand, trade agreements also can work against environmental protection. The World Trade Organization (WTO) was established to make international trade more fair and to encourage development. It has been used, however, to weaken national environmental laws. In 1990, after decades of public protests and boycotts, the United States banned the import of tuna caught using methods that killed thousands of dolphins each year. Shrimp caught with nets that kill endangered sea turtles were also banned. Mexico filed a complaint with the WTO, contending that dolphin-safe tuna laws represented an illegal barrier to trade. Thailand, Malaysia, India, and Pakistan filed a similar suit over turtle-friendly shrimp laws. The WTO ordered the United States to allow the import of both tuna and shrimp from countries that allow fisheries to kill dolphins and turtles. Environmentalists point out that the WTO has never ruled against a corporate suit, in part because rules are decided by a committee composed mainly of appointed industry leaders, rather than by elected officials representing a spectrum of political and economic interests.

The North American Free Trade Agreement (NAFTA) has also been used to undermine national and local environmental laws. The Canadian company Methanex has sued to force California to overturn its ban on MTBE, a carcinogenic gasoline additive that has contaminated drinking water in thousands of cities and towns. The company seeks to recover nearly a billion dollars in lost MTBE sales and damages, as well as to force California to allow its continued use. In a similar NAFTA lawsuit, the Ethyl Corporation of the United States won a suit against Canada for banning the manganese-based gasoline additive, MMT, which is suspected to be a neurotoxin. And log exports from Canada to the United States facilitated by NAFTA are controversial because of their environmental effects in Canada and their economic impacts in the U.S. (fig. 15.19).

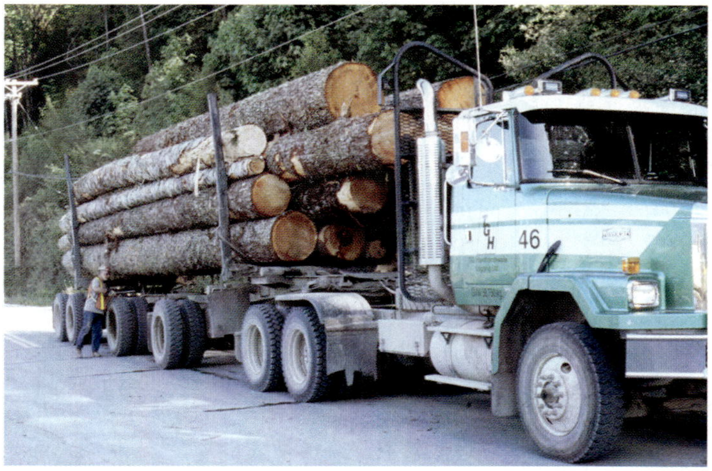

FIGURE 15.19 *Trade agreements can weaken environmental protection as countries compete to market their resources. NAFTA, for example, encourages logging in British Columbia for U.S. markets.*

DISPUTE RESOLUTION AND COMMUNITY-BASED PLANNING

The adversarial approach of our current legal system often fails to find good solutions for many complex environmental problems. Identifying and punishing an enemy for transgressions often seem more important to us than finding win/win compromises. Gridlocks occur in which conflicts between adversaries breed mutual suspicion and decision paralysis. The results can be continuing ecosystem deterioration, economic stagnation, and growing incivility and confrontation. The complexity of many environmental problems arises from the fact that they are not purely ecological, economic, or social but a combination of all three. They require an understanding of the interrelations between nature and people. Are there ways to break these logjams and find creative solutions? In this section we will look at some new developments in mediation, dispute resolution, and alternative procedures for environmental decision making.

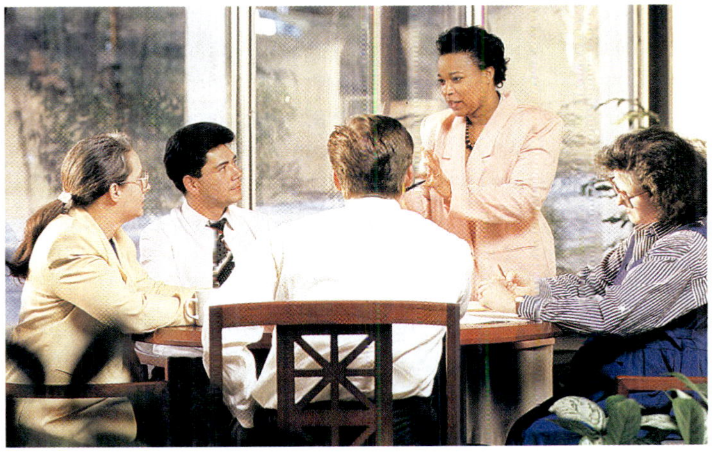

FIGURE 15.20 *Mediation encourages stakeholders to discuss issues and try to find a workable compromise.*

Arbitration and Mediation

Litigation and administrative challenges tend to be highly adversarial. You may win a battle but end up hardening the opposition to your ideas. Increasingly used to avoid the time, expense, and winner-take-all confrontation inherent in our legal system, arbitration and mediation encourage compromise and workable solutions with which everyone can live.

Arbitration is a formal process of dispute resolution somewhat like a trial. There are stringent rules of evidence and cross-examination of witnesses, and the process results in a legally binding decision. The arbitrator takes a more active role than a judge, however, and is not as constrained by precedent. The arbitrator is more interested in resolving the dispute than in strict application of the law. Arbitrators must have formal training and be certified by the Federal Mediation and Conciliation Service or the American Arbitration Association. Arbitration is usually an attractive prospect if you don't think you could win a formal lawsuit, but why would people agree to arbitration if they think they can win the whole enchilada in court? They might take this route just to avoid disagreeable surprises. Juries can be fickle. Furthermore, they might want to get an unpleasant process over with sooner rather than later. In addition, arbitration often is written into contracts so that the disputants have no choice in the matter.

There are disadvantages to arbitration, however. It doesn't create a legally binding precedent, something that often is the main motivation for a lawsuit. There is less opportunity to appeal if you don't like the decision you get. There also is less protection from self-incrimination, false witnesses, or evidence you didn't expect. You don't generate nearly as much publicity because the proceedings and record are not public. For some litigants, the publicity generated by a trial is more valuable than the settlement itself. Finally, you are less likely to win the whole thing. Some sort of compromise is the most likely outcome.

Mediation is a process in which disputants are encouraged to sit down and talk to see if they can come up with a solution by themselves (fig. 15.20). The mediator makes no final decision but is simply a facilitator of communication. This process is especially useful in complex issues where there are multiple stakeholders with different interests, as is often the case in environmental controversies. There are both benefits and perils of mediation. It can be quicker and cheaper than court battles. It can lead to compromise and understanding that will lead to further cooperation, and that will solve problems faster than endless appeals. And it may find creative solutions that satisfy multiple parties and interests. On the other hand, no one can be forced to mediate or to do so in good faith. Rancorous participants can tie up the process in long, pointless arguments that only make others more angry. Ultimately, there can be a tyranny of the minority. A single person can veto an agreement that everyone else wants. Furthermore, mediation represses or denies certain irreconcilable structural conflicts, giving the impression of equality between disputants when none really exists. Unequal negotiating skills of the participants can lead to unfair outcomes and even more rancor and paranoia than before the mediation was attempted. As is the case with arbitration, mediation doesn't generate the publicity and complete victory that some groups desire.

Collaborative Approaches to Community-Based Planning

Over the past several decades, natural resource managers have come to recognize the value of **community-based planning** that incorporates holistic, adaptive, pluralistic approaches. Involving all stakeholders and interest groups early in the planning process can help avoid the "train wrecks" in which adversaries become entrenched in nonnegotiable positions. Working with local communities can tap into traditional knowledge and gain acceptance for management plans that finally emerge from policy planning. This approach is especially important in nonlinear, nonequilibrium systems and "wicked" problems. Among the more important reasons to use collaborative approaches are:

- The way "wicked" problems are formulated depends on your worldview. Incorporating a variety of perspectives early in the process is more likely to lead to the development of acceptable solutions in the end.

- People have more commitment to plans they have helped develop. The first stage is therefore to identify those involved and to engage them in the process.
- There is truth in the old adage that "two heads are better than one." Involving multiple stakeholders and multiple sources of information enriches the process.
- Community-based planning provides access to situation-specific information and experience that can often only be obtained by active involvement of local residents.
- Participation is an important management tool. Project-threatening resistance on the part of certain stakeholders can be minimized by inviting active cooperation of all stakeholders throughout the planning process.
- The knowledge and understanding needed by those who will carry out subsequent phases of a project can only be gained through active participation.

A good example of community-based planning can be seen in the Atlantic Coastal Action Programme (ACAP) in eastern Canada. The purpose of this project is to develop blueprints for the restoration and maintenance of environmentally degraded harbors and estuaries in ways that are both biologically and socially sustainable (fig. 15.21). Officially established under Canada's Green Plan and supported by Environment Canada, this program created 13 community groups, some rural and some urban, with membership in each dominated by local residents. Federal and provincial government agencies are represented primarily as nonvoting observers and resource people. Each community group is provided with core funding for full-time staff who operate an office in the community and facilitate meetings. To cope with the complex biological and social problems affecting coastlines, ACAP is bringing together different stakeholders to create comprehensive plans for ecological, economic, and social sustainability. Through citizen monitoring and adaptive management, the community builds social capital (knowledge, cooperative spirit, trust, optimism, working relations), develops a sense of ownership in the planning process, and eliminates some of the fears and factional rivalry that often divide local groups, outsiders, and government agents.

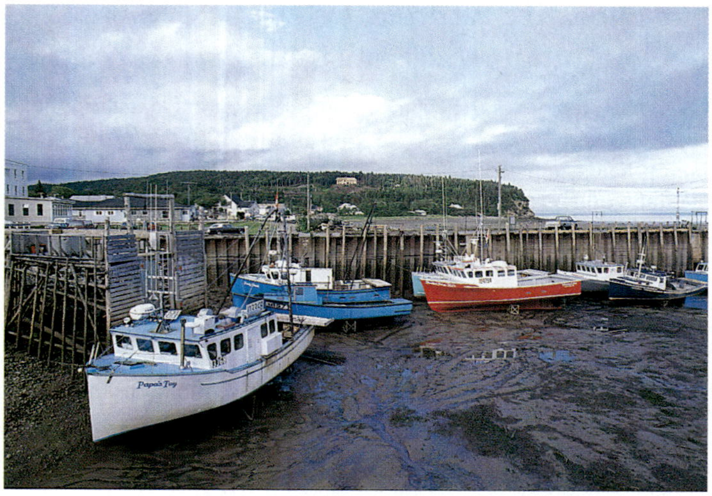

FIGURE 15.21 *The Bay of Fundy is the site of an innovative community-based environmental planning process.*

CITIZEN PARTICIPATION

There are many things that individuals can do to live in a more sustainable manner. In nearly every chapter in this book, you can find a "What Can You Do?" box that lists some simple steps for living more lightly on the earth. Taking personal responsibility for our environmental impact can have many benefits. Recycling, buying "green" products, and other environmental actions set good examples for your friends and neighbors. They also strengthen your sense of involvement and commitment in valuable ways. There are limits, however, to how much we can do individually through our buying habits and personal actions to bring about the fundamental changes needed to save the earth. Green consumerism generally can do little about larger issues of global equity, chronic poverty, oppression, and the suffering of millions of people in the Third World. There is a danger that exclusive focus on such problems as whether to choose paper or plastic bags will divert our attention from the greater need to change basic institutions.

Environmentally concerned citizens have many opportunities to influence government policies. Get to know the positions of your state legislators, congressional representatives, and senators. Be active in party politics. Going to your district, county, and state political conventions gives you a voice in choosing candidates and establishing party platforms. Individuals can also contact legislators directly. You would probably be surprised at how little mail most legislators get from their constituents. Even on controversial issues, a representative might receive fewer than 100 personal letters or telephone calls. Since each congressional district includes about half a million people, the legislator tends to assume that each letter represents the views of 5,000 to 10,000 people. Your voice can have great impact. A single, well-written letter can make a difference in whether important legislation gets passed.

All legislators now have email access, but it isn't clear how many of them read Internet messages or how much attention they pay to them. Emails may fall in the category of form letters and petitions. Individually, they don't count for much, but if a decision maker gets a million of them, he or she probably will notice. If you don't have time to write, a telephone call to the local or Washington, D.C. office of your senator or representative can be effective. Follow the same steps in formulating your argument that you would use in a letter. You probably won't talk directly to the senator or representative, but your opinion will be registered by an aide. A well-organized, factual argument can be very persuasive and may change the position of your legislator.

Don't forget that many important decisions also are made at the local level. Your city planning and zoning board, county commissioners, state departments of natural resources or environmental protection, and a host of other agencies have power to establish many significant policies. These bodies are much more accessible

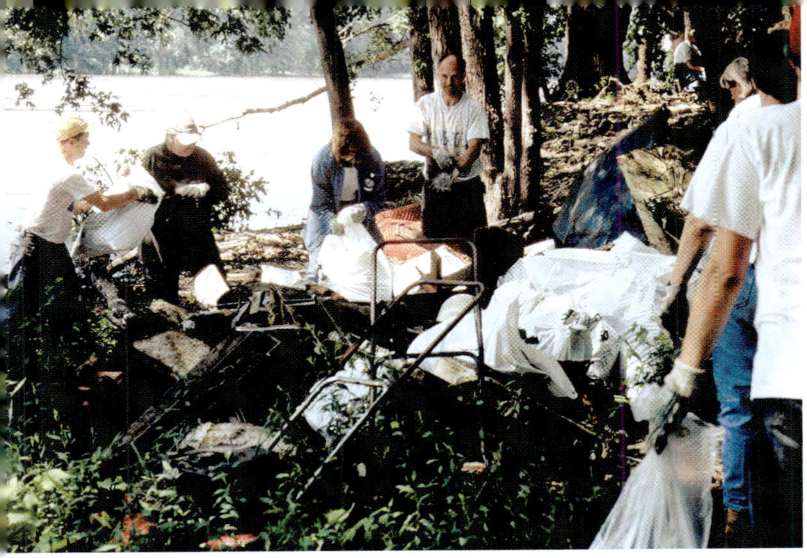

FIGURE 15.22 *Volunteers cleaned up 25 tons of trash from the banks of the Mississippi River in 2003. Each of us can help improve the quality of our local environment.*

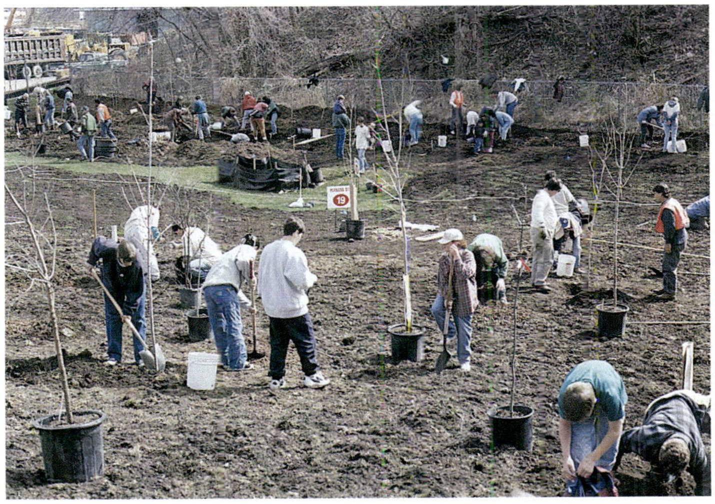

FIGURE 15.23 *Student volunteers plant native trees and bushes in a watershed protection project. Working together on a practical problem can be enjoyable and productive.*

to ordinary citizens. You might even run for a seat on a local board. What better way to ensure that local actions are sustainable than to become a policymaker yourself? Participating in practical environmental projects, such as litter cleanup or restoration projects, can help build a sense of community, be educational, and do good (fig. 15.22).

COLLECTIVE ACTION

Collective action multiplies individual power. You get encouragement and useful information from meeting regularly with others who share your interests. It's easy to get discouraged by the slow pace of change; having a support group helps maintain your enthusiasm. You should realize, however, that there is a broad spectrum of environmental and social action groups. Some will suit your particular interests, preferences, or beliefs more than others. In this section, we will look at some environmental organizations, as well as options for getting involved.

Student Environmental Groups

A number of organizations have been established to teach ecology and environmental ethics to elementary and secondary school students, as well as to get them involved in active projects to clean up their local community. Groups such as Kids Saving the Earth or Eco-Kids Corps are an important way to reach this vital audience. Family education results from these efforts as well (fig. 15.23). In a World Wildlife Fund survey, 63 percent of young people said they "lobby" their parents about recycling and buying environmentally responsible products.

Organizations for secondary and college students often are among our most active and effective groups for environmental change. The largest student environmental group in North America is the Student Environmental Action Coalition (SEAC). Formed in 1988 by students at the University of North Carolina at Chapel Hill, SEAC has grown rapidly to more than 30,000 members in some 500 campus environmental groups. SEAC is both an umbrella organization and grassroots network that functions as an information clearinghouse and a training center for student leaders. Member groups undertake a diverse spectrum of activities, ranging from politically neutral recycling promotion to confrontational protests of government or industrial projects. National conferences bring together thousands of activists who share tactics and inspiration while also having fun. If there isn't a group on your campus, why not look into organizing one?

Another important student organizing group is the network of Public Interest Research Groups (PIRGs) active on most campuses in the United States. While not focused exclusively on the environment, the PIRGs usually include environmental issues in their priorities for research. By becoming active, you could probably introduce environmental concerns to your local group if it is not already working on problems of importance to you.

One of the most important skills that you are likely to learn in SEAC or other groups committed to social change is how to organize. Organizing is a dynamic process in which you must constantly adapt to changing conditions. Some basic principles apply in most situations, however (table 15.7). Remember that you are not alone. Others share your concerns and want to work with you to bring about change; you just have to find them.

Mainline Environmental Organizations

Among the oldest, largest, and most influential environmental groups in the United States are the National Wildlife Federation, the World Wildlife Fund, the Audubon Society, the Sierra Club, the Izaak Walton League, Friends of the Earth, Greenpeace, Ducks Unlimited, the Natural Resources Defense Council, and The Wilderness Society. Sometimes known as the "group of 10," these organizations are criticized by radical environmentalists for their tendency to compromise and cooperate with the establishment.

TABLE 15.7 Organizing an Environmental Campaign

1. What do you want to change? Are your goals realistic, given the time and resources you have available?
2. What and who will be needed to get the job done? What resources do you have now, and how can you get more?
3. Who are the stakeholders in this issue? Who are your allies and constituents? How can you make contact with them?
4. How will your group make decisions and set priorities? Will you operate by consensus, majority vote, or informal agreement?
5. Have others already worked on this issue? What successes or failures did they have? Can you learn from their experience?
6. Who has the power to give you what you want or to solve the problem? Which individuals, organizations, corporations, or elected officials should your campaign target?
7. What tactics will be effective? Using the wrong tactics can alienate people and be worse than taking no action at all.
8. Are there social, cultural, or economic factors that should be recognized in this situation? Will the way you dress, talk, or behave offend or alienate your intended audience? Is it important to change your appearance or tactics to gain support?
9. How will you know when you have succeeded? How will you evaluate the possible outcomes?
10. What will you do when the battle is over? Is yours a single-issue organization, or will you want to maintain the interest, momentum, and network you have established?

Source: Based on material from "Grassroots Organizing for Everyone" by Claire Greensfelder and Mike Roselle from *Call to Action,* 1990 Sierra Book Club Books.

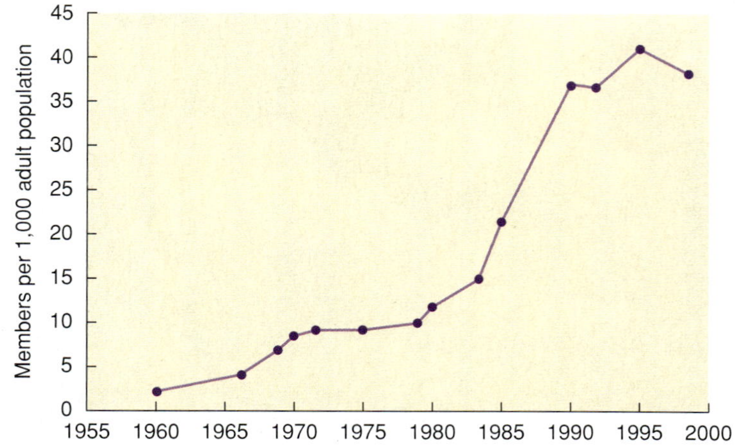

FIGURE 15.24 *Growth of national environmental organizations in the United States.*
Source: Robert Putnam, 2000.

Although many of these groups were militant— even extremist—in their formative stages, they now tend to be more staid and conservative. Members are mostly passive and know little about the inner workings of the organization, joining as much for publications or social aspects as for their stands on environmental issues. Collectively, these groups grew rapidly during the 1908s (fig. 15.24), but many of their new members had little contact with them beyond making a one-time donation.

Still, these groups are powerful and important forces in environmental protection. Their mass membership, large professional staffs, and long history give them a degree of respectability and influence not found in newer, smaller groups. The Sierra Club, for instance, with about half a million members and chapters in almost every state, has a national staff of about 400, an annual budget over $20 million, and 20 full-time professional lobbyists in Washington, D.C. These national groups have become a potent force in Congress, especially when they band together to pass specific legislation, such as the Alaska National Interest Lands Act or the Clean Air Act.

In a survey that asked congressional staff and officials of government agencies to rate the effectiveness of groups that attempt to influence federal policy on pollution control, the top five were national environmental organizations. In spite of their large budgets and important connections, the American Petroleum Institute, the Chemical Manufacturers Association, and the Edison Electric Institute ranked far behind these environmental groups in terms of influence.

Although much of the focus of the big environmental groups is in Washington, Audubon, Sierra Club, and Izaak Walton have local chapters, outings, and conservation projects. This can be a good way to get involved. Go to some meetings, volunteer, offer to help. You may have to start out stuffing envelopes or some other unglamorous job, but if you persevere, you may have a chance to do something important and fun. It's a good way to learn and meet people.

Some environmental groups, such as the Environmental Defense Fund (EDF), The Nature Conservancy (TNC), the National Resources Defense Council (NRDC), and the Wilderness Society (WS), have limited contact with ordinary members except through their publications. They depend on a professional staff to carry out the goals of the organization through litigation (EDF and NRDC), land acquisition (TNC), or lobbying (WS). Although not often in the public eye, these groups can be very effective because of their unique focus. TNC buys land of high ecological value that is threatened by development. With more than 3,200 employees and assets around $3 billion, TNC manages 7 million acres in what it describes as the world's largest private sanctuary system (fig. 15.25). Still, the Conservancy is controversial for some of its management decisions, such as gas and oil drilling in some reserves, and including executives from some questionable companies on its governing board and advisory council. The Conservancy replies that it is trying to work with these companies to bring about change rather than just criticize them.

Radical Environmental Groups

A striking contrast to the mainline conservation organizations are the direct action groups, such as Earth First!, Sea Shepherd, and a

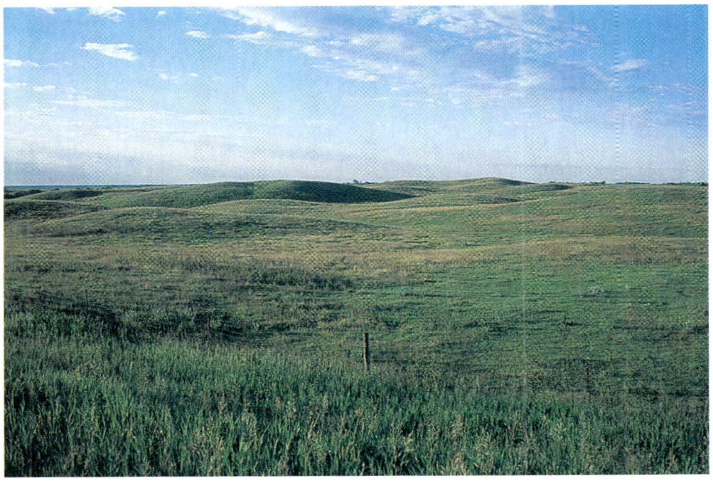

FIGURE 15.25 *The Nature Conservancy buys land, such as this short-grass prairie in Montana, to protect it from misuse and development.*

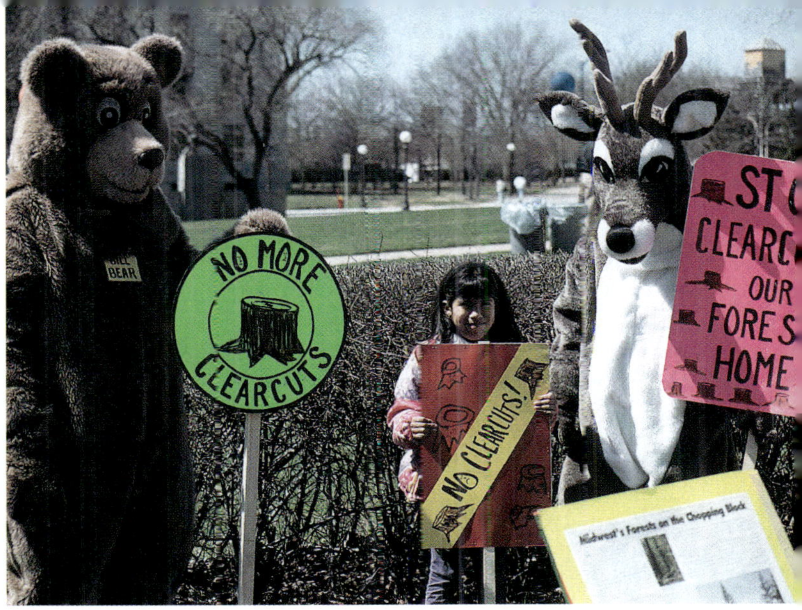

FIGURE 15.26 *Street theater can be a humorous yet effective, way to convey a point in a nonthreatening manner. Confrontational tactics get attention, but they may alienate those who might be your allies and harden your opposition.*

few other groups that form either the "cutting edge" or the "radical fringe" of the environmental movement, depending on your outlook. Often associated with the deep ecology philosophy and bioregional ecological perspective, the strongest concerns of these militant environmentalists tend to be animal rights and protection of wild nature. Their main tactics are civil disobedience and attention-grabbing actions, such as picketing, protest marches, road blockades, and other demonstrations. Some of these actions are humorous and lighthearted, such as street theater that gets a point across in a nonthreatening way (fig. 15.26). Many of these techniques are borrowed from the civil rights movement and Mahatma Gandhi's nonviolent civil disobedience. While often more innovative than the mainstream organizations, pioneering new issues and new approaches, the tactics of these groups can be controversial.

Members of Earth First! chained themselves to a giant tree-smashing bulldozer to prevent forest clearing in Texas and blockaded roads being built into wilderness areas. In one remarkable case, a 25-year-old activist named Julia "Butterfly" Hill spent more than two years sitting on a small, tarp-covered platform 55 m (180 ft) up in a redwood tree in northern California. She was protesting the clear-cutting of the Headwaters Forest by the Maxxam/Pacific Lumber Company. She came down from her perch in 1999 when her supporters raised $50,000 to buy the tree from Maxxam. While some people regard this direct action as heroic and noble, others see it as dangerous and counterproductive. What do you think? Are there circumstances in which it is appropriate or effective to use confrontation rather than cooperation and compromise to achieve your goals? Would you ever break a law to protect nature?

International Nongovernmental Organizations

The rise in international environmental organizations in recent years has been phenomenal. At the Stockholm Conference in 1972, only a handful of environmental groups attended, almost all from First World countries. Twenty years later, at the Rio Earth Summit, more than 30,000 individuals representing several thousand environmental groups, many from the Third World, held a global Ecoforum to debate issues and form alliances for a better world. We call these groups working for social change **nongovernmental organizations (NGOs).** They have become a powerful aspect of environmental protection.

Some NGOs are located primarily in the more highly developed countries of the north and work mainly on local issues. Others are headquartered in the north but focus their attention on the problems of developing countries in the south. Still others are truly global, with active groups in many different countries. A few are highly professional, combining private individuals with representatives of government agencies on quasi-government boards or standing committees with considerable power. Others are on the fringes of society, sometimes literally voices crying in the wilderness. Many work for political change, more specialize in gathering and disseminating information, and some undertake direct action to protect a specific resource.

Public education and consciousness-raising using protest marches, demonstrations, civil disobedience, and other participatory public actions and media events are generally important tactics for these groups. Greenpeace, for instance, carries out well-publicized confrontations with whalers, seal hunters, toxic waste dumpers, and others who threaten very specific and visible resources. Greenpeace may well be the largest environmental organization in the world, claiming some 2.5 million contributing members.

In contrast to these highly visible groups, others choose to work behind the scenes, but their impact may be equally important. Conservation International has been a leader in debt-for-nature swaps to protect areas particularly rich in biodiversity. It also has some interesting initiatives in economic development, seeking products made by local people that will provide income along with environmental protection (fig. 15.27).

The famous anthropologist Margaret Meade once wrote, "Never doubt that a small group of thoughtful, committed people can change the world; indeed it is the only thing that can." We hope that in this book you have found the inspiration and tools to make a positive change in our shared world.

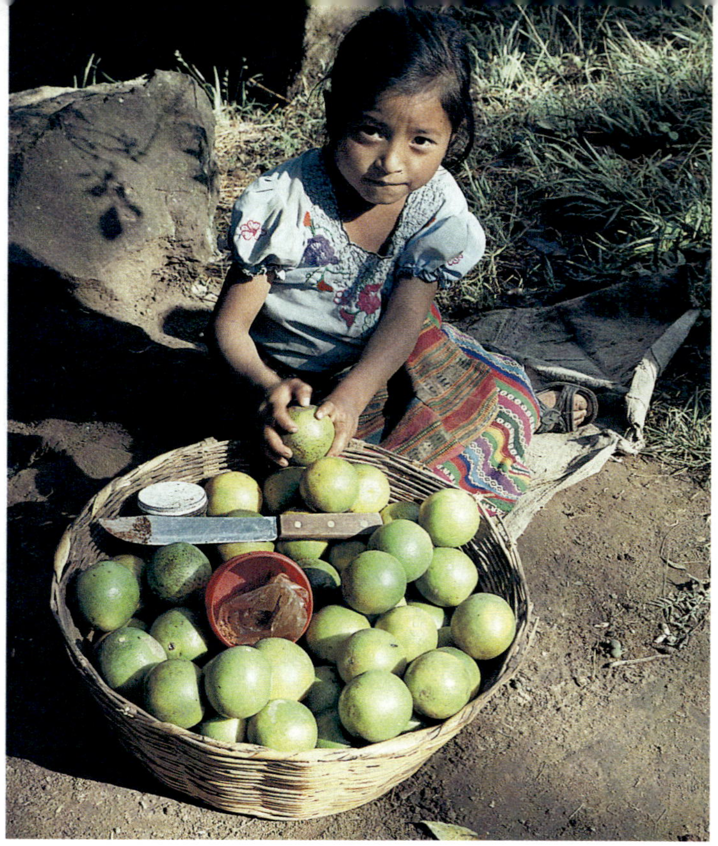

FIGURE 15.27 *International conservation groups often initiate economic development projects that provide local alternatives to natural resource destruction.*

SUMMARY

- Throughout this book we've studied a variety of serious environmental problems. Science can help us understand why these problems occur and what we might do about them, but for many complex issues—sometimes called "wicked" problems because they have no single, clear answer—we can't wait until all possible evidence is gathered. We must make reasoned judgments based on the best available evidence.
- Learning from ecological systems, we see that some of the main goals for environmental policy and planning might be the precautionary principle and adaptive management. Citizen-science provides hands-on experience in environmental science and provides information to policymakers that can help them make informed decisions.
- Environmental education and literacy are important if we are to manage our natural resources for long-term sustainability. There are many opportunities for environmental careers in both natural and social sciences.
- Although "policy" can have multiple meanings, in this chapter, environmental policy is taken to mean both public opinion as well as official rules and regulations concerning our environment. The policy cycle describes the steps by which problems are identified and defined and solutions are proposed, debated, enacted into law, and monitored.
- The National Environmental Policy Act (NEPA) forms the cornerstone of both environmental policy and law in the United States. One of its most important provisions is the requirement of Environmental Impact Statements (EIS) for all major federal projects and programs. Laws are rules established through legislation (statutes), judicial decisions (case law), or executive decisions (administrative law).
- Lobbying, litigation, and administrative interventions have been among environmentalists' most effective ways to shape policy and protect the environment. Individuals can play important roles in these processes, but often it is more effective to work collectively.

- There are many different environmental organizations, and their philosophies and tactics range from quiet, behind-the-scene negotiations with decision makers to public protests and radical activism. Everyone should be able to find a group that fits his or her outlook.
- Although many international treaties and conventions have been passed to protect our global environment, most are vague or toothless. Some innovative measures have been devised to compel compliance. Some alternatives to adversarial litigation include arbitration, mediation, and community-based planning. These techniques are useful in complex, unpredictable, multistakeholder, multivalue issues.

QUESTIONS FOR REVIEW

1. Describe adaptive management and the conditions necessary for its implementation.
2. What are "wicked" problems? Why are they difficult?
3. List two goals and four potential outcomes of environmental education.
4. What environmental career might you find rewarding and compatible with your interests?
5. What is the policy cycle, and how does it work?
6. Describe the three important provisions of NEPA (National Environmental Policy Act).
7. Discuss the differences and similarities among statutory, case, and administrative law.
8. List some of the major U.S. environmental legislation, as well as some important international environmental conventions and treaties.
9. Why have some international environmental treaties and conventions been effective, while most have not? Describe two such treaties.
10. What is collaborative, community-based planning?

THINKING SCIENTIFICALLY

1. Table 15.1 lists some important environmental questions. What would you add to this list? Which of these questions would you tackle first if you were head of a major foundation or research institute?
2. Think of an example of a "wicked" environmental problem. What makes it complex and difficult? What institutional changes could we implement to make this issue less wicked?
3. Which of the many environmental issues you have read about in this book are most interesting to you? Which laws in tables 15.5 or 15.6 pertain to those issues?
4. What fields of science help us understand or resolve the issues in question 3? What science classes could you take that would help you understand them or contribute to creative solutions? Which nonscience classes are also essential to understanding these issues?
5. As you read in chapter 1, scientists try to remain skeptical of evidence and rarely consider theories "proven." Why is this? How can politicians and lawyers make firm rules using scientific evidence when there is always uncertainty in scientific data?
6. Which is the most important step in the policy cycle (fig. 15.8)? If you were leader of a major environmental group, where would you put your efforts in establishing policy?
7. Do you believe that trees, wild animals, rocks, or mountains should have legal rights and standing in the courts? Why or why not? Are there partial rights or some other form of protection you would favor for nature?
8. It's sometimes difficult to determine whether a lawsuit is retaliatory or based on valid reason. How would you define a SLAPP suit and differentiate it from a legitimate case?
9. Under what conditions do you think mediation, arbitration, or collaborative planning could be more effective than litigation or confrontation? If you were planning a campaign to solve the problem you considered in question 2, which of these approaches would you use?
10. Try creating a list of arguments for and against an international body with power to enforce global environmental laws. Can you see a way to create a body that could satisfy both reasons for and against this power?

KEY TERMS

adaptive management 354
agency rule-making 365
arbitration 369
case law 363
citizen science 358
community-based planning 369
criminal law 364
environmental law 361
environmental literacy 356
environmental policy 358
federal laws (statutes) 361
international treaties and conventions 367
legal standing 363
lobbying 362
mediation 369
National Environmental Policy Act (NEPA) 360
nongovernmental organizations (NGOs) 373
policy cycle 359
precautionary principle 355
Strategic Lawsuits against Political Participation (SLAPP) 365
"wicked" problems 355

SUGGESTED READINGS

Campbell, L. M., and Vainio-Mattila. 2003. "Participatory development and community-based conservation: opportunities missed for lessons learned." *Human Ecology* 3(3):417–37.

Dombeck, Michael P., Christopher A. Wood, and Jack E. Williams. 2003. *From Conquest to Conservation: Our Public Lands Legacy.* Island Press.

Fischman, Robert L. 2004. *The National Wildlife Refuges: Coordinating a Conservation System Through Law.* Island Press.

National Wildlife Federation. 2004. *Conservation Directory 2004: The Guide to Worldwide Environmental Organizations.* Island Press.

Orr, David. 2004. "Law of the Land." *Orion* 23(1):18–25.

Putnam, Robert D. 2000. *Bowling Alone: The Collapse and Revival of American Community.* Simon & Schuster.

Roberts, Jane. 2002. *Environmental Policy: Theory and Practice.* Routledge Press.

Speth, James G., ed. 2003. *Worlds Apart: Globalization and the Environment.* Island Press.

Tickner, Joel A. 2002. *Precaution, Environmental Science, and Preventive Public Policy.* Island Press.

Train, Russell E. 2004. *Politics, Pollution, and Pandas: An Environmental Memoir.* Island Press.

Welcome to McGraw-Hill's Online Learning Center

http://www.mhhe.com/cunningham3e

WEB EXERCISE

Environmental Scorecard

Find out how the U.S. Congress voted on key environmental issues by going to the webpage of the League of Conservation Voters (LCV) at http://scorecard.lcv.org/. You can download the entire scorecard in PDF format or view the full Senate or full House vote online. To find out how your own senators and congressional representative voted, search by state, enter the name of a specific member, or enter your zip code and click on *go*. Look at the descriptions of the specific issues on which the rating was based to learn more about them and to see if you agree with the assessment offered by this scorecard. The LCV may regard voting in a particular way to be pro- or antienvironmental, but do you agree? Note that an absence during a specific vote is recorded as negative, even if the absence was for illness or some other valid reason. Under the Overview section in the left frame on the scorecard page, you can learn more about the issues discussed by Congress.

To keep up to date on current issues, you can visit the websites of specific groups, such as the Natural Resources Defense Council (www.nrdc.org/legislation/legwatch.asp) or the Endangered Species Coalition (www.stopextinction.org/). The Thomas website of the U.S. Library of Congress (http://thomas.loc.gov/) allows you to find the latest action in Congress.

Finding an Environmental Organization

To learn more about environmental organizations, go to www.webdirectory.com/, which describes itself as the "world's biggest search engine." You'll find thousands of listings there. Many of the websites are for institutions and agencies, but you'll also find public groups in almost any environmental issue. Choose a general category that appeals to you and investigate a group that seems interesting. What are the goals and tactics of this group? How long has it been in existence? Do you agree (or disagree) with its principles and practices, as far as you can discern these from what's published on the website?

If you can't find an environmental organization that gives useful information about itself in the categories listed in the Environmental Organization Web directory, try searching for one of the "big 10" organizations described in this chapter. What do they tell you about themselves? Would you consider joining them? Why or why not?

Although the Environmental Working Group no longer updates its Clearinghouse on Environmental Advocacy and Research (CLEAR) website, you still may be able to find useful information about antienvironmental groups at www.ewg.org/pub/home/clear/clear.html. Click on your home state (if you're from the United States) or choose a western state to find out about some of these groups and their activities.

APPENDIXES

Vegetation

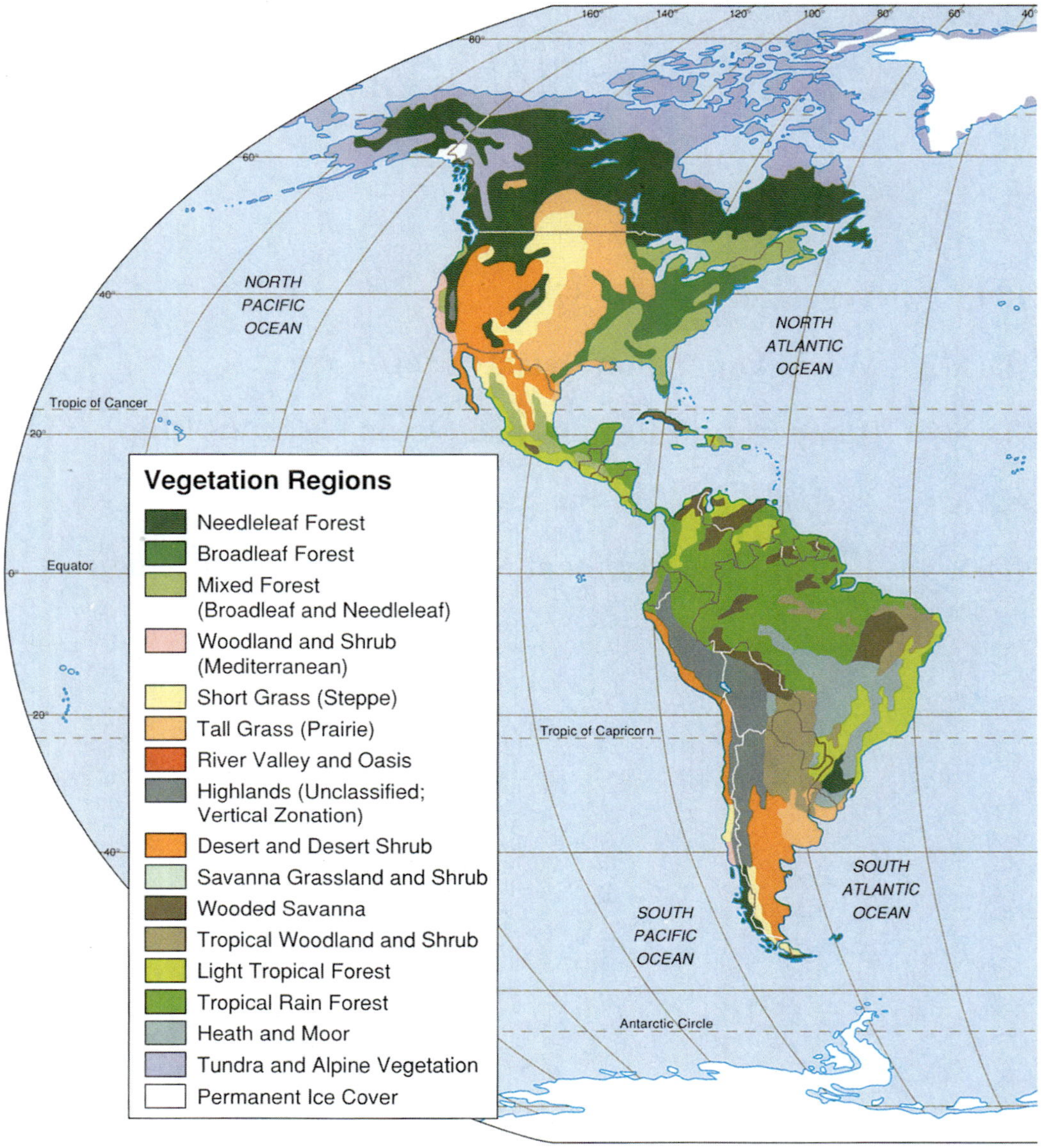
160°
140°
120°
100°
80°
60°
40°
NORTH PACIFIC OCEAN
NORTH ATLANTIC OCEAN
Tropic of Cancer
Equator
Tropic of Capricorn
SOUTH PACIFIC OCEAN
SOUTH ATLANTIC OCEAN
Antarctic Circle
Vegetation Regions
Needleleaf Forest
Broadleaf Forest
Mixed Forest (Broadleaf and Needleleaf)
Woodland and Shrub (Mediterranean)
Short Grass (Steppe)
Tall Grass (Prairie)
River Valley and Oasis
Highlands (Unclassified; Vertical Zonation)
Desert and Desert Shrub
Savanna Grassland and Shrub
Wooded Savanna
Tropical Woodland and Shrub
Light Tropical Forest
Tropical Rain Forest
Heath and Moor
Tundra and Alpine Vegetation
Permanent Ice Cover

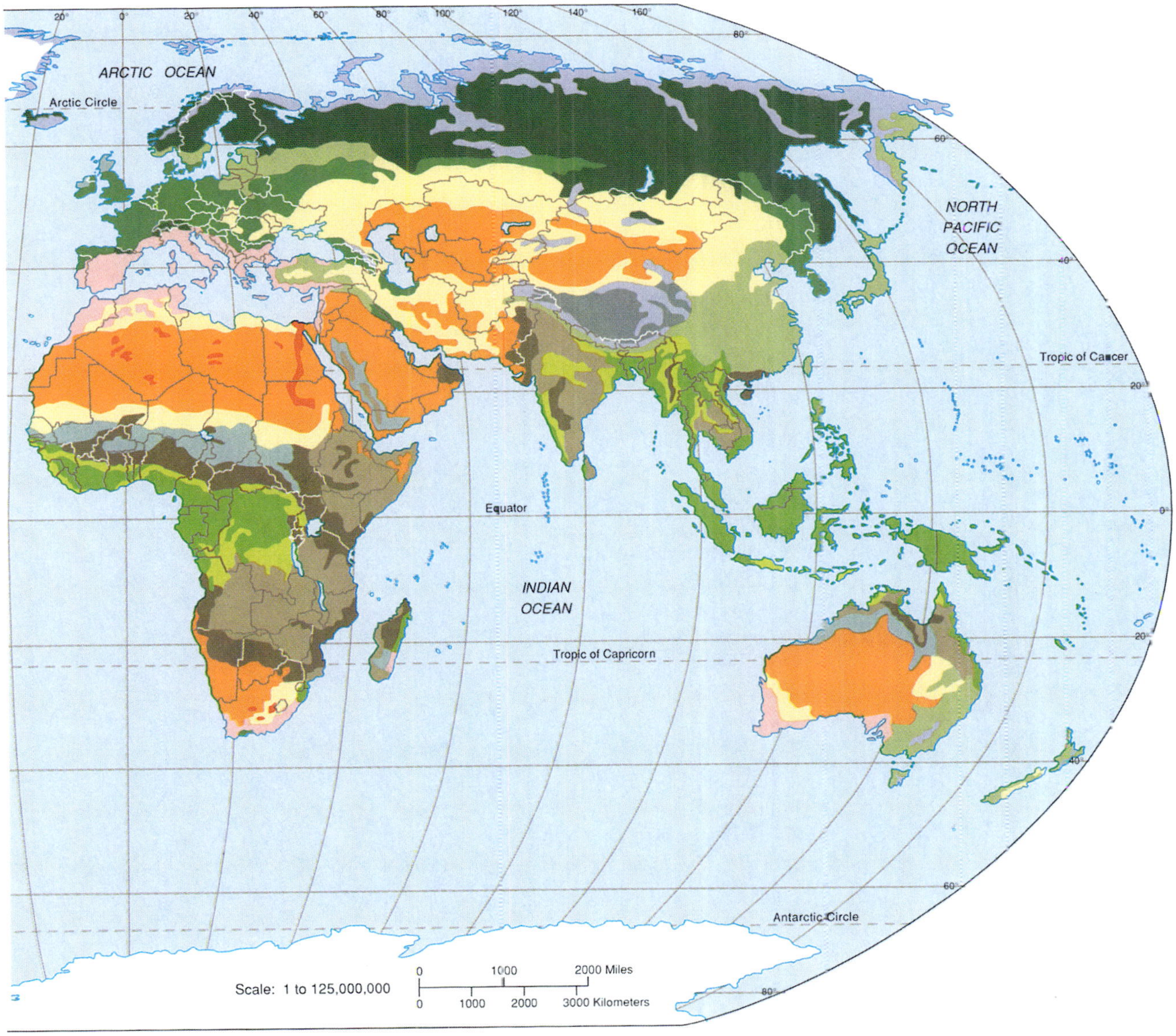

Vegetation is the most visible consequence of the distribution of temperature and precipitation. The global distribution of vegetation types and the global distribution of climate are closely related. But not all vegetation types are the consequence of temperature and precipitation or other climatic variables. Many types of vegetation, in many areas of the world, are the consequence of human activities, particularly the grazing of domesticated livestock, burning, and forest clearance.

World Population Density

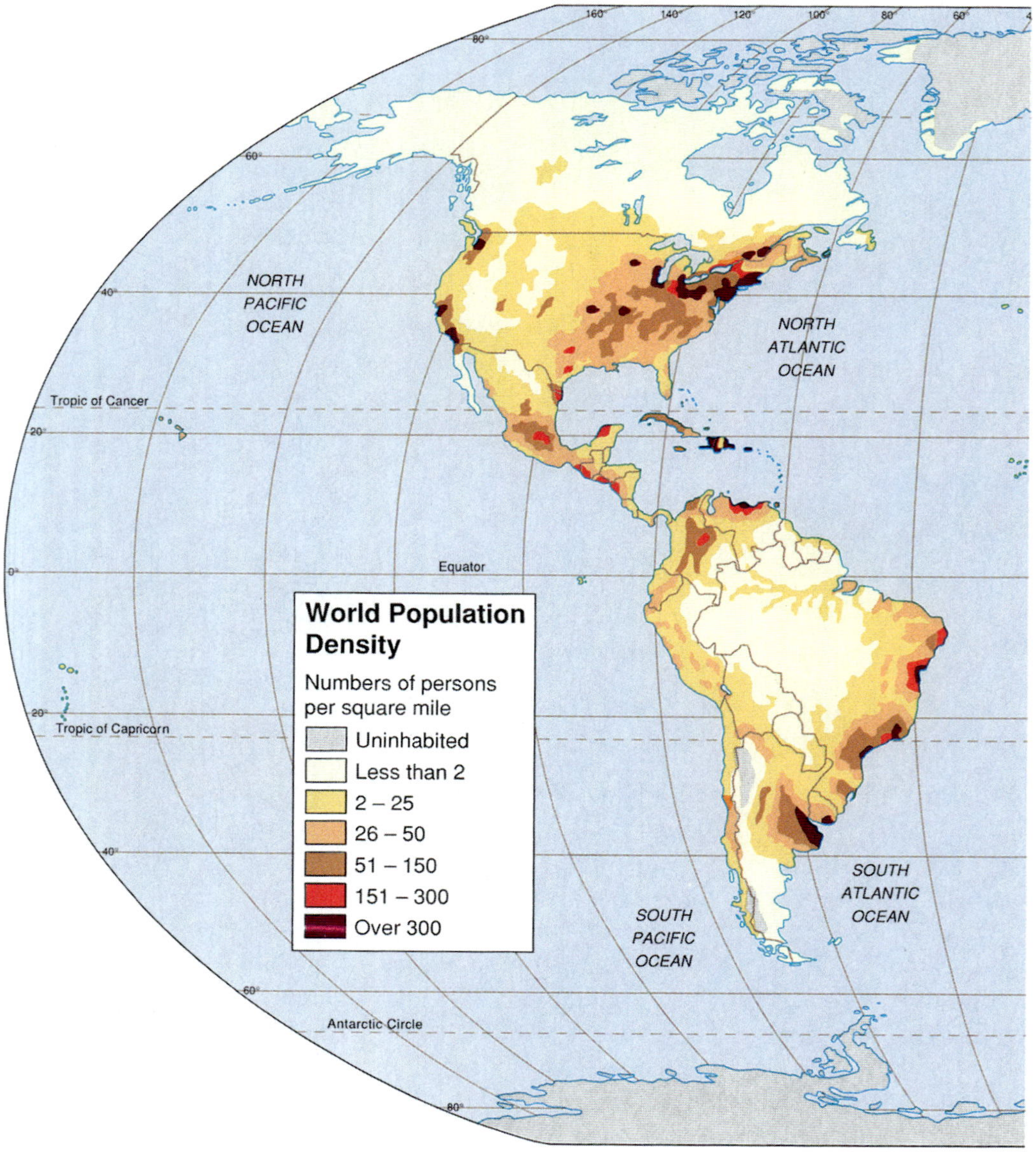

No feature of human activity is more reflective of environmental conditions than where people live. In the areas of densest population, a mixture of natural and human factors have combined to allow maximum food production, maximum urbanization, and especially concentrated economic activity. Three such great concentrations appear on the map—East Asia, South Asia, and Europe—with a fourth lesser concentration in eastern North America (the "Megalopolis" region of the United States and Canada). One of these great population clusters —South Asia—is still growing rapidly and can be expected to become even more densely populated by the beginning of the twenty-first century. The other concentrations are likely to remain about as they are now. In

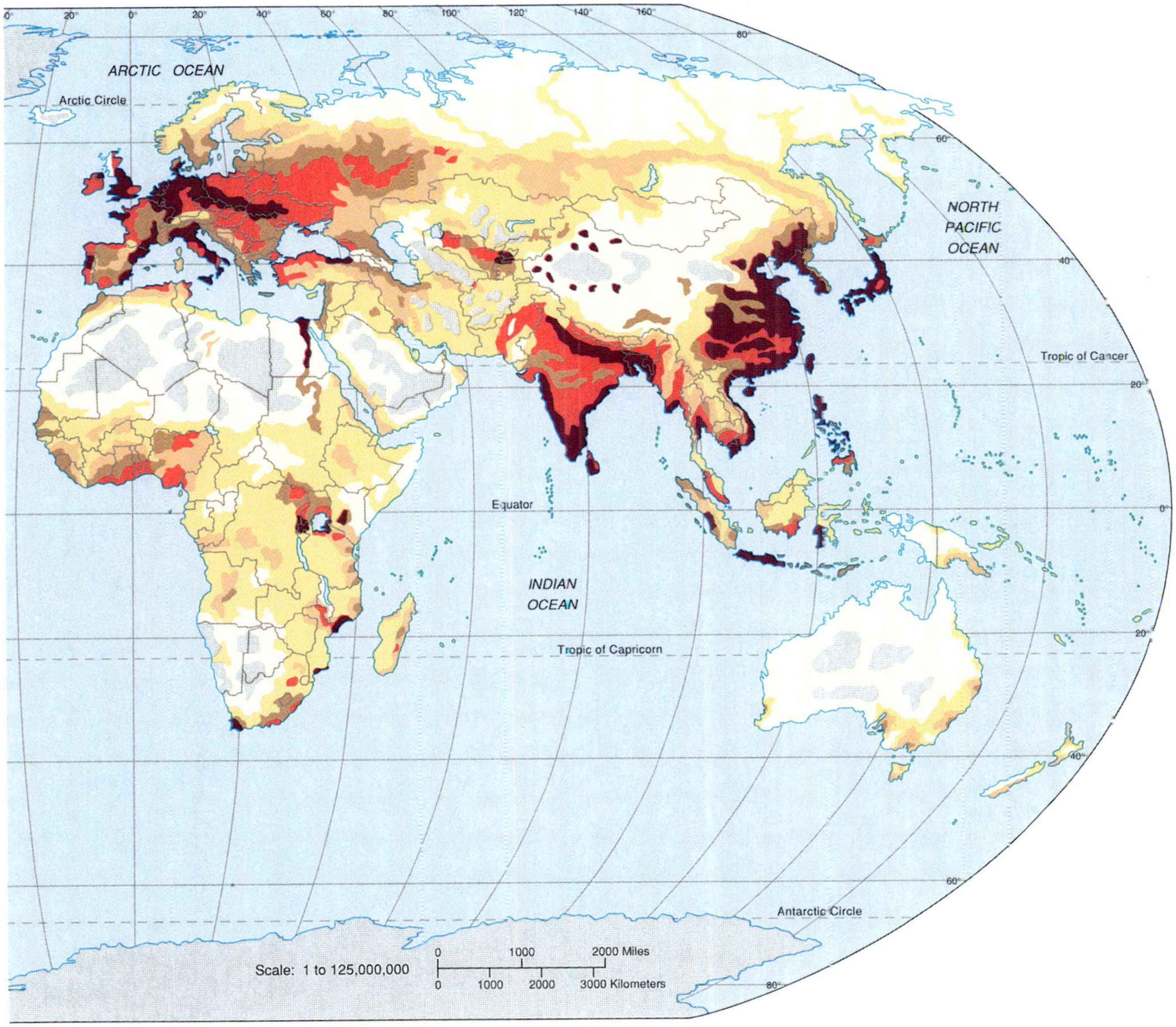

Europe and North America, this is the result of economic development that has caused population growth to level off during the last century. In East Asia, population has also begun to grow more slowly. In the case of Japan and the Koreas, this is the consequence of economic development; in the case of China, it is the consequence of government intervention in the form of strict family planning. The areas of future high density (in addition to those already existing) are likely to be in Middle and South America and Africa, where population growth rates are well above the world average. Population that is extremely dense or growing at an excessive rate when measured against a region's habitability is one of the greatest indicators of environmental deterioration.

Temperature Regions and Ocean Currents

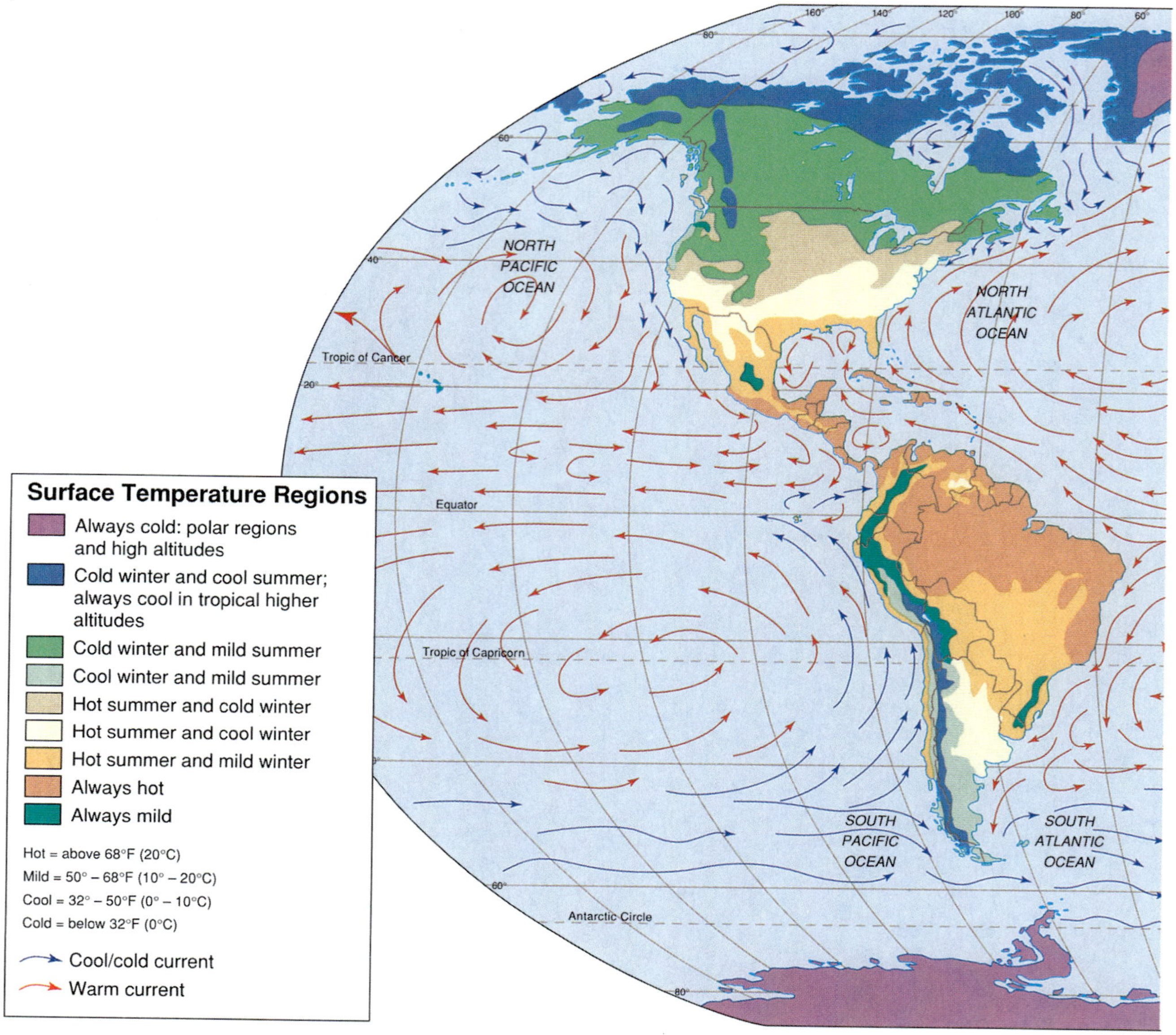

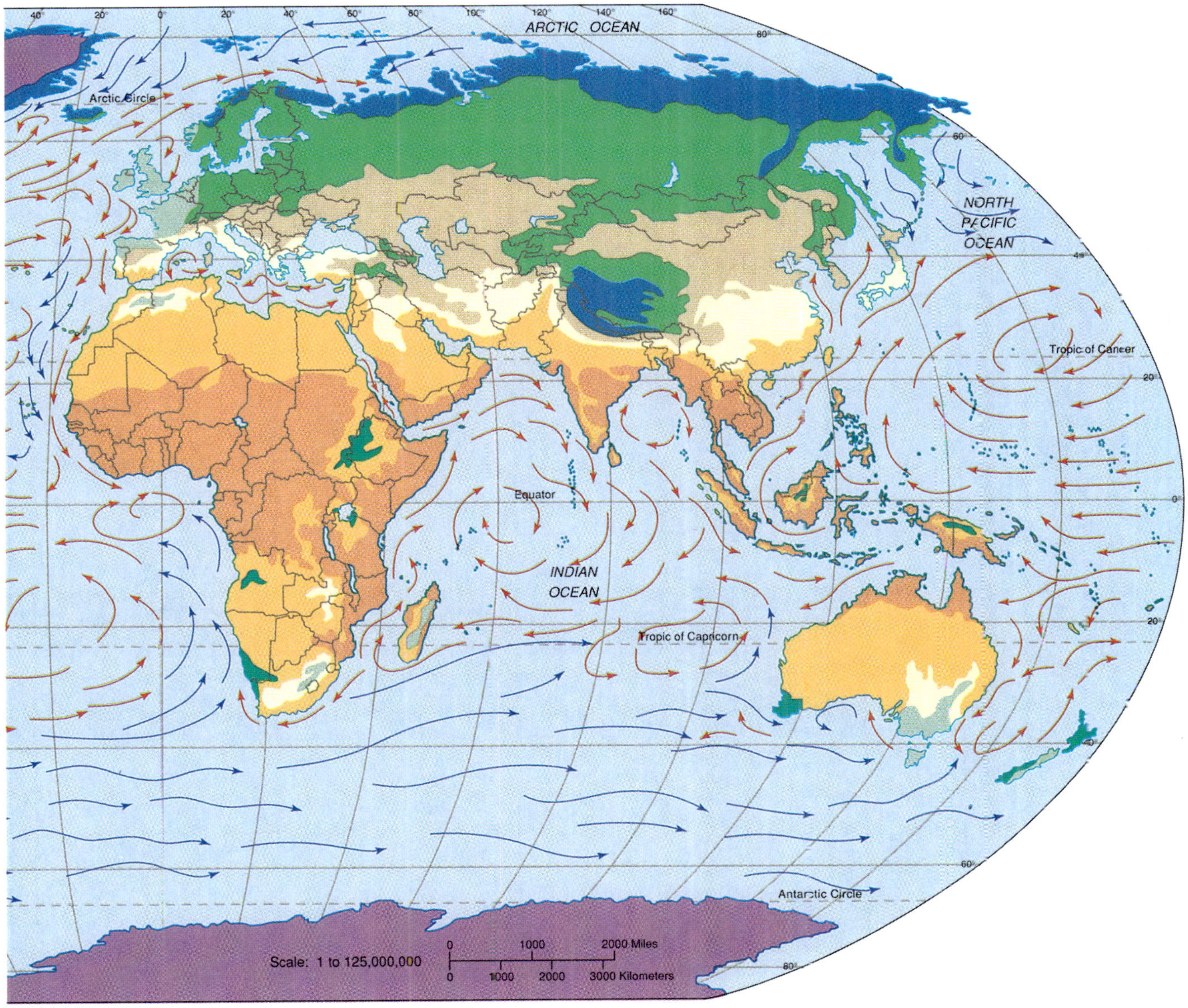

Along with precipitation, temperature is one of the two most important environmental variables, defining the climatic conditions so essential for the distribution of human activities and the human population. Ocean currents exert a significant influence over the climate of adjacent continents and are the most important mechanism for redistributing surplus heat from the equatorial region into middle and high latitudes.

Periodic Table of the Elements

Key

1 Hydrogen **H** 1.0079	Atomic number Name Symbol Atomic weight

- Metals
- Metalloids
- Nonmetals
- Lanthanides
- Actinides

Period	IA	IIA	IIIB	IVB	VB	VIB	VIIB	VIIIB	VIIIB	VIIIB	IB	IIB	IIIA	IVA	VA	VIA	VIIA	VIIIA
1	1 Hydrogen **H** 1.0079																	2 Helium **He** 4.0026
2	3 Lithium **Li** 6.941	4 Beryllium **Be** 9.0122											5 Boron **B** 10.811	6 Carbon **C** 12.0112	7 Nitrogen **N** 14.0067	8 Oxygen **O** 15.9994	9 Fluorine **F** 18.9984	10 Neon **Ne** 20.179
3	11 Sodium **Na** 22.989	12 Magnesium **Mg** 24.305											13 Aluminum **Al** 26.9815	14 Silicon **Si** 28.086	15 Phosphorus **P** 30.9738	16 Sulfur **S** 32.064	17 Chlorine **Cl** 35.453	18 Argon **Ar** 39.948
4	19 Potassium **K** 39.098	20 Calcium **Ca** 40.08	21 Scandium **Sc** 44.956	22 Titanium **Ti** 47.90	23 Vanadium **V** 50.942	24 Chromium **Cr** 51.996	25 Manganese **Mn** 54.938	26 Iron **Fe** 55.847	27 Cobalt **Co** 58.933	28 Nickel **Ni** 58.71	29 Copper **Cu** 63.546	30 Zinc **Zn** 65.38	31 Gallium **Ga** 69.723	32 Germanium **Ge** 72.59	33 Arsenic **As** 74.992	34 Selenium **Se** 78.96	35 Bromine **Br** 79.904	36 Krypton **Kr** 83.80
5	37 Rubidium **Rb** 85.468	38 Strontium **Sr** 87.62	39 Yttrium **Y** 88.905	40 Zirconium **Zr** 91.22	41 Niobium **Nb** 92.906	42 Molybdenum **Mo** 95.94	43 Technetium **Tc** (99)	44 Ruthenium **Ru** 101.07	45 Rhodium **Rh** 102.905	46 Palladium **Pd** 106.4	47 Silver **Ag** 107.868	48 Cadmium **Cd** 112.40	49 Indium **In** 114.82	50 Tin **Sn** 118.69	51 Antimony **Sb** 121.75	52 Tellurium **Te** 127.60	53 Iodine **I** 126.904	54 Xenon **Xe** 131.30
6	55 Cesium **Cs** 132.905	56 Barium **Ba** 137.34	*57 Lanthanum **La** 138.91	72 Hafnium **Hf** 178.49	73 Tantalum **Ta** 180.948	74 Tungsten **W** 183.85	75 Rhenium **Re** 186.2	76 Osmium **Os** 190.2	77 Iridium **Ir** 192.2	78 Platinum **Pt** 195.09	79 Gold **Au** 196.967	80 Mercury **Hg** 200.59	81 Thallium **Tl** 204.37	82 Lead **Pb** 207.19	83 Bismuth **Bi** 208.980	84 Polonium **Po** (209)	85 Astatine **At** (210)	86 Radon **Rn** (222)
7	87 Francium **Fr** (223)	88 Radium **Ra** (226)	**89 Actinium **Ac** (227)	104 Rutherfordium **Rf** (261)	105 Hahnium **Ha** (262)	106 Seaborgium **Sg** (263)	107 Neilsbohrium **Ns** (261)	108 Hassium **Hs** (265)	109 Meitnerium **Mt** (266)									

58 Cerium **Ce** 140.12	59 Praseodymium **Pr** 140.907	60 Neodymium **Nd** 144.24	61 Promethium **Pm** 144.913	62 Samarium **Sm** 150.35	63 Europium **Eu** 151.96	64 Gadolinium **Gd** 157.25	65 Terbium **Tb** 158.925	66 Dysprosium **Dy** 162.50	67 Holmium **Ho** 164.930	68 Erbium **Er** 167.26	69 Thulium **Tm** 168.934	70 Ytterbium **Yb** 173.04	71 Lutetium **Lu** 174.97
90 Thorium **Th** 232.038	91 Protactinium **Pa** (231)	92 Uranium **U** 238.03	93 Neptunium **Np** (237)	94 Plutonium **Pu** 244.064	95 Americium **Am** (243)	96 Curium **Cm** (247)	97 Berkelium **Bk** (247)	98 Californium **Cf** 242.058	99 Einsteinium **Es** (254)	100 Fermium **Fm** 257.095	101 Mendelevium **Md** 258.10	102 Nobelium **No** 259.10	103 Lawrencium **Lr** 260.105

The periodic table arranges elements by atomic number (number of protons). The rows and columns are organized to show groups of similar chemical characteristics. For example, the right-most column contains "noble" gases that do not react readily with other elements, and the next column to the left (F, Cl, Br, I, At) includes highly reactive elements known as halogens.

Units of Measurement
Metric/English Conversions

Length

1 meter = 39.4 inches = 3.28 feet = 1.09 yard
1 foot = 0.305 meters = 12 inches = 0.33 yard
1 inch = 2.54 centimeters
1 centimeter = 10 millimeters = 0.394 inch
1 millimeter = 0.001 meter = 0.01 centimeter = 0.039 inch
1 fathom = 6 feet = 1.83 meters
1 rod = 16.5 feet = 5 meters
1 chain = 4 rods = 66 feet = 20 meters
1 furlong = 10 chains = 40 rods = 660 feet = 200 meters
1 kilometer = 1,000 meters = 0.621 miles = 0.54 nautical miles
1 mile = 5,280 feet = 8 furlongs = 1.61 kilometers
1 nautical mile = 1.15 mile

Area

1 square centimeter = 0.155 square inch
1 square foot = 144 square inches = 929 square centimeters
1 square yard = 9 square feet = 0.836 square meters
1 square meter = 10.76 square feet = 1.196 square yards = 1 million square millimeters
1 hectare = 10,000 square meters = 0.01 square kilometers = 2.47 acres
1 acre = 43,560 square feet = 0.405 hectares
1 square kilometer = 100 hectares = 1 million square meters = 0.386 square miles = 247 acres
1 square mile = 640 acres = 2.59 square kilometers

Volume

1 cubic centimeter = 1 milliliter = 0.001 liter
1 cubic meter = 1 million cubic centimeters = 1,000 liters
1 cubic meter = 35.3 cubic feet = 1.307 cubic yards = 264 US gallons
1 cubic yard = 27 cubic feet = 0.765 cubic meters = 202 US gallons
1 cubic kilometer = 1 million cubic meters = 0.24 cubic mile = 264 billion gallons
1 cubic mile = 4.166 cubic kilometers
1 liter = 1,000 milliliters = 1.06 quarts = 0.265 US gallons = 0.035 cubic feet
1 US gallon = 4 quarts = 3.79 liters = 231 cubic inches = 0.83 imperial (British) gallons
1 quart = 2 pints = 4 cups = 0.94 liters
1 acre foot = 325,851 US gallons = 1,234,975 liters = 1,234 cubic meters
1 barrel (of oil) = 42 US gallons = 159 liters

Mass

1 microgram = 0.001 milligram = 0.000001 gram
1 gram = 1,000 milligrams = 0.035 ounce
1 kilogram = 1,000 grams = 2.205 pounds
1 pound = 16 ounces = 454 grams
1 short ton = 2,000 pounds = 909 kilograms
1 metric ton = 1,000 kilograms = 2,200 pounds

Temperature

Celsius to Fahrenheit ° F = (°C × 1.8) + 32
Fahrenheit to Celsius ° C = (° F – 32) ÷ 1.8

Energy and Power

1 erg = 1 dyne per square centimeter
1 joule = 10 million ergs
1 calorie = 4.184 joules
1 kilojoule = 1,000 joules = 0.949 British Thermal Units (BTU)
1 megajoule = MJ = 1,000,000 joules
1 kilocalorie = 1,000 calories = 3.97 BTU = 0.00116 kilowatt-hour
1 BTU = 0.293 watt-hour
1 kilowatt-hour = 1,000 watt-hours = 860 kilocalories = 3,400 BTU
1 horsepower = 640 kilocalories
1 quad = 1 quadrillion kilojoules = 2.93 trillion kilowatt-hours

Quantitative Prefixes

Large Numbers	Description	Small Numbers
exa 10^{18}	quintillion	atto 10^{-18}
peta 10^{15}	quadrillion	femto 10^{-15}
tera 10^{12}	trillion	pico 10^{-12}
giga 10^{9}	billion	nano 10^{-9}
mega 10^{6}	million	micro 10^{-6}
kilo 10^{3}	thousand	milli 10^{-3}

(e.g., a kilogram = 1,000 gm; a milligram = one-thousandth of a gram)

GLOSSARY

A

acid precipitation Acidic rain, snow, or dry particles deposited from the air due to increased acids released by anthropogenic or natural resources.

acids Substances that release hydrogen atoms in water.

active solar systems Mechanical systems that use moving substances to collect and transfer solar energy.

acute effects A sudden onset of symptoms or effects of exposure to some factor.

acute poverty Insufficient income or access to resources needed to provide the basic necessities for life, such as food, shelter, sanitation, clean water, medical care, and education.

adaptation Physical changes that allow organisms to survive in a given environment.

adaptive management A management plan designed from the outset to "learn by doing" and to actively test hypotheses and adjust treatments as new information becomes available.

administrative law Executive orders, administrative rules and regulations, and enforcement decisions by administrative agencies and special administrative courts.

aerosols Minute particles or liquid droplets suspended in the air.

agency rule-making The formal process of establishing rules and standards by administrative agencies.

albedo A description of a surface's reflective properties.

allergens Substances that activate the immune system and cause an allergic response; may not be directly antigenic themselves but may make other materials antigenic.

ambient air The air immediately around us.

analytical thinking A way of systematic analysis that asks, "How can I break this problem down into its constituent parts?"

anemia Low levels of hemoglobin due to iron deficiency or lack of red blood cells.

anthropocentric Believing that humans hold a special place in nature; being centered primarily on humans and human affairs.

antigens Substances that stimulate the production of, and react with, specific antibodies.

aquifers Porous, water-bearing layers of sand, gravel, and rock below the earth's surface; reservoirs for groundwater.

arbitration A formal process of dispute resolution resulting in a legally binding decision that all parties must obey.

arithmetic growth A pattern of growth that increases at a constant amount per unit time, such as 1, 2, 3, 4 or 1, 3, 5, 7.

atmospheric deposition Sedimentation of solids, liquids, or gaseous materials from the air.

atom The smallest particle that exhibits the characteristics of an element.

atomic number The characteristic number of protons per atom of an element.

autotroph An organism that synthesizes food molecules from inorganic molecules by using an external energy source, such as light energy.

B

barrier islands Low, narrow, sandy islands that form offshore from a coastline.

bases Substances that readily bond with hydrogen ions in an aqueous solution.

Batesian mimicry Evolution by one species to resemble another species that is protected from predators by a venomous stinger, bad taste, or some other defensive adaptation.

benthic The bottom of a sea or lake.

bioaccumulation The selective absorption and concentration of molecules by cells.

biocentric preservation A philosophy that emphasizes the fundamental right of living organisms to exist and to pursue their own ends.

biocentrism The belief that all creatures have rights and values; being centered on nature rather than humans.

biochemical oxygen demand (BOD) A standard test for measuring the amount of dissolved oxygen utilized by aquatic microorganisms.

biodegradable plastics Plastics that can be decomposed by microorganisms.

biodiversity The genetic, species, and ecological diversity of the organisms in a given area.

biogeochemical cycles Movement of matter within or between ecosystems; caused by living organisms, geologic forces, or chemical reactions. The cycling of nitrogen, carbon, sulfur, oxygen, phosphorus, and water are examples.

biogeographical area A region or an ecosystem with characteristic biological, water, and land resources.

biological community The populations of plants, animals, and microorganisms living and interacting in a certain area at a given time.

biological controls Use of natural predators, pathogens, or competitors to regulate pest populations.

biomagnification Increase in concentration of certain stable chemicals (for example, heavy metals or fat-soluble pesticides) in successively higher trophic levels of a food chain or web.

biomass The accumulated biological material produced by living organisms.

biomass fuel Organic material produced by plants, animals, or microorganisms that can be burned directly as a heat source or converted into a gaseous or liquid fuel.

biomass pyramid A metaphor or diagram that explains the relationship between the amounts of biomass at different trophic levels.

biomes Broad, regional types of ecosystems characterized by distinctive climate and soil conditions and distinctive kinds of biological community adapted to those conditions.

bioremediation Use of biological organisms to remove pollution or restore environmental quality.

biosphere The zone of air, land, and water at the surface of the earth that is occupied by organisms.

biosphere reserves World heritage sites identified by the IUCN as worthy for national park or wildlife refuge status because of high biological diversity or unique ecological features.

biota All organisms in a given area.

biotic potential The maximum reproductive rate of an organism, given unlimited resources and ideal environmental conditions. Compare with environmental resistance.

birth control Any method used to reduce births, including celibacy, delayed marriage, contraception; devices or medications that prevent implantation of fertilized zygotes and induced abortions.

blind experiments A design in which researchers don't know which subjects were given experimental treatment until after data have been gathered and analyzed.

bogs Areas of waterlogged soil that tend to be peaty; fed mainly by precipitation; low productivity; some bogs are acidic.

boreal forest A broad band of mixed coniferous and deciduous trees that stretches across northern North America (and Europe and Asia); its northernmost edge, the taiga, intergrades with the arctic tundra.

brownfields Abandoned or underused urban areas in which redevelopment is blocked by liability or financing issues related to toxic contamination.

C

cancer Invasive, out-of-control cell growth that results in malignant tumors.

capital Any form of wealth, resources, or knowledge available for use in the production of more wealth.

carbohydrate An organic compound consisting of a ring or chain of carbon atoms with hydrogen and oxygen attached; examples are sugars, starches, cellulose, and glycogen.

carbon cycle The circulation and reutilization of carbon atoms, especially via the processes of photosynthesis and respiration.

carbon management Projects to reduce carbon dioxide emissions from fossil fuel or to ameliorate their effects.

carbon monoxide Colorless, odorless, nonirritating but highly toxic gas produced by incomplete combustion of fuel, incineration of biomass or solid waste, or partially anaerobic decomposition of organic material.

carbon sink Places of carbon accumulation, such as in large forests (organic compounds) or ocean sediments (calcium carbonate).

carcinogens Substances that cause cancer.

carnivores Organisms that mainly prey upon animals.

carrying capacity The maximum number of individuals of any species that can be supported by a particular ecosystem on a long-term basis.

case law Precedents from both civil and criminal court cases.

cellular respiration The process in which a cell breaks down sugar or other organic compounds to release energy used for cellular work; may be anaerobic or aerobic, depending on the availability of oxygen.

chain reaction A self-sustaining reaction in which the fission of nuclei produces subatomic particles that cause the fission of other nuclei.

chaparral A biological community characterized by thick growth of thorny, evergreen shrubs typical of a Mediterranean climate.

chemical bond The force that holds molecules together.

chemical compounds Molecules made up of two or more kinds of atoms held together by chemical bonds.

chemical energy Potential energy stored in chemical bonds of molecules.

chlorofluorocarbons Chemical compounds with a carbon skeleton and one or more attached chlorine and fluorine atoms. Commonly used as refrigerants, solvents, fire retardants, and blowing agents.

chloroplasts Chlorophyll-containing organelles in eukaryotic organisms; sites of photosynthesis.

chronically undernourished Receiving less than 90 percent of the minimum caloric intake needed for normal growth and development and a healthy, productive life.

chronic effects Long-lasting results of exposure to a toxin; can be a permanent change caused by a single, acute exposure or a continuous, low-level exposure.

citizen science Projects in which trained volunteers work with scientific researchers to answer real-world questions.

city A differentiated community with a sufficient population and resource base to allow residents to specialize in arts, crafts, services, and professional occupations.

civil law A body of laws regulating relations between individuals or between individuals and corporations concerning property rights, personal dignity and freedom, and personal injury.

classical economics Modern, Western economic theories of the effects of resource scarcity, monetary policy, and competition on supply and demand of goods and services in the marketplace. This is the basis for the capitalist market system.

clear-cutting Cutting every tree in a given area, regardless of species or size; an appropriate harvest method for some species; can be destructive if not carefully controlled.

climate A description of the long-term pattern of weather in a particular area.

closed-canopy A forest where tree crowns spread over 20 percent of the ground; has the potential for commercial timber harvests.

cloud forests High mountain forests where temperatures are uniformly cool and fog or mist keeps vegetation wet all the time.

coevolution The process in which species exert selective pressure on each other and gradually evolve new features or behaviors as a result of those pressures.

cogeneration The simultaneous production of electricity and steam or hot water in the same plant.

cold front A moving boundary of cooler air displacing warmer air.

coliform bacteria Bacteria that live in the intestines (including the colon) of humans and other animals; used as a measure of the presence of feces in water or soil.

commensalism A symbiotic relationship in which one member is benefited and the second is neither harmed nor benefited.

common law The body of court decisions that constitutes a working definition of individual rights and responsibilities where no formal statutes define these issues.

communal resource management systems Resources managed by a community for long-term sustainability.

community-based planning Involving community stakeholders in pluralistic, adaptive, inclusive, proactive planning.

community ecology The study of interactions of all populations living in the ecosystem of a given area.

competitive exclusion A theory that no two populations of different species will occupy the same niche and compete for exactly the same resources in the same habitat for very long.

complexity The number of species at each trophic level and the number of trophic levels in a community.

composting The biological degradation of organic material under aerobic (oxygen-rich) conditions to produce compost, a nutrient-rich soil amendment and conditioner.

conifer A needle-bearing tree that produces seeds in cones.

conservation of matter In any chemical reaction, matter changes form; it is neither created nor destroyed.

conspicuous consumption A term coined by economist and social critic Thorstein Veblen to describe buying things we don't want or need to impress others.

consumers Organisms that obtain energy and nutrients by feeding on other organisms or their remains. See also *heterotroph.*

consumption The fraction of withdrawn water that is lost in transmission or that is evaporated, absorbed, chemically transformed, or otherwise made unavailable for other purposes as a result of human use.

contour plowing Plowing along hill contours; reduces erosion.

controlled studies Comparisons made between two populations that are identical (as far as possible) in every factor except the one being studied.

control rods Neutron-absorbing material inserted into spaces between fuel assemblies in nuclear reactors to regulate fission reaction.

convection currents Rising or sinking air currents that stir the atmosphere and transport heat from one area to another. Convection currents also occur in water.

conventional (criteria) pollutants The seven substances (sulfur dioxide, carbon monoxide, particulates, hydrocarbons, nitrogen oxides, photochemical oxidants, and lead) that make up the largest volume of air quality degradation; identified by the Clean Air Act as the most serious threat of all pollutants to human health and welfare.

convergent evolution Species evolve from different origins but under similar environmental conditions to have similar traits.

coral reefs Prominent oceanic features composed of hard, limy skeletons produced by coral animals; usually formed along edges of shallow, submerged ocean banks or along shelves in warm, shallow, tropical seas.

core The dense, intensely hot mass of molten metal, mostly iron and nickel, thousands of kilometers in diameter at the earth's center.

Coriolis effect The tendency for air above the earth to appear to be deflected to the right (in the Northern Hemisphere) or the left (in the South) because of the earth's rotation.

corridors Strips of natural habitat that connect two adjacent nature preserves to allow migration of organisms from one place to another.

cost-benefit analysis (CBA) An evaluation of large-scale public projects by comparing the costs and benefits that accrue from them.

cover crops Plants, such as rye, alfalfa, or clover, that can be planted immediately after harvest to hold and protect the soil.

creative thinking Original, independent thinking that asks, "How might I approach this problem in new and inventive ways?"

criminal law A body of court decisions based on federal and state statutes concerning wrongs against persons or society.

criteria pollutants See *conventional pollutants*.

critical factor The single environmental factor closest to a tolerance limit for a given species at a given time.

critical thinking An ability to evaluate information and opinions in a systematic, purposeful, efficient manner.

crude birth rate The number of births in a year divided by the midyear population.

crude death rate The number of deaths per thousand persons in a given year; also called crude mortality rate.

crust The cool, lightweight, outermost layer of the earth's surface that floats on the soft, pliable underlying layers; similar to the "skin" on a bowl of warm pudding.

cultural eutrophication An increase in biological productivity and ecosystem succession caused by human activities.

D

debt-for-nature swaps Forgiveness of international debt in exchange for nature protection in developing countries.

deciduous Trees and shrubs that shed their leaves at the end of the growing season.

decline spiral A catastrophic deterioration of a species, community, or whole ecosystem; accelerates as functions are disrupted or lost in a downward cascade.

decomposer Fungus or bacterium that breaks complex organic material into smaller molecules.

deductive reasoning "Top down" reasoning in which we start with a general principle and derive a testable prediction about a specific case.

deep ecology A philosophy that calls for a profound shift in our attitudes and behavior based on rejection of anthropocentric attitudes; a belief in the sacredness of nature; direct personal action to protect nature.

delta Fan-shaped sediment deposit found at the mouth of a river.

demanufacturing Disassembly of products so components can be reused or recycled.

demographic transition A pattern of falling death rates and birth rates in response to improved living conditions; could be reversed in deteriorating conditions.

demography The statistical study of human populations relating to growth rate, age structure, geographic distribution, etc., and their effects on social, economic, and environmental conditions.

dependency ratio The number of nonworking members compared with working members for a given population.

desalinization (or desalination) Removal of salt from water by distillation, freezing, or ultrafiltration.

desertification Denuding and degrading a once fertile land, initiating a desert-producing cycle that feeds on itself and causes long-term changes in soil, climate, and biota of an area.

deserts Biomes characterized by low moisture levels and infrequent and unpredictable precipitation. Daily and seasonal temperatures fluctuate widely.

detritivore Organisms that consume organic litter, debris, and dung.

dew point The temperature at which condensation occurs for a given concentration of water vapor in the air.

dieback A sudden population decline; also called a population crash.

disability-adjusted life years (DALYs) A health measure that assesses the total burden of disease by combining premature deaths and loss of a healthy life that result from illness or disability.

discharge The amount of water that passes a fixed point in a given amount of time; usually expressed as liters or cubic feet of water per second.

discount rate The amount we discount or reduce the value of a future payment. When you borrow money from the bank at 10 percent annual interest, you are in effect saying that having the money now is worth 10 percent more to you than having the same amount one year from now.

disease A deleterious change in the body's condition in response to destabilizing factors, such as nutrition, chemicals, or biological agents.

dissolved oxygen (DO) content Amount of oxygen dissolved in a given volume of water at a given temperature and atmospheric pressure; usually expressed in parts per million (ppm).

divergent evolution Separation of a species into new types.

diversity The number of species present in a community (species richness), as well as the relative abundance of each species.

DNA Deoxyribonucleic acid; the long, double-helix molecule in the nucleus of cells that contains the genetic code and directs the development and functioning of all cells.

double-blind design Neither the subject (participant) nor the experimenter knows which participants are receiving the experimental or the control treatments until after data have been gathered and analyzed.

drip irrigation Uses pipe or tubing perforated with very small holes to deliver water one drop at a time directly to the soil around each plant.

E

earth charter A set of principles for sustainable development, environmental protection, and social justice developed by a council appointed by the United Nations.

earthquakes Sudden, violent movement of the earth's crust.

ecocentric (ecologically centered) A philosophy that claims moral values and rights for both organisms and ecological systems and processes.

ecofeminism A pluralistic philosophy of respect for nature based on feminist philosophies of justice and egalitarianism.

ecological development A gradual process of environmental modification by organisms.

ecological economics Application of ecological insights to economic analysis; incorporating ecological principles and priorities into economic accounting systems.

ecological niche The functional role and position of a species in its ecosystem, including what resources it uses, how and when it uses the resources, and how it interacts with other species.

ecological services Processes or materials, such as clean water, energy, climate regulation, and nutrient cycling, provided by ecosystems.

ecological succession The process by which organisms gradually occupy a site, alter its ecological conditions, and are eventually replaced by other organisms.

ecology The scientific study of relationships between organisms and their environment. It is concerned with the life histories, distribution, and behavior of individual species as well as the structure and function of natural systems at the level of populations, communities, and ecosystems.

economic development A rise in real income per person; usually associated with new technology that increases productivity or resources.

economic growth An increase in the total wealth of a nation; if population grows faster than the economy, there may be real economic growth, but the share per person may decline.

ecosystem A specific biological community and its physical environment interacting in an exchange of matter and energy.

ecosystem management An integration of ecological, economic, and social goals in a unified systems approach to resource management.

ecosystem restoration To reinstate an entire community of organisms to as near its natural condition as possible.

ecotones Boundaries between two types of ecological communities.

ecotourism A combination of adventure travel, cultural exploration, and nature appreciation in wild settings.

edge effects A change in species composition, physical conditions, or other ecological factors at the boundary between two ecosystems.

electron A negatively charged subatomic particle that orbits around the nucleus of an atom.

element A substance that cannot be broken into simpler units by chemical means.

El Niño A climatic change marked by shifting of a large warm water pool from the western Pacific Ocean toward the east. Wind direction and precipitation patterns are changed over much of the Pacific and perhaps around the world.

emergent disease A new disease or one that has been absent for at least 20 years.

emigration The movement of members from a population.

emission standards Regulations for restricting the amounts of air pollutants that can be released from specific point sources.

endangered species A species considered to be in imminent danger of extinction.

endemism A state in which species are restricted to a single region.

endocrine hormone disrupters Chemicals that interfere with the function of endocrine hormones such as estrogen, testosterone, thyroxine, adrenaline, or cortisone.

energy The capacity to do work, such as moving matter over a distance.

energy recovery The incineration of solid waste to produce useful energy.

environment The circumstances or conditions that surround an organism or a group of organisms as well as the complex of social or cultural conditions that affect an individual or a community.

environmental ethics A search for moral values and ethical principles in human relations with the natural world.

environmental health The science of external factors that cause disease, including elements of the natural, social, cultural and technological worlds in which we live.

environmental impact statement (EIS) An analysis of the effects of any major program or project planned by a federal agency; required by provisions in the National Environmental Policy Act of 1970.

environmental indicators Organisms or physical factors that serve as a gauge for environmental changes. Indicator organisms, which cannot survive beyond certain environmental limits, are known as bioindicators.

environmental justice Fair access to a clean, healthy environment, regardless of class, race, income level, or other status.

environmental law Legal rules, decisions, and actions concerning environmental quality, natural resources, and ecological sustainability.

environmental literacy A basic understanding of ecological principles and the ways society affects, or responds to, environmental conditions.

environmental policy The official rules or regulations concerning the environment adopted, implemented, and enforced by some government agency.

environmental racism Decisions that unfairly expose people to polluted or degraded environments on the basis of race.

environmental resistance All the limiting factors that tend to reduce population growth rates and set the maximum allowable population size or carrying capacity of an ecosystem.

environmental science The systematic, scientific study of our environment as well as our role in it.

enzymes Molecules, usually proteins or nucleic acids, that act as catalysts in biochemical reactions.

epidemiology The study of the distribution and causes of disease and injuries in human populations.

epiphyte A plant that grows on a substrate other than the soil, such as the surface of another organism.

equilibrium community Also called a disclimax community; a community subject to periodic disruptions, usually by fire, that prevent it from reaching a climax stage.

estuaries Bays or drowned valleys where a river empties into the sea.

eutrophic Rivers and lakes rich in organic material (*eu* = well; *trophic* = nourished).

evolution A theory that explains how random changes in genetic material and competition for scarce resources cause species to change gradually.

exhaustible resources Materials present in fixed amounts in the environment, especially the earth's geologic endowment: minerals, nonmineral resources, fossil fuels.

exotic organisms Alien species introduced by human agency into biological communities where they would not naturally occur.

exponential growth Growth at a constant rate of increase per unit of time; can be expressed as a constant fraction or exponent. See also *geometric growth.*

externalizing costs Shifting expenses, monetary or otherwise, to someone other than the individuals or groups who use a resource.

extinction The irrevocable elimination of species; can be a normal process of the natural world as species outcompete or kill off others or as environmental conditions change.

extirpate To destroy totally; extinction caused by direct human action, such as hunting, trapping, etc.

F

family planning Controlling reproduction; planning the timing of birth and having only as many babies as are wanted and can be supported.

famines Acute food shortages characterized by large-scale loss of life, social disruption, and economic chaos.

fauna All of the animals present in a given region.

fecundity The physical ability to reproduce.

federal laws (statutes) Laws passed by the federal legislature and signed by the chief executive.

fens Wetlands fed mainly by groundwater.

feral A domestic animal that has taken up a wild existence.

fertility The actual number of offspring produced through sexual reproduction; usually described in terms of number of offspring of females, since paternity can be difficult to determine.

fetal alcohol syndrome A tragic set of permanent physical, mental, and behavioral birth defects that result when mothers drink alcohol during pregnancy.

fire-climax community An equilibrium community maintained by periodic fires; examples include grasslands, chaparral shrubland, and some pine forests.

first law of thermodynamics States that energy is conserved; that is, it is neither created nor destroyed under normal conditions.

First World The industrialized capitalist or market-economy countries of Western Europe, North America, Japan, Australia, and New Zealand.

flood An overflow of water onto land that normally is dry.

floodplains Low lands along riverbanks, lakes, and coastlines subjected to periodic inundation.

flora All of the plants present in a given region.

food chain A linked feeding series; in an ecosystem, the sequence of organisms through which energy and materials are transferred, in the form of food, from one trophic level to another.

food security The ability of individuals to obtain sufficient food on a day-to-day basis.

food web A complex, interlocking series of individual food chains in an ecosystem.

fossil fuels Petroleum, natural gas, and coal created by geologic forces from organic wastes and dead bodies of formerly living biological organisms.

fragmentation Disruption of habitat into small, isolated fragments.

freshwater ecosystems Ecosystems in which the fresh (nonsalty) water of streams, rivers, ponds, or lakes plays a defining role.

fuel assembly A bundle of hollow metal rods containing uranium oxide pellets; used to fuel a nuclear reactor.

fuel cells Mechanical devices that use hydrogen or hydrogen-containing fuel, such as methane, to produce an electric current. Fuel cells are clean, quiet, and highly efficient sources of electricity.

fugitive emissions Substances that enter the air without going through a smokestack, such as dust from soil erosion, strip mining, rock crushing, construction, and building demolition.

fungi Nonphotosynthetic, eukaryotic organisms with cell walls, filamentous bodies, and absorptive nutrition.

fungicide A chemical that kills fungi.

G

gamma rays Very short wavelength forms of the electromagnetic spectrum.

gap analysis A biogeographical technique of mapping biological diversity and endemic species to find gaps between protected areas that leave endangered habitats vulnerable to disruption.

gasohol A mixture of gasoline and ethanol.

gene A unit of heredity; a segment of DNA nucleus of the cell that contains information for the synthesis of a specific protein, such as an enzyme.

general fertility rate Crude birth rate multiplied by the percentage of reproductive-age women.

genetic assimilation The disappearance of a species as its genes are diluted through crossbreeding with a closely related species.

genetically modified organisms (GMOs) Organisms created by combining natural or synthetic genes using the techniques of molecular biology.

genetic engineering Laboratory manipulation of genetic material using molecular biology.

genuine progress index (GPI) An alternative to GNP or GDP for economic accounting that measures real progress in quality of life and sustainability.

geometric growth Growth that follows a geometric pattern of increase, such as 2, 4, 8, 16, etc. See also *exponential growth.*

geothermal energy Energy drawn from the internal heat of the earth, either through geysers, fumaroles, hot springs, or other natural geothermal features or through deep wells that pump heated groundwater.

global environmentalism The extension of modern environmental concerns to global issues.

grasslands Biomes dominated by grasses and associated herbaceous plants.

greenhouse effect Trapping of heat by the earth's atmosphere, which is transparent to incoming visible light waves but absorbs outgoing long-wave infrared radiation.

greenhouse gas A gas that traps heat in the atmosphere.

green plans Integrated national environmental plans for reducing pollution and resource consumption while achieving sustainable development and environmental restoration.

green political parties Political organizations based on environmental protection, participatory democracy, grassroots organization, and sustainable development.

green pricing Plans in which consumers can voluntarily pay premium prices for renewable energy.

green revolution Dramatically increased agricultural production brought about by "miracle" strains of grain; usually requires high inputs of water, plant nutrients, and pesticides.

gross domestic product (GDP) The total economic activity within national boundaries.

gross national product (GNP) The sum total of all goods and services produced in a national economy. Gross domestic product (GDP) is used to distinguish economic activity within a country from that of offshore corporations.

groundwater Water held in gravel deposits or porous rock below the earth's surface; does not include water or crystallization held by chemical bonds in rocks or moisture in upper soil layers.

gully erosion Removal of layers of soil, creating channels or ravines too large to be removed by normal tillage operations.

H

habitat The place or set of environmental conditions in which a particular organism lives.

habitat conservation plans Agreements under which property owners are allowed to harvest resources or develop land as long as habitat is conserved or replaced in ways that benefit resident endangered or threatened species in the long run. Some incidental "taking" or loss of endangered species is generally allowed in such plans.

half-life The time required for one-half of a sample to decay or change into some other form.

hazardous waste Any discarded material containing substances known to be toxic, mutagenic, carcinogenic, or teratogenic to humans or other life-forms; ignitable, corrosive, explosive, or highly reactive alone or with other materials.

health A state of physical and emotional well-being; the absence of disease or ailment.

heap-leach extraction A technique for separating gold from extremely low-grade ores. Crushed ore is piled in huge heaps and sprayed with a dilute alkaline-cyanide solution, which percolates through the pile to extract the gold, which is separated from the effluent in a processing plant. This process has a high potential for water pollution.

heat Total kinetic energy of atoms or molecules in a substance not associated with the bulk motion of the substance.

herbicide A chemical that kills plants.

herbivores Organisms that eat only plants.

heterotroph An organism that is incapable of synthesizing its own food and, therefore, must feed upon organic compounds produced by other organisms.

high-level waste repository A place where intensely radioactive wastes can be buried and remain unexposed to groundwater and earthquakes for tens of thousands of years.

high-quality energy Intense, concentrated, and high-temperature energy that is considered high-quality because of its usefulness in carrying out work.

HIPPO Habitat destruction, Invasive species, Pollution, Population (human), and Overharvesting, the leading causes of extinction.

holistic science The study of entire, integrated systems rather than isolated parts. Often takes a descriptive or an interpretive approach.

homeostasis A dynamic, steady state in a living system maintained through opposing, compensating adjustments.

humus Sticky, brown, insoluble residue from the bodies of dead plants and animals; gives soil its structure, coating mineral particles and holding them together; serves as a major source of plant nutrients.

hurricanes Large cyclonic oceanic storms with heavy rain and winds exceeding 119 km/hr (74 mph).

hydrologic cycle The natural process by which water is purified and made fresh through evaporation and precipitation. This cycle provides all the freshwater available for biological life.

hypothesis A conditional explanation that can be verified or falsified by observation or experimentation.

I

igneous rocks Crystalline minerals solidified from molten magma from deep in the earth's interior; basalt, rhyolite, andesite, lava, and granite are examples.

inbreeding depression In a small population, an accumulation of harmful genetic traits (through random mutations and natural selection) that lowers viability and reproductive success of enough individuals to affect the whole population.

inductive reasoning "Bottom-up" reasoning in which we study specific examples and try to discover patterns and derive general explanations from collected observations.

industrial revolution Advances in science and technology that have given us power to understand and change our world.

infiltration The process of water percolation into the soil and pores and hollows of permeable rocks.

inherent value Ethical values or rights that exist as an intrinsic or essential characteristic of a particular thing or class of things simply by the fact of their existence.

inholdings Private lands within public parks, forests, or wildlife refuges.

insecticide A chemical that kills insects.

insolation Incoming solar radiation.

instrumental value The value or worth of objects that satisfy the needs and wants of moral agents. Objects that can be used as a means to some desirable end.

intangible resources Factors such as open space, beauty, serenity, wisdom, diversity, and satisfaction that cannot be grasped or contained. Ironically, these resources can be both infinite and exhaustible.

integrated pest management (IPM) An ecologically based pest-control strategy that relies on natural mortality factors, such as natural enemies, weather, cultural control methods, and carefully applied doses of pesticides.

Intergovernmental Panel on Climate Change (IPCC) A large group of scientists from many nations and a wide variety of fields assembled by the United Nations Environment Program and World Meteorological Organization to assess the current state of knowledge about climate change.

internalizing costs Planning so that those who reap the benefits of resource use also bear all the external costs.

international treaties and conventions Agreements between nations on important issues.

interspecific competition In a community, competition for resources between members of different species.

intraspecific competition In a community, competition for resources among members of the same species.

invasive species Organisms that thrive in new territory where they are free of predators, diseases or resource limitations that may have controlled their population in their native habitat.

ionizing radiation High-energy electromagnetic radiation or energetic subatomic particles released by nuclear decay.

ionosphere The lower part of the thermosphere.

ions Electrically charged atoms that have gained or lost electrons.

irruptive growth See *Malthusian growth.*

island biogeography The study of rates of colonization and extinction of species on islands or other isolated areas based on size, shape, and distance from other inhabited regions.

isotopes Forms of a single element that differ in atomic mass due to a different number of neutrons in the nucleus.

J

J curve A growth curve that depicts exponential growth; called a J curve because of its shape.

jet streams Powerful winds or currents of air that circulate in shifting flows; similar to oceanic currents in extent and effect on climate.

joule A unit of energy. One joule is the energy expended in 1 second by a current of 1 amp flowing through a resistance of 1 ohm.

K

***K*-adapted species** Organisms whose population growth is regulated by internal (or intrinsic) as well as external factors. Large animals, such as whales and elephants, as well as top predators, generally fall in this category. They have relatively few offspring and often stabilize their population size near the carrying capacity of their environment.

keystone species A species whose impacts on its community or ecosystem are much larger and more influential than would be expected from mere abundance. This could be a top predator, a plant that shelters or feeds other organisms, or an organism that plays a critical ecological role.

kinetic energy Energy contained in moving objects, such as a rock rolling down a hill, the wind blowing through the trees, or water flowing over a dam.

kwashiorkor A widespread human protein deficiency disease resulting from a starchy diet low in protein and essential amino acids.

Kyoto Protocol An international treaty adopted in Kyoto, Japan, in 1997, in which 160 nations agreed to roll back CO_2, methane, and nitrous oxide emissions to reduce the threat of global climate change.

L

landscape ecology The study of the reciprocal effects of spatial pattern on ecological processes.

landslides Mass wasting or mass movement of rock or soil downhill. Often triggered by seismic events or heavy rainfall.

latent heat Stored energy in a form that is not sensible (detectable by ordinary senses).

LD50 A chemical dose lethal to 50 percent of a test population.

legal standing The right to take part in legal proceedings.

life expectancy The average age that a newborn infant can expect to attain in a particular time and place.

life span The longest period of life reached by a type of organism.

limiting factors Chemical or physical factors that limit the existence, growth, abundance, or distribution of an organism.

limits to growth A belief that the world has a fixed carrying capacity for humans.

lobbying Using personal contacts, public pressure, or political action to persuade legislators to vote in a particular manner.

logical thinking A rational way of thought that asks, "How can orderly, deductive reasoning help me think clearly?"

logistic growth Growth rates regulated by internal and external factors that establish an equilibrium with environmental resources. See also *S curve*.

longevity The length or duration of life; compare with survivorship.

low-quality energy Diffuse, dispersed energy at a low temperature that is difficult to gather and use for productive purposes.

LULUs Locally Unwanted Land Uses, such as toxic waste dumps, incinerators, smelters, airports, freeways, and other sources of environmental, economic, or social degradation.

M

magma Molten rock from deep in the earth's interior; called lava when it spews from volcanic vents.

malnourishment A nutritional imbalance caused by lack of specific dietary components or inability to absorb or utilize essential nutrients.

Malthusian growth A population explosion followed by a population crash; also called irruptive growth.

Man and Biosphere (MAB) program A design for nature preserves that divides protected areas into zones with different purposes. A highly protected core is surrounded by a buffer zone and peripheral regions in which multiple-use resource harvesting is permitted.

mangrove forests Diverse groups of salt-tolerant trees and other plants that grow in intertidal zones of tropical coastlines.

mantle A hot, pliable layer of rock that surrounds the earth's core and underlies the cool outer crust.

marasmus A widespread human protein deficiency disease caused by a diet low in calories and protein or imbalanced in essential amino acids.

marginal costs The cost to produce one additional unit of a good or service.

marshes Wetlands without trees; in North America, this type of land is characterized by cattails and rushes.

mass burn The incineration of unsorted solid waste.

matter Anything that takes up space and has mass.

mean Average.

mediation An informal dispute resolution process in which parties try to reach agreement through discussion and compromise; often used as an alternative to resolving disputes through lawsuits.

Mediterranean climate areas Regions defined by warm, dry summers and cool, wet winters; these areas may have distinctive and endemic species.

megacities See *megalopolis.*

megalopolis Also known as a megacity or supercity; megalopolis indicates an urban area with more than 10 million inhabitants.

megawatt (MW) Unit of electrical power equal to 1,000 kilowatts or 1 million watts.

mesosphere The atmospheric layer above the stratosphere and below the thermosphere; the middle layer; temperatures are usually very low.

metabolism All the energy and matter exchanges that occur within a living cell or organism; collectively, the life processes.

metamorphic rocks Igneous and sedimentary rocks modified by heat, pressure, and chemical reactions.

methane hydrate Small bubbles or individual molecules of methane (natural gas) trapped in a crystalline matrix of frozen water.

midoceanic ridges Mountain ranges on the ocean floor where magma wells up through cracks and creates new crust.

Milankovitch cycles Periodic variations in tilt, eccentricity, and wobble in the earth's orbit; Milutin Milankovitch suggested these are responsible for cyclic weather changes.

mineral A naturally occurring, inorganic, crystalline solid with definite chemical composition, a specific internal crystal structure, and characteristic physical properties.

minimum viable population The number of individuals needed for long-term survival of rare and endangered species.

mitigation Repairing or rehabilitating a damaged ecosystem or compensating for damage by providing a substitute or replacement area.

modern environmentalism A fusion of conservation of natural resources and preservation of nature with concerns about pollution, environmental health, and social justice.

molecules Combinations of two or more atoms.

monitored, retrievable storage Holding wastes in underground mines or secure surface facilities, such as dry casks, where they can be watched and repackaged, if necessary.

monoculture forestry Intensive planting of a single species; an efficient wood production approach, but one that encourages pests and disease infestations and conflicts with wildlife habitat or recreation uses.

monsoons Sasonal reversals of wind patterns caused by the different heating and cooling rates of the oceans and continents.

montane coniferous forests Coniferous forests of the mountains consisting of belts of different forest communities along an altitudinal gradient.

morals A set of ethical principles that guides our actions and relationships.

morbidity Illness or disease.

more-developed countries (MDC) Industrialized nations characterized by high per capita incomes, low birth and death rates, low population growth rates, and high levels of industrialization and urbanization.

mortality Death rate in a population, such as number of deaths per thousand people per year.

mulch Protective groundcover that protects the soil, saves water, and prevents weed growth; often straw, seaweed, leaves, or synthetic materials, such as heavy paper or plastic.

Müllerian (or Muellerian) mimicry Evolution of two species, both of which are unpalatable and have poisonous stingers or some other defense mechanism, to resemble each other.

multiple use Many uses that occur simultaneously; used in forest management; limited to mutually compatible uses.

mutagens Agents, such as chemicals or radiation, that damage or alter genetic material (DNA) in cells.

mutation A change, either spontaneous or by external factors, in the genetic material of a cell; mutations in the gametes (sex cells) can be inherited by future generations of organisms.

mutualism A symbiotic relationship between individuals of two different species in which both species benefit from the association.

N

National Environmental Policy Act (NEPA) The law that established the Council on Environmental Quality and that requires environmental impact statements for all federal projects with significant environmental impacts.

natural increase Crude death rate subtracted from crude birth rate.

natural resources Goods and services supplied by the environment.

natural selection The mechanism for evolutionary change in which environmental pressures cause certain genetic combinations in a population to become more abundant; genetic combinations best adapted for present environmental conditions tend to become predominant.

negative feedbacks Factors that result from a process and, in turn, reduce that same process.

neo-classical economics The branch of economics that attempts to apply the principles of modern science to economic analysis in a mathematically rigorous, noncontextual, abstract, predictive manner.

neo-Malthusians Those who believe that the world is characterized by scarcity and competition in which too many people fight for too few resources. Named for Thomas Malthus, who predicted a dismal cycle of misery, vice, and starvation as a result of human overpopulation.

net energy yield Total useful energy produced during the lifetime of an entire energy system minus the energy used, lost, or wasted in making useful energy available.

neurotoxins Toxic substances, such as lead or mercury, that specifically poison nerve cells.

neutron A subatomic particle, found in the nucleus of the atom, that has no electromagnetic charge.

NIMBY Not-In-My-Back-Yard: the position of those opposed to LULUs.

nitrogen cycle The circulation and reutilization of nitrogen in both inorganic and organic phases.

nitrogen-fixing bacteria Bacteria that convert nitrogen from the atmosphere or soil solution into ammonia that can then be converted to plant nutrients by nitrite- and nitrate-forming bacteria.

nitrogen oxides Highly reactive gases formed when nitrogen in fuel or combustion air is heated to over 650°C (1,200°F) in the presence of oxygen or when bacteria in soil or water oxidize nitrogen-containing compounds.

noncriteria pollutants See *unconventional pollutants*.

nongovernmental organizations (NGOs) Pressure and research groups, advisory agencies, political parties, professional societies, and other groups concerned about environmental quality, resource use, and many other issues.

nonpoint sources Scattered, diffuse sources of pollutants, such as runoff from farm fields, golf courses, and construction sites.

nonrenewable resources Minerals, fossil fuels, and other materials present in essentially fixed amounts (within human time scales) in our environment.

nuclear fission The radioactive decay process in which isotopes split apart to create two smaller atoms.

nuclear fusion A process in which two smaller atomic nuclei fuse into one larger nucleus and release energy; the source of power in a hydrogen bomb.

nucleic acids Large organic molecules made of nucleotides that function in the transmission of hereditary traits, in protein synthesis, and in control of cellular activities.

nucleus The center of the atom; occupied by protons and neutrons. In cells, the organelle that contains the chromosomes (DNA).

numbers pyramid A diagram showing the relative population sizes at each trophic level in an ecosystem; usually corresponds to the biomass pyramid.

O

obese Pathologically overweight, having a body mass greater than 30 kg/m^2, or roughly 30 pounds above normal for an average person.

offset allowances A controversial component of air quality regulations that allows a polluter to avoid installation of control equipment on one source with an "offsetting" pollution reduction at another source.

oil shales Fine-grained sedimentary rock rich in solid organic material called kerogen. When heated, the kerogen liquefies to produce a fluid petroleum fuel.

old-growth forests Forests free from disturbance for long enough (generally 150 to 200 years) to have mature trees, physical conditions, species diversity, and other characteristics of equilibrium ecosystems.

oligotrophic Condition of rivers and lakes that have clear water and low biological productivity (*oligo* = little; *trophic* = nourished); are usually clear, cold, infertile headwater lakes and streams.

omnivores Organisms that eat both plants and animals.

open access system A commonly held resource for which there are no management rules.

open canopy A forest where tree crowns cover less than 20 percent of the ground; also called woodland.

open system A system that exchanges energy and matter with its environment.

organic compounds Complex molecules organized around skeletons of carbon atoms arranged in rings or chains; includes biomolecules, molecules synthesized by living organisms.

overharvesting Harvesting so much of a resource that it threatens its existence.

overnutrition Receiving too many calories.

overshoots The extent to which a population exceeds the carrying capacity of its environment.

oxygen sag Oxygen decline downstream from a pollution source that introduces materials with high biological oxygen demands.

ozone A highly reactive molecule containing three oxygen atoms; a dangerous pollutant in ambient air. In the stratosphere, however, ozone forms an ultraviolet absorbing shield that protects us from mutagenic radiation.

P

paradigms Overarching models of the world that shape our worldviews and guide our interpretation of how things are.

parasite An organism that lives in or on another organism, deriving nourishment at the expense of its host, usually without killing it.

parsimony A principle that says where two equally plausible explanations for a phenomenon are possible, we should choose the simpler one (also known as Ockham's razor).

particulate material Atmospheric aerosols, such as dust, ash, soot, lint, smoke, pollen, spores, algal cells, and other suspended materials; originally applied only to solid particles but now extended to droplets of liquid.

parts per billion (ppb) Number of parts of a chemical found in 1 billion parts of a particular gas, liquid, or solid mixture.

parts per million (ppm) Number of parts of a chemical found in 1 million parts of a particular gas, liquid, or solid mixture.

parts per trillion (ppt) Number of parts of a chemical found in 1 trillion parts of a particular gas, liquid, or solid mixture.

passive heat absorption The use of natural materials or absorptive structures without moving parts to gather and hold heat; the simplest and oldest use of solar energy.

pastoralists People who live by herding domestic animals.

patchiness Within a larger ecosystem, the presence of smaller areas that differ in some physical conditions and thus support somewhat different communities; promotes diversity in a system or area.

pathogens Organisms that produce disease in host organisms, disease being an alteration of one or more metabolic functions in response to the presence of the organisms.

peat Deposits of moist, acidic, semidecayed organic matter.

pelagic Zones in the vertical water column of a water body.

perennial species Plants that grow for more than two years.

permafrost A permanently frozen layer of soil that underlies the arctic tundra.

permanent retrievable storage Placing waste storage containers in a secure location where they can be inspected periodically and retrieved, if necessary, for repacking or for transfer if a better means of disposal or reuse is developed.

persistent organic pollutants (POPs) Chemical compounds that persist in the environment and retain biological activity for a long time.

pest Any organism that reduces the availability, quality, or value of a useful resource.

pesticide Any chemical that kills, controls, drives away, or modifies the behavior of a pest.

pesticide treadmill A need for constantly increasing doses or new pesticides to prevent pest resurgence.

pest resurgence Rebound of pest populations due to acquired resistance to chemicals and nonspecific destruction of natural predators and competitors by broadscale pesticides.

pH A value that indicates the acidity or alkalinity of a solution on a scale of 0 to 14, based on the proportion of H^+ ions present.

phosphorus cycle The movement of phosphorus atoms from rocks through the biosphere and hydrosphere and back to rocks.

photochemical oxidants Products of secondary atmospheric reactions. See also *smog*.

photodegradable plastics Plastics that break down when exposed to sunlight or to a specific wavelength of light.

photosynthesis The biochemical process by which green plants and some bacteria capture light energy and use it to produce chemical bonds. Carbon dioxide and water are consumed while oxygen and simple sugars are produced.

photovoltaic cell An energy-conversion device that captures solar energy and directly converts it to electrical current.

phytoplankton Microscopic, free-floating, autotrophic organisms that function as producers in aquatic ecosystems.

pioneer species In primary succession on a terrestrial site, the plants, lichens, and microbes that first colonize the site.

plankton Primarily microscopic organisms that occupy the upper water layers in both freshwater and marine ecosystems.

plasma A hot, electrically neutral gas of ions and free electrons.

poaching Hunting wildlife illegally.

point sources Specific locations of highly concentrated pollution discharge, such as factories, power plants, sewage treatment plants, underground coal mines, and oil wells.

policy A societal plan to statement of intentions intended to accomplish some social or economic goal.

policy cycle The process by which problems are identified and acted upon in the public arena.

pollution To make foul, unclean, dirty; any physical, chemical, or biological change that adversely affects the health, survival, or activities of living organisms or that alters the environment in undesirable ways.

pollution charges Fees assessed per unit of pollution based on the "polluter pays" principle.

population All members of a species that live in the same area at the same time.

population crash A sudden population decline caused by predation, waste accumulation, or resource depletion; also called a dieback.

population explosion Growth of a population at exponential rates to a size that exceeds environmental carrying capacity; usually followed by a population crash.

population momentum A potential for increased population growth as young members reach reproductive age.

positive feedbacks Factors that result from a process and, in turn, increase that same process.

potential energy Stored energy that is latent but available for use. A rock poised at the top of a hill or water stored behind a dam are examples of potential energy.

power The rate of energy delivery; measured in horsepower or watts.

precautionary principle The rule that we should leave a margin of safety for unexpected developments. This principle implies that we should strive to prevent harm to human health and the environment even if risks are not fully understood.

precedent An act or a decision that can be used as an example in dealing with subsequent similar situations.

predator An organism that feeds directly on other organisms in order to survive; live-feeders, such as herbivores and carnivores.

primary pollutants Chemicals released directly into the air in a harmful form.

primary producers Photosynthesizing organisms.

primary productivity Synthesis of organic materials (biomass) by green plants using the energy captured in photosynthesis.

primary standards Regulations of the 1970 Clean Air Act; intended to protect human health.

primary succession Ecological succession that begins in an area where no biotic community previously existed.

primary treatment A process that removes solids from sewage before it is discharged or treated further.

principle of competitive exclusion A result of natural selection whereby two similar species in a community occupy different ecological niches, thereby reducing competition for food.

probability The likelihood that a situation, a condition, or an event will occur.

producer An organism that synthesizes food molecules from inorganic compounds by using an external energy source; most producers are photosynthetic.

productivity The amount of biomass (biological material) produced in a given area during a given period of time.

prokaryotic Cells that do not have a membrane-bounded nucleus or membrane-bounded organelles.

pronatalist pressures Influences that encourage people to have children.

prospective study A study in which experimental and control groups are identified before exposure to some factor. The groups are then monitored and compared for a specific time after the exposure to determine any effects the factor may have.

proteins Chains of amino acids linked by peptide bonds.

proton A positively charged subatomic particle found in the nucleus of an atom.

proven-in-place reserves Energy sources that have been thoroughly mapped and are likely to be economically recoverable with available technology.

pull factors Conditions that draw people from the country into the city.

push factors Conditions that force people out of the country and into the city.

R

***r*-adapted species** Organisms whose population growth is regulated mainly by external factors. They tend to have rapid reproduction and high mortality of offspring Given optimum environmental conditions, they can grow exponentially. Many "weedy" or pioneer species fit in this category.

radioactive decay A change in the nuclei of radioactive isotopes that spontaneously emit high-energy electromagnetic radiation and/or subatomic particles while gradually changing into another isotope or different element.

rainforest A forest with high humidity, constant temperature, and abundant rainfall (generally over 380 cm [150 in.] per year); can be tropical or temperate.

rain shadow Dry area on the downwind side of a mountain.

rangeland Grasslands and open woodlands suitable for livestock grazing.

rational choice Public decision making based on reason, logic, and science-based management.

reasoned judgment Thoughtful decisions based on careful, logical examination of available evidence.

recharge zones Areas where water infiltrates into an aquifer.

reclamation Chemical, biological, or physical cleanup and reconstruction of severely contaminated or degraded sites to return them to something like their original topography and vegetation.

recycling Reprocessing of discarded materials into new, useful products; not the same as reuse of materials for their original purpose, but the terms are often used interchangeably.

red tide A population explosion, or "bloom," of single-celled marine organisms called dinoflagellates. Billions of these cells can accumulate in protected bays where the toxins they contain can poison other marine life.

reduced tillage systems Farming methods that preserve soil and save energy and water through reduced cultivation; includes minimum till, conserve-till, and no-till systems.

reflective thinking A thoughtful, contemplative analysis that asks, "What does this all mean?"

reformer A device that strips hydrogen from fuels such as natural gas, methanol, ammonia, gasoline, or vegetable oil so they can be used in a fuel cell.

refuse-derived fuel Processing of solid waste to remove metal, glass, and other unburnable materials; organic residue is shredded, formed into pellets, and dried to make fuel for power plants.

regenerative farming Farming techniques and land stewardship that restore the health and productivity of the soil by rotating crops, planting ground cover, protecting the surface with crop residue, and reducing synthetic chemical inputs and mechanical compaction.

regulations Rules established by administrative agencies; regulations can be more important than statutory law in the day-to-day management of resources.

rehabilitation Rebuilding basic structure or function in an ecological system without necessarily achieving complete restoration to its original condition.

relative humidity At any given temperature, a comparison of the actual water content of the air with the amount of water that could be held at saturation.

relevé A rapid assessment of vegetation types and biodiversity in an area.

remediation Cleaning up chemical contaminants from a polluted area.

renewable resources Resources normally replaced or replenished by natural processes; resources not depleted by moderate use; examples include solar energy, biological resources such as forests and fisheries, biological organisms, and some biogeochemical cycles.

renewable water supplies Annual freshwater surface runoff plus annual infiltration into underground freshwater aquifers that are accessible for human use.

reproducibility Making an observation or obtaining a particular result consistently.

residence time The length of time a component, such as an individual water molecule, spends in a particular compartment or location before it moves on through a particular process or cycle.

resilience The ability of a community or ecosystem to recover from disturbances.

resistance (inertia) The ability of a community to resist being changed by potentially disruptive events.

resource partitioning In a biological community, various populations sharing environmental resources through specialization, thereby reducing direct competition. See also *ecological niche*.

resources In economic terms, anything with potential use in creating wealth or giving satisfaction.

restoration To bring something back to a former condition. Ecological restoration involves active manipulation of nature to re-create conditions that existed before human disturbance.

restoration ecology Seeks to repair or reconstruct ecosystems damaged by human actions.

retrospective study A study that looks back in history at a group of people (or other organisms) who suffer from some condition to try to identify something in their past life that the whole group shares but that is not found in the histories of a control group as near as possible to those being studied but who do not suffer from the same condition.

riders Amendments attached to bills in conference committee, often completely unrelated to the bill to which they are added.

rill erosion The removing of thin layers of soil as little rivulets of running water gather and cut small channels in the soil.

risk The probability that something undesirable will happen as a consequence of exposure to a hazard.

risk assessment Evaluation of the short-term and long-term risks associated with a particular activity or hazard; usually compared with benefits in a cost-benefit analysis.

rock A solid, cohesive aggregate of one or more crystalline minerals.

rock cycle The process whereby rocks are broken down by chemical and physical forces; sediments are moved by wind, water, and gravity; sedimented and reformed into rock; and then crushed, folded, melted, and recrystallized into new forms.

rotational grazing Confining grazing animals in a small area for a short time to force them to eat weedy species as well as the more desirable grasses and forbes.

runoff The excess of precipitation over evaporation; the main source of surface water and, in broad terms, the water available for human use.

S

salinity The amount of dissolved salts (especially sodium chloride) in a given volume of water.

salinization A process in which mineral salts accumulate in the soil, killing plants; occurs when soils in dry climates are irrigated profusely.

saltwater intrusion The movement of saltwater into freshwater aquifers in coastal areas where groundwater is withdrawn faster than it is replenished.

sample To analyze a small but representative portion of a population to estimate the characteristics of the entire class.

sanitary landfills Landfills in which garbage and municipal waste are buried every day under enough soil or fill to eliminate odors, vermin, and litter.

scientific method A systematic, precise, objective study of a problem. Generally this requires observation, hypothesis development and testing, data gathering, and interpretation.

scientific theory An explanation or idea accepted by a substantial number of scientists.

S curve A curve that depicts logistic growth; called an S curve because of its shape.

secondary pollutants Chemicals modified to a hazardous form after entering the air or that are formed by chemical reactions as components of the air mix and interact.

secondary succession Succession on a site where an existing community has been disrupted.

secondary treatment Bacterial decomposition of suspended particulates and dissolved organic compounds that remain after primary sewage treatment.

second law of thermodynamics States that, with each successive energy transfer or transformation in a system, less energy is available to do work.

secure landfills Solid waste disposal sites lined and capped with an impermeable barrier to prevent leakage or leaching.

sedimentary rocks Rocks composed of accumulated, compacted mineral fragments, such as sand or clay; examples include shale, sandstone, breccia, and conglomerates.

sedimentation The deposition of organic materials or minerals by chemical, physical, or biological processes.

selective cutting Harvesting only mature trees of certain species and size; usually more expensive than clear-cutting but less disruptive for wildlife and often better for forest regeneration.

selective pressure Limited resources or adverse environmental conditions that tend to favor certain adaptations in a population. Over many generations, this can lead to genetic change, or evolution.

shade-grown coffee and cocoa Plants grown under a canopy of taller trees, which provides habitat for birds and other wildlife.

sheet erosion Peeling off thin layers of soil from the land surface; accomplished primarily by wind and water.

shelterwood harvesting Mature trees are removed from the forest in a series of two or more cuts, leaving young trees and some mature trees as a seed source for future regeneration.

sick house syndrome A cluster of allergies and other illnesses caused by sensitivity to molds, synthetic chemicals, or other harmful compounds trapped in insufficiently ventilated buildings.

significant numbers Meaningful data that can be measured accurately and reproducibly.

sinkholes A large surface crater caused by the collapse of an underground channel or cavern; often triggered by groundwater withdrawal.

sludge A semisolid mixture of organic and inorganic materials that settles out of wastewater at a sewage treatment plant.

smart growth The efficient use of land resources and existing urban infrastructure that encourages in-fill development, provides a variety of affordable housing and transportation choices, and seeks to maintain a unique sense of place by respecting local cultural and natural features.

smelting Roasting ore to release metals from mineral compounds.

smog The combination of smoke and fog in the stagnant air of London; now often applied to photochemical pollution.

social justice Equitable access to resources and the benefits derived from them; a system that recognizes inalienable rights and adheres to what is fair, honest, and moral.

soil A complex mixture of weathered rock material, partially decomposed organic molecules, and a host of living organisms.

soil horizons Horizontal layers that reveal a soil's history, characteristics, and usefulness.

southern pine forest United States coniferous forest ecosystem characterized by a warm, moist climate.

species All the organisms genetically similar enough to breed and produce live, fertile offspring in nature.

species diversity The number and relative abundance of species present in a community.

species recovery plan A plan for restoration of an endangered species through protection, habitat management, captive breeding, disease control, and other techniques that increase populations and encourage survival.

specific heat The amount of heat energy needed to change the temperature of a body. Water has a specific heat of 1, which is higher than most substances.

sprawl Unlimited, unplanned growth of urban areas that consumes open space and wastes resources.

stability In ecological terms, a dynamic equilibrium among the physical and biological factors in an ecosystem or a community; relative homeostasis.

stable runoff The fraction of water available year-round; usually more important than total runoff when determining human uses.

Standard Metropolitan Statistical Area (SMSA) An urbanized region with at least 100,000 inhabitants with strong economic and social ties to a central city of at least 50,000 people.

statistics Mathematical analysis of the collection, organization, and interpretation of numerical data.

statutory law Rules passed by a state or national legislature.

steady-state economy Characterized by low birth and death rates, use of renewable energy sources, recycling of materials, and emphasis on durability, efficiency, and stability.

stewardship A philosophy that holds that humans have a unique responsibility to manage, care for, and improve nature.

Strategic Lawsuits against Public Participation (SLAPP) Lawsuits that have no merit but are brought merely to intimidate and harass private citizens who act in the public interest.

strategic metals and minerals Materials a country cannot produce itself but that it uses for essential materials or processes.

stratosphere The zone in the atmosphere extending from the tropopause to about 50 km (30 mi) above the earth's surface; temperatures are stable or rise slightly with altitude; has very little water vapor but is rich in ozone.

stress Physical, chemical, or emotional factors that place a strain on an animal. Plants also experience physiological stress under adverse environmental conditions.

strip-cutting Harvesting trees in strips narrow enough to minimize edge effects and to allow natural regeneration of the forest.

strip-farming Planting different kinds of crops in alternating strips along land contours; when one crop is harvested, the other crop remains to protect the soil and prevent water from running straight down a hill.

strip-mining Extracting shallow mineral deposits (especially coal) by scraping off surface layers with giant earth-moving equipment; creates a huge open pit; an alternative to underground or deep open-pit mines.

subsidence Settling of the ground surface caused by the collapse of porous formations that result from withdrawal of large amounts of groundwater, oil, or other underground materials.

subsoil A layer of soil beneath the topsoil that has lower organic content and higher concentrations of fine mineral particles; often contains soluble compounds and clay particles carried down by percolating water.

sulfur cycle The chemical and physical reactions by which sulfur moves into or out of storage and through the environment.

sulfur dioxide A colorless, corrosive gas directly damaging to both plants and animals.

Superfund A fund established by Congress to pay for containment, cleanup, or remediation of abandoned toxic waste sites. The fund is financed by fees paid by toxic waste generators and by cost recovery from cleanup projects.

surface mining Some minerals are also mined from surface pits. See also *strip-mining*.

surface tension The tendency for a surface of water molecules to hold together, producing a surface that resists breaking.

survivorship The percentage of a population reaching a given age or the proportion of the maximum life span of the species reached by any individual.

sustainability Ecological, social, and economic systems that can last over the long term.

sustainable agriculture (regenerative farming) Ecologically sound, economically viable, socially just agricultural system. Stewardship, soil conservation, and integrated pest management are essential for sustainability.

sustainable development A real increase in well-being and standard of life for the average person that can be maintained over the long term without degrading the environment or compromising the ability of future generations to meet their own needs.

sustained yield Utilization of a renewable resource at a rate that does not impair or damage its ability to be fully renewed on a long-term basis.

swamps Wetlands with trees, such as the extensive swamp forests of the southern United States.

symbiosis The intimate living together of members of two species; includes mutualism, commensalism, and, in some classifications, parasitism.

synergism When an injury caused by exposure to two environmental factors together is greater than the sum of exposure to each factor individually.

T

taiga The northernmost edge of the boreal forest, including species-poor woodland and peat deposits; intergrading with the arctic tundra.

tailings Mining waste left after mechanical or chemical separation of minerals from crushed ore.

taking The unconstitutional confiscation of private property.

tar sands Geologic deposits composed of sand and shale particles coated with bitumen, a viscous mixture of long-chain hydrocarbons.

tectonic plates Huge blocks of the earth's crust that slide around slowly, pulling apart to open new ocean basins or crashing ponderously into each other to create new, larger landmasses.

temperate rainforest The cool, dense, rainy forest of the northern Pacific coast; enshrouded in fog much of the time; dominated by large conifers.

temperature A measure of the speed of motion of a typical atom or molecule in a substance.

teratogens Chemicals or other factors that specifically cause abnormalities during embryonic growth and development.

terracing Shaping the land to create level shelves of earth to hold water and soil; requires extensive hand labor or expensive machinery, but it enables farmers to farm very steep hillsides.

tertiary treatment The removal of inorganic minerals and plant nutrients after primary and secondary treatment of sewage.

thermal pollution Artificially raising or lowering of the temperature of a water body in a way that adversely affects the biota or water quality.

thermocline In water, a distinctive temperature transition zone that separates an upper layer that is mixed by the wind (the epilimnion) and a colder deep layer that is not mixed (the hypolimnion).

thermodynamics The branch of physics that deals with transfers and conversions of energy.

thermosphere The highest atmospheric zone; a region of hot, dilute gases above the mesosphere extending out to about 1,600 km (1,000 mi) from the earth's surface.

Third World Less-developed countries that are not capitalistic and industrialized (First World) or centrally planned socialist economies (Second World); not intended to be derogatory.

thorn scrub A dry, open woodland or shrubland characterized by sparse, spiny shrubs.

threatened species While still abundant in parts of its territorial range, this species has declined significantly in total numbers and may be on the verge of extinction in certain regions or localities.

tolerance limits See *limiting factors.*

topsoil The first true layer of soil; layer in which organic material is mixed with mineral particles; thickness ranges from a meter or more under virgin prairie to zero in some deserts.

total fertility rate The number of children born to an average woman in a population during her entire reproductive life.

total growth rate The net rate of population growth resulting from births, deaths, immigration, and emigration.

total maximum daily loads (TMDL) The amount of particular pollutant that a water body can receive from both point and nonpoint sources and still meet water quality standards.

Toxic Release Inventory A program created by the Superfund Amendments and Reauthorization Act of 1984 that requires manufacturing facilities and waste handling and disposal sites to report annually on releases of more than 300 toxic materials. You can find out from the EPA whether any of these sites are in your neighborhood and what toxics they release.

toxins Poisonous chemicals that react with specific cellular components to kill cells or to alter growth or development in undesirable ways; often harmful, even in dilute concentrations.

tradable permits Pollution quotas or variances that can be bought or sold.

"The Tragedy of the Commons" An inexorable process of degradation of communal resources due to selfish self-interest of "free riders" who use or destroy more than their fair share of common property. See *open access system.*

transpiration The evaporation of water from plant surfaces, especially through stomates.

trophic level Step in the movement of energy through an ecosystem; an organism's feeding status in an ecosystem.

tropical rainforests Forests near the equator in which rainfall is abundant—more than 200 cm (80 in.) per year—and temperatures are warm to hot year-round.

tropical seasonal forests Semievergreen or partly deciduous forests tending toward open woodlands and grassy savannas dotted with scattered, drought-resistant trees.

tropopause The boundary between the troposphere and the stratosphere.

troposphere The layer of air nearest to the earth's surface; both temperature and pressure usually decrease with increasing altitude.

tundra Treeless arctic or alpine biome characterized by cold, dark winters; a short growing season; and potential for frost any month of the year; vegetation includes low-growing perennial plants, mosses, and lichens.

U

unconventional pollutants Toxic or hazardous substances, such as asbestos, benzene, beryllium, mercury, polychlorinated biphenyls, and vinyl chloride, not listed in the original Clean Air Act because they were not released in large quantities; also called noncriteria pollutants.

urbanization An increasing concentration of the population in cities and a transformation of land use to an urban pattern of organization.

urban renewal Programs to revitalize old, blighted sections of inner cities.

utilitarian conservation The philosophy that resources should be used for the greatest good for the greatest number for the longest time.

V

values An estimation of the worth of things; a set of ethical beliefs and preferences that determines our sense of right and wrong.

vertical stratification The vertical distribution of specific subcommunities within a community.

visible light A portion of the electromagnetic spectrum that includes the wavelengths used for photosynthesis.

vitamins Organic molecules essential for life that we cannot make for ourselves; we must get them from our diet; they act as enzyme cofactors.

volatile organic compounds Organic chemicals that evaporate readily and exist as gases in the air.

volcanoes Vents in the earth's surface through which molten lava (magma), gases, and ash escape to create mountains.

vulnerable species Naturally rare organisms or species whose numbers have been so reduced by human activities that they are susceptible to actions that could push them into threatened or endangered status.

W

warm front A long, wedge-shaped boundary caused when a warmer advancing air mass slides over neighboring cooler air parcels.

waste stream The steady flow of varied wastes, from domestic garbage and yard wastes to industrial, commercial, and construction refuse.

water cycle The recycling and reutilization of water on earth, including atmospheric, surface, and underground phases and biological and nonbiological components.

waterlogging Water saturation of soil that fills all air spaces and causes plant roots to die from lack of oxygen; a result of overirrigation.

watershed The land surface and groundwater aquifers drained by a particular river system.

water table The top layer of the zone of saturation; undulates according to the surface topography and subsurface structure.

weather The physical conditions of the atmosphere (moisture, temperature, pressure, and wind).

weathering Changes in rocks brought about by exposure to air, water, changing temperatures, and reactive chemical agents.

wetlands Ecosystems of several types in which rooted vegetation is surrounded by standing water during part of the year. See also *swamps, marshes, bogs, fens.*

"wicked" problems Problems with no simple right or wrong answer where there is no single, generally agreed upon definition of or solution for the particular issue.

wilderness An area of undeveloped land affected primarily by the forces of nature; an area where humans are visitors who do not remain.

wildlife refuges Areas set aside to shelter, feed, and protect wildlife; due to political and economic pressures, refuges often allow hunting, trapping, mineral exploitation, and other activities that threaten wildlife.

wind farms Large numbers of windmills concentrated in a single area; usually owned by a utility or large-scale energy producer.

Wise Use Movement A coalition of ranchers, loggers, miners, industrialists, hunters, off-road vehicle users, land developers, and others who call for unrestricted access to natural resources and public lands.

withdrawal A description of the total amount of water taken from a lake, a river, or an aquifer.

woodland A forest where tree crowns cover less than 20 percent of the ground; also called open canopy forest.

work The application of force through a distance; requires energy input.

world conservation strategy A proposal for maintaining essential ecological processes, preserving genetic diversity, and ensuring that utilization of species and ecosystems is sustainable.

World Trade Organization (WTO) An association of 135 nations organized to regulate international trade.

X

X ray Very short wavelength in the electromagnetic spectrum; can penetrate soft tissue; although it is useful in medical diagnosis, it also damages tissue and causes mutations.

Z

zero population growth (ZPG) A condition in which births and immigration in a population just balance deaths and emigration.

zone of aeration Upper soil layers that hold both air and water.

zone of leaching The layer of soil just beneath the topsoil where water percolates, removing soluble nutrients that accumulate in the subsoil; may be very different in appearance and composition from the layers above and below it.

zone of saturation Lower soil layers where all spaces are filled with water.

CREDITS

PHOTOS

Chapter 1

Opener: David L. Hansen, University of Minnesota Agriculture Experiment Station; 1.1: Courtesy of Keene Engineering; 1.2: © Earth Imaging/Stone/Getty Images; 1.3: © Vol. 6/Corbis; 1.5: Courtesy of Monumenti Mussei E. Gallerie Pontificie; 1.6, 1.8: David L. Hansen, University of Minnesota Agriculture Experiment Station; 1.10: © PhotoDisc; 1.11: Courtesy of Grey Towers National Historic Landmark; 1.12: Courtesy of the Bancroft Library at the University of California, Berkeley; 1.13: AP/Wide World Photos; 1.14: © Norbert Schiller/The Image Works; 1.16: © The McGraw-Hill Companies, Inc./Barry Barker, photographer; 1.17: © William P. Cunningham; 1.18: © The McGraw-Hill Companies, Inc./Barry Barker, photographer; 1.21: © William P. Cunningham.

Chapter 2

Opener: William P. Cunningham; 2.2: William P. Cunningham; 2.8: © G.I. Bernard/Animals Animals/Earth Scenes; 2.9: Greg Slater, Montana State University; p. 35: The SeaWIFS Project, NASA/Goddard Space Flight Center and ORBIMAGE; 2.21: © David Dennis/Tom Stack & Assoc.

Chapter 3

Opener: © John Warden/Stone/Getty Images; 3.1: Portrait of Charles Darwin, 1840 by George Richmond (1809–96). Down House, Downe, Kent, UK/Bridgeman Art Library; 3.3: William P. Cunningham; 3.4: © Vol. 86 /Corbis; 3.6, 3 9: William P. Cunningham; 3.10: © Ray Coleman/Photo Researchers, Inc.; 3.11: © D.P. Wilson/Photo Researchers, Inc.; 3.12: William P. Cunningham; 3.13: © PhotoDisc; 3.14: © Michael Fogden/Animals Animals/Earth Scenes; 3.15a,b: © Edward S. Ross; 3.16: © Randy Morse/Tom Stack & Associates; 3.17: National Museum of Natural History, © Smithsonian Institution; p. 66: Courtesy of David Tilman; 3.24: © Fred Bavendam/Peter Arnold, Inc.; 3.25: © Vol. 262/Corbis; 3.28: © William P. Cunningham; 3.29: © William P. Cunningham; 3.30: © Gerald Lacz/Peter Arnold, Inc.

Chapter 4

Opener: © The McGraw-Hill Companies, Inc./Barry Barker, photographer; 4.1: Courtesy of John Cunningham; 4.6, 4.10: © William P. Cunningham; 4.15: © The McGraw-Hill Companies, Inc./Bob Coyle, photographer.

Chapter 5

Opener: © Corbis Royalty Free; 5.4: © William P. Cunningham; 5.5, 5.6: © Mary Ann Cunningham; 5.7: © William P. Cunningham; 5.8: © Vol. 90/Corbis; 5.9: © William P. Cunningham; 5.10: © Vol. 6/Corbis; 5.11: © William P. Cunningham; 5.12: Courtesy of Sea WIFS/NASA; 5.14: © The McGraw-Hill Companies, Inc./Barry Barker, photographer; 5.15: © William P. Cunningham; 5.16: © Stephen Rose/Gamma Liaison International; 5.18: © William P. Cunningham; 5.19: © The McGraw-Hill Companies, Inc./Barry Barker, photographer; 5.21, 5.22: © William P. Cunningham; p. 113: David L. Hansen, University of Minnesota Agriculture Experiment Station; 5.26: © Vol. 5/Corbis; 5.27: Printed with permission from the Bell Museum of Natural History at the University of Minnesota; 5.28: © William P. Cunningham; 5.29: © Lynn Funkhouser/Peter Arnold, Inc.; 5.30: © Vol. 6/Corbis.

Chapter 6

Opener: © Corbis Royalty Free; 6.4, 6.5, 6.7: © William P. Cunningham; 6.8: © Steven P. Lynch; 6.9: © Greg Vaughn/Tom Stack & Assoc.; 6.10: © Gary Braasch/Stone/Getty Images; 6.11: Courtesy of John McColgan, Alaska Fires Service/Bureau of Land Management; p. 133: © Martos Hoffman, photographer; 6.12: © William P. Cunningham; 6.14: Tom Finkle; 6.15: David L. Hansen, University of Minnesota Agriculture Experiment Station; 6.16: © William P. Cunningham; 6.17: © Corbis Royalty Free; 6.18: © William P. Cunningham; 6.19: © Richard Hamilton Smith/Corbis; 6.20: © American Heritage Center, University of Wyoming; p. 139: © Gary Milburn/Tom Stack & Associates; 6.24: Courtesy of R.O. Bierregaard; 6.25: © The McGraw-Hill Companies, Inc./Barry Barker, photographer; 6.27: © William P. Cunningham; 6.28: © The McGraw-Hill Companies, Inc./Barry Barker, photographer.

Chapter 7

Opener: © Vol. 16/PhotoDisc. 7.1: National Renewable Energy Lab; 7.5: © Norbert Schiller/The Image Works; 7.20: © Corbis Royalty Free; 7.7: © Lester Bergman/Corbis; 7.8: © Scott Daniel Peterson/Gamma Liaison International; 7.10: © William P. Cunningham; 7.11: © Vol. 102/Corbis; 7.12: Food and Agriculture Organization photo/H. Zhang; 7.15: Food and Agriculture Organization photo/R. Faidutti; 7.17: Photo by Lynn Betts, courtesy of USDA Natural Resources Conservation Service; 7.18: Photo by Jeff Vanuga, courtesy of USDA Natural Resources Conservation Center; 7.19: © William P. Cunningham; 7.21: © Vol. 120/Corbis; 7.22: © William P. Cunningham; 7.24: © Michael Rosenfeld/Stone/Getty Images; 7.26: Photo by Lynn Betts, courtesy of USDA Natural Resources Conservation Service; 7.27: © The McGraw-Hill Companies, Inc./Barry Barker, photographer; p. 170: © William P. Cunningham; 7.28: Courtesy of Dave Hansen, College of Agriculture Experiment Station, University of Minnesota; 7.29: © Tom Sweeny/Minneapolis Star Tribune; 7.30: © William P. Cunningham.

Chapter 8

Opener: AP photo/Avant Givon; 8.2: © William P. Cunningham; 8.3a: © Vol. 40/Corbis; 8.3b: Courtesy of Stanley Erlandsen, University of Minnesota; 8.3c: Courtesy of Donald R. Hopkins; 8.6: © Vol. 72/Corbis; p. 188: © William P. Cunningham.

Chapter 9

Opener: © Vol. 44/PhotoDisc; 9.4: © Vol. 188/Corbis; 9.6: Image produced by Hal Pierce, Laboratory for Atmospheres, NASA Goddard Space Flight Center/NOAA; 9.8: © Vic Englebert/Photo Researchers, Inc.; p. 211(both): National Snow and Ice Data Center/University of Colorado/NOAA; 9.16: © William P. Cunningham; 9.18: National Renewable Energy Lab; 9.19: Courtesy of Dr. Delbert Swanson; 9.20: © William P. Cunningham; 9.22: © Guang Hui Xie/Image Bank/Getty Images; 9.24: NASA; 9.26, 9.28: © William P. Cunningham; 9.29: © John D. Cunningham/Visuals Unlimited; 9.32: © William P. Cunningham.

Chapter 10

Opener: Courtesy of Kathleen Smith; 10.4, 10.7: © William P. Cunningham; 10.10: © Vol. 120/Corbis; 10.11: © William P. Cunningham; 10.12: Courtesy of National Renewable Energy Laboratory/NREL/PIX; 10.14: Courtesy of USDA/NRCS/ Photo by Lynn Betts; 10.15: Courtesy of Tim McCabe, Soil Conservation Service, USDA; 10.16: © William P. Cunningham; 10.18: © Simon Fraser/SPL/Photo Researchers, Inc.; 10.19: © Joe McDonald/Animals Animals/Earth Scenes; 10.21: © William P. Cunningham; 10.22: © Lawrence Lowry/Photo Researchers, Inc.; 10.25: © Les Stone/Sygma/Corbis; 10.27: © Frans Lanting/Photo Researchers, Inc.; 10.30: National Renewable Energy Lab.

Chapter 11

Opener: Department of Energy; 11.8: © Vol. 16/PhotoDisc; 11.10: © Bryan F. Peterson; 11.11: © AP Photo/Bob Bird; 11.13: © Joseph Nettis/Photo Researchers, Inc.; 11.14: © Reuter/Sankei Shimbum; 11.15: Courtesy of Chris G. Newhall/U.S. Geological Survey; 11.17: © James Shaffer; 11.18: © Los Angeles Times Photo by Al Seib; 11.19: © Stephen Rose.

Chapter 12

Opener: © Ytre Stengrund/ Windpowerphotos.com; 12.6: © James P. Blair/National Geographic Image Collection; 12.9, 12.11: © Vol. 160/Corbis; p. 290: Courtesy of Toyota; 12.15: National Renewable Energy Lab; 12.16: Courtesy of Carolyn Roberts/A House of Straw; 12.18: Courtesy of Capstone Microtubules; 12.20: © William P. Cunningham; 12.21: © The McGraw-Hill Companies, Inc./Doug Sherman, photographer; 12.23: National Renewable Energy Lab; 12.24: © Vol. 160/Corbis; 12.26: © William P. Cunningham; 12.27: Courtesy of Dr. Douglas Pratt; 12.28: National Renewable Energy Lab; 12.30, 12.32: © William P. Cunningham.

Chapter 13

Opener: © Ray Pfortmer/Peter Arnold, Inc.; 13.3: © Fred McConnaughey/Photo Researchers, Inc.; 13.4: © Vol. 31/PhotoDisc; p. 312: © Barbara Gauntt/The Clarion-Ledger, Jackson, MS; 13.7: © William P. Cunningham; 13.8: David L. Hansen, University of Minnesota Agriculture Experiment Station; 13.12: Basel Action Network (www.ban.org); 13.13: Courtesy of Urban Ore, Inc. Berkeley, CA; 13.15: © Michael Greenlar/The Image Works; 13.19: © William P. Cunningham; 13.20: © Piet Van Lier.

Chapter 14

Opener: © William P. Cunningham; 14.4: © Vol. 6/Corbis; 14.10: © The McGraw-Hill Companies, Inc./Barry Barker, photographer; 14.11: © Mark Luthringer; 14.13: © The McGraw-Hill Companies, Inc./Barry Barker, photographer; 14.17: © John Chiasson/Gamma Liaison International/Getty Images; 14.18: © William P. Cunningham; 14.19: © psihoyos.com; 14.20: Courtesy of Kathleen Smith; 14.21: © William P. Cunningham; 14.22: © 2003 Regents of the University of Minnesota. All rights reserved. Used with permission of the Design Center for American Urban Landscape; 14.23: © William P. Cunningham; 14.24,14.26, p. 328: © William P. Cunningham; p. 349: © Bob Boyer/Shoot The Works.

Chapter 15

Opener: Courtesy of Dave Hansen, College of Agriculture Experiment Station, University of Minnesota; 15.1: Courtesy of Dave Hansen, College of Agriculture Experiment Station, University of Minnesota; 15.2: © William P. Cunningham; 15.4: Courtesy of Dave Hansen, College of Agriculture Experiment Station, University of Minnesota; 15.5, 15.6, 15.7: © William P. Cunningham; 15.9: Courtesy of Tom Finkle; 15.11: © Vol. 160/Corbis; 15.12: © Bob Daemmrich/The Image Works; 15.13: © William P. Cunningham; 15.14: © Carr Clifton; 15.17, 15.19: © William P. Cunningham; 15.20: © Jon Riley/Stone/Getty Images; 15.21: © Phil Degginger/Animals Animals/Earth Scenes; 15.22, 15.23, 15.25, 15.26, 15.27: © William P. Cunningham.

LINE ART

Chapter 1

1.19: From United Nations (U.N.) Critical Trends: Global Change and Sustainable Development, 1997, p. 58: Growing Disparities in Incomes Among Regions.

Chapter 3

3.26: From Verner, J. et al. *Wildlife 2000.* © 1986. Reprinted by permission of The University of Wisconsin Press.

Chapter 4

4.2: Figure redrawn with permission from *Population Bulletin,* vol. 18, no. 1, 1985. Population Reference Bureau; 4.4: From Thomas Merrick, with PRB staff, "World Population in Transition," *Population Bulletin,* vol. 41, no. 2 (reprinted 1991).

Chapter 7

Table 7.2: *Source:* Based on 14 years of data from Missouri Experiment Station, Columbia, Missouri.

Chapter 12

12.13: Courtesy of Northern States Power Company. Minneapolis, Minn.

Chapter 14

14.6 and 14.7: Reprinted from *Beyond the Limits,* copyright © 1992 by Meadows, Meadows, and Randers. With permission from Chelsea Green Publishing Co., White River Junction, Vermont; 14.25: From Randall Arenct, "Creating Open Space Networks" in *Environment & Development,* May/June 1996, American Planning Association, Chicago, IL. Reprinted by permission.

Chapter 15

15.3: From *Better Environmental Decisions* by Ken Sexton et al., eds. Copyright © 1999 by Island Press. Reproduced by permission of Island Press, Washington, D.C.; 15.10: *Source:* Data from PEW Research Center. Used by permission of Public Agenda Online; 15.24: Reprinted with the permission of Simon & Schuster Adult Publishing Group as it appears in *Bowling Alone: The Collapse and Revival of American Community* by Robert D. Putnam. Copyright © 2000 by Robert D. Putman.

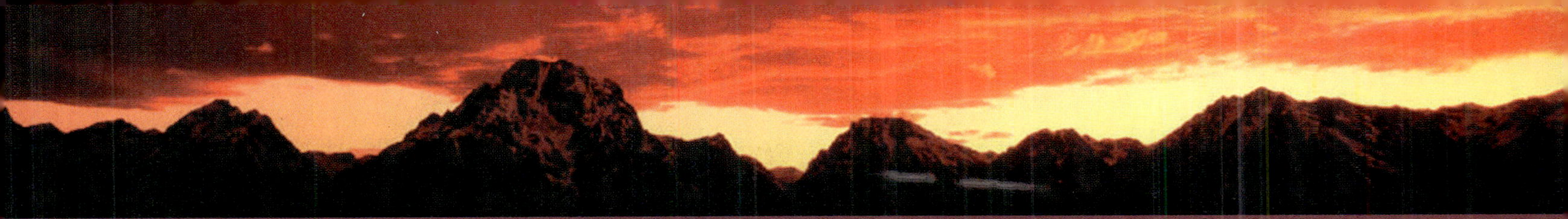

INDEX

A

B

C

E

F

G

H

I

J

K

N

O

P

Q

R

S

T

U

V

W

X

Y

Z

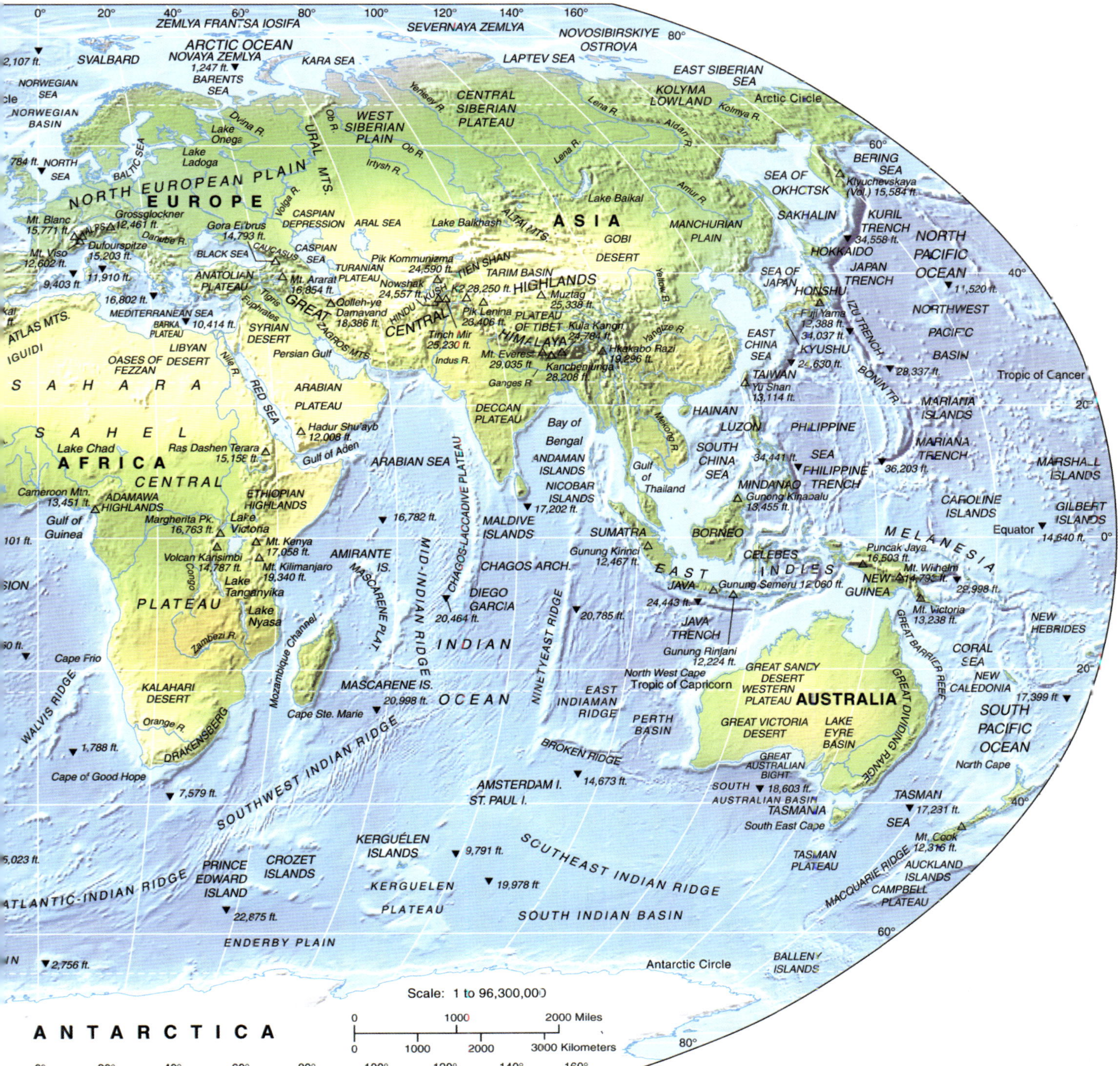
0°
20°
40°
60°
80°
100°
120°
140°
160°
ZEMLYA FRANTSA IOSIFA
SEVERNAYA ZEMLYA
NOVOSIBIRSKIYE OSTROVA
ARCTIC OCEAN
SVALBARD
NOVAYA ZEMLYA
1,247 ft.
KARA SEA
LAPTEV SEA
EAST SIBERIAN SEA
BARENTS SEA
NORWEGIAN SEA
NORWEGIAN BASIN
CENTRAL SIBERIAN PLATEAU
KOLYMA LOWLAND
Arctic Circle
WEST SIBERIAN PLAIN
Lake Onega
Lake Ladoga
URAL MTS.
NORTH SEA
BALTIC SEA
NORTH EUROPEAN PLAIN
EUROPE
ASIA
BERING SEA
SEA OF OKHOTSK
Klyuchevskaya (Vol.) 15,584 ft.
Lake Baikal
CASPIAN DEPRESSION
ARAL SEA
Lake Balkhash
ALTAI MTS.
GOBI DESERT
MANCHURIAN PLAIN
SAKHALIN
KURIL TRENCH
34,558 ft.
NORTH PACIFIC OCEAN
Mt. Blanc 15,771 ft.
ALPS
Grossglockner 12,461 ft.
Gora El'brus 18,510 ft.
CAUCASUS
BLACK SEA
CASPIAN SEA
Dufourspitze 15,203 ft.
Mt. Viso 12,602 ft.
11,910 ft.
9,403 ft.
ANATOLIAN PLATEAU
Mt. Ararat 16,854 ft.
TURANIAN PLATEAU
Pik Kommunizma 24,590 ft.
TIEN SHAN
TARIM BASIN
HIGHLANDS
HOKKAIDO
JAPAN TRENCH
SEA OF JAPAN
HONSHU
11,520 ft.
16,802 ft.
MEDITERRANEAN SEA
BARKA PLATEAU
10,414 ft.
ATLAS MTS.
SYRIAN DESERT
Qolleh-ye Damavand 18,386 ft.
Nowshak 24,557 ft.
K2 28,250 ft.
Muztag 25,338 ft.
Pik Lenina 23,406 ft.
PLATEAU OF TIBET
Kula Kangri 24,784 ft.
Fuji Yama 12,388 ft.
34,037 ft.
IZU TRENCH
NORTHWEST PACIFIC BASIN
LIBYAN DESERT
OASES OF FEZZAN
Persian Gulf
GREAT ZAGROS MTS.
HINDU KUSH
CENTRAL
Tirich Mir 25,230 ft.
HIMALAYA
Mt. Everest 29,035 ft.
Kanchenjunga 28,208 ft.
Hkakabo Razi 19,296 ft.
EAST CHINA SEA
KYUSHU
28,337 ft.
BONIN TR.
Tropic of Cancer
SAHARA
ARABIAN PLATEAU
RED SEA
Indus R.
Ganges R.
TAIWAN
Yu Shan 13,114 ft.
MARIANA ISLANDS
SAHEL
Hadur Shu'ayb 12,008 ft.
DECCAN PLATEAU
Bay of Bengal
HAINAN
LUZON
PHILIPPINE SEA
Lake Chad
Ras Dashen Terara 15,158 ft.
Gulf of Aden
ARABIAN SEA
ANDAMAN ISLANDS
SOUTH CHINA SEA
MARIANA TRENCH
36,203 ft.
MARSHALL ISLANDS
AFRICA
CENTRAL
ETHIOPIAN HIGHLANDS
CHAGOS-LACCADIVE PLATEAU
NICOBAR ISLANDS
Gulf of Thailand
34,441 ft.
PHILIPPINE TRENCH
MINDANAO
Cameroon Mtn. 13,451 ft.
ADAMAWA HIGHLANDS
16,782 ft.
17,202 ft.
Gunong Kinabalu 13,455 ft.
CAROLINE ISLANDS
GILBERT ISLANDS
Gulf of Guinea
Margherita Pk. 16,763 ft.
Lake Victoria
MALDIVE ISLANDS
SUMATRA
BORNEO
Equator
14,640 ft.
MELANESIA
Mt. Kenya 17,058 ft.
Volcan Kansimbi 14,787 ft.
Mt. Kilimanjaro 19,340 ft.
AMIRANTE IS.
MID-INDIAN RIDGE
CHAGOS ARCH.
Gunung Kirinci 12,467 ft.
CELEBES
EAST INDIES
Puncak Jaya 16,503 ft.
Mt. Wilhelm
NEW GUINEA
22,998 ft.
Lake Tanganyika
MASCARENE PLAT.
DIEGO GARCIA
JAVA
Gunung Semeru 12,060 ft.
PLATEAU
Lake Nyasa
20,464 ft.
NINETYEAST RIDGE
20,785 ft.
24,443 ft.
JAVA TRENCH
Mt. Victoria 13,238 ft.
NEW HEBRIDES
Zambezi R.
Mozambique Channel
INDIAN
GREAT BARRIER REEF
Cape Frio
Gunung Rinjani 12,224 ft.
CORAL SEA
WALVIS RIDGE
KALAHARI DESERT
MASCARENE IS.
20,998 ft.
OCEAN
EAST INDIAMAN RIDGE
North West Cape
Tropic of Capricorn
GREAT SANDY DESERT
WESTERN PLATEAU
AUSTRALIA
NEW CALEDONIA
17,399 ft.
Orange R.
DRAKENSBERG
Cape Ste. Marie
PERTH BASIN
GREAT VICTORIA DESERT
LAKE EYRE BASIN
GREAT DIVIDING RANGE
SOUTH PACIFIC OCEAN
1,788 ft.
SOUTHWEST INDIAN RIDGE
BROKEN RIDGE
GREAT AUSTRALIAN BIGHT
North Cape
Cape of Good Hope
7,579 ft.
AMSTERDAM I.
ST. PAUL I.
14,673 ft.
SOUTH AUSTRALIAN BASIN
18,603 ft.
TASMANIA
TASMAN SEA
17,231 ft.
South East Cape
KERGUÉLEN ISLANDS
9,791 ft.
SOUTHEAST INDIAN RIDGE
Mt. Cook 12,316 ft.
PRINCE EDWARD ISLAND
CROZET ISLANDS
TASMAN PLATEAU
MACQUARIE RIDGE
AUCKLAND ISLANDS
CAMPBELL PLATEAU
ATLANTIC-INDIAN RIDGE
KERGUELEN PLATEAU
19,978 ft.
22,875 ft.
SOUTH INDIAN BASIN
ENDERBY PLAIN
60°
2,756 ft.
Antarctic Circle
BALLENY ISLANDS
Scale: 1 to 96,300,000
0
1000
2000 Miles
3000 Kilometers
ANTARCTICA
80°

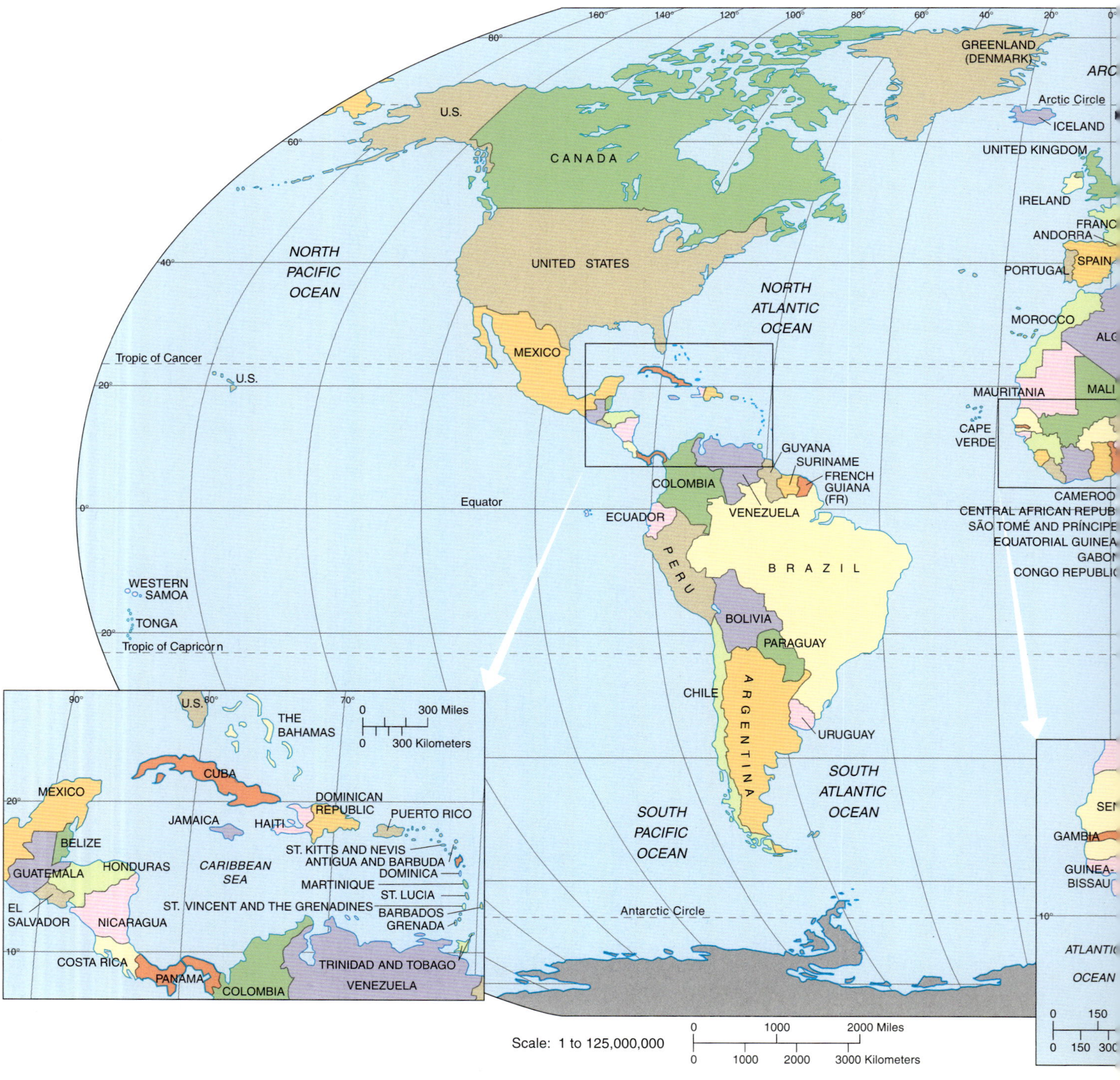

GREENLAND (DENMARK)
Arctic Circle
ICELAND
UNITED KINGDOM
IRELAND
ANDORRA
PORTUGAL
SPAIN
U.S.
CANADA
UNITED STATES
NORTH PACIFIC OCEAN
NORTH ATLANTIC OCEAN
MOROCCO
MEXICO
Tropic of Cancer
MAURITANIA
MALI
CAPE VERDE
GUYANA
SURINAME
FRENCH GUIANA (FR)
COLOMBIA
Equator
ECUADOR
VENEZUELA
PERU
BRAZIL
WESTERN SAMOA
TONGA
Tropic of Capricorn
BOLIVIA
PARAGUAY
CHILE
ARGENTINA
URUGUAY
SOUTH ATLANTIC OCEAN
SOUTH PACIFIC OCEAN
Antarctic Circle
THE BAHAMAS
CUBA
DOMINICAN REPUBLIC
JAMAICA
HAITI
PUERTO RICO
BELIZE
GUATEMALA
HONDURAS
CARIBBEAN SEA
ST. KITTS AND NEVIS
ANTIGUA AND BARBUDA
DOMINICA
MARTINIQUE
ST. LUCIA
ST. VINCENT AND THE GRENADINES
BARBADOS
GRENADA
EL SALVADOR
NICARAGUA
COSTA RICA
PANAMA
TRINIDAD AND TOBAGO
300 Miles
300 Kilometers
GAMBIA
GUINEA-BISSAU
Scale: 1 to 125,000,000
0 1000 2000 Miles
0 1000 2000 3000 Kilometers

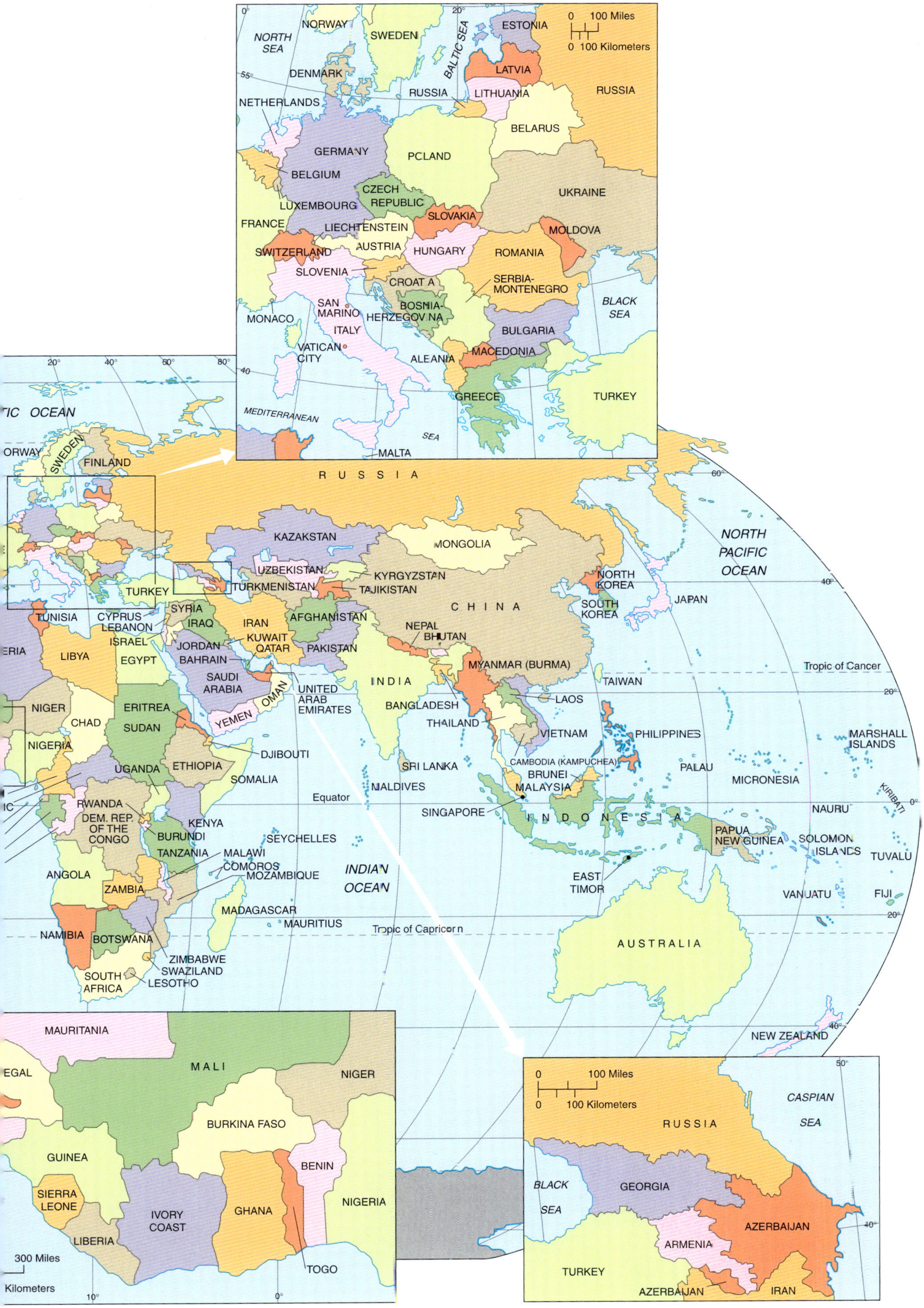

NORWAY
NORTH SEA
SWEDEN
BALTIC SEA
ESTONIA
0 100 Miles
0 100 Kilometers
DENMARK
LATVIA
RUSSIA
LITHUANIA
NETHERLANDS
BELARUS
GERMANY
PCLAND
BELGIUM
CZECH REPUBLIC
UKRAINE
LUXEMBOURG
SLOVAKIA
FRANCE
LIECHTENSTEIN
MOLDOVA
SWITZERLAND
AUSTRIA
HUNGARY
ROMANIA
SLOVENIA
CROAT A
SERBIA-MONTENEGRO
SAN MARINO
BOSNIA-HERZEGOV NA
BLACK SEA
MONACO
ITALY
BULGARIA
VATICAN CITY
ALE ANIA
MACEDONIA
GREECE
TURKEY
MEDITERRANEAN SEA
MALTA
IC OCEAN
ORWAY
SWEDEN
FINLAND
R U S S I A
NORTH PACIFIC OCEAN
KAZAKSTAN
MONGOLIA
UZBEKISTAN
KYRGYZSTAN
NORTH KOREA
TURKMENISTAN
TAJIKISTAN
TURKEY
C H I N A
SOUTH KOREA
JAPAN
TUNISIA
CYPRUS
SYRIA
LEBANON
IRAQ
IRAN
AFGHANISTAN
ISRAEL
KUWAIT
NEPAL
BHUTAN
ERIA
LIBYA
JORDAN
QATAR
PAKISTAN
EGYPT
BAHRAIN
MYANMAR (BURMA)
Tropic of Cancer
SAUDI ARABIA
INDIA
TAIWAN
OMAN
UNITED ARAB EMIRATES
LAOS
NIGER
ERITREA
BANGLADESH
YEMEN
CHAD
SUDAN
THAILAND
MARSHALL ISLANDS
VIETNAM
PHILIPPINES
NIGERIA
DJIBOUTI
CAMBODIA (KAMPUCHEA)
UGANDA
ETHIOPIA
SRI LANKA
PALAU
SOMALIA
BRUNEI
MICRONESIA
MALDIVES
MALAYSIA
KIRIBATI
Equator
RWANDA
NAURU
SINGAPORE
I N D O N E S I A
DEM. REP. OF THE CONGO
KENYA
BURUNDI
SEYCHELLES
PAPUA NEW GUINEA
SOLOMON ISLANDS
TUVALU
TANZANIA
MALAWI
COMOROS
INDIAN OCEAN
ANGOLA
MOZAMBIQUE
EAST TIMOR
ZAMBIA
VANUATU
FIJI
MADAGASCAR
MAURITIUS
Tropic of Capricorn
NAMIBIA
BOTSWANA
AUSTRALIA
ZIMBABWE
SWAZILAND
SOUTH AFRICA
LESOTHO
NEW ZEALAND
MAURITANIA
MALI
NIGER
EGAL
BURKINA FASO
GUINEA
BENIN
SIERRA LEONE
IVORY COAST
GHANA
NIGERIA
LIBERIA
300 Miles
Kilometers
TOGO
0 100 Miles
0 100 Kilometers
CASPIAN SEA
RUSSIA
BLACK SEA
GEORGIA
AZERBAIJAN
ARMENIA
TURKEY
AZERBAIJAN
IRAN

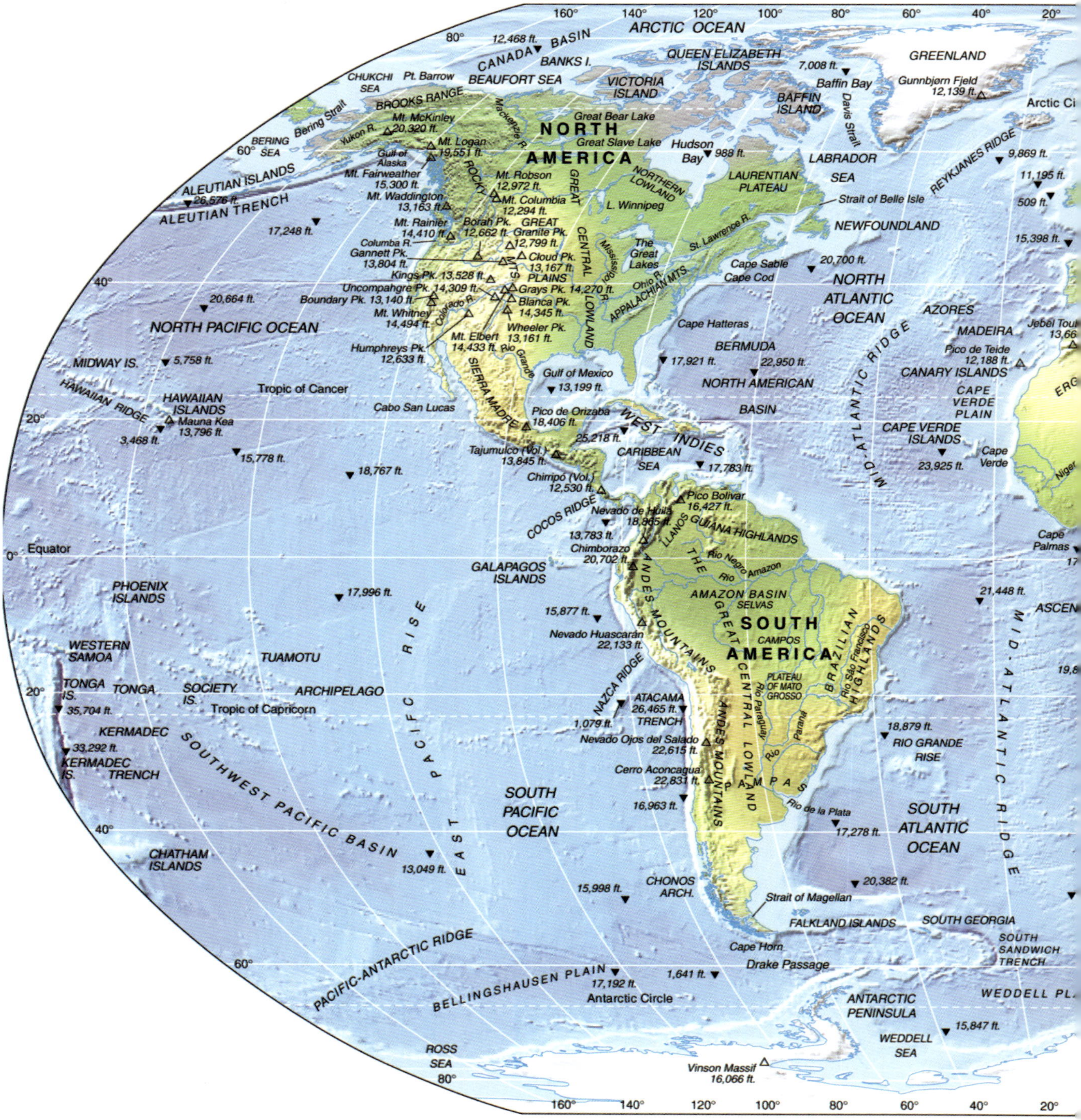

ARCTIC OCEAN
CANADA BASIN
12,468 ft.
BANKS I.
QUEEN ELIZABETH ISLANDS
GREENLAND
CHUKCHI SEA
Pt. Barrow
BEAUFORT SEA
VICTORIA ISLAND
7,008 ft.
Baffin Bay
Gunnbjørn Fjeld 12,139 ft.
BROOKS RANGE
BAFFIN ISLAND
Davis Strait
Arctic Ci
Bering Strait
Mt. McKinley 20,320 ft.
Yukon R.
Great Bear Lake
NORTH AMERICA
BERING SEA
Mt. Logan 19,551 ft.
Mackenzie R.
Great Slave Lake
Hudson Bay
988 ft.
LABRADOR SEA
REYKJANES RIDGE
9,869 ft.
Gulf of Alaska
Mt. Fairweather 15,300 ft.
ROCKY
Mt. Robson 12,972 ft.
GREAT
NORTHERN LOWLAND
LAURENTIAN PLATEAU
11,195 ft.
ALEUTIAN ISLANDS
26,576 ft.
ALEUTIAN TRENCH
Mt. Waddington 13,163 ft.
Mt. Columbia 12,294 ft.
L. Winnipeg
Strait of Belle Isle
509 ft.
17,248 ft.
Mt. Rainier 14,410 ft.
Borah Pk. 12,662 ft.
GREAT PLAINS
Granite Pk. 12,799 ft.
CENTRAL LOWLAND
Mississippi R.
NEWFOUNDLAND
St. Lawrence R.
Columba R.
Gannett Pk. 13,804 ft.
Cloud Pk. 13,167 ft.
The Great Lakes
15,398 ft.
Kings Pk. 13,528 ft.
MTS.
Ohio R.
Cape Sable
20,700 ft.
Uncompahgre Pk. 14,309 ft.
Grays Pk. 14,270 ft.
APPALACHIAN MTS.
Cape Cod
NORTH ATLANTIC OCEAN
Boundary Pk. 13,140 ft.
Blanca Pk. 14,345 ft.
20,664 ft.
Colorado R.
Mt. Whitney 14,494 ft.
AZORES
NORTH PACIFIC OCEAN
Wheeler Pk. 13,161 ft.
Cape Hatteras
MADEIRA
Jebel Toub
Mt. Elbert 14,433 ft.
BERMUDA
Humphreys Pk. 12,633 ft.
Rio Grande
Pico de Teide 12,188 ft.
MIDWAY IS.
5,758 ft.
SIERRA MADRE
17,921 ft.
22,950 ft.
MID-ATLANTIC RIDGE
CANARY ISLANDS
Gulf of Mexico
HAWAIIAN RIDGE
13,199 ft.
NORTH AMERICAN BASIN
Tropic of Cancer
HAWAIIAN ISLANDS
CAPE VERDE PLAIN
Cabo San Lucas
Pico de Orizaba 18,406 ft.
Mauna Kea 13,796 ft.
WEST INDIES
3,468 ft.
25,218 ft.
CAPE VERDE ISLANDS
Tajumulco (Vol.) 13,845 ft.
CARIBBEAN SEA
Cape Verde
15,778 ft.
17,783 ft.
23,925 ft.
18,767 ft.
Niger
Chirripó (Vol.) 12,530 ft.
Pico Bolívar 16,427 ft.
COCOS RIDGE
Nevado de Huila 18,865 ft.
GUIANA HIGHLANDS
LLANOS
13,783 ft.
Cape Palmas
Equator
Chimborazo 20,702 ft.
Rio Negro
Amazon
GALAPAGOS ISLANDS
THE
Rio
PHOENIX ISLANDS
AMAZON BASIN
SELVAS
17,996 ft.
21,448 ft.
ASCEN
15,877 ft.
ANDES MOUNTAINS
SOUTH AMERICA
GREAT
Nevado Huascarán 22,133 ft.
CAMPOS
WESTERN SAMOA
TUAMOTU
EAST PACIFIC RISE
BRAZILIAN HIGHLANDS
Rio São Francisco
TONGA IS.
TONGA
SOCIETY IS.
ARCHIPELAGO
NAZCA RIDGE
ATACAMA TRENCH 26,465 ft.
PLATEAU OF MATO GROSSO
Rio Paraguay
CENTRAL LOWLAND
35,704 ft.
Tropic of Capricorn
1,079 ft.
Paraná
18,879 ft.
KERMADEC
Nevado Ojos del Salado 22,615 ft.
RIO GRANDE RISE
33,292 ft.
KERMADEC IS.
TRENCH
SOUTHWEST PACIFIC BASIN
Cerro Aconcagua 22,831 ft.
Rio
PAMPAS
SOUTH PACIFIC OCEAN
16,963 ft.
Río de la Plata
SOUTH ATLANTIC OCEAN
17,278 ft.
CHATHAM ISLANDS
13,049 ft.
CHONOS ARCH.
20,382 ft.
15,998 ft.
Strait of Magellan
FALKLAND ISLANDS
SOUTH GEORGIA
PACIFIC-ANTARCTIC RIDGE
Cape Horn
SOUTH SANDWICH TRENCH
Drake Passage
BELLINGSHAUSEN PLAIN
17,192 ft.
1,641 ft.
Antarctic Circle
ANTARCTIC PENINSULA
WEDDELL PL.
15,847 ft.
WEDDELL SEA
ROSS SEA
Vinson Massif 16,066 ft.
160°
140°
120°
100°
80°
60°
40°
20°